Introduction to the Cellular and Molecular Biology of Cancer

Margaret A. Knowles
Peter J. Selby
Cancer Research UK Clinical Centre, St James's University Hospital, Leeds

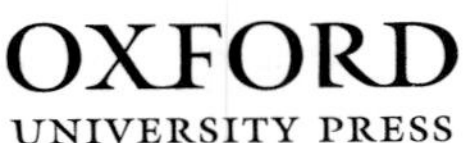

OXFORD
UNIVERSITY PRESS

Great Clarendon Street, Oxford OX2 6DP

Oxford University Press is a department of the University of Oxford.
It furthers the University's objective of excellence in research, scholarship,
and education by publishing worldwide in

Oxford New York

Auckland Cape Town Dar es Salaam Hong Kong Karachi
Kuala Lumpur Madrid Melbourne Mexico City Nairobi
New Delhi Shanghai Taipei Toronto

With offices in

Argentina Austria Brazil Chile Czech Republic France Greece
Guatemala Hungary Italy Japan Poland Portugal Singapore
South Korea Switzerland Thailand Turkey Ukraine Vietnam

Oxford is a registered trade mark of Oxford University Press
in the UK and in certain other countries

Published in the United States
by Oxford University Press Inc., New York

Fourth edition first published 2005

British Library Cataloguing in Publication Data

(Data available)

Library of Congress Cataloging in Publication Data

Knowles, Margaret A.
Introduction to the cellular and molecular biology of cancer / Margaret A. Knowles, Peter J. Selby.
p. cm.
ISBN 0-19-852563-X (alk. paper) — ISBN 0-19-856853-3 (alk. paper) 1. Cancer—Molecular aspects.
2. Cancer cells. I. Selby, P. (Peter) II. Title.
RC268.5.K56 2005
616.99′4071—dc22

2004030576

Typeset by Newgen Imaging Systems (P) Ltd., Chennai, India
Printed in Great Britain
on acid-free paper by
Antony Rowe, Chippenham

ISBN 0-19-856853-3 (Hbk) 978-0-19-856853-7
ISBN 0-19-852563-X (Pbk) 978-0-19-852563-9

10 9 8 7 6 5 4 3 2 1

Preface to the fourth edition

The first edition of this book, published in 1985 was a testimony to the dramatic molecular revolution that was taking place in biology and consequently in cancer research at that time. The book evolved from a series of introductory lectures developed to help new students and research fellows that came to work at the Imperial Cancer Research Fund Laboratories in London to assimilate the rapidly evolving body of knowledge on cancer. These popular talks were designed to give the non-expert a background to related areas of research and were given by experts from within the Imperial Cancer Research Fund, many of whom subsequently contributed chapters to the first edition of the book. Twenty years later, the need for a comprehensive introduction to this broad field is even more apparent and the introductory lectures at what is now the Cancer Research UK London Research Institute continue and are as popular as ever. Today, laboratory science has begun to have a real impact on clinical medicine and it is of utmost importance that scientists have not only a broad view of laboratory cancer research but also a good understanding of the most up to date treatment options. Similarly, it is essential that clinicians treating the various types of neoplastic disease are aware of developments in basic science and can apply these appropriately. It is our view that only when determined attempts to bridge the gap between the laboratory and clinic are made by both clinicians and scientists that rapid translation will take place. Our objective has been to facilitate acquisition of basic information on all aspects of cancer research to facilitate this process.

Inevitably over the years, many authors of this book have changed, some topics have become less relevant and new topics have been added. However, we are delighted that the initiator of the series and one of the editors of the first three editions of the book has given advice during the planning of this fourth edition and has again contributed to the first chapter of the book. Sammy Franks was Ph.D. supervisor to one of us (MK) and throughout his career has encouraged young scientists to look beyond the topic of their personal Ph.D. or post-doctoral project to encompass the wider picture. His care in selection of topics and authors for the earlier editions of the book generated a comprehensive and readable text that has been used extensively. In preparing this new edition we have tried to keep his original goals in mind.

Our task in updating this has not been easy, not least because of the unprecedented developments in many areas of biology. There are many more relevant and indispensable topics than before and this creates a conflict with the size limitations for a textbook of this kind. Perhaps the most difficult aspect of modern biology, however, is the complexity of current knowledge that seems to defy simplification to the level of the 'non-expert'. Inevitably, this is more apparent in some areas than in others and we are aware that the factual content of the book has increased enormously. The modern cell or molecular biologist faces a challenging initiation into the field of cancer research. Ultimately, however, the dramatic increase in knowledge provides young scientists today with the power to understand and manipulate the fundamental processes of life as never before. We believe, and hope, that the reader will find, that the obvious benefits in understanding complex biological problems far outweigh the effort required to assimilate the increased information content of this volume.

We have expanded the number of chapters from 22 to 30 to include chapters that cover some of the new technologies such as global analyses of the genome, transcriptome, and proteome and more recent concepts and discoveries in cell biology such as the process of apoptosis, the rapid advances made in understanding the finite or infinite proliferative capacity of somatic cells and the epigenome. Huge strides have been made in our understanding of genomic alterations in cancer cells and these are reflected in an extensively updated chapter on molecular cytogenetics. All chapters with similar titles to the previous edition have been completely rewritten or extensively updated. On reviewing the final content of the book, one of the most striking changes is the general acceptance by authors of the identity of the key genes affecting the processes they seek to elucidate. No longer is identification of genes a critical issue but the (almost entire) sequence of the human genome now allows biologists to focus on biological processes rather than detective work designed to find genes. One of the striking observations is the diversity of types of genes involved in cancer development that is reflected in several chapters. Similarly, developments in novel cancer therapies now draw on many areas of molecular biology and several are now represented as separate chapters. This is indeed a period of plenty in terms of what is known and what is possible and the scope for new scientists and clinicians to draw on this is unprecedented. Authorship for this edition continues to represent experts in each field of research but this now extends beyond the confines of a single organization to draw on expertise from around the world. The assembly of such an impressive group of experts in such a fast-moving area of research ensures that the content is as up-to-date as possible and we are indebted to all contributors for their efforts. Inevitably, there will be omissions and imbalances that will be felt more acutely by some readers than others and we encourage readers to comment and make suggestions for any future editions of the book.

Leeds M. A. K.
January 2005 P. J. S.

Preface to the third edition

Successive editions of this book have mirrored developments in cancer research and we hope that this new edition will achieve our original objective of providing a relatively brief but comprehensive introduction to the initiation, development, and treatment of cancer. On this background we have tried to provide an introduction to the results and new developments in the field using the current techniques of cell and molecular biology. A fuller understanding of the detail in some chapters needs a basic knowledge of molecular biology which can be found in several textbooks (e.g. Lodish et al., 1995) but the general principles in each chapter should be comprehensible without this. This edition has allowed us to bring up-to-date information in fields in which there has been great activity and even some achievement. In particular, the chapters concerned with epidemiology, genetic and chromosome changes, oncogenes, chemical and radiation carcinogenesis, growth factors, the biology of human leukaemia, and hormones and cancer, and the Glossary have been rewritten or extensively revised. Other chapters have been brought up-to-date and new chapters on cytokines and cancer, the molecular pathology of cancer, cancer prevention, and screening have been added.

Gene nomenclature may cause some confusion since although there is now a standardized format it is not yet generally accepted by all workers in the field. Many of the genes and oncogenes described by some earlier workers have retained their original format for historical reasons. Some genes were discovered in mouse cells, others in humans, and still others in viruses, and different names were given to genes which are now known to be essentially the same. Genes described for human cells are now usually written in upper case, italic type and their protein products in roman type. Mouse genes are often given in lower case italic type, their products as for those of human genes; those from *Drosophilia* are italicized with only the first letter capitalized. Specific oncogenes may be cited by a lower case first letter (c for cellular, v for viral), followed by a hyphen, and then the gene name in italic type. However, there may be further modifier terms. For the most part, we have tried to maintain some degree of consistency but in some chapters we have retained the original format if this is still used by many workers.

The apparently inevitable increase in girth that seems to accompany middle age has had its effect on the book which is somewhat larger than its predecessors but we hope that the increase in information will compensate.

As one of the philosophers in The Crock of Gold (Stephens 1931) commented 'Perfection is finality; finality is death. Nothing is perfect. There are lumps in it.'* No doubt there are lumps, and errors, and omissions in this new edition. We should be pleased to have comments and suggestions for their correction.

References

Lodish, H., Baltimore, D., Berk, A., Zipursky, S. L., Matsudaira, P., Darnell, J. (1995). *Molecular Cell Biology*. Scientific American Books, W. H. Freeman, New York.

Stephens, J. (1931). *The Crock of Gold*. Macmillan, London.

London *L. M. F.*
June 1996 *N. M. T.*

* He was complaining to his wife about his porridge. She hit him on the head.

Preface to the second edition

The second edition of this book—prepared sooner than we had expected—has given us an opportunity to correct some of the faults and errors pointed out by our readers and reviewers, as well as allowing us to bring the book up-to-date in a number of areas in which there have been rapid developments. In particular the chapters on the genetic and chromosomal changes, growth factors, immunotherapy, and epidemiology have been expanded and more information on viral and chemical carcinogenesis added to the appropriate sections. We have also clarified and added new information to most of the other chapters.

At some stage all authors and editors of introductory textbooks are faced with the awful choice of deciding what to leave out. When does completeness conflict with comprehension? Is the omission of this and that piece of information really a mortal sin or could the distinguished reviewer who pointed it out just happen to have been told about it by a passing graduate student? In the end of course we did what all editors must do and made our own choice.

We hope that this second edition will continue to be of use to its readers as an introduction to cancer studies and as a source of further information either in key references or in specialized reviews such as *Cancer Surveys*.

We should still appreciate comments and suggestions for further improvement.

London *L. M. F.*
January 1990 *N. M. T.*

Preface to the first edition

Cancer holds a strange place in modern mythology. Although it is a common disease and it is true to say that one person in five will die of cancer, it is equally true to say that four out of five die of some other disease. Heart disease, for example, a much more common cause of death, does not seem to carry with it the gloomy overtones, not always justifiable, of a diagnosis of cancer. This seems to stem largely from the fact that we had so little knowledge of the cause of a disease which seemed to appear almost at random and proceed inexorably. At the turn of the century, when the ICRF was founded (in 1902), the clinical behaviour and pathology of the more common tumours was known but little else. Over the years clinicians, laboratory scientists and epidemiologists established a firm database. The behaviour patterns of many tumours, and in some cases even the causal agents, were known but how these agents transformed normal cells and influenced tumour cell behaviour remained a mystery.

The development of molecular biology opened up a major new approach to the molecular analysis of normal and tumour cells. We can now ask and begin to answer questions particularly about the genetic control of cell growth and behaviour that have a bearing on our understanding not only of the family of diseases that we know as cancer but of the whole process of life itself. It is this, as much as finding a cause and cure for the disease, that gives cancer research its importance.

The initiating event which ultimately led to the publication of this book was the realization that many graduate students and research fellows who came to work in our Institute, although highly specialized in their own fields, had relatively little knowledge of cancer and there were few suitable textbooks to which they could be referred. Consequently, regular introductory courses were organized for new staff members at which 'experts' were asked to give a general introduction to their particular field of study. The talks were designed to give a background for the non-expert, as for example, molecular biology for the morphologist or cell biology for the protein chemist. The courses proved to be very popular. This book follows a similar pattern and has many of the same contributors—hence the fact that most are, or have been, connected with the Imperial Cancer Research Fund.

After a general introduction describing the pathology and natural history of the disease, each section gives a more detailed, but nevertheless general, survey of its particular area. We have tried to present principles rather than a mass of information, but inevitably some chapters are more detailed than others. Each chapter gives a short list of recommended reading which provides a source for seekers of further knowledge.

The topics covered have been selected with some care. Although some, particularly those concerned with treatment, may not at first glance appear to be directly related to cell and molecular biology, we feel that a knowledge of the methods used must give a wider understanding of the practical problems which may ultimately prove to be solvable by the application of modern scientific technology. On the other hand, knowledge of inherent cell behaviour (e.g. radiosensitivity, cell cycling, development of drug resistance, etc.) is important for the design of novel therapeutic approaches that rely less on empirical considerations.

Despite differences in the levels of technical details presented in some chapters, we hope that all are comprehensible. We have provided a fairly comprehensive glossary so that if some terms are not explained adequately in the text, do try the glossary. Finally, the editors would appreciate any comments, suggestions or corrections should a second edition prove desirable.

London | *L. M. F.*
December 1985 | *N. M. T.*

Contents

Contributors

Naomi Allen, Cancer Research UK, Epidemiology Unit, University of Oxford, Gibson Building, Radcliffe Infirmary, Oxford OX2 6HE, naomi.allen@cancer.org.uk

Frances Balkwill, Translational Oncology Laboratory, Barts and the London, Queen Mary's School of Medicine and Dentistry, The John Vane Science Centre, Charterhouse Square, London EC1M 6BQ, frances.balkwill@cancer.org.uk

Emily Banks, National Centre for Epidemiology & Population Health, Australian National University, Canberra, ACT 0200, Australia, emily.banks@anu.edu.au

Rosamonde Banks, Cancer Research UK Clinical Centre, St James's University Hospital, Beckett Street, Leeds LS9 7TF, r.banks@leeds.ac.uk

Amy Berrington de Gonzalez, Cancer Research UK Epidemiology Unit, University of Oxford, Oxford OX2 6HE, amy.berringtondegonzalez@cancer.org.uk

Anton Berns, The Netherlands Cancer Institute, Division of Molecular Genetics, Plesmanlaan 121, 1066 CX Amsterdam, The Netherlands, a.berns@nki.nl

Charlotte Bevan, Department of Cancer Medicine, Imperial College London, 5th Floor Laboratories, MRC Cyclotron Building, Du Cane Road, London W12 0NN, charlotte.bevan@imperial.ac.uk

Peter Beverley, The Edward Jenner Institute for Vaccine Research, Compton, Newbury, Berkshire RG20 7NN, peter.beverley@jenner.ac.uk

Roy Bicknell, Cancer Research UK, Angiogenesis Laboratory, Weatherall Institute of Molecular Medicine, John Radcliffe Hospital, Headley Way, Headington, Oxford OX3 9DS, roy.bicknell@cancer.org.uk

Tim Bishop, Cancer Research UK, Genetic Epidemiology, St. James's University Hospital, Beckett Street, Leeds LS9 7TF, t.bishop@cancer.org.uk

Ross Camidge, Edinburgh Cancer Centre, Western General Hospital, Edinburgh EH4 2XU, ross.camidge@ed.ac.uk

Jonathan Cheng, USC/Norris Cancer Center, 1441 Eastlake Avenue, Los Angeles, CA 9033, USA, jonathcc@usc.edu

John Chester, Cancer Research UK Clinical Centre, St James's University Hospital, Beckett Street, Leeds LS9 7TF, j.d.chester@cancermed.leeds.ac.uk

Rachel Craven, Cancer Research UK Clinical Centre, St James's University Hospital, Beckett Street, Leeds LS9 7TF, r.craven@cancermed.leeds.ac.uk

Tatjana Crnogorac-Jurcevic, Barts and the London, Queen Mary's School of Medicine and Dentistry, Charterhouse Square, London EC1M 6BQ, t.c.jurcevic@qmul.ac.uk

Jack Cuzick, Cancer Research UK, Centre for Epidemiology, Mathematics and Statistics, Wolfson Institute for Preventive Medicine, Barts and the London, Queen Mary's School of Medicine and Dentistry, Charterhouse Square, London EC1M 6BQ, jack.cuzick@cancer.org.uk

Silvana Debernardi, Department of Medical Oncology, Barts and The London, Queen Mary's School of Medicine and Dentistry, Charterhouse Square, London EC1M 6BQ, silvana.debernardi@cancer.org.uk

Paul Farrell, Ludwig Institute for Cancer Research, Department of Virology, Imperial College, St. Mary's Campus, Norfolk Place, London W2 1PG, p.farrell@imperial.ac.uk

Dean Fennell, Northern Ireland Thoracic Oncology Research Group, Cancer Research Centre, University Floor, Belfast City Hospital, Lisburn Road, Belfast BT9 7AB, Northern Ireland, d.fennel@qub.ac.uk

Ian Fentiman, Academic Oncology, 3rd Floor, Thomas Guy House, Guy's Hospital, St. Thomas Street, London SE1 9RT, ian.fentiman@cancer.org.uk

L. M. Franks, 13 Allingham Street, London, N1 8NX, sammyfranks@onetel.com

Tom Geldart, Cancer Research UK Oncology Unit, Cancer Sciences Division, Southampton University School of Medicine, Southampton General Hospital, Southampton SO16 6YD, trg@soton.ac.uk

Martin Glennie, Tenovus Laboratory, Cancer Sciences Division, Southampton University School of Medicine, Southampton General Hospital, Southampton SO16 6YD, m.j.glennie@soton.ac.uk

Mel Greaves, Institute of Cancer Research, Chester Beatty Laboratories, 237 Fulham Road, London SW3 6JB, mel.greaves@icr.ac.uk

Jane Green, Cancer Research UK Epidemiology Unit, University of Oxford, Oxford OX2 6HE, jane.green@cancer.org.uk

Ian Hart, Department of Tumour Biology, Barts and The London, Queen Mary's School of Medicine and Dentistry, John Vane Science Centre, Charterhouse Square, London EC1M 6BQ, ian.hart@cancer.org.uk

Andrew Jackson, Genitourinary Cancer Immunotherapy Program, Duke University Medical Centre, Durham, NC2 7710, USA, aj40@duke.edu

Duncan Jodrell, University of Edinburgh Cancer Research Centre, Crewe Road South, Edinburgh EH4 2XR, duncan.jodrell@cancer.org.uk

Peter Johnson, Cancer Research UK Oncology Unit, Cancer Sciences Division, Southampton University School of Medicine, Southampton General Hospital, Southampton SO16 6YD, johnsonp@soton.ac.uk

Peter Jones, USC/Norris Cancer Center, 1441 Eastlake Avenue, Los Angeles, CA 90033, USA, jones_p@ccnt.hsc.usc.edu

Jos Jonkers, The Netherlands Cancer Institute, Division of Molecular Biology, Plesmanlaan 121, 1066 CX Amsterdam, The Netherlands, j.jonkers@nki.nl

Timothy Key, Cancer Research UK, Epidemiology Unit, Gibson Building, Radcliffe Infirmary, Oxford OX2 6HE, timothy.key@cancer.org.uk

Anne Kiltie, Cancer Research UK Clinical Centre, St James's University Hospital, Beckett Street, Leeds LS9 7TF, anne.kiltie@cancer.org.uk

Margaret Knowles, Cancer Research UK Clinical Centre, St. James's University Hospital, Beckett Street, Leeds LS9 7TF, margaret.knowles@cancer.org.uk

Beate Köberle, University of Pittsburgh Cancer Institute, Hillman Cancer Center, 5117 Centre Avenue, Research Pavilion, Suite 2.6, Pittsburgh, Pa, 15213-1863, USA, bmk27@pitt.edu

Sonia Laín, Department of Surgery and Molecular Oncology, Nine Wells Hospital Medical School, University of Dundee, Dundee DD1 9SY, s.lain@dundee.ac.uk

David Lane, Department of Surgery and Molecular Oncology, Nine Wells Hospital Medical School, University of Dundee, Dundee DD1 9SY, d.p.lane@dundee.ac.uk

Nicholas Lemoine, Cancer Research UK, Molecular Oncology Unit, Barts and the London, Queen Mary's School of Medicine and Dentistry, Charterhouse Square, London EC1M 6BQ, Nick.Lemoine@cancer.org.uk

Robert Newbold, Brunel Institute of Cancer Genetics and Pharmacogenomics, Brunel University, Uxbridge UB8 4SP, robert.newbold@brunel.ac.uk

Robert Newton, Cancer Research UK Epidemiology Unit, University of Oxford, Oxford OX2 6HE, rob.newton@cancer.org.uk

Chris Norbury, Sir William Dunn School of Pathology, University of Oxford, South Parks Road, Oxford OX1 3RE, chris.norbury@path.ox.ac.uk

Joanne Porte, Department of Reproductive Endocrinology, University of North Carolina, Chapel Hill, NC27599, USA

Richard Poulsom, In Situ Hybridisation Service Histopathology Unit, Cancer Research UK, 44 Lincoln's Inn Fields, London, WC2A 3PX, richard.poulsom@cancer.org.uk

Sally Prigent, Department of Biochemistry, Room 201E, Adrian Building, University of Leicester, University Road, Leicester LE1 7RH Sap8@leicester.ac.uk

Peter Sasieni, Cancer Research UK, Centre for Epidemiology, Mathematics and Statistics, Wolfson Institute for Preventive Medicine, Barts and the London, Queen Mary's School of Medicine and Dentistry, Charterhouse Square, London EC1M 6BQ, peter.sasieni@cancer.org.uk

Peter Selby, Cancer Research UK Clinical Centre, St. James's University Hospital, Beckett Street, Leeds LS9 7TF, peter.selby@cancer.org.uk

Denise Sheer, Cancer Research UK London Research Institute, Human Cytogenetics Laboratory, Lincoln's Inn Fields Laboratories, 44 Lincoln's Inn Fields, London WC2A 3PX, denise.sheer@cancer.org.uk

Janet Shipley, Molecular Cytogenetics, The Institute of Cancer Research, 15 Cotswold Road, Belmont, Sutton, Surrey SM2 5NG, janet.shipley@icr.ac.uk

Peter Szlosarek, Translational Oncology Laboratory, Cancer Research UK, Barts and The London, Queen Mary's School of Medicine and Dentistry, Charterhouse Square, London EC1M 6BQ, peter.szlosarek@cancer.org.uk

Kiki Tahtis, Cancer Research UK, Angiogenesis Laboratory, Weatherall Institute of Molecular Medicine, John Radcliffe Hospital, Headley Way, Headington, Oxford OX3 9DS, kiki.tahtis@cancer.org.uk

John Wittschieben, University of Pittsburgh Cancer Institute, Hillman Cancer Center, 5117 Centre Avenue, Research Pavilion, Suite 2.6, Pittsburgh, Pa, 15213-1863, USA, jpw31@pitt.edu

Richard Wood, University of Pittsburgh Cancer Institute, Hillman Cancer Center, 5117 Centre Avenue, Research Pavilion, Suite 2.6, Pittsburgh, Pa, 15213-1863, USA, rdwood@pitt.edu

Bryan Young, Department of Medical Oncology, Barts and The London, Queen Mary's School of Medicine and Dentistry, Charterhouse Square, London EC1M 6BQ, bryan.young@cancer.org.uk

CHAPTER 1

What is cancer?

Leonard M. Franks and Margaret A. Knowles

1.1 Introduction

Cancer has been known since human societies first recorded their activities. It was well known to the ancient Egyptians and to succeeding civilizations but, as most cancers develop in the latter decades of life, until the expectation of life began to increase from the middle of the nineteenth century onwards, the number of people surviving to this age was relatively small. Now that the infectious diseases, the major causes of death in the past, have been controlled by improvements in public health and medical care, the proportion of the population at risk of cancer has increased dramatically. Although diseases of the heart and blood vessels are still the main cause of death in our ageing population, cancer is now a major problem. At least one in three will develop cancer and one in four men and one in five women will die from it. For this reason, cancer prevention and control are major health issues. However, cancer research has wider significance.

Cancer is not confined to man and the higher mammals but affects almost all multicellular organisms, plants as well as animals. Since it involves disturbances in cell proliferation, differentiation, and development, knowledge of the processes underlying this disease help us to understand the very basic mechanisms of life.

About 140 years ago a German microscopist, Johannes Mueller, showed that cancers were made up of cells, a discovery which began the search for changes which would help to pinpoint the specific differences between normal and cancer cells. In the intervening period a huge amount of information has been acquired about the cancer cell. In the past two decades in particular, rapid technological progress has allowed us to begin to dissect the cancer genome, transcriptome, and proteome in unprecedented detail and today there seems no limit to the amount of information that can be obtained. However, this does not naturally answer all of the questions posed by those early cancer biologists. Some fundamental questions remain unanswered, despite our technical prowess and the availability of commercial 'kits' for most basic assays. Even the most advanced technology is of no value if it is not applied appropriately and it is still too early for the benefits of some recent technical advances to be clear. In the past, some of the major questions for the cancer biologist concerned what types of experiments were possible and the development of new techniques to extend these possibilities formed a major part of the work done. Now that almost anything seems technically possible, the key issue for the twenty-first century biologist is to identify the right questions to ask. This can make the difference between a deluge of uninterpretable data and a real improvement in understanding. This book does not aim to identify what these 'right' questions are but to provide an introduction to current understanding of cancer, its causes, biology, and treatment. However, we do indicate areas in which new and exciting discoveries are being made and those in which key questions remain unanswered.

Cancer is a disorder of cells and although it usually appears as a tumour (a swelling) made up of a mass of cells, the visible tumour is the end result of a whole series of changes which may have taken many years to develop. In this chapter, we discuss in general terms what is known about the changes that take place during the process of tumour development, consider tumour diagnosis and nomenclature, and provide some definitions. Succeeding chapters deal with specific aspects in more detail.

1.2 Normal cells and tissues

The tissues of the body can be divided into four main groups: the general supporting tissues collectively known as mesenchyme; the tissue-specific cells—epithelium; the 'defence' cells—the haemato-lymphoid system; and the nervous system. The mesenchyme consists of connective tissue—fibroblasts which make collagen fibres and associated proteins, bone, cartilage, muscle, blood vessels, and lymphatics. The epithelial cells are the specific, specialized cells of the different organs, for example, skin, intestine, liver, glands, etc. The haemato-lymphoid system consists of a wide group of cells, mostly derived from precursor cells in the bone marrow which give rise to all the red and white blood cells. In addition, some of these cells (lymphocytes and macrophages) are distributed throughout the body either as free cells or as fixed constituents of other organs, for example, in the liver, or as separate organs such as the spleen and lymph nodes. Lymph nodes are specialized nodules of lymphoid cells, which are distributed throughout the body and act as filters to remove cells, bacteria, and other foreign matter. The nervous system is made up of the central nervous system (the brain and spinal cord and their coverings) and the peripheral nervous system, which is comprised of nerves leading from these central structures. Thus, each tissue has its own specific cells, usually several different types, which maintain the structure and function of the individual tissue. Bone, for example, has one group of cells responsible for bone formation and a second group responsible for bone resorption and remodelling when the need arises, as in the repair of fractures. The intestinal tract has many different epithelial cell types responsible for the different functions of the bowel, and so on.

The specific cells are grouped in organs which have a standard pattern (Figure 1.1). There is a layer of epithelium, the tissue-specific cells, separated from the supporting mesenchyme by a semi-permeable basement membrane. The supporting tissues (or stroma) are made up of connective tissue (collagen fibres) and fibroblasts (which make collagen), which may be supported on a layer of muscle and/or bone depending on the organ. Blood

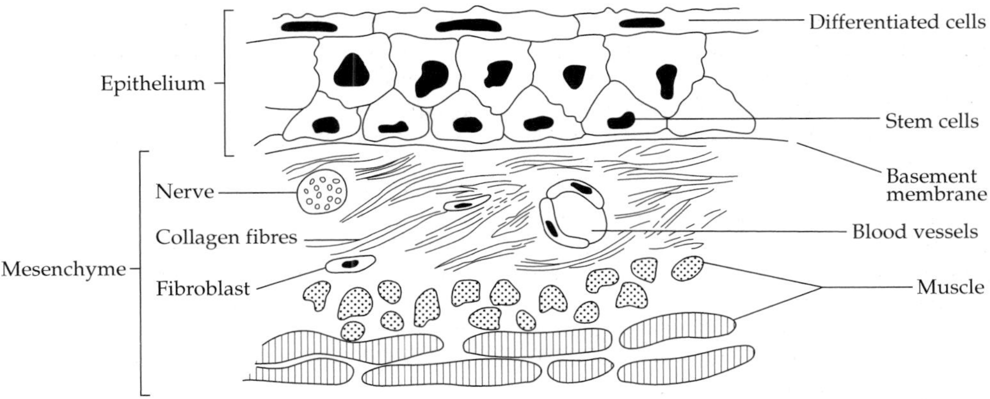

Figure 1.1 A typical tissue showing epithelial and mesenchymal components.

vessels, lymphatic vessels, and nerves pass through the connective tissue and provide nutrients and nervous control among other things for the specific tissue cells. In some instances, for example, the skin and intestinal tract, the epithelium which may be one or more cells thick depending on the tissue, covers surfaces. In others it may form a system of tubes (e.g. in the lung or kidney), or solid cords (e.g. liver), but the basic pattern remains the same. Different organs differ in structure only in the nature of the specific cells and the arrangement and distribution of the supporting mesenchyme.

1.3 Control of growth in normal tissues

The mechanism of control of cell growth and proliferation is one of the most intensively studied areas in biology. It is important to make the distinction between the terms 'growth' and 'proliferation'. Growth is used here to refer to an increase in size of a cell, organ, tissue, or tumour and proliferation to an increase in the number of cells by division. 'Growth' is often used as a loose term for both of these processes but the distinction is particularly important now that factors controlling both of these processes are becoming clear. In normal development and growth there is a very precise mechanism that allows individual organs to reach a fixed size, which for all practical purposes, is never exceeded. If a tissue is injured, the surviving cells in most organs begin to divide to replace the damaged cells. When this has been completed, the process stops, that is, the normal control mechanisms persist throughout life. Although most cells in the embryo can proliferate, not all adult cells retain this ability. In most organs there are special reserve or stem cells, which are capable of dividing in response to a stimulus such as an injury to replace organ-specific cells. The more highly differentiated a cell is, for example, muscle or nerve cells, the more likely it is to have lost its capacity to divide. In some organs, particularly the brain, the most highly differentiated cells, the nerve cells, can only proliferate in the embryo, although the special supporting cells in the brain continue to be able to proliferate. A consequence of this, as we shall see later, is that tumours of nerve cells are only found in the very young and tumours of the brain in adults are derived from the supporting cells.

In other tissues there is a rapid turnover of cells, particularly in the small intestine and the blood and immune system. A great deal of work has been done on the control of stem cell growth in the red and white cells (haemopoietic system), and the relationship of the factors involved in this process to tumour development (Chapter 18). For reasons that are still unclear, rapid cell division itself is not necessarily associated with an increased risk of tumour development, for example, tumours of the small intestine are very rare.

In the embryo there is a range of stem cells, some cells capable of reproducing almost any type of cell and others with a limited potential for producing more specific cells, for example, liver or kidney. In the adult, there is now unequivocal evidence for the existence of stem cells capable of perpetuating themselves through self-renewal to generate specialized cells of particular tissues. Striking parallels exist between the properties of stem cells and cancer cells. This, together with the potential for the use of human stem cells in various types of regenerative medicine, makes this a very active area of research (Reya et al., 2001).

Control of organ or tissue size is achieved via a fine balance between stimulatory and inhibitory stimuli. When the balance is shifted, for example, when the tissue is damaged and repair is needed, when a specific physiological stimulus is applied, for example, hormonal stimulation or because extra work is required from an organ, the component cells may respond in one of two ways to achieve these objectives. This may be by hypertrophy, that is, an increase in size of individual components, usually of cells which do not normally divide. An example is the increase in size of particular muscles in athletes. The alternative is hyperplasia, that is, an increase in number of the cells. When the stimulus is removed, commonly the situation returns to the *status quo* as exemplified by the rapid loss of muscle mass in the lapsed athlete. Some of the stimuli that lead to these compensatory responses are well-known growth factors and hormones that are discussed in more detail in Chapters 11, 14, and 15. Recent work on the insulin/IGF (insulin-like growth factor) system, particularly in the fruit fly *Drosophila*, has demonstrated that this plays a pivotal role in the control of organ and organism size (Oldham and Hafen, 2003). It is of note that several molecules involved in these processes are known to act as oncogenes or to be dysregulated in cancer. For example, IGFs are commonly overexpressed and the phosphoinositide 3-kinase (PI3K) pathway, which is activated by insulin/IGF signalling, is functionally disrupted in various ways in cancer cells (Vivanco and Sawyers, 2002).

1.4 The cell cycle

The way in which cells increase in number is similar for all somatic cells and involves the growth of all cell components (increase in cell mass) followed by division to generate two daughter cells. Although the structural changes which take place during this process, the cell cycle, have been known for many years, our current detailed knowledge of the molecular basis of the process has only been acquired in the past two decades. Four stages are recognized: G1, S, G2, and M. Following a proliferative stimulus, G1 is a gap or pause after stimulation where little seems to be happening. However, if the cell is destined to divide, there is much biochemical activity in G1 in preparation for DNA replication. S is the phase of DNA synthesis, where the chromosomes are replicated and other cell components also increase. G2 is a second gap period following DNA synthesis and M is the stage of mitosis in which the nuclear membrane breaks down and the condensed chromosomes can be visualized as they pair and divide prior to division of the cytoplasm to generate two daughter cells. A further cell cycle phase is recognized, G0, which is a resting phase in which non-cycling cells rest with a G1 DNA content. Progression through the cell cycle is now known to be restricted at specific checkpoints, one in G1 and others in S and G2/M. These provide an opportunity for cells to be diverted out of the cycle or to programmed cell death (apoptosis) if, for example, there is DNA damage or inappropriate expression of oncogenic proteins. Disruption of these cell cycle checkpoints or alterations to key cell cycle proteins are found in many, if not all, cancers. A detailed discussion of the cell cycle, its regulation and disruption in cancer is given in Chapter 9.

1.5 Tumour growth or neoplasia

It is not possible to define a tumour cell in absolute terms. Tumours are usually recognized by the fact that the cells have shown abnormal proliferation, so that a reasonably acceptable definition is that tumour cells differ from normal cells in their lack of response to normal control mechanisms. Since there are almost certainly many different factors involved, the altered cells may still respond to some but not to others. A further complication is that some tumour cells, especially soon after the cells have been transformed from the normal, may not be dividing at all. In the present state of knowledge any definition must be 'operational'. Given these qualifications we can classify tumours into three main groups:

(1) Benign tumours may arise in any tissue, grow locally, and cause damage by local pressure or obstruction. However, the common feature is that they do not spread to distant sites.

(2) *In situ* tumours usually develop in epithelium and are usually but not invariably, small. The cells have the morphological appearance of cancer cells but remain in the epithelial layer. They do not invade the basement membrane and supporting mesenchyme. Various degrees of dysplasia, that is, epithelial irregularity but not identifiable as cancer *in situ* are recognized in some tissues and these may sometimes precede cancer *in situ*. Theoretically, cancers *in situ* may arise also in mesenchymal, haemato-lymphoid, or nervous tissue but they have not been recognized.

(3) Cancers are fully developed (malignant) tumours with a specific capacity to invade and destroy the underlying mesenchyme (local invasion). The tumour cells need nutrients via the bloodstream and produce a range of proteins that stimulate the growth of blood vessels into the tumour, thus allowing continuous growth to occur (Chapter 17). The new vessels are not well formed and are easily damaged so that the invading tumour cells may penetrate these and lymphatic vessels. Tumour fragments may be carried in these vessels to local lymph nodes or to distant organs where they may produce secondary tumours (metastases) (Chapter 16). Cancers may arise in any tissue. Although there may be a progression from benign to malignant, this is far from invariable. Many benign tumours never become malignant. Some of these problems of definition may be more easily understood if we consider the whole process of tumour induction and development (carcinogenesis).

1.6 The process of carcinogenesis

Carcinogenesis (the process of cancer development) is a multistage process (Figure 1.2). In an animal, the application of a cancer-producing agent (carcinogen) does not lead to the immediate production of a tumour. Cancers arise after a long latent period and multiple carcinogen treatments are more effective than a single application. Experiments carried out on mouse skin in the 1940s by Berenblum and Shubik (reviewed by Yuspa, 1994) indicated that at least three major stages are involved. The first was termed initiation and was found to involve mutagenic effects of the carcinogen on skin stem cells. The second stage, which can be induced by a variety of agents that are not directly carcinogenic in their own right, was termed promotion. Following chronic treatment of carcinogen-initiated mouse skin with promoting agents, papillomas (benign skin tumours) arise. The major effect of promoters seems to be their ability to promote clonal expansion of initiated cells. Finally in the third stage, progression, some of these benign tumours either spontaneously or following additional treatment with carcinogens, progress to invasive tumours. The terms coined to describe this animal model are still commonly applied to describe the process of carcinogenesis in man.

The mouse skin model indicated that carcinogenesis is a multistep process and clearly this is

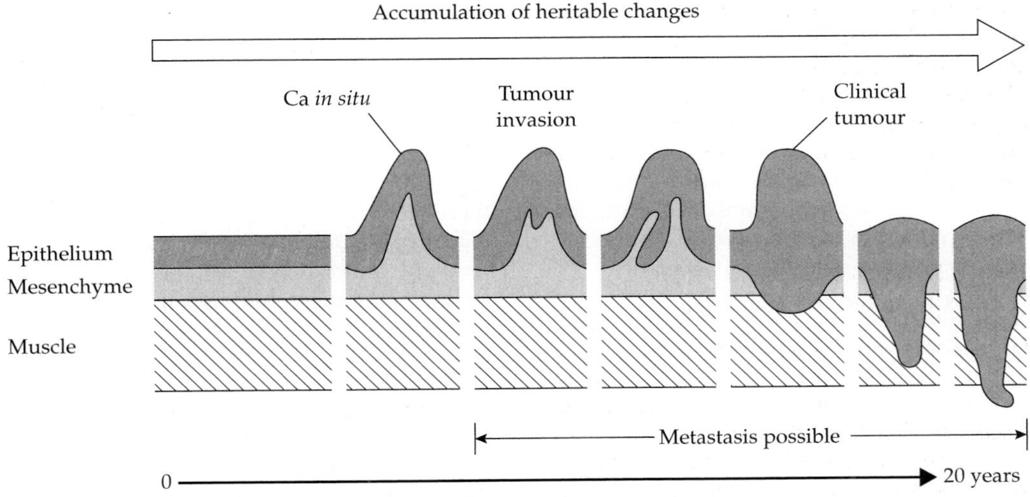

Figure 1.2 Tumour development showing progression from normal to invasive tumour via accumulation of heritable changes over a long period of time. The rate of acquisition of these changes will be influenced by environmental exposures and host response.

also the case for human cancer. For example, most solid tumours of adults arise in the later decades of life, usually a long time after exposure to a specific carcinogenic insult or after a long period of continuous exposure and this can be explained in terms of the requirement for several distinct heritable changes. The nature of some of these changes is now known in detail and is discussed at length in several of the following chapters. These include genetic alterations to proto-oncogenes and tumour suppressor genes (Chapters 7 and 8) and epigenetic alterations (Chapter 5). Histopathological observations also provide evidence for a long preneoplastic period, sometimes with morphologically identifiable lesions such as benign tumours or *in situ* dysplasia, which may persist for many years and within which a malignant tumour eventually arises.

The latent period between initiation and the appearance of tumours is great. In man, after exposure to industrial carcinogens, it may take over 20 years before tumours develop. Even in animals given massive doses of carcinogens, it may take up to a quarter or more of the total lifespan before tumours appear. The requirement for acquisition of multiple events is the likely explanation for this. In the tumour that finally emerges, most of the genetic and epigenetic changes seen are clonal, that is they are present in the entire population of cells. It is likely that a series of selective phases of clonal expansion takes place in the tumour such that after each event, there is outgrowth of a clone of cells with a selective advantage. Evidence for this has come from studies on many tissues and particularly where areas of surrounding tissue or multiple related lesions can be sampled at surgery. In these circumstances, it is common to find several shared clonal events in different lesions and occasionally in the apparently 'normal' surrounding epithelium and additional events in the most histopathologically advanced lesion (see Section 1.8.1).

1.6.1 Genes involved in carcinogenesis

Several types of genes are now known to contribute to the development of cancer. The discovery that the oncogenes of tumour-producing retroviruses are related to cellular genes (proto-oncogenes) (Chapter 7) has led to intensive research into the role of these genes in normal and tumour cell growth, proliferation, and differentiation. Many cellular genes can act as oncogenes when expressed inappropriately or mutated. These genes act in a dominant way at the cellular level to drive proliferation or prevent normal differentiation. This dominant mode of action makes oncogenes attractive potential targets for specific cancer therapies and there is currently a huge effort to inhibit the activity of specific oncogenes using a variety of approaches, some of which are already bearing fruit (Druker and Lydon, 2000). An interesting question in this regard concerns the role of such genes in the initiation, progression, and maintenance of tumours. In mouse skin, for example, mutational activation of a *ras* oncogene is an initiating event and subsequent tumour progression and metastasis appear to depend on sequential incremental levels of expression of the gene which is clearly required for tumour maintenance. Similarly it has been shown in mouse models of melanoma that expression of a *ras* transgene is required for tumour maintenance. However, in this model, examples of escape of tumours in which *ras* gene expression had been switched off (Chin and DePinho, 2000), raises the possibility that not all genetic events required early in tumour development may be required later in the process, a fact that represents a caveat in the design of oncogene-targeted therapies.

Genes that provide negative regulatory signals in the normal cell are also implicated in the development of cancer. If such a gene requires loss or inactivation to contribute to the transformation process, then it is likely that both copies of the gene must be altered and that such tumour suppressor genes would be genetically recessive at the cellular level. It was proposed by Knudson that two independent mutations are needed for the development of inherited cancers. In such cases of inherited (familial) tumour predisposition, the first mutation is present in the germ cells (sperm or ovum) and is therefore inherited by every cell in the body (Chapter 3). Only one further somatic mutation is required for complete gene inactivation in these cases. In the more common non-familial cancers, two somatic mutations in the gene are required and the chances of this happening in the same cell are much less. Many tumour suppressor genes have now been identified and many appear to conform to Knudson's so-called 'Two-hit hypothesis' (reviewed in Knudson, 1996). Several mechanisms of inactivation of the two alleles have been described and these are discussed in detail in Chapters 5 and 8. Not surprisingly however, there are exceptions to this rule and there are several examples where loss of function of one allele of a tumour suppressor gene is sufficient to generate an altered cell phenotype that can contribute to transformation. This is termed haploinsufficiency and as discussed in Chapter 8, the levels of protein required for adequate function may vary from gene to gene, leading to the prediction that some genes will be more strongly haploinsufficient than others.

In normal cells, the requirement for efficient repair mechanisms is clear. In the absence of such repair capacity, it is difficult to see how long-lived species such as man could survive daily exposure to environmental carcinogens without severe toxicity and inevitably a high cancer rate. The mechanisms of repair of different types of DNA damage have now been elucidated in great detail both in lower organisms and in mammalian systems. There are several familial syndromes in which components of the DNA repair machinery are mutated in the germline and these have provided valuable tools for discovery of the mechanisms of repair of different types of DNA lesions. One of the consequences of altered repair capacity is an increased risk of cancer. This class of cancer-causing genes can be referred to as 'mutator' genes as their altered function leads to an increased capacity for mutation of other genes. Any alteration in the function of such genes, however small, has the capacity to alter an individual's lifetime risk of cancer. However, in contrast to the tumour suppressor genes, replacement of the function of these genes has no direct effect on tumour phenotype. There is currently much interest in identifying not only highly penetrant mutations in DNA repair and carcinogen-metabolizing genes but also the less penetrant polymorphisms that affect each individual's response to environmental damage. DNA repair and its relationship to cancer development are discussed in detail in Chapter 4.

Other mutator genes include genes involved in regulation of the mitotic apparatus which can also affect the rate of acquisition of other mutations. An example is aurora kinase A (*AURKA*) also known as *STK15*, a gene whose product associates with the centrosome in S phase and appears to play a role in centrosome separation, duplication, and maturation. This gene is amplified and overexpressed in several types of cancer and this is associated with the generation of aneuploidy (deviation from the normal diploid number of chromosomes) (Dutertre et al., 2002). Other genes which also lead to aneuploidy when altered include the mitotic checkpoint genes *BUB1* and *BUBR1* both of which can be classified as tumour suppressor genes as inactivation is required for phenotypic effect.

This last example indicates that some subdivision within the large grouping of tumour suppressor genes is possible. This has led to invention of the terms 'gatekeeper' and 'caretaker' to describe these different suppressor roles (Kinzler and Vogelstein, 1998). Gatekeeper genes are defined as rate-limiting for a step in the pathway of tumour development. Thus, the adenomatous polyposis coli gene *APC* is considered to be an initiation gatekeeper as its inactivation is required early in colorectal carcinogenesis. Caretaker genes include those which when functionally inactivated lead to defective DNA repair or other loss of function that leads to mutation, for example, some DNA repair genes, *BUB1* and *BUBR1*.

Finally, the ability of the immune system to detect and destroy altered cells that are identified as 'non-self' (immune surveillance) may have an impact on cancer incidence. For some time it has been proposed that tumour cells expressing antigens that are recognized by the immune system will be eradicated at an early, preclinical stage and only those cells not eliciting such a response can survive to generate a clinically detectable tumour. This may be reflected in the difficulty in prompting a patient to mount a response against their tumour. However, it is still not clear how much impact this theoretical effect has on tumour incidence, nor whether specific defects in the immune system have a major impact (see Chapters 20 and 27).

1.7 Factors influencing the development of cancers

Many factors are involved in the development of cancer. These include both endogenous factors such as inherited predisposition and exogenous factors such as exposure to environmental carcinogens and infectious agents. All of these factors are discussed in depth in Chapters 2, 3 and 13.

Another factor not discussed in detail elsewhere in the book and which has a clear influence on the type of cancer which develops is age. In fact, age is the biggest risk factor for developing cancer (Figure 1.3). There is an age-associated, organ-specific tumour incidence. Most cancers in man

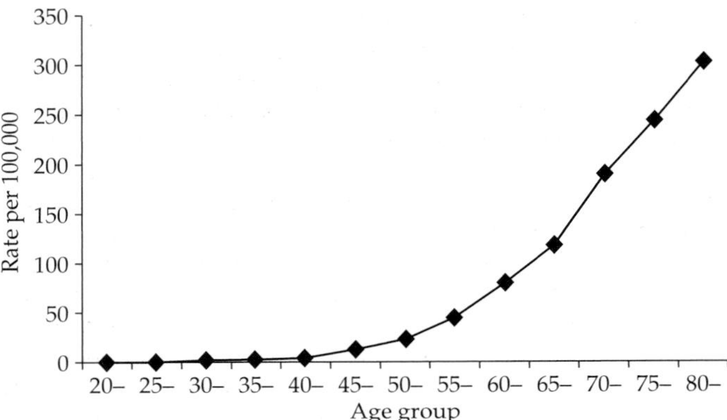

Figure 1.3 An example of age-specific cancer incidence rate. Colon cancer incidence in men in England in 1999.

and experimental animals can be divided into three main groups depending on their age-specific incidence:

(1) Embryonic tumours, for example, neuroblastoma (tumours of embryonic nerve cells), embryonal tumours of kidney (Wilms' tumours), retinoblastoma, etc.
(2) Tumours found predominantly in the young, for example, some leukaemias, tumours of the bone, testis, etc.
(3) Those with an increasing incidence with age, for example, tumours of prostate, colon, bladder, skin, breast, etc.

The juvenile onset of some cancers such as some leukaemias and those described as embryonal, is believed to reflect the requirement for only a limited number of alterations. Some of them such as familial retinoblastoma, originate in cells that already contain one inherited genetic defect and if only one or two further events is required for tumorigenicity of a target cell (e.g. inactivation of the second allele of *RB*), tumour development becomes almost inevitable given the large number of essentially initiated cells present.

There are several possible molecular and physiological explanations for the last group of age-associated tumours (group 3) which include the most common adult human cancers. First, in the normal individual there is continuous exposure throughout life to low levels of exogenous carcinogens and it is likely that it is both the time required for accumulation of multiple genetic changes and for multiple phases of clonal selection that results in tumours only later in life. This is probably a major factor in determining the age association of most epithelial tumours.

A second possibility is that with age there are changes in the cellular environment that are more permissive for outgrowth of altered clones or which allow or encourage neoplastic change to take place, for example, alterations in the immune or hormonal systems or changes in the tissue microenvironment. The relationship of tumour development in endocrine-sensitive organs such as the breast or prostate to age-associated hormonal changes in the patient is still to be completely defined but seems likely to be involved in the rate of growth of these tumours. One of the roles of hormones is to stimulate division of hormone-sensitive cells, that is, these may act as a promoting agent (Chapter 15). There is some debate about whether the relative decline in function of the immune system in old age plays a role and this is discussed in Chapter 20. Interestingly, there is also recent evidence that senescence-associated changes that occur in mesenchymal cells can affect adjacent epithelial cells and this may have a promoting effect. Senescent fibroblasts express several enzymes involved in extracellular matrix remodelling, for example, MMP-9 and stromelysin and it has been hypothesized that the ageing stroma may contribute to epithelial carcinogenesis in this way (Krtolica and Campisi, 2003). Some elegant experiments have been carried out by Cunha and colleagues which identify important effects of tumour stromal cells. They studied the effect of stromal cells derived from prostate tumours or from normal prostate on the *in vivo* growth of pre-neoplastic prostate epithelial cells in tissue recombination experiments. In combination with tumour stroma, the preneoplastic epithelium was able to form carcinomas, whereas when combined with normal stroma, only normal ductular structures were formed indicating that, even though non-tumorigenic themselves, stromal cells derived from the tumour microenvironment had lost the ability to exert their normal inhibitory control over the epithelial component of the tissue. Thus, normal age-associated changes and acquired changes in the tumour stroma can contribute to epithelial carcinogenesis.

Finally, it is possible that there are age-associated changes in some cells which increase their susceptibility to neoplastic transformation. Age-associated decline in DNA repair capacity with associated increase in mutation rate could be considered as such a factor. Although certain mutations can themselves alter this capacity, it is not clear whether changes in basal mutation rate can account in any significant measure for the age-associated increase in tumour incidence. There is some evidence that certain types of damage are repaired less efficiently by cells derived from old tissues. For example, UV-induced damage is repaired less efficiently by skin fibroblasts from old donors than from young donors. These differences may make a minor contribution to carcinogenesis in the old but are clearly not the major drivers. There is some experimental evidence for an increased sensitivity to carcinogen-induced neoplastic change in tissue cultures and in transplants derived from some organs from old animals, but it is not clear how much this is related to the presence of cells in old tissues which have already sustained genetic damage.

Interestingly, tumours that develop in aged laboratory mice are more frequently haematological and mesenchymal cell tumours than the epithelial types seen in man. Until recently this has been an unexplained observation. However, recent results provide a highly plausible explanation. As described in Chapter 10, the ends of mammalian chromosomes contain telomeric repeat sequences that with each normal round of DNA replication, lose some sequence due to the 'end-replication' problem. Thus, telomere length decreases with successive divisions and with age. It is now known that normal human cells, which show a finite lifespan *in vitro*, enter a phase commonly known as 'crisis' when they are stimulated by certain viral oncogenes (for example, SV40 large T) to continue proliferation beyond their normal senescence limit. At crisis, telomere length is severely shortened, rendering the telomeres vulnerable to end-to-end fusion and subsequent chromosomal breakage at mitosis. This can generate some of the typical cytogenetic abnormalities seen in epithelial tumours. Such tumours therefore bear the cytogenetic hallmarks of telomere attrition. Escape from crisis occurs only when cells begin to express telomerase, the specialized reverse transcriptase that allows them to maintain telomere length. The likely explanation for the species-specific age-associated tumour spectrum is that mice have very long telomeres which unlike human telomeres never undergo critical shortening within the lifespan of the organism, nor within the additional proliferative lifespan required for tumour development. Somatic mouse tissues also express telomerase. Hence the tumours that develop do not show major chromosomal rearrangements. So why do they develop mesenchymal tumours and leukaemias? The answer may lie in the requirement for fewer genetic events for transformation of these cell types.

1.8 Genetic instability, clonal selection, and tumour evolution

Our recent ability to dissect the cancer genome at both the gross chromosomal and nucleotide level has revealed extensive genetic change. Often this is complex, particularly in advanced epithelial cancers and is commonly referred to as genetic or genomic instability. Recent studies have revealed that genetic instability can take distinct forms and a debate has arisen over whether these represent cause or effect.

One type of instability is that which results from inactivation of mismatch repair (MMR) genes such as *MSH2* and *MLH1* (Chapter 4). Defects in MMR lead to numerous changes in short simple sequence repeats spread throughout the genome (called microsatellites; MMR is also termed microsatellite instability, MIN). MIN is characteristic of tumours found in patients with hereditary non-polyposis colorectal cancer (HNPCC) who inherit mutations in *MSH2* or *MLH1*. Interestingly, MIN tumours usually have a diploid karyotype which contrasts with non-MIN epithelial cancers which commonly show complex karyotypic abnormalities, commonly termed chromosomal instability (CIN). The causes of CIN have been less obvious. There are several possibilities including alterations in mitotic checkpoint genes or genes involved in centrosome function or chromosomal segregation as discussed above. Already some tumours have been found to contain this type of alteration. It is also possible that once a cell has become aneuploid by chance, this in itself predisposes it to become even more aneuploid. This might happen, for example, at mitosis where segregation of aberrant or large numbers of chromosomes is more error-prone. A final mechanism is the inherent CIN which is generated in cells at senescence when chromosomes have severe telomere attrition. As indicated above, shortening of telomeres in advance of re-expression of telomerase can lead to severe chromosomal rearrangement via end-to-end fusion followed by breakage at segregation. There is evidence for all of these mechanisms and it is likely that one or more may contribute to the development of any given tumour and that the mechanism that is active will shape the genome in specific and recognizable ways that may well be tissue or tumour type specific. More detailed analysis of tissue samples taken throughout the course of tumour development should help to clarify these issues in the next few years.

While it is clear that tumours often have MIN or CIN, it is not yet clear whether this is an early event in the process, nor whether it is necessary for tumour development. It has been argued that the probability of tumours acquiring the necessary number of genetic alterations is too low without some additional mutator effect. This type of calculation is difficult and to date no clear answer is apparent, though there is no doubt that some tumour cells have this phenotype while others, particularly early in their development, have little genomic alteration that can be identified. It is probable however, that the level of generation of mutations is critical and that too much instability is likely to impede tumour development rather than promote it. Already it is known that the type of genetic instability present in the tumour cell has an effect on the type of mutation found. Thus, for example, MIN colorectal tumours tend to inactivate the two alleles of the *APC* gene via two point mutations, whereas CIN tumours tend to have one point mutation and one allele lost by deletion.

Two recent reviews explore these concepts in depth using what is known about colorectal carcinogenesis, possibly the best-studied model system, as an example (Rajagopalan et al., 2003; Sieber et al., 2003).

1.8.1 Selection of altered clones

The process by which cancer cells develop and spread involves not only mutation but also selection of altered clones. These processes are the drivers of tumour evolution. It is thought that repeated rounds of mutation and selection occur during somatic evolution of a tumour. As the lineage evolves, the tumour cells acquire increased autonomy and eventually the capacity for metastasis. This is often compared to Darwinian evolution where in this case the fittest cell survives and multiplies. The low rate of mutation, calculated as 2×10^{-7} per gene per cell division for cultured human cells (Oller et al., 1989) precludes the acquisition by a single cell of multiple mutations simultaneously. Even when large carcinogen doses are applied, the large number of potentially lethal mutations sustained at the same time as any set of mutations with potential advantage is likely to lead to cell death rather than instant tumorigenicity. Thus the expectation is that events occur singly and in a particular sequence in each cancer. This is frequently referred to as a genetic pathway or progression pathway and for several cancer types attempts have been made to map the pathway in genetic terms. As indicated above, colorectal cancer is arguably the best elucidated model in this regard (Ilyas et al., 1999). In the colon, mutation of the *APC* gene is the initiating event. The resulting 'early' adenoma then commonly acquires mutations in *KRAS*, *SMAD4*, and *TP53*, respectively as it progresses histopathologically via 'intermediate' and 'late' adenoma to carcinoma. The frequency of each of these changes in each of the lesion types suggests that there is a preferred order of events in this case but this does not appear to be invariable. Results from other tumour types where samples can be obtained from lesions at different stages in the process, or from cancers with different malignant potential, also show shared lesions and temporal ordering of events in some cases. There is also evidence that alternative pathways can lead to the same result, and in different tissues specific mechanisms may dominate. For example, many tumours show inactivation of *TP53* via mutation while some others show amplification of the negative regulator of p53, *MDM2*. In the Rb pathway, some tumours show direct mutation of *RB* while others show inactivation of the pathway via inactivation of the negative regulator p16. The order of events may differ in different tissues. For example, mutations of *TP53* are found frequently in lung cancer but patients with a germline mutation in *TP53* (Li–Fraumeni syndrome) do not develop lung cancer as part of the syndrome. Possibly this reflects inability of loss of p53 function to act early in the pathway to lung cancer but its suitability as an early event in the other tumours that develop in these Li–Fraumeni patients.

The ultimate result of clonal evolution is escape from the normal growth restraints imposed on the cell in its normal tissue milieu. It follows therefore that the way in which this is achieved will depend to a great extent on what those growth restraints are. Hence the finding of tissue- and cell type-specific genetic alterations, different timing of alterations, etc.

It is easy to envisage selection of mutations that increase proliferation or allow resistance to apoptosis or any of the other key features of cancer cells. However, mutations that increase mutation frequency such as those that generate CIN or MIN do not in themselves confer an immediate advantage to the cell. At present, it is not clear how such a phenotype is selected. One plausible explanation is that such mutations may occur rarely in the same cell as a second mutation that does confer an immediate advantage and thus are selected as 'passenger' or 'bystander' events.

Many forms of treatment, for example, radiation and chemotherapy may provide additional mutagenic and selective stimuli and may precipitate the emergence of more aggressive variants. An obvious example is the destruction of X-ray-sensitive cells by X-ray treatment. If the tumour also contains X-ray-resistant cells, the cancer cells which are left after treatment will be X-ray resistant. Although progression is usually towards greater malignancy, this is not invariably so. There are a number of cases, unfortunately small, in which rapidly growing tumours have ceased to grow or even disappeared completely. Although we do not yet have a full explanation for this, some studies indicate that this may be related to the development of anti-tumour immunity in the host.

Thus, a series of changes occur in a cell as carcinogenesis proceeds. As the tumour progresses, more and more normal characteristics are lost and it is common to observe what has been described as dedifferentiation within the tumour tissue. This refers to the loss of normal structure and cellular functions characteristic of the tissue. Specialized products of the cell, for example, secretions or structural components may no longer be produced as the cell begins to take on new characteristics. The loss of normal differentiated features is referred to by a pathologist as anaplasia and the degree of such changes identified in tissue sections is used by the pathologist to 'grade' tumours. In general, less well-differentiated tumours have a poorer prognosis than those that retain the differentiated characteristics of the normal tissue. As a rule, there is an approximate correlation between tumour grade and growth rate. The most differentiated tumours (low grade, i.e. Grade I) tend to be more slow-growing and the most anaplastic (high grade, i.e. III or IV) the more rapidly growing. Human breast cancers are graded in this way and it has been shown that about 80% of patients with well-differentiated Grade I breast cancers will be alive and well at five years (and often much longer) but only 20% of patients with Grade IV tumours will survive for this time. It is of course equally obvious from these figures that although 80% of patients with Grade I cancers survive, 20% with the same structural type of tumour do not. Tumour growth and progression is influenced by factors other than tumour structure, and these may range from the rate of mutation and type of mutation they contain to the reaction of the patient's own defence mechanisms. In recent years much effort has been made to identify additional tests that can be carried out in the pathology laboratory at the time of tumour diagnosis to add both diagnostic and prognostic (predictive) information and the search for molecular markers (proteins or DNA changes) that can supplement the repertoire of morphological tests is intense. These are discussed at length in Chapter 21. In fact, there are many examples of success in identifying such markers for use in tumour classification, prediction of prognosis or response to therapy, disease monitoring, and markers that can be used as therapeutic targets. These are described in several of the other chapters of this book. Possibly, the identification of such markers has been the earliest and most clinically applicable result of the intense effort of the past two decades to characterize human tumours at the molecular level. More successes will undoubtedly follow.

1.8.2 Tumour clonality

We have alluded to clonal evolution during tumour development but what of the origin of the tumour? Tumour clonality refers to the cellular origin of cancers. A monoclonal tumour develops from a single progenitor cell and a polyclonal tumour develops from multiple cells. In many tissues, a solitary primary tumour is the norm and this may or may not recur or progress. In this circumstance the question of clonality concerns only this single tumour and its direct descendents. However, in some tissues the situation is more complex and when the structure of the organ is examined in detail widespread abnormal pathology may be found. In such a tissue multicentric tumours are sometimes found. Could there be many cells involved in the generation of a tumour or does each tumour arise from a single initiated cell?

The appearance of multiple preneoplastic lesions in a tissue has been described as a 'field change'. Figures 1.4 and 1.5 illustrate such a possible field effect. These tissues show a gradation from benign to malignant (as in Figure 1.2) but here the 'progression' is in space rather than time. This has been particularly described in tissues such as the bladder, colon, oesophagus, and oral mucosa where there is a large epithelial surface available for study and in which essentially all of the cells have received similar exposure to environmental agents. Here the question of clonality can be addressed to each individual tumour that arises, that is, tumour clonality, but of equal interest both to biologist and clinician, is the relationship between all the lesions in a single patient. This can be referred to as the clonality of the disease. With the advent of molecular genetic techniques there has been an explosion of information concerning the genetic relationship of such synchronous lesions.

There are several possibilities based on the clonality of each lesion and of the overall disease in the patient:

(1) Each individual tumour consists of lineages derived from multiple normal parent cells. Such

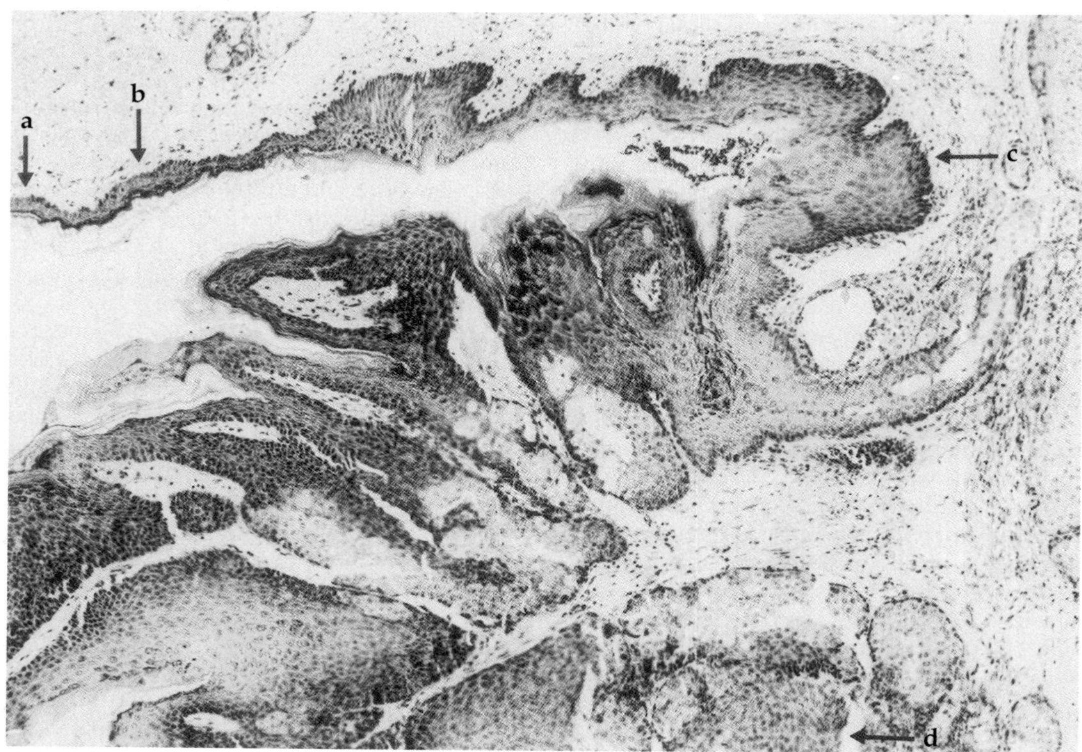

Figure 1.4 Section of the edge of a squamous cell carcinoma of skin, with normal skin (a) on the left and increasing dysplasia (b) and (c) leading into the main mass of the tumour (d) below right. Stained with haematoxylin and eosin (×50).

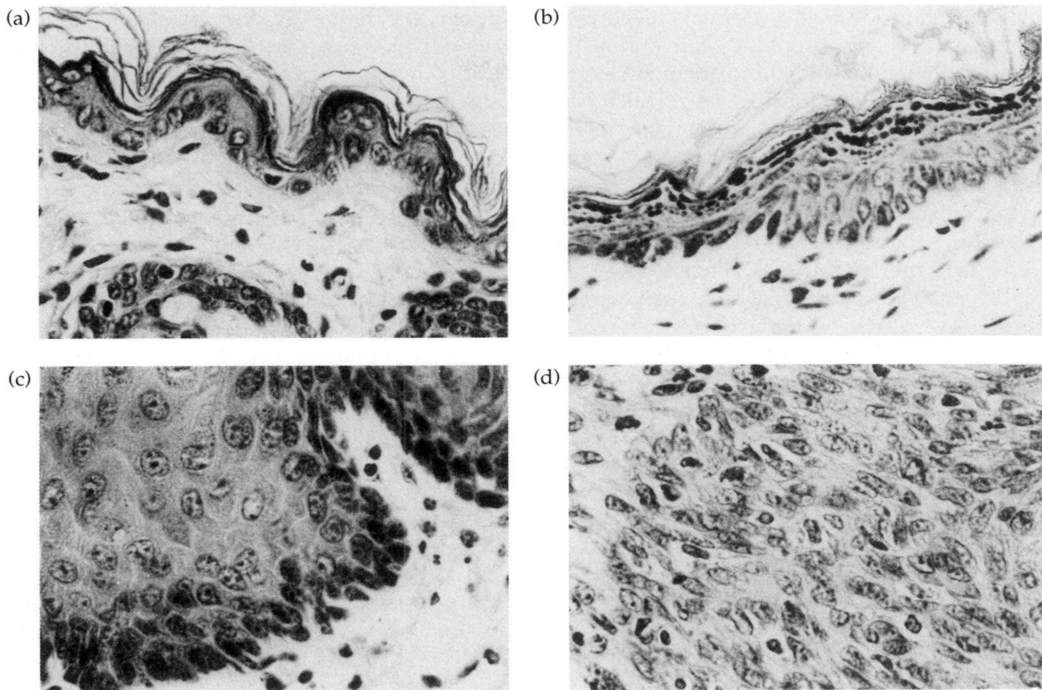

Figure 1.5 Detail of the areas marked in Figure 1.4 at higher magnification. (a) Normal skin (compare with Figure 1.1) showing mesenchyme below covered by normal epithelium with basal cells, more differentiated superficial cells and on top, layers of keratin formed from the superficial cells (×360), (b) Dysplastic skin. There is an increase in the number of basal cells, which are more irregular than in the normal and there is a disturbance in the formation of keratin, which is clumped into an irregular dark mass in the surface layer instead of the more regular sheets in (a), that is, differentiation is disturbed, (c) Cell overgrowth. The cells themselves are abnormal; they vary in shape and size, the nuclei are much larger than normal and some are deeply stained. The usually distinct separation between epithelium and stroma is not seen, suggesting that invasion may be taking place. The cells are still recognizable as skin cells. This would be diagnosed as a moderately well-differentiated squamous carcinoma (×360). (d) The centre of the tumour is made up of a mass of irregular spindle-shaped cells with no recognizable skin features. This would be diagnosed as an anaplastic (undifferentiated) carcinoma (×360).

a tumour would be described as polyclonal. A tumour derived from a few parent cells would be termed oligoclonal.

(2) Each tumour has a single parental cell of origin and multiple tumours in the same organ arise via seeding or direct spread of cells. Each is therefore a monoclonal tumour and this is monoclonal disease.

(3) The disease is polyclonal, that is, more than one initiated cell progresses to generate multiple tumours each of which is derived from a single cell (monoclonal).

There is in fact evidence for all three situations, though the majority of human cancers are solitary tumours of monoclonal origin and there is ongoing debate over whether true polyclonal tumours do exist (Garcia et al., 2000).

The methods most commonly used to assess tumour clonality are X-chromosome inactivation and loss of heterozygosity (LOH) analysis by microsatellite typing. During the course of embryonic development in females, genes on one of the X chromosomes are silenced by methylation of cytosine residues in the promoter (Chapter 5). Such methylation is heritably maintained and prevents transcriptional activation within the promoter region. This process is random and in any tissue, 50% of cells have methylation of each copy of X. A monoclonal tumour will therefore have inactivation of any gene on only one of its X chromosomes and this can be detected at the molecular level.

Polymorphisms in X-linked genes have been used to identify individual parental alleles and when assessed in combination with the use of methylation-sensitive restriction endonucleases, which cut only non-methylated DNA, assays for allele-specific methylation can be developed. Several X-chromosome loci have been used including glycerophosphate kinase (*PGK*), hypoxanthine phosphoribosyltransferase (*HPRT*), and the androgen receptor gene (*HUMARA*) (Vogelstein et al., 1987). Such analyses are restricted to female tissues and to those women who are heterozygous at the locus of choice, namely those that have distinguishable maternal and paternal alleles. While there are some problems in interpretation of X-inactivation assays for clonality, these assays have the significant advantage that the feature studied is not itself part of the neoplastic process.

Microsatellite typing uses the polymerase chain reaction (PCR) reaction to amplify short DNA products containing simple sequence repeats that are highly polymorphic in the human genome. Because the repeat length varies, alleles inherited from each parent are frequently distinguishable by size. In a tumour with genomic deletion, for example, deletion of one copy of a tumour suppressor gene, loss of one allele (LOH, loss of heterozygosity) at nearby microsatellite repeats is commonly found in the tumour. Indeed this method has been widely used to map the locations of novel tumour suppressor genes. However, the use of this assay or any tumour-specific molecular alteration to assess clonality per se is somewhat restricted. For example, LOH analysis cannot detect true cellular polyclonality since LOH in a mixed population is difficult to detect.

When tumour-specific genetic markers are used for clonality analysis, it is predicted that in related monoclonal tumours, markers associated with changes that occurred early in tumour development will show greatest concordance and those that occur later in tumour development may show divergence in related tumours that have undergone clonal evolution. This latter observation can be referred to as sub-clonal evolution. LOH analysis has been used to assess the temporal sequence of genetic events that has taken place during the

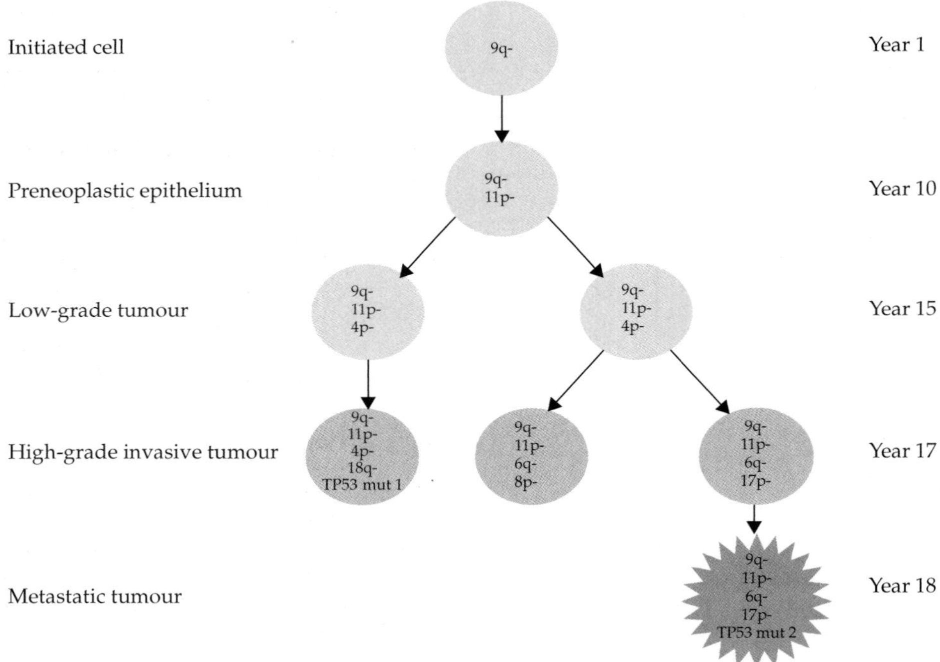

Figure 1.6 Example of possible evolution of a metastatic tumour from a single initiated cell, over the course of many years. Changes shown are common deletions that may be identified by LOH analysis and different mutations in *TP53* (*TP53* mut 1 and 2). 9q-, 11p-, etc. denote deletions of the long (q) or short (p) arms of different chromosomes. Sub-clonal evolution within the population may lead to several distinct but spatially related tumours that differ in some but not all genetic changes. A final event in one cell may allow a metastatic clone to evolve.

evolution of a tumour from a series of temporally or spatially related lesions. Examples of such studies include the elucidation of neoplastic lineages in Barrett oesophagus (Barrett et al., 1999) and in synchronous and metachronous bladder cancer (Takahashi et al., 1998). An example of the type of lineage deduced from such studies is shown in Figure 1.6.

Not only does information about the relationships between such lesions give valuable biological information about disease development but it also provides information with potential clinical application. For example, the presence of multiple different tumour clones within an epithelium may show a relationship to tumour recurrence rate or time to recurrence and may indicate a need for more vigilant monitoring. In the future, as targeted therapies become available, knowledge of the specific molecular characteristics of all tumours present, may influence choice of therapy and polyclonal tumours may be more difficult to target in this way.

By the time a tumour is detectable clinically, whether it has arisen from one or many cells, it has been present for a long time and the cells have had to go through a large number of cell divisions. A tumour of about 0.5 cm in diameter, which is just detectable, may contain over 500 million cells. Within such a population, even if deemed monoclonal by X-inactivation and other genetic assays, it is likely that at any point in time a large tumour could contain many potential new sub-clones with potential to evolve and some already forming sizeable sub-clones. Certainly, tumours show morphological differences in different regions and these can be accompanied by changes in protein expression detected by immunohistochemistry or other assays.

1.9 Tumour diagnosis

There are no absolute methods for diagnosing and assessing the degree of malignancy of tumours. Microscopic examination of tissue is still the mainstay for routine use and the role of the pathologist at the time of diagnosis is critical. The pathologist has to decide whether the structure of the cells in the tissue is sufficiently removed from the normal to allow a diagnosis of neoplasia and if so, whether the tumour is benign or malignant, its probable cell of origin, its degree of differentiation, and its extent of spread. For practical purposes, the two techniques used are tumour grading and tumour staging. Tumour grading attempts to measure the degree of dedifferentiation in tumours and is based on histological and cytological criteria (Figures 1.4 and 1.5). Histological differentiation is concerned with alterations in the structure of the tissue, that is, the relationship of cells to each other and to their underlying stroma. Cytological grading is based on the application of similar criteria to the structure of the specific tumour cells. Tumour staging assesses the extent of spread of tumours. Ideally, a range of objective molecular markers that can be added to this routine morphological assessment is highly desirable. To date such objective markers do not exist for all applications. However, as discussed in Chapters 6 and 21 there has been great progress in recent years in adding to the routine morphological assessment, a variety of assays based on our accumulating knowledge of the molecular biology of cancer. Many such tests are still at the experimental stage but some are in widespread application in the pathology or cytogenetics laboratory. For example, the differential diagnosis of many haematological malignancies routinely uses specific antibody panels for immunohistochemistry and/or the detection of specific chromosomal translocations in the genome. More details of these and other assays are given in Chapters 6 and 21 and here we will only discuss morphological assessment which is applicable to all neoplasms.

Several papers have been written on tumour diagnosis by international panels of tumour pathologists. The following brief survey will only give a guide. We have chosen some of the examples, not because they are common, but because they illustrate particular points more clearly than the more common tumours.

1.9.1 Benign tumours

Benign tumours usually resemble their tissue of origin but every tissue component need not be involved and the cells may or may not be in their normal relationship. Benign tumours arise in most tissues, increase in size, but do not invade. They are usually separated from the surrounding normal tissue by a capsule of connective tissue. Cytologically, the specific tumour cells do not differ substantially from the structure of the normal organ cells. Benign tumours of bone or cartilage may produce nodules of bone or cartilage indistinguishable from normal tissues. In epithelial tissues, groups of cells may also form local benign tumours made up of all tissue components. The covering or lining tissues of skin, intestinal tract, bladder, etc. may produce wart-like outgrowths containing all the tissue components (a papilloma). The common wart is a local outgrowth of all skin components. In other situations only one constituent cell may give rise to a benign tumour. The pituitary, for example, is a small gland at the base of the brain which produces many different hormones, each produced by a different type of cell, arranged in solid cords. Benign tumours of one of these cell types may then produce an excess of one particular hormone. Other benign tumours of the pituitary may contain more than one cell type, or produce more than one hormone, and some may be derived from non-hormone-producing cells. The cells in all these tumours are arranged in solid cords as in the normal gland. The benign tumours do not invade the surrounding tissue but, if they increase in size, they may press on and damage the remaining normal cells or overlying nervous tissue or press on the optic nerves which pass nearby and lead to blindness. So, although these pituitary tumours themselves are benign, they may cause serious disturbances by local pressure, or may continue to produce excessive amounts of their normal product, which may in itself cause severe symptoms. Benign tumours of any other hormone-producing gland such as the thyroid, adrenal, etc. may have similar effects. Alternatively, benign tumours may damage the remaining normal cells and cause a loss of normal function.

Benign epithelial tumours arise in many organs. There is a different pattern of tumour growth in organs with a tubular structure. Both the kidney and breast, for example, consist of tubular structures with the epithelial tubules lined by several different epithelial cell types and surrounded by connective tissue. Benign tumours in these organs are made up of tubules, usually with one, or less commonly two, different epithelial cell types, together with a variable amount of connective tissue.

1.9.2 Malignant tumours

Malignant tumours show two characteristic features; cellular abnormalities (dyskaryosis), sometimes slight, and invasion of surrounding tissues. When both features are present, diagnosis is easy. The standard cellular criteria include a local increase in cell number, loss of the normal regular arrangement of cells, variation in cell shape and size, increase in nuclear size and density of staining (both of which often reflect an increase in DNA content), an increase in mitotic activity (increased cell division), and the presence of abnormal mitoses and chromosomes. The diagnosis of carcinomas (malignant epithelial tumours) *in situ* depends on the recognition of these cellular changes in an area of epithelium, usually on a surface such as the cervix of the uterus, skin, or bladder, but it may occur in other organs. The changes only involve the epithelium and there is no invasion of underlying tissues, that is, the neoplastic cells remain where they began, *in situ*.

The only definite evidence of malignancy is invasion of underlying tissues. In most cases this is easily recognized as the tumour cells destroy and replace the normal tissues. Malignant tumours have no well-defined capsule and the tumour cells grow in a much more disorganized form than is found in benign tumours. The same criteria apply to all malignant tumours, whatever their tissue of origin. Sometimes, tumour cells may be found invading blood or lymphatic vessels; they may then be carried to other parts of the body in blood or lymph and develop into secondary tumours (metastases) in these distant sites. This type of spread is characteristic of malignant tumours and is the major problem in treatment since a tumour that remains localized to its site of origin is more easily removed surgically or destroyed by radiation. The problem of metastasis is discussed in Chapter 16.

1.10 Tumour nomenclature

Although the precise nomenclature (naming) of tumours may seem to be an academic exercise, it is of great practical importance in deciding on treatment for each individual patient. Obviously, it is important for each pathologist, surgeon, and oncologist to use the same name for the same type of tumour. Inevitably, there is still variation between laboratories and even after many years of effort by international organizations, there is still some confusion about names. However, for most tumour types, more or less agreed systems of nomenclature are in general use. A more important point is that knowledge of the type of tumour cell and the extent of spread are essential in planning treatment. Some tumours are known to be sensitive to particular drugs, hormones, or X-rays but others are resistant. Knowing the extent of spread will help to define the area for treatment by radiation or surgery or even whether surgery is possible. For these reasons, the surgeon will usually remove a piece, or the whole tumour if it is readily accessible, for examination by a pathologist. The tissue removed, (a biopsy), is preserved by a chemical fixative and thin sections are prepared for examination under the microscope.

Although the names given to tumours may at first seem confusing, there is a simple logical basis to tumour nomenclature. The terms tumour, growth, or neoplasm can be used to describe a malignant tumour. Tumours are described by a generic name which specifies the general tissue of origin, that is, mesenchyme, epithelium, or haemato-lymphoid, and whether the tumour is benign or malignant. This generic name is qualified by the specific tissue of origin, for example, kidney, breast, and this too may be qualified by further terms describing the cell of origin (if identifiable) and the pattern of growth. Some examples will make this clearer; a list is given in Table 1.1.

1.10.1 Tumours of epithelium

Benign tumours

Benign tumours of epithelium are usually described by their growth pattern and tissue of origin. Benign tumours of skin may be papillary (a warty outgrowth or papilloma) or solid. A benign skin tumour derived from squamous (flattened) epithelium could be described as a squamous cell papilloma of skin. Benign tumours of glandular tissues are called adenomas and may be solid or papillary, for example, solid or papillary adenoma of thyroid.

Malignant tumours

The generic name for malignant tumours of epithelium is carcinoma, for example, carcinoma of skin. The common skin carcinomas may appear to arise from the differentiated squamous cells or from the less-differentiated basal cells, so that skin carcinomas may be described as squamous cell carcinomas or basal cell carcinomas. They may grow as flat (sessile) plaques or as warty (papillary) outgrowths. So a tumour may, for example, be described as a papillary squamous cell carcinoma of skin. Its grade and the extent of invasion may also be given. The final pathologist's report may read 'moderately well differentiated (Grade II) squamous carcinoma of skin. The structure is mainly papillary but there is invasion of the underlying connective tissue; muscle is not involved'. This report tells the surgeon and oncologist that the tumour is made up of squamous cells which are known to be sensitive to X-irradiation and that the extent of spread is limited, that is, it could easily be removed by local surgery. The final decision on treatment would then depend on the exact position of the tumour and among other factors, whether surgery or irradiation would be easier or leave less scarring.

Malignant tumours of glandular tissues are also carcinomas but are sometimes described as adenocarcinomas, for example, adenocarcinoma of breast, implying that the tumour has a glandular structure. As with the skin tumours, the cell type can be described (e.g. columnar cell or cuboidal) and if the cell of origin is known, this too can be added (e.g. ductal cuboidal cell adenocarcinoma of breast). The gross pattern of growth (sessile or papillary) and extent of spread can also be defined. Adenocarcinomas have a wider range of cellular patterns than tumours of covering epithelium. The cells may be arranged as large or small tubules or solid cords (trabeculae) or masses and this pattern will also be described. In some cases the tumour grade can be assessed.

Most tumours retain some of the structural features of the cells from which they have arisen and, as we have seen, this allows the pathologist to make a rough assessment of the degree of malignancy, by the extent to which the tumours have departed from the normal (grading); it also may allow the source of a secondary tumour to be established. However, there are still problems. Some tumours may be so undifferentiated that they no longer retain any structure which indicates the tissue of origin. In others, some cells may differentiate in an abnormal way. A common event is that tumour cells from a glandular organ such as the breast, which are normally columnar in structure, may develop into squamous cells resembling those in skin tumours. This process is known as metaplasia and although confusing, does not as a rule influence the degree of malignancy. A final point is that in many tumours, the structure is not homogeneous and more than one cell type, growth pattern, or grade of tumour may be present.

Table 1.1 Nomenclature of common tumours

Tissue	Cell type	Benign tumour	Malignant tumour
Epithelium			
Skin	Squamous epithelium	Squamous cell papilloma	Squamous carcinoma Basal cell carcinoma
	Melanocytes	Melanocytic naevus	Malignant melanoma
Upper aero-digestive tract			
Nose, mouth, pharynx, larynx, and oesophagus	Squamous epithelium	Squamous cell papilloma	Squamous carcinoma
Alimentary tract			
Stomach, small and large bowel	Columnar epithelium	Adenoma	Adenocarcinoma
Lungs	Respiratory epithelium		Squamous carcinoma Adenocarcinoma Small cell carcinoma Undifferentiated carcinoma
Urinary system			
Ureters and bladder	Urothelium (transitional epithelium)	Transitional cell papilloma	Transitional cell carcinoma
Solid epithelial organs			
Liver, pancreas, kidney, prostate, etc.	Specific epithelium	Adenoma	Adenocarcinoma
Gonads			
Ovary	Surface epithelium	Serous cystadenoma Mucinous cystadenoma	Serous cystadenocarcinoma Mucinous cystadenocarcinoma
Ovary	Germ cells	Teratoma	Dysgerminoma Yolk sac tumour Embryonal carcinoma Choriocarcinoma
Testis	Germ cells		Seminoma Teratoma Yolk sac tumour Choriocarcinoma
Mesenchyme			
Fibrous tissue	Fibroblasts	Fibroma	Fibrosarcoma
Fat	Adipocytes	Lipoma	Liposarcoma
Bone	Osteocytes	Osteoma	Osteosarcoma
Cartilage	Chondrocytes	Chondroma	Chondrosarcoma
Smooth muscle	Smooth muscle cells	Leiomyoma	Leiomyosarcoma
Striated muscle	Striated muscle cells	Rhadbomyoma	Rhabdomyosarcoma
Blood vessels	Endothelial cells	Haemangioma	Angiosarcoma
Peripheral nerve	Schwann cells	Schwannoma Neurofibroma	Malignant peripheral nerve sheath tumour
Haemato-lymphoid			
Haemopoietic system	Red cells, leukocytes, and platelets		Acute myeloid leukaemia Chronic myeloid leukaemia Myeloproliferative disorders
Immune system	Lymphoid cells		Acute lymphoblastic leukaemia Chronic lymphocytic leukaemia Non-Hodgkin lymphoma Hodgkin lymphoma Multiple myeloma
Central Nervous System			
Glial cells	Astrocytes and oligodendrocytes		Glioma—Astrocytoma and oligodendroglioma
Meninges	Meningothelial cells	Meningioma	Anaplastic (malignant) meningioma
Embryonal	Neurones		Medulloblastoma and primitive neuroectodermal tumour

1.10.2 Tumours of mesenchyme

Benign tumours

Benign tumours of mesenchyme are described by the cellular tissue from which they arise (see Table 1.1). Benign tumours of fibrous tissue are fibromas, benign tumours of bone may be described as osteomas and benign tumours of blood vessels as angiomas.

Malignant tumours

The generic name for malignant tumours of mesenchyme is sarcoma and as with carcinomas, this is qualified by the cell of origin and growth patterns. Thus a malignant tumour of bone cells is called a bone sarcoma or osteosarcoma but this can be qualified to describe behaviour. A tumour made of cells forming bone could be described as an osteogenic sarcoma and one with bone-destroying cells described as an osteolytic sarcoma. Tumours derived from blood vessels are angiosarcomas, and so on. The extent of spread of sarcomas can also be defined and in principle sarcomas may also be graded in the same way as carcinomas, depending on the degree of dedifferentiation. In practice, however, this is rarely done since most of the sarcomas are very rapidly growing and require aggressive treatment.

1.10.3 Tumours of the haemato-lymphoid system

This is a complicated field encompassing a huge variety of malignant tumours with a wide range of biological and clinical diversity (Chapter 18). Broadly speaking, these tumours may be subdivided into those that arise from stem cells that produce blood cells (haematopoietic stem cells) which involve the peripheral blood and bone marrow and are termed leukaemia, and those that arise from cells of the immune system which form solid tumours of lymph nodes and extranodal lymphatic tissue which are termed lymphoma.

The leukaemias may show myeloid or lymphoid differentiation which is determined by their cellular morphology, cytochemical characteristics, and phenotype. They may also be subdivided into acute and chronic forms; the acute leukaemias show little evidence of differentiation to mature haemopoietic cells such as neutrophils, red cells and platelets or lymphocytes. The chronic leukaemias show variable degrees of terminal differentiation but always contain large numbers of mature blood cells. The leukaemias are characterized by circulating malignant cells in the peripheral blood and to a variable extent evidence of bone marrow failure in the form of an absence of normal blood components. Rarely, leukaemias may form solid tumour deposits or infiltrate and compromise the function of visceral organs such as the liver.

The lymphomas are traditionally subdivided into Hodgkin's and non-Hodgkin's types. Although both arise from cells of the lymphoid system, there are profound biological and clinical differences between them. Hodgkin's lymphoma is a disease of germinal centre B lymphocytes which only affects lymph nodes and the thymus and typically presents in young adults with enlarged lymph nodes. The non-Hodgkin's lymphomas may be of T or B lymphoid lineage, affect a wide age range (but are much commoner in older people) and may begin in lymph nodes or extranodal sites such as the stomach, thyroid, or salivary glands. There are a large number of distinctive disease entities included under the term non-Hodgkin's lymphoma which range from indolent but incurable diseases to those that are rapidly progressive but potentially curable in some patients. Some non-Hodgkin's lymphomas may have a leukaemic phase with circulating lymphoma cells in the peripheral blood and thus, within tumours of the lymphoid system, the distinction between lymphoma and leukaemia is not absolutely clear-cut.

1.10.4 Tumours of the nervous system

Tumours of the nervous system may arise in peripheral nerves, the autonomic nervous system, or the central nervous system (CNS).

Tumours of peripheral nerves are most commonly benign and comprise two broad categories, schwannomas and neurofibromas. Schwannomas are encapsulated tumours which arise from the perineurium of the nerve and are composed of masses of proliferating Schwann cells. Neurofibromas may be solitary or multiple and may affect the skin or visceral organs. They are derived from the endoneurium and although clonal, contain a variety of components including Schwann cells and small nerve fibres. The syndrome of type 1 neurofibromatosis is associated with mutations of the *NF1* gene located at 17q11.2. The syndrome includes the occurrence of multiple neurofibromas and abnormal patches of skin and iris pigmentation.

There is a risk of malignant transformation in the neurofibromas of *NF1* patients estimated to be a 2% lifetime risk. Malignant tumours of peripheral nerve sheath are, in general, high-grade soft tissue sarcomas with high metastatic potential and a poor survival.

Tumours of the autonomic nervous system include neoplasms of adrenaline and noradrenaline secreting structures, the paraganglia. Tumours of the adrenal medulla are termed phaeochromocytomas and tumours occurring outside the adrenal are termed extra-adrenal paragangliomas. They are histologically identical. Approximately 10% are malignant and metastasise. Neuroblastomas are tumours of primitive neuroectodermal origin which are destined to develop into catecholamine-secreting paraganglionic cells. Neuroblastomas most frequently arise in the adrenal medulla of children under five. Extra-adrenal, paraganglionic sites occur in approximately 10% of cases. They are composed of primitive 'round blue cells' and are highly malignant.

Tumours of the CNS may be derived from embryonic neuronal stem cells or supporting cells of the CNS termed glial cells. Tumours of embryonic neuronal stem cells form highly malignant undifferentiated tumours such as retinoblastoma, medulloblastoma, and primitive neuroectodermal tumour. These occur predominantly in childhood and spread via the cerebrospinal fluid and by direct invasion of the brain. Tumours of glial cells are termed gliomas. They may arise from astrocytic cells and form astrocytomas, oligodendroglial cells to form oligodendrogliomas and from cells lining the ventricular system, ependymal cells to form ependymomas. Gliomas are tumours of adult life and rarely occur in children. They are all malignant and their degree of malignancy ranges from slow-growing indolent tumours to rapidly growing destructive tumours, termed glioblastoma multiforme, whose median survival is less than six months. Gliomas invade the substance of the brain but do not metastasise outside the CNS.

Tumours of the covering of the brain, the meninges, are termed meningiomas. The majority of these are benign and come to clinical attention because of pressure effects on the CNS.

1.10.5 Germ cell tumours

A variety of tumours arise from germ cells in both males and females. The majority occur within the ovary and testis but extragonadal locations are also seen along the course of germ cell migration during foetal development.

Germ cell tumours that resemble primitive germ cells and show no differentiation towards other structures are termed seminoma in the testis and dysgerminoma in the ovary. These are both malignant tumours but have a high cure rate because of their sensitivity to radio- and chemotherapy.

Germ cell tumours that differentiate towards ectoderm, endoderm, and mesenchyme are called teratomas. These may contain fully mature or undifferentiated elements. In the ovary, differentiated teratomas are usually cystic and are termed mature cystic teratoma or dermoid cyst; they are benign. Ovarian teratomas containing immature or undifferentiated elements have malignant potential.

All testicular teratomas are regarded as malignant with a spectrum of malignant behaviour dependent on the presence of undifferentiated elements. Some teratomas will show evidence of extra-embryonic differentiation and form structures resembling foetal yolk sac or trophoblast of the developing placenta. Extra-embryonic differentiation in teratomas is associated with secretion of proteins which may be detected in the serum of patients and prove useful as tumour markers in following the course of the disease. Alpha-fetoprotein is secreted by yolk sac tumours and the beta subunit of human chorionic gonadotrophin by tumours showing trophoblastic differentiation.

1.10.6 Tumours showing divergent differentiation

Rarely, tumours may show divergent differentiation and contain both epithelial and mesenchymal elements which are clonally related. In these tumours both elements may be benign such as the ovarian adenofibroma, one element may be malignant, for example, the endometrial adenosarcoma where the epithelial component is benign and the mesenchymal component malignant or both may be malignant as in the carcinosarcoma. The mesenchymal component in these mixed tumours may show a variety of differentiation patterns and form muscle, cartilage, bone, and fat, or a mixture.

1.10.7 Tumour staging and the spread of tumours (metastasis)

Tumour metastasis is the major practical problem and a common cause of death in clinical cancer. Tumours invade the surrounding tissues and may grow out of the organ in which they arise and involve surrounding tissues (Figure 1.2). During this local invasion, tumour cells may penetrate the lymphatics and be carried to the regional lymph nodes where they are arrested. Some are destroyed but others may grow and produce new tumours. If tumour cells get into blood vessels, they may be carried to any organ in the body. Again, many are destroyed but others grow into secondary tumours. There are many unexplained problems. Carcinomas often involve lymph nodes but sarcomas rarely do. Some tumours give rise to secondary deposits more frequently in particular organs than in others. Metastases in the lungs, liver, and bones are common but other organs, like muscle and spleen are rarely the site of tumour deposits. The relative importance of the seed (the tumour cells) and the soil (the destination organs involved) are discussed in more detail in Chapter 16.

Tumour staging is used to give an assessment of the extent of spread of tumours. One of the more commonly used systems is that established by the International Union Against Cancer. This TNM system is based on an assessment of the primary tumour (T), the regional lymph nodes (N), and the presence or absence of metastases (M). Each of these categories is qualified by a number which indicates the precise extent of involvement according to clearly defined criteria. An additional code, R, has now been suggested to reflect the amount of residual tumour after treatment (Wittekind et al., 2002).

1.11 How tumours present: some effects of tumours on the body

Tumours are usually diagnosed when they produce some effects. Tumours of the skin or of organs which can be easily examined such as breast, often present as a noticeable lump. Many cells in tumours die and these dead cells release enzymes which damage the overlying tissues so that a non-healing ulcer may form. Blood vessels at the base of the ulcer are damaged so that bleeding occurs. In the bowel or the urinary system, blood may be present in the stools, or in the urine, so that bleeding is a common presenting symptom in these organs. Many of the effects produced by tumours are due to the position of the tumour which may press on or destroy surrounding tissues or affect nerves and cause pain. Tumours in the bowel, for example, may cause obstruction either because the tumour mass grows into the cavity of the bowel, or by growing into the wall and destroying the muscle which normally moves the contents down the intestine. Tumours of the brain may present with headache caused by increased pressure inside the skull; tumours involving the bile ducts leading from the liver may cause jaundice and so on. The physical effects obviously depend on the exact site of the tumour. Some tumours, particularly those which arise from hormone-producing organs, may cause effects either by producing an excess of the hormones which the normal organ produces or they may cause a hormone deficiency by damaging the remaining normal gland cells. Less commonly they may produce abnormal hormones or hormones may be produced in tumours of organs which do not normally produce these substances (ectopic expression), for example, some lung tumours may produce hormones normally produced by the pituitary gland. Anaemia due to bleeding from the tumour or due to some toxic effects on the bone marrow is a not uncommon presenting symptom. As well as these effects, many tumours may cause general wasting and loss of appetite (tumour cachexia), sometimes even though the primary tumour is still fairly small. The cause is unknown but it may be due to some toxic product of the tumour, possibly a growth factor.

1.12 How does cancer kill?

As we have seen, many cancers develop in older people and a substantial number of patients do not die as a consequence of the disease but of some unrelated condition such as heart disease or incidental infections. Tumour-related events may cause death directly or indirectly depending on the site of the tumour and the extent of spread. A common cause of death is involvement of vital organs, either by direct local invasion or from distant metastases, for example, in the brain, lung, or liver. Rarely, death may be due to haemorrhage. More often, anaemia and unexplained wasting may lead to decreased resistance to infection so that terminal bronchopneumonia or infection of the urinary tract (pyelonephritis) is common. In many cases it is not possible to establish the immediate cause of death.

1.13 Treatment of cancer

The aim of an ideal cancer treatment is the removal or destruction of all cancer cells and ideally of areas already predisposed to tumour development. Currently, treatment can involve a large repertoire of techniques ranging from those that have been standard treatments for the past several decades (surgery, radiation, chemotherapy) through to novel treatments involving biological agents, immunotherapy, and new highly specific small molecules. This range of therapies is discussed in Chapters 23–28. What is clear at the beginning of the twenty-first century is that laboratory science and hospital medicine are now very closely entwined in the effort to develop new agents to treat cancer.

However, we are only at a relatively early stage in the application of these more novel approaches. In many cases, treatment may not be possible because the tumour has involved vital organs or has spread throughout the body. Although theoretically unsatisfactory since tumour spread may take place at a very early stage in the disease, local surgical removal of the primary tumour remains a very effective method of treatment in many cases. The scalpel is still the surgeon's best weapon but attempts to improve on this are being developed using laser-induced energy, or cryosurgery using liquid nitrogen probes, to coagulate tumour cells *in situ*. One experimental technique is to give photosensitizing drugs that may be concentrated in the tumour and activated by the local application of laser energy of the appropriate wavelength. Radiation therapy is another widely used method for destroying tumour cells but there are often problems in applying a high dose to kill tumour cells without destroying the surrounding normal tissues. Some tumour cells are also resistant to radiation-induced damage. Currently, new approaches are successfully combining radiation with other agents including radiosensitizers (Chapter 25). Chemotherapy remains a mainstay of treatment for disseminated cancer (Chapter 24). Some long-standing single- or multiple-agent treatment regimes are still used but there has been much recent progress in the optimization of use of 'old' agents and the introduction of many new agents, including small molecules that target specific gene products or the vasculature in the tumour. Other novel agents include biological molecules such as antibodies (Chapter 26) and biological response modifiers such as cytokines (Chapter 14). Similarly, great progress in our ability to harness the host's immune system is reflected in many new approaches to immunotherapy (Chapter 27).

Not only are new approaches using cancer-specific markers as targets for drug design, but knowledge about the molecular changes in the cancer cell also provides information that can be used in the development of various forms of gene therapy (Chapter 28). Many approaches are being tested, ranging from attempts at direct replacement of defective gene function (tumour suppressor genes, e.g. *p53*, *Rb*) to a plethora of approaches for the design of vectors for delivery of prodrugs or other therapeutic molecules and tumour targeting of both vectors and expression of the therapeutic genes they contain.

Two major problems for these various forms of therapy are delivery of the therapeutic agents to disseminated tumour cells and specificity, that is, restricting toxic effects of the agent to tumour cells only, without damage to normal tissues. The identity of absolute tumour-specific markers would allow an approach to this and should allow the development of specific antitumour antibodies. Some relatively tumour-specific molecules have indeed been identified in the past few years and studies are in progress to develop therapies based on them. Even if absolute markers are not available for all tumours, it may still be possible to use antibodies against normal tissues if the tissue-specific determinants are only exposed where tissue architecture is disturbed in tumours. Molecular biological research is currently fuelling huge efforts in these fields.

1.14 Cancer prevention and screening

Since at least one in four people will develop cancer at some time in their lives, prevention seems an obvious approach. However, 70% of all cancers develop in people over 60 years old and even the prevention of all cancers would not have a substantial effect on the total lifespan. The rationale for prevention and effective treatment is to improve the quality of life.

Prevention is based mainly on the avoidance of cancer-producing agents. Since lung cancer alone is responsible for about a quarter of all cancer deaths the avoidance of smoking and other tobacco products would make a more dramatic reduction in cancer than almost any other measure known at present. The reduction of other environmental hazards and the effects of diet would play a lesser role and the identity of dietary factors is still not clear. Research in these areas is discussed in Chapter 2.

Common sense also suggests that early treatment should lead to a better end result and for this reason massive (and expensive) screening programmes have been set up to try to identify tumours before they produce symptoms. Screening for the presence of cancer has been carried out for cancers of the uterine cervix, breast, colon, ovary, prostate, and in areas of high incidence, stomach (Japan and China) and liver (Southern Africa). Ideally, screening should help to reduce mortality and morbidity from cancer and for some cancers screening is believed to be beneficial (e.g. breast and cervix). However, benefits are not clear in all cases. For example, some claim that screening may detect small tumours that would never cause any symptoms of disease. Cancers can be found in the prostate in at least 30–40% of men dying of unrelated disease. Since 30–40% of men do not die from prostate cancer it is believed that most of these tumours would not have killed their host. Similar latent tumours can be found in many other organs although not at such high frequency. These and other issues related to screening are discussed in Chapter 29.

1.15 Experimental methods in cancer research

Much of our knowledge of the development and growth of tumours has come from the study of cancers in patients by clinicians and pathologists. Although much is still to be gained from the application of current technology to direct studies of human cancer in the patient or in the setting of a pathology laboratory, such studies are largely observational and extensive experimental manipulation in man is not possible. Thus, the development of techniques that allow experimental manipulation of cells and tumours and increase the scope for identification of the molecules they contain has been pivotal. A wide range of methods and approaches is now available. This is both exciting and quite daunting. A detailed discussion of what is available now would encompass aspects of a broad range of disciplines including the clinical sciences, biology, physics, and chemistry and is beyond the scope of this book. Many approaches are referred to and discussed in some detail in subsequent chapters and the reader is referred to the excellent series of practical guides to methods entitled *Current Protocols (Current Protocols in Molecular Biology*, etc. published by John Wiley and Sons) for guidance on choice of methods and experimental protocols.

The unanswered questions in cancer research today demand a wide range of skills from the biologist and clinical scientist. For example, examination of tumour samples using expression microarrays, which in itself may present both laboratory and bioinformatic challenges, may lead rapidly to the examination of a range of 'candidate genes' that requires isolation of gene sequences, expression analyses, raising of antibodies, cell culture, modulation of gene expression both in cultured cells and in model organisms and almost inevitably to complete the circle, direct studies of the genes in human cancers. Though it is unlikely that all of these activities will be carried out by an individual researcher, they are commonly undertaken by a single research team and their close collaborators. This requirement for such diverse approaches highlights an important point—that collaboration and communication may be the most important skills or tools for cancer research in the future.

1.16 Conclusions

Cancer is a complex disease and it is apparent from this brief overview that although many of the underlying molecular processes are now yielding their secrets to modern technologies, there are still unanswered questions for the future. The succeeding chapters describe our current state of knowledge in more detail and identify more precisely where some of these key questions lie.

References and further reading

Barrett, M. T., Sanchez, C. A., Prevo, L. J., Wong, D. J., Galipeau, P. C., Paulson, T. G. et al. (1999). Evolution of neoplastic cell lineages in Barrett oesophagus. *Nat Genet*, **22**, 106–9.

Chin, L. and DePinho, R. A. (2000). Flipping the oncogene switch: illumination of tumor maintenance and regression. *Trends Genet*, **16**, 147–50.

Druker, B. J. and Lydon, N. B. (2000). Lessons learned from the development of an abl tyrosine kinase inhibitor for chronic myelogenous leukemia. *J Clin Invest*, **105**, 3–7.

Dutertre, S., Descamps, S., and Prigent, C. (2002). On the role of aurora-A in centrosome function. *Oncogene*, **21**, 6175–83.

Garcia, S. B., Novelli, M., and Wright, N. A. (2000). The clonal origin and clonal evolution of epithelial tumours. *Int J Exp Pathol*, **81**, 89–116.

Ilyas, M., Straub, J., Tomlinson, I. P., and Bodmer, W. F. (1999). Genetic pathways in colorectal and other cancers. *Eur J Cancer*, **35**, 335–51.

Kinzler, K. W. and Vogelstein, B. (1998). Landscaping the cancer terrain. *Science*, **280**, 1036–7.

Knudson, A. G. (1996). Hereditary cancer: two hits revisited. *J Cancer Res Clin Oncol*, **122**, 135–40.

Krtolica, A. and Campisi, J. (2003). Integrating epithelial cancer, aging stroma and cellular senescence. *Adv Gerontol*, **11**, 109–16.

Oldham, S., and Hafen, E. (2003). Insulin/IGF and target of rapamycin signaling: a TOR de force in growth control. *Trends Cell Biol*, **13**, 79–85.

Oller, A. R., Rastogi, P., Morgenthaler, S., and Thilly, W. G. (1989). A statistical model to estimate variance in long term-low dose mutation assays: testing of the model in a human lymphoblastoid mutation assay. *Mutat Res*, **216**, 149–61.

Rajagopalan, H., Nowak, M. A., Vogelstein, B., and Lengauer, C. (2003). The significance of unstable chromosomes in colorectal cancer. *Nat Rev Cancer*, **3**, 695–701.

Reya, T., Morrison, S. J., Clarke, M. F., and Weissman, I. L. (2001). Stem cells, cancer, and cancer stem cells. *Nature*, **414**, 105–11.

Sieber, O. M., Heinimann, K., and Tomlinson, I. P. (2003). Genomic instability—the engine of tumorigenesis? *Nat Rev Cancer*, **3**, 701–8.

Takahashi, T., Habuchi, T., Kakehi, Y., Mitsumori, K., Akao, T., Terachi, T. et al. (1998). Clonal and chronological genetic analysis of multifocal cancers of the bladder and upper urinary tract. *Cancer Res*, **58**, 5835–41.

Vivanco, I. and Sawyers, C. L. (2002). The phosphatidylinositol 3-kinase AKT pathway in human cancer. *Nat Rev Cancer*, **2**, 489–501.

Vogelstein, B., Fearon, E. R., Hamilton, S. R., Preisinger, A. C., Willard, H. F., Michelson, A. M. et al. (1987). Clonal analysis using recombinant DNA probes from the X-chromosome. *Cancer Res*, **47**, 4806–13.

Wittekind, C., Compton, C. C., Greene, F. L., and Sobin, L. H. (2002). TNM residual tumor classification revisited. *Cancer*, **94**, 2511–16.

Yuspa, S. H. (1994). The pathogenesis of squamous cell cancer: lessons learned from studies of skin carcinogenesis—Thirty-third G. H. A. Clowes Memorial Award Lecture. *Cancer Res*, **54**, 1178–89.

Textbooks

DeVita, V.E., Hellman, S., and Rosenberg, S.A. (eds.) (2001). *Cancer: Principles and Practice of Oncology*, 6th edn. Lippincott Williams and Wilkins, Philadelphia, PA.

Lodish, H., Berk, A., Zipursky, S. L., Matsudaira, P., Baltimore, D., and Darnell, J. E. (eds.) (2000). *Molecular Cell Biology*, 4th edn. W.H. Freeman and Co., New York.

Underwood, J. C. E. (2004) *General and Systematic Pathology*. Churchill Livingstone, London.

CHAPTER 2

The causes of cancer

Naomi Allen, Robert Newton, Amy Berrington de Gonzalez, Jane Green, Emily Banks, and Timothy J. Key

2.1 Epidemiology of cancer

2.1.1 Burden of cancer

In the year 2000, cancer was diagnosed in 10 million people worldwide and caused 6.2 million deaths, an increase of about 22% since 1990 (Ferlay et al. 2001). Cancer causes 10% of all deaths worldwide and is second only to cardiovascular disease as the main cause of death in developed countries. Although cancer is usually regarded as a problem of the developed world, about two-thirds of all cancer occurs in the three-quarters of the world's population who live in developing countries. Worldwide, there are about 22 million people living with cancer at any one time. Further, the number of cases of cancer worldwide is predicted to increase by 5 million to 15 million new cases each year by 2020 (World Health Organization, 2003). This is largely due to the increasing longevity of many populations, to medical advances in the treatment of other non-communicable diseases, and also to current trends in the prevalence of smoking and unhealthy lifestyles leading to an increase in the incidence of certain forms of cancer.

2.1.2 Descriptive epidemiology of the most common cancers

Figure 2.1 shows the numbers of cancers diagnosed and the number of deaths from cancer for the most common cancer sites worldwide. Lung cancer is the most common type of cancer, whether considered in terms of number of cases (1.2 m) or deaths (1.1 m), and accounts for approximately 12% of all cancers diagnosed (17% of all cancers in men and 7% in women). Breast cancer is the second-most common cancer diagnosed worldwide, with just over 1 million incident cases per year, and accounts for 10% of all cancers. Among women, breast cancer accounts for 28% of all cancers diagnosed each year, although it contributes to a lower proportion of cancer deaths (14% in women; 6% overall), due to a relatively favourable prognosis. Cancers of the colorectum (large bowel), stomach, liver, and prostate are also very common worldwide and

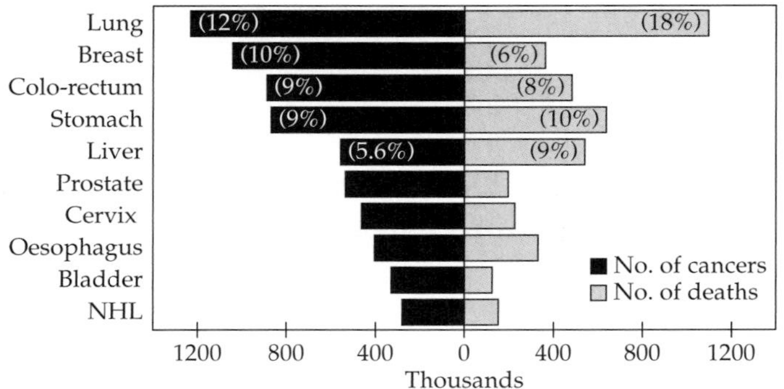

Figure 2.1 Numbers of worldwide cancer cases and deaths each year for the ten most common cancer sites.

Source: Ferlay et al. (2001).

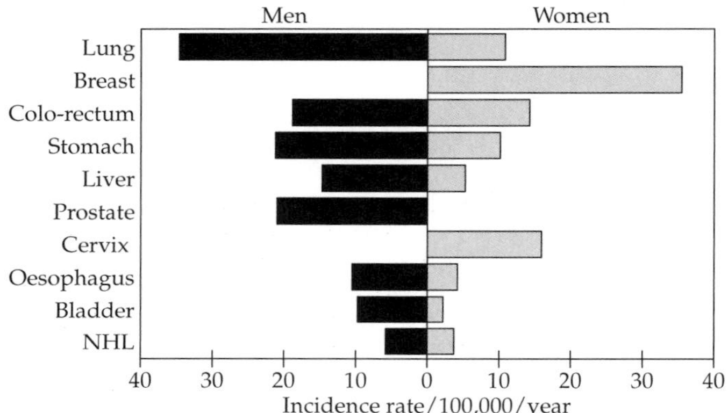

Figure 2.2 Cancer incidence rates in men and women of the most common cancer sites. Rates are age-standardized to the World population.

Source: Ferlay et al. (2001).

each have over 500,000 new cases diagnosed each year; cancers of the cervix, oesophagus, bladder, and non-Hodgkin lymphoma (NHL) each have over 200,000 new cases diagnosed each year worldwide. Figure 2.2 shows the incidence rates of the most common cancers in men and women separately. Cancers of the lung, stomach, liver, oesophagus, and bladder are more common in men than in women, which largely reflect differences in exposure to the main risk factors rather than differences in susceptibility to the disease.

Geographical variation in cancer rates

A comparison of age-standardized incidence rates between populations shows that most types of cancer are much more common in some countries than in others. Figures 2.3(a) and (b) show the incidence rates for the 10 most common cancers in countries classified as 'more developed' (i.e. North America, Europe, Australasia) and 'less developed' (i.e. Africa, India, Asia, South America), for men and women separately. For men (Figure 2.3(a)), the rates of cancers of the prostate, colorectum, and bladder are four-to sixfold higher, while rates of cancers of the liver and oesophagus are twofold lower in more developed countries than in less developed countries. For women (Figure 2.3(b)), rates of cancers of the breast, colorectum, ovary, and non-Hodgkin's lymphoma are two-to threefold higher, while rates of cancers of the liver, oesophagus, and cervix are two- to fourfold lower in more developed countries than in less developed countries. Overall, the age-standardized incidence rate of all cancers (excluding non-melanoma skin cancer) is about 2.5 times higher in more developed countries, although there are more people diagnosed with cancer in developing countries because most of the world's population lives in these areas. The disparities in the distribution of cancer rates between developed and developing countries suggest that certain cancers (i.e. those of the lung, colorectum, breast, and prostate) are caused by factors that relate to Westernization (such as earlier onset of smoking, Western diet, and/or sedentary lifestyle). However, with increasing Westernization of societies in many less developed countries, the cancer burden in these

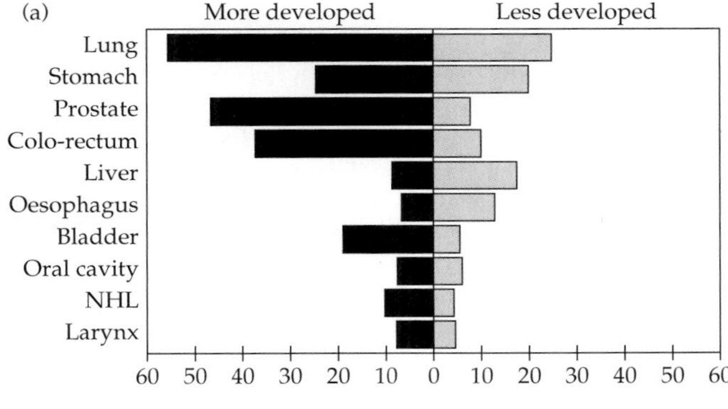

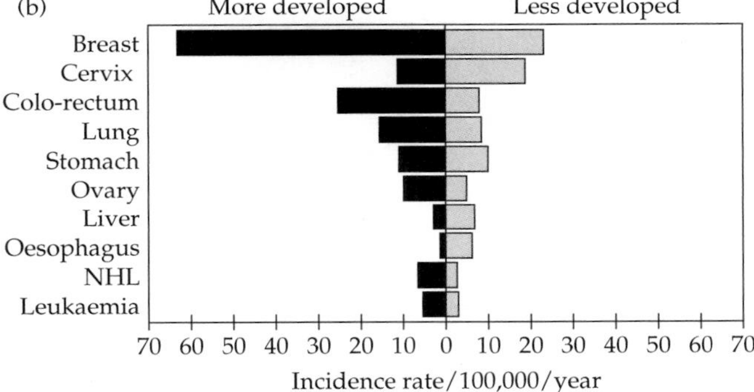

Figure 2.3 (a) Incidence rates for the 10 most common cancers in men in more and less developed countries. (b) Incidence rates for the 10 most common cancers in women in more and less developed countries. Rates are age-standardized to the world population.
Source: Ferlay et al. (2001).

areas is set to increase, making cancer an important global public health problem.

Temporal variation in cancer rates

Within populations, a comparison of age-standardized incidence and mortality rates over time shows that the rates of many common cancers have changed over the last 50 years. This further supports the conclusion that most cancers are caused by environmental factors (here defined as behavioural, reproductive, and lifestyle factors) and are therefore, at least in principle, preventable.

Figure 2.4 shows the age-standardized incidence rates of breast cancer in selected populations between 1975 and 1990. The rates vary by more than threefold, being lowest in Asia and South America and highest in North America. Incidence rates have increased throughout the world over the last 30 years, by over 1% per year in high-incidence countries such as North America and Europe and by over 5% per year in former low-incidence countries, such as Japan and Singapore. These increases may be partly due to more complete cancer registration or increased detection, but the large increases reported in the former low-risk countries are mostly due to a real increase in incidence rates.

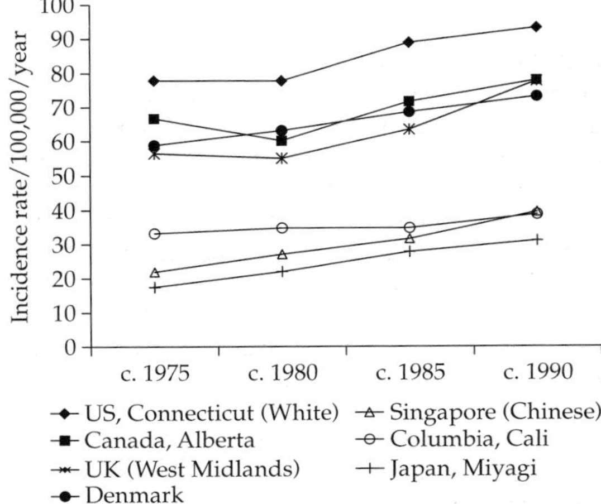

Figure 2.4 Breast cancer incidence rates in selected registries, 1975–90. Rates are age-standardized to the World population.
Source: *Cancer Incidence in Five Continents*, volumes IV, V, VI, and VII.

In contrast, although stomach cancer is still the fourth most common cancer worldwide, both incidence and mortality rates have been declining steadily over the last 50 years in former high-incidence and low-incidence countries. For example, in Japan stomach cancer mortality rates have declined by more than half since the 1950s, with an average reduction of 1% per year, although they are still among the highest in the world. Stomach cancer mortality rates have also declined in other formerly high-incidence countries, such as in Northern and Eastern Europe, as well as in low-incidence countries such as the United States (Figure 2.5) (World Health Organization, 2001). The reasons for these large reductions in mortality rates are not fully understood, but are thought to be related to changes in dietary patterns and methods of preserving foods (see section on dietary-related

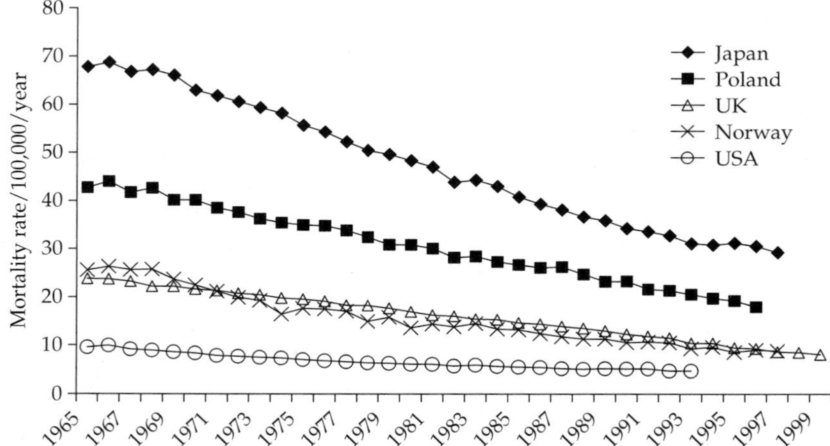

Figure 2.5 Stomach cancer mortality rates in men in selected countries, 1951–99. Rates are age-standardized to the World population.
Source: World Health Organization, 2001.

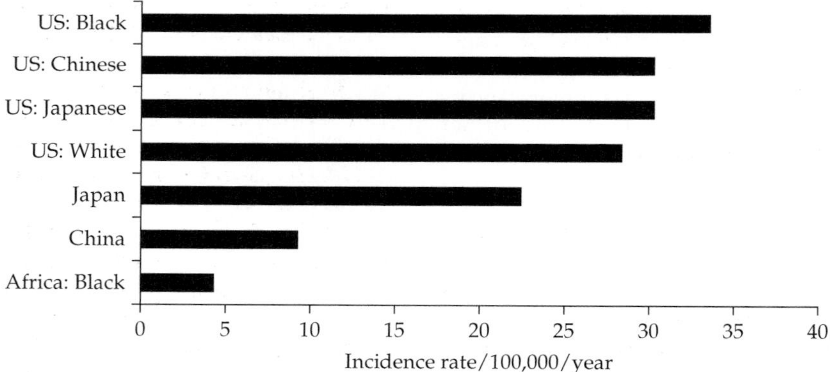

Figure 2.6 Incidence rates for colon cancer in men in different populations (c. 1990). Rates are age-standardized to the World population.

Notes: For US: black, weighted means of rates from 8 US registries (Atlanta, Central Louisiana, Connecticut, Detriot, Los Angeles, New Orleans, San Francisco, SEER).
For US: Chinese and Japanese, weighted means of rates from 3 registries (Los Angeles, San Francisco, Hawaii).
For US: white, weighted means of rates from 11 US registries (Atlanta, Central California, Central Louisiana, Connecticut, Detriot, Hawaii, Los Angeles, New Mexico, New Orleans, San Francisco, SEER).
For Japan, weighted means of rates from 6 Japanese registries (Hiroshima, Miyagi, Nagasaki, Osaka, Sagi, Yamagata).
For China, weighted means of rates from 3 Chinese registries (Shanghai, Tianjin, Qidong).
For Africa: black, weighted means of rates from 3 African registries (Mali Bamako, Uganda Kyadondo, Zimbabwe Harare).

Source: Parkin et al. (1997).

factors), together with a reduction in the prevalence of infection with *Helicobacter pylori* (see section on infections).

Migrant studies

A comparison of age-standardized incidence rates in populations who migrate from a country of low cancer incidence to one with a high incidence (or vice versa) is another way of assessing whether the changes in exposure to environmental factors that accompany cultural assimilation have an impact on cancer rates. For breast cancer, Japanese women in Japan have a rate that is a quarter of that of US whites, whereas Japanese women who have migrated to the United States now have rates similar to those of US whites. These dramatic effects of migration show that environmental factors are major determinants of breast cancer risk and that the differences in breast cancer rates between Japan and the United States cannot simply be attributable to differences in genetic susceptibility. Indeed, for most cancers, the pattern of disease among migrants comes to resemble that of their host country after a few generations presumably as they adopt the local lifestyle. As can be seen in Figure 2.6, incidence rates of colon cancer in African-, Chinese-, and Japanese-American men are much higher than among those who live in their country of origin (Parkin et al. 1997). Indeed, rates of colon cancer among these migrants are now higher than the rates seen among white American men, indicating that lifestyle changes, such as adoption of a Western-type diet, have a strong effect on the development of colon cancer.

2.2 Risk factors for cancer

The large differences in the pattern of cancer incidence between different populations and over time suggest that cancer might be largely avoided if the environmental and/or behavioural factors responsible for the wide variation in the rates of site-specific cancers could be identified and modified.

Table 2.1 summarizes the main risk factors for major cancer sites. The contribution to total cancer incidence and mortality gives an indication of the relative importance of each cancer, and the male to female mortality ratio gives an indication of the importance of sex-specific risk factors. Major risk factors for each cancer (i.e. that account for 25% or more of the total number of cases of that particular cancer) have been listed separately from other, more minor risk factors, to reflect their relative importance to the total cancer burden of that cancer site. What is clear from this summary is that although the major and specific causes of some cancers are known, most notably smoking for lung cancer, reproductive factors for breast cancer, and human papillomavirus infection for cervical cancer, little is yet understood about the causes of other common cancers, such as those of the colorectum and prostate.

2.2.1 Tobacco

It is estimated that tobacco use causes about 4 million deaths each year, corresponding to about a third of all deaths in men aged 35–69 years in North America and Europe and between 12 and 20% of all deaths in the rest of the world (World Health Organization, 2003). Tobacco causes a range of fatal diseases, of which the most important are ischaemic heart disease, chronic obstructive lung disease, and cerebrovascular disease. Tobacco consumption is also the major preventable cause of cancer. It is estimated that tobacco smoking accounts for about a third of all cancers in Western populations, including a large proportion of cancers of the lung, pancreas, bladder, kidney, larynx, mouth, pharynx (except nasopharynx), and oesophagus. Several other types of cancers, such as stomach, liver, cervix, nasal cavities, and myeloid leukaemia are also associated with smoking (World Cancer Research Fund, 1997). Chewing betel quid and tobacco is also an important risk factor for cancer of the mouth and pharynx in some parts of South-East Asia. Tobacco is therefore a direct and avoidable cause of an enormous cancer burden.

Over 60 carcinogens have been identified in cigarette smoke. The main compounds thought to cause cancer in humans are the polycyclic aromatic hydrocarbons and aromatic amines, although other compounds including *N*-nitrosamines and heavy metals may also be involved.

Smoking accounts for 80–90% of the 900,000 cases of lung cancer diagnosed in men and 55–80% of the 330,000 cases diagnosed in women each year worldwide. Because the disease takes a long time to develop (i.e. it has a long latency period), rates of lung cancer are a reflection of the patterns of cigarette smoking that occurred several decades before. Smoking among men in Europe and North America became increasingly popular after the First World War, and in the 1950s several case-control

Table 2.1 The contribution to total cancer incidence and mortality, male to female mortality ratio, and environmental risk factors for major sites of cancer in the world, 2000[a]

Site of cancer (in order of decreasing proportion of all cancers)	Proportion of all incident cancers[b](%)	Proportion of all cancer deaths[b](%)	Male/female mortality ratio	Risk factors		
				Major[c] established	Other[c] established	Likely (probable) but unproven
Lung	12.3	17.8	1.7 : 1	Smoking	Radon Asbestos Coal tar combustion products Arsenic Nickel refining Chromates Bischloromethyl ether Air pollution (polycyclic aromatic hydrocarbons)	Low intake of fruit and vegetables
Breast	10.4	6.0	0.006 : 1	Female sex Reproductive/hormonal factors[d] Post-menopausal obesity	Alcohol consumption Ionizing radiation	Western-style diet
Colorectum	9.4	7.9	1.1 : 1	Obesity and low physical activity (colon) *S. japonicum*	Aspirin (protective)	Western-style diet (especially low fibre intake, high meat intake)
Stomach	8.7	10.4	1.7 : 1	*H. pylori* High intake of salt-preserved foods	Smoking	Low intake of fruit and vegetables
Liver	5.6	8.8	2.3 : 1	Cirrhosis Hepatitis B and C viruses	Liver flukes Aflatoxin Excessive intake of alcohol Smoking Vinyl chloride Arsenic Anabolic steroids	
Prostate	5.4	3.3	—	Black race		Endogenous hormones Western-style diet
Cervix	4.7	3.8	—	Certain human papillomavirus strains	High parity Smoking	Genital hygiene
Oesophagus	4.1	5.4	2.1	Smoking Alcohol Obesity (adenocarcinoma)	Oral contraceptives	Vitamin deficiency
Bladder	3.3	2.1	3 : 1	Smoking *S. haematobium* (squamous cell carcinoma)	Aromatic amines Cyclophosphamide Chlornaphazine	

Non-Hodgkin lymphoma	2.9	2.6	1.4 : 1	Immunosuppression	EBV HIV HTLV–1	
Oral cavity	2.7	2.1	1.7 : 1	Smoking Alcohol Very hot drinks	Oral tobacco Betel quid chewing and reversed smoking	Certain HPV strains
Leukaemia	2.6	3.1	1.3 : 1		Population mixing (childhood leukaemia) Smoking (myeloid leukaemia) Ionizing radiation Benzene Certain anticancer drugs HTLV	
Pancreas	2.2	3.4	1 : 1	Smoking Obesity	Diabetes	
Ovary	1.9	1.8	—	Low parity Oral contraceptives (protective)		
Kidney (including renal pelvis)	1.9	1.5	1.7 : 1	Smoking Obesity	Aromatic amines Phenacetin	
Endometrium	1.9	0.7	—	Low parity Exogenous oestrogens Combined oral contraceptives (protective) Obesity	Early menarche and late menopause Tamoxifen	
Brain and other central nervous system	1.8	2.1	1.3 : 1		Ionizing radiation	
Skin (melanoma)	1.3	0.6	1 : 1	Sun or other ultraviolet light Benign melanocytic naevi White race	Xeroderma pigmentosa Immune impairment	
Skin (non-melanoma)	Not accurately known[e]	Not accurately known[e]	1.2 : 1	Sun or other ultraviolet light White race HIV and immunosuppression (Kaposi's sarcoma)	Ionizing radiation Arsenic Polycyclic aromatic hydrocarbons Xeroderma pigmentosa	Tropical ulcers
Multiple myeloma	0.7	0.9	1.1 : 1	Black race		
Hodgkin's disease	0.6	0.4	1.7 : 1	EBV		
Nasopharynx	0.6	0.6	2.4	EBV	Chinese-style salted fish	
Thyroid	0.5	<0.5	0.5 : 1		Ionizing radiation	
Larynx	0.5	<0.5	3.7 : 1			
Testis	0.5	<0.5	—	White race Undescended testis		Early puberty

(*Continued*)

Table 2.1 (*Continued*)

Site of cancer (in order of decreasing proportion of all cancers)	Proportion of all incident cancers[b](%)	Proportion of all cancer deaths[b](%)	Male/female mortality ratio	Risk factors		
				Major[c] established	Other[c] established	Likely (probable) but unproven
Gallbladder and bile ducts	<0.5	<0.5	0.6 : 1	Obesity Gallstones		
Pleura and peritoneum	<0.5	<0.5	5.6 : 1	Asbestos (some types)		
Bone	<0.5	<0.5	1.5 : 1		Ionizing radiation Paget's disease	
Penis and other genital organs	<0.5	<0.5	—	Certain HPV strains Circumcision (protective)		
Anus	<0.5	<0.5	0.8 : 1	Certain HPV strains		
Vagina and vulva	<0.5	<0.5	—	Certain HPV strains Diethylstilboestrol (in utero exposure)	Smoking	
Lip	<0.5	<0.5	0.8 : 1	Smoking (esp. pipe) Sun or other ultraviolet light		
Nasal cavities	<0.5	<0.5	1.7 : 1		Nickel refining Hardwood furniture Leather manufacture Isopropyl alcohol production Formaldehyde Smoking	

Notes:

[a] Non-modifiable risk factors such as age and inherited susceptibility are common to all cancers (to a greater or lesser extent) and are therefore not included in this table.

[b] Excluding non-melanoma skin cancer.

[c] A 'major' risk factor is defined as a factor that may account for more than 25% of all cases of a particular cancer; 'other' risk factors account for less than 25% of all cases of a particular cancer.

[d] Reproductive factors include early age at menarche, late first birth, low parity, lack of breast-feeding, late menopause, hormone replacement therapy use, and oral contraceptive use, (see text for details).

[e] The proportion of cancers due to non-melanoma skin cancer is known to be under-reported, but registered cases account for 15–20% of all cancers in Western countries.

studies conducted in the United Kingdom and the United States suggested that smoking was the main cause of lung cancer. On the basis of this, the first large, modern prospective study on smoking and lung cancer was initiated among British doctors. The results of this study have shown that lung cancer mortality rates in smokers of 1–14, 15–24, and 25 or more cigarettes per day are 8-, 15-, and 25-fold higher respectively, than those of non-smokers (Doll et al. 1994). The risk of lung cancer increases rapidly among current smokers, being highest in those who begin to smoke at an early age and who continue to smoke throughout life. Exposure to environmental tobacco smoke (passive smoking) is also carcinogenic; non-smokers whose spouses smoke cigarettes have an approximately 30% increased risk of developing lung cancer compared with non-smoking spouses (US Environmental Protection Agency, 1992).

Stopping smoking has a rapid beneficial effect on lung cancer risk and people who stop smoking even well into middle age avoid most of their subsequent risk of lung cancer. Indeed, people who stop smoking before the age of 35 avoid more than 90% of the risk attributable to tobacco smoking (Peto et al. 2000). With the reduction in the prevalence of smoking, at least in Western countries, lung cancer mortality rates are beginning to fall. For example, lung cancer mortality rates in British men fell by 40% between 1968 and 1997, while reductions in the United States started 20 years later. However, on a global scale, cigarette consumption and hence lung cancer rates are increasing. For example, in Eastern Europe and in some Asian countries, male lung cancer mortality rates have doubled over the last 30 years (Figure 2.7). Because of the rising prevalence of smoking in less developed countries, it has been estimated that there may be up to 3 million smoking-related lung cancer deaths per year by 2025, compared with about 1 million annual deaths that occurred in the mid-1990s (Peto et al. 1996). However, if smoking rates could be halved, we would avoid 20–30 million premature deaths from all causes by the year 2025 and about 150 million deaths by 2050 (World Health Organization, 2003). Efforts to reduce tobacco consumption are therefore of the utmost importance for preventing premature death, not only from cancer but from other tobacco-related diseases.

2.2.2 Infections

Collectively, infectious agents are the most important *established* cause of cancer after tobacco. Approximately 18% of cancers worldwide (about 1.6 million cases per year) are attributable to viral (13%), bacterial (5%), and helminth (0.1%) infections (World Health Organization, 2003), the majority of which occur in the developing world. In theory, if these infectious diseases were controlled, up to one in four cancers in developing countries, and 1 in 10 cancers in developed countries could be prevented.

Human papillomaviruses

More cancer cases are attributable to human papillomavirus (HPV) infection than to any other transmissible agent. It is well established that this

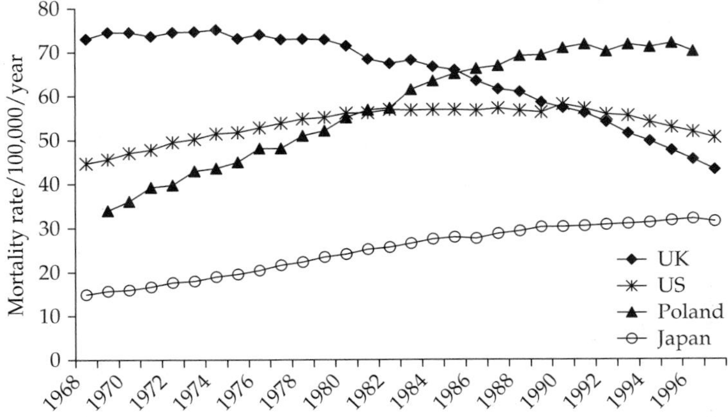

Figure 2.7 Lung cancer mortality rates in men in selected countries, 1968–97. Rates are age-standardized to the World population.
Source: World Health Organization, 2001.

sexually transmitted virus is the major causative agent for invasive cervical cancer. Epidemiological studies have shown very large relative risks (of the order of 50) in association with infection with certain HPV subtypes. The most common HPV subtypes identified are HPV16, 18, 31, 33, and 45, although in some Asian countries the subtypes HPV52 and 58 are more common. The same subtypes also account for up to 80% of cancers of the anus and approximately one-third of cancers of the penis, vagina, and vulva. HPV infection may also cause some cancers of the head and neck (particularly cancers of the oral cavity) and squamous cell carcinomas of the skin. It has been suggested that HPV infection may also be related to cancers of the bladder and prostate, although the evidence remains scant.

In developed countries, cervical cancer-screening programmes that rely on the detection, by exfoliative cervical cytology, of treatable pre-cancerous lesions, are established and are effective at reducing both the incidence and mortality of invasive cervical cancer. However, in many developing countries, screening procedures do not yet exist and incidence and mortality rates are still very high. Vaccination against the main HPV sub-types at an early age holds the most promise to substantially reduce the incidence of this cancer and preliminary results from trials have shown very promising results.

Hepatitis viruses

Chronic infection with the hepatitis B virus is responsible for causing up to 250,000 liver cancers (specifically hepatocellular carcinoma) each year, which corresponds to about 60% of all primary liver cancers across the world. Approximately 10% of the population in parts of sub-Saharan Africa, China, and South-East Asia are infected with the hepatitis B virus. Transmission can occur from a mother to her child, from person to person during childhood, and via sexual or parenteral transmission during adulthood. About two-thirds of these people will develop chronic hepatitis, and a quarter of these will eventually die from primary liver cancer or cirrhosis, making liver cancer one of the most common cancers in these areas.

Prospects for the prevention of hepatitis B virus associated liver cancer are good. In developed countries, screening of blood and organ donors has reduced the spread of infection among adults. In areas where infection is most prevalent, however, the best hope for prevention lies with mass vaccination against the hepatitis B virus. Although it will be many years before an effect on the incidence of liver cancer is demonstrated in adults, the introduction of mass vaccination in Taiwan has already been associated with a sharp decline in the incidence of liver cancer in children.

The unrelated hepatitis C virus is also involved in the aetiology of hepatocellular carcinoma and may cause about 25% of all liver cancers, with particularly high proportions in Africa (41%), Japan (36%), and Oceania (33%). The prevalence of hepatitis C virus infection is estimated to be about 1–1.5% in Europe and North America, about 3% in Japan and Oceania (excluding Australia and New Zealand), and up to 3.6% in Africa. Transmission is commonly via the parenteral route, although sexual and perinatal transmission can also occur. However, almost half of all hepatitis C infected individuals have no identifiable risk factors. Although a vaccine is not currently available, screening programmes have greatly reduced transmission of hepatitis C via blood transfusions.

Herpesviruses

Infection with the Epstein Barr virus is involved in the aetiology of several types of lymphoma (including Burkitt's lymphoma, Hodgkin's disease, and immunosuppression-related lymphomas) and nasopharyngeal carcinoma and may contribute up to 100,000 cancers per year worldwide. The Epstein Barr virus infects more than 90% of the world's population and is usually acquired during childhood. It is transmitted orally in saliva and establishes a latent infection with life-long persistence in the infected host. The overgrowth of virally transformed B cells is controlled by specific cytotoxic T-cell responses, the absence of which (in allograft recipients and others with impaired T-cell function) can result in lymphoma.

Human herpesvirus-8 (HHV-8), or Kaposi's sarcoma-associated herpesvirus, is closely related to the Epstein Barr Virus and is considered the principal cause of Kaposi's sarcoma. HHV-8 also causes a rare type of lymphoma (primary effusion lymphoma) and a lymphoproliferative B cell disorder (Castleman's disease). HHV-8 is most prevalent in populations at highest risk of developing Kaposi's sarcoma, such as homosexual men infected with the human immunodeficiency virus in Western countries and in African populations where the tumour has long been endemic.

Human T-Cell leukaemia virus-type 1

Human T-cell leukaemia virus type 1 (HTLV-1) is a causal agent of adult T-cell leukaemia/lymphoma. It is estimated that there are about 15–20 million individuals infected with HTLV-1 worldwide, predominantly in Japan, the Caribbean, South America, and Central Africa. Adult T-cell leukaemia/lymphoma develops in about 2–5% of HTLV-1 infected individuals and is especially frequent among those infected early in life. Perinatal transmission has been greatly reduced in Japan by avoidance of prolonged breast-feeding (i.e. more than 6 months) and several countries have introduced universal screening of blood donors. Passive and active immunization is effective in animal models but no preventive vaccine is yet available for humans.

Human immunodeficiency virus

There is little evidence that the human immunodeficiency virus (HIV) has a direct oncogenic effect. Instead, its immunosuppressive effect appears to facilitate the development of Kaposi's sarcoma, non-Hodgkin lymphoma, squamous cell carcinoma of the conjunctiva, and probably also Hodgkin's disease and leiomyosarcoma in children. In areas of sub-Saharan Africa where HIV infection is highly prevalent, the incidence of Kaposi's sarcoma has increased about 20-fold with the spread of HIV, such that in Uganda and Zimbabwe it is now the most common cancer in males and among the most common in females.

The first cases of HIV disease were reported in 1981. The epidemic continues to escalate and an estimated 38 million people are infected, the majority in sub-Saharan Africa (World Health Organization, 2003). Transmission is primarily sexual, and from mother to child, but parenteral transmission is also important. There is evidence of a reduction in the increase in risk of both Kaposi's sarcoma and non-Hodgkin lymphoma among those on anti-retroviral therapy for HIV. However, in the developing world, where such treatment is prohibitively expensive and therefore not widely available, the incidence of HIV-associated cancers is likely to increase with the spread of the HIV epidemic. Screening programmes have greatly reduced transmission of HIV via blood banks and transfusions, but in the absence of an effective vaccine, changes in sexual activity are still the most important method of controlling the epidemic.

Helicobacter pylori

About half of the world's population is chronically infected with the bacterium *Helicobacter pylori*. This bacterium colonizes the stomach lining and, although many people remain asymptomatic, some go on to develop gastric or duodenal ulcers. In a very small proportion of infected individuals, gastric adenocarcinoma, and to a lesser extent, gastric non-Hodgkin lymphoma may develop. Although it is clear that *H. pylori* infection plays a role in the development of stomach cancer, other factors, such as diet, are also involved.

The prevalence of infection is highest in developing countries and increases rapidly during the first two decades of life, such that 80–90% of the population may be infected by early adulthood; in most developed countries, the prevalence of infection is now substantially lower. Rates of infection with *H. pylori* have fallen over the last few decades, and this could explain much of the parallel decline in stomach cancer rates seen in most countries. This may be due to improvements in living conditions and trends towards a smaller family size, both of which are risk factors for *H. pylori* infection. Although antibiotics are effective in eradicating *H. pylori* in about 80% of cases, this has proved to be difficult to implement on a large scale and re-infection is common.

Helminths

Infestation with the water-borne trematode, *Schistosoma haematobium*, which causes schistosomiasis (bilharzia), is associated with an increased risk of squamous cell carcinoma of the bladder, and is the predominant cause of this cancer in tropical and sub-tropical areas. Schistosomiasis affects approximately 200 million people worldwide and is endemic in Northern Africa and the Middle East; in these areas, over half of the population is at risk of infection from contaminated water supplies (lakes, rivers, swamps) that contain the larvae. There is also some evidence that *Schistosoma japonicum* and to a lesser extent, *Schistosoma mansoni* is related to the development of cancers of the liver and colorectum in China. Although treatable, preventative measures focusing on reducing contact with contaminated water supplies are currently the best method of reducing infection.

Food-borne trematodes (liver flukes), such as *Opisthorchis viverrini*, *Opisthorchis felineus* and *Clonorchis sinensis* are an established cause of cancer of the bile ducts (cholangiocarcinoma) in parts of

South-East Asia, due to consumption of raw or undercooked freshwater fish that contain the infective stage of the fluke. Control of infection has been achieved in some areas by a combination of chemotherapy, health education, and improved sanitation. However, eradication programmes have, as yet, had little effect on the incidence of cholangiocarcinoma in these areas and a vaccine is not yet available.

2.2.3 Dietary-related factors

The possible role of diet in the aetiology of cancer was highlighted in the 1970s, when it was noted that Western countries that have diets high in animal products, fat, and sugar, have high rates of cancers of the colorectum, breast, and prostate. In contrast, developing countries with diets that are typically based on one or two starchy staple foods, with low intakes of animal products, fat, and sugar have low rates of these cancers. These observations suggested that the diets of different populations might partly explain their different cancer rates. Since then, dietary factors have been the subject of much epidemiological research and there is a consensus that dietary changes could have a major impact on some of the most common cancers, including cancers of the colorectum and stomach and possibly cancers of the breast, prostate, and lung. Recent estimates suggest that about a quarter of cancer deaths in the United Kingdom might be avoidable by dietary change, with a margin of uncertainty ranging from 15% to 35% (Doll et al. 2003). Dietary factors are thought to account for about 20% of cancer in developing countries, but this proportion is set to increase with growing urbanization and the corresponding 'Westernization' of dietary patterns.

Several dietary factors, such as fat and meat, have been suggested to increase cancer risk, while other factors, such as fruit, vegetables and fibre, have been hypothesized to decrease risk. However, despite extensive research over the last two decades, few specific dietary determinants of cancer risk have been established, even for cancers such as colorectal cancer where dietary factors are the most obvious candidate risk factors. This is due to various reasons, the most important being the difficulty in accurately measuring dietary intake in epidemiological studies. Other problems with epidemiological studies of diet and cancer include the relatively narrow range of dietary exposures within one population, and the changes in dietary patterns over time, so that it is very difficult to determine whether dietary habits at a young age may affect cancer risk later in life. The best prospects for improving our understanding of the relationship between diet and cancer appear to lie with very large prospective studies that are now underway, together with randomized trials of promising candidate factors. Despite these problems, some diet-related risk factors, most notably overweight/obesity and an accompanying sedentary lifestyle, and consumption of alcohol, have been clearly established as risk factors for specific cancers, perhaps because they can be measured reasonably easily and accurately.

Overweight/obesity

Overweight and obesity is usually measured in terms of an individual's body mass index (BMI) (weight in kilograms/height in metres^2) where a BMI of greater than 25 kg/m^2 is considered overweight and a BMI of greater than 30 kg/m^2 is considered obese. Overweight and obesity increase the risk of colon cancer by about a third and increase the risk of breast cancer in post-menopausal (but not pre-menopausal) women by about a half. Overweight and obesity is associated with an approximate threefold increased risk of endometrial cancer in both pre- and post-menopausal women, and may account for up to 40% of endometrial cancer worldwide. Overweight and obesity also increases the risk of cancers of the kidney and gallbladder and of adenocarcinoma (but not squamous cell carcinoma) of the oesophagus. It has been estimated that overweight and obesity account for about 5% of all cancers in Europe, most of which are cancers of the colon, endometrium, and breast. Thus, up to 36,000 cases of cancer could be prevented each year if the prevalence of overweight and obesity in Europe was halved (Bergstrom et al. 2001). In countries such as the United States, where the prevalence of obesity is higher than in Europe, an even higher proportion of cancers may be attributable to being overweight. Furthermore, the prevalence of obesity is increasing in both developed and developing countries, and is therefore expected to lead to a greater burden of cancers in the future.

Physical activity

Related to the effects of BMI and diet is the effect of physical activity on cancer risk. High amounts of physical activity are associated with a reduced risk of colon (but not rectal) cancer, with average risk reductions of between 40 and 50% in most studies. A protective effect for physical activity has also been observed for breast cancer, although the data are less consistent than for colon cancer.

Alcohol

A high intake of alcoholic beverages increases the risk of cancers of the upper respiratory and digestive tracts (oral cavity, tongue, pharynx, larynx, and oesophagus). These cancers are also caused by smoking, and the increase in risk is particularly great for people who both smoke and drink heavily. Heavy and prolonged alcohol consumption is also associated with liver cancer via the development of cirrhosis and alcoholic hepatitis.

Cancers of the upper gastro-intestinal tract are particularly associated with excessive alcohol consumption, although a moderate intake of 10 g of alcohol per day (approximately one drink) has been shown to increase the risk of breast cancer by around 7%. Given the high proportion of women who drink moderate amounts of alcohol and the high incidence of breast cancer in some populations, these results suggest that about 4% of breast cancers in developed countries may be caused by alcohol (Collaborative Group on Hormonal Factors in Breast Cancer, 2002).

Foods and nutrients

Very few foods or nutrients have been established as being associated with an increased or reduced cancer risk. The only clearly established dietary-related risk factors are consumption of known chemical carcinogens. For example, aflatoxin-contaminated foods contribute to the causation of liver cancer in some tropical countries, and consumption of nitrosamine-rich foods such as chinese-style salted fish is a cause of nasopharyngeal cancer. In both these cases, the dietary carcinogens appear to act largely in association with viral infections.

Certain foods and nutrients are believed to be associated with an increased risk of several common cancers, namely cancers of the stomach, colorectum, prostate, breast, and lung, but the specific factors in these foods have not been identified and the epidemiological evidence is not entirely consistent. Stomach cancer is common in most parts of Asia, but cancers of the colorectum, prostate, breast, and lung are often considered Western diseases and have been, to a greater or lesser extent, attributed to some aspect of a Western-style diet that is high in animal and saturated fats and low in cereals and other plant foods rich in fibre.

For stomach cancer, there is substantial evidence that diet is important and dietary changes are implicated in the recent decline in stomach cancer incidence rates in many countries (Figure 2.5). Epidemiological evidence suggests that risk is increased by high intake of some traditionally preserved salted foods, especially meats and pickles, and with salt *per se*, and that risk is reduced by high intakes of fruit and vegetables, perhaps due to their vitamin C content.

For colorectal cancer, there is almost universal agreement that some aspect of a Western diet is a major determinant of risk. International correlation studies show a strong association between *per capita* consumption of meat and colorectal cancer mortality. A recent systematic review concluded that preserved meat is associated with an increased risk for colorectal cancer but that fresh meat is not, whereas most studies have not observed positive associations with poultry or fish (Norat et al. 2002). The evidence is not conclusive but suggests that high consumption of preserved and red meat probably increases the risk for colorectal cancer. Many case-control studies of colorectal cancer have observed moderately lower risk in association with high consumption of fruits and vegetables and/or dietary fibre, but the results of recent large prospective studies have been inconsistent. At present, the evidence currently available suggests that fruit, vegetables, and foods rich in fibre probably reduce the risk for colorectal cancer.

For prostate cancer, although red meat, dairy products, and animal fat have been suggested as risk factors, the data from epidemiological studies are inconsistent. Randomized controlled trials have provided strong evidence that supplements of β-carotene (largely found in green-yellow vegetables) do not protect against prostate cancer. Other nutrients, such as vitamin E, selenium, and lycopene are under investigation as potential protective agents, although no firm conclusions can yet be made.

For breast cancer, much of the international variation in incidence rates is due to differences in established reproductive risk factors (see section on reproductive and hormonal factors), but differences in dietary habits may also contribute. In fact, age at menarche is partly determined by dietary factors, in that restricted dietary intake during childhood and adolescence leads to delayed menarche. Adult height is also weakly positively associated with breast cancer risk, and is partly determined by dietary factors during childhood and adolescence. However, the only dietary factors which have been established to increase breast cancer risk are obesity and alcohol (see above sections). Studies of other dietary factors including fat, meat, dairy products, fruit and vegetables, fibre and phyto-oestrogens on breast cancer risk are inconsistent.

For lung cancer, numerous observational studies have found that cases generally report a lower intake of fruits, vegetables, and related nutrients than healthy individuals. However, only β-carotene has been tested in randomized trials, which have failed to find any reduction in risk among those given a supplement for up to 12 years. The possible effect of diet on lung cancer risk remains controversial, and the apparent protective effect of fruit and vegetables may be largely due to residual confounding by smoking, since smokers generally consume less fruit and vegetables than non-smokers. In public health terms, the overriding priority for preventing lung cancer is to reduce the prevalence of smoking.

2.2.4 Reproductive and hormonal factors

Hormonal and reproductive factors play a crucial role in the aetiology of breast cancer, with an early age at menarche, low parity, a late age at first birth and a late age at menopause being established risk factors. Taken together, about 15% of all cancer deaths in the United Kingdom are believed to be attributable to reproductive factors (Doll et al. 2003). For example, a delay in the age at menarche reduces breast cancer risk by around 5% per year and a delay in menopause increases risk by about 3% per year (Collaborative Group on Hormonal Factors in Breast Cancer, 1996). Childbearing seems to have a dual effect on breast cancer risk, with risk being transiently increased shortly after pregnancy, but which exerts an overall protective effect over the long-term. Compared with nulliparous women (women with no children), the risk of breast cancer in women who have had at least one child is reduced by about a quarter; women with five or more children have about half the risk of nulliparous women. Irrespective of the number of children a woman has, the earlier a woman has her first birth, the greater the reduction in risk, so that women with a first birth under the age of 20 have about half the risk of nulliparous women. Breast-feeding has a small protective effect on breast cancer risk, but this may have a larger impact in developing countries where a woman's cumulative lifelong exposure of breast-feeding may be longer, as a result of a large number of children and of breast-feeding each child for a long time.

Many of these reproductive factors suggest that cumulative exposure to oestrogens during a woman's lifetime increase the risk of breast cancer. It is now known that high circulating levels of oestrogens are directly associated with breast cancer risk, at least in post-menopausal women (Endogenous Hormones and Breast Cancer Collaborative Group, 2002). Further evidence for a role of hormones comes from consistent observations that current users of exogenous hormones, either in the form of oral contraceptives (OCs) or hormone-replacement therapy (HRT), have a 25–35% higher risk of developing breast cancer than never-users (Collaborative Group on Hormonal Factors in Breast Cancer, 1996). However, this risk appears to be transient and has largely disappeared after 10 years since stopping.

Recent trials have shown that tamoxifen, an anti-oestrogenic drug used to treat breast cancer, can reduce the risk of invasive breast cancer by about 40% among women who have an elevated risk for the disease. Thus, drugs such as tamoxifen, that block or reduce oestrogen exposure, could potentially be used as chemopreventative agents for breast cancer. However, the effects of tamoxifen on other hormone-sensitive cancers and other diseases needs to be evaluated; indeed, tamoxifen has been associated with an increased risk of endometrial cancer.

As with breast cancer, reproductive factors that increase exposure to oestrogens also increase the risk for endometrial cancer. However, unlike breast cancer, the observations that parity and OC use have a strong protective effect indicates that the mitogenic effect of oestrogen is counter-balanced by the presence of progestagens. Women who are long-term users of oestrogen-only HRT preparations have up to a ninefold increased risk of developing endometrial cancer and the use of combined (oestrogen plus progestagen) HRT preparations is associated with a much smaller increase in risk than those that contain oestrogen only.

Reproductive factors are also strongly related to ovarian cancer and, as for endometrial cancer, the most established protective factors are parity and use of OCs. In general, a first-term pregnancy is associated with about a 40% reduction in risk, with a smaller reduction in risk with each term pregnancy thereafter. Combination OCs are associated with up to a halving of risk after 5 years of use, which persists up to at least 15–20 years after cessation of use. The risk of ovarian cancer in relation to HRT use is unclear, but most data point to no association or a weak positive effect. Although it is clear that hormonal factors are involved in some way in the aetiology of ovarian cancer, little is known about the association between endogenous hormone levels and ovarian cancer.

For cancer of the cervix, the most established reproductive factors are an increased number of sexual partners and an early age at first intercourse, both of which are related to the infectious aetiology of this cancer (see section on infections). Recent studies also suggest that long-term use of OCs increases the risk of cervical cancer, so that women who have used OCs for 10 years or longer have about a twofold increased risk. High parity has also been associated with an increased risk in some, but not all studies and may be related to the hormonal changes in pregnancy or to cervical trauma during childbirth. Other reproductive factors such as age at menarche and age at menopause have not been consistently associated with cervical cancer.

Reproductive and hormonal factors may play a role in some cancers in men, notably prostate cancer and possibly cancer of the testes. However, the evidence from epidemiological studies that endogenous androgen levels are related to an increased risk of prostate cancer is inconsistent. There is a hypothesis that sexual activity is associated with an increased risk, acting either as a marker for endogenous androgen levels or due to a sexually transmitted agent; although there is some evidence to support both these hypotheses, the data are not conclusive. The development of testicular cancer may also depend on hormones, but apart from the increased risk among boys with an undescended testis, and some evidence for an increase in risk with early puberty, no behavioural or reproductive factor is strongly related to cancer risk.

2.2.5 Radiation

Much of our knowledge of the potential carcinogenic effects of radiation exposure is derived from the observed effects of large doses of radiation received by the survivors of the atomic bombs that were dropped on Hiroshima and Nagasaki in 1945. Other populations that have been studied for the effects of radiation include those exposed for medical reasons (both therapeutic and diagnostic), and occupational groups such as radiologists, nuclear power workers, and uranium miners exposed to radon.

The most recent estimates suggest that all types of radiation (ionizing and non-ionizing) may cause about 6% of cancer deaths in the United Kingdom (Doll et al. 2003). Radiation can cause cancer in almost any tissue or organ in the body, although the red bone marrow, breast and thyroid are the most sensitive. Excess cancers continue to occur at least 40 years after radiation exposure and the risk is often greater among those exposed at younger ages. To date, there is no convincing evidence for the existence of a 'threshold dose' (i.e. below which radiation is considered safe). Although most research has focused on the effects of ionizing radiation, largely from indoor radon gas or from medical procedures, most of the radiation-induced cancers are caused by non-ionizing radiation in the form of ultraviolet light. There is little evidence that other forms of non-ionizing radiation, such as extremely low frequency electromagnetic fields emitted from electrical appliances and mobile phones, are related to cancer risk.

Ultraviolet radiation

It is well established that high exposure to non-ionizing radiation in the form of sunlight is the principal cause of non-melanoma and malignant melanoma skin cancer and accounts for 80–90% of these tumours. Non-melanoma skin cancer has the highest incidence of all cancers, accounting for between 15 and 20% of all cancers diagnosed in Western countries each year. The actual number of cases may be somewhat higher than this because this type of cancer tends to be under-reported as most cases are easily treated and cured. Malignant melanoma is a less common type of skin cancer, but accounts for substantially more deaths than that of non-melanoma skin cancer. Both types of skin cancer have been increasing in many Western countries in recent years, primarily as a result of increased sun exposure. Among Caucasian populations around the world, rates of skin cancer increase with proximity to the equator, where the intensity of sunlight is strongest. Rates of skin cancer are more than 10 times higher in whites than in blacks due to lower amounts of melanin, the pigment in skin, which absorbs ultraviolet radiation rays before they can damage DNA. Public health measures aimed at increasing awareness of the dangers of prolonged and intense sunlight are the most effective way of reducing the incidence of both non-melanoma and malignant melanoma skin cancer.

Radon

Exposure to ionizing radiation from radon gas is a well-established lung carcinogen, as shown by studies conducted among underground uranium miners, where high concentrations of radon gas can occur. Relatively high concentrations can also occur in homes that are built on rock that contains uranium, and in some parts of the United Kingdom exposure to radon gas contributes about half the total dose from all forms of radiation. Indoor radon gas escaping from the ground or from building materials has been found to cause lung cancer in current smokers; whether exposure to radon gas increases the risk of lung cancer among non-smokers is unclear. Based on risk projections from studies conducted in underground miners, it has been estimated that residential radon may account for about 1–3% of all cancers (excluding non-melanoma skin cancer) and 6% of lung cancer, making it the second biggest cause of lung cancer after smoking. Exposure to radon gas can be prevented however, and in some countries (notably Sweden, Germany, the United States and the United Kingdom), building guidelines have been recently introduced in the most affected parts of these countries to reduce levels of radon gas in new homes.

Medical radiation exposures

The use of ionizing radiation for medical diagnosis and therapy is widespread throughout the world. In general, its use is confined to an anatomical region of interest and, although designed to directly benefit the individual, these exposures will inevitably involve some risk of cancer, given the consensus that there is no safe dose. Although the dose of a single diagnostic X-ray is low, their widespread and frequent use makes them the largest man-made source of radiation exposure. It has been estimated that radiation exposure from diagnostic X-rays may account for up to 2% of all cancer deaths in some developed countries, where X-rays are a common procedure.

Radiotherapy is used to treat some cancers, notably cancers of the cervix, breast, ovary, and Hodgkin's disease. However, its use can also cause damage to neighbouring healthy tissue and, in a very small proportion of patients, may cause a second cancer to develop. For example, between 5 and 10% of children treated for a first malignancy (i.e. Hodgkin's disease, leukaemia) will go on to develop radiation-induced second tumours in adulthood. The cancer sites most affected are the thyroid, brain, bone, and soft tissue sarcomas and non-melanoma skin cancer.

2.2.6 Occupational carcinogens

The majority of chemicals established as human carcinogens have been identified because workers have been exposed to these agents at very high levels for many years. In 1775, black soot was identified as the first known occupational carcinogen, following the observation by Percival Potts that chimney sweeps had a high risk of developing cancer of the scrotum. In 1895, the carcinogenic effect of synthetic chemicals was identified when bladder cancer was reported in German dye manufacturers following the introduction of synthetic aromatic amine dyes in the 1870s. However, it was not until the 1950s that the possible long-term dangers of exposures in the workplace in relation to subsequent cancer risk were widely examined in epidemiological studies.

Established carcinogens that occur mainly in occupational settings are not usually considered major risk factors (Table 2.1), although for workers in the relevant industries they may be of great importance. For example, bladder cancer is related to occupational exposure to aromatic amines, chiefly found in the textile, rubber, and printing industries. Exposure to these agents may account for up to 20% of all bladder cancers in men worldwide. Other established associations include the combustion of coal tar with lung cancer, and exposure to nickel compounds with cancer of the nasal sinuses. Most of these chemicals are either inhaled or absorbed through the skin during routine use and have been found to be mutagenic *in vitro* and carcinogenic in animals.

Exposure levels for many industrial hazards have been progressively reduced in Western countries following improvements in health and safety. It is now estimated that less than 4% of cancers in men and less than 1% of cancers in women are attributable to occupational factors. However, exposure to chemicals that occurred several decades ago may still contribute to today's cancer burden. In particular, the huge increase in mesothelioma in the 1990s (a rare form of cancer of the pleura and peritoneum) among many builders was caused by exposure to certain types of asbestos fibres between the 1950s and 1970s. Because it takes 30–40 years for the disease to develop, the number of men dying from mesothelioma in Western Europe is set to double each year, with approximately 250,000 deaths over the next 35 years (Peto et al., 1999).

2.2.7 Medical carcinogens (non-radiation)

Some chemicals used to treat cancer (chemotherapy) have been associated with an increased risk of cancers at other sites. The most established of these are the use of chlornaphazine (now discontinued) and cyclophosphamide, which are associated with a large increase in the risk for bladder cancer. Immunosuppressive drugs given to transplant recipients are also related to an increased risk of some cancers, most notably non-Hodgkin lymphoma, for which the risk is increased by 50-fold or more (usually occurring within a year or two of the transplant).

Other, more common medications, such as phenacetin-containing analgesics are also suspected human bladder carcinogens and are associated with an increased risk of cancer of the renal pelvis (kidney). Conversely, there is evidence that use of non-steroidal anti-inflammatory drugs such as aspirin can protect against colorectal cancer; data on whether aspirin protects against any other cancers are less consistent.

2.2.8 Environmental pollution

It is very difficult to quantify the role of environmental pollution (defined here as environmental contaminants) in relation to cancer risk, because of the exposure of the general population to ubiquitous pollutants at very low levels. Pollution of air, water, and soil is estimated to account for between 1 and 4% of all cancers worldwide (World Health Organization, 2003). The most established association between environmental pollution and cancer risk is that of air pollution with lung cancer risk. It is estimated that air pollution may account for about 3% of lung cancer worldwide, occurring mostly in areas where domestic burning of wood and coal and vehicle exhaust emissions are not well controlled. However, because air pollution is a complex mixture of soot, particulate, and volatile organic compounds, the specific constituents that are causally related to lung cancer have not been firmly established.

There has also been much interest in whether environmental exposure to aromatic organochlorines found in many pesticides, combustion, and industrial products increases the risk for some cancers. Most concern has focused on a possible association with breast cancer risk because experimental studies have shown some of these chemicals to have weak oestrogenic effects. However, current evidence from epidemiological studies does not support such an association.

2.2.9 Genetic predisposition

Exploration of the human genome has presented new opportunities to identify the genetic basis underlying cancer development. As discussed elsewhere in this book, cancer is essentially a genetic disease in that genetic alterations (mutations) cause the breakdown of the regulatory mechanisms that govern normal cell behaviour, leading to loss of normal function, aberrant or uncontrolled cell growth, and eventual spread to other parts of the body. Specific mutations that activate genes involved in cell growth and proliferation (oncogenes), or inactivate genes involved in cell senescence and apoptosis (tumour suppressor genes), are often associated with carcinogenesis. Mutations in genes involved in DNA repair are also associated with carcinogenesis, with inadequate DNA repair leading to replication of mutations, DNA adduct formation, and subsequent cancer development. As will be discussed below, mutations in specific genes that are inherited (germline mutations) have been implicated in a variety of human cancers.

Family history and high-risk mutations

The evidence for a genetic predisposition to cancer derives originally from observations of cancer clustering in families. Most cancers show some degree of familial clustering and, in general, a person who has a sibling or a parent with cancer has about a 50% increased risk of also developing that cancer. A family history of cancer may be partly due to common exposure to environmental agents, as well as shared genetic susceptibility. Some affected families may have an increased susceptibility to several types of cancer; for example, those with multiple endocrine neoplasia syndrome have a substantially increased risk for developing cancers of the pituitary, parathyroid, adrenal, pancreas, and other endocrine tissues. However, it should be noted that family history does not account for the majority of cases of cancer. For example, 87% of breast cancers occur in women without a family history of the disease and 85% of women with a family history will never develop breast cancer (Collaborative Group on Hormonal Factors in Breast Cancer, 2001).

Clustering of relatively large number of cases of cancer within families may indicate that an inherited mutation in one gene is sufficient to substantially increase risk and, in several cases, specific germline mutations in these genes have been identified through cytogenetic and molecular analyses of affected family members. Examples include the *TP53* gene and Li–Fraumeni cancer syndrome, which predisposes to childhood sarcomas and brain tumours as well as early-onset breast and/or ovarian cancer; the *ATM* gene and ataxia telangiectasia, which increases susceptibility to lymphomas, T-cell leukaemias and breast cancer, and mutations in the *RB* gene, which predispose to retinoblastoma. Germline mutations in *BRCA1* and *BRCA2* genes, both of which are involved in DNA repair, have also been identified as increasing susceptibility to ovarian and breast cancers. Although these high-penetrance germline mutations substantially increase the risk of developing a specific cancer, the vast majority of people who develop cancer do not possess these mutations. Overall, the proportion of cancer classified as being attributable to dominantly inherited high-risk genes is estimated to be between 5 and 10% of all cancer that occurs in the general population.

Most cancers are therefore sporadic (i.e. not associated with an inherited germline mutation). However, the observation that identical twins of people with cancer have an increased risk of developing cancer at the same site suggests that inherited genetic factors are involved, particularly for cancers of the stomach, colorectum, lung, breast, and prostate. Much laboratory and epidemiological research over the last decade has focused on identifying genetic variants that have a smaller effect on cancer risk than the high-risk genetic variants that manifest themselves in a strong family history. This may have important implications because these mutations are much more common and so may exert a more substantial effect on cancer risk at a population level.

Low-risk genetic polymorphisms

It is well known that people differ in their ability to metabolize drugs; we now know that this is chiefly related to individual (genetic) differences that affect the function of the enzymes involved. Since many chemical carcinogens require metabolism to exert their carcinogenic effects, common variants in genes that encode for drug-metabolizing enzymes may influence cancer development. In particular, there is growing interest in whether differences in environmental exposure have different effects on cancer risk according to common metabolic genotypes (often termed 'gene-environment interaction'). One of the best-studied examples is the *N*-acetyltransferase (*NAT*s) genes that encode for a large family of enzymes involved in metabolizing drugs and other exogenous substances. Individuals with a 'slow' variant of the *NAT2* gene, which results in a reduced ability to metabolize aromatic amines, appear to have a moderately increased risk of bladder cancer, which may be seen particularly in smokers and in people occupationally exposed to aromatic amines. In general however, the epidemiological evidence of an association between such low-risk genes and cancer risk is limited and inconsistent, although the literature is continually growing (Human Genome Epidemiology Network, 2003). Future large-scale studies are required to determine whether common genetic variants, either on their own, or in combination with other genetic and environmental factors, are important in cancer development at a population level.

2.2.10 Mutagens and mutational spectra in relation to cancer types

In addition to investigating inherited mutations, much research has been done to identify somatic mutations in known oncogenes (e.g. *ras*, c-*myc*), tumour suppressor genes (e.g. *TP53*, *APC*, *RB*, *Ras*, *MYC*, *CDKN2A*), and DNA repair genes (e.g. *XPD*, *BRCA1*, *BRCA2*) in relation to sporadic cancers. Other genes related to chromosome instability, cell cycle control, signal transduction, and immune function are also of interest. To date, the *TP53* tumour suppressor gene, involved in the cellular response to DNA damage, is the most extensively studied. Mutations in this gene are found in about half of all human cancers.

Many mutagens produce specific DNA changes in certain regions of a gene, either directly or indirectly by reacting with DNA and binding to nucleotides (usually guanine) to form DNA adducts; formation of DNA adducts can then induce specific mutations that may subsequently lead to cancer. Because mutagens bind to specific parts of DNA a given exposure can create a characteristic 'mutation signature' in that gene. Identification of such mutational spectra can be used to strengthen the argument for a causal association between a suspected mutagen and cancer risk. A complementary approach is to directly quantify the levels of DNA adducts in human tissues. These can be used both as a marker of the biologically effective dose of carcinogens and as a marker of genetic damage, because they are considered directly related to tumour formation. For example, aflatoxin-DNA adducts and their specific associated *TP53* gene mutations are found in over half of all liver cancers (hepatocellular carcinoma) associated with high exposure to dietary aflatoxin. It was not until molecular studies of this type were conducted that aflatoxin was considered a causative agent for liver cancer and independent of hepatitis B virus infection. Increased levels of polycyclic aromatic hydrocarbon-DNA adducts have also been associated with an increased risk of lung cancer in smokers and among workers in the coal and gas production/cleaning industries, where exposure to such chemicals may be high. The presence of high levels of 4-aminobiphenyl-haemoglobin adducts in bladder tumours that occur in smokers has also strengthened the evidence that aromatic amines in cigarette smoke are an important cause of bladder cancer in smokers.

2.3 Implications for cancer prevention

Based on current epidemiological evidence, it is clear that the majority of cancers can, in theory, be prevented. It is now well established that tobacco consumption is the main avoidable cause of cancer, accounting for about 30% of all cancer deaths. Dietary modifications could perhaps potentially prevent about the same number of cancer deaths as smoking cessation, but it is still not clear which specific dietary constituents are related to cancer risk. Chemoprevention, for example, in the form of vitamin supplementation, has been investigated in several clinical trials, but results have, to date, been largely negative. Nevertheless, eliminating overweight and obesity may prevent between 5 and 10% of all cancers, at least in developed countries where the prevalence of obesity is high. Infectious agents are thought to cause about 18% of all cancers worldwide, and although most of these could be prevented through vaccination or early treatment of infection, such medical interventions are often not available to the people who might benefit from them most. In some developing countries, vaccination programmes may actually be more easily implemented than other public health interventions aimed at lifestyle changes. Ultraviolet radiation is another important avoidable cause of cancer and public health initiatives that aim to educate individuals on protective measures against excessive exposure to sunlight have been implemented in most Western countries where the incidence of skin cancer is high. Occupational exposure to established carcinogens has been substantially reduced in recent years and is now estimated to contribute no more than 4% of the global cancer burden, and may be even lower in developed countries where rigorous health and safety legislation applies. In comparison with these factors, the contribution of other avoidable risk factors to cancer risk, such as environmental pollution, medical drugs, etc. is small.

Screening also plays an important role in reducing the burden of cancer death by aiming to provide early detection and early treatment of the disease. Population-based screening procedures for cancers of the cervix and breast are well established in most developed countries and have led to significant reductions in cancer-specific mortality. For colorectal cancer, several available screening options are currently under investigation, including faecal occult blood testing, sigmoidoscopy and colonoscopy which detect pre-cancerous adenomatous polyps, but the most effective and acceptable screening tool remains to be determined. A blood test to measure prostate-specific antigen levels as a marker of early prostate cancer is widely available in many countries, but is unlikely to be implemented in an organized screening programme until a reduction in cancer mortality has been demonstrated in randomized trials.

Although the early detection and treatment of cancer remains an important strategy to reduce the cancer burden in many countries, the main focus of public health must be to prevent cancer from developing in the first place. The large geographical differences in cancer incidence make it clear that there is enormous potential for preventing cancer by removing the effects of smoking, known infections, alcohol, ultraviolet radiation, occupational carcinogens, inactivity and obesity and by making changes to our diet. Indeed, it is estimated that the projected five million increase in the number of annual cancer cases by the year 2020 could be reduced by a third if all available preventative measures were implemented; thus up to 2 million cases of cancer could be prevented in the next 20 years (World Health Organization, 2003). Public health measures aimed at achieving behavioural changes on a population level, and that are compatible with preventative measures for other non-communicable diseases, are therefore the most important factor for reducing the future cancer burden.

References and further reading

Bergstrom, A., Pisani, P., Tenet, V., Wolk, A., and Adami, H. O. (2001). Overweight as an avoidable cause of cancer in Europe. *Int J Cancer*, **91**, 421–30.

Collaborative Group on Hormonal Factors in Breast Cancer (1996). Breast cancer and hormonal contraceptives: collaborative reanalysis of individual data on 53 297 women with breast cancer and 100 239 women without breast cancer from 54 epidemiological studies. *Lancet*, **347**, 1713–27.

Collaborative Group on Hormonal Factors in Breast Cancer (2001). Familial breast cancer: collaborative reanalysis of individual data from 52 epidemiological studies including 58,209 women with breast cancer and 101,986 women without the disease. *Lancet*, **358**, 1389–99.

Collaborative Group on Hormonal Factors in Breast Cancer (2002). Alcohol, tobacco and breast cancer: collaborative reanalysis of individual data from 53 epidemiological studies, including 58 515 women with breast cancer and 95 067 women without the disease. *Br J Cancer*, **87**, 1234–45.

Doll, R. and Peto, R. (2003). Epidemiology of cancer. In: *Oxford Textbook of Medicine, 4th edition* (ed. D. A. Warell, T. M. Cox, and J. D. Firth), Oxford University Press, New York, pp. 194–216.

Doll, R., Peto, R., Wheatley, K., Gray, R., and Sutherland, I. (1994). Mortality in relation to smoking: 40 years' observations on male British doctors. *Br Med J*, **309**, 901–11.

Endogenous Hormones and Breast Cancer Collaborative Group (2002). Endogenous sex hormones and breast cancer in postmenopausal women: reanalysis of nine prospective studies. *J National Cancer Inst*, **94**, 606–16.

Ferlay, J., Bray, F., Pisani, P., and Parkin, D. M. (2001). Globocan 2000: Cancer incidence, mortality and prevalence worldwide, version 1.0. www-iarc.f/globocan/globocan.html.

Human Genome Epidemiology Network (2003). HuGENet. www.cdc.gov/genomic/hugenet/default.htm.

Norat, T., Lukanova, A., Ferrari, P., and Riboli, E. (2002). Meat consumption and colorectal cancer risk: dose-response meta-analysis of epidemiological studies. *Int J Cancer*, **98**, 241–56.

Parkin, D. M., Whelan, S. L., Ferlay, J., Raymond, L., and Young, J. (1997). *Cancer Incidence in Five Continents. Vol II*. IARC Scientific Publication No. 143. International Agency for Research on Cancer, Lyon, France.

Peto, R., Lopez, A. D., Boreham, J., Thun, M., Heath, C. J., and Doll, R. (1996). Mortality from smoking worldwide. *Br Med Bull*, **52**, 12–21.

Peto, J., Decarli, A., La Vecchia, C., Levi, F., and Negri, E. (1999). The European mesothelioma epidemic. *Br J Cancer*, **79**, 666–72.

Peto, R., Darby, S., Deo, H., Silcocks, P., Whitley, E., and Doll, R. (2000). Smoking, smoking cessation, and lung cancer in the UK since 1950: combination of national statistics with two case-control studies. *Br Med J*, **321**, 323–9.

US Environmental Protection Agency (1992)., In *Respiratory health effects of passive smoking: lung cancer and other disorders*. Office of Research and Development, Office of Health and Environmental Assessment, Washington, DC, EPA 600/6-90/006F.

World Cancer Research Fund (1997). *Food, Nutrition and the Prevention of Cancer: A Global Perspective*. American Institute for Cancer Research, Washington DC, USA.

World Health Organization (2001). World Health Statistics Annual, WHO Mortality Database. www.who.in/whosis.

World Health Organization (2003). *World Cancer Report*. (ed. B. W. Stewart & P. Kleihues), IARC Press, Lyon.

CHAPTER 3

Inherited susceptibility to cancer

D. Timothy Bishop

Chapter 2 describes the evidence regarding a number of different exposures such as diet and radiation on a person's risk of cancer. Responses to such exposures may well be defined by the person's genetic makeup while genetic factors themselves could be the major determinant of risk. This chapter focuses on the evidence relating to inheritance and cancer risk.

The most direct evidence for a role of genetic susceptibility to cancer comes from the clinical identification of relatively rare but clearly characterized inherited diseases in which the role of inheritance is unequivocal. Some of these diseases are observed in the presence of particular exposures capable of causing genetic damage and are associated with a failure of DNA repair following this exposure. The inherited susceptibility is then the failure to repair this damage either correctly or completely. Some of these susceptibilities are recessively determined, meaning that a person with such a syndrome has two defective copies of the same gene, one inherited from each parent. The parent has only one copy of the defective gene and may therefore have either complete or marginally defective DNA repair capabilities which translates into only minimal extra cancer risk, if any at all.

Other syndromes are associated with dominant inheritance meaning that only a single copy of the defective gene is inherited but this is sufficient to increase the risk of cancer in both the parent carrying such a mutation and, on average, one half of their offspring who inherit this mutation. These syndromes are identifiable by the pattern of disease expression in family members (termed the 'phenotype'). For instance, one such syndrome, familial adenomatous polyposis (FAP), is associated with susceptibility to large numbers of colorectal adenomatous polyps which are benign but premalignant lesions. Other syndromes are associated with increased risk of cancer but lack a distinctive phenotype.

Since the first human genetic map in 1987, the capability to identify the critical genes in susceptibility to these syndromes has improved dramatically so that the critical gene or genes for many of these syndromes, and certainly the commonest recognized syndromes, are now known. These technological and informational improvements have also clearly identified the precise genes for a number of syndromes including those associated with susceptibility to common cancer. For many years, families had been documented showing family members with cancer at one or more of a limited number of cancer sites within each family. Some of these families had been systematically followed over many generations and the increased risk was apparent for each of those generations. For instance, Dr Eldon Gardner in Utah, recorded families with breast cancer, initially identified in the late 1940s. Every 10 years, he updated the cancer incidence in these families showing the continued dominant pattern of inheritance across distinct branches of the same family among members unknown to each other and with notably early ages of onset. While the clinical observation provided clear evidence of an inherited susceptibility, the identification of the precise gene involved is essential both to confirm the genetic basis of the disease and to understand the mechanism by which the cancer develops.

The identification of these genes is the starting point for a number of distinct areas of research such as defining the role of the wild-type gene, determining the risk associated with carrying mutations, applying this information to clinical management and the potential approaches to risk reduction. Epidemiological studies suggest that even after accounting for known genes associated with inherited susceptibility to common cancers, there is still clear evidence that close relatives of cases have an increased risk of the same cancer suggesting that other factors must explain this family aggregation. This could, of course, be other genes or lifestyle factors or the combination of the two perhaps interacting in some way. More modest genetic effects are not characterized by extended families with many affected members and the method of identifying the responsible gene differs accordingly. Such studies are based on comparing the genetic makeup of persons with the disease and those without the disease and are termed 'association studies'.

3.1 Dominantly inherited susceptibility

The clearest evidence for the role of genes in cancer has come from the identification of families with numerous cases of the same cancer. These families have been recognized clinically for almost 200 years. For instance, Pierre Paul Broca, the neurologist, reported in the mid-nineteenth century a family with more than ten breast cancer deaths among his wife's relatives. Such a high number of cancer cases within one family does not occur by chance and Broca speculated that inheritance could play a role (reported in Lynch et al., 1972).

The reasons that these families have been recognized is varied but can be summarized as:

(1) Families with multiple cases of the same common cancer (e.g. breast cancer) with average age of onset considerably younger than that seen in the general population.

(2) Families with an associated phenotype which is clearly genetically determined including bowel adenomas in patients with FAP. FAP patients have a greatly increased risk of colorectal cancer later in life.

(3) Families with several cases of rare cancers or in which the observation of multiple families with the same tumours is particularly notable.

While the initial observations date back to the 1800s, more detailed and systematic observational studies did not occur until the 1950s when the work especially of Dr David Anderson (Texas, USA), Dr Eldon Gardner (among the Mormon families of Utah) and Prof. Henry Lynch (Iowa, USA) documented large numbers of families. At this stage, it was apparent that such families were not the single case reports as had appeared previously but rather involved clinically meaningful numbers of families and persons (Lynch et al., 1972). Chief among the observations made were that within many of these families, inheritance was consistent with that of a single mutated gene within each family. It took until the 1990s to begin to identify the precise genes involved.

The recognition of such families presented physicians with a need to plan their clinical management. An NIH committee produced the following guidelines 'Guidelines for identifying individuals who merit genetic evaluation' and identified six criteria by which persons and families with such apparent inheritance could be recognized. The six criteria were:

(1) Cancer occurring in both of paired organs that is thought not to be the result of metastases (e.g. cancer in both breasts).

(2) More than one focus of cancer in a single organ (e.g. multiple retinoblastomas in one eye).

(3) Two or more distinct primary cancers (e.g. breast and ovarian cancers).

(4) Cancer that has occurred:
- **(a)** at an atypical age (e.g. breast or ovarian cancer at age less than 40 years), Wilms' tumour in an adult;
- **(b)** at an atypical site;
- **(c)** in the less usually affected sex (e.g. breast cancer in a man).

(5) Cancers associated with other conditions:
- **(a)** birth defects (e.g. mental retardation);
- **(b)** a single gene disorder known to complicated by neoplasia;
- **(c)** precursor lesions;

(d) other diseases.
(6) Unusual or rare cancers.

The delineation of syndromes as described above is to a great extent an issue of statistics and biology. The assessment of the number of cancers likely to be seen in each family requires a statistical calculation; the fact that many families have more cases than statistically plausible by chance is convincing evidence of the existence of a causative factor. The occurrence of cancers at different anatomical sites in relatives may not be statistically significant but may identify a plausible biological link. In either case, the hypothesis of inherited susceptibility can only be proven by finding the precise gene in each family.

3.1.1 Linkage mapping

The majority of the genes associated with an inherited susceptibility to cancer have been identified though linkage mapping (also termed 'positional cloning'). The approach is based on the observation that within each family, inheritance of a single mutation is consistent with the pattern of disease among relatives. The procedure behind linkage analysis is not new, having been suggested 80 years ago by Thomas Hunt Morgan and with statistical methods described soon after (Fisher, 1935). The informativeness of the procedure, however, changed entirely with the Human Genome Project, and especially the identification of genetic variants across the genome which can be routinely assayed (Botstein et al., 1980). The publication of a genetic map of the genome in 1992 (NIH/CEPH Collaborative Mapping Group, 1992) marked the time when such studies could be conducted with a reasonable chance of success. This map showed a set of genetic variants in the genome which could be assayed in any person's DNA. If family members had a genetically determined trait then, with a large enough pedigree, the inheritance of the trait should be tracked by the inheritance of one or more of these variants.

The first step in the process of mapping the critical gene involves identifying families with multiple cases of cancer which are informative; informativity relates to the structure of the family including the genetic relationships among the affected persons and the strength of evidence that the family disease does not represent a chance occurrence. Informativity also means that germline DNA samples are available from both affected and unaffected family members. These DNA samples are then typed for a panel of genetic variants. A number of commercially available panels have been produced. Typically for first-round screening, the panel consists of 300–400 markers approximately equally spaced at 10 cM intervals (of the order of 10 Mb apart on average). These markers are simply sites of known population variation and have typically involved repeats of the CA sequence which are found in sufficient numbers across the genome. Assays of each marker have been produced based on the polymerase chain reaction (PCR). These genetic markers are then typed in family members and markers identified which track with disease segregation within families. Figure 3.1 shows such a pattern.

Genotyping of these variants in families such as Figure 3.1 limits the size of the genetic region containing the susceptibility gene. For instance, person V:12 has inherited only part of the critical DNA segment from her mother indicating that the susceptibility gene must lie below DNA marker D17S857. Such an observation reflects a genetic recombination event in the production of the egg which formed V:12 occurring between genetic markers D17S857 and D17S846. Examination of this and other families with the same genetic aetiology can reduce the region before proceeding with molecular approaches examining the genes within the critical region for causative mutations. Identification of several distinct mutations in the same gene are indicative that the causative gene has been found. This latter component has been greatly enhanced by the availability of more detailed sequence information over the last five years.

Linkage analysis has been impressively successful in localizing genes for a number of cancer syndromes, as described in the following sections. The major limitations of linkage analysis are (1) the availability of sufficient numbers of extended families with many affected persons, which can be identified and sampled as the basis of the linkage analysis and (2) the proportion of these families, which are due to each specific gene. The second requirement for successful genotyping requires that significant numbers of families are attributable to each gene and in fact, for genetic studies of common cancers, remarkably few genes have explained the majority of the high-risk predisposition. For many cancer sites, two genes at most have been identified and these genes are the predominant cause of high-penetrance susceptibility to that

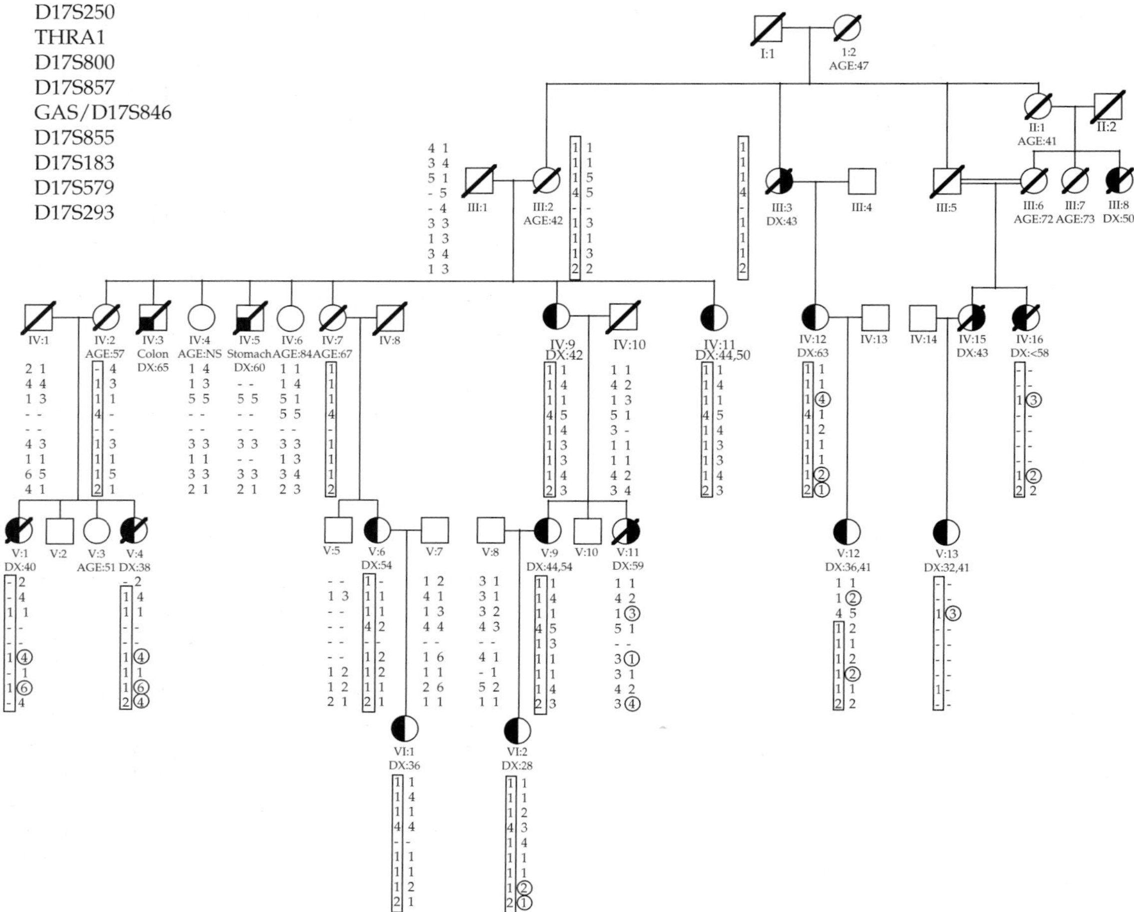

Figure 3.1 This figure shows a family with dominantly inherited susceptibility to breast and ovarian cancer. Males are shown by squares in the pedigree, females by circles. Left-half shading indicates a woman with breast cancer; right-half shading depicts ovarian cancer. Left-lower quarter shading depicts cancer other than breast or ovarian cancer. Ages of onset are shown as DX: 'age' beneath each affected family member. Oblique lines indicate family member deceased. The set of genetic variants assayed for each family member are shown in the top left of the figure. These markers are in their order along chromosome 17. The variants carried by each person are shown under that person's symbol on the pedigree (-symbol implies that no genotype could be determined). The set of variants transmitted in conjunction with the disease mutation are boxed (the 'haplotype') indicating the genomic region inherited intact among family members and carried by most women who developed breast or ovarian cancer. Person V:11 is an exception having not inherited the high-risk haplotype but developing ovarian cancer indicative of the fact that within such families, not all affected family members are carriers of the high-risk mutation. Genetic variants circled have been shown to be somatically deleted in the tumour, in keeping with the susceptibility gene (*BRCA1*) being a tumour suppressor gene. In tumours examined in this way, genetics variants not circled could not be definitively scored for deletion status.

cancer. For instance, for breast cancer two genes, *BRCA1* and *BRCA2*, are the major cause but there is still evidence that there are further genes to be identified. The difficulty in identifying these other genes may simply reflect the fact that the remaining families are in fact attributable to a number of different genes or simply to chance aggregation of disease in families.

3.1.2 Gene characterization

The successful cloning of a susceptibility gene by linkage mapping or other technique permits the identification of the precise genetic mutations in particular families. This knowledge also provides a basis for placing the cloned gene into a population context, essentially applying the usual techniques of epidemiology to understand the contribution of each gene to cancer incidence in the general population. By the nature of linkage mapping, the approach is likely to identify the genes and mutations which are associated with highest risk of disease. Thus, it is by no means clear that all mutations will be associated with same risk of disease. This process has been termed 'gene characterization' and includes:

(1) evaluating the mutation spectrum for each gene;
(2) defining the characteristics of families in which mutations are more likely to be found (e.g. by numbers of cases of cancer, ages of onset, combinations of tumours found among mutation carriers);
(3) estimating the penetrance of each gene and/or each mutation to determine future risks of cancer in persons currently unaffected;
(4) identifying the proportion of cancer cases carrying a mutation in this gene by age of onset and, where appropriate, gender;
(5) estimating the proportion of persons in the general population carrying such a mutation.

Once cloning has been achieved, the familial mutation can be sought by examining one or a couple of the affected family members. For the syndromes discussed above, such investigations indicate that for the majority of the cloned genes, there are many distinct mutations of each of these genes. For instance, the database of *BRCA1* and *BRCA2* mutations shows over 1000 distinct mutations across the two genes to date. Such investigations can also be performed on population-based samples, selected entirely at random or stratified, for instance, by age or family history. Investigations of such systematic collections provide estimates of the contribution of each of the susceptibility genes to cancer incidence in the general population. In general, we expect that these mutations explain only a small proportion of all cancer in the general population, as the families required to perform linkage mapping have typically been particularly notable for the numbers of cancers diagnosed within the families. However, such families may represent the totality of high-risk predisposition or the tip of an iceberg if, for instance, not all mutations had the same risk of cancer associated with them. Under these circumstances, the population-based samples might be expected to contain a significant proportion of mutations with lesser effects on risk (lower penetrance variants).

3.1.3 Examples of dominant syndromes

Various autosomal dominant syndromes have been identified in this manner. Tables 3.1 and 3.2 show details of some of these syndromes.

Retinoblastoma

Retinoblastoma is a rare cancer of childhood which affects about 1 in 20,000 children (Sanders et al., 1988). Cancer occurs in the retinoblasts of the eye. Usually diagnosis is made in the first five years of life. Most cases are unilateral (involving only one eye) and have a single focus within the eye (Hodgson and Maher, 1993). Family studies showed that bilateral and multifocal cases were more likely to have a family history than unilateral cases. Several authors including Knudson speculated that the majority of lesions occur in persons without any apparent susceptibility and that the malignancy develops as a consequence of somatic mutation events in one or more genes. With inherited susceptibility, one or more of these genetic events is inherited so that all cells are at risk of progressing to malignancy. On this basis, statistical estimates suggest that 60% of cases are unilateral and non-hereditary, 15% are unilateral and hereditary while the remaining 25% are bilateral and hereditary (Knudson, 1971). The recognition that some of the multifocal cases had a microscopically visible deletion adjacent to the esterase D locus led to the cloning of the *RB* gene (Ward et al., 1984).

In his statistical analysis, Knudson considered the nature of inherited and somatic mutations and postulated a relationship between these germline (inherited) and somatic changes. He argued that when a mutation in a critical gene involved in the initiation or progression of cancer is present in the germline, all of the somatic cells of that person would also inherit this particular mutation. This would increase the rate at which progression occurred so that genetically predisposed persons should be at greatly increased risk of cancer as there would be an increased chance that a second event which eliminated the wild-type copy of the gene would occur. The molecular characterization of tumours arising in persons not genetically predisposed showed frequent acquired homozygosity of an *RB* mutation which was achieved by a somatic mutation followed by non-disjunction and duplication of the mutant chromosome, confirming that *RB* also played a significant role

Table 3.1 Genes associated with predisposition to common cancers[a]

Primary cancer	Syndrome	Genes	Normal function of gene	Locations	Types of lesions (malignancy unless otherwise specified)
Breast	Breast and breast/ovarian	*BRCA1*	DNA repair	17q21	Ovary (36–66%), pancreas (RR = 2.3), uterus (RR = 2.7), cervix (RR = 3.7)
		BRCA2	DNA repair	13q12.3	Prostate (RR = 4.7), pancreas (RR = 3.5), gallbladder (RR = 5.0), stomach (RR = 2.6), melanoma (RR = 2.6)
	Li–Fraumeni	*TP53*	Cell cycle regulation, apoptosis, transcription factor	17p13.1	Soft tissue sarcoma, brain tumours, adrenocortical tumours, leukaemia (overall cancer RR = 41)
		CHEK2	DNA repair	22q12.1	
	Cowden syndrome	*PTEN*	Protein tyrosinase phosphatase	10q23.31	Thyroid, endometrium
Bowel	Familial adenomatous polyposis	*APC*	Cell proliferation, adhesion	5q21–q22	Colorectal neoplasia, papillary thyroid cancers
	Hereditary non-polyposis colorectal cancer	*hMSH2*	DNA mismatch repair	2p22–p21	Colorectal cancer, endometrial cancer, ovarian cancer + other malignancies
		hMSH6	DNA mismatch repair	2p16	As above
		hMLH1	DNA mismatch repair	3p21.3	As above
		hPMS1	DNA mismatch repair	2q31–q33	As above
		hPMS2	DNA mismatch repair	7p22	As above
	Juvenile Polyposis Coli	*SMAD4*	Serine/threonine kinase	18q21.1	Gastrointestinal juvenile polyps
		BMPR1A	Serine/threonine kinase receptor	10q22.3	
	Peutz–Jeghers	*STK11*	Serine/threonine kinase	19p13.3	Breast, hamartomatous polyps
Skin	Familial melanoma	*CDKN2A*	Cell cycle regulation	9p21	Melanoma (67%), Pancreas (RR = 1.6)
		CDK4	Cell cycle regulation	12q14	
	Nevoid cell carcinoma	*PTCH*	Regulator of cell division	9q22.3	Basal cell carcinoma

[a] Table shows syndrome names, the role of the critical gene, the genetic location and the estimated risk of cancer (where known) given as a lifetime risk (%) or as a risk relative to that of the general population (RR) so RR = 2.0 implies that a mutation carrier has twice the risk of that cancer as a person without that mutation. All estimates have 'best guess' at this time.

outside the familial syndrome (Cavenee et al., 1983). This remains the clearest example of Knudson's ideas regarding the relationship between somatic and germline mutations. Such loci have been termed 'tumour suppressor genes' (more details can be found in Chapter 8). *RB* is now known to be involved in cell cycle control.

Breast cancer syndromes

Breast and breast-ovarian syndrome. This syndrome is characterized by early onset breast cancer which, in many families, is predominantly premenopausal, as well as an increased risk of ovarian cancer in some families. Many families with this syndrome are notable for the number of cancer cases (for an example of a family now known to be due to a mutation, see Figure 3.1). In the early 1990s, the first gene for this syndrome was mapped and subsequently cloned (*BRCA1*) (Miki et al., 1994). At the time of this mapping, analysis of families showed that an estimated 45% of such breast cancer families was due to this gene but that predominant among these families were those in which one or more relatives had been diagnosed with ovarian cancer (Easton et al., 1993). Other families which involved a male with breast cancer were not due to this gene and a subsequent analysis involving such families identified the *BRCA2* gene

Table 3.2 Genes associated with predisposition to cancer and with lesions affecting multiple organs [a]

Syndrome	Gene	Types of lesions (malignancy unless otherwise specified)	Genetic location
Hereditary papillary renal cell carcinoma	*MET*	Papillary renal cell	7q31
Hereditary paraganglioma and phaeochromocytoma	*SDHD*	Paraganglioma, phaeochromocytoma	11q23
	SDHC		1q21
	SDHB		1p36.1–p35
Multiple endocrine neoplasia type 1	*MEN1*	Parathyroid glands, anterior pituitary, pancreatic islet cells	11q13
Multiple endocrine neoplasia type 2	*RET*	Medullary thyroid carcinoma, phaeochromocytoma, and parathyroid adenomas	10q11.2
Neurofibromatosis type 1	*NF1*	Neurofibromas, optic glioma, neurofibrosarcoma, gliomas, phaeochromocytoma, leukaemia	17q11
Neurofibromatosis type 2	*NF2*	Bilateral vestibular schwannomas, meningiomas	22q12
Retinoblastoma	*RB*	Retinal tumours, osteogenic sarcoma	13q14
Tuberous sclerosis	*TSC1*	Hamartomas, astrocytomas, renal cell carcinoma, phaeochromocytoma	9q34
	TSC2		16p13
von Hippel Lindau	*VHL*	Retinal angioma, haemangioblastoma, renal cell carcinoma,	3p25
Wilms' tumour	*WT*	Kidney tumours	11p13

[a] A more complete discussion can be found elsewhere ((Hodgson and Maher, 1993) or at http://www.ncbi.nlm.nih.gov:80/entrez/query.fcgi?db = OMIM).

(Wooster et al., 1995). These two genes are the commonest high-penetrance genes for susceptibility to breast cancer but the search for further genes continues.

Mutations in *BRCA1* and *BRCA2* are predominantly protein truncating. Research has begun to elucidate the function of *BRCA1* and *BRCA2* as well as to describe in more detail the effect of germline mutations on cancer risk within the general population. Both *BRCA1* and *BRCA2*-associated tumours are found to be of significantly higher grade than tumours in the general population, with *BRCA1* tumours most likely to be grade III (Breast Cancer Linkage Consortium, 1997).

Several studies of breast cancer predisposition through *BRCA1* and *BRCA2* have now been published. The issue of the risk of cancer in mutation carriers has been problematic with early small studies showing considerable variation in the estimated risk. Soon after the cloning of *BRCA1* and *BRCA2*, only families with multiple cases of breast cancer were screened for mutations in *BRCA1* and *BRCA2*. As the families are identified because of the particular constellation of cancer within the family, statistical estimation of the risk has to take into account the way in which the families have been identified (ascertained). This estimation procedure leads to estimates with a wide confidence interval indicating the inherent imprecision in the estimate. The published estimates of risk from families with multiple cases of breast and/or ovarian cancer are 54% by age 60 years for breast cancer and 30% for ovarian cancer among *BRCA1* mutation carriers and 84% and 27% for *BRCA2* to age 70 with suggestions that breast cancer risks are lower to age 50 than for *BRCA2* (Easton et al., 1995; Ford et al., 1998). More recently estimates have been obtained from population-based studies which involve examining the germline of persons with newly diagnosed breast cancer, identifying those with mutations and estimating the risk of breast cancer in their relatives by mutation carrier status. In a review of 22 studies comprising 500 persons with breast cancer and a germline *BRCA1* or *BRCA2* mutation, the estimated risk of breast cancer in *BRCA1* mutation carriers was 65% by age 70 years (95% confidence interval (CI) 44–78%) for breast cancer, 39% (95% CI 18–54%) by the same age for ovarian cancer as compared to 45% (95% CI 31–56%) for breast cancer and 11% (95% CI 2.4–19%) for ovarian cancer (Antoniou et al., 2003). This latter study found evidence that mutations in particular regions of both *BRCA1* and *BRCA2* are associated with higher ovarian cancer risks and that relatives of early onset cases were more likely to be affected than relatives of older onset probands indicating that there may be an interplay with other factors.

Estimates have been obtained for the proportion of all breast cancer cases and the proportion of the general public carrying *BRCA1* or *BRCA2* mutations. Among UK breast cancer cases, 5.95% of women diagnosed before age 36 had *BRCA1* or *BRCA2* mutations, 4.1% diagnosed between ages 36 and 45 years (Peto et al., 1999). These figures suggest that in the United Kingdom, an estimated 3.1% of women with breast cancer have a *BRCA1* mutation and 3.0% have a *BRCA2* mutation with the earlier onset cases being more likely to have a mutation. The study also estimated that 1 in 500 of the general population has a *BRCA1* or *BRCA2* mutation making this one of the more common dominant disease-associated genes known. This study also showed that *BRCA1* and *BRCA2* only explained a small proportion of familial risk, meaning that other familial factors must also be important for risk.

The low prevalence of mutations in the UK population is not replicated in the Ashkenazi Jewish population. In that population, three specific mutations are common together implying that about 2.7% of this population carries one or more of the mutations (Roa et al., 1996). This observation is consistent with founder effects where generations ago, the population size was small and, by chance, several members of the population carried these mutations.

Li–Fraumeni syndrome. Li and Fraumeni described this syndrome after identifying families with similar constellations of cancers involving breast cancer and other neoplasms including soft tissue sarcomas, brain tumours, childhood rhabdomyosarcoma, osteosarcoma, leukaemia and adrenocortical carcinoma (Li and Fraumeni, 1969). A gene for this syndrome was hypothesized to be *TP53* on the basis of the wide variety of somatic mutations of *TP53* found in these tumours and this was indeed confirmed (Malkin et al., 1990). It has been estimated that 90% of mutation carriers develop cancer by the age of 70 and that female *TP53* mutation carriers have a relative risk of about 40 for cancer at any site (i.e. 40 times the risk for a person without such a mutation) (Hwang et al., 2003). Many families have phenotypic features of this syndrome but a definitive diagnosis is not possible so the term Li–Fraumeni-syndrome-variant has been coined. An estimated 20% of such families have *TP53* mutations but among the remainder some heterozygous mutations in *CHEK2* have also been found (Bell et al., 1999). *CHEK2* is a homologue of yeast RAD53 which is a protein kinase required for DNA damage and replication checkpoints.

Cowden syndrome. Cowden syndrome is characterized by multiple hamartomatous lesions of the skin, mucinous membranes, breast, and thyroid (Hodgson and Maher, 1993). About 50% of carriers show polyps in the gastrointestinal and urinary tracts while 50% of female carriers suffer from fibrocystic disease of the breast. Overall the risk of breast cancer has been estimated to be about 30%. The syndrome was mapped to chromosome 10 in 1995 and when subsequently the *PTEN* gene was mapped to the same chromosomal region, germline mutations in these families were identified (Li et al., 1997; Liaw et al., 1997).

Bowel cancer syndromes

Familial adenomatous polyposis. Familial adenomatous polyposis is a dominantly inherited syndrome characterized by the development of hundreds of adenomatous polyps in the bowel starting during adolescence with a prevalence of about 1 in 8000. Over time these polyps grow and increase in levels of dysplasia. The number of lesions and their increasing dysplasia means that the risk of malignancy increases. As a result, surgical removal of the bowel becomes necessary to prevent the development of malignancy which, in the absence of surgery, occurs before age 40 years (Hodgson and Maher, 1993).

A gene for FAP, *APC*, was mapped following the identification of a person with the colon characteristics and mental retardation, who was subsequently shown to have a germline deletion of chromosome 5 (Herrera et al., 1986; Bodmer et al., 1987). Detailed analysis of the region around the deletion was also involved in colorectal cancer (in the general population) with the observation of somatic deletions in tumours (Solomon et al., 1987), showing that *APC* is a tumour suppressor gene. It is now recognized that the majority of colorectal tumours have one or more mutations or deletions of the *APC* gene.

Investigation of *APC* in families with early-onset colorectal cancer indicates that some mutations do not produce the florid polyposis in the bowel. Such forms are termed 'attenuated FAP' and are associated with mutations at the 5′ end of the gene (Foulkes, 1995). By comparison, mutations in the middle of the gene are associated with the more florid phenotype. Also, a proportion of persons with FAP but without a family history have been found to have new mutations, that is, their mutation arose in a parent (Nugent et al., 1994). The location of the primary site for such mutations explains the association with large numbers of polyps in the bowel in such persons.

Hereditary non-polyposis colorectal cancer (HNPCC). Hereditary non-polyposis colorectal cancer is another form of dominantly inherited susceptibility to colorectal cancer. It was named to distinguish the syndrome from FAP and to indicate the lack of polyposis. While there is a lack of polyposis, there are certainly adenomatous polyps. The literature is unclear as to whether persons with HNPCC have more or less polyps than the general population but indicates similarity to the general population. The suggestion is that the adenomas progress to malignancy at a faster rate than in the general population so that polyps which take 15 years to progress to cancer in a person without HNPCC instead take only one or two years in a person with the syndrome. Cancer onset is, on average, in the early forties (Hodgson and Maher, 1993).

Persons with HNPCC are at increased risk of other cancers, most notably in women with a significantly increased risk of endometrial cancer as well as an increased risk of ovarian cancer. The mapping of an HNPCC family to chromosome 2p was followed within months by the cloning of the first gene for HNPCC and the recognition that tumours from family members showed a novel phenotype associated with a specific type of genetic alteration affecting repeat sequences (Aaltonen et al., 1993). This pattern of change was recognized as being indicative of a DNA mismatch repair error and on this basis, two genes for HNPCC were cloned (Kolodner et al., 1994). The lifetime risk of developing colorectal cancer has been shown to be significantly greater for males than for females (an estimated 74% versus 30%) while the risk of uterine cancer (42%) exceeded that for colorectal cancer in females (Dunlop et al., 1997).

Melanoma

The syndrome is characterized by the observation of multiple cases of melanoma within a family. Susceptibility is inherited as an autosomal dominant with incomplete penetrance. Within some families, relatives also have increased numbers of melanocytic naevi (Newton Bishop et al., 1998). Initial reports of melanoma families suggested that the phenotype of the abnormal naevus phenotype was a consistent component of the syndrome but more recent studies indicate that the naevus phenotype is observed in some families only. Linkage analysis mapped a locus to 9p21 and germline mutations were subsequently identified in the *CDKN2A* gene (Cannon-Albright et al., 1994). The *CDKN2* locus codes for two proteins, p16 coded for by *CDKN2A* and p14ARF coded for by a separate exon 1 together with exon 2 of *CDKN2A*, read in an alternative reading frame (ARF). Both p16 and p14ARF are involved in cell cycle regulation but in different pathways; p16 is in the Rb pathway while p14ARF is in the p53 pathway. The majority of mutations in *CDKN2A* are missense mutations or germline deletions affecting p16 but not p14ARF. Mutations in *CDK4* have also been found in a few families worldwide; *CDK4* binds to *CDKN2A* and this binding is impaired by the *CDK4* mutations (Hayward, 2003).

Mutations in *CDKN2A* have been found in families with multiple cases of melanoma worldwide. The penetrance of these mutations has been estimated to be 0.30 (95% CI 0.12–0.62%) by age 50 years, and 0.67 (95% CI 0.31–0.96%) by age 80 years (Bishop et al., 2002). This penetrance varied across geographical locations with lifetime penetrances being higher in Australia than in the United States and higher in Sweden than in the remainder of Europe, consistent with the ranking of melanoma incidence rates in the general population. The analysis suggests that UV exposure increases the risk of melanoma to a similar extent to that identified in the general population. The most notable risk of cancer within these families besides melanoma is for pancreatic cancer. Finally, a few mutations have now been identified in p14ARF. Families with p14ARF deletions removing the whole of the coding region of the alternative exon 1, exon 1β, have been associated with the melanoma–neural system tumour syndrome while a germline deletion has been observed in Spanish melanoma families. Finally, a further melanoma locus has been mapped to 1p22 (Hayward, 2003).

Other syndromes and issues

There are a number of cancers for which linkage attempts have been less successful to date. These include, for example, prostate cancer where the average age of onset limits the informativeness of families. The older age of onset means that there is more opportunity for genetically predisposed persons to die of other causes making such families carrying mutations less notable. To date, at least six genomic regions have been postulated as being the locations of predisposing genes but the studies have not been substantiated (Schaid, 2004).

The successful mapping and cloning of the genes described above through linkage analysis indicates the power of the approach in the correct circumstances but the approach has made less of a contribution in other circumstances. For instance, for a number of cancer sites the high rate of mortality after onset and the small number of extended families available have limited the informativeness of linkage mapping studies. Examples of such studies include those of pancreatic cancer, ovarian cancer, and lung cancer.

The power of the approach depends upon the availability of informative families but also the proportion of families attributable to each gene (not each mutation). For breast cancer, bowel cancer, and melanoma, the most common causes of susceptibility in the dominant families with convincing evidence of this susceptibility have been important to substantial proportions of families (25–50%). This, however, may not be the case for other cancers or syndromes in which many different genes could contribute to family aggregation and each of which only explains a small proportion of families. Such loci will be exceedingly difficult to map because the approach requires adequate numbers of sufficiently informative families to be due to the same gene to have any power for a mapping study. The completion of the human gene map has made genetic linkage studies more efficient and can now be considered in circumstances previously beyond the scope of this approach. Such studies are in progress for several cancer predispositions such as prostate cancer.

Family studies of such dominant syndromes often exhibit considerable variation in phenotype either in terms of ages of onset or in the severity of the phenotype. Causes of such variation include allelic variation, indicating that particular mutations may have different associated risks. Thus, for *BRCA2*, mutations in the 'ovarian cluster region' of the gene are associated with much higher ovarian cancer risks than mutations outside that region (Thompson and Easton, 2002). Variations within families cannot be explained by this effect. Potential explanations for variation are, of course, chance events or effects of other genes or lifestyle. In such circumstances, knowledge of the modifying factors, whether genetic or environmental (lifestyle) could be relevant to defining approaches to risk reduction among those with a high-risk predisposition. Identification of genetic modifiers of penetrance has not been a successful area of research to date, due, to a great extent, to the difficulties of recruiting sufficient numbers of persons in which to conduct these studies. Studies of lifestyle factors which might influence risk have produced some positive, but not convincing, effects to date. For instance, the use of oral contraceptives in *BRCA1* or *BRCA2* mutation carriers has been suggested as being both a risk factor and also protective.

Finally, the recognition that high-penetrance predisposition does not explain the majority of family aggregation indicates that other factors remain to be identified. Among the possibilities is the contribution of genes with more modest effect on risk which would also produce family aggregation but not extended pedigrees such as that depicted in Figure 3.1.

3.2 Recessively inherited susceptibility

Recessively inherited syndromes, as indicated above, require that each parent transmit a mutated copy of the same critical gene to an offspring who is therefore deficient for the product of this gene. The syndromes discussed in this section are all related to DNA repair deficiencies. The biology of DNA repair is discussed in more detail in Chapter 4.

3.2.1 Examples of recessive syndromes

Bloom syndrome

Bloom syndrome is characterized by low birth weight, growth deficiency, an abnormal face with a relatively large nose, and an adult height usually less than 150 cm but with normal intelligence (Bloom, 1966). Recessive persons develop an erythematous rash in their first year of life which becomes more noticeable in UV-exposed body parts and which worsens with increasing sun exposure. Both hypo- and hyperpigmentation of the skin are common features (Hodgson and Maher, 1993). Cases have a severe immunodeficiency and cancer incidence and mortality rates are high. Cancer incidence starts at young ages with persons in their twenties developing common cancers such as cancer of the bowel and the breast, 40 years before the average age of onset in the general population (German, 1997). The distribution of cancers is similar to that of the general population with the exception a particularly notable increase in rates of leukaemia and lymphoma (German, 1997).

At the cellular level, Bloom's patients show both an elevated frequency of chromosomal breaks as well as an increase in sister chromatid exchange rates and an abnormal distribution of DNA replication intermediates (Lonn et al., 1990). The Bloom syndrome gene, *BLM*, was shown to encode a DNA helicase related to the bacterial RecQ helicase and the *Saccharomyces cerevisiae SGS1* gene product (Ellis et al., 1995).

Bloom's is notably more common among those of Ashkenazi Jewish decent and this has been shown to be due to an ancestral mutation with a carrier frequency of 0.85%; no increase in cancer risk has been found for persons carrying a single copy of the common Ashkenazi mutation (Cleary et al., 2003).

Xeroderma pigmentosum

Xeroderma pigmentosum (XP) is the general term for a group of related recessive disorders associated with a defect in nucleotide excision repair. Clinically, XP is characterized by hypersensitivity to UV and a high incidence of UV-induced skin cancers (Cohen and Levy, 1989). The affected patients show onset in symptoms in the first few years of life (Hodgson and Maher, 1993). These early symptoms include an abnormal reaction to UV exposure. XP patients develop both malignant and benign neoplasms, primarily basal cell or squamous cell carcinoma with about 5% of patients developing melanoma; lesions primarily occur in sun-exposed sites. In one study, the median age of onset of skin neoplasm was estimated as eight years of age and the frequency of skin neoplasms was estimated at 2000 times the frequency of that in the general population for the under 20 years of age group while internal malignancies (such as cancers of the lung, uterine, breast) were increased at least tenfold over the general population under the age of twenty years (Kraemer et al., 1994).

Excision repair is the process required to correct a wide variety of DNA damage which has been induced by exposure to UV, X-rays or chemicals. Nucleotide excision repair (NER) is a specific form of excision repair which takes single stranded, damaged DNA and replaces the damage with a new sequence using the intact strand as a template (see Chapter 4 for more details). The association between XP and defective NER was made in 1968 (Cleaver, 1968). Cancer predisposition is then thought to be due to the inability or reduced ability of XP cells to repair DNA damage.

Ataxia–telangiectasia

Ataxia–telangiectasia (AT) is an autosomal recessive disorder identified by progressive cerebral ataxia with onset between the ages of one and three years (Gatti et al., 1991). The prevalence of AT has been estimated at 1 in 40,000 to 1 in 100,000 live births. The clinical features of the syndrome are broad and include neurological, immunological, developmental, and neoplastic disorders. The progressive cerebral ataxia is the most obvious characteristic of the AT syndrome. Although the children begin to walk on a normal time scale they then develop a stagger, which increases to the extent that by 10 years of age they are unable to walk. Over a third of AT patients develop malignancy during their lifetimes. Approximately 85% of these malignancies are either leukaemia or lymphoma. The acute lymphocytic leukaemia is often of T cell origin. With improved survival of AT patients various non-lymphoid cancers have been observed such as those of the breast, stomach and ovary, and melanoma. There has also been a suggestion that AT heterozygotes are at increased risk of cancer especially of the breast with a relative risk of 3.8 by comparison with the general population (Easton, 1994). Linkage analysis of 176 families showed that the *ATM* gene was located on chromosome 11q22–23. The *ATM* gene was isolated from this region (Savitsky et al., 1995). To date over 250 mutations in the *ATM* gene have been identified. *ATM* appears to play a major role as an intracellular signal transducer that is involved in indicating DNA damage requiring repair. *ATM* therefore, is involved in cell cycle checkpoints. However, it is presently unclear how defects in the DNA damage response can account for all of the clinical features of AT.

3.3 Association studies

Linkage analysis provides the basis for identifying genes associated with susceptibility to disease in the absence of any prior concepts of mechanism. Genotyping more families and using more genetic polymorphisms decreases the size of the plausible region containing the gene, which allows the identification of the causative gene in the sampled families. Successful linkage analysis does not require that all families are due to the same mutation and, in fact, the evidence that a particular gene is causative is strengthened by the observation of numerous different mutations within the same gene. For instance, there is convincing evidence for *BRCA1* as the chromosome 17 locus for susceptibility to breast cancer obtained by showing the large numbers of distinct truncating mutations within the same coding sequence, that is, that the critical gene had been identified. This is, however, not true for association studies.

Association studies involve comparing the genotypic distribution of a series of cases diagnosed with a particular cancer and comparing this genotype distribution with that of a set of controls. These controls are chosen from the general population to have characteristics similar to those of the cases (in terms of age, gender, geographical location, race, ethnicity), but to be unaffected with that cancer. Many epidemiology studies choose to identify such controls through population registers. For instance, within the United Kingdom, identifying controls have often been accomplished through a register of individuals maintained by the GP of each case. In the most informative association studies, cases are recruited soon after diagnosis of cancer, so that the case series represented is not modified in any way by issues of survival.

The linkage analysis approach allowed the genotyping of large numbers of markers across the genome to identify the critical region, followed by localization and eventual identification of the critical gene. Association studies currently require that attention focuses on postulated causative mechanisms for susceptibility. For instance, as there is clear evidence that factors related to hormones influence the risk of breast cancer, many such studies have focused on genes with a known role in hormone synthesis. Typically, a number of different genes within a particular pathway are genotyped and then the genotypic distribution compared between cases and controls; that is, one or more variants within a gene are assayed and the proportion of all cases that carry each variant is compared with the proportion of controls carrying the same variant. In terms of specific mutations within genes, there are two distinct approaches which can be taken. The first involves identifying functional or presumed functional variants of the gene under consideration and comparing the distribution of this variant between cases and controls. Analyses are conducted for each specific variant within the critical gene. The second approach is based more on genetic history and takes advantage of the fact that the ancestry of particular components of each genetic region can be identified. In many studies of disease-associated genes, it has been found that approximately five common haplotypes explained the majority of all haplotypes within a given population. The particular variants which are critical to identifying these specific haplotypes of each case and control can then be typed and the distribution of haplotypes compared between cases and controls. This approach has the advantage of taking into account the extent of linkage disequilibrium across the genome.

The linkage analysis approach has proved to be robust, in that few regions have been identified which have subsequently been found not to harbour a disease gene. The same cannot be said of association studies, for which results to date have been inconsistent. This inconsistency arises in that particular studies have found differences in the frequency of a particular variant between cases and controls, but subsequent studies have failed to validate this difference. There are a number of potential explanations for this. The first is that the initial study was simply a false-positive result and there is truly no association between the presence of the variant and risk of disease. Statistical analyses are usually based on p-values or significance levels, which indicates the probability that a particular observation would have been seen by chance if there was truly no effect. So a p-value of 0.05 implies that 5% of all tests conducted when there was truly no effect would in fact give evidence suggesting that there was an effect. Thus we can reasonably expect that some positive findings (around 5% of all conducted analyses as distinct from the proportion of reported analyses) will in fact be false. Investigators may however increase the nominal rate of false-positive findings by not taking into account the number of statistical tests that they perform. So, dividing and subdividing the data and analysing each particular subset of data will eventually lead to false-positive findings. The second option is that in fact that there may indeed be effect, but this effect differs between populations.

Finally, the power of such studies can be increased by selecting cases more likely to be attributable to a genetic effect. Thus for instance, in such studies, one design is to recruit cases that also have a family history, thereby enriching for all genetic causes and hopefully for the specific genetic cause under analysis. In the following section, we describe various association studies that have been conducted on common cancers and these examples have been chosen to illustrate association studies.

Table 3.3 shows the estimated sample sizes required to conduct a case–control study when, genetically, the population can be divided into two groups, one which is at 'standard' risk and the other at increased risk. This table shows the size of study that would be required to test the hypothesis of the involvement of one genetic variant. Studies which investigate rare genetic variants or small increases in risk are not logistically feasible, while studies searching for more major effects can realistically be achieved.

3.3.1 Examples of association studies

CHEK2 *and breast cancer*

High-penetrance mutations have been found in *CHEK2* in Li–Fraumeni syndrome (see earlier). Arguing that some variants in this gene might be associated with increased risk of breast cancer, a recent study looking at the *CHEK2* gene showed a difference between cases and controls. Cases were breast cancer cases selected for those with a family history, while controls came from the general population. This study showed a significant effect of a *CHEK2* variant 1100delC on risk of breast cancer essentially doubling the risk of breast cancer in women (Meijers-Heijboer et al., 2002). In this study about 1.1% of the general population carried this variant.

Table 3.3 Sample size requirements. Number of cases needed to achieve 80% power in a case–control study with equal number of controls, using a two-sided 5% significance level

Odds ratio	Population frequency of those at increased risk (%)					
	1	5	10	20	50	70
1.5	7954	1687	910	534	387	499
1.8	3487	746	407	244	187	250
2.0	2394	515	282	171	136	185
2.5	1245	271	151	94	80	114
3.0	803	177	99	64	58	85
4.0	448	100	58	38	38	59
10.0	112	27	17	14	18	32
50.0	20	7	6	6	12	23

ATM *and breast cancer*

The prevalence of an *ATM* mutation is about 1 in 40,000 live births, implying that about 1% of the population are heterozygous (see previous section). An increased risk of breast cancer has been observed in female A–T heterozygotes with an estimated risk of 3.8 times that of the general population (Easton, 1994). On this basis, about 3.5% of all breast cancer should occur in the 1% of heterozygous women. Studies have been conducted to assess the accuracy of this estimate using the case–control approach. The difficulty with attempting this study is that if these figures were correct, such a study would require minimally 750 cases and 750 controls (if all mutations were detected) to have high statistical power and the complexity of mutation detection makes such studies logistically challenging (Bishop and Hopper, 1997). If only 75% of mutations could be detected then the sample size would need to be 1000 cases and 1000 controls, indicative of the difficulty of performing association studies for such rare variants.

APC *I1307K and bowel cancer*

Germline mutations in the *APC* gene are associated with FAP (see earlier). The *APC* gene variant I1307K is common in the Ashkenazi population with about 6% of the population carrying this variant (Gryfe et al., 1999). Studies are inconsistent as to the effect of this mutation on risk with some studies finding an effect (Gryfe et al., 1999) while others do not (Strul et al., 2003) so that further research is required. The variant is of interest because it appears to be associated with an increased rate of somatic changes in the *APC* gene (Laken et al., 1997), which suggests that as *APC* is a tumour suppressor gene, it would increase the risk of neoplasia.

MC1R *and melanoma*

The major genetic determinant of susceptibility to melanoma is skin colour, as melanoma is predominantly a cancer of white skinned peoples. Within white populations, the highest incidence is in countries nearest to the equator as sun exposure is the major environmental factor for melanoma (Armstrong, 1988). It is probable therefore, that skin colour itself is important in predisposition to skin cancer generally. That is, that the genes which control melanin production and its deposition in the cell, are probably important aetiologically

(Boissy, 2003). There are two types of melanin, eumelanin, and pheomelanin. Pheomelanin is produced particularly in people with red hair and freckles. This type of melanin is functionally different to eumelanin, being less photoprotective. The ratio of pheomelanin to eumelanin produced by the melanocyte is modulated by the melanocortin receptor *MC1R* (Suzuki et al., 1996). The *MC1R* gene at chromosome 16q is highly polymorphic and some variants are shown to be associated with red hair (Valverde et al., 1995) and freckles (Bastiaens et al., 2001). Predictably inheritance of those variants which are highly correlated with red hair such as Asp84Glu has been shown to be a risk factor for melanoma (Valverde et al., 1996) but predisposition was also shown to be independent of skin type and hair colour in some individuals.

General comments

The examples shown above indicate the typical studies conducted to date involving genes with a biologically plausible role and variants with a functional significance. Studies involving genetic variants without a clear functional role have also been conducted on the basis that such variants may be in linkage disequilibrium with functionally relevant variants (i.e. that at some stage in the past an unrecognized functional variant occurred on a chromosome carrying another recognized but non-functional variant). While the studies described above show some positive but largely inconclusive evidence of an association, many other studies do not provide such evidence. For instance, the role of genes involved in the metabolism of aromatic and heterocyclic amines (which are present in food) are candidates for being associated with colorectal cancer risk but without any clear proof at this time (Houlston and Tomlinson, 2001).

3.3.2 Discussion

The linkage mapping approach has been remarkably successful for cloning genes for syndromes associated with cancer, especially those in which the mutation carrier status is clear before cancer onset, such as FAP. Diseases without such an overt marker of genetic status have proved more challenging but the magnitude of the penetrance has meant that some of these genes have been found. The successful studies have resulted from situations in which a small number of genes have been responsible for the high-penetrance susceptibility. The fewer the number of genes involved in susceptibility, the more homogeneity of susceptibility will be present in families identified because of the high number of affected persons, and hence the more informative will be the linkage mapping studies. At this time, it is not clear why for the successfully mapped syndromes so few genes contribute to the majority of high-penetrance predisposition. This must depend upon the particular pathway that is impaired, the number of other genes within the pathway, their proclivity to mutation and the impact of such mutations on survival and development. For prostate cancer and other syndromes there remains the possibility that many different genes can cause susceptibility and none of them is a 'common' cause. Having multiple genes for susceptibility is a feature of other syndromes such as renal cell cancer where at least five genes are known including *VHL* and *MET* while two more are postulated (Pavlovich and Schmidt, 2004). However, for a number of these genes, the syndrome is identifiable by other phenotypic characteristics.

The efforts to find high-penetrance genes are in progress, especially for prostate cancer. For breast cancer, where the epidemiology is most advanced, it is clear that these genes explain only a small portion of the family aggregation. Other factors such as genes with lesser effects are postulated and there is some supportive evidence as described earlier. However, many of the studies reported to date have either been unsuccessful or have produced equivocal results. There are a number of potential technical reasons for this such as sample sizes of studies and the manner in which they were conducted (e.g. by choice of controls) or the choice of candidate loci may be at fault. There remains the potential that susceptibility may be due to many different factors, each of which is only relevant in a small proportion of people which would make such mapping studies extremely low in power. However, even this situation could be overcome if, for instance, the critical genes were all within a single pathway.

References

Aaltonen, L. A., Peltomäki, P., Leach, F. S., Sistonen, P., Pylkkänen, L., Mecklin, J.-P. et al. (1993). Clues to the pathogenesis of familial colorectal cancer. *Science*, **260**, 812–16.

Antoniou, A., Pharoah, P. D., Narod, S., Risch, H. A., Eyfjord, J. E., Hopper, J. L. et al. (2003). Average risks of breast and ovarian cancer associated with BRCA1 or BRCA2 mutations detected in case Series unselected for family history: a combined analysis of 22 studies. *Am J Hum Genet*, **72**, 1117–30.

Armstrong, B. K. (1988). Epidemiology of malignant melanoma: intermittent or total accumulated exposure to the sun? *J Dermatol Surg Oncol*, **14**, 835–49.

Bastiaens, M., ter Huurne, J., Gruis, N., Bergman, W., Westendorp, R., Vermeer, B. J. et al. (2001). The melanocortin-1-receptor gene is the major freckle gene. *Hum Mol Genet*, **10**, 1701–8.

Bell, D. W., Varley, J. M., Szydlo, T. E., Kang, D. H., Wahrer, D. C., Shannon, K. E., et al. (1999). Heterozygous germline hCHK2 mutations in Li-Fraumeni syndrome. *Science*, **286**, 2528–31.

Bishop, D. T. and Hopper, J. (1997). AT-tributable risks? *Nat Genet*, **15**, 226.

Bishop, D. T., Demenais, F., Goldstein, A. M., Bergman, W., Bishop, J. N., Bressac-de Paillerets, B. et al. (2002). Geographical variation in the penetrance of CDKN2A mutations for melanoma. *J Natl Cancer Inst*, **94**, 894–903.

Bloom, D. (1966). The syndrome of congenital telangiectatic erythema and stunted growth. *J Paed*, **68**, 103–13.

Bodmer, W. F., Bailey, C. J., Bodmer, J., Bussey, H. J., Ellis, A., Gorman, P. et al. (1987). Localization of the gene for familial adenomatous polyposis on chromosome 5. *Nature*, **328**, 614–6.

Boissy, R. E. (2003). Melanosome transfer to and translocation in the keratinocyte. *Exp Dermatol*, **12**(Suppl. 2), 5–12.

Botstein, D., White, R. L., Skolnick, M., and Davis, R. W. (1980). Construction of a genetic linkage map in man using restriction fragment length polymorphisms. *Am J Hum Genet*, **32**, 314–31.

Breast Cancer Linkage Consortium (1997). Pathology of familial breast cancer: differences between breast cancers in carriers of BRCA1 or BRCA2 mutations and sporadic cases. *Lancet*, **349**, 1505–10.

Cannon-Albright, L., Goldgar, D., Neuhausen, S., Gruis, N., Anderson, D., Lewis, C. et al. (1994). Localization of the 9p melanoma susceptibility locus (MLM) to a 2-cM region between D9S736 and D9S171. *Genomics*, **23**, 265–8.

Cavenee, W. K., Dryja, T. P., Phillips, R. A., Benedict, W. F., Godbout, R., Gallie, B. L. et al. (1983). Expression of recessive alleles by chromosomal mechanisms in retinoblastoma. *Nature*, **305**, 779–84.

Cleary, S. P., Zhang, W., Di Nicola, N., Aronson, M., Aube, J., Steinman, A. et al. (2003). Heterozygosity for the BLM(Ash) mutation and cancer risk. *Cancer Res*, **63**, 1769–71.

Cleaver, J. E. (1968). Defective repair replication of DNA in xeroderma pigmentosum. *Nature*, **218**, 652–6.

Cohen, M. M. and Levy, H. P. (1989). Chromosome instability syndromes. *Adv Hum Genet*, **18**, 43–149.

Dunlop, M. G., Farrington, S. M., Carothers, A. D., Wyllie, A. H., Sharp, L., Burn, J. et al. (1997). Cancer risk associated with germline DNA mismatch repair gene mutations. *Hum Mol Genet*, **6**, 105–10.

Easton, D. F. (1994). Cancer risks in A-T heterozygotes. *Int J Radiat Biol*, **66**, S177–82.

Easton, D. F., Ford, D., and Bishop, D. T. (1995). Breast and ovarian cancer incidence in BRCA1-mutation carriers. Breast Cancer Linkage Consortium. *Am J Hum Genet*, **56**, 265–71.

Easton, D. F., Bishop, D. T., Ford, D., and Crockford, G. P. (1993). Genetic linkage analysis in familial breast and ovarian cancer: results from 214 families. The Breast Cancer Linkage Consortium. *Am J Hum Genet*, **52**, 678–701.

Ellis, N. A., Groden, J., Ye, T. Z., Straughen, J., Lennon, D. J., Ciocci, S. et al. (1995). The Bloom's syndrome gene product is homologous to RecQ helicases. *Cell*, **83**, 655–66.

Fisher, R. A. (1935). The detection of linkage with 'dominant' abnormalities. *Ann Eugenics*, **6**, 187–201.

Ford, D., Easton, D. F., Stratton, M., Narod, S., Goldgar, D., Devilee, P. et al. (1998). Genetic heterogeneity and penetrance analysis of the BRCA1 and BRCA2 genes in breast cancer families. The Breast Cancer Linkage Consortium. *Am J Hum Genet*, **62**, 676–89.

Foulkes, W. D. (1995). A tale of four syndromes: familial adenomatous polyposis, Gardner syndrome, attenuated APC and Turcot syndrome. *QJM*, **88**, 853–63.

Gatti, R. A., Boder, E., Vinters, H. V., Sparkes, R. S., Norman, A., and Lange, K. (1991). Ataxia-telangiectasia: an interdisciplinary approach to pathogenesis. *Medicine (Baltimore)*, **70**, 99–117.

German, J. (1997). Bloom's syndrome. XX. The first 100 cancers. *Cancer Genet Cytogenet*, **93**, 100–6.

Gryfe, R., Di Nicola, N., Lal, G., Gallinger, S., and Redston, M. (1999). Inherited colorectal polyposis and cancer risk of the APC I1307K polymorphism. *Am J Hum Genet*, **64**, 378–84.

Hayward, N. K. (2003). Genetics of melanoma predisposition. *Oncogene*, **22**, 3053–62.

Herrera, L., Kakati, S., Gibas, L., Pietrzak, E., and Sandberg, A. A. (1986). Gardner syndrome in a man with an interstitial deletion of 5q. *Am J Med Genet*, **25**, 473–6.

Hodgson, S. V. and Maher, E. R. (1993). *A Practical Guide to Human Cancer Genetics*. Cambridge University Press, Cambridge.

Houlston, R. S. and Tomlinson, I. P. (2001). Polymorphisms and colorectal tumor risk. *Gastroenterology*, **121**, QJ;282–301.

Hwang, S. J., Lozano, G., Amos, C. I., and Strong, L. C. (2003). Germline p53 mutations in a cohort with childhood sarcoma: sex differences in cancer risk. *Am J Hum Genet*, **72**, 975–83.

Knudson, A. G., Jr. (1971). Mutation and cancer: statistical study of retinoblastoma. *Proc Natl Acad Sci USA*, **68**, 820–3.

Kolodner, R. D., Hall, N. R., Lipford, J., Kane, M. F., Rao, M. R. S., Morrison, P. et al. (1994). Structure of the human MSH2 locus and analysis of two Muir-Torre kindreds for msh2 mutations. *Genomics*, **24**, 516–26.

Kraemer, K., Lee, M.-M., Andrews, A., and Lambert, W. (1994). The role of sunlight and DNA repair in melanoma and nonmelanoma skin cancer. The xeroderma pigmentosum paradigm. *Arch Dermatol*, **130**, 1018–21.

Laken, S. J., Petersen, G. M., Gruber, S. B., Oddoux, C., Ostrer, H., Giardiello, F. M. et al. (1997). Familial colorectal cancer in Ashkenazim due to a hypermutable tract in APC. *Nat Genet*, **17**, 79–83.

Li, F. P. and Fraumeni, J. F., Jr. (1969). Soft-tissue sarcomas, breast cancer, and other neoplasms. A familial syndrome? *Ann Intern Med*, **71**, 747–52.

Li, J., Yen, C., Liaw, D., Podsypanina, K., Bose, S., Wang, S. I. et al. (1997). PTEN, a putative protein tyrosine phosphatase gene mutated in human brain, breast, and prostate cancer. *Science*, **275**, 1943–7.

Liaw, D., Marsh, D. J., Li, J., Dahia, P. L., Wang, S. I., Zheng, Z. et al. (1997). Germline mutations of the PTEN gene in Cowden disease, an inherited breast and thyroid cancer syndrome. *Nat Genet*, **16**, 64–7.

Lonn, U., Lonn, S., and Nylen, U. (1990). An abnormal profile of DNA replication intermediates in Bloom's syndrome. *Cancer Res*, **50**, 3141–45.

Lynch, H. T., Krush, A. J., Lemon, H. M., Kaplan, A. R., Condit, P. T., and Bottomley, R. H. (1972). Tumor variation in families with breast cancer. *J Am Med Assoc*, **222**, 1631–5.

Malkin, D., Li, F. P., Strong, L. C., Fraumeni, J. F., Jr., Nelson, C. E., Kim, D. H. et al. (1990). Germline p53 mutations in a familial syndrome of breast cancer, sarcomas, and other neoplasms. *Science*, **250**, 1233–8.

Meijers-Heijboer, H., van den Ouweland, A., Klijn, J., Wasielewski, M., de Snoo, A., Oldenburg, R. et al. (2002). Low-penetrance susceptibility to breast cancer due to CHEK2(*)1100delC in noncarriers of BRCA1 or BRCA2 mutations. *Nat Genet*, **31**, 55–9.

Miki, Y., Swensen, J., Shattuck-Eidens, D., Futreal, P. A., Harshman, K., Tavtigian, S. et al. (1994). A strong candidate for the breast and ovarian cancer susceptibility gene BRCA1. *Science*, **266**, 66–71.

Newton Bishop, J. A., Harland, M., and Bishop, D. T. (1998). The genetics of melanoma: the UK experience. *Clin Exp Dermatol*, **23**, 158–61.

NIH/CEPH Collaborative Mapping Group (1992). A comprehensive genetic linkage map of the human genome. *Science*, **258**, 67–86.

Nugent, K. P., Phillips, R. K., Hodgson, S. V., Cottrell, S., Smith-Ravin, J., Pack, K. et al. (1994). Phenotypic expression in familial adenomatous polyposis: partial prediction by mutation analysis. *Gut*, **35**, 1622–3.

Pavlovich, C. P. and Schmidt, L. S. (2004). Searching for the hereditary causes of renal-cell carcinoma. *Nat Rev Cancer*, **4**, 381–93.

Peto, J., Collins, N., Barfoot, R., Seal, S., Warren, W., Rahman, N. et al. (1999). Prevalence of BRCA1 and BRCA2 gene mutations in patients with early-onset breast cancer. *J Natl Cancer Inst*, **91**, 943–9.

Roa, B. B., Boyd, A. A., Volcik, K., and Richards, C. S. (1996). Ashkenazi Jewish population frequencies for common mutations in BRCA1 and BRCA2. *Nat Genet*, **14**, 185–7.

Sanders, B. M., Draper, G. J., and Kingston, J. E. (1988). Retinoblastoma in Great Britain 1969–80: incidence, treatment, and survival. *Br J Ophthalmol*, **72**, 576–83.

Savitsky, K., Sfez, S., Tagle, D. A., Ziv, Y., Sartiel, A., Collins, F. S. et al. (1995). The complete sequence of the coding region of the ATM gene reveals similarity to cell cycle regulators in different species. *Hum Mol Genet*, **4**, 2025–32.

Schaid, D. J. (2004). The complex genetic epidemiology of prostate cancer. *Hum Mol Genet*, **13**(Spec. No. 1), R103–21.

Solomon, E., Voss, R., Hall, V., Bodmer, W. F., Jass, J. R., Jeffreys, A. J. et al. (1987). Chromosome 5 allele loss in human colorectal carcinomas. *Nature*, **328**, 616–9.

Strul, H., Barenboim, E., Leshno, M., Gartner, M., Kariv, R., Aljadeff, E. et al. (2003). The I1307K adenomatous polyposis coli gene variant does not contribute in the assessment of the risk for colorectal cancer in Ashkenazi Jews. *Cancer Epidemiol Biomarkers Prev*, **12**, 1012–5.

Suzuki, I., Cone, R. D., Im, S., Nordlund, J., and Abdel-Malek, Z. A. (1996). Binding of melanotropic hormones to the melanocortin receptor MC1R on human melanocytes stimulates proliferation and melanogenesis. *Endocrinology*, **137**, 1627–33.

Thompson, D. and Easton, D. (2002). Variation in BRCA1 cancer risks by mutation position. *Cancer Epidemiol Biomarkers Prev*, **11**, 329–36.

Valverde, P., Healy, E., Jackson, I., Rees, J., and Thody, A. (1995). Variants of the melanocyte-stimulating hormone receptor gene are associated with red hair and fair skin in humans. *Nature Genetics*, **11**, 328–30.

Valverde, P., Healy, E., Sikkink, S., Haldane, F., Thody, A. J., Carothers, A. et al. (1996). The Asp84Glu variant of the melanocortin 1 receptor (MC1R) is associated with melanoma. *Human Molec Genet*, **5**, 1663–6.

Ward, P., Packman, S., Loughman, W., Sparkes, M., Sparkes, R., McMahon, A. et al. (1984). Location of the retinoblastoma susceptibility gene(s) and the human esterase D locus. *J Med Genet*, **21**, 92–5.

Wooster, R., Bignell, G., Lancaster, J., Swift, S., Seal, S., Mangion, J. et al. (1995). Identification of the breast cancer susceptibility gene BRCA2. *Nature*, **378**, 789–92.

CHAPTER 4

DNA repair and cancer

Beate Köberle, John P. Wittschieben, and Richard D. Wood

This chapter concentrates on the main DNA repair mechanisms operating in human cells and the relationship of DNA repair to cancer. There are several pathways for repairing damaged DNA (Lindahl et al., 1997; Hoeijmakers, 2001). More than 125 human gene products are involved in DNA repair (see http://www.cgal.icnet.uk/DNA_Repair_Genes.html) and (Wood et al., 2001). Owing to space limitations, in-depth reviews are largely cited below, which should be consulted for more complete references.

4.1 Direct reversal

Direct reversal is the simplest mechanism of DNA repair. It involves a single enzyme reaction for the removal of certain types of damage directly from the DNA. The best studied example is removal of the miscoding alkylation lesion O^6-methylguanine (O^6-meG). This lesion is potentially mutagenic mainly due to the tendency of O^6-meG to pair with thymine during replication, resulting in a GC to AT base pair transition. DNA methylation can occur through exposure to methylating agents or by endogenously generated reactive cellular catabolites. In human cells, O^6-methylguanine-DNA methyltransferase (MGMT) is a 22 kDa protein that removes O^6-meG through transfer of the methyl group to one of its own cysteine residues in a rapid and error-free repair process. During this process MGMT is inactivated, and is subsequently degraded through ubiquitination pathways. Cells and tissues are reported to vary greatly in MGMT expression. MGMT activity in tumours correlates inversely with sensitivity to agents that form O^6-alkylguanine DNA adducts, such as carmustine (BCNU), temozolomide, streptozotocin, and dacarbazine (Gerson, 2002).

This may be important in successful treatment of gliomas.

The adducts 1-methyladenine and 3-methylcytosine are repaired by oxidative demethylation, another mechanism of repair by direct reversal. In *Escherichia coli*, oxidative demethylation is carried out by AlkB (Trewick et al., 2002). Recently, human homologues of AlkB have been identified (Duncan et al., 2002).

4.2 Nucleotide excision repair

Nucleotide excision repair (NER) acts on a wide variety of potentially toxic and mutagenic helix-distorting DNA lesions like UV-light induced photolesions, bulky chemical adducts and DNA intrastrand-crosslinks. NER requires the action of around 30 polypeptides which then function by the stepwise assembly of several complexes at the site of the DNA damage (Volker et al., 2001). Two NER sub-pathways can be distinguished: global genome NER (GG-NER) and transcription-coupled NER (TC-NER). GG-NER surveys the entire genome for DNA damage. TC-NER removes DNA lesions significantly faster from the transcribed strand of genes than from the non-transcribed strand or the bulk of DNA. The two sub-pathways differ only in the damage recognition step of NER.

In the NER pathway the DNA damage is first recognized. Incisions are then made 5′ and 3′ of the lesion, followed by excision of the damage-containing oligonucleotide. NER is completed by DNA synthesis to replace the excised oligonucleotide and ligation of the repair patch (Figure 4.1). In GG-NER the first step of damage recognition involves XPC-HR23B-centrin 2. The 106 kDa XPC protein forms a complex with its 43 kDa partner HR23B and centrin 2. This complex binds single-stranded DNA and has a preference for distortions in DNA. XPC is restricted to GG-NER and is dispensable for transcription-coupled NER. In addition to XPC-complex, the DNA damage binding

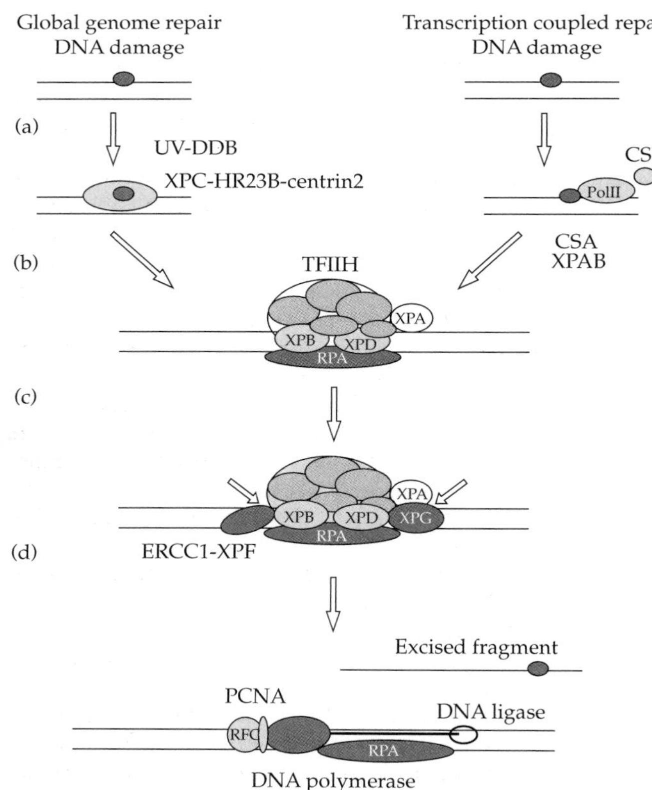

Figure 4.1 Nucleotide excision repair consists of (a) distortion recognition, (b) formation of an open structure and recognition of the damaged strand, (c) dual incisions made by structure-specific endonucleases, and (d) excision, DNA repair synthesis, and ligation.

protein (UV-DDB) complex appears to have an important function for GG-NER *in vivo*, perhaps assisting DNA damage recognition in chromatin (Wittschieben and Wood, 2003).

Transcription-coupled NER appears to be initiated when RNA polymerase II halts at a lesion in DNA. This could serve as a damage-recognition signal resulting in recruitment of other NER factors. This initial step in TC-NER requires CSA, CSB, and XAB2 proteins. CSB has been shown to interact with RNA polymerase II (van Gool et al., 1997). It is suggested that CSB recruits NER proteins *in vivo* when RNA polymerase II is stalled at damage on the transcribed strand.

The next steps in GG-NER and TC-NER are the same. Initial distortion recognition is followed by the formation of an open complex which requires local unwinding of the DNA helix. The unwinding of the helix is brought about by the helicase activity of the basal transcription factor TFIIH. TFIIH is a ten-subunit protein complex containing the XPB and XPD helicases among its subunits (Giglia-Mari et al., 2004). TFIIH mediates strand separation at the site of the lesion where XPB can translocate DNA in the 3′ to 5′ direction and XPD in the opposite direction, a process that most likely takes place in the presence of XPG. The open, unwound complex spans a region of up to 24–32 bp around the lesion. Other core NER factors are required for the formation of a functional repair complex, including XPA and the single-stranded DNA-binding protein A (RPA). XPA is a DNA and protein-binding factor in the NER complex and it is believed that XPA helps position the repair machinery correctly around the lesion (de Laat et al., 1999). Replication protein A (RPA) is thought to bind to the single-stranded region of the undamaged strand, stabilizing the opened DNA complex and assisting in positioning the XPG and ERCC1-XPF endonucleases around the lesion. Incisions are then made sequentially on the damaged strand. XPG cuts on the 3′ side two to nine phosphodiester bonds from the lesion. This usually occurs before ERCC1-XPF cuts 16–25 phosphodiester bonds on the 5′ side. The 24–32mer oligonucleotide containing the damage is then released, possibly still bound by one of the damage recognition proteins. The gap is filled by a proliferating cell nuclear antigen (PCNA)-dependent DNA polymerase δ or ε holoenzyme and sealed by a DNA ligase to regenerate the intact DNA structure.

4.2.1 Human syndromes with defects in NER genes

In humans, at least three different rare, inherited syndromes are associated with defects in NER: xeroderma pigmentosum (XP), Cockayne syndrome (CS), and trichothiodystrophy (TTD), all three associated with extreme sensitivity to sunlight (Bootsma et al., 2002). XP is characterized by numerous skin abnormalities ranging from excessive freckling to multiple skin cancers. These abnormalities are caused by the inability to repair DNA damage induced by sunlight. Individuals suffering from XP have at least a 1000-fold greater risk of developing skin cancer than normal individuals. They also have a small increased risk of developing several types of internal cancers. Some XP patients suffer progressive neurological abnormalities due to neuronal degeneration. When cells derived from XP patients were used in cell-fusion studies, this led to the identification of 7 NER-deficient complementation groups, XP-A to XP-G, each reflecting a defect in a single protein required for the incision step of NER. Differences in sun sensitivity and repair defects among the different XP groups have been observed. The most marked clinical abnormalities with severe skin changes and neurological abnormalities at an early age are seen in patients from XP-A. XP-C cells are less sensitive to UV than XP-A or XP-D cells and have a residual repair synthesis of up to 30% due to TC-NER. XP-E cells show the mildest defect in NER of all XP groups, with about 50% of normal repair capacity.

Cockayne syndrome is characterized by dwarfism, microcephaly, mental retardation, retinal and skin abnormalities. CS patients, however, show no predisposition to develop skin cancer. That may be explained by the fact that CS cells are particularly sensitive to lesion-induced apoptosis (Hanawalt, 2000) and therefore protected against tumorigenesis. There are rare cases of individuals with the combined symptoms of XP and CS (XP/CS), though most cases do not have the clinical features of XP. Patients with combined XP and CS phenotype belong to the XP-B, XP-D or XP-G genotype. Cells derived from CS patients are sensitive to UV light, are unable to carry out TC-NER but have normal GG-NER.

Trichothiodystrophy is characterized by brittle hair which is caused by reduced content of cysteine rich matrix proteins in the hair shaft. In addition, TTD patients show mental retardation, unusual facies, ichthyotic skin, and reduced stature. About 50% of patients with TTD are sensitive to sunlight, but their cancer incidence is not increased. The NER defect in different TTD individuals is heterogenous, ranging from very severe to no defect at all in those individuals who are not sensitive to sunlight. Cell fusion experiments have shown that three genes are involved in TTD: *XPB*, *XPD*, and *TTDA* (Stefanini et al., 1993; Giglia-Mari et al., 2004). Most repair defective TTD cell lines are assigned to the XP-D group.

Mutations in *XPD* can give rise to all three diseases XP, XP/CS, and TTD. This can be explained by the fact that XPD is subunit of TFIIH. TFIIH is necessary not only for NER but for general initiation of mRNA transcription in cells. Therefore it is the site of the mutation that determines the phenotype. Mutations may affect the NER function of TFIIH resulting in photosensitivity and cancer development in XP patients, but may also affect the basal transcription function of TFIIH, accounting for the typical TTD and CS phenotypes (Lehmann, 2001).

4.3 Base excision repair

Base excision repair (BER) is the main pathway dealing with damage induced by cellular metabolites (Lindahl and Wood, 1999). BER removes lesions such as uracil (arising by spontaneous deamination of cytosine) by employing specific DNA glycosylase enzymes to excise the altered base. Connections of BER deficiency with cancer susceptibility are just beginning to be identified. Some families with multiple colorectal carcinomas have inherited inactivating mutations in *MYH*, a DNA glycosylase that excises A residues when paired with 8-hydroxyguanine residues (Al-Tassan et al., 2002). 8-hydroxyguanine is a common oxidation product of guanine and replicative DNA polymerases occasionally misinsert A opposite this adduct. The disabling of MYH activity causes an increased spontaneous mutation frequency, including GC to TA mutations in the *APC* (adenomatous polyposis coli) gene.

4.4 Mismatch repair

The mismatch repair (MMR) system is the major pathway that corrects single base mispairs or looped intermediates which arise during DNA replication and as a result of damage to DNA. The MMR process consists of recognition of the mismatch, identification and degradation of the mismatched strand, and resynthesis of the excised strand (Figure 4.2) (Kolodner and Marsischky, 1999; Jiricny, 2000; Karran, 2001).

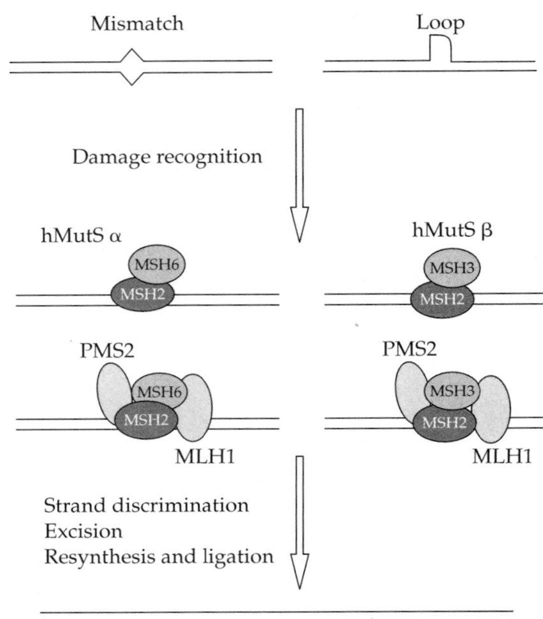

Figure 4.2 Mismatch repair is initiated by recognition and binding of the damage by MSH2-MSH6 or MSH2-MSH3 followed by recruitment of MLH1-PMS2. Repair is completed by removal of the damage, resynthesis, and ligation.

Identification and binding of the mismatched DNA is carried out in humans by one of two known mismatch recognition complexes, hMutSα and hMutSβ. hMutSα, a heterodimer of hMSH2 and hMSH6, preferentially binds most single base mispairs and loops of up to two bases. The second heterodimer, hMutSβ which consists of hMSH2 and hMSH3, binds more effectively to loops of three and four bases. In human cells, hMutSα appears to be the predominant mismatch binding activity. Following the recognition step by hMutSα and hMusSβ, the next step most probably involves the heterodimer hMutLα. This consists of hMLH1 and hPMS2 and is the primary MutL activity for mismatch correction in human cells. There seem to be at least two other hMLH1 containing heterodimers in human cells, namely hMLH1-hPMS1 and hMLH1-hMLH3, but only the heterodimer of hMLH1-hPMS2 has been shown to be involved in MMR so far (Jiricny and Nyström-Lahti, 2000).

hMutLα interacts with the MSH2-containing heterodimers which are already bound to the mispaired bases as well as with other factors to assemble a functional repair complex. A stretch of DNA containing the mismatch is removed, resynthesized and ligated to complete the repair. Although this process is not entirely understood, a number of the factors involved have been identified. These include the endo/exonucleases EXO1 and FEN1, the replication factors PCNA, RPA, and RFC. Although it is not known exactly how eukaryotic cells determine which strand should be repaired, PCNA is implicated in this process (Umar et al., 1996). Both hMutSα and hMutSβ heterodimers bind PCNA through a conserved motif found in hMSH3 and hMSH6. In one model, hMutSα binds to PCNA loaded onto newly replicated DNA and is transferred from PCNA to mispaired bases in DNA (Lau and Kolodner, 2003). EXO1 and FEN1 are reported to be involved in the excision of the damaged strand. The resynthesis step in human mismatch repair appears to be performed by DNA polymerase δ and possibly DNA polymerase ε. The DNA ligase that completes the MMR reaction remains to be identified.

Genetic defects in mismatch repair genes play an important role in common cancer-susceptibility syndromes such as hereditary non-polyposis colon cancer (HNPCC), Turcot's syndrome and Muir–Torre syndrome. HNPCC has been described in Chapter 3. Turcot's syndrome is characterized by predisposition to colon and brain tumours. Germline mutations in *hPMS2* can result in Turcot's syndrome (Hamilton et al., 1995; De Rosa et al., 2000). Muir–Torre syndrome is a subtype of HNPCC. Individuals with Muir–Torre syndrome are at increased risk for cancers seen in HNPCC, but they also can develop skin tumours. A germline mutation in *hMSH2* has been reported as a cause of Muir–Torre syndrome (Suspiro et al., 1998).

4.5 Double-strand break repair

Double-strand breaks (DSB) in DNA may arise as a consequence of exposure of cells to harmful DNA damaging agents such as ionizing radiation or some 'chemical' agents, or through errors in cellular functions, such as collapse of DNA replication forks at sites of blockage. Unrepaired or misrepaired DSBs are highly cytotoxic lesions that disrupt the genomic integrity of a cell and can lead to mutations and cancer. Therefore repair mechanisms that efficiently remove DSBs are important for the maintenance of genomic stability and prevention of cancer. There are two general types of DSB repair pathways: homologous recombination (HR) and non-homologous end-joining (NHEJ) (Haber, 2000). HR is used by both bacteria and higher organisms. In mammalian somatic cells, the major pathway for repairing DSBs is NHEJ.

ATM is the 'master regulator' protein kinase responsible for coordinating cellular responses to repair DNA DSBs (Shiloh, 2003). The kinase activity of ATM is autoactivated following DSB formation. Although it is currently unknown if ATM interacts with DNA, ATM localizes to DSB sites known as repair foci. Activated ATM phosphorylates a large number of substrates, some of which arrest the cell cycle to allow time for repair and include p53, Mdm2, Chk2, and RAD9. Other targets of ATM are either directly or indirectly involved in DNA repair, among which are H2AX, NBS1, BRCA1, BLM, and FANCD2. These repair factors are discussed in more detail in this chapter. Human cells lacking ATM are very sensitive to DSB-inducing agents and have increased levels of DSBs following irradiation (Cornforth and Bedford, 1985). Radioresistant DNA synthesis results from checkpoint failure and contributes to elevated mutagenesis and chromosome instability.

Loss or mutation of *ATM* results in the disorder ataxia telangiectasia (AT) (Becker-Catania and Gatti, 2001). This disease is defined by early-onset cerebellar degeneration and small blood vessel dilation in facial skin and sclera. Additional manifestations are sterility and immunodeficiency due to defective processing of the programmed DSBs generated during gametogenesis and immune system diversification. The incidence of cancer is increased ~100-fold, 75% of which are lymphomas and T-cell leukaemias with the remainder being solid tumours of various types. Heterozygous carriers of *ATM* missense mutations (rather than a truncated allele) have an increased cancer susceptibility (Spring et al., 2002).

NBS1 is a target for the action of ATM. It forms a complex with MRE11-RAD50 nuclease and recruits these proteins to the site of the DSB. It appears that this complex is involved in both pathways of DSB repair. The assumed function of RAD50-MRE11-NBS1 complex in NHEJ and HR is discussed later in the chapter. As for *ATM*, mutations in *NBS1 and MRE11* result in inherited diseases, which are also characterized by chromosomal instability and cancer predisposition. Defects in NBS1 give rise to Nijmegen breakage syndrome (NBS), a rare recessive condition with only about 70 families affected worldwide. Mutations in *MRE11* are associated with an AT-like disorder (AT-LD), characterized by developmental defects, radiosensitivity and an increased risk of lymphoid tumour development.

4.6 Non-homologous end-joining

Non-homologous end-joining (NHEJ) is a major pathway for repairing DSBs in human cells. This process involves the rejoining of the broken DNA ends with little or no base-pairing at the junction (Figure 4.3) (Haber, 2000). NHEJ is often prone to error, and small sequence deletions can be introduced. Several of the genes involved in NHEJ have been identified and their protein products characterized. A key role in the NHEJ process is played by the DNA-dependent protein kinase (DNA-PK). DNA-PK has a primary DSB recognition role and facilitates the recruitment and activation of other components involved in the NHEJ process. DNA-PK consists of Ku and a 460 kDa catalytic subunit (DNA-PKcs). Ku, a heterodimer of Ku70 and Ku80 proteins, exhibits a high affinity for DNA ends and appears to be the primary damage sensor in the NHEJ process. After a DSB has been formed, both DNA ends are bound by Ku, which recognizes both blunt ends and those with overhangs. The crystal structure of Ku bound to DNA has been reported (Walker et al., 2001). After Ku is bound to the DNA ends it recruits the 460 kDa catalytic subunit DNA-PKcs which subsequently is activated. Following binding by Ku and DNA-PKcs, the DNA ends are processed, aligned, and ligated. This step requires XRCC4 and DNA ligase IV. In addition, the Artemis endonuclease appears to be involved in trimming the DNA ends. The endonucleolytic activity of Artemis depends on the presence of and phosphorylation by DNA-PKcs. Upon phosphorylation Artemis acquires endonucleolytic activity for 5′ and 3′ overhang processing in NHEJ. XRCC4 and DNA ligase IV are then recruited to the DSB and complete NHEJ by ligation. *XRCC4* encodes a 38 kDa protein that stabilizes and stimulates DNA ligase IV. The end-joining step catalysed by DNA ligase IV seems to be stimulated by Ku. Experiments with yeast suggest as an additional factor for the NHEJ process the RAD50-MRE11-XRS2 complex, the yeast homologue of the human RAD50-MRE11-NBS1 (Usui et al., 1998). RAD50-MRE11-NBS1 binds to DNA DSBs and it has been proposed that it acts as a sensor of DNA damage (Nelms et al., 1998). In addition RAD50-MRE11-NBS1 has exonuclease and helicase activities and might be involved in nucleolytic processing of the DSBs before they are repaired by NHEJ. In yeast, the Rad50-Mre11-Xrs2 complex interacts directly with the yeast homologue of XRCC4-ligase IV and specifically enhances ligation activity by the complex (Chen et al., 2001).

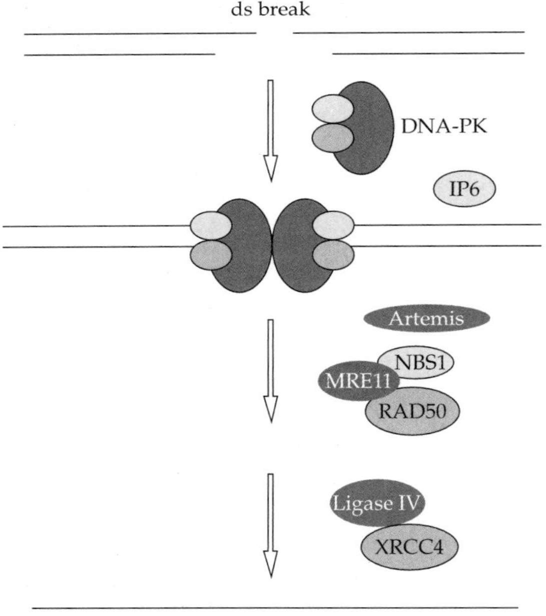

Figure 4.3 Non-homologous end-joining. DNA-PK binds to the ends of a double-strand break. Repair is completed by Ligase IV and XRCC4. Other factors (IP6, Artemis, RAD50/MRE11/NBS1) are also involved in NHEJ.

Genetic defects in NHEJ genes can result in clinical disorders and sporadic cancers. A mutation in the DNA ligase IV gene has been described in LIG4 syndrome, which is associated with immunodeficiency and growth developmental delay (O'Driscoll et al., 2001). The syndrome RS-SCID (radiosensitive severe combined immunodeficiency syndrome) is characterized by the development of severe infections and increased lymphoma incidence. This syndrome occurs among southwestern native Americans. Mutations in the Artemis gene can result in RS-SCID in humans (Moshous et al., 2001).

4.7 Homologous recombination

The second pathway by which DNA DSBs are repaired is by homologous recombination (HR). Although the total number of DSBs repaired by HR is less than the number repaired by NHEJ in mammalian cells, this pathway is preferentially used when a damaged cell is in S or G2 phase (Takata et al., 1998). While processing of ends by NHEJ may result in loss or gain of nucleotides at the break site, the benefit of repair by this pathway is that HR faithfully restores the original sequence of the broken chromosome. During HR, it is the sister chromatid that most often functions as an undamaged template for synthesizing the DNA sequence found at the break on the damaged chromatid. Although recombination between chromosome homologues does occur, it is not favoured (Johnson and Jasin, 2000). The drawback of homologous recombination between chromosomes is loss of heterozygosity through replication of the allelic chromosome. However, DSB repair by interhomologue recombination may still be preferable to repair by NHEJ, which may generate translocations if more than one DSB occurs simultaneously.

Following introduction of a DSB, the ATM kinase is activated and an early event is phosphorylation of serine 139 of histone H2AX (Shiloh, 2003). NBS1 interacts with phospho-H2AX, suggesting a mechanism to target the RAD50-MRE11-NBS1 complex to the break. NBS1 is phosphorylated by ATM to facilitate DNA repair and also to activate an intra-S phase cell cycle checkpoint. The RAD50-MRE11-NBS1 complex prepares a 3′ tail for the RAD51 nucleoprotein filament that will invade the homologous duplex (Figure 4.4). Phospho-H2AX foci co-localize with RAD51 foci and are believed to be DNA repair sites. RAD52 is believed to assist in the formation of the RAD51 nucleoprotein filament. RAD54 assists in the homologous sequence search and in joint molecule formation. A strand transfer reaction occurs whereby the strand that is the copy of the invading strand is displaced by the 3′ end of the invading sequence. Strand invasion may be either one-ended, where a single 3′ end invades the homologous duplex, or two-ended where both 3′ ends of the original DSB are converted to RAD51 nucleofilaments and both invade the homologous sequence

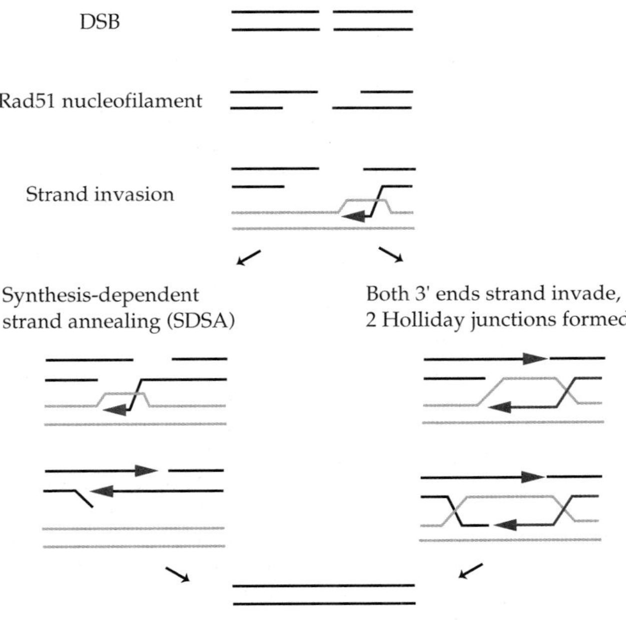

Figure 4.4 DNA DSB repair by homologous recombination. Following introduction of a DSB, ATM phosphorylates H2AX, and the RAD50-MRE11-NBS1 complex generates 3′ ends for the RAD51 nucleoprotein filament. Two possible homologous recombination strand invasion pathways are shown. In the synthesis-dependent strand annealing pathway (left pathway), DNA synthesis follows one-ended nucleofilament invasion. Both 3′ nucleofilaments may also invade the repair template (right pathway), leading to the formation of two Holliday junctions. Details of the pathways are described in the text.

(Haber, 2000). In the synthesis-dependent strand annealing pathway (Figure 4.4, left pathway), DNA synthesis follows one-ended nucleofilament invasion. At some point, the newly synthesized DNA dissociates from the repair template and reanneals to the broken duplex. The remaining gap is filled in and ends are processed for DNA ligation. A variation of SDSA called break-induced replication occurs when lagging strand replication follows the initial D-loop DNA synthesis. Both 3′ nucleofilaments may also invade the repair template (Figure 4.4, right pathway) and this leads to the formation of two Holliday junctions and branch migration. DNA synthesis at newly formed 3′ primer termini begins and continues for a distance that extends beyond the sequence of the broken duplex end. Completion of recombination occurs when enzymes capable of cleaving Holliday junctions (known as resolvases) separate the two chromosomes and a DNA ligase seals the newly recombined chromosomes. Proteins proposed to participate in branch migration and resolution of Holliday junctions include the RAD51 paralogues (XRCC2, XRCC3, RAD51B, RAD51C, RAD51D) (Liu et al., 2004) and the Mus81 nuclease complex (Blais et al., 2003).

The BRCA1 and BRCA2 proteins function in the homologous recombination process (Venkitaraman, 2002). BRCA1 binds branched DNA preferentially and may function in HR by co-localizing with other DNA repair factors at sites of DSB damage through direct interaction with RAD50. Both proteins are phosphorylated by ATM. Absence of BRCA1 decreases the efficiency of RAD51 localization at these foci and this may explain the decreased HR levels found in *BRCA1* mutant cells. Although BRCA1 does not interact directly with RAD51, it does interact with BRCA2, which has been shown to bind directly to RAD51. BRCA1 may also function in DNA checkpoint pathways and in a signalling capacity as a transcription factor for a diverse set of genes. BRCA2 binds single strand DNA and stimulates a RAD51-mediated *in vitro* recombination reaction (Yang et al., 2002).

A familial predisposition to breast and ovarian cancer arises from germline mutation of either *BRCA1* or *BRCA2* and ~5% of breast cancers are due to these autosomal dominant susceptibility alleles (Martin and Weber, 2000). *BRCA1* mutation leads to a higher incidence of ovarian cancer than does *BRCA2* mutation. For male breast cancer the reversed relationship has been observed as *BRCA2* mutation leads to a higher incidence of male breast cancer than *BRCA1* mutation. Loss of the remaining allele invariably occurs, suggesting a tumour suppressor function that is supported by mutant *Brca1* and *Brca2* mouse models (Moynahan, 2002). Although mutation of these two genes is rare in non-familial sporadic cancers, a number of studies have documented decreased expression of BRCA1 mRNA in sporadic breast tumours (Mueller and Roskelley, 2002).

Probably less essential for the core homologous recombination reaction in mammals, yet clearly having some function in DSB repair, are the Fanconi anaemia (FA) gene products (D'Andrea and Grompe, 2003). FA is a rare and clinically heterogenous syndrome that requires cytogenetic confirmation of sensitivity to a cross-linking agent for accurate diagnosis (Tischkowitz and Hodgson, 2003). Common features are pancytopenia, hypopigmentation, and limb/thumb abnormalities. Other organs may also show abnormal development. Fertility is decreased. Although many types of cancer have been documented, clonal chromosome abnormalities in blood progenitor cells lead to leukaemia (particularly AML) with high frequency.

At least nine separate complementation groups comprise FA and the genes for seven groups have been identified (FA-A, B, C, D1, D2, E, F, G, and L). A major cellular phenotype of FA cells is hypersensitivity to chemicals that create DNA interstrand cross-links. Although similarities between FA and BRCA mutant cell phenotypes and clinical features exist, the finding that the *FANCD1* gene is identical to *BRCA2* has linked the two pathways (Howlett et al., 2002). A key protein of the group appears to be FANCD2. A complex of the FA-A, C, E, F, G, and L group gene products function to monoubiquitinate FANCD2 (Meetei et al., 2004) which then is relocated to DNA repair foci containing FANCD1/BRCA2, BRCA1, and RAD51. FANCD2 is a substrate for the ATM kinase and is potentially involved in checkpoint and processing events at DSBs.

4.8 DNA damage tolerance

One of the least well-understood areas within the DNA repair field is the process of DNA damage tolerance. DNA damage tolerance is necessary if DNA damage has not been repaired by the completion of S-phase and this may be especially important for damage that is not efficiently recognized by a DNA repair pathway (e.g. cyclobutane pyrimidine dimers). All cells can complete DNA replication in the presence of unrepaired DNA damage. NER-deficient XP-A cells cannot remove pyrimidine dimers from DNA, yet following UVC irradiation, 50% of cells with ~30,000 dimers in their genomes survive and continue dividing. DNA damage tolerance can be subdivided into two pathways, recombination-dependent replication and translesion DNA synthesis. Both processes begin when cellular DNA replication is impeded by a discontinuity in either a base or the phosphodiester backbone of the template strand. Both depend on S-phase checkpoints to allow time for what are undoubtedly complex protein–DNA interactions to occur (Tercero and Diffley, 2001). Choice of the DNA damage tolerance pathway utilized is likely to be controlled by ubiquitin and SUMO modifications of the DNA polymerase sliding clamp PCNA, and other proteins (Hoege et al., 2002).

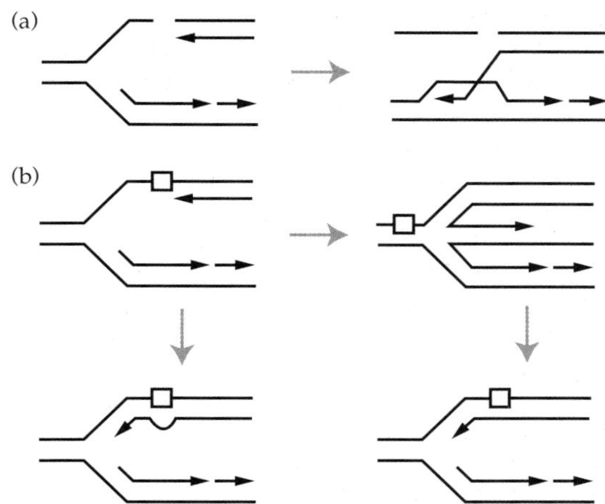

Figure 4.5 DNA damage tolerance pathways. (a) Recombination-dependent replication due to a leading strand DNA break. The nucleoprotein filament is generated by all or a subset of homologous recombination factors (see Figure 4.4 and text). Following DNA synthesis, the invading strand dissociates and reanneals to the original broken strand (Figure 4.4, SDSA pathway). A similar mechanism would operate at a lagging strand break. (b) Two possible mechanisms for tolerating DNA damage on the leading strand. The replication fork reversal mechanism (rightward pathway) uses the undamaged template for DNA synthesis. Alternatively (leftward pathway), the DNA damage may be bypassed by translesion synthesis.

4.9 Recombination-dependent replication

The main features of the pathways described below is that they attempt to avoid DNA damage during DNA replication through use of an undamaged template strand and that they are probably more error-free than translesion synthesis mechanisms. DNA strand breaks are strong blocks to DNA replication and all cells possess mechanisms to tolerate this situation. When a replication fork encounters a strand break, the newly synthesized daughter DNA duplex containing the broken DNA strand is converted into a DSB (Figure 4.5). Co-ordinated leading and lagging strand synthesis stops due to collapse of one of the arms, but synthesis on the undamaged strand may continue. DSBs which form at DNA replication forks activate the ATR kinase, an enzyme related to the global DNA break-responsive ATM kinase (Shiloh, 2003). ATR phosphorylates H2AX at replication fork breaks and this form of H2AX may recruit the RAD50-MRE11-NBS1 complex to process the ends of the break. A RAD51 nucleoprotein filament is created by homologous recombination factors. Following the formation of a D-loop structure by strand invasion of the newly replicated sister chromatid, leading or both leading and lagging strand DNA synthesis occurs and a replication fork may be created (Holmes and Haber, 1999). At some point, the invading strand dissociates and reanneals to the original broken strand. If the replication fork encounters breaks in both DNA strands (a DSB), then both leading and lagging strand synthesis will collapse and three potentially cytotoxic and mutagenic DSBs could arise. Repair using the homologous chromosome may be necessary in such instances and translocations may result if recombination occurs at a site other than at the allelic locus.

There are also less severe types of DNA replication blocking structures which retain an intact backbone, such as a damaged or missing DNA base. In these instances, current models propose that the replication fork is more likely to temporarily stall than to completely collapse. The mechanisms used to tolerate the DNA damage depend on whether the damage is on the leading or lagging strand (McGlynn and Lloyd, 2002).

When a block is on the lagging strand, the DNA replication fork can continue unimpeded because lagging strand synthesis is discontinuous. Instead of synthesizing DNA up to the RNA primer of the previous Okazaki fragment, the lagging strand polymerase dissociates at the damaged site and begins synthesis at the next Okazaki initiation site. The 3′ terminus left at the site of DNA damage is processed to invade the newly replicated sister chromatid to fill in the lagging strand gap by a homologous recombination-mediated process.

There are two main models for replication reactivation when damage is on the leading strand and these are less proven in mammals. One mechanism requires that the stalled fork be processed by an endonuclease such as Mus81-Eme1 (Blais et al., 2003) to yield a DSB at the DNA replication fork. Reactivation of DNA replication could continue by a pathway of break-induced replication discussed in connection with homologous recombination (Figure 4.4). The other leading strand replication reactivation pathway does not involve nuclease activity and possibly not the HR pathway either. Upon stalling at a leading strand block, DNA replication fork uncoupling can occur, with the lagging strand continuing for at least some distance (Figure 4.5). The parental template strands are then reannealed and the replication fork reversed in a DNA helicase-mediated process. The newly synthesized lagging strand is extruded and free to anneal with the 3′ terminus of the blocked leading strand when it is met by the reversal reaction. A Holliday junction structure, known as the 'chicken foot intermediate', is formed and DNA synthesis can occur on this template until the sequence where lagging strand synthesis terminated is encountered. Another DNA helicase would function to move the Holliday junction in the 'forward' direction until the branched DNA replication fork structure is re-established and DNA replication can resume. Alternatively, fork reversal moves the DNA damage away from the replication fork and back into a DNA duplex structure that may be now recognized by a DNA repair pathway.

Three human syndromes have been identified with defects in enzymes believed to process Holliday junctions formed during DNA recombination or DNA replication fork reversal (van Brabant et al., 2000). Both Bloom syndrome and Werner syndrome patients are characterized by increased incidences of cancer, skeletal abnormalities and decreased fertility but some notable differences exist. Bloom syndrome patients (with mutations in the *BLM* gene) are distinguished by proportional dwarfism, immunodeficiency, and skin photosensitivity while Werner syndrome patients (with mutations in the *WRN* gene) age prematurely, have different skeletal abnormalities and are not immunodeficient or photosensitive. Loss of BLM results in a strong increase in cancers of all types while WRN deficiency predisposes individuals to soft tissue sarcomas. At the cellular level, both disorders are characterized by genetic instability. However, mutant BLM cells have a 10-fold increased incidence of sister chromatid exchanges while WRN mutant cells do not. A third cancer predisposition syndrome that is also marked by skin and skeletal abnormalities is Rothmund–Thomson syndrome. Mutation of the *RECQ4* gene has been identified for some cases of this syndrome but little is known regarding DNA repair defects or genomic instability in such cells.

The BLM and WRN proteins are members of the *E. coli* RecQ family of 3′ to 5′ helicases, enzymes that function to unwind duplex DNA (Hickson, 2003). Helicase function is necessary to migrate DNA branch or Holliday junction structures during some DNA replication and repair processes. Both helicases are able to promote migration of these structures over long distances *in vitro*. Either enzyme could also possibly act on abnormal DNA structures that may block progression of DNA replication. One proposed function for the BLM helicase is to reverse-migrate Holliday junctions that may form at replication forks to allow DNA damage bypass in order to resume normal DNA replication. In the absence of this activity, these stalled forks may be subject to recombination repair, consistent with the elevated number of sister chromatid exchanges and DNA breaks observed. Proteins found to interact with that BLM helicase include RPA, RAD51, topoisomerase III, and p53. The WRN helicase is also believed to operate at Holliday junctions, but may be more likely to participate in the resolution of DNA recombination intermediates particularly those at telomeres, rather than to restore the replication fork. In addition to helicase function, the WRN protein is also a 3′–5′ exonuclease. WRN interacts with Ku heterodimer and is phosphorylated by DNA-PKcs, strongly suggesting a role for this enzyme in NHEJ.

4.10 Translesion synthesis

Mechanisms by which DNA replication can directly bypass DNA lesions exist and, due to disruption of correct base-pairing, can create mutations. Almost all types of DNA damage block DNA polymerases alpha, delta, and epsilon, the enzymes responsible for replicating most of the eukaryotic genome (Hübscher et al., 2002). Biochemical and genetic data suggest that replication past DNA lesions is performed by a specialized group of enzymes known as DNA damage bypass polymerases. The damaged template base may vary from a base with a large bulky adduct to no base at all (an AP site).

Some translesion polymerases are specialized for specific types of DNA base damage such that they function to insert a correct base opposite a lesion and are considered to be 'error-free' (Goodman, 2002). Other polymerases have more relaxed template specificity and will insert an incorrect base opposite a lesion to create a mutation. Complete bypass may be catalysed by a single enzyme or may occur by a mechanism where one enzyme incorporates a base opposite a lesion, dissociates from the template and another DNA polymerase more capable of extending a 3′ mispaired primer completes the bypass. At least six DNA polymerases (zeta, eta, iota, kappa, mu and theta) are capable of translesion synthesis, suggesting that lesion bypass is a high priority in mammals, at least at certain times and in some cell types. Important features of a polymerase with a direct link to a cancer-prone syndrome and an enzyme with a possible influence on carcinogenesis are presented here.

DNA polymerase zeta is relatively error-free during bypass of a *cis-syn* thymine–thymine dimer because it preferentially and efficiently inserts two adenines (Masutani et al., 2000). The enzyme interacts with PCNA to localize the enzyme to the primer terminus and to enhance the catalytic activity of DNA polymerase eta. Cells lacking DNA polymerase eta display increased UV-sensitivity and an increased frequency of mutagenesis, demonstrating that it normally functions to correctly bypass UV lesions.

Loss of DNA polymerase zeta also results in DNA damage sensitivity (Lawrence, 2002). Absence of DNA polymerase zeta, however, causes a large decrease in the number of UV-induced basepair and frameshift mutations. This indicates that the majority of mutagenic UV-bypass events involve DNA polymerase zeta in yeast and mammalian cells. DNA polymerase zeta is able to efficiently extend mispaired termini left by other DNA polymerases at different types of DNA damage. It may therefore function to 'fix' mutations rather than to perform initial misincorporations. Mammalian pol zeta is necessary for normal embryonic development, for reasons that are not yet understood (Wittschieben et al., 2000).

The importance of DNA damage replication bypass in humans is underlined by the identification of the xeroderma pigmentosum variant (XP-V) protein as DNA polymerase eta (Masutani et al., 2000). The XP-V complementation group is clinically indistinguishable from other XP groups, with an increased incidence of skin cancer, but nucleotide excision repair is functional in XP-V cells. XP-V cells have a reduced rate of nascent DNA strand elongation following UV-induced DNA damage and are hypermutable. XP-V is currently the only known human pathology attributable to loss or malfunction of a DNA polymerase. Other DNA damage bypass polymerases, such as iota and zeta, may play an important part in the XP-V phenotype, by substituting as the translesion synthesis polymerase(s) responsible for the elevated mutability of XP-V.

4.11 DNA repair and approaches to understanding cancer incidence and improving cancer therapy

4.11.1 Variation in DNA repair between individuals

Does the capacity for DNA repair vary significantly between individuals? Inherited syndromes associated with dramatic defects in various DNA repair processes are examples of extreme variations. But do smaller variations in activity exist that might affect cancer risk?

A major difficulty at present is the lack of methods to easily and reliably measure DNA repair activities in different individuals. Ideally, one would like to measure the activity of as many DNA repair pathways as possible using readily obtained biological material, such as a blood sample. Assays with either whole cells or cell extracts might also be envisaged. *In vitro* assays with cell extracts, however, are still not precise enough. For example, assays for measuring NER typically have inherent variations of twofold or so, even when extracts are made from the ample material available from cell lines. A twofold difference in NER activity between individuals could be significant, but impossible to detect with current assays.

Because of its inherent interest, the epidemiology of DNA repair and susceptibility to cancer has nevertheless been investigated by a number of approaches (Berwick and Vineis, 2000). Examining DNA repair in individuals by single cell gel electrophoresis or 'comet' assays has become popular. Although this technique has the advantage of requiring only a small amount of easily obtained material, it is a gross measurement that uses only DNA breaks as an endpoint together with undefined mechanisms of chromatin disassembly and compaction. Another approach that has received some attention is the use of plasmid host–cell reactivation assays in human lymphocytes. Damaged plasmids, transfected into cells, contain a selectable marker such as chloramphenicol acetyl transferase or luciferase. DNA recovered from the cells is assayed for reactivation of the marker gene as a measure of repair. The method requires considerable care but has been validated with repair-defective cells in some cases. In one study series, lower DNA repair capacity was associated with increased skin cancer incidence (Grossman and Wei, 1995). Overall, tests in human populations seem to yield modest associations between DNA repair capacity measurements and cancer occurrence (Berwick and Vineis, 2000). However, the relevance of measurements in human lymphocytes to repair in human tumour cells from the same patient has been questioned (Hemminki et al., 2000), partly because of strong selective forces in tumours.

4.11.2 Polymorphisms in DNA repair genes

There are many single-nucleotide differences between individuals (polymorphisms), and it is relatively easy to use PCR and DNA sequencing methods to assay for the presence or absence of a known polymorphism. It is conceivable that some polymorphisms in DNA repair genes, such as aminoacid substitutions, will cause differences in DNA repair capacity (Mohrenweiser et al., 2003). Some relatively common DNA repair gene polymorphisms have been examined for possible correlations with cancer incidence or success in treatment. In this type of study, it is always possible that a polymorphism serves as a genetic marker indicating linkage to another gene that is responsible for the outcome being measured. Haplotyping can clarify this issue.

Further development of this field will require the discovery of relatively common polymorphisms that have significant effects on DNA repair activity *in vivo*. A systematic effort to catalogue polymorphisms is part of the environmental genome project sponsored by the NIEHS in the United States. This venture includes a survey of human genes related to DNA repair, cell cycle control, cell signalling, cell division, homeostasis, and metabolism. The initial aim to re-sequence the DNA in about 200 such genes from about 450 unrelated, ethnically diverse individuals has been completed. A web resource integrates the resulting gene, sequence, and polymorphism data into individually annotated gene models and is available at http://www.genome.utah.edu/genesnps/.

As an example, in the gene for the MGMT protein, a non-conservative substitution of L residue 84 for F (L84F) is found in around 20% of individuals. This substitution has no measurable effect on MGMT function as a purified enzyme or in cells (Inoue et al., 2000). Another rare polymorphism in MGMT, W65C, is reported to give rise to an unstable MGMT protein (Inoue et al., 2000). As assays develop, the most interesting course of action will be to concentrate on those polymorphisms that alter protein function, and to assess their relevance to cancer incidence or curability. Two common polymorphisms in the *XPD* gene, D312N and K751Q, have received most attention in published studies. Both occur at evolutionarily diverged positions in the protein, away from functional motifs, and neither seems likely to have any significant effect on NER or transcription activity.

4.11.3 Variation in DNA repair between different types of tumours

Because of differences in gene expression between cells in specific tissues, it is possible that tumours could vary in their DNA repair capacity according to tissue or cell type of origin. Unusually for metastatic cancer, testicular germ cell tumours are particularly curable by chemotherapy based on cisplatin or related compounds. Several DNA repair pathways may influence cellular sensitivity to cisplatin. NER-defective cells are cisplatin sensitive and NER is the only known repair pathway which actually excises the major cisplatin adducts from DNA. Recombinational mechanisms are also important in tolerance of cisplatin-induced DNA damage (Zdraveski et al., 2000). Cells with defects in recombination pathway genes such as *XRCC2* and *XRCC3* are cisplatin-sensitive (Liu et al., 1998). Several specialized DNA polymerases are also able to overcome the DNA replication block presented by cisplatin adducts using translesion synthesis. Further, mismatch recognition proteins can also bind to DNA containing cisplatin adducts (Mello et al., 1996), and it has been argued that variations in levels of proteins such as MSH2 can influence repair of cisplatin adducts to some extent. In a model system with A2780 ovarian carcinoma cells, inactivation of mismatch repair was not found to be a frequent route for escape from cisplatin toxicity (Massey et al., 2003).

Direct measurements of removal of cisplatin-induced DNA damage have been made in testis tumour lines in comparison with other less-responsive tumour cell lines, with the finding that the testis tumour lines examined have, on the whole, a reduced rate of removal of cisplatin-DNA lesions (Masters and Köberle, 2003). By *in vitro* analysis of NER repair capacity, it was found that two testis tumour cell extracts had low levels of NER for a 1,3 dGpTpG cisplatin adduct. Immuno-blotting analysis showed that the testis tumour cell lines had lower than normal (about 25%) levels of XPA, ERCC1, and XPF proteins (Köberle et al., 1999). Levels of other NER proteins were not reduced. Addition of XPA protein to the extracts was able to restore repair activity to the extracts, indicating that XPA is rate-limiting in these extracts. A relative deficiency in XPA appears to be a general feature of testis tumour cell lines (Welsh et al., 2004). The reasons for any lower amounts of XPA, ERCC1, and XPF proteins remain to be elucidated.

4.11.4 DNA repair and drug resistance

In too many instances after an initially successful response to chemotherapy, a tumour will reappear, typically months or years after the initial treatment. The recurring tumour is often resistant to the chemotherapeutic agent used previously, because of the strong selective pressure of the toxic treatment. One possibility that receives ongoing consideration is that drug-resistant tumours might have enhanced DNA repair in comparison with the original tumour or normal cells. Conclusive evidence for functionally increased NER in resistant tumours has not been presented. In an A2780 ovarian cancer model system, however, a threefold increase in NER activity in a cisplatin-resistant cell line was reported (Ferry et al., 2000). A different approach has been to assess levels of DNA repair proteins via mRNA levels and attempt to correlate these with intrinsic cellular sensitivity to DNA damage or response to therapy. Evidence usually has not been obtained as to whether variations in mRNA levels give rise to correlated changes in amounts of the encoded protein. For example, ERCC1 expression in ovarian cancer samples was postulated to correlate with clinical response (Dabholkar et al., 1994), but the reverse transcription polymerase chain reaction (RT-PCR) method used to measure mRNA levels was not quantitative. Further, it is known that ERCC1 mRNA levels do not correlate with ERCC1 protein levels. ERCC1 is a subunit of the ERCC1-XPF nuclease and when ERCC1 is overexpressed, it is readily degraded in the absence of its XPF partner. Consequently, even large changes in ERCC1 expression level in mammalian cells do not lead to increases in ERCC1 protein (Sijbers et al., 1996; Yagi et al., 1998), because there is no concomitant change in XPF level.

4.11.5 Mismatch recognition and resistance to alkylating agents

An intriguing interplay between DNA repair pathways is exemplified by the fact that a mismatch recognition complex involving MSH2, MSH6, MLH1, and PMS1 recognizes some DNA adducts as mismatches. O^6-meG in DNA is apparently recognized as a mismatch, even when paired to the 'correct' base, cytosine. Attempted mismatch repair of a base pair containing O^6-meG often removes the C and replaces it with another base, leaving the O^6-meG in DNA and setting off another round of futile repair. Apparently such futile repair is a toxic event, because mismatch repair-defective cells are considerably more tolerant to methylating agents that produce O^6-meG such as *N*-methyl-*N*-nitrosourea, temozolomide, and dacabazine (Modrich and Lahue, 1996; O'Driscoll et al., 1998).

These observations raise the possibility that tumour cells with defects in mismatch repair might be unusually resistant to treatment with methylating agents such as temozolimide. Sporadic loss of mismatch repair protein expression is found in a number of human tumours (Friedman et al., 1997) and in general it appears that such tumours are more resistant to methylating agents (Fink et al., 1998; Gerson, 2002). Mice with defects in MGMT and MLH1 are resistant to the toxic but not the tumorigenic effects of *N*-methyl-*N*-nitrosourea (Kawate et al., 1998). A study of mouse tumours indicated that inactivation of *msh2* allowed better proliferation of gastrointestinal tract cells damaged by methylating agents (Colussi et al., 2001). In human cells, *MSH2* heterozygous (+/−) lymphoblastoid cell lines are on average about fourfold more tolerant than wild-type cells to killing by the methylating agent temozolomide (Marra et al., 2001). Further research will reveal whether these observations in mismatch repair-compromised cells are relevant to induction of human tumours by methylation, and their treatment with such agents.

Methotrexate is used in cancer chemotherapy as an agent to inhibit dihydrofolate reductase (DHFR) and cripple pyrimidine biosynthesis in tumour cells. *DHFR* and *MSH3* are adjacent on the same chromosome and are transcribed divergently from a shared promoter. Methotrexate resistance in cell lines can arise by gene amplification of DHFR, concomitantly amplifying the *MSH3* locus. MutS alpha (*MSH2-MSH6*) and *MutS* beta (MSH2-MSH3) share a common component, *MSH2*. Under conditions of *Msh3* amplification, *MutS* beta forms at the expense of *MutS* alpha. Because *MutS* alpha is the principal recognition factor for base–base mismatches, the mutation rate in tumour cell lines with *DHFR* and *MSH3* amplification can rise more than 100-fold (Drummond et al., 1997). The implications for cancer chemotherapy include a potential increase in mutability when tumours are treated with methotrexate, by reducing mismatch repair in the tumour.

4.12 DNA repair-based approaches for improving therapy

4.12.1 Chemical inhibitors of DNA repair

One approach to improve chemotherapy may be to develop drugs that cause DNA damage which is poorly recognized or repaired. For example, intercalating interstrand DNA crosslinkers that lie in the minor groove may be repaired poorly (Brooks et al., 2000). Specific chemical inhibitors of DNA repair enzymes may also be envisaged. For instance, methoxyamine binds and reacts with AP sites, which are intermediates in the BER process. Using a human colon cancer xenograft model in nude mice, methoxyamine was found to enhance the antitumour effect of the alkylating agent temozolomide (Liu et al., 2002). Specific inhibitors of BER that affect DNA polymerase beta could also be useful (Sobol and Wilson, 2001). As another example, an inhibitor of MGMT, O^6-benzylguanine, depletes MGMT in human tumours without associated toxicity and is in phase II clinical trials (Gerson, 2002). Inhibition of NER also seems a possible approach but specific targeted inhibitors have not yet been reported. The kinase inhibitor 7-hydroxystaurosporine has been reported to inhibit repair of UV-induced DNA damage (Jiang and Yang, 1999).

4.12.2 Gene therapy approaches

Gene therapy approaches involving DNA repair are being tested in animal models. For example, chloroethylnitrosourea alkylating agents are commonly used for cancer chemotherapy, but are limited by bone marrow toxicity. A retroviral vector expressing the human *MGMT* gene has been used to reconstitute mouse bone marrow with genetically modified, MGMT-expressing hematopoietic stem cells. This confers considerable resistance to the cytotoxic effects of BCNU. Further, mutations within the active site region of the *MGMT* gene render the protein resistant to O^6-benzylguanine inactivation. As a result, mutant *MGMT* gene transfer into hematopoietic stem cells can selectively protect the marrow from the combination of an alkylating agent and BG, while at the same time sensitizing tumour cells (Kleibl and Margison, 1998, Roth and Samson, 2000, Gerson, 2002).

The preceding discussion makes it clear that DNA repair is highly relevant to oncology for two main reasons. First, DNA repair is a front-line defence against cancer. When a DNA repair pathway is disabled, surviving cells accumulate mutations and genomic alterations that lead to an increased incidence of tumours. Second, many agents used for cancer therapy are DNA damaging agents and induce DNA damage in tumour cells. This consideration leads to the possibility that cancer therapy with DNA damaging agents could be improved by developing specific inhibitors of DNA repair that could be directed towards tumour cells and used as adjuvants with radiotherapy or some chemotherapies.

References

Al-Tassan, N., Chmiel, N. H., Maynard, J., Fleming, N., Livingston, A. L., Williams, G. T. et al. (2002). Inherited variants of MYH associated with somatic G : C-- > T : A mutations in colorectal tumors. *Nat Genet*, **30**, 227–32.

Becker-Catania, S. G. and Gatti, R. A. (2001). Ataxia-telangiectasia. *Adv Exp Med Biol*, **495**, 191–8.

Berwick, M. and Vineis, P. (2000). Markers of DNA repair and susceptibility to cancer in humans: an epidemiologic review. *J Natl Cancer Inst*, **92**, 874–97.

Blais, V., Gao, H., Elwell, C. A., Boddy, M. N., Gaillard, P. H., Russell, P. et al. (2003). RNAi inhibition of Mus81 reduces mitotic recombination in human cells. *Mol Biol Cell*, 10.1091/mbc.E03-08-0586.

Bootsma, D., Kraemer, K. H., Cleaver, J. E., and Hoeijmakers, J. H. (2002). Nucleotide excision repair syndromes: xeroderma pigmentosum, Cockayne syndrome, and trichothiodystrophy. In *The Metabolic and Molecular Bases of Inherited Disease* (Eds., C. R. Scriver, A. L. Beaudet, D. Vaile, W. S. Sly, B. Vogelstein, B. Childs, and K. W. Kinzler) McGraw-Hill Companies, Section 4, Chapter 28, http://genetics.accessmedicine.com/server-java/Arknoid/amed/mmbid/co_chapters/ch02/ch028_p01.html.

Brooks, N., McHugh, P. J., Lee, M., and Hartley, J. A. (2000). Alteration in the choice of DNA repair pathway with increasing sequence selective DNA alkylation in the minor groove. *Chem Biol*, **7**, 659–68.

Chen, L., Trujillo, K., Ramos, W., Sung, P., and Tomkinson, A. E. (2001). Promotion of Dnl4-catalyzed DNA end-joining by the Rad50/Mre11/Xrs2 and Hdf1/Hdf2 complexes. *Mol Cell*, **8**, 1105–15.

Colussi, C., Fiumicino, S., Giuliani, A., Rosini, S., Musiani, P., Macri, C. et al. (2001). 1,2-Dimethylhydrazine-induced colon carcinoma and lymphoma in msh2(−/−) mice. *J Natl Cancer Inst*, **93**, 1534–40.

Cornforth, M. N. and Bedford, J. S. (1985). On the nature of a defect in cells from individuals with ataxia-telangiectasia. *Science*, **227**, 1589–91.

D'Andrea, A. D. and Grompe, M. (2003). The Fanconi anaemia/BRCA pathway. *Nat Rev Cancer*, **3**, 23–34.

Dabholkar, M., Vionnet, J., Bostick-Bruton, F., Yu, J. J., and Reed, E. (1994). Messenger RNA levels of XPAC and ERCC1 in ovarian cancer tissue correlate with response to platinum-based chemotherapy. *J Clin Invest*, **94**, 703–8.

de Laat, W. L., Jaspers, N. G., and Hoeijmakers, J. H. (1999). Molecular mechanism of nucleotide excision repair. *Genes Dev*, **13**, 768–85.

De Rosa, M., Fasano, C., Panariello, L., Scarano, M. I., Belli, G., Iannelli, A. et al. (2000). Evidence for a recessive inheritance of Turcot's syndrome caused by compound heterozygous mutations within the PMS2 gene. *Oncogene*, **19**, 1719–23.

Drummond, J. T., Genschel, J., Wolf, E., and Modrich, P. (1997). DHFR/MSH3 amplification in methotrexate-resistant cells alters the hMutSalpha/hMutSbeta ratio and reduces the efficiency of base-base mismatch repair. *Proc Natl Acad Sci USA*, **94**, 10144–9.

Duncan, T., Trewick, S. C., Koivisto, P., Bates, P. A., Lindahl, T., and Sedgwick, B. (2002). Reversal of DNA alkylation damage by two human dioxygenases. *Proc Natl Acad Sci USA*, **99**, 16660–5.

Ferry, K. V., Hamilton, T. C., and Johnson, S. W. (2000). Increased nucleotide excision repair in cisplatin-resistant ovarian cancer cells: role of ERCC1-XPF. *Biochem Pharmacol*, **60**, 1305–13.

Fink, D., Aebi, S., and Howell, S. B. (1998). The role of DNA mismatch repair in drug resistance. *Clin Cancer Res*, **4**, 1–6.

Friedman, H. S., Johnson, S. P., Dong, Q., Schold, S. C., Rasheed, B. K., Bigner, S. H. et al. (1997). Methylator resistance mediated by mismatch repair deficiency in a glioblastoma multiforme xenograft. *Cancer Res*, **57**, 2933–6.

Gerson, S. L. (2002). Clinical relevance of MGMT in the treatment of cancer. *J Clin Oncol*, **20**, 2388–99.

Giglia-Mari, G., Coin, F., Ranish, J. A., Hoogstraten, D., Theil, A., Wijgers, N. et al. (2004). A new, tenth subunit of TFIIH is responsible for the DNA repair syndrome trichothiodystrophy group A. *Nature Genetics*, **36**, 714–19.

Goodman, M. F. (2002). Error-prone repair DNA polymerases in prokaryotes and eukaryotes. *Annu Rev Biochem*, **71**, 17–50.

Grossman, L. and Wei, Q. Y. (1995). DNA-repair and epidemiology of basal-cell carcinoma. *Clin Chem*, **41**, 1854–63.

Haber, J. E. (2000). Partners and pathways repairing a double-strand break. *Trends Genet*, **16**, 259–64.

Hamilton, S. R., Liu, B., Parsons, R. E., Papadopoulos, N., Jen, J., Powell, S. M. et al. (1995). The molecular basis of Turcot's syndrome. *N Engl J Med*, **332**, 839–47.

Hanawalt, P. C. (2000). DNA repair. The bases for Cockayne syndrome. *Nature*, **405**, 415–6.

Hemminki, K., Xu, G. G., and LeCurieux, F. (2000). Re: Markers of DNA repair and susceptibility to cancer in humans: an epidemiologic review. *J Natl Cancer Inst*, **92**, 1536–37.

Hickson, I. D. (2003). RecQ helicases: caretakers of the genome. *Nat Rev Cancer*, **3**, 169–78.

Hoege, C., Pfander, B., Moldovan, G. L., Pyrowolakis, G., and Jentsch, S. (2002). RAD6-dependent DNA repair is linked to modification of PCNA by ubiquitin and SUMO. *Nature*, **419**, 135–41.

Hoeijmakers, J. H. (2001). Genome maintenance mechanisms for preventing cancer. *Nature*, **411**, 366–74.

Holmes, A. M. and Haber, J. E. (1999). Double-strand break repair in yeast requires both leading and lagging strand DNA polymerases. *Cell*, **96**, 415–24.

Howlett, N. G., Taniguchi, T., Olson, S., Cox, B., Waisfisz, Q., De Die-Smulders, C. et al. (2002). Biallelic inactivation of BRCA2 in Fanconi anemia. *Science*, **297**, 606–9.

Hübscher, U., Maga, G., and Spadari, S. (2002). Eukaryotic DNA polymerases. *Annu Rev Biochem*, **71**, 133–63.

Inoue, R., Abe, M., Nakabeppu, Y., Sekiguchi, M., Mori, T., and Suzuki, T. (2000). Characterization of human polymorphic DNA repair methyltransferase. *Pharmacogenetics*, **10**, 59–66.

Jiang, H. and Yang, L. Y. (1999). Cell cycle checkpoint abrogator UCN-01 inhibits DNA repair: association with attenuation of the interaction of XPA and ERCC1 nucleotide excision repair proteins. *Cancer Res*, **59**, 4529–4534.

Jiricny, J. (2000). Mediating mismatch repair. *Nat Genet*, **24**, 6–8.

Jiricny, J. and Nyström-Lahti, M. (2000). Mismatch repair defects in cancer. *Curr Opin Genet Dev*, **10**, 157–61.

Johnson, R. D. and Jasin, M. (2000). Sister chromatid gene conversion is a prominent double-strand break repair pathway in mammalian cells. *Embo J*, **19**, 3398–407.

Karran, P. (2001). Mechanisms of tolerance to DNA damaging therapeutic drugs. *Carcinogenesis*, **22**, 1931–7.

Kawate, H., Sakumi, K., Tsuzuki, T., Nakatsuru, Y., Ishikawa, T., Takahashi, S., et al. (1998). Separation of killing and tumorigenic effects of an alkylating agent in mice defective in two of the DNA repair genes. *Proc Natl Acad Sci USA*, **95**, 5116–20.

Kleibl, K. and Margison, G. P. (1998). Increasing DNA repair capacity in bone marrow by gene transfer as a prospective tool in cancer therapy. *Neoplasma*, **45**, 181–6.

Köberle, B., Masters, J. R., Hartley, J. A., and Wood, R. D. (1999). Defective repair of cisplatin-induced DNA damage caused by reduced XPA protein in testicular germ cell tumours. *Curr Biol*, **9**, 273–6.

Kolodner, R. D. and Marsischky, G. T. (1999). Eukaryotic DNA mismatch repair. *Curr Opin Genet Dev*, **9**, 89–96.

Lau, P. J. and Kolodner, R. D. (2003). Transfer of the MSH2. MSH6 complex from proliferating cell nuclear antigen to mispaired bases in DNA. *J Biol Chem*, **278**, 14–7.

Lawrence, C. W. (2002). Cellular roles of DNA polymerase zeta and Rev1 protein. *DNA Repair (Amst)*, **1**, 425–35.

Lehmann, A. R. (2001). The xeroderma pigmentosum group D (XPD) gene: one gene, two functions, three diseases. *Genes Dev*, **15**, 15–23.

Lindahl, T. and Wood, R. D. (1999). Quality control by DNA repair. *Science*, **286**, 1897–905.

Lindahl, T., Karran, P., and Wood, R. D. (1997). DNA excision repair pathways. *Curr Opin Genet Dev*, **7**, 158–69.

Liu, L., Nakatsuru, Y., and Gerson, S. L. (2002). Base excision repair as a therapeutic target in colon cancer. *Clin Cancer Res*, **8**, 2985–91.

Liu, N., Lamerdin, J. E., Tebbs, R. S., Schild, D., Tucker, J. D., Shen, M. R. et al. (1998). XRCC2 and XRCC3, new human RAD51-family members, promote chromosome stability and protect against DNA cross-links and other damages. *Mol Cell*, **1**, 783–93.

Liu, Y., Masson, J.-Y., Shah, R., O'Regan, P., and West, S. C. (2004). RAD51C is required for Holliday junction processing in mammalian cells. *Science*, **303**, 243–6.

Marra, G., D'Atri, S., Corti, C., Bonmassar, L., Cattaruzza, M. S., Schweizer, P. et al. (2001). Tolerance of human MSH2 +/− lymphoblastoid cells to the methylating agent temozolomide. *Proc Natl Acad Sci USA*, **98**, 7164–9.

Martin, A. M. and Weber, B. L. (2000). Genetic and hormonal risk factors in breast cancer. *J Natl Cancer Inst*, **92**, 1126–35.

Massey, A., Offman, J., Macpherson, P., and Karran, P. (2003). DNA mismatch repair and acquired cisplatin resistance in *E. coli* and human ovarian carcinoma cells. *DNA Repair (Amst)*, **2**, 73–89.

Masters, J. R. and Köberle, B. (2003). Curing metastatic cancer: lessons from testicular germ-cell tumours. *Nat Rev Cancer*, **3**, 517–25.

Masutani, C., Kusumoto, R., Yamada, A., Yuasa, M., Araki, M., Nogimori, T. et al. (2000). Xeroderma pigmentosum variant: from a human genetic disorder to a novel DNA polymerase. *Cold Spring Harb Symp Quant Biol*, **65**, 71–80.

McGlynn, P. and Lloyd, R. G. (2002). Recombinational repair and restart of damaged replication forks. *Nat Rev Mol Cell Biol*, **3**, 859–70.

Meetei, A. R., Yan, Z., Wang, W. (2004). FANCL replaces BRCA1 as the likely ubiquitin ligase responsible for FANCD2 monoubiquitination. *Cell Cycle*, **3**, 179–81.

Mello, J. A., Acharya, S., Fishel, R., and Essigmann, J. M. (1996). The mismatch-repair protein hMSH2 binds selectively to DNA-adducts of the anticancer drug cisplatin. *Chem Biol*, **3**, 579–89.

Modrich, P. and Lahue, R. (1996). Mismatch repair in replication fidelity, genetic-recombination, and cancer biology. *Annu Rev Biochem*, **65**, 101–133.

Mohrenweiser, H. W., Wilson, D. M., III, and Jones, I. M. (2003). Challenges and complexities in estimating both the functional impact and the disease risk associated with the extensive genetic variation in human DNA repair genes. *Mutat Res*, **526**, 93–125.

Moshous, D., Callebaut, I., de Chasseval, R., Corneo, B., Cavazzana-Calvo, M., Le Deist, F. et al. (2001). Artemis, a novel DNA double-strand break repair/V(D)J recombination protein, is mutated in human severe combined immune deficiency. *Cell*, **105**, 177–86.

Moynahan, M. E. (2002). The cancer connection: BRCA1 and BRCA2 tumor suppression in mice and humans. *Oncogene*, **21**, 8994–9007.

Mueller, C. R. and Roskelley, C. D. (2002). Regulation of BRCA1 expression and its relationship to sporadic breast cancer. *Breast Cancer Res*, **5**, 45–52.

Nelms, B. E., Maser, R. S., MacKay, J. F., Lagally, M. G, and Petrini, J. H. (1998). In situ visualization of DNA double-strand break repair in human fibroblasts. *Science*, **280**, 590–2.

O'Driscoll, M., Humbert, O., and Karran, P. (1998). DNA mismatch repair. In *Nucelic Acids and Molecular Biology*, Vol. 12 (Eds., F. Eckstein and D. M. J. Lilley) Springer-Verlag, Berlin Heidelberg, 173–97.

O'Driscoll, M., Cerosaletti, K. M., Girard, P. M., Dai, Y., Stumm, M., Kysela, B. et al. (2001). DNA ligase IV mutations identified in patients exhibiting developmental delay and immunodeficiency. *Mol Cell*, **8**, 1175–85.

Roth, R. B. and Samson, L. D. (2000). Gene transfer to suppress bone marrow alkylation sensitivity. *Mutat Res*, **462**, 107–20.

Shiloh, Y. (2003). ATM and related protein kinases: safeguarding genome integrity. *Nat Rev Cancer*, **3**, 155–68.

Sijbers, A. M., van der Spek, P. J., Odijk, H., van den Berg, J., van Duin, M., Westerveld, A. et al. (1996). Mutational analysis of the human nucleotide excision repair gene *ERCC1*. *Nucleic Acids Res.*, **24**, 3370–80.

Sobol, R. W. and Wilson, S. H. (2001). Mammalian DNA beta-polymerase in base excision repair of alkylation damage. *Prog Nucleic Acid Res Mol Biol*, **68**, 57–74.

Spring, K., Ahangari, F., Scott, S. P., Waring, P., Purdie, D. M., Chen, P. C. et al. (2002). Mice heterozygous for mutation in Atm, the gene involved in ataxia-telangiectasia, have heightened susceptibility to cancer. *Nat Genet*, **32**, 185–90.

Stefanini, M., Vermeulen, W., Weeda, G., Giliani, S., Nardo, T., Mezzina, M. et al. (1993). A new nucleotide-excision-repair gene associated with the disorder trichothiodystrophy. *Am J Hum Genet*, **53**, 817–21.

Suspiro, A., Fidalgo, P., Cravo, M., Albuquerque, C., Ramalho, E., Leitao, C. N. et al. (1998). The Muir-Torre syndrome: a rare variant of hereditary nonpolyposis colorectal cancer associated with hMSH2 mutation. *Am J Gastroenterol*, **93**, 1572–4.

Takata, M., Sasaki, M. S., Sonoda, E., Morrison, C., Hashimoto, M., Utsumi, H. et al. (1998). Homologous recombination and non-homologous end-joining pathways of DNA double-strand break repair have overlapping roles in the maintenance of chromosomal integrity in vertebrate cells. *Embo J*, **17**, 5497–508.

Tercero, J. A. and Diffley, J. F. (2001). Regulation of DNA replication fork progression through damaged DNA by the Mec1/Rad53 checkpoint. *Nature*, **412**, 553–7.

Tischkowitz, M. D. and Hodgson, S. V. (2003). Fanconi anaemia. *J Med Genet*, **40**, 1–10.

Trewick, S. C., Henshaw, T. F., Hausinger, R. P., Lindahl, T., and Sedgwick, B. (2002). Oxidative demethylation by *Escherichia coli* AlkB directly reverts DNA base damage. *Nature*, **419**, 174–8.

Umar, A., Buermeyer, A. B., Simon, J. A., Thomas, D. C., Clark, A. B., Liskay, R. M. et al. (1996). Requirement for PCNA in DNA mismatch repair at a step preceding DNA resynthesis. *Cell*, **87**, 65–73.

Usui, T., Ohta, T., Oshiumi, H., Tomizawa, J., Ogawa, H., and Ogawa, T. (1998). Complex formation and functional versatility of Mre11 of budding yeast in recombination. *Cell*, **95**, 705–16.

van Brabant, A. J., Stan, R., and Ellis, N. A. (2000). DNA helicases, genomic instability, and human genetic disease. *Annu Rev Genomics Hum Genet*, **1**, 409–59.

van Gool, A. J., Citterio, E., Rademakers, S., van Os, R., Vermeulen, W., Constantinou, A. et al. (1997). The Cockayne syndrome B protein, involved in transcription-coupled DNA repair, resides in an RNA polymerase II-containing complex. *Embo J*, **16**, 5955–65.

Venkitaraman, A. R. (2002). Cancer susceptibility and the functions of BRCA1 and BRCA2. *Cell*, **108**, 171–82.

Volker, M., Mone, M. J., Karmakar, P., van Hoffen, A., Schul, W., Vermeulen, W. et al. (2001). Sequential assembly of the nucleotide excision repair factors *in vivo*. *Mol Cell*, **8**, 213–24.

Walker, J. R., Corpina, R. A., and Goldberg, J. (2001). Structure of the Ku heterodimer bound to DNA and its implications for double-strand break repair. *Nature*, **412**, 607–14.

Welsh, C., Day, R., McGurk, C., Masters, J. R., Wood, R. D., and Köberle, B. (2004). Reduced levels of XPA, ERCC1 and XPF DNA repair proteins in testis tumor cell lines. *Int J Cancer*, **110**, 352–61.

Wittschieben, B. Ø. and Wood, R. D. (2003). DDB Complexities. *DNA Repair*, **2**, 1065–9.

Wittschieben, J., Shivji, M. K. K., Lalani, E.-N., Jacobs, M. A., Marini, F., Gearhart, P. J. et al. (2000). Disruption of the developmentally regulated *Rev3l* gene causes embryonic lethality. *Current Biology*, **10**, 1217–1220.

Wood, R. D., Mitchell, M., Sgouros, J., and Lindahl, T. (2001). Human DNA repair genes. *Science*, **291**, 1284–9.

Yagi, T., Katsuya, A., Koyano, A., and Takebe, H. (1998). Sensitivity of group-F xeroderma-pigmentosum cells to UV and mitomycin-c relative to levels of XPF and ERCC1 overexpression. *Mutagenesis*, **13**, 595–9.

Yang, H., Jeffrey, P. D., Miller, J., Kinnucan, E., Sun, Y., Thoma, N. H. et al. (2002). BRCA2 function in DNA binding and recombination from a BRCA2-DSS1-ssDNA structure. *Science*, **297**, 1837–48.

Zdraveski, Z. Z., Mello, J. A., Marinus, M. G., and Essigmann, J. M. (2000). Multiple pathways of recombination define cellular responses to cisplatin. *Chem Biol*, **7**, 39–50.

CHAPTER 5

Epigenetic events in cancer

Jonathan C. Cheng and Peter A. Jones

5.1 Introduction

The diverse cell types in multicellular organisms have identical genotypes but are functionally and morphologically different. This is due to differences in gene expression patterns which are established during development and are subsequently retained through mitosis. Stable alterations of this kind are known as epigenetic modifications, which are defined as heritable, but potentially reversible changes in gene expression that occur without alterations in the DNA sequence. In this chapter, we will focus on two key epigenetic phenomena that seemingly impact each other: DNA methylation and chromatin inheritance. Accumulating evidence indicates that alterations in DNA methylation and chromatin structure are linked to various human diseases, such as cancer and mental retardation syndromes. Elucidation of the epigenetic regulation of chromatin structure, DNA methylation and gene expression in development and in cancer can provide us with insights into the underlying causes of such diseases.

5.2 DNA methylation

5.2.1 CpG islands

DNA methylation involves the addition of a methyl ($-CH_3$) group to the 5′ -carbon on a cytosine in DNA and is a major contributor to the stability of gene expression states (Figure 5.1). The majority of 5-methylcytosine (5mC) in mammalian DNA is present in the context of the CpG dinucleotide (Riggs and Jones, 1983). However, non-CpG sequences such as CpNpG (Clark et al., 1995) or

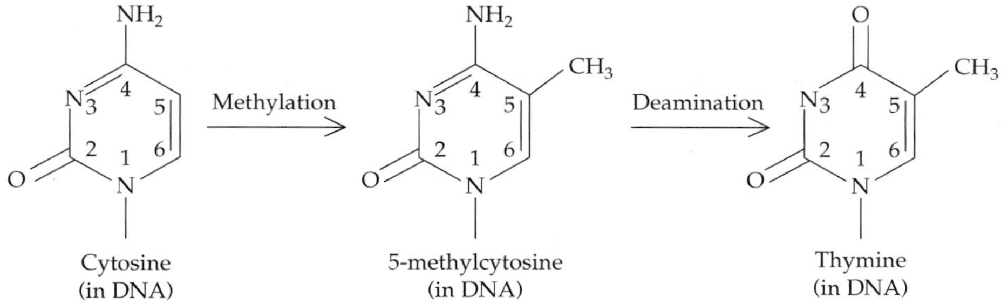

Figure 5.1 Cytosine methylation and spontaneous deamination. A methyl group is added to the 5-carbon position of cytosine residues in DNA to become 5-methylcytosine (5mC) in the DNA. 5mC can undergo spontaneous hydrolytic deamination to cause cytosine to thymine transition mutations in DNA.

non-symmetrical CpA and CpT sequences may also exhibit methylation, but generally at a much lower frequency. Non-CpG methylation is more prevalent in mouse embryonic stem cells than in somatic cells, plants, and fungi.

The distribution of 5mC and of the CpG dinucleotide itself are neither uniform nor random. CpG is the only dinucleotide to be severely under-represented in the human genome, and this is thought to be due to the decreased efficiency of repairing thymine (T) rather than uracil (U), the spontaneous deamination products of 5mC and cytosine (C), respectively (Figure 5.1). Approximately 70% of the CpGs that are present in the genome are methylated, whereas the majority of unmethylated CpGs occur in small clusters known as CpG islands, which are often found within or near promoters and first exons of genes (Bird, 1986). CpG islands, which comprise 1–2% of the genome, are sequences of approximately 0.5–4 kb in length, with a GC content [(number of C bases + number of G bases)/sequence length] of over 55% (in contrast to a genome wide average of about 40%), and an observed/expected ratio for the occurrence of CpG $\geq$ 0.65 {[number of CpG sites/(number of C bases $\times$ number of G bases)]} (Gardiner-Garden and Frommer, 1987, Takai and Jones, 2002.). There are an estimated 45,000 CpG islands in the genome, and approximately 50–60% of all genes contain a promoter-associated CpG island (Antequera and Bird, 1993*a,b*). While most CpG islands are unmethylated and associated with transcriptionally active genes, such as 'housekeeping' genes, certain CpG islands are methylated, including those associated with imprinted genes and genes on the inactive X chromosome in females. Since the promoter CpG islands of most genes are generally unmethylated in the germline, they are less susceptible to deamination and thus have retained the expected frequency of CpG dinucleotides. Conversely, the methylation of cytosines in the majority of the genome makes them more susceptible to mutation, which thereby reduces the overall frequency of CpGs in the bulk genome (Bird, 1992).

5.2.2 Maintenance of DNA methylation

DNA methylation in mammals is carried out by at least three DNA methyltransferase (DNMT) enzymes known to be catalytically active out of a family of five known members, DNMT1, DNMT2, DNMT3A, DNMT3B, and DNMT3L (Bestor, 2000; Robertson, 2002). These enzymes exhibit two distinct functions but vary in their abilities to perform one or the other. Maintenance methyltransferase activity is responsible for copying methylation patterns onto newly synthesized strands of DNA based on the methylation status of the template parent strand (Figure 5.2). Thus a pattern of methylated and unmethylated CpGs along a DNA strand tends to be copied, and this provides a way for passing epigenetic information between cell generations. The second function, *de novo* methylation, is responsible for the methylation of CpG sites that were previously unmethylated (Figure 5.2). DNMT1 is believed to be primarily a maintenance methyltransferase, whereas *de novo* methylation of DNA sequences is mediated by DNMT3A and 3B. These methyltransferases have also been shown to exhibit cooperativity in the methylation of certain classes of DNA repeats. Despite extensive *in vitro* and *in vivo* analysis of the various DNMTs, the mechanisms by which specific

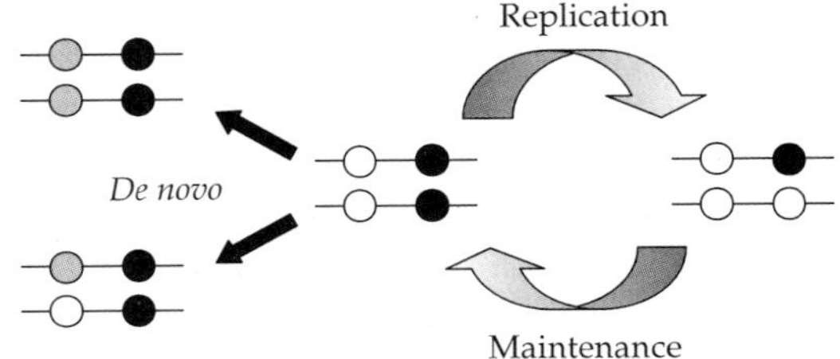

Figure 5.2 Maintenance of cytosine methylation patterns. During DNA replication, the methylation patterns are copied onto the newly synthesized strands of DNA based on the template parental strand by DNA methyltransferase (DNMT). *De novo* methylation involves the addition of methyl groups on previously unmethylated CpG sites. Each circle represents a CpG dinucleotide. Open circles are unmethylated CpGs, while black circles are methylated CpGs. Grey circles represent *de novo* methylated CpGs which can occur on either one or both strands, the mechanism of which is still unclear. Interestingly, DNMT3A was recently demonstrated to be a strand asymmetric hemi-methylase by preferentially methylating one strand of DNA without concurrent methylation of the CpG site on the complementary strand.

DNA sequences are targeted for methylation by the various DNMTs remain poorly understood (Jones and Baylin, 2002).

In the adult, the amount and pattern of methylation are tissue- and cell type-specific, and ageing-related methylation changes in CpG islands, such as in the oestrogen receptor gene and *MYOD1*, have been demonstrated. Variations in the methylation patterns of certain genomic regions appear tissue-specific and are reproducible after transmission through the germline, suggesting that distinct blueprints for the tissue-specific regulation of methylation may exist in the homologous chromosomes. The establishment and maintenance of methylation patterns are hence regulated both temporally and spatially. Disruption of proper DNA methylation has been shown in several human disorders, including ATRX (X-linked alpha-thalassaemia and mental retardation), Fragile X, and ICF (Immune deficiency, Centromeric instability, and Facial anomalies) syndromes (Robertson, 2002).

5.2.3 Role in development

DNA methylation is essential for mammalian embryogenesis and methylation patterns are established during defined phases of development. The methylation profile of the early embryo shows an initial wave of genome wide demethylation, which removes most of the pre-existing patterns of methylation inherited from parental DNA, from fertilization until the eight-cell stage of blastocyst formation (Reik and Walter, 2001). This is followed after implantation by a wave of *de novo* methylation.

The importance of DNMTs in development has been clearly established by the generation of null mice as well as by the study of the human ICF syndrome. *Dnmt1*$^{-/-}$ mice die early in embryonic development, and exhibit severe genomic hypomethylation. Furthermore, conditional deletion of *Dnmt1* from mouse fibroblasts results in *p53*-dependent apoptosis and massive dysregulation of gene expression. Mouse embryos having homozygous *Dnmt3A* deletions die approximately four weeks after birth. *Dnmt3B*$^{-/-}$ mice also die early in embryonic development with a pronounced loss of genomic DNA methylation in pericentromeric heterochromatin repeats. This defect is similar to that seen in lymphocytes of ICF syndrome patients who have immune defects that frequently lead to death at an early age. Mutations of *DNMT3B* have been found in the majority of patients with ICF syndrome. Loss of DNMT3B function results in hypomethylation and chromatin decondensation of the repetitive satellite DNA in pericentromeric heterochromatin regions on chromosomes 1, 9, and 16, as well as changes in gene expression (Robertson, 2002; Geiman and Robertson, 2002). It is clear from these observations that DNA methylation plays a critical role in development, and that the disruption of methylation can have detrimental consequences.

5.2.4 Functions of DNA methylation in normal cells

DNA methylation serves as an essential mechanism for permanent, heritable silencing of gene transcription in mammalian development, most notably exhibited in genomic imprinting, transcriptional silencing of parasitic sequence elements, and X-chromosome inactivation (Walsh et al., 1998; Jones and Baylin, 2002) (Figure 5.3).

An important regulatory role of DNA methylation has been established in genomic imprinting. Differential DNA methylation is a critical signal for mammalian gene imprinting, leading to monoallelic expression of these genes (Plass and Soloway, 2002). The functional differences between the paternal and maternal genomes are attributed to the differential expression of the respective alleles of several dozen imprinted genes during development. In many clusters of imprinted genes, one allele is highly methylated and the other unmethylated or

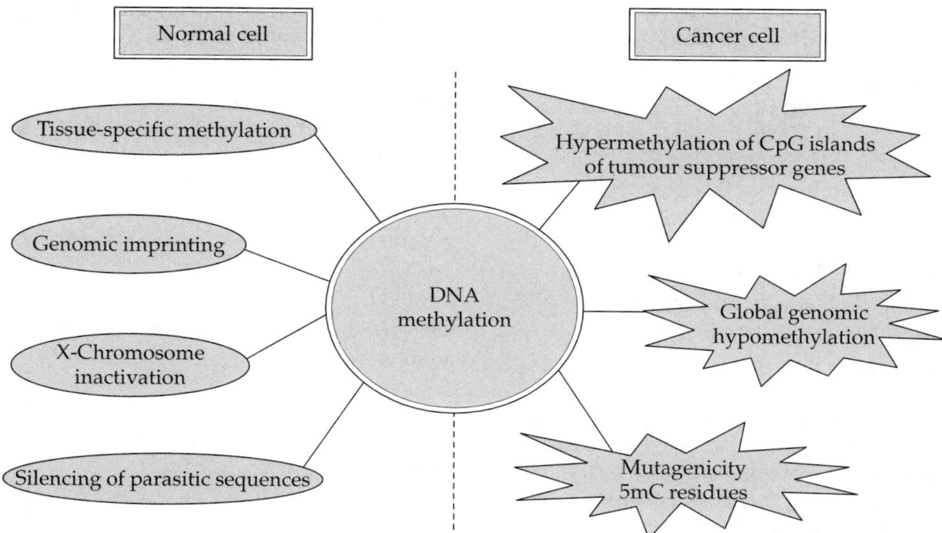

Figure 5.3 DNA methylation in normal and cancer cells. In normal cells, DNA methylation is known to play important roles in tissue-specific methylation, genomic imprinting, X-chromosome inactivation, and silencing of parasitic sequences. On the other hand, cancer cells are usually found to be associated with hypermethylation of CpG islands of tumour suppressor genes, global genomic hypomethylation and increased mutagenicity due to spontaneous deamination of 5mC residues.

methylated at only a small percentage of CpGs in a 1–5 kb CpG-rich differentially methylated region (DMR). The methylation patterns of DMRs exhibit gamete-specific differences, which are usually partially retained during embryogenesis and appeared generally to be the primary imprinting mark (Ehrlich, 2003). The paternal alleles of the *H19* (transforming-suppressing RNA) and *Rasgrf1* (guanine nucleotide exchange factors) genes are methylated in their 5′ upstream regions in the male germ cells during embryogenesis, whereas the other known imprinted genes, such as *Igf2r* (anti-apoptotic growth factor) and *Snrpn* (encodes Smn protein involved in RNA splicing), acquire their methylation imprints from the oocyte. Deletion of such differentially methylated regions results in the loss of imprinting (Li, 2002). The importance of methylation in genomic imprinting has been well demonstrated in homozygous mice with a targeted disruption of *Dnmt1*, which can result in decreased global methylation levels and major perturbations in the expression of several imprinted genes. In mutant embryos, the normally silent paternal allele of the *H19* gene is activated, whereas the normally active paternal allele of the *Igf2* gene and the active maternal allele of the *Igf2r* gene are repressed (Li, 2002). These results suggest that a normal level of DNA methylation is required to control differential expression of the paternal and maternal alleles of imprinted genes.

A prominent example of transcriptional regulation by DNA methylation in genomic imprinting involves the role of the CTCF protein at the *H19*/*Igf2* in mice (Feinberg, 1999; Takai et al., 2001; Bird, 2002). CTCF, associated with transcriptional domain boundaries, can safeguard a promoter from being affected by remote enhancers. When CTCF binds between the promoter and a downstream enhancer, the maternally derived copy of the *Igf2* gene becomes transcriptionally silent. In contrast, these CpG-rich binding sites are methylated at the paternal locus, which prevents CTCF from binding and thus allows the activation *Igf2* expression by the downstream enhancer. Although the *H19*/*Igf2* imprinting may involve additional processes, the role of CTCF represents one of the clearest examples of transcriptional regulation by DNA methylation (Bird, 2002).

Methylation has also been implicated as a possible genome defence mechanism against mobile genetic elements. CpG dinucleotides found outside CpG islands are mostly methylated and many of these CpGs reside within repetitive DNA sequences or retrotransposons, such as endogenous retroviruses, *L1* and *Alu* sequences (Yoder et al., 1997; Robertson and Wolffe, 2000). Since these repetitive sequences comprise almost 40% of the human genome, it has been proposed that DNA methylation may have evolved as a genomic defence system to suppress these sequences and prevent their spread through the genome. DNA retrotransposons may pose a significant threat to the integrity and stability of the genome by mediating recombination between non-allelic repeats, which can cause chromosome rearrangements or translocations, and actively integrating into and disrupting genes (Robertson and Wolffe, 2000). Many retrotransposons have potentially active promoters that, if integrated within a transcriptional unit, could result in internal initiation. Depending on the orientation of the integration, the consequences can vary and be quite harmful (Yoder et al., 1997; Robertson and Wolffe, 2000). The mobility of these retrotransposons depends on the expression of their encoded genes. However, the transcription of these genes has been shown to be silenced by the methylation of retrotransposon promoters. Apparently, methylation of the promoters of intragenomic parasites can function to inactivate these sequences and moreover, the mutagenicity of 5mC can introduce C to T transition mutations resulting in the disabling of many retrotransposons.

In female mammals, dosage compensation is mainly achieved by X-chromosome inactivation, a process that silences one of the two X chromosomes during embryogenesis. An X chromosome is converted from active euchromatin into transcriptionally silenced and highly condensed heterochromatin during inactivation through a sequence of events that include the coating of the X chromosome by *XIST* (X inactive specific transcript) RNA, DNA methylation and histone modification (Avner and Heard, 2001; Li, 2002). Recently, it was shown that histone H3 lysine 9 (H3-K9) methylation is a very early event in the process of X inactivation. The choice of the inactive X chromosome and initiation of the inactivation process also depend on the expression of *XIST* RNA (a non-coding transcript that originates at the X inactivation centre (XIC)), accumulation of this transcript, and then spreading to coat the entire inactive X chromosome (Avner and Heard, 2001; Li, 2002). This ultimately leads to chromosome wide transcriptional silencing, condensation and the late replication of the inactive X. The expression of the *XIST* gene appears to correlate with the methylation status of its promoter, but *XIST* is unmethylated and expressed from the inactive X, and methylated and silent on the active X. In fact, in *DNMT1*$^{-/-}$ embryonic stem cells, the normally silenced *XIST* gene on the active X chromosome in males became reactivated (Costello and Plass, 2001). It is still unclear whether DNA methylation initiates the process *in vivo* or if methylation is a secondary effect following the formation of transcriptionally inactive chromatin. Nevertheless, X-chromosome inactivation is an important process which is mediated and controlled by *XIST* RNA, DNA methylation, as well as histone modification which will be discussed in greater detail.

5.2.5 DNA methylation and transcriptional repression

There are several ways by which DNA methylation may repress transcription (Karpf and Jones, 2002). One mechanism involves DNA methylation sterically hindering the binding of activating transcription factors to gene promoters. Another mechanism involves the activities of methyl-CpG binding domain (MBD) proteins, which bind specifically to methylated DNA and prevent subsequent binding of transcription factors. Several members of this protein family (MBD1, MBD2, and MeCP2) have been shown to recruit transcriptional co-repressors, including histone deacetylases (HDAC1 and 2) and chromatin-remodelling activities (Sin3A and Mi-2), to methylated DNA (Karpf and Jones, 2002). The last mechanism of methylation silencing involves a non-enzymatic transcriptional repression by DNMT proteins (Karpf and Jones, 2002). Most DNMTs (DNMT1, 3A and 3B) have been shown to contain transcriptional repressor domains. Furthermore, similar to MBDs, each of these DNMTs can recruit HDACs and/or other co-repressor proteins to DNA (Robertson and Wolffe, 2000; Karpf and Jones, 2002). Apparently, DNMTs and MBDs can also function as direct repressors to help form transcriptionally repressive chromatin structures.

5.3 Methods for detection of DNA methylation

5.3.1 Methylation-sensitive restriction enzymes for detection of DNA methylation

Methylation-sensitive and -insensitive restriction endonucleases are widely used for studying DNA methylation patterns of specific regions of DNA.

One of the restriction enzymes of the isoschizomer pair cleaves the DNA only when its target is unmethylated, whereas the other is insensitive to methylated cytosines. The most common isoschizomers used are the *Hpa*II/*Msp*I pair. Both enzymes cleave the DNA at the CCGG target, but *Hpa*II is unable to cut when the second cytosine is methylated (CmCGG) in a double-stranded DNA template. After the DNA has been digested with methylation-sensitive endonucleases, the methylation status of a gene can subsequently be identified using Southern blot hybridization or polymerase chain reaction (PCR) procedures (Fraga and Esteller, 2002).

These methods for the quantification of DNA methylation patterns are simple, rapid, and can be used for any known sequence genomic DNA region. Despite the fact that these methods are extremely specific, their limitation to specific restriction sites reduces their value.

5.3.2 Bisulfite methods for detection of DNA methylation

Southern blot analysis of DNA digested with methylation-sensitive restriction endonucleases has previously been an indispensable tool in the study of DNA methylation. However, they are unable to provide the critical information required for a complete understanding of the role of methylcytosine in a more specific sequence context. These isoschizomer-based methods have now been replaced by PCR methods that are based on initial modification of DNA with bisulfite. Bisulfite modification of the DNA selectively deaminates cytosine residues into uracil in genomic DNA, whereas the methylated cytosine residues are resistant to this modification. This bisulfite-modified DNA can then be used as a template in a standard PCR using primers specific for the gene of interest. Bisulfite genomic sequencing of the resulting PCR product provides an accurate display of methylated cytosines, but may be technically difficult and labour intensive. Various PCR methods have been developed, including methylation-specific PCR (MSP), methylation-sensitive single nucleotide primer extension (Ms-SNuPE), real-time PCR-based MethyLight, and methods based on the use of restriction endonucleases, which are simple to use but all suffer from the drawback that only a limited number of CpG sites can be analysed in each assay (Fraga and Esteller, 2002; Dahl and Guldberg, 2003). Different methods which are commonly used to detect DNA methylation are compared in Table 5.1. It is important to note that there is no one technique or general approach that is universally superior to the others, since the ultimate goals of quantitative accuracy, sensitive detection, high local or global informational content, compatibility with formalin-fixed tissues and compatibility with automation are not all found in a single or specific technique (Laird, 2003). Therefore, the method of choice will depend on the desired application.

5.3.3 Techniques for global detection of hypermethylated genes

In the past, the lack of sequence information and the presence of multiple candidate genes in amplified or deleted regions have hampered the rapid identification of novel cancer genes. Fortunately, with the availability of the human genome sequence, the large insert genomic clone resources, and the development of various new genomic scanning techniques, there is now growing interest in the discovery of novel cancer genes. Since most cancers are associated with abnormally hypermethylated genes, a large number of techniques have been developed to screen the cancer cell genome for these genes (Table 5.1). Some of these techniques are aimed specifically at identifying genes by discovering aberrantly hypermethylated CpG islands, since the identification of these CpG islands will allow the discovery of those genes disrupted during tumour progression. Other techniques are aimed at identifying regions of abnormal methylation per se rather than specific genes (Table 5.1). The search for differences between tumour tissue and equivalent histologically normal tissue from the same patient, as well as different stages of disease progression from various patients, has often been of great interest to researchers. This type of screening approach can lead to identification of methylation markers that are useful for the sensitive detection of disease or markers associated with disease progression (Laird, 2003).

5.4 Chromatin inheritance

5.4.1 Histone modification and 'histone code'

Transcription in mammalian cells does not occur on naked DNA, but instead occurs in the context of chromatin. The basic repeat unit of chromatin, the

Table 5.1 Methods for detection of methylation patterns and methylation profiles

Technology	Methylation discrimination principle	Quantitative/ qualitative	Application	Disadvantages
Methylation patterns				
MSP[a]	Bisulfite conversion	Qualitative	Rapid sensitive detection of methylation at specific sequences	Poor resolution at the nucleotide level
Ms-SNUPE	Bisulfite conversion/ radioactive incorporation	Quantitative	Detect specific CpG methylation at specific sequences	PCR bias/difficulty with high CpG-rich regions
MethyLight	Bisulfite conversion/ fluorescence-based, real-time PCR	Quantitative	Rapid high throughput analysis of methylation at specific sequences	Inability to distinguish in detail different methylation patterns in present at the same location
COBRA	Bisulfite conversion/ restriction enzyme digestion	Semi-quantitative	Analysis of methylation status at specific regions in any DNA sample	Confined to restriction targets
Bisulfite-SSCP	Bisulfite conversion/ SSCP	Semi-quantitative	Sensitive detection of high-resolution polymorphisms in human coding loci	Detection of single-base changes requires a minimal level of alteration
In-tube fluorescence melting curve	Bisulfite conversion/ melting analysis	Quantitative	Detection of overall methylation status of a CpG island	No information is provided on the methylation status of individual cytosines
Bisulfite genomic sequencing	Bisulfite conversion/cloning	Qualitative	Positive identification and localization of 5mC in genomic DNA	Possible clonal selection bias
Methylation profiles				
RLGS	Restriction digestion/2D fractional electrophoresis	Qualitative	Genomewide scan for changes in DNA methylation in CpG islands	CpG island detection are sometimes not in the promoter regions of genes
MS AP-PCR	Restriction digestion/arbitrarily primed PCR	Qualitative	Rapid identification of CpG islands that are differentially methylated in different tissues	Most CpG islands detected are not in the promoter regions of genes
DMH	Restriction digestion/CpG island array hybridization	Qualitative	Identification of hypermethylated sequences in tumour cells	Defining exact transcriptional start site can be laborious
Gene re-expression arrays	Drug agent activation (5-Aza-CdR, TSA)/cDNA microarray analysis	Qualitative	Detection of hypermethylated sites is linked to the transcriptional status of genes	Identifying hypermethylated CpG island, which is associated with the gene promoter, requires genomic databases
MSO	Bisulfite conversion/ oligonucleotide microarray analysis	Quantitative	Rapid screening of multiple CpG sites in many gene promoters	Possible cross-hybridization between imperfect-match probes and targets
ICEAMP	Methyl-CpG binding column/subtractive hybridization	Qualitative	Identification methylation changes in genomic regions during tumorigenesis	Possible PCR amplification bias; may not detect all methylation changes in or near a repetitive element
MCA-RDA	Restriction digestion/subtractive hybridization	Qualitative	Detect large numbers of CpG islands which are mostly associated with genes	Defining exact transcriptional start site can be laborious

[a] MSP = methylation-sensitive PCR; Ms-SNUPE = methylation-sensitive single nucleotide primer extension; COBRA = combined bisulfite restriction analysis; Bisulfite-SSCP = bisulfite single-strand conformation polymorphism; RLGS = restriction landmark genomic scanning; MS AP-PCR = methylation-sensitive arbitrarily primed polymerase chain reaction; MSO = methylation-specific oligonucleotide; ICEAMP = identification of CGI exhibiting altered methylation patterns; MCA-RDA = methylated CpG island amplification/representational difference analysis.

nucleosome, includes two copies of each of the four core histones H2A, H2B, H3, and H4 wrapped by 146 bp of DNA. Chromatin is not uniform with respect to gene distribution and transcriptional activity and is packaged as heterochromatin and euchromatin. Heterochromatin represents a tightly packed, condensed conformation and is usually associated with transcriptional inactivity. On the other hand, euchromatin contains less condensed regions of chromosomal DNA and is generally associated with transcriptional activity. Histones are basic proteins consisting of a globular domain and a 'tail' that protrudes out of the nucleosome. Epigenetic processes, such as histone modifications on the N-terminal tails and chromatin remodelling, have recently been shown to cooperate to control chromatin structure and ultimately cellular processes such as gene expression and DNA methylation itself. These histone tails are targets for diverse post-translational modifications, which include acetylation, phosphorylation, methylation, ubiquitination, and ADP-ribosylation (Geiman and Robertson, 2002; Lachner et al., 2003). The roles of acetylation, phosphorylation, and methylation of various amino residues on histones H3 and H4 have been described (Lachner et al., 2003).

The acetylation and deacetylation of conserved lysine residues present in histone tails has long been linked to transcriptional activity and has been the most studied histone modification. Histone acetyltransferases (HATs) acetylate lysine residues to create an accessible and open chromatin configuration that facilitates transcriptional activity, whereas histone deacetylases (HDACs) remove acetyl groups to facilitate chromatin compaction that leads to transcription repression. Histone deacetylase inhibitors, such as trichostatin A (TSA), can activate the transcription of certain genes. Methylation of lysine residues on the histone tails of H3 and H4 appears to provide an additional layer of control over the chromatin structure, and ultimately over gene expression. A group of histone methyltransferases (HMTase) is responsible for catalysing histone lysine methylation (Lachner and Jenuwein, 2002). Members of this group contain a conserved SET domain that is flanked by cysteine-rich regions. Some of the more prominent histone tail modifications include the acetylation of lysine 9 and methylation of lysine 4 (specifically, trimethylation of lysine 4; Santos-Rosa et al., 2002) of histone H3, both of which were shown to be associated with an open chromatin configuration. In contrast, methylation of lysine 9 of H3 (H3-K9) is a marker of condensed, inactive chromatin as with the inactive X-chromosome and is also found to be associated with aberrant gene silencing in cancer cells. The link between H3-K9 methylation and repressive chromatin is clearly evident, however this heterochromatin is shown to be associated with lack of transcriptional initiation but not inhibition of elongation by RNA polymerase II (Nguyen et al., 2002).

It is becoming increasingly apparent that characteristic modification patterns, or combinations thereof, constitute a code that defines actual or potential transcriptional states (Wu and Grunstein, 2000; Jenuwein and Allis, 2001). The histone code hypothesis predicts that a pre-existing modification affects subsequent modifications on histone tails, and that these modifications act as marks for the recruitment of different proteins or protein complexes to regulate various chromatin functions, such as gene expression, chromosome segregation, and DNA replication (Strahl and Allis, 2000). In order to realize its full information carrying potential, the code must use various combinations of modifications. This requires not only proteins that can read such combined modifications, but also mechanisms by which they can be initiated and maintained. This intricate interplay between various covalent modifications occurring in different sites on the histone tails appears to ultimately impact gene expression.

5.4.2 Chromatin remodelling and DNA methylation

DNA methylation and histone modification are vital to the control of gene expression. However, chromatin remodelling proteins also play a crucial role in the regulation of this process. The SNF2 family of chromatin remodelling proteins, which utilize adenosine triphosphate (ATP) to alter the structure of chromatin through the disruption of the histone/DNA contacts, acts in various cellular processes such as gene expression, replication, DNA repair and recombination (Geiman and Robertson, 2002). Depending on the SNF2 factor and the proteins with which it interacts, SNF2 family members function in transcriptional activation as well as repression. Some of these family members have been connected recently to the process of maintaining proper DNA methylation patterns in organisms as diverse as *Arabidopsis thaliana* and humans (Geiman and Robertson, 2002).

The first connection between a member of the SNF2 helicase/ATPase family and DNA methylation was the *A. thaliana* protein DDM1 (decrease in DNA methylation). Mutation of this gene results in a 70% reduction in global DNA methylation levels, which becomes more pronounced with successive generations. In *DDM1* mutants, this loss of DNA methylation altered the expression and mobility of transposable elements, most likely by disrupting the formation of silent heterochromatin. The *DDM1* gene is closely related to the mammalian lymphoid specific helicase (*Lsh*) (*Hells, PASG*) gene, which was first identified as an SNF2 helicase family member highly expressed in fetal thymus and activated lymphocytes. Mice with a homozygous deletion of *Lsh* show perinatal lethality and global defects in the level of DNA methylation, both in repetitive elements and single copy genes. Chromatin remodellers, such as *DDM1* and *Lsh*, appeared to be important in the control of genomic DNA methylation levels, as evidenced by the substantial loss of methylation in both *DDM1* and *Lsh* mutants (Robertson, 2002; Geiman and Robertson, 2002).

Another member of the SNF2 family of chromatin remodelling proteins is ATRX, the gene for which is mutated in alpha-thalassaemia mental retardation, x-linked (ATRX) syndrome (Gibbons et al., 2000). Mutation of the *ATRX* gene on the X chromosome leads to an unusual form of thalassaemia, presumably due to a 30–60% decrease in alpha globin gene expression levels. Even though there are no changes in the methylation pattern of the alpha globin gene in ATRX patients, both hyper- and hypomethylation changes in highly repetitive elements such as satellite DNA have been demonstrated (Gibbons et al., 2000; Geiman and Robertson, 2002).

Apparently, both of these chromatin remodelling family members are essential for proper DNA methylation. However, the mechanisms by which they function may differ, probably due to a different complement of interacting proteins. This connection between chromatin remodelling and DNA methylation supports the notion that there are multiple layers of epigenetic modifications to heritably modulate gene expression.

Chromatin structure is closely linked to gene expression, and deregulation of chromosome-remodelling activity may thus interfere with many critical cellular processes, resulting in development of disease (Luo and Dean, 1999). A classic example demonstrating the cancer-chromatin connection is the fact that a well-known tumour suppressor, retinoblastoma gene (*RB*), is closely linked to histone deacetylation. Most *RB* mutants found in cancers affect the integrity of the pocket, which is the region that binds to HDAC1 and HDAC2. Hence, *RB* mutants are no longer able to recruit histone deacetylases to maintain a repressed chromatin structure. Another example is acute promyelocytic leukaemia which is caused by a chimeric mutant of the retinoic acid receptor associated with HDAC1. Treatment of patients with acute promyelocytic leukaemia with a histone deacetylase inhibitor and retinoic acid re-induced remission (Robertson, 2000). Finally, the finding that dermatomyositis-specific autoantigen Mi2 is a component of a complex containing histone deacetylase and nucleosome remodelling activities further demonstrates the broad spectrum of diseases associated with deregulation of chromatin structure (Zhang et al., 1998; Luo and Dean, 1999).

5.4.3 Link between DNA methylation and chromatin structure

Cytosine methylation changes the interactions between proteins and DNA, leading to alterations in chromatin structure and either a decrease or an increase in the rate of transcription. The processes of histone deacetylation and DNA methylation are tightly linked through protein complexes containing DNMTs and HDACs. This link provides a plausible mechanism between DNA methylation and histone deacetylation in transcriptional repression, since the recruitment of DNMTs and their associated HDACs to methylated DNA would cause local deacetylation of core histone tails, thereby resulting in tight chromatin compaction and limited access of transcription factors to their binding sites (Robertson and Wolffe, 2000).

Recently, four of the methyl-CpG binding domain-containing proteins MeCP2, MBD1, MBD2, and MBD3, have been associated with aspects of the chromatin remodelling machinery in addition to HDACs. In *Xenopus* eggs, for instance, MBD3 is a component of the Mi-2 chromatin remodelling complex which also includes Rpd3 (*Xenopus* HDAC1/2) and two Rb-associated histone-binding proteins, RbAp46/48 (Robertson and Wolffe, 2000). The mechanistic link between DNA methylation and histone deacetylation has also been supported by combination treatment of tumour cells with the DNA methyltransferase inhibitor, 5-aza-2-deoxycytidine (5-Aza-CdR), and the histone deacetylation inhibitor, trichostatin A (TSA). Treatment of cells with low doses of 5-Aza-CdR resulted in a low level of gene re-expression and minimal demethylation of hypermethylated CpG-island-associated genes. Interestingly, a combination of 5-Aza-CdR and TSA resulted in robust activation of these same genes, whereas TSA alone had no effect. This supports the idea that DNA methylation and histone deacetylation worked co-operatively to silence gene transcription.

Histone methylation provides another crucial link to associations between DNA methylation and chromatin modification processes. In *Neurospora crassa*, mutations of the *DIM-5* (defective in methylation 5) gene, which encodes a SET domain-containing H3-K9 methyltransferase, result in the complete loss of genomic DNA methylation (Tamaru and Selker, 2001). When wild-type *Neurospora* H3-K9 is replaced by H3 with an altered amino acid at position 9 that cannot be methylated, the genomic DNA methylation is also reduced. Specifically, it was shown that trimethylated H3-K9, not dimethylated H3-K9, marks the chromatin regions for cytosine methylation and that DIM-5 is the enzyme responsible for creating this mark (Geiman and Robertson, 2002). Similar observations were made in *A. thaliana*, in which mutations of an H3-K9 methyltransferase [encoded by *kryptonite* (*kyp*)] abolished methylation of CpNpG sites, but not CpG sites. Furthermore, the loss of DNA methylation in DDM1 mutants in *Arabidopsis* may be a consequence of reduced H3-K9 methylation in heterochromatin. Interestingly, the DNMT chromomethylase 3 (CMT3) was also shown in *Arabidopsis* to interact with the methyl–lysine binding protein, heterochromatin protein 1 (HP1), thereby providing a specific mechanism for directing DNA methylation to regions of the genome marked by histone methylation (Jackson et al., 2002; Geiman and Robertson, 2002). In both of these organisms, it appears that the establishment and maintenance of DNA methylation is dependent upon histone H3-K9 methylation and may represent a common epigenetic mechanism in eukaryotes (Figure 5.4).

Histone H3 lysine 9 methylation and DNA methylation are generally both associated with transcriptionally silent heterochromatin. Methylated lysine 9 of histone H3 is a binding site for

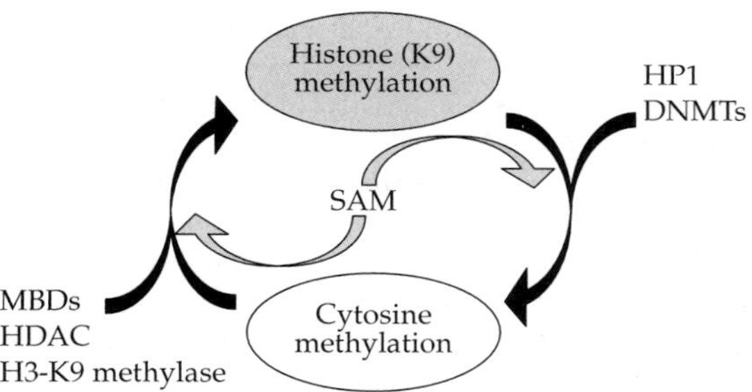

Figure 5.4 Complex interplay between two epigenetic marks of heterochromatin: histone H3 lysine 9 methylation and cytosine methylation. The establishment of permanent, heritable silencing of gene transcription and heterochromatin involves the intimate connection between histone H3 lysine 9 methylation and cytosine methylation, irrespective of which comes first. Recent evidence from *N. crassa* and *A. thaliana* suggests that histone H3 lysine 9 methylation, specifically trimethylated lysine 9, drives cytosine methylation, presumably through heterochromatin protein 1 (HP1) and DNA methyltransferases (DNMTs). The mechanism by which this occurs in mammalian cells is still unclear. Cytosine methylation may also facilitate histone H3 lysine 9 methylation through methyl-CpG binding domain proteins (MBDs), histone deacetylases (HDACs), and histone H3 lysine 9 methylase (H3-K9 methylase), thereby reinforcing the repressive function of these two distinct epigenetic markers.

HP1, and the histone H3 lysine 9 methyltransferase SUV39H1 co-localizes and interacts with HP1 in regions of heterochromatin (Lachner et al., 2001). As a major component of heterochromatin, HP1 contributes to the establishment and maintenance of the transcriptionally repressed state of heterochromatin. In murine embryonic stem cells, it is interesting to find that DNMT3 proteins co-localize with HP1 to pericentromeric heterochromatin regions, indicating that DNA methylation may be targeted to heterochromatic sites through HP1 (Geiman and Robertson, 2002). Therefore, in addition to methylation abilities, DNA methyltransferases may function as transcriptional repressors and serve as scaffolds to direct other chromatin-modifying activities in establishing heterochromatin. MeCP2 was also recently demonstrated to be associated with H3-K9 methylation *in vitro* as well as *in vivo*, thereby providing another mechanistic bridge between DNA methylation and histone methylation in establishing the repressed state. Furthermore, MBD1, which possesses an MBD involved in mediating DNA methylation-dependent transcriptional repression, was shown to direct SUVH1–HP1 complex to methylated DNA regions, suggesting a potential pathway from DNA methylation to histone methylation for epigenetic gene regulation. To further corroborate the idea that cytosine methylation directs H3-K9 methylation, it was shown that DNA methylation precedes and controls H3-K9 methylation and heterochromation in *Arabidopsis* using *DDM1* and *MET1* (encodes a maintenance methyltransferase) mutants. Even though this appeared to contradict previous results in *Neurospora crassa* and *Arabidopsis*, which show that DNA methylation is dependent on H3-K9 methylation, this discrepancy may be due to differences in the function between the methylases involved (Robertson, 2002; Geiman and Robertson, 2002).

Together, these data provide new insights into the link identified between DNA methylation and histone methylation and open up new avenues by which DNA methylation might be connected to the chromatin structure to bring about gene silencing. Nevertheless, the mechanism by which histone methylation regulates CpG methylation in mammalian cells is still unknown. It is also yet to be determined whether the maintenance of DNA methylation patterns depends on histone methylation or vice versa in mammalian cells. Since mammalian cells contain several CpG methyltransferases and H3-K9 methyltransferases, the interaction is likely to be more complicated than that in *Neurospora* and *Arabidopsis*. The molecules that target histone methyltransferases and DNA methyltransferases to specific genomic loci also remain to be elucidated (Geiman and Robertson, 2002).

5.5 Cancer epigenetics

Aberrant patterns of cytosine methylation have been found to be associated with an increasing number of cancers over the past few decades. Two distinct patterns have been well described: (1) global genomic hypomethylation (loss of methylation at normally methylated sequences) and (2) localized hypermethylation (gain of methylation) usually in normally unmethylated CpG islands (Jones and Laird, 1999; Jones and Baylin, 2002). These disparities can be found together in a single tumour, yet the overall effect is commonly a drop in total methylation levels. It is currently unknown whether genomic hypomethylation and CpG island hypermethylation are linked by a common underlying mechanism or result from distinct abnormalities in the cancer cell. However, both of these changes in methylation patterns can precede malignancy, suggesting that they are not simply a consequence of the malignant state (Costello and Plass, 2001). In addition, the mutagenicity of 5mC and secondary effects of DNA methylation can also influence tumorigenesis via different mechanisms (Figure 5.3).

5.5.1 CpG island hypermethylation in tumour suppressor genes

CpG island hypermethylation in the promoter regions of cancer-related or tumour suppressor genes has been commonly associated with their silencing. Since methylation of the associated CpG islands corresponds with inactivation of these genes in the tumours, hypermethylation has been included as an alternative mechanism to genetic mutation and/or deletion in eliciting allelic gene silencing of tumour suppressor genes in cancer (Jones and Laird, 1999). Abnormal methylation of CpG islands can efficiently repress transcription of the associated gene in a manner similar to mutations and deletions, thereby acting as one of the 'hits' in the Knudsen two-hit hypothesis for tumour generation (Jones and Laird, 1999; Baylin and Herman, 2000; Jones and Baylin, 2002). Biallelic inactivation of a tumour suppressor or cancer-related gene may result from either genetic and epigenetic mechanisms alone or combinations thereof. Interestingly, demethylating agents are capable of restoring gene activity and tumour suppressor function in cultured tumour cells. Numerous genes involved in fundamental pathways, such as cell cycle regulation, DNA repair, drug resistance and detoxification, differentiation, apoptosis, angiogenesis, metastasis, and invasion, have been shown to be inappropriately silenced by methylation (Table 5.2) (Momparler and Bovenzi, 2000; Costello and Plass, 2001; Esteller, 2002; Das and Singal, 2004). It is clear that hypermethylation is a significant alteration in the cancer genome but the mechanisms responsible for eliciting this change are not well understood.

Two models have been suggested for the abnormal CpG island methylation of various tumour-suppressor genes in cancer (Costello and Plass, 2001; Jones and Baylin, 2002). One proposed mechanism involves the loss of protective factors that normally bind to CpG islands and prevent them from methylation. The protective factors, such as structural proteins or transcription factors, could compete with DNMTs for sites within the CpG island to prevent methylation. An example

Table 5.2 Genes abnormally methylated in human cancers

Function	Gene abbreviation(s)	Genes	Tumour type(s)	Location
Apoptosis	*DAPK*	Death associated protein kinase	Uterine, cervix, lymphoma, colon, lung	9q34.1
	CASP8	Caspase 8	Primary PNET/ medulloblastoma	2q33-34
	TMS1	Target of methylation induced silencing	Breast	16p11.2-12.1
Angiogenesis Cell cycle	*THBS1*	Thrombospondin-1	Glioblastoma multiforme	15q15
	RB	Retinoblastoma	Glioblastomas	13q14
	p14ARF	p14 Alternative reading frame of *CDKN2A*	Colorectal, stomach, kidney	9p21
	CDKN2A/p16INK4a	Cyclin-dependent kinase 2A	Solid tumors	9p21
	CDKN2B/p15INK4b	Cyclin-dependent kinase 2B	Haematological malignancies	9p21
	p27	p27/KIP1	Melanoma	12p13
	TP73, p73	p73 (TP73)	Lymphomas	1p36
	SFN/ 14–3–3–σ	Stratifin	Breast, gastric, colorectal, hepatocellular	1p
Differentiation	*MYOD*	Myogenic differentiation antigen-1	Colorectal	11p15.4
	PAX6	Paired box gene 5	Colon, bladder	11p13
	RAR β2	Retinoic acid receptor	Nasopharyngeal	3p24
	WT1	Wilms' tumour 1	Wilms' Tumour	11p13
DNA repair	*hMLH1*	Human MutL homologue 1	Colon, gastric	3p23–p21.3
	O^6-MGMT	O-6-methylguanine-DNA methyltransferase	Colon, gastric, lymphoma	10q26
Detoxification/drug resistance	*GSTP1*	Glutathione S-transferase π	Breast, prostate, kidney	11q13
	MDR1	Multi-drug resistance 1	Human T cell leukaemia	7q21.1
Invasion/metastasis	*CDH1*	E-cadherin	Breast, gastric, leukaemia	16q22.1
	CDH13	*H-cadherin*	Colorectal, breast, lung	16q24
	TIMP-3	Tissue inhibitor of metalloproteinase 3	Colon, renal	22q12.3
	Maspin/ PI5	Maspin (protease inhibitor 5)	Breast	18q21.3
	PR	Progesterone receptor	Breast, prostate	11q22
	RASSF1A	Ras association domain family member 1	Nasopharyngeal, ovarian, renal	3p21.3
	STK11/LKB1	Serine/threonine protein kinase 11	Colon, breast	19p13.3
Signal transduction	*APC*	Adenomatous polyposis of the colon	Colon, gastric	5q21–22
	PTEN	Phosphatase and tensen homologue deleted on chromosome 10	Prostate	10q23.3
	AR	Androgen receptor	Prostate	Xq11-12
	ESR1	Estrogen receptor 1	Breast	6q25.1
	PR	Progesterone receptor	Breast, prostate	11q22
	RASSF1A	Ras association domain family member 1	Nasopharyngeal, ovarian, renal	3p21.3
	STK11/LKB1	Serine/threonine protein kinase 11	Colon, breast, lung	19p13.3
Transcription/transcription factors	*VHL*	Von Hippel-Lindau syndrome	Renal, haemangioblastoma	3p26–p25
	HIC-1	Hypermethylated in cancer	Breast	17p13.3
	BRCA1	Breast cancer, type1	Breast, ovarian	17q21
	SRBC	BRCA1-binding protein	Breast, lung	1p15
	SYK	Spleen tyrosine kinase	Breast, lymphoblastic leukaemia	9q22
	SOCS-1	Suppressor of cytokine signalling 1	Hepatoblastomas; multiple myeloma	16p13.13
Other	*CD44*	CD44 antigen	Prostate	11pter–p13
	COX2	Cyclo-oxygenase 2	Colon, gastric	1q25.2-25.3
	CACNA1G	Calcium channel, voltage dependent, T type, alpha-1G subunit	Colorectal, gastric	17q22
	CALCA	Calcitonin	Chronic myelogenous leukaemia	11p15.2-15.1
	FHIT	Fragile histidine triad gene	Oesophageal, cervical, breast	3p14.2
	TERT	Telomerase reverse transcriptase	Colorectal	5p15.33
	TPEF/HPP1	Transmembrane protein containing epidermal growth factor and follistatin domains	Bladder, colon	2q33
	CSPG2	Chondroitin sulphate proteoglycan 2	Colon	5q12-14
	RIZ1	Retinoblastoma protein -interacting zinc finger	Breast, liver, Nasopharyngeal	1p36

supporting this mechanism is the SP1 transcription factor, whose recognition sites for binding are usually found within most CpG islands, and mutation of its site in transgenic mice resulted in methylation of the associated transgene CpG island. Nevertheless, in *SP1*$^{-/-}$ mouse embryos, CpG islands remain unmethylated. Undoubtedly other transcription factors may function in a similar matter. However, the fact that even CpG islands from non-expressed genes remain unmethylated in normal cells suggests that factors other than those associated with active transcription may also function to protect some CpG islands from methylation (Costello and Plass, 2001).

In human tumour cells, the loss of protective factors may provide a mechanism by which methylation can spread into the CpG island from flanking densely methylated sequences that often contain *Alu* elements. Even though most CpG islands of tumour suppressor genes are unmethylated in normal tissues, these islands are embedded between heavily methylated flanking regions containing multiple *Alu* repeats. Together, these findings suggest that abnormal CpG island methylation in cancer can possibly result from the loss of protective factors and the encroachment of methylation from flanking methylated regions through the boundaries that apparently exist at both ends of the unmethylated CpG island (Costello and Plass, 2001).

Another model suggests that aberrant CpG island methylation is an active process and functions primarily to maintain gene silencing (Clark and Melki, 2002). There is considerable evidence showing the overexpression of all DNMTs at the mRNA level in several cancers, and increased DNMT1 expression in normal human fibroblasts cause aberrant *de novo* methylation of CpG islands and promote cellular transformation in NIH3T3 cells. Conversely, low levels of DNMT1 appear to have protective effects. For instance, hypomorphic alleles of *Dnmt1* lead to the complete suppression of intestinal polyp formation in *Min* mice, which are genetically predisposed to colonic polyp formation. Furthermore, inhibition of the methyltransferase using an antisense to *DNMT1* reduces the tumorigenicity of murine adrenocortical tumour cells. However, other reports indicate that there is no correlation between CpG island hypermethylation and DNMT1 levels. Alterations in DNA function will result in gains and losses in DNA methylation as well as cause variations in DNA methylation pattern (Costello and Plass, 2001).

5.5.2 Global genomic hypomethylation

Malignant cells can have 20–60% less genomic 5mC than their normal counterparts (Lapeyre and Becker, 1979; Gama-Sosa et al., 1983). Global DNA hypomethylation has also been reported in almost every human malignancy. Interestingly, the majority of hypomethylation events occur in repetitive elements localized in satellite sequences or centromeric regions, which are normally methylated. In tumours, the extent of genome wide hypomethylation parallels closely the degree of malignancy, although this may be tumour type-dependent. In various tumours, such as breast, cervical, ovarian, and brain tumours, hypomethylation increases progressively with increasing tumour grade (Gama-Sosa et al., 1983; Costello and Plass, 2001). In addition, another study on breast lesions demonstrated a significant correlation between the extent of hypomethylation and disease stage, tumour size, and degree of malignancy (Soares et al., 1999). Hence, hypomethylation may have prognostic use as a biological marker.

DNA hypomethylation can contribute to tumorigenesis in several ways. Loss of methylation in cancers could induce expression of the normally repressed transposons scattered throughout the genome, leading to deleterious transposition events (Yoder et al., 1997). There is evidence that cancer-related hypomethylation results in increased expression of some of these elements, but whether this increased expression is harmful to the genome either directly or through transposition of the elements is not clear. Secondly, genomic hypomethylation in cancer has been linked to chromosome instability, and may favour mitotic recombination leading to loss of heterozygosity (LOH), as well as promoting karyotypically detectable rearrangements. Though genomic demethylation may be protective against some cancers such as intestinal tumours in the *Apc*^{Min} mouse model (Laird et al., 1995), it may act as a double-edged sword by also promoting chromosome instability and LOH, as well as increasing the risk of cancer in other tissues, as seen in hypomethylated mutant mice (Chen et al., 1998). Thirdly, although evidence for activation of oncogenes by specific gene demethylation in cancer is poor, hypomethylation has been reported in the coding regions of some oncogenes, including *MYC* and *HRAS*. Hypomethylation has also been reported to be responsible for the activation of *MAGE* and related genes. These genes are germline-specific and their promoters are normally methylated and silent in all adult somatic tissue but can become aberrantly activated in a number of tumours. Finally, the loss of methyl groups can affect imprinted genes, such as the *H19/IGF2* locus, where the disturbance of methylation may cause overexpression of *IGF2* and loss of *H19* in certain childhood tumours (Feinberg, 1999). All four mechanisms mentioned above are possible means in which hypomethylation can contribute to tumorigenesis (Esteller and Herman, 2002).

5.5.3 Mutagenesis of 5-methylcytosine

Cytosine methylation can also influence tumorigenicity via mechanisms other than through hypo- and hypermethylation. 5mC can undergo spontaneous hydrolytic deamination to cause C to T transition mutations and an estimated 31% of germline mutations which lead to genetic disorders can be attributed to 5mC to T transitions at methylated CpG dinucletotides. Moreover, a high incidence of C to T transition mutations occurring at methylated cytosines was also observed in the human *TP53* tumour suppressor gene in somatic cells (Jones and Baylin, 2002).

The spontaneous deamination of 5mC to T generates a G/T mismatch, which can be recognized and repaired by G/T mismatch thymine DNA glycosylase. This type of transition mutation may also arise from the spontaneous deamination of cytosine to uracil, generating a G/U mismatch, which can be recognized by uracil DNA glycosylase. An accumulation of either G/U or G/T mismatches, which are not appropriately repaired by their respective enzymes, uracil- (or thymine) DNA glycosylases, will increase the frequencies of C to T transition mutations in the genome (Bender et al., 1998). Studies have shown that bacterial methyltransferases can enhance C to T transition mutations by blocking the repair of G/U mismatches by uracil DNA glycosylase, and can mediate 5mC to T transition mutations at CpG dinucleotides under specific conditions which include increased DNMT expression or decreased cellular *S*-adenosylmethionine (SAM) levels. There is, however, no evidence as yet that this particular SAM-deficient mechanism plays a significant role in inducing mutation in human cells. The major cause of the high mutation rate at CpG dinucleotides is still likely to be spontaneous deamination of 5mC (Laird and Jaenisch, 1994; Bender et al., 1998; Pfeifer et al., 2000).

There are other causes for mutation induction secondary to DNA methylation. For instance, the UV absorption wavelength of cytosine is shifted by methylation into the range of incident sunlight, thereby increasing CC to TT mutations that commonly occur in skin cancers. In addition, methylated CpG dinucleotides show enhanced binding of benzo[a]pyrene diol epoxide and other carcinogens found in tobacco smoke, which causes DNA adduct formation and G to T transversion mutations. Methylation can therefore directly contribute to the induction of mutations that cause cancer (Jones and Baylin, 2002).

5.6 Reversal of epigenetic modifications as a cancer therapy

Inactivation of tumour suppressor genes by genetic and epigenetic mechanisms are functionally equivalent in many ways. However, there are some fundamental differences between these two pathways that may be potentially important for anticancer therapy. Genetic hits confer a fixed, irreversible state of gene inactivation, whereas epigenetic events do not change the information content of the affected genes and are potentially reversible. This feature makes epigenetic modifications good targets for therapeutic interventions in cancer patients. Epigenetic silencing may be alleviated at two different levels: inhibition of DNA methylation and inhibition of chromatin modification. Many inhibitors of DNA methylation or histone deacetylase are available that can modulate gene transcription *in vitro* and *in vivo* (Worm and Guldberg, 2002).

A potent specific inhibitor of DNA methylation, 5-Aza-CdR, has been widely used as a demethylating agent *in vitro*. 5-Aza-CdR is specific inhibitor of DNA methyltransferase, which forms an irreversible covalent complex with the enzyme after incorporation into DNA (Christman, 2002). 5-Aza-CdR exhibits promising activity as an anticancer agent, and is used clinically in the treatment of acute leukaemias and myelodysplasia. However, this demethylating agent and its ribo analogue, 5-azacytidine (5-Aza-CR), are unstable in neutral aqueous solutions and quite toxic, thereby complicating their clinical use. Zebularine, a cytidine analogue, was shown recently to be a stable, minimally toxic demethylating agent capable of reactivating an epigenetically silenced gene by oral administration in tumours grown in nude mice (Cheng et al., 2003). Other drugs include the antihypertensive and antiarrhythmic agents, hydralazine and procainamide respectively, both of which are non-nucleoside analogues that have been shown to inhibit DNA methylation and reactivate silenced genes in cultured cells and in mice. Inhibition of DNA methylation as a target for cancer therapy is further supported by the interesting observation that antisense to DNMT1 shows *in vitro* antitumour activity and some potential to reverse the malignant phenotype. This antisense oligonucleotide also inhibits tumour growth in an animal model. Likewise, cell culture experiments have shown that histone deacetylase inhibitors (i.e. butyrates, suberoylanilide hydroxamic acid (SAHA), valproic acid (VPA)) can reactivate a range of epigenetically silenced genes, and several of these agents are now in clinical trials (Marks et al., 2001). Unfortunately, a major problem of drugs targeting the DNA methylation or histone methylation machineries is the lack of specificity (Worm and Guldberg, 2002). The potential activation of genes that are normally silenced, but contribute to tumour initiation or progression in the activated state, may significantly limit the beneficial effects of these drugs. Future studies need to address these concerns and to focus on developing better strategies to reactivate specific genes.

5.7 Conclusions

DNA methylation is critical for the permanent, heritable silencing of gene transcription in mammals. Exciting new observations point to the importance of multiple layers of epigenetic modifications in the control of chromatin structure and gene expression. The complexities of the silencing process are just beginning to be elucidated in relation to other epigenetic mechanisms, and the complex interplay between these various epigenetic mechanisms will need to be investigated further.

With all the recent discoveries related to the interactions between DNMTs with various proteins or protein complexes, the roles of the methylation machinery in transcriptional regulation, chromatin structure, DNA repair, and genome stability will become a significant focus in the methylation field. By characterizing these interactions, the nature of methylation defects in cancer cells is likely to be clarified, with the potential of finding novel therapies to reverse aberrant methylation patterns and restore growth control in cancers. Investigation of the complex interaction between various epigenetic modulators can potentially shed new light on the fundamentals of various epigenetic processes, and the problems associated with their deregulation as they pertain to inherited human disorders and cancer.

Acknowledgements

We would like to thank Dr Daniel Weisenberger and Dr Gangning Liang for helpful discussions and critical reading of the manuscript. We also like to thank Dr Carvell T. Nguyen for help with the figure.

References

Antequera, F. and Bird, A. (1993*a*). CpG islands. *Experientia Supplementum*, **64**, 169–85.

Antequera, F. and Bird, A. (1993*b*). Number of CpG islands and genes in human and mouse. *Proc Natl Acad Sci USA*, **90**, 11995–9.

Avner, P. and Heard, E. (2001). X-chromosome inactivation: counting, choice and initiation. *Nat Rev Genet*, **2**, 59–67.

Baylin, S. B. and Herman, J. G. (2000). DNA hypermethylation in tumorigenesis: epigenetics joins genetics. *Trends Genet*, **16**, 168–74.

Bender, C. M., Zingg, J. M., and Jones, P. A. (1998). DNA methylation as a target for drug design. *Pharm Res*, **15**, 175–87.

Bestor, T. H. (2000). The DNA methyltransferases of mammals. *Hum Mol Genet*, **9**, 2395–402.

Bird, A. (1992). The essentials of DNA methylation. *Cell*, **70**, 5–8.

Bird, A. (2002). DNA methylation patterns and epigenetic memory. *Genes Dev*, **16**, 6–21.

Bird, A. P. (1986). CpG-rich islands and the function of DNA methylation. *Nature*, **321**, 209–13.

Chen, R. Z., Pettersson, U., Beard, C., Jackson-Grusby, L., and Jaenisch, R. (1998). DNA hypomethylation leads to elevated mutation rates. *Nature*, **395**, 89–93.

Cheng, J. C. (2003). Characterization of zebularine as an inhibitor of DNA methylation. *Department of Biochemistry and Molecular Biology*. USC/Keck School of Medicine, Los Angeles.

Cheng, J. C., Matsen, C. B., Gonzales, F. A., Ye, W., Greer, S., Marquez, V. E., Jones, P. A., and Selker, E. U. (2003). Inhibition of DNA methylation and reactivation of silenced genes by zebularine. *J Natl Cancer Inst*, **95**, 399–409.

Christman, J. K. (2002). 5-Azacytidine and 5-aza-2′-deoxycytidine as inhibitors of DNA methylation: mechanistic studies and their implications for cancer therapy. *Oncogene*, **21**, 5483–95.

Clark, S. J. and Melki, J. (2002). DNA methylation and gene silencing in cancer: which is the guilty party? *Oncogene*, **21**, 5380–7.

Clark, S. J., Harrison, J., and Frommer, M. (1995). CpNpG methylation in mammalian cells. *Nat Genet*, **10**, 20–7.

Costello, J. F. and Plass, C. (2001). Methylation matters. *J Med Genet*, **38**, 285–303.

Dahl, C., and Guldberg, P. (2003). DNA methylation analysis techniques. *Biogerontology*, **4**, 233–50.

Das, P. M., and Singal, R. (2004). DNA methylation and cancer. *J Clin Oncol*, **22**, 4632–42.

Ehrlich, M. (2003). Expression of various genes is controlled by DNA methylation during mammalian development. *J Cell Biochem*, **88**, 899–910.

Esteller, M. (2002). CpG island hypermethylation and tumor suppressor genes: a booming present, a brighter future. *Oncogene*, **21**, 5427–40.

Esteller, M., and Herman, J. G. (2002). Cancer as an epigenetic disease: DNA methylation and chromatin alterations in human tumours. *J Pathol*, **196**, 1–7.

Feinberg, A. P. (1999). Imprinting of a genomic domain of 11p15 and loss of imprinting in cancer: an introduction. *Cancer Res*, **59**, 1743s–46s.

Fraga, M. F. and Esteller, M. (2002). DNA methylation: a profile of methods and applications. *Biotechniques*, **33**, 632, 634, 636–49.

Gama-Sosa, M. A., Slagel, V. A., Trewyn, R. W., Oxenhandler, R., Kuo, K. C., Gehrke, C. W. et al. (1983). The 5-methylcytosine content of DNA from human tumors. *Nucleic Acids Res*, **11**, 6883–94.

Gardiner-Garden, M. and Frommer, M. (1987). CpG islands in vertebrate genomes. *J Mol Biol*, **196**, 261–82.

Geiman, T. M. and Robertson, K. D. (2002). Chromatin remodeling, histone modifications, and DNA methylation-how does it all fit together? *J Cell Biochem*, **87**, 117–25.

Gibbons, R. J., McDowell, T. L., Raman, S., O'Rourke, D. M., Garrick, D., Ayyub, H. et al. (2000). Mutations in ATRX, encoding a SWI/SNF-like protein, cause diverse changes in the pattern of DNA methylation. *Nat Genet*, **24**, 368–71.

Jackson, J. P., Lindroth, A. M., Cao, X., and Jacobsen, S. E. (2002). Control of CpNpG DNA methylation by the KRYPTONITE histone H3 methyltransferase. *Nature*, **416**, 556–60.

Jenuwein, T. and Allis, C. D. (2001). Translating the histone code. *Science*, **293**, 1074–80.

Jones, P. A. and Baylin, S. B. (2002). The fundamental role of epigenetic events in cancer. *Nat Rev Genet*, **3**, 415–28.

Jones, P. A. and Laird, P. W. (1999). Cancer epigenetics comes of age. *Nat Genet*, **21**, 163–7.

Karpf, A. R. and Jones, D. A. (2002). Reactivating the expression of methylation silenced genes in human cancer. *Oncogene*, **21**, 5496–503.

Lachner, M. and Jenuwein, T. (2002). The many faces of histone lysine methylation. *Curr Opin Cell Biol*, **14**, 286–98.

Lachner, M., O'Sullivan, R. J., and Jenuwein, T. (2003). An epigenetic road map for histone lysine methylation. *J Cell Sci*, **116**, 2117–24.

Lachner, M., O'Carroll, D., Rea, S., Mechtler, K., and Jenuwein, T. (2001). Methylation of histone H3 lysine 9 creates a binding site for HP1 proteins. *Nature*, **410**, 116–20.

Laird, P. W., and Jaenisch, R. (1994). DNA methylation and cancer. *Hum Mol Genet* 3 Spec No: 1487–95.

Laird, P. W. (2003). The power and the promise of DNA methylation markers. *Nat Rev Cancer*, **3**, 253–66.

Laird, P. W., Jackson-Grusby, L., Fazeli, A., Dickinson, S. L., Jung, W. E., Li, E. et al. (1995). Suppression of intestinal neoplasia by DNA hypomethylation. *Cell*, **81**, 197–205.

Lapeyre, J. N. and Becker, F. F. (1979). 5-Methylcytosine content of nuclear DNA during chemical hepatocarcinogenesis and in carcinomas which result. *Biochem Biophys Res Commun*, **87**, 698–705.

Li, E. (2002). Chromatin modification and epigenetic reprogramming in mammalian development. *Nat Rev Genet*, **3**, 662–73.

Luo, R. X. and Dean, D. C. (1999). Chromatin remodeling and transcriptional regulation. *J Natl Cancer Inst*, **91**, 1288–94.

Marks, P., Rifkind, R. A., Richon, V. M., Breslow, R., Miller, T., and Kelly, W. K. (2001). Histone deacetylases and cancer: causes and therapies. *Nat Rev Cancer*, **1**, 194–202.

Momparler, R. L., and Bovenzi, V. (2000). DNA methylation and cancer. *J Cell Physiol*, **183**, 145–54.

Nguyen, C. T., Weisenberger, D. J., Velicescu, M., Gonzales, F. A., Lin, J. C., Liang, G., and Jones, P. A. (2002). Histone H3-lysine 9 methylation is associated with aberrant gene silencing in cancer cells and is rapidly reversed by 5-aza-2′-deoxycytidine. *Cancer Res*, **62**, 6456–61.

Pfeifer, G. P., Tang, M., and Denissenko, M. F. (2000). Mutation hotspots and DNA methylation. *Curr Top Microbiol Immunol*, **249**, 1–19.

Plass, C. and Soloway, P. D. (2002). DNA methylation, imprinting and cancer. *Eur J Hum Genet*, **10**, 6–16.

Reik, W. and Walter, J. (2001). Genomic imprinting: parental influence on the genome. *Nat Rev Genet*, **2**, QJ;21–32.

Riggs, A. D. and Jones, P. A. (1983). 5-methylcytosine, gene regulation, and cancer. *Adv Cancer Res*, **40**, 1–30.

Robertson, K. D. (2002). DNA methylation and chromatin—unraveling the tangled web. *Oncogene*, **21**, 5361–79.

Robertson, K. D. and Wolffe, A. P. (2000). DNA methylation in health and disease. *Nat Rev Genet*, **1**, 11–9.

Rountree, M. R., Bachman, K. E,. and Baylin, S. B. (2000). DNMT1 binds HDAC2 and a new co-repressor,

DMAP1, to form a complex at replication foci. *Nat Genet*, **25**, 269–77.

Santos-Rosa, H., Schneider, R., Bannister, A. J., Sherriff, J., Bernstein, B. E., Emre, N. C. et al. (2002). Active genes are tri-methylated at K4 of histone H3. *Nature*, **419**, 407–11.

Soares, J., Pinto, A. E., Cunha, C. V., Andre, S., Barao, I., Sousa, J. M., and Cravo, M. (1999). Global DNA hypomethylation in breast carcinoma: correlation with prognostic factors and tumor progression. *Cancer*, **85**, 112–8.

Strahl, B. D. and Allis, C. D. (2000). The language of covalent histone modifications. *Nature*, **403**, 41–5.

Takai, D. and Jones, P. A. (2002). Comprehensive analysis of CpG islands in human chromosomes 21 and 22. *Proc Natl Acad Sci USA*, **99**, 3740–5.

Takai, D., Gonzales, F. A., Tsai, Y. C., Thayer, M. J., and Jones, P. A. (2001). Large scale mapping of methylcytosines in CTCF-binding sites in the human H19 promoter and aberrant hypomethylation in human bladder cancer. *Hum Mol Genet*, **10**, 2619–26.

Tamaru, H. and Selker, E. U. (2001). A histone H3 methyltransferase controls DNA methylation in *Neurospora crassa*. *Nature*, **414**, 277–83.

Walsh, C. P., Chaillet, J. R., and Bestor, T. H. (1998). Transcription of IAP endogenous retroviruses is constrained by cytosine methylation. *Nat Genet*, **20**, 116–7.

Worm, J. and Guldberg, P. (2002). DNA methylation: an epigenetic pathway to cancer and a promising target for anticancer therapy. *J Oral Pathol Med*, **31**, 443–9.

Wu, J. and Grunstein, M. (2000). 25 years after the nucleosome model: chromatin modifications. *Trends Biochem Sci*, **25**, 619–23.

Yoder, J. A., Walsh, C. P., and Bestor, T. H. (1997). Cytosine methylation and the ecology of intragenomic parasites. *Trends Genet*, **13**, 335–40.

Zhang, Y., LeRoy, G., Seelig, H. P., Lane, W. S., and Reinberg, D. (1998). The dermatomyositis-specific autoantigen Mi2 is a component of a complex containing histone deacetylase and nucleosome remodeling activities. *Cell*, **95**, 279–89.

CHAPTER 6

Molecular cytogenetics of cancer

Denise Sheer and Janet M. Shipley

6.1 Introduction

Cancer arises from the accumulation of genetic changes which confer a selective advantage to the cells in which they occur. These changes consist of mutations, and numerical and structural chromosome aberrations. They usually occur in somatic cells, but certain genetic changes can be inherited and cause a predisposition to cancer (Lengauer et al., 1998; Balmain et al., 2003; see also Chapter 3).

Recurrent and sometimes highly specific chromosome aberrations are present in different types of cancer. Molecular genetic analysis of these aberrations has identified numerous genes which contribute to tumorigenesis, opening new avenues of research into regulatory pathways in the cell. Chromosome aberrations are increasingly playing a role in clinical management of cancer patients, since they can provide critical diagnostic and prognostic information. Tumour-specific chromosome aberrations act as tumour markers and can be used to monitor the effectiveness of therapy. Identification of genes affected by these aberrations have started to provide novel targets for innovative cancer therapy.

Human somatic cells normally have 46 chromosomes and are described as diploid. Chromosome analysis is conventionally carried out on cells during the metaphase stage of mitosis (cell division) when the chromosomes become visible as distinct entities. After each chromosome in a cell is identified by its characteristic size, shape, and staining properties, a karyotype displaying the full chromosome complement of the cell can be prepared.

The first recurrent chromosome aberration to be described in a human tumour was the 'Philadelphia chromosome', an unusually small chromosome found in chronic myeloid leukaemia (CML) in 1960 by Nowell and Hungerford in Philadelphia. This discovery aroused considerable interest in cancer cytogenetics as it gave the first direct evidence for a consistent genetic alteration in a tumour.

The search that followed for abnormalities in other tumour types was hampered by difficulties in defining chromosome aberrations using current staining methodology, by the apparent variation in chromosome abnormalities from one tumour to the next, and by the finding of aneuploidy (abnormal chromosome numbers) and multiple rearrangements (abnormal breakage and rejoining of chromosomes) in many tumours.

The introduction of chromosome banding techniques in 1970 revolutionized cancer cytogenetics. Consistent chromosome aberrations were shown in other types of tumours. Chromosome aberrations in different cells of a tumour were found to be related to one another, and further aberrations were shown to occur during tumour progression. Methods for improving yields of dividing cells and for high resolution banding of elongated chromosomes were developed in the 1980s. Developments in fluorescence *in situ* hybridization (FISH) and molecular genetic analysis have led to more precise definition of rearrangements as well as the identification of previously undetected rearrangements.

Our current understanding of the significance of consistent chromosome aberrations in cancer will be reviewed below. Evidence that these aberrations are non-random has come from cytogenetic analysis of large numbers of human tumours. These have been catalogued in the Mitelman Database of Chromosome Aberrations in Cancer, which can be accessed via the 'Cancer Genome Anatomy Project' website, (http://cgap.nci.nih.gov/). Another excellent website is the 'Atlas of Genetics and Cytogenetics in Oncology and Haematology' (http://www.infobiogen.fr/services/chromcancer/).

6.2 Methodology

6.2.1 Cytogenetic analysis

Methods and theoretical background to cytogenetic and FISH analysis of tumours can be found in Rooney et al. (2001). Ideally, cytogenetic studies are performed before a patient has undergone radiotherapy or chemotherapy as these treatments generate secondary genetic instability. Leukaemias are analysed from bone marrow aspirates, or peripheral blood samples if the white cell count is high, by immediate processing (direct preparation) or after *in vitro* culture for 24–72 h. The cells in solid tumours often have to be physically or enzymatically separated and may have a low mitotic index. Direct preparations, short- or long-term cultures, and cell lines from solid tumours are all used as sources of metaphase spreads. However, direct preparations are preferable to avoid difficulties in distinguishing aberrations generated *in vivo* from those generated *in vitro*.

Chromosomes are conventionally examined during or just prior to the metaphase stage of mitosis when they become condensed and can easily be seen under the microscope. DNA replication occurs before mitosis so that each chromosome consists of two identical sister chromatids held together at the centromere. When making chromosome preparations, colchicine or a related agent is added to the tumour cells to arrest them in metaphase. The cells are then swollen in a hypotonic solution, fixed in methanol–acetic acid, and metaphase 'spreads' prepared by dropping the fixed cells onto microscope slides. Chromosomes can be identified by staining techniques which produce a characteristic series of bands along the chromosomes, or by using FISH as described below.

6.2.2 Fluorescence *in situ* hybridization

Fluorescence *in situ* hybridization has become an essential tool for gene mapping and characterization of chromosome aberrations. DNA probes which are specific for single loci, chromosomal regions or whole chromosomes are chemically modified, usually by incorporation of biotin and/or digoxygenin, and are then hybridized to complementary sequences in denatured metaphase chromosomes. After removal of unbound probe by washing, hybridized sequences are detected using avidin, which binds strongly to biotin, and/or antibodies to digoxygenin, coupled to fluorescein isothiocyanate (FITC), Texas red, or another fluorochrome. As the target DNA remains intact, unlike in molecular genetic analysis, information is obtained directly about the positions of probes in relation to chromosome bands or to other hybridized probes, enabling chromosome aberrations to be defined.

Spectral karyotyping (SKY) or multiplex-FISH (M-FISH) techniques have recently provided a means for unambiguous identification of all chromosomes within a metaphase spread. FISH is performed simultaneously with paint probes for each chromosome labelled with unique combinations of fluorochromes.

It is often difficult to obtain chromosome spreads from solid tumours. FISH performed on interphase nuclei from tumour biopsies or cultured tumour cells allows cytogenetic aberrations to be visualized without the need for chromosome preparations. This procedure is called 'interphase cytogenetics', and is useful for rapid detection of aberrations which give diagnostic or prognostic information. Another approach which does not rely on tumour chromosome preparations is termed comparative genomic hybridization (CGH). CGH has been used extensively to identify chromosomal regions of loss, gain and amplification (http://www.ncbi.nlm.nih.gov/sky/). Control and tumour DNA samples are labelled with two different fluorochromes and co-hybridized to normal human metaphase chromosomes. The ratios of fluorochromes are then measured along each target chromosome. Regions with non-equivalent fluorescence ratios are thus identified as regions of chromosomal gain or loss in the tumour, enabling the whole genome to be screened in one experiment.

6.3 Terminology and types of chromosome aberrations in tumours

Karyotypes are described according to an International System for Human Cytogenetic Nomenclature (Mitelman, 1995). The total chromosome number is listed first, then the sex chromosomes, then gains and losses of whole chromosomes, and finally structural rearrangements. The short and long arms of chromosomes are represented by 'p' and 'q', respectively. Gains and losses of whole chromosomes are identified by a ' + ' or a ' − ' before the chromosome number. 46,XY and 46,XX represent normal diploid male and female karyotypes, respectively. 47,XX, + 8 represents a female karyotype with an extra copy of chromosome 8.

Translocations are common structural chromosome aberrations in tumours and are derived from the interchange of segments from different chromosomes. They may be balanced (reciprocal), or unbalanced resulting in loss or gain of genetic material. Translocations are signified by 't'; the chromosomes involved are enclosed within a first set of brackets and the translocation breakpoints are enclosed within a second set of brackets. For example, t(9;22)(q34;q11) represents a reciprocal translocation between chromosomes 9 and 22 at bands 9q34 and 22q11, respectively. Outstanding reviews on chromosome translocations in cancer are found in Rabbitts (1994; 2001, see also other papers in the same issue of the journal).

Other structural aberrations include deletions, which may be interstitial or terminal, inversions, and isochromosomes. Deletions are signified by 'del', followed by the chromosome in one set of brackets and the breakpoint(s) in a second set of brackets. Thus, del(5)(q13q32) represents an interstitial deletion of bands 5q13 to 5q32, with breakage and rejoining of these bands. del(5)(q32) represents a terminal deletion of chromosome 5 from band 5q32 to the telomere. Inversions are signified by 'inv', so that inv(16)(p13;q22) represents an inversion within chromosome 16, with breakpoints occurring in bands p13 and q22. This inversion is present in acute myelomonocytic leukaemia with abnormal eosinophils (AML-M4Eo). Isochromosomes are derived from loss of either the long or the short arm of the chromosome with the duplication of the other arm. They are signified by an 'i'. Thus an i(17)(q10) or i(17q), which is frequently seen in many types of tumour, consists of the duplicated long arm of chromosome 17.

Amplified chromosomal regions often manifest as homogeneously staining regions (HSRs) or small acentric (centromere-lacking) chromosomes known as double minute (DM) chromosomes. Thus, hsr(2)(q31) in a karyotype represents a homogeneously staining region in band 2q31. DM chromosomes are signified by 'dmin' after descriptions of other chromosome aberrations.

Only clonal chromosome aberrations are reviewed here. Clonal structural aberrations and chromosome gains are conventionally defined as being seen in at least two cells of a tumour. Clonal chromosome loss (monosomy) is defined as being seen in at least three cells. Although these may seem very few cells to be considered definitive, both the presence of normal cells in tumour preparations and the difficulty of getting metaphase spreads from tumours can hamper karyotype analysis from large numbers of tumour cells.

6.4 Mechanisms underlying chromosome aberrations

A central feature of many malignancies is the presence of aneuploidy. Abnormal chromosome segregation during mitosis results in gain or loss of chromosomes. This can occur sporadically, which is likely to be the case in leukaemias that have relatively stable karyotypes. However, defects in proteins associated with the mitotic machinery, such as centrosomes, microtubules, and kinetochores, may lead to continuous chromosome missegregation resulting in aneuploidy and chromosome instability (Pihan and Doxsey, 1999). Abnormal centrosomes are often found in carcinomas. For example, the *AuRKA* gene, whose product is associated with centrosome regulation, is mutated in breast and colorectal carcinomas. Defects in genes involved in mitotic checkpoints that sense whether chromosomes and the spindle are correctly aligned are also proposed to contribute to aneuploidy (Jallepalli and Lengauer, 2001). Examples of these are the *BUB* and *MAD* genes, which are mutated in different tumour types including lung and colorectal carcinomas.

The rate at which chromosome aberrations occur is also influenced by internal and external agents which damage DNA, or affect repair, replication, or recombination processes (Hoeijmakers, 2001). A major contributor to chromosome instability is telomere dysfunction (Hahn, 2003). Telomeres are protective caps at the ends of chromosomes which consist of long tandem arrays of the sequence TTAGGG. These telomeric sequences act, together with telomere-binding proteins, as a buffer against the progressive loss of DNA that inevitably occurs during replication of chromosome ends due to lagging strand synthesis. At each cell division, telomeres gradually become shorter, finally triggering the damage-response pathway and replicative senescence (growth arrest). Tumours bypass the damage-response pathway (e.g. from *TP53* mutation), enabling chromosome instability to arise (Felsder et al., 2003). Another mechanism for achieving immortalization in tumour cells is to turn on expression of telomerase, a dedicated reverse transcriptase that synthesizes telomeric sequences, but is normally not found in human cells (see Chapter 10).

In B and T lymphoid cells, the Ig or *TCR* genes normally recombine during lymphocyte development. Translocations involving these genes are frequently found in B- and T-cell malignancies, where they are thought to be mediated by the enzymes, RAG1 and RAG2, that normally initiate V(D)J recombination (reviewed in Klein, 2000). In other tumour types, however, there is little evidence that recombinase enzymes are involved. Instead, the mis-repair of double-strand breaks leading to non-homologous end-joining is likely to play a role. The presence of small insertions, deletions, duplications, and inversions at certain breakpoints supports this proposal (Weimels and Greaves, 1999). Regions of the genome may be more susceptible to breakage or recombination events due to the presence of certain sequence motifs at or near translocation breakpoints. For example, Alu sequences, which are interspersed throughout the genome, have been associated with chromosomal rearrangements (Kolomietz et al., 2002). The possible significance of topoisomerase II binding sites close to the breakpoints in the *MLL* gene is discussed below.

Several models have been proposed for the development of gene amplification from molecular genetic analysis of sequences in the amplicon (Schwab, 1999). One of these, the 'breakage–fusion–bridge' mechanism, has been described for amplification of the *MET* oncogene in gastric sarcoma (Hellman et al., 2002). When a double-stranded break occurs, such as at a fragile site, this can lead to an uncapped chromatid carrying the selected gene. After replication, a dicentric chromosome is formed from the fusion of the uncapped sister chromatids. The chromosomal material forming a bridge between the two centromeres breaks during anaphase as the centromeres move to opposite poles. If the break occurs centromeric to the gene, duplication of the region between the breaks would occur in one of the daughter cells. Recurrent rounds of this process under appropriate selective conditions would lead to intrachromosomal amplification.

6.5 Molecular consequences of chromosome aberrations in tumours

Genes which are directly affected by chromosome aberrations can be grouped into two broad classes: cellular oncogenes and tumour suppressor genes (Chapters 7 and 8). The protein products of cellular oncogenes generally promote cell growth and division, inhibit differentiation or block apoptosis. They transmit signals to the genome via multiple regulatory pathways. When oncogenes become inappropriately activated, they stimulate cells to multiply relentlessly, forming a tumour. The protein products of tumour suppressor genes, on the other hand, normally constrain cell growth and division. Their removal or inactivation from the genome also results in relentless cell multiplication. The general principles of the roles played by chromosome aberrations in activating oncogenes and removing or inactivating tumour suppressor genes are given below.

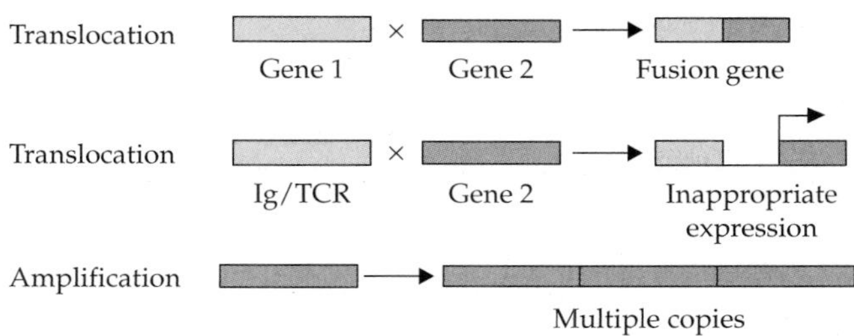

Figure 6.1 Chromosomal mechanisms of oncogene activation.

6.5.1 Activation of oncogenes

Chromosome aberrations and mutations activate cellular oncogenes in a dominant fashion. This means that only one activated oncogene is required to exert a tumorigenic effect. There are three basic chromosomal mechanisms for activating oncogenes (Figure 6.1):

(1) Fusion of the oncogene with a second gene at a translocation or inversion junction generating a chimaeric gene, mRNA, and protein. This mechanism is found predominantly in leukaemias, lymphomas, and sarcomas.
(2) Juxtaposition of the oncogene to regulatory elements in immunoglobulin or T-cell receptor genes in B- and T-lymphocyte malignancies, respectively, leading to inappropriate expression of the oncogene.
(3) Gene amplification (i.e. the generation of multiple gene copies), in DMs or HSRs, leading to overexpression. Gene amplification is a common feature of solid tumours, but is only occasionally seen in haematological malignancies.

6.5.2 Deletion of tumour suppressor genes

Analysis of constitutional deletions of chromosome 13 associated with hereditary retinoblastoma led to the development of the 'two-hit' model of tumorigenesis (Knudson, 1971). This model predicted that certain genes, which were later called 'tumour suppressor genes', exert a tumorigenic effect when both alleles become inactivated by mutation or chromosomal deletion. The first allele is inactivated either in the germ cells, where it confers dominant familial susceptibility to cancer, or in the somatic cells. The second allele is inactivated in the somatic cells. The mutation or deletion which is inherited as a dominant trait is thus recessive at the cellular level. This model was validated for retinoblastoma when the *RB* gene was cloned and shown to be mutated or deleted in a wide variety of malignancies. Since then, molecular studies of chromosome deletions and regions showing loss of heterozygosity (LOH) in a variety of hereditary and sporadic tumours have led to the discovery of other tumour suppressor genes, as described in Chapter 8.

6.6 Leukaemias and lymphomas

Leukaemias and lymphomas usually have few chromosome rearrangements. Chromosome numbers are in the diploid range, except for Hodgkin's disease which usually has chromosomes in the triploid–tetraploid range. The chromosome rearrangements are therefore relatively easy to define. Diagnosis of acute myeloid (AML) and lymphoid (ALL) leukaemias is usually based on the French–American–British (FAB) classification system that distinguishes morphological features of the leukaemic cells (Bennett et al., 1985). Consistent and, in some cases, highly specific chromosome aberrations have been found in the different forms of leukaemia and lymphoma (Tables 6.1–6.3) (Kuppers and Dalla-Favera, 2001; Kelly et al., 2002). For this reason, and also because certain aberrations are associated with different prognostic categories, chromosome aberrations have been integrated more recently into the WHO classification of leukaemia and lymphoma (Harris et al., 1999). Translocations and inversions in these tumours result in inappropriate activation of cellular oncogenes, many of which encode transcription factors that play essential roles in haemopoiesis (Look, 1998; Scandura et al., 2002). The presence of recurrent chromosome deletions as the sole visible chromosome changes, or in combination with other changes, indicates the involvement of tumour suppressor genes as well (Krug et al., 2002). Trisomies are sometimes the only visible aberrations in leukaemias. Mutations involving

Table 6.1 Examples of recurrent chromosome aberrations in myeloid malignancies

Malignancy	Chromosome aberration	Affected genes
CML	t(9;22)(q34;q11)	*ABL, BCR*
CML blast crisis	(9;22)(q34;q11), +8, +Ph, +19, or i(17q)	*ABL, BCR, TP53*
AML-M2	t(8;21)(q22;q22)	*ETO, AML1*
APL-M3, M3V	t(15;17)(q22;q11.2)	*PML, RARA*
AMMoL-M4Eo	inv(16)(p13q22) or t(16;16)(p13;q22)	*MYH11, CBFB*
AMMoL-M4/M5	t(4;11)(q21;q23)	*AF4, MLL*
	t(6;11)(q27;q23)	*AF6, MLL*
	t(9;11)(p22;q23)	*AF9, ML*
	t(10;11)(p12;q23)	*AF10, MLL*
	t(11;17)(q23;q21)	*AF17, MLL*
	t(11;19)(q23;p13)	*ENL, MLL*
AML-M7 (infants)	t(1;22)(p13;q13)	*OTT, MAL*
AML	t(6;9)(p23;q34)	*DEK, CAN*
	t(3;21)(q26;q22)	*EAP/EVI1/MDS1, AML1*[a]
	−5 or del(5q), −7 or del(7q), +8, t(12p) or del(12p)	
Therapy-related AML	t(3;21)(q26;q22)	*EAP/EVI1/MDS1, AML1*[a]
	t(9;11)(p22;q23)	*AF9, MLL*
	−5 or del(5q)	
	−7 or del(7q)	

[a] In this translocation, the *AML1* gene can fuse with either the *EAP, EVI1*, or *MDS1* genes at 3q26.

Table 6.2 Examples of prognostic associations in myeloid and lymphoid malignancies

	Prognosis		
Malignancy	Good	Intermediate	Poor
CML blast crisis			+Ph, +8, i(17q), or +19
AML	t(8;21) t(15;17) inv(16)	del(7q), del(9q), abn 11q23, +22, Other structural and numerical abnormalities, No abnormality	abn 3q, −5 or del(5q), −7, complex karyotypes, +8[a], +11[a], +13[a], +21[a]
ALL	>50 chromosomes t(12;21), t(10;14) +4, +10	47–50 chromosomes	<47 chromosomes ~96 chromosomes t(9;22), t(8;14)[b] t(1;19)[b] t(4;11), t(11;19)

Adapted from Grimwade et al. (1998), Farag et al. (2002), and Ferrando and Look (2000).

[a] These trisomies are associated with poor prognosis when they are the sole chromosome change.

[b] Although these translocations are markers of poor prognosis, recent therapeutic advances have greatly improved the outlook for patients with leukaemias carrying them.

the *FLT3, RAS*, and *KIT* genes have been recognized as playing an essential role in leukaemogenesis (Kelly et al., 2002). Their occurrence, together with specific chromosome aberrations in some leukaemias, indicates that they constitute the 'second hit' during transformation.

6.6.1 Myeloid malignancies

Different subtypes of AML carry consistent and in some cases highly specific chromosome aberrations, some of which are described below and shown in Table 6.1. Prognostic associations of these aberrations are shown in Table 6.2. The most common numerical change in myeloid malignancies is trisomy 8, occurring together with other aberrations in about 9% of cases, and as a sole change in about 5–7% of cases (Paulsson et al., 2001). The significance of trisomy 8 is underscored by the presence of distinct expression profiles in AML with trisomy 8 and AML with normal karyotypes (Virtaneva et al., 2001).

Table 6.3 Examples of recurrent chromosome rearrangements in lymphoid malignancies (excluding Ig and TCR rearrangements)

Malignancy	Chromosome aberration	Afffected genes
pre-B ALL	t(1;19)(q23;p13.3)	*PBX1, E2A*
pro-B ALL	t(17;19)(q22;p13.3)	*HLF, E2A*
ALL	t(9;22)(q34;q11)	*ABL, BCR*
	t(1;11)(p32;q23)	*EPS15, MLL*
	t(4;11)(q21;q23)	*AF4, MLL*
	t(6;11)(q27;q23)	*AF6, MLL*
	t(9;11)(p22;q23)	*AF9, MLL*
	t(11;17)(q23;q21)	*AF17, MLL*
	t(11;19)(q23;p13)	*ENL, MLL*
	t(X;11)(q13;q23)	*AFX1, MLL*
	del(9p)	CDKN2A/B
	del(6q)	
	del(11q), del(12p)	
CLL	+12	

See text for references.

Both myelodysplastic syndrome (MDS) and myeloproliferative disease (MPD) can evolve to an acute leukaemia indistinguishable clinically from *de novo* AML, but are more refractory to treatment. Certain chromosome deletions are common to MPD, MDS, and AML, reflecting the poor definition of boundaries between these conditions (Mauritzson et al., 2002). MDS and AML can arise as a late complication of cytotoxic therapy. Deletions or monosomy of chromosomes 5 and/or 7 are present in the majority of secondary AMLs which arise after therapy with alkylating agents, compared to an incidence of only 16% in patients with *de novo* AML. These deletions are also present in AML following exposure to pesticides and organic solvents (Cuneo et al., 1992). The putative tumour suppressor genes in the deleted regions of chromosomes 5 and 7 have not yet been identified. Many MDS and AML arising following therapy with topoisomerase II inhibitors have aberrations involving the *MLL* gene at band 11q23 or the *AML1* gene at band 21q22 (Pedersen-Bjergaard et al., 2002).

The Philadelphia chromosome—BCR–ABL *fusion*

Virtually all patients with CML have the Philadelphia (Ph) chromosome, resulting from the translocation of chromosomes 9 and 22, in their leukaemic cells (Figures 6.2 and 6.3). Approximately 70–80% of patients entering blast crisis show further chromosome abnormalities (Shet et al., 2002). These secondary changes are usually an extra Ph chromosome, trisomy 8, i(17q), or trisomy 19. A change in karyotype in CML is a grave prognostic sign, with death usually occurring within a few months. At a molecular level, the most frequent abnormality during blast crisis is mutation of the *TP53* gene associated with rearrangements of chromosome 17. About half of CML patients with a lymphoid blast crisis have homozygous deletions of the *CDKN2A* gene on chromosome 9.

The t(9;22)(q34;q11), which generates the Ph chromosome, results in the fusion of the *BCR* gene at band 22q11 with the cellular oncogene, *ABL*, at band 9q34 (reviewed in Laurent et al., 2000) The Ph chromosome also occurs in ALL (Section 6.5.2). *BCR* is a large gene of 130 kb containing many exons. It encodes a serine kinase. The ABL protein is a tyrosine kinase that contains a DNA binding domain. It appears to function as a negative regulator of cell growth, since overexpression causes cell cycle arrest. The translocation breakpoints in *BCR* usually occur in either of two introns within a small region, but in *ABL* they occur over a large distance of more than 200 kb. One of two alternative first exons normally used by the *ABL* gene becomes replaced by *BCR* sequences, generating a fused mRNA.

The BCR–ABL protein has constitutive tyrosine kinase activity and is present in the cytoplasm. It activates numerous signalling pathways, including the Ras, PI3K/AKT, and STAT pathways, leading to resistance to apoptosis, expansion of the malignant clone, and cell adhesion alterations. Experiments with mouse models have shown that the primary causal event in the chronic phase of CML is the formation of the fusion BCR–ABL protein. Additional, less consistent events are needed for blast crisis. A major development in the treatment of CML in recent years is the use of a potent inhibitor of BCR–ABL kinase activity, called Gleevec, Imatinib, or STI571 (Clarkson et al., 2003). The drug is highly effective against CML in the chronic phase, but not in the acute phase. However, some patients on long-term treatment have developed drug resistance due to the presence of additional genetic aberrations.

t(8;21)(q22;q22)—AML1–ETO *fusion*

This translocation occurs in about 40% of all cases of AML-M2, and at a lower frequency in AML-M1 and -M4. AML-M2 patients with the translocation have a higher remission rate than those without it. The chimaeric gene generated from the *AML1* gene at 21q22 and the *ETO* gene at 8q22 greatly enhances self-renewal of the haemopoietic stem cell

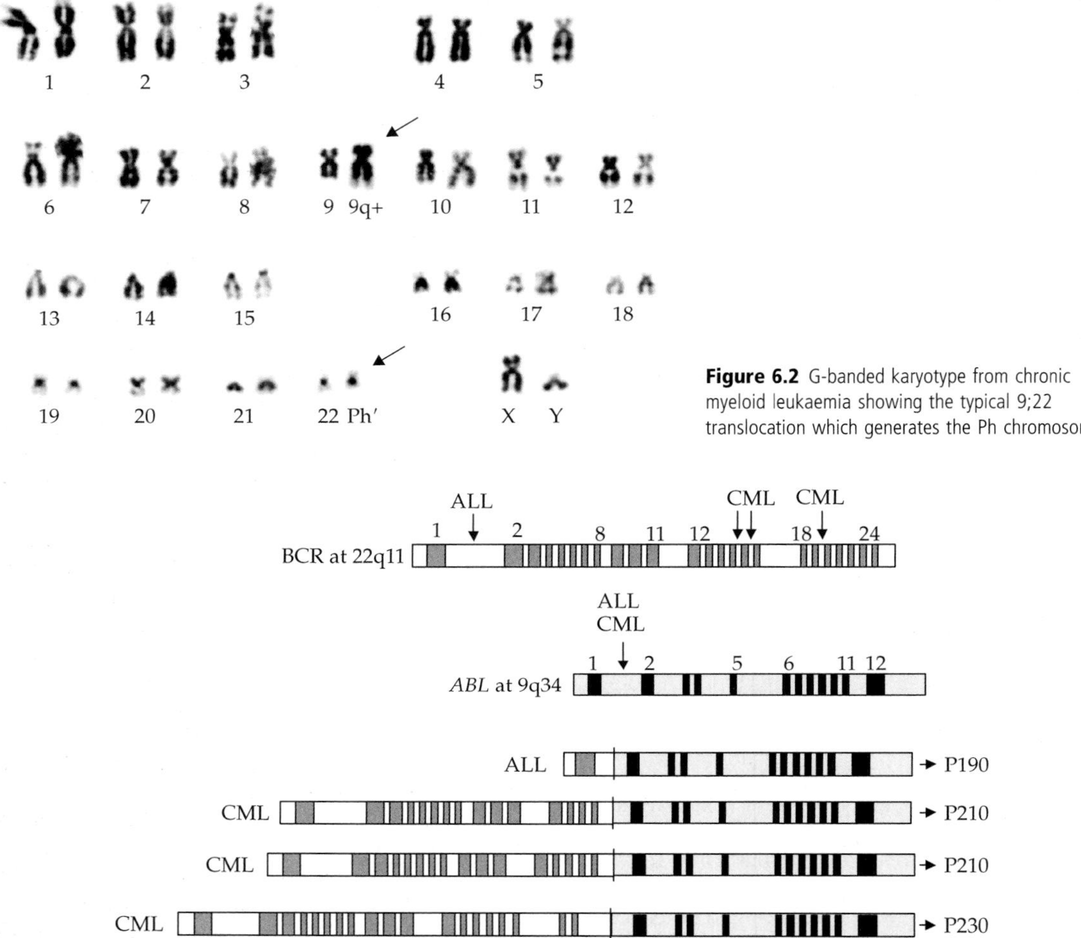

Figure 6.2 G-banded karyotype from chronic myeloid leukaemia showing the typical 9;22 translocation which generates the Ph chromosome.

Figure 6.3 Translocations of the *BCR* and *ABL* genes in chronic myeloid leukaemia (CML) and acute lymphoblastic leukaemia (ALL) generate fusion genes of different configurations. The sizes of the proteins encoded by each of the fusion genes is given on the right (adapted from Heisterkamp and Groffen, 2002).

population and blocks differentiation of committed progenitor cells (Mulloy et al., 2002).

The *AML1/RUNX1/CBFA2* gene encodes a transcription factor that is critical for haemopoiesis and is expressed constitutively in all haemopoietic cell lines studied so far. The AML1 protein contains a DNA- and protein-binding region which is homologous both to the CBFA (PEBP2a) component of the mouse core binding factor (CBF), and to the Drosophila segmentation gene *runt*. CBF in the mouse binds to the core site of polyomavirus and to the enhancers of T-cell receptor genes. The *ETO* gene is not normally expressed in myeloid cells. It has two putative zinc finger-DNA binding domains and a transcriptional activation domain. The AML1–ETO fusion protein contains the DNA-binding domain of *AML1*, but not its transcriptional activation domain, and almost the entire length of *ETO*.

The importance of the *AML1* gene in leukaemia is emphasized by the variety of aberrations that subvert its activity. For example, loss of function mutations of the gene are present in AML-M2, AML-M0, and in AML or MDS in Down's syndrome patients. A translocation between *AML1* and the *TEL* gene on chromosome 12 is found in *ALL* (Section 6.2 and Chapter 18). The gene encoding the second component of the core binding factor (CBFB) is a target of chromosome 16 inversions and translocations in AML.

t(15;17)(q22;q11.2–12)—PML–RARA *fusion*

This translocation is only found in acute promyelocytic leukaemia, AML-M3. The translocation breakpoints occur within the retinoic acid receptor alpha (*RARA*) gene on chromosome 17 and the *PML* gene on chromosome 15, generating a chimaeric *PML–RARA* gene (Melnick and Licht, 1999). In normal cells, the PML protein forms distinct nuclear bodies which contain other proteins involved in diverse pathways. In APL cells, a fine granular pattern is present in the nucleus instead of PML nuclear bodies. The PML protein has a set of zinc fingers known as the B-box and RING finger domains, which are involved in protein–protein interactions and are necessary for PML nuclear body formation. Other domains include a coiled-coil region and a nuclear localization signal. Despite intensive research, definitive functions for PML have remained unclear.

RARα is a transcription factor that normally binds to all-*trans* retinoic acid (ATRA). The protein has a zinc finger region, with which it binds to retinoic acid response elements (RARE) in the promotors of many genes, and a transcriptional activation domain. RARα is involved in myeloid differentiation through its ability to activate transcription via RAREs. The PML–RARA fusion protein retains most of the functional domains of the RARA and PML proteins, and blocks haemopoietic differentiation. Variant translocations have been described in APL, all involving the *RARA* gene. A dramatic advance in the treatment of APL has come from the use of retinoic acid which induces terminal differentiation of APL blasts into mature granulocytes, accompanied by the formation of PML nuclear bodies. When combined with anthracyclin-based chemotherapy, complete remission can be achieved in about 70% of cases (Mistry et al., 2003).

t(11q23)—MLL fusions

Reciprocal translocations affecting the *MLL* gene (mixed lineage leukaemia, also called the *ALL-1*, *HTRX* gene) at chromosome band 11q23 are present in about 10% of all *de novo* AMLs and ALLs (reviewed in Rowley, 1998), and in about 80% of AML and ALL arising in infants. *MLL* translocations are also found in almost all secondary AMLs in patients who have received chemotherapeutic drugs that inhibit topoisomerase II, such as etoposide for a primary tumour. Over 50 different translocations have been identified, and the fusion partners in about half of these have been cloned and sequenced. The most frequent translocation is the t(4;11)(q21;q23), which is found in about 4% of childhood pro-B ALL. *MLL* translocations are generally associated with a very poor prognosis.

The *MLL* gene is a large gene spanning 100 kb (Figure 6.4), which encodes a protein of 3968 amino acids. The N-terminal half has three AT hooks, which bind to the minor groove of DNA, the SNL1 and SNL2 subnuclear localization regions, a methyltransferase region, and a zinc finger domain, called a plant homologous domain (PHD). Transactivation and SET domains are located at the C-terminal end. During embryogenesis, the protein maintains the correct expression of *HOX* genes, probably by controlling chromatin structure through its methyltransferase activity and its ability to assemble a large complex of chromatin modifying proteins (Nakamura et al., 2002). Translocation breakpoints are clustered in the PHD region, resulting in the AT hooks, methyltransferase, SNL1 and SNL2 regions being retained in the chimaeric protein, but most of the the PHD and the C-terminal half including the SET domain being replaced by sequences from the partner gene.

Many of the partner genes have roles in transcription, encoding transcription factors and transcriptional co-activators. Analysis of translocations involving these partner genes has shown that they provide heterologous transcriptional effector properties to the fusion genes (Ayton and Cleary, 2001). Other partner genes which encode cytoplasmic proteins have no known roles in transcriptional regulation. Two of the translocations have been shown to exert their oncogenic effect by homo- or oligomerization of the fusion proteins mediated by coiled-coil interaction domains in the partner genes (So et al., 2003). In mouse cells this leads to upregulation of the *Hoxa7*, *-a9*, and *-a10* genes, and the Hox co-factor gene *Meis1*, which are normally repressed in myeloid progenitor cells. This is significant since this upregulation of *HOX* genes is reported as a key outcome in *MLL* fusions involving partner genes encoding proteins involved in transcriptional regulation (Armstrong et al., 2002; So et al., 2003). Furthermore, upregulation of *Hoxa7* and *HoxA9* has been shown to be essential for transformation of myeloid progenitors by MLL fusion proteins (Ayton and Cleary, 2003).

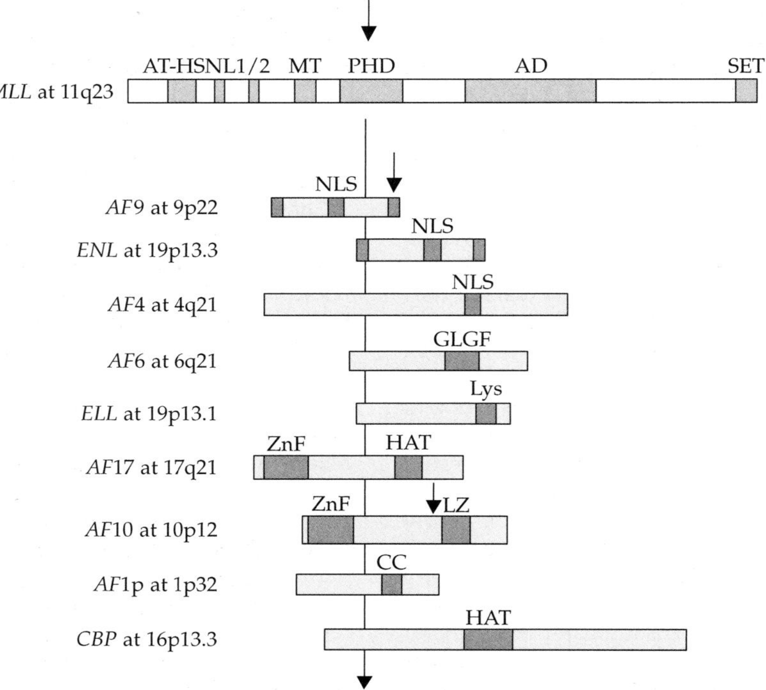

Figure 6.4 Translocations between *MLL* and partner genes in leukaemias are depicted by showing the breaks (arrowed) on the proteins encoded by the genes. In each translocation, the AT hooks, subnuclear localization signal domains, the methyltransferase domain and part of the PHD domain of *MLL* are fused to the region to the right of the vertical arrow on each translocation partner. Domains are shown as follows: AT-H: AT hook; SNL1/2: subnuclear localization domains 1 and 2; MT: methyltransferase; PHD: plant homeodomain; TA: transactivation; SET: SETdomain; NLS: nuclear localization; GLGF: GLGF; Lys: lysine-rich; ZnF: Zinc finger; HAT: histone acetyltransferase; CC: coiled coil; LZ: leucine zipper (adapted from Rowley, 1998).

Several Alu repeat sequences, a DNA hypersensitive site, and a topoisomerase II cleavage site have been found close to the breakpoint region in the *MLL* gene (Strissel et al., 1998). Topoisomerase II plays an essential role in untangling chromatids after DNA replication, first making a double-strand break in the DNA, unwinding the strands, and then re-ligating them. Topoisomerase II inhibiting drugs prevent re-ligation, resulting in double-strand breaks and possibly joining of non-homologous chromosomes. Patients with secondary leukaemia who have been treated with these drugs might have specific sensitivity in this region of the *MLL* gene for breakage.

6.6.2 Lymphoid malignancies

Recurrent chromosome aberrations in lymphoid malignancies include translocations, inversions, and deletions, as well as numerical abnormalities (Look, 1998; Ferrando and Look., 2000; Takeuchi et al., 2003). The translocations and inversions can either generate chimaeric genes (Table 6.3), or cause overexpression of oncogenes as a result of juxtaposition with adjacent regulatory sequences from immunoglobulin or T-cell receptor genes, which are normally highly active in lymphoid cells. Examples are given below.

The prognosis for children with ALL has improved dramatically, with the majority of patients being cured with intensive therapy. Chromosome aberrations in ALL are of particular importance as they are clear indicators of prognosis in both adults and children (Table 6.2). A hyperdiploid karyotype (51–59 chromosomes) is usually present in ALL in young children. The prognosis in this category is good, and over 75% of patients achieve long-term survival following treatment. Hypodiploidy in ALL is relatively rare but indicates a very poor prognosis as does the translocation, t(9;22) (q34;q12). This translocation is present in about 30% of adult ALL and about 5% of childhood ALL, where it generates a chimaeric *BCR–ABL* gene, with a smaller segment of *BCR* than in CML (Figure 6.3). The t(4;11)(q21;q23), resulting in fusion of the *MLL* gene, is found primarily in very immature, pre-B ALL in infants where it is associated with an extremely poor prognosis.

t(12;21)(p13;q22)—TEL–AML1 *fusion*

The t(12;21)(p13;q22) causes a fusion between the *TEL* gene on chromosome 12 and the *AML1* gene at 21q22, which has been described above. This translocation occurs in about 25% of all childhood ALL, often occurs *in utero*, as described in Chapter 18, and is associated with a good response to therapy. The second *TEL* allele is commonly deleted at a later time from cells with the translocation. The TEL protein is a basic helix–loop–helix (bHLH) transcription protein of the ETS family. The fusion product has the HLH domain of TEL joined to all the functional domains of the AML1 protein, including the DNA binding and transactivation domains. The role of the fusion protein in malignant transformation is thus likely to involve subversion of normal TEL and AML1 transcriptional activities.

t(1;19)(q23;p13)—E2A–PBX1 *fusion*

This translocation occurs in about 25% of childhood and 5% of adult pre-B ALL. The E2A protein normally heterodimerizes with other bHLH transcription factors to regulate gene expression during development. PBX-1 is normally involved in cell differentiation and development through its interactions with HOX proteins. The resulting *E2A–PBX1* chimaeric gene has the transactivator domains of *E2A* fused to the DNA-binding homeodomain of *PBX-1*. The fusion protein has been shown to block differentiation and induce cell proliferation. Although the translocation has been associated with a poor prognosis, the use of more intensive therapy has led to an improvement in outcome for these patients. A variant translocation in pre-B ALL, t(17;19)(q22;p13), similarly generates an *E2A–HLF* fusion gene in which the transactivator domains of E2A are fused to the DNA binding and protein dimerization bZIP (leucine zipper) domain of *HLF*. The fusion protein is suggested to interfere with the normal sensitivity of lymphoid cells to apoptotic stimuli.

Activation by the immunoglobulin and T-cell receptor loci

B-lymphocytes are responsible for immunoglobulin (Ig) mediated immunity, while T-lymphocytes play a role in cellular immunity after conditioning in the thymus. During B-lymphocyte maturation, somatic recombination of the Ig heavy (IgH) chain, and the *k* and *l* light chain loci precedes Ig production. Newly synthesized Ig molecules are retained in the cytoplasm and, only after further cellular maturation, are expressed on the cell surface. The *IgH*, *IgLκ*, and *IgLλ* loci are present on chromosome bands 14q32, 12p12, and 22q11, respectively. The T-cell receptor molecules are encoded by the *TCRα*, -β and -γ chain loci located at bands 14q11.2, 7q35, and 7p15, respectively.

In B- and T-cell malignancies, specific translocations and inversions place cellular oncogenes under the control of regulatory elements of the *Ig* or *TCR* loci (Figure 6.5) (Rabbitts, 1994; Klein, 2000; Willis and Dyer, 2000). These rearrangements are thought to arise from errors in the recombination process, as mentioned above. The primary effect of these translocations is dysregulated expression of the

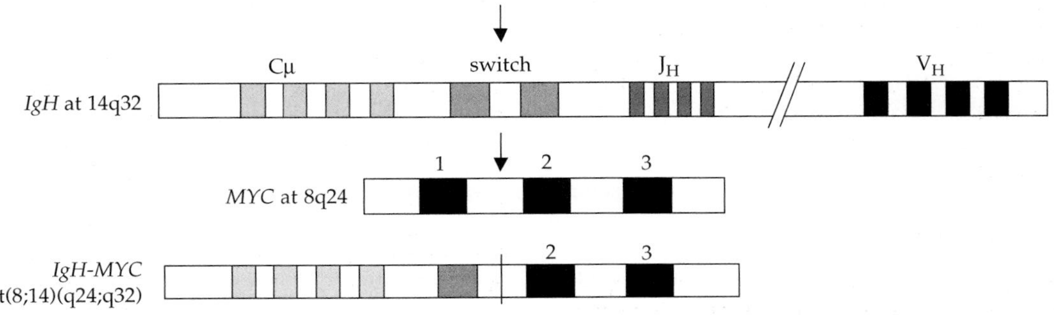

Figure 6.5 Activation of the *MYC* gene by juxtaposition with sequences from the *IgH* gene in Burkitt's lymphoma and B-cell ALL.

oncogene under the influence of the adjacent *Ig* or *TCR* sequences which may result in abnormally high expression levels. In some cases, the oncogene is also mutated.

Translocations involving the Ig genes are present in all Burkitt's lymphoma and also in other B-cell malignancies. The translocation t(8;14)(q24;q32), which is the most common, juxtaposes the *MYC* gene at band 8q24 and the *IgH* chain locus. In the other translocations, t(2;8)(p12;q24) and t(8;22)(q24;q11), *MYC* becomes juxtaposed to either the *IgLκ* or *λ* genes, respectively. Each of these rearrangements results in the constitutive expression of *MYC* throughout the cell cycle, instead of in early G1. As described in Chapter 7, *MYC* is a bHLH transcription factor which can function as both an activator and repressor, and plays a role in apoptosis and proliferation.

Approximately 80% of follicular lymphomas have a translocation in which the *IgH* locus at band 14q32 juxtaposes with the *BCL2* gene located at band 18q21, resulting in its constitutive high expression. *BCL2* encodes a small GTP-binding protein which is a key modulator of apoptosis. Overexpression of *BCL2* thus drives the cell through a continuous proliferative state. The *CCND1* gene at 11q13 is also activated by translocation with the *IgH* gene, leading to acceleration of the cell cycle through G1 phase. Another example is *BCL3*, encoding an Iκ-B type protein that regulates the rel/NF-κ-B family of transcription factors.

In T-cell lymphomas and acute leukaemias, specific translocations with TCR genes result in dysregulated expression of transcription factors which regulate haemopoiesis but are not normally expressed in T-lymphoid cells. These include the b-HLH genes, *TAL1/SCL, TAL2/SCL2*, and *LYL1* at bands 1p32, 9q32.1, and 19p13 respectively. Expression of MYC is similarly dysregulated in T-cell tumours. Other types of genes activated by juxtaposition with TCR sequences are *LMO1 (RBTN1), LMO2* (*RBTN2)*, and *HOX11* at bands 11p13, 11p15, and 10q24, respectively. The LMO1 and LMO2 proteins contain two LIM zinc finger-like domains that function in protein–protein interactions. LMO1 is normally expressed in the central nervous system. LMO2 is essential for yolk sac erythropoiesis and adult haemopoiesis. The LMO2 protein forms a transcriptional complex with TAL1 in several lineages, including erythroid, and in mouse T-cell leukaemias induced by these dysregulated genes. *HOX11*, which encodes a homeodomain transcription factor, is present in a variety of different tissues and is essential for development of the spleen. Translocations of HOX11 are associated with a favourable outcome in T-ALL.

6.7 Chromosomes in solid tumours

Identification of recurrent chromosome aberrations in solid tumours has been relatively slow. It is often difficult to obtain good metaphase preparations where each chromosome can be recognized by banding alone. The application of molecular cytogenetic techniques such as M-FISH/SKY and CGH has therefore been highly productive for these tumour types (Albertson et al., 2003) (Figure 6.6). Examples of recurrent chromosome aberrations found in solid tumours are described below and shown in Tables 6.4–6.6. The identification of some of these aberrations can be of direct benefit to the patient as it can enable an accurate diagnosis to be made, as well as an assessment of prognosis (Mitelman et al., 1997).

6.7.1 Sarcomas

Sarcomas are a heterogeneous group of mesenchymal tumours that display differentiated features of the various supporting tissues of the body. Although they constitute only a small proportion of all malignant tumours, great interest has been shown in their genetic aberrations (Bennicelli and Barr, 2002; Mackall et al., 2002) (Table 6.4). Many sarcomas have specific translocations that result in the formation of chimaeric genes encoding transcription factors which retain the DNA binding domain from one gene and the transcriptional transactivating domain from the other. Simple gain-of-function models focusing on transactivation were proposed initially for these rearrangements, but more recent evidence supports multiple and complex effects which are specific to the fusion genes. Examples of rearrangements in sarcomas are described below.

t(22q12)—EWS *fusions*

The *EWS* gene on chromosome 22 participates in specific translocations in at least five types of sarcomas (Figure 6.7). In each translocation analysed so far, the partner gene encodes a transcription factor. *EWS* itself encodes a ubiquitously expressed RNA binding protein consisting of two main functional domains. The N-terminal region contains a transcriptional transactivation domain, while the

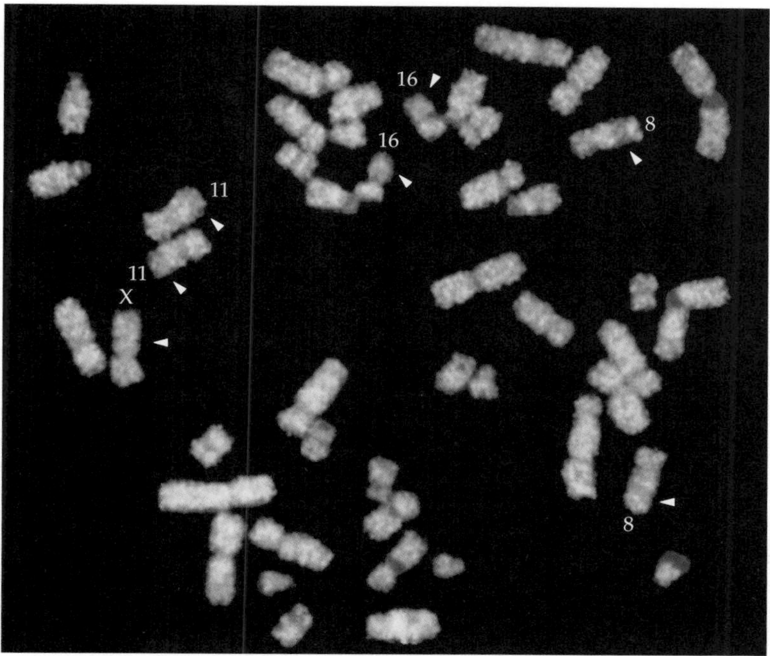

Figure 6.6 Comparative genomic hybridization experiment to determine genomic copy number changes in a primitive neuroectodermal tumour from a two-year old boy. Tumour and female control DNA were labelled with fluorescenin isothiocyanate (FITC) and Texas red, respectively. Regions of deletion are visualized in red (arrowed). The X-chromosome acts as an internal control as it appears red when male DNA (green) and female DNA (red) are co-hybridized to male metaphase chromosomes (See also plate 1).

C-terminal region contains an RNA binding domain. The common theme in all these translocations is that the chimaeric gene formed contains the transcriptional transactivating domain of *EWS* and the DNA binding domain of the partner gene.

The most common *EWS* translocation is the t(11;22)(q24;q12) present in virtually all Ewing's sarcomas and in peripheral neuroepitheliomas, also known as peripheral primitive neuroectodermal tumours (pPNET) (Ladanyi 2002). These malignancies, which affect children and adolescents, are believed to be of neuroectodermal origin and show varying degrees of neuronal differentiation. As a result of the 11;22 translocation, the *EWS* gene fuses with the *ETS*-related gene, *FLI-1*, on chromosome 11. Variant translocations are also present in a small proportion of pPNETs, resulting in the fusion of *EWS* with other *ETS*-related genes, such as *ETV1* or *ERG*. The fusion EWS–FLI-1 protein is able to transform mesenchyme-derived NIH3T3 cells, while inhibition of expression prevents tumorigenesis and leads to decreased cell proliferation. Several genes involved in cell cycle control and mitogenic signalling are emerging as targets of the EWS–FLI-1 fusion protein. These include *TGFBR2, CCND1*, and *MYC*. There is also evidence that EWS–FLI-1 and related proteins interfere with normal splicing processes. The p53 pathway is disrupted in about 30% of Ewing's sarcomas, either by *CDKN2A* deletion or *TP53* mutation. Patients showing these changes usually have a very poor outcome, possibly linked to the inability to launch an apoptotic response in cells carrying an EWS translocation.

t(X;18)(p11.2;q11.2)—SYT–SSX *fusions in synovial sarcoma*

Synovial sarcomas occur predominantly in adolescents and young adults and usually affect the extremities in the vicinity of the joints, such as the knee and lower thigh region. A specific translocation t(X;18)(p11.2;q11.2) is present in almost all cases, and fuses the *SYT* gene on chromosome 18 to one of the *SSX* genes on the X chromosome (Crew et al. 1995; dos Santos et al. 2001). SSX proteins co-localize in the nucleus with polycomb group proteins, while SYT interacts and colocalizes with

Table 6.4 Examples of recurrent chromosome aberrations in sarcomas

Tumour	Chromosome aberration	Affected genes
Benign tumours		
Lipoma	t(3;12)(q27–28;q13–14)	*HMGA2*
	t/ins(1;12)(p32–34;q13–15)	
	t/ins(12;21)q13–15;q21–22)	
	t(2;12)(p21–23;q13–14)	
	del(13)(q12q22)	
Uterine leiomyoma	del(7)(q22q32)	
	t(12;14)(q14–15;q23–24)	*HMGA2*
	−22	
	+12	
Malignant tumours		
Ewing's sarcoma and pPNET	t(11;22)(q24;q12)	*FLI-1, EWS*
	t(2;22)(q33;q12)	*FEV, EWS*
	t(7;22)(p22;q12)	*ETV1, EWS*
	t(17;22)(q21;q12)	*ETV4, EWS*
	t(21;22)(q22;q12)	*ERG, EWS*
Ewing's sarcoma	t(1;16)(q11–25;q11–24)	
Clear cell sarcoma	t(12;22)(q13;q12)	ATF1, *EWS*
Intra-abdominal small cell sarcoma	t(11;22)(p13;q12)	*WT1, EWS*
Extraskeletal myxoid chondrosarcoma	t(9;22)(q22;q12)	*DDIT3, EWS*
Alveolar rhabdomyosarcoma	t(2;13)(q35–37;q14)	*PAX3, FKHR*
Synovial sarcoma	t(X;18)(p11.2;q11.2)	*SSX1/SSX2/SSX4, SYT*
Myxoid liposarcoma	t(12;16)(q13;p11)	*CHOP, TLS/FUS*
Dermatofibrosarcoma protruberans	t(17;22)(q22;q13)	*COL1A, PDGFB*
Congenital fibrosarcoma	t(2;15)(p13;q25)	*ETV6, NTRK3*
Alveolar soft part sarcoma	t(X;17)(p11.2;q25)	*ASPL, TFE3*

Adapted from Sreekantaiah et al. (1994); Mackall et al. (2002).

the BRM protein. Tumours with the *SYT–SSX1* fusion gene are more likely than those with the *SYT-SSX2* to exhibit biphasic histology with both epithelial and spindle cell components. They also show a higher rate of proliferation and are associated with a poorer clinical outcome.

Aberrations in rhabdomyosarcoma

Rhabdomyosarcoma (RMS) is the most common soft tissue tumour in children. The alveolar form occurs in adolescents and young adults, while the embryonal form occurs in infants. Histologically, RMS resembles foetal skeletal muscle. The alveolar and embryonal forms have distinct genetic aberrations that can be used for diagnosis when it is not possible to use standard criteria, such as features of differentiation. Alveolar RMS usually have a t(2;13)(q35–37;q14) or, occasionally, variant translocations such as the t(1;13)(1p36.1;q14) (Anderson et al., 1999; Merlino and Helman, 1999). In these translocations, the forkhead transcription factor gene (FKHR) at 13q14, becomes fused with the transcription factor genes *PAX3* or *PAX7*, respectively. Both PAX3 and PAX7 have been found to play critical roles in muscle development. The resulting fusion proteins are more potent transcriptional activators than the wild-type PAX proteins, thereby causing dysregulation of downstream targets of PAX leading to aberrant myogenesis. It is remarkable that NIH-3T3 cells transfected with the *PAX3–FKHR* gene show upregulation of genes involved in myogenesis and muscle development, many of which are also highly expressed in RMS (Khan et al., 1999). Embryonal RMS do not have a specific translocation but almost invariably have allele loss at band 11p15 (Merlino and Helman, 1999). This region includes imprinted genes implicated in tumorigenesis, such as *IGF2* and *H19*. Both forms of RMS show disruption of genes in the p53 and Rb pathways.

Other aberrations in sarcomas

Other aberrations are frequently found together with specific translocations in sarcomas. These additional changes are likely to contribute to the

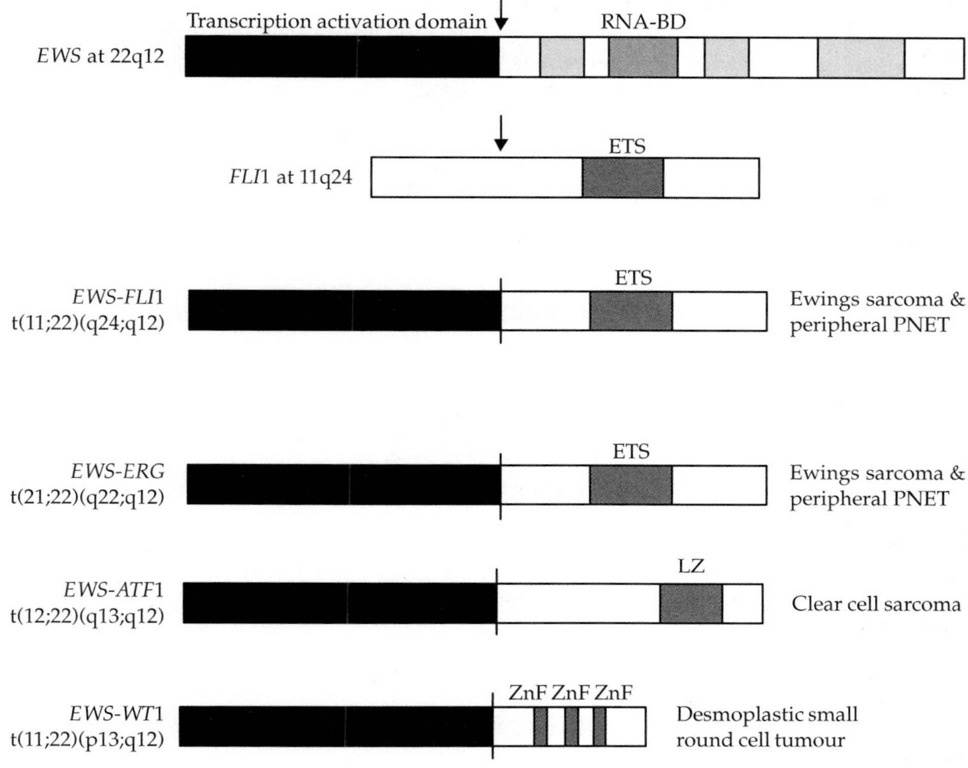

Figure 6.7 Diagram showing the EWS protein, the FLI-1 protein, and fusion proteins generated by translocations in Ewing's sarcoma and other soft tissue tumours. Domains are shown as follows: RNA-BD: RNA-binding domain, ETS: ETS domain, LZ: leucine zipper, ZnF: Zinc finger.

phenotype of the tumours and may indeed be essential for tumour development (Deneen and Denny, 2001). Several types of sarcomas, such as leiomyosarcomas and osteosarcomas do not have specific translocations but have complex and heterogeneous karyotypes. The *MDM2* gene which maps to band 12q13 is frequently co-amplified in sarcomas with several other genes from this band, including *CDK4*, *GLI*, *SAS*, and *CHOP* (Table 6.6). Overexpression of MDM2 or p53 in soft tissue tumours correlates with poor prognosis and short survival times. The CDK4 protein, when complexed with cyclin D1, governs progression through G1 of the cell cycle by phosphorylating the RB protein.

The recent finding of *KIT* mutations in gastrointestinal stromal tumours (GISTs) has identified these tumours as a distinct entity and facilitated a targeted approach to treatment. The tyrosine kinase inhibitor STI571 has been described above for treatment of CML. The clinical efficacy of the drug against the mutated *KIT* gene product in GISTs has been described (Tuveson et al., 2001). In addition, STI571 has been shown to inhibit the *COL1A1–PDGFB* fusion gene product associated with dermatofibrosarcoma protruberans, and may in time constitute an effective treatment strategy in these tumours.

6.7.2 Carcinomas

Carcinomas often have gross aneuploidy, many chromosome rearrangements, and considerable variability from cell-to-cell within the same tumour and between tumours of the same type. It is thus important to karyotype substantially more cells than for other tumour types and from different regions of the tumour if possible, in order to derive a representative genetic profile. However, whole genome techniques, such as CGH and analysis of LOH, have played a major role in the identification of recurrent genetic aberrations, particularly genomic gains and losses. Chromosome deletions are often large, possibly indicating the presence of multiple tumour suppressor genes. Gene mutations are prevalent, as described in Chapters 7 and 8. Gene inactivation by methylation has also been recognized. Gene amplification is common in carcinomas and is often associated with advanced stages of malignancy. Examples of recurrent genetic aberrations in carcinomas are presented in Tables 6.5 and 6.6 and Figure 6.8.

In colorectal carcinomas, the well-defined progression from premalignant adenoma to metastatic carcinoma was shown to correlate with distinct genetic aberrations (Fearon and Vogelstein, 1990). Since then, several inter-related genetic pathways to colorectal cancer have been analysed in detail (Ilyas et al., 1999). Sporadic colorectal cancer can arise via the pathway originally described by Fearon and Vogelstein, with *APC* mutation occurring as an early event, followed by *KRAS, DCC, SMAD2/4*, and *TP53* mutations. Another pathway involves either sporadic or inherited mutation of the DNA mismatch repair genes, giving rise to replication error positive (RER+) tumours. Colorectal tumours

Table 6.5 Examples of recurrent chromosome aberrations in epithelial tumours

Malignancy	Chromosome aberration	Affected genes
Colorectal adenocarcinoma	+7, +13, −14, −18, +20, +X	*DCC* (chrom 18)
	del(5)(q22–35)	*APC*
	del(8)(p11–23)	
	del(10(q22–26)	*PTEN*
	del(17)(p11–13)	*TP53*
Breast adenocarcinoma	+7, −X, +18, −18, +20	
	der(1;16)(q10;p10)	
	i(1)(q10),	
	del(1)(q11–12)	
	del(3)(p14–23)	
	del(6)(q21–27)	
	t(8p12)	*NRG1*
Ovarian adenocarcinoma	+7, +8, +12, −13, −17, −18, −X	
	del(6)(q15–25)	
	del(11)(p11–15)	
	del(11)(q23–25)	*OPCML*
	del(1)(q21–44)	
	del(1)(p31–36)	
	del(3)(q13–23)	
Non-small cell undifferentiated lung carcinoma	del(3)(p14–23)	*FHIT*
	del(15)(p10–11)	
	del(9)(p21–23)	
	del(17)(p11–13)	
	del(11)(p11–15)	
	del(1)(p32–36)	
	del(7)(p11–13)	
Papillary thyroid carcinoma	inv(10)(q11.2q21)	*RET, H4*
	inv(10)(q11.2q11.2)	*RET, ELE1*
	t(10;17)(q11.2;q23)	*RET, PRKAR1A*
	t(8;10)(p21–22;q11.2)	*PCM1,RET*
Paediatric renal cell carcinoma	t(X;1)(p11.2;q21)	*TFE3, PRCC*
	t(X;17)(p11.2;q25)	*TFE3, PRCC2*
	t(X;1)(p11.2;p34)	*TFE3, PSF*
	inv(X)(p11.2;q12)	*TFE3, NONO*
	t(X;17)(p11.2;q23)	*TFE3,CLTC*
Poorly differentiated carcinoma	t(15;19)(q13;p13.1)	*NUT, BRD4*

Table 6.6 Examples of gene amplification in cancer

Gene	Location of normal allele	Malignancy
MYC	8q24	Breast, colorectal, lung carcinoma, and many other solid tumours
MYCN	2p24	Neuroblastoma, retinoblastoma, small cell lung carcinoma
MYCL1	1p34	Small cell lung carcinoma
PDGFRA	4q12	Glioblastoma
PDGFRB	5q33–35	Glioblastoma
EGFR	7p11–13	Squamous cell carcinoma, astrocytoma
IGFR-1	15q25–26	Breast carcinoma
MYB	6q22–23	Colorectal carcinoma
ERBB-2	17q12	Breast, ovarian, gastric carcinoma, and many other solid tumours
CCND1 *FGF3* *FGF4*	11q13	Breast, oesophageal carcinoma squamous carcinoma, and many other solid tumours
GLI *SAS* *CDK4* *MDM2*	12q13	Soft tissue sarcoma, glioma
AR	Xq11–13	Prostate carcinoma

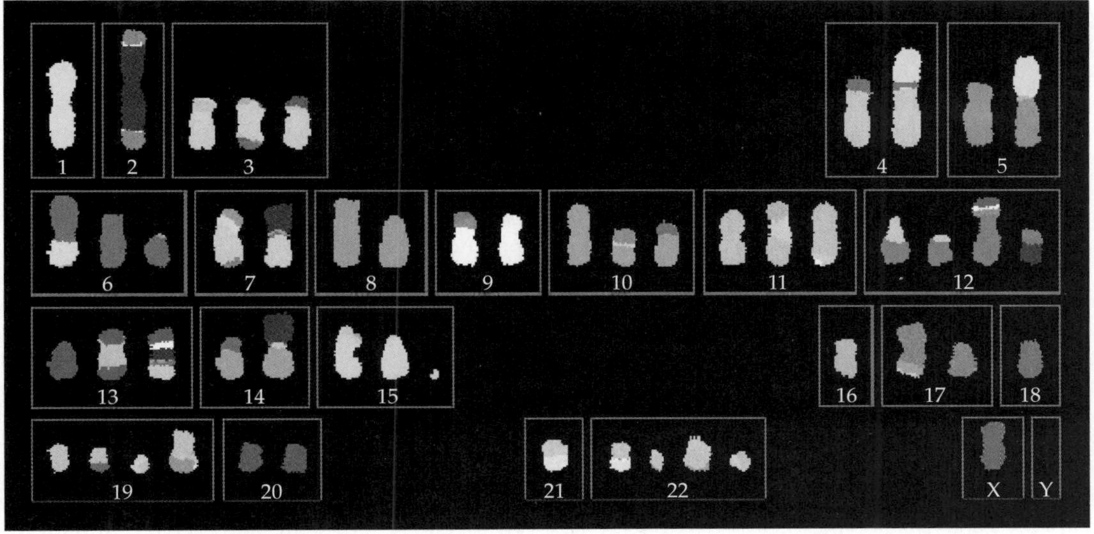

Figure 6.8 Spectral karyotype (SKY) from breast carcinoma cell line showing multiple chromosome rearrangements (Courtesy: Mira Grigorova and Paul Edwards) (See also plate 2).

with and without functional mismatch repair mechanisms have very different karyotypes. RER – tumours show aneuploidy and evidence of chromosomal instability, while RER + tumours show relatively simple, stable karyotypes with few aberrations.

Breast carcinomas are an example of a tumour type showing considerable cell-to-cell heterogeneity.

In spite of this, analysis of short-term cultures from a large series of primary breast carcinomas has revealed non-random primary and secondary chromosome aberrations (Texeira et al., 2002). Most of the structural aberrations are unbalanced rearrangements, such as deletions, isochromosomes and amplification in the form of HSRs. Careful consideration by the authors of their finding that ~70% of breast carcinomas have cytogenetically unrelated clones, leads them to the conclusion that a significant proportion of breast carcinomas are polyclonal. An interesting recent discovery is that 8p11–21 rearrangements in breast adenocarcinomas target the *NRG1* gene (Adélaïde et al., 2003). *NRG1* encodes multiple isoforms of an epidermal growth factor-like ligand for the ERBB/EGFR family. Since *ERBB2* is commonly amplified or overexpressed without amplification in breast tumours, this finding highlights the importance of disruption to specific pathways in cancer.

Gene fusions have been described so far in only a few carcinomas and adenomas. For example, in papillary thyroid carcinomas the *RET* oncogene at band 10q11.2 is activated by fusion with other genes, such as *H4*, *ELE*1, and the gene encoding the R1α regulatory subunit of protein kinase A. Examination of different cell populations within thyroid tumours has revealed that RET is activated in small focal regions within benign thyroid nodules, suggesting that it is an early event in malignant transformation (Fusco et al., 2002). Paediatric renal cell carcinomas carry translocations in which the *TFE3* gene, encoding a transcription factor, fuses with one of several genes. These include *PRCC2, NONO,* and *PSF*, all encoding splicing factors, and *CLTC* encoding a major subunit of clathrin (Argani et al., 2003). Poorly differentiated carcinomas can have a t(15;19)(q13;p13.1), in which the bromodomain gene *BRD4* becomes fused with a novel gene, *NUT*, of unknown function (French et al., 2003). The presence of this translocation is associated with a highly aggressive, invariably lethal phenotype.

6.7.3 Germ cell tumours

Germ cell tumours of various histological subtypes occur in childhood, adolescents/young adults and older men. The variability in presentation and genetic aberrations in tumours arising at different ages suggest differences in their underlying aetiology. The most consistent cytogenetic finding is an isochromosome of the short arm of chromosome 12 in about 80% of adolescent/adult testicular germ cell tumours. In testicular germ cell tumours without the i(12p), gain of 12p material occurs as a result of other rearrangements, including amplification of subregions of 12p. Gain of 12p material has also been identified in some non-testicular germ cell tumours, enabling a germ cell tumour to be identified in extragonadal cases that are difficult to diagnose using morphological criteria. The i(12p) has also been found in germ cell tumours of the ovary. The putative precursor lesion of testicular germ cell tumours is carcinoma *in situ* (intratubular germ cell neoplasia). CGH analysis of carcinoma *in situ* failed to find gain of 12p, suggesting that the formation of this aberration is critical in the progression to invasive disease (Summersgill et al., 2001). Other aberrations are occasionally present in germ cell tumours of different types, including gain of material from chromosomes 4, 21 and X and 12q in adolescent/adult testicular germ cell tumours, and distal 1p losses and translocations of 6q in childhood cases.

6.7.4 Neuroblastoma

Neuroblastoma is the most common extracranial solid malignant tumour of children. It is included in this consideration of solid tumours since genetic aberrations are of particular importance in the clinic. Neuroblastoma patients fall into two broad prognostic categories, which have been correlated with distinct clinical, biological, and genetic factors (Brodeur, 2003). Favourable prognosis neuroblastoma is associated with young age and early stage (1, 2a, or 4s), triploid karyotype, absence of 1p abnormalities or *MYCN* gene amplification. This type has an excellent outcome with little or no therapy. Unfavourable prognosis neuroblastoma is associated with older age, advanced stage (2b, 3, or 4), pseudodiploid and tetraploid karyotypes, 1p deletions, 17q gain, and MYCN amplification (Figure 6.9). The outcome is generally poor in these patients despite aggressive multi-agent chemotherapy and, in some cases, marrow ablative treatment and bone marrow transplantation. The presence of del(1p), gain of 17q, *MYCN* amplification, or pseudodiploidy/tetraploidy can thus be used at diagnosis to identify patients who need to be given intensive treatment.

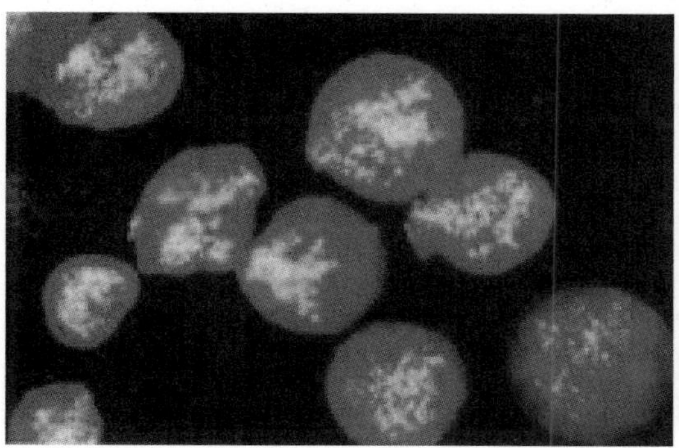
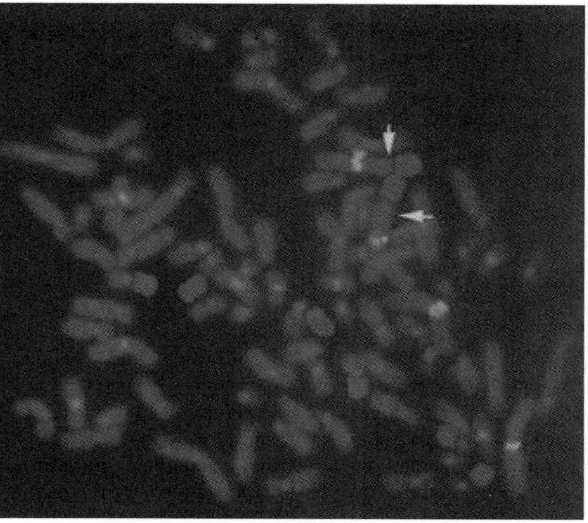

Figure 6.9 Detection by fluorescence *in situ* hybridization (FISH) of prognostic markers in neuroblastoma. Left: Interphase FISH on nuclei showing multiple copies of *MYCN* labelled yellow. Right: Metaphase spread from neuroblastoma cell line with deleted 1p (arrowed), and additional copies of 17q labelled red. Centromeres of chromosome 1 are labelled green (See also plate 3).

6.8 Conclusions and future prospects

It is apparent that chromosomal aberrations play a central role in tumorigenesis and tumour progression. Basic chromosomal mechanisms for oncogene activation and tumour suppressor gene inactivation have been identified from cytogenetic and molecular genetic analysis of large numbers of aberrations. These studies have been accompanied by functional analysis of these genes which has revealed numerous regulatory pathways concerned with signal transduction, cell cycle control, differentiation, and apoptosis.

Major differences have emerged from these studies in the types of aberrations observed in different malignancies. For example, leukaemias, lymphomas, and sarcomas generally have few aberrations with near-diploid karyotypes, whereas carcinomas often have many aberrations and gross aneuploidy. Amplification is a common feature of sarcomas and carcinomas, but has hardly ever been seen in leukaemias and lymphomas. Leukaemias, lymphomas, and sarcomas often have oncogene activation by gene fusion, whereas in carcinomas this mechanism has been confirmed so far in only a few types. The complexity of chromosome aberrations may simply be hampering the identification of gene fusions and gene rearrangements in other forms of carcinoma (Mitelman et al., 2004).

There are several factors to consider when examining the aetiology of tumorigenic aberrations. Exposure to external or intracellular mutagens, such as cosmic radiation, dietary factors, or endogenous metabolites, is well known to play a major role in DNA damage. However, other factors also need to be considered, such as increased susceptibility resulting from an inherited DNA repair defect or an inactivated tumour suppressor gene. Presumably most genetic aberrations are not tumorigenic and are detected by the damage-response pathway resulting in apoptosis unless repaired. Those aberrations which confer a proliferative advantage, and do not result in apoptosis (either because they are not detected by p53 or because p53 is not functional) allow clonal expansion of the cells carrying them.

Numerous examples have been given here of the clinical applications of cytogenetic aberrations. Treatment strategies for cancer are critically dependent on accurate diagnosis. In cases where conventional histopathology is insufficient to determine the tumour type, further investigations including cytogenetic analysis may then become necessary. For example, small round cell tumours of childhood which include Ewing's sarcoma, pPNET, neuroblastoma, and rhabdomyosarcoma may be difficult to distinguish from each other when they are undifferentiated, but as described above, these tumours have distinctive chromosome aberrations that enable their precise diagnosis.

Identification of aberrations may also be important prognostically. The presence of those associated with poor prognosis may indicate that intensive therapy should be started as soon as possible to optimize the patient's likelihood of survival. On the other hand, the presence of those that are associated with good prognosis may indicate that less intensive therapy can be used or therapy even avoided altogether. Once the genetic aberrations in a tumour are identified, they can be used as tumour markers for serial sampling of blood or bone marrow, as in the case of leukaemia and lymphoma, to examine a patient's response to treatment and to monitor the clinical course in the longer term.

Future research on chromosome aberrations in cancer will undoubtedly focus on several issues. All the targeted genes have to be identified and their roles in normal and tumour cells understood. There is an urgent need to develop efficient procedures to analyse carcinomas, for which a disproportionately small number of cases has been examined so far. Another question is why certain translocations are so specific to particular tumour types (Barr, 1998). An improved understanding of lineage-specific transcription should emerge from functional studies of the abnormal genes generated by these translocations. These studies will all give rise to fundamental knowledge of the biological processes that govern tumorigenesis and tumour progression, and will hopefully lead to prevention of some cancers and the development of new, more effective forms of therapy.

References

Adélaïde, J., Huang, H. E., Murati, A., Alsop, A. E., Orsetti, B., Mozziconacci, M. J. et al. (2003). A recurrent chromosome translocation breakpoint in breast and pancreatic cancer cell lines targets the neuregulin/NRG1 gene. *Genes Chrom Cancer*, **37**, 333–45.

Albertson, D., Collins, C., McCormick, F., and Gray, J. W. (2003). Chromosome aberrations in solid tumours. *Nat Genet*, **34**(4), 369–76.

Anderson, J., Gordon, A., Pritchard-Jones, K and Shipley, J. (1999). Genes, chromosomes, and rhabdomyosarcoma. *Genes Chrom Cancer*, **26**(4) 275–85.

Argani, P., Lui, M. Y., Couturier, J., Bouvier, R., Fournet, J. C., and Ladanyi, M. (2003). A novel CLTC-TFE3 gene fusion in pediatric renal adenocarcinoma with t(X;17)(p11.2;q23). *Oncogene*, **22**(34), 5374–8.

Armstrong, S. A., Staunton, J. E., Silverman, L. B., Pieters, R., den Boer, M. L., Minden, M. D. et al. (2002). MLL translocations specify a distinct gene expression profile that distinguishes a unique leukemia. *Nat Genet*, **30**(1), 41–7.

Ayton, P. M. and Cleary, M. L. (2001). Molecular mechanisms of leukemogenesis mediated by MLL fusion proteins. *Oncogene*, **20**, 5695–707.

Ayton, P. M. and Cleary, M. L. (2003). Transformation of myeloid progenitors by MLL oncoproteins is dependent on *Hoxa7* and *Hoxa9*. *Genes Dev*, **17**, 2298–307.

Balmain, A., Gray, J., Ponder, B. (2003). The genetics and genomics of cancer. *Nat Genet*, **33** (Suppl.), 238–44.

Barr, F. G. (1998). Translocations, cancer and the puzzle of specificity. *Nature Genetics*, **19**, 121–4.

Bennett, J. M., Catovsky, D., Daniel, M.-T., Flandrin, G., Galton, D. A. G., Gralnick, H. R. et al. (1985). Proposed revised criteria for the classification of acute myeloid leukemia. *Ann Int Med*, **103**, 626–9.

Bennicelli, J. L. and Barr, F. G. (2002). Chromosomal translocations and sarcomas. *Curr Opin Oncol*, **14**, 412–19.

Brodeur, G. M. (2003). Neuroblastoma: Biological insights into a clinical enigma. *Nat Rev Cancer*, **3**, 203–16.

Clarkson, B., Strife, A., Wisniewski, D., Lambek., C. L., and Liu, C. (2003). Chronic myelogenous leukemia as a paradigm of early cancer and possible curative strategies. *Leukemia*, **17**, 1211–62.

Crew, A. J., Clark, J., Fisher, C., Gill, S., Grimer, R., Chand, A. et al. (1995). Fusion of syt to 2 genes, ssx1 and ssx2, encoding proteins with homology to the kruppel-associated box in human synovial sarcoma. *EMBO J*, **14**, 2333–40.

Cuneo, A., Fagioli, F., Pazzi, I., Tallarico, A., Previati, R., Piva, N. et al. (1992). Morphologic, immunological and cytogenetic studies in acute myeloid-leukemia following occupational exposure to pesticides and organic-solvents. *Leukemia Res*, **16**, 789–96.

Deneen, B. and Denny, C. T. (2001). Loss of p16 pathways stabilizes EWS/FLI1 expression and complements EWS/FLI1 mediated transformation. *Oncogene*, **20**, 6731–41.

dos Santos, N. R, de Bruijn, D. R., and van Kessel, A. G. (2001). Molecular mechanisms underlying human synovial sarcoma development. *Genes Chrom Cancer*, **30**(1), 1–14.

Farag, S. S., Archer, K. J., Mrozek, K., Vardiman, J. W., Carroll, A. J., Pettenati, M. J. et al. (2002). Isolated trisomy of chromosomes 8, 11, 13 and 21 is an adverse prognostic factor in adults with de novo acute myeloid leukemia: results from Cancer and Leukemia Group B 8461. *Int J Oncol*, **21**(5), 1041–51.

Fearon, E. R. and Vogelstein, B. (1990). A genetic model for colorectal tumorigenesis. *Cell*, **61**, 759–67.

Felsder, D. M., Hackett, J. A., and Greider, C. W. (2003). Telomere dysfunction and the initiation of genome instability. *Nat Rev Cancer*, **3**, 1–5.

Ferrando, A. A. and Look, A. T. (2000). Clinical implications of recurring chromosomal and associated molecular abnormalities in acute lymphoblastic leukemia. *Sem Hematol*, **37**, 381–95.

French, C. A., Miyoshi, I., Kubonishi, I., Grier, H. E., Perez-Atayde, A. R., and Fletcher, J. A. (2003). BRD4-NUT fusion oncogene: a novel mechanism in aggressive carcinoma. *Canc Res*, **63**(2), 304–7.

Fusco, A., Chiappetta, G., Hui, P., Garcia-Rostan, G., Golden, L., Kinder, B. K. et al. (2002). Assessment of RET/PTC oncogene activation and clonality in thyroid nodules with incomplete morphological evidence of papillary carcinoma: a search for the early precursors of papillary cancer. *Am J Pathol*, **160**(6), 2157–67.

Grimwade, D., Walker, H., Oliver, F., Wheatley, K., Harrison, C., Harrison, G. et al. (1998). The importance of diagnostic cytogenetics on outcome in AML: analysis of 1,612 patients entered into the MRC AML 10 trial. The Medical Research Council Adult and Children 's Leukaemia Working Parties. *Blood*, **92**, 2322–33.

Hahn, W. C. (2003). Role of telomeres and telomerase in the pathogenesis of human cancer. *J Clin Oncol*, **21**, 2034–43.

Harris, N. L., Jaffe, E. S., Diebold, J., Flandrin, G., Muller-Hermelink, H. K., Vardiman, J. et al. (1999). World Health Organization classification of neoplastic diseases of the hematopoietic and lymphoid tissues: report of the Clinical Advisory Committee meeting-Airlie House, Virginia, November 1997. *J Clin Oncol*, **17**(12), 3835–49.

Heisterkamp, N., and Groffen, J. (2002). Philadelphia-positive leukemia: a personal perspective. *Oncogene*, **21**(56), 8536–40.

Hellman, A., Zlotorynski, E., Scherer, S. W., Cheung, J., Vincent, J. B., Smith, D. I. et al. (2002). A role for common fragile site induction in amplification of human oncogenes. *Cancer Cell*, **1**(1), 89–97.

Hoeijmakers, J. H. J. (2001). Genome maintenance mechanisms for preventing cancer. *Nature*, **411**, 366–74.

Ilyas, M., Straub, J., Tomlinson, I. P., and Bodmer, W. F. (1999). Genetic pathways in colorectal and other cancers. *Eur J Cancer*, **35**(14), 1986–2002.

Jallepalli, P.V. and Lengauer C. (1999). Chromosome segregation and cancer: cutting through the mystery. *Nat Rev Cancer*, **1**, 109–17.

Kelly, L., Clark, J., and Gilliland, D. G. (2002). Comprehensive genotypic analysis of leukemia: clinical and therapeutic implications. *Curr Opin Oncol*, **14**, 10–18.

Khan, J., Bittner, M. L., Saal, L. H., Teichmann, U., Azorsa, D.O., Gooden, G.C. et al. (1999). cDNA microarrays detect activation of a myogenic transcription program by the PAX3-FKHR fusion oncogene. *Proc Natl Acad Sci USA*, **96**(23), 13264–9.

Klein, G. (2000). Dysregulation of lymphocyte proliferation by chromosomal translocations and sequential genetic changes. *Bioessays*, **22**, 414–22.

Knudson, A. G. (1971). Mutations and cancer: statistical study of retinoblastoma. *Proc Natl Acad Sci USA*, **68**, 820–3.

Krug, U., Ganser, A., and Koeffler, H. P. (2002). Tumor suppressor genes in normal and malignant hematopoiesis. *Oncogene*, **21**(21), 3475–95.

Kolomietz, E., Meyn, M. S., Pandita, A., and Squire, J. A. (2002). The role of *Alu* repeat clusters as mediators of recurrent chromosomal aberrations in tumours. *Genes Chrom Cancer*, **35**, 97–112.

Kuppers, R. and Dalla-Favera, R. (2001). Mechanisms of chromosomal translocations in B cell lymphomas. *Oncogene*, **20**, 5580–94.

Ladanyi, M. (2002). EWS-FLI1 and Ewing's sarcoma: recent molecular data and new insights. *Cancer Biol Ther*, **1**(4), 330–6.

Laurent, E., Talpaz, M., Kantarjian, H., and Kurzrock, R. (2000). The BCR gene and Philadelphia chromosome-positive leukemogenesis. *Cancer Res*, **61**, 2343–55.

Lengauer, C., Kinzler, K. W., and Vogelstein, B. (1998). Genetic instabilities in human cancers. *Nature*, **396**, 643–9.

Look, A. T. (1998). Genes altered by chromosomal translocations in leukemia cells and lymphomas. In Genetic Basis of Human Cancer. (Eds. B. Vogelstein and K. W. Kinzler). McGraw-Hill, New York, pp. 109–41.

Mackall C. L., Melzer, P. S., and Helman, L. J. (2002). Focus on sarcomas. *Cancer Cell*, **2**, 175–8.

Mauritzson, N., Albin, M., Rylander, L., Billstrom, R., Ahlgren, T., Mikoczy, Z. et al. (2002). Pooled analysis of clinical and cytogenetic features in treatment-related and de novo adult acute myeloid leukemia and myelodysplastic syndromes based on a consecutive series of 761 patients analyzed 1976–1993 and on 5098 unselected cases reported in the literature 1974–2001. *Leukemia*, **16**(12), 2366–78.

Melnick, A. and Licht, J. D. (1999). Deconstructing a disease: RARalpha, its fusion partners, and their roles in the pathogenesis of acute promyelocytic leukemia. *Blood*, **93**, 3167–215.

Merlino, G. and Helman L. J. (1999). Rhabdomyosarcoma—working out the pathways. *Oncogene*, **18**, 5340 –48.

Mistry, A. R., Pedersen, E. W., Solomon, E., Grimwade, D. (2003). The molecular pathogenesis of acute promyelocytic leukaemia: implications for the clinical management of the disease. *Blood Rev*, **17**(2), 71–97.

Mitelman, F. (ed.) (1995). International System for Human Cytogenetic Nomenclature (ISCN). *Guidelines for Cancer Cytogenetics (Suppl)*. S. Karger, Basel.

Mitelman, F., Johansson, B., Mandahl, N., and Mertens, F. (1997). Clinical significance of cytogenetic findings in solid tumours. *Cancer Genet Cytogenet*, **95**, 1–8.

Mitelman, F., Johansson, B., and Mertens, F. (2004). Fusion genes and rearranged genes as a linear function of chromosome aberrations in cancer. *Nat Gent*, **36**(4), 331–4.

Mulloy, J. C., Cammenga, J., MacKenzie, K. L., Berguido, F. J., Moore, M. A. S., Nimer, S. D. (2002). The AML1-ETO fusion protein promotes the expansion of hematopoietic stem cells. *Blood*, **99**, 15–23.

Nakamura, T., Mori, T., Tada, S., Krajewski, W., Rozovskaia, T., Wassell, R. et al. (2002). ALL-1 is a histone methyltransferase that assembles a supercomplex of proteins involved in transcriptional regulation. *Mol Cell*, **10**, 1119–28.

Paulsson, K., Sall, T., Fioretos., T., Mitelman, F., and Johansson., B. (2001). The incidence of trisomy 8 as a sole chromosomal aberration in myeloid malignancies varies in relation to gender, age, prior iatrogenic genotoxic exposure, and morphology. *Cancer Genet Cytogenet*, **130**(2), 160–5.

Pedersen-Bjergaard, J., Christiansen, D. H., Andersen, M. K., and Skovby, F. (2002). Causality of myelodysplasia and acute myeloid leukemia and their genetic abnormalities, *Leukemia*, **16**, 2177–84.

Pihan, G. A. and Doxsey, S. J.(1999). The mitotic machinery as a source of genetic instability in cancer. *Semin Cancer Biol*, **9**(4), 289–302.

Rabbitts, T. H. (1994). Chromosomal translocations in human cancer. *Nature*, **372** (6502), 143–9.

Rabbitts, T. H. (2001). Chromosomal translocation master genes, mouse models and experimental therapeutics. *Oncogene*, **20** (40), 5763–77.

Rooney, D. E. (ed.) (2001). *Human Cytogenetics: Malignancy and Acquired Abnormalities: A Practical Approach*, 3rd edn. Oxford University Press, Oxford.

Rowley, J. D. (1998). The critical role of chromosome translocations in human leukemias. *Ann Rev Genet*, **32**, 495–519.

Scandura, J. M., Boccucini, P., Cammenga, J., and Nimer, S. D. (2002). Transcription factor fusions in acute leukemia: variations on a theme. *Oncogene*, **21**, 3422–44.

Schwab, M. (1999). Oncogene amplification in solid tumours. *Sem Cancer Biol*, **9**, 319–25.

Shet, A. S., Jahagirdar, B. N., and Verfaillie, C. M. (2002). Chronic myelogenous leukemia: mechanisms underlying disease progression. *Leukemia*, **16**, 1402–11.

So, C. W., Karsunky, H., Passegue, E., Cozzio, A., Weissman, I. L., and Cleary, M.L. (2003). MLL –GAS7 transforms multipotent hematopoietic progenitors and induces mixed lineage leukemias in mice. *Cancer Cell*, **3**, 161–71.

Sreekantaiah, C., Ladanyi, M., Rodriguez, E., and Chaganti, R. S. (1994). Chromosomal aberrations in soft tissue tumors. Relevance to diagnosis, classification, and molecular mechanisms. *Am J Pathol*, **144**(6), 1121–34.

Strissel, P. S., Strick, R., Rowley, J. D., and Zeleznik-Le, N. (1998). An in vivo topoisomerase II cleavage site and a DNase hypersensitive site co-localize near exon 9 in the MLL breakpoint cluster region. *Blood*, **92**, 3793–803.

Summersgill, B., Osin, P., Lu, Y. J., Huddart, R., and Shipley, J. (2001). Chromosomal imbalances associated with carcinoma in situ and associated testicular germ cell tumours of adolescents and adults. *Br J Cancer*, **85**(2), 213–20.

Takeuchi, S., Tsukasaki, K., Bartram, C. R., Seriu, T., Zimmermann, M., Schrappe, M. et al. (2003). Long-term study of the clinical significance of loss of heterozygosity in childhood actue lymphoblastic leukemia. *Leukemia*, **17**, 149–54.

Teixeira, M. R., Pandis, N., and Heim, S. (2002). Cytogenetic clues to breast carcinogenesis. *Genes Chrom Cancer*, **33**(1) 1–16.

Tuveson, D. A., Willis, N. A., Jacks, T., Griffin, J. D., Singer, S., Fletcher, C. D. et al. (2001). STI571 inactivation of the gastrointestinal stromal tumor c-KIT oncoprotein: biological and clinical implications. *Oncogene*, **20**(36), 5054–8.

Virtaneva, K., Wright, F. A., Tanner, S. M., Yuan, B., Lemon, W. J., Caligiuri, M. A. et al. (2001). Expression profiling reveals fundamental biological differences in acute myeloid leukemia with isolated trisomy 8 and normal cytogenetics. *Proc Natl Acad Sci USA*, **98**(3), 1124–9.

Wiemels, J. L. and Greaves, M. (1999). Structure and possible mechanisms of TEL-AML1 gene fusions in childhood acute lymphoblastic leukemia. *Cancer Res*, **59**, 4075–82.

Willis, T. G. and Dyer, M. J. S. (2000). The role of immunoglobulin translocations in the pathogenesis of B-cell malignancies. *Blood*, **96**, 808–22.

CHAPTER 7

Oncogenes

Margaret A. Knowles

The involvement of multiple genetic events in the generation of human cancers has been discussed in previous chapters and the terms oncogene and tumour suppressor gene have been used to describe the two major classes of cellular genes that are genetically or epigenetically altered. In this section we will examine the discovery and characterization of those genes classified as 'oncogenes' and will consider their role in the process of carcinogenesis and their potential use as therapeutic targets.

Initially, oncogene was coined as a generic term to describe any gene capable of causing cancer. Subsequently, as tumour suppressor genes were identified and it became clear that these contributed via loss of function, use of the term oncogene was restricted to those genes that contribute to tumorigenesis via gain of function, and are dominant at the cellular level.

7.1 Retroviral transduction: the discovery of transforming genes

The concept that certain genes can induce cancer came initially from studies of animal viruses. Several viruses capable of inducing tumours in animals and birds were identified in the first half of the twentieth century. They fall into two major groups, the double-stranded DNA tumour viruses and the RNA tumour viruses or retroviruses. Both groups are described in more detail in Chapter 13 but some discussion of the retroviruses is relevant here as these viruses provided the first clues to the identity of the genes that can contribute to the development of human cancer and have provided a wealth of information on the ways in which alterations of cellular genes can drive the process of transformation. Detailed information on retroviruses can be found in the excellent book edited by Coffin and colleagues (Coffin et al., 1997).

Studies of tumour induction by retroviruses in animals revealed two distinct patterns of tumour development (Varmus, 1988). In some cases, for example, leukaemia viruses and murine mammary tumour virus, tumours arose after a long latent period (months), suggesting that some form of *in vivo* selection was required during the process of tumour induction. These viruses are commonly known as chronic or slow tumour viruses. Other retroviruses showed a dramatically short latent period for tumour induction (days or weeks) and these isolates were able to alter or 'transform' cultured cells, implying that each virion carried information that had a direct and dominant effect on cells. The resulting tumours are therefore polyclonal in contrast to those induced by the chronic retroviruses that are monoclonal. Examination of the genome of these two types of retrovirus revealed that the chronic viruses contained only the usual *gag*, *pol*, and *env* genes required for replication (see Chapter 13) but that the acutely transforming viruses contained novel sequences in place of some of this genetic information. These acute retroviruses were therefore replication defective and required complementation by wild-type virus for productive replication.

7.1.1 Transduction of normal cellular genes by retroviruses

The new sequences contained within the viral genome were designated viral oncogenes (*v-oncs*) and rapidly during the 1970s and 1980s, more than 30 viral oncogenes were distinguished. Where did these novel sequences come from and what was their role in the transformation process? It was shown by hybridizing the *v-onc* sequences to DNA extracted from the host species, that these oncogenic sequences were closely related to cellular genes. Furthermore, these sequences were highly conserved evolutionarily and found in all higher vertebrates. Many have also now been shown to have homologous sequences in lower organisms. In each case, a rare recombination event had resulted in the acquisition by the retrovirus of cellular DNA, a process known as transduction, and this had conferred new properties on the virus. A wide range of genes was identified and these were shown to be genes that are not silent but expressed in normal cells. Clearly in this normal cellular context they did not act as oncogenes and there was much speculation about what the difference between the viral and cellular genes might be. Possibilities included expression in an abnormal context, expression at high level from the strong viral promoters and enhancers or that the genes might be altered in some way in the virus. A range of genes was identified including growth factors, receptors, signal transduction molecules and transcription factors (Table 7.1). As DNA sequencing became routine and the *v-oncs* were compared with their cellular counterparts, it became clear that in many cases the viral genes contained alterations predicted to confer novel properties or regulatory alterations on the genes. Their cellular counterparts were thus termed proto-oncogenes or cellular oncogenes to denote this.

For example, the ras oncogenes captured by retroviruses contain point mutations in codon 12, a position later shown to activate the signalling function of the protein (see below). Commonly, *v-oncs* encoding receptor tyrosine kinases show loss of sequences that encode the ligand-binding domain and this renders the receptor constitutively active e.g. v-erbB, v-sea, v-ros, v-kit. In v-fms, the viral counterpart of the colony stimulating factor 1 (CSF1) receptor, there is a mutation in the ligand-binding domain that causes altered conformation of the protein, mimicking the effect of ligand binding.

Myc is transduced by several retroviruses and here it is altered levels of expression that are critical, though some mutations do enhance the transforming ability. Normally, expression of cellular *myc* is very tightly regulated and it is only expressed in particular phases of the cell cycle. When transduced by a retrovirus, the strong promoter and enhancer elements of the viral long terminal repeat sequences (LTRs) override these normal controls (Figure 7.1).

7.1.2 Insertional activation by replication competent retroviruses

Work on the replication competent tumour-inducing retroviruses revealed that although these did not transduce cellular genes, the mechanism by which they exerted their effect was by proviral insertion in specific regions of the genome. The retroviral life cycle involves initial release of RNA from the viral particle in the cytoplasm, followed by reverse transcription of the RNA to generate a double-stranded DNA form that enters the nucleus and inserts into the host chromosomal DNA. The inserted form is known as the provirus. Following integration, viral RNA is transcribed, packaged into viral particles and released from the cell. Integration into the host genome is a more or less random process and occasionally, insertional events occur that place the viral LTRs in a position that allows high-level expression of a cellular gene to occur, driven by these strong promoter and enhancer sequences.

Table 7.1 Retroviral oncogenes: cellular genes transduced by retroviruses

Function	Oncogene	Virus[a]	Species and tissue of origin
Non-receptor tyrosine kinase	*src*	RSV	Chicken sarcoma
	fps	Fu-SV	Chicken sarcoma
	fes	GA-SV	Cat sarcoma
	yes	Y73-ASV	Chicken sarcoma
	fgr	GR-FeSV	Cat sarcoma
	abl	Ab-MLV	Mouse pre-B lymphoma
Receptor tyrosine kinase	*ros*	UR2-ASV	Chicken sarcoma
	erbB	AEV-ES4	Chicken erythroblastosis
	fms	SM-FeSV	Cat sarcoma
	kit	HZ4-FeSV	Cat sarcoma
	sea	S13-AEV	Chicken erythroblastosis
	eyk	RPL30	Chicken sarcoma
Cytokine receptor	*mpl*	MPLV	Mouse myeloproliferative disease
G protein	*ras^K*	Ki-MSV	Rat sarcoma/erythroleukaemia
	ras^H	Ha-MSV	Rat sarcoma/erythroleukaemia
Serine/threonine kinase	*raf*	3611-MSV	Mouse sarcoma
	mil	MH2	Chicken sarcoma/carcinoma
	akt	AKT8	Mouse T cell lymphoma
	mos	Mo-MSV	Mouse sarcoma
Growth factor	*sis*	SSV	Monkey sarcoma
Adapter protein	*cbl*	Cas NS-1	Mouse pre-B lymphoma/myeloid leukaemia
	crk	ASV-1	Chicken sarcoma
Transcription factor	*ski*	SKV-ASV	Chicken carcinoma
	erbA	AEV-ES4	Chicken erythroblastosis
	jun	ASV-17	Chicken sarcoma
	fos	FBJ-MSV	Mouse osteosarcoma
	myc	MC29	Chicken myelocytoma/carcinoma
	myb	BAI-AMV	Chicken myeloblastosis
	rel	REV-T	Turkey reticuloendotheliosis
	ets	E26-AMV	Chicken erythroblastosis/myeloblastosis
	maf	AS42	Chicken sarcoma
	qin	ASV-31	Chicken sarcoma

[a] Only one example of a retrovirus carrying each gene is given. For comprehensive lists see Coffin et al. (1997).

By definition, every integration event is an insertional mutation and it can be envisaged that these not only activate transcription of cellular genes on occasion but perhaps more commonly may cause cellular gene inactivation by disruption. The genes that might be targets for this latter type of mutation are the tumour suppressor genes. However, these typically require inactivation of both alleles for phenotypic effect (Chapter 8) and as retroviral insertional mutation is always monoallelic, the many predicted insertional inactivations are not predicted to affect cell phenotype.

The first example of insertional activation came from B cell lymphomas induced by avian leukaemia viruses (ALVs). RNA transcripts in the induced tumour cells contained both viral LTR sequences and cellular sequences. The cellular gene was the *Myc* gene, also found in acutely transforming viruses. Retroviral insertion placed the coding region of *myc* downstream of the powerful viral LTR, again resulting in high levels of expression (Figure 7.1). Subsequent identification of the insertion sites of other proviruses in animal tumours revealed that several of the cellular genes targeted and activated by these events were the same as those transduced by the acutely transforming retroviruses, including *Myc, Mos, Myb, Hras, Kras, ErbB1,* and *Fms.* Some other genes were also

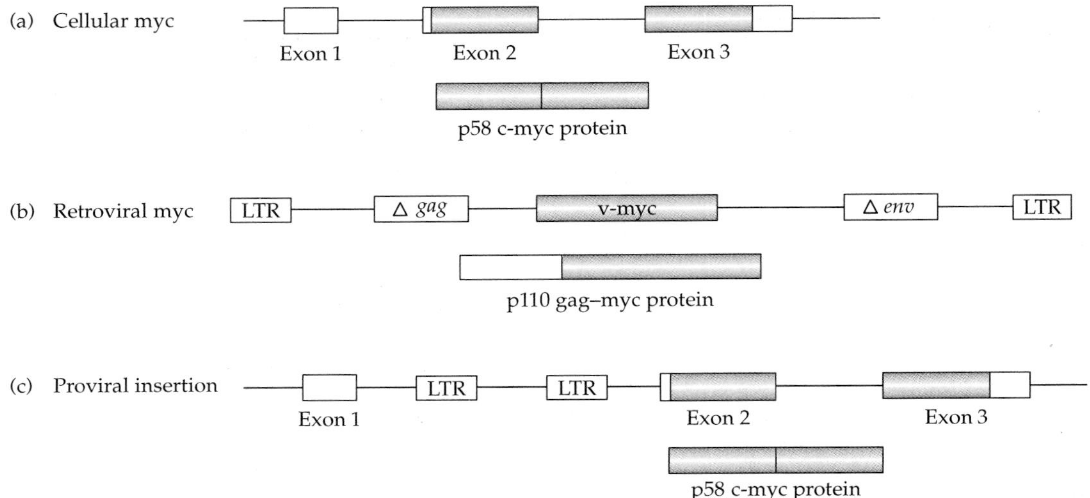

Figure 7.1 (a) Normal c-myc locus. There are three exons, two of which are coding (grey) which give rise to a 58 kDa protein product. (b) The transduced *myc* gene of MC29 is inserted between the retroviral *gag* and *env* genes and gives rise to a transforming gag–myc fusion protein of 110 kDa from a translational start site within *gag*. (c) An example of proviral insertion into the c-myc locus. The provirus is inserted between exon one and the coding exons and drives high-level expression of a normal 58 kDa myc protein.

identified, for example *IL2, IL3* and genes activated by insertional mutagenesis in murine mammary tumour virus (MMTV)-induced tumours, known originally as the Int genes. Int1, Int2, Int3, and Int4 are the cellular genes *Wnt1, Fgf3, Notch4,* and *Wnt3* respectively. These latter genes are not normally expressed in mammary cells and are therefore genes that act as oncogenes by virtue of inappropriate expression. Examples of genes activated by insertional mutagenesis are listed in Table 7.2.

This ability of retroviral insertion to select rare cancer causing mutations has led in recent years to the use of retroviruses as mutagens in systematic approaches to identify oncogenes that can be activated in this way. The use of polymerase chain reaction (PCR) and current knowledge of the sequence of both human and mouse genomes has greatly facilitated the identification of genes adjacent to the integration sites. An example is an elegant study by Suzuki and co-workers, where the induction of mouse leukaemia by retroviruses was used in conjunction with an inverse polymerase chain reaction (PCR)-based strategy to identify several hundred proviral integration sites (Suzuki et al., 2002). These included many of the known suspects and a large number of novel genes. This and other animal-based approaches to oncogene discovery are discussed in more detail in Chapter 19.

7.2 Identification of cellular oncogenes

If cellular genes can cause cancer when transduced by a virus, it would not be surprising if alterations to the same genes within the host cell could have a similar effect. This indeed proved to be the case and numerous cellular genes have now been shown to act as oncogenes in human tumours. Currently more than 100 mammalian genes have been reported to act as oncogenes when expressed inappropriately or altered by mutation.

Several approaches have been used to identify cellular genes that contribute as dominant oncogenes in human and animal tumours. In the early 1980s, a functional assay to screen tumour DNA was developed and widely used (Shih et al., 1979). This is known as the NIH-3T3 transformation assay and involves the introduction into the immortal murine cell line NIH-3T3 of tumour-derived DNA by means of a process known as transfection (Weinberg, 1981). Currently there are many possible ways of introducing DNA into cultured cells and the NIH-3T3 assay used in the 1980s employed a method known as calcium phosphate precipitation. Following introduction of DNA, the cells were maintained at confluence and examined for the presence of colonies or 'foci' of piled up, morphologically altered, transformed cells (Figure 7.2).

Table 7.2 Cellular genes activated by retroviral insertional mutagenesis

Function[a]	Locus	Virus[b]	Species and tissue of origin
Growth factor/cytokine	*FGF3/Int2*	MMTV	Mouse mammary carcinoma
	FGF4/Hst1	MMTV	Mouse mammary carcinoma
	FGF8/AIGF	MMTV	Mouse mammary carcinoma
	CSF-1	MLV	Mouse myeloid leukaemia
	GM-CSF	IAP	Mouse myeloid cell lines
	IL2	GaLV	Ape T cell leukaemia cell line
	IL3	IAP	Mouse myeloid cell lines
	WNT3/Int4	MMTV	Mouse mammary carcinoma
	WNT1/Int1		Mouse mammary carcinoma
Receptor tyrosine kinase	*ErbB*	RAV-1	Chicken erythroblastosis
	Fms	Fr-MLV	Mouse myeloblastic leukaemia
	Int3/Notch4	MMTV	Mouse mammary carcinoma
	IL2 receptor	IAP	Mouse T cell lymphoma cell line
	Prlr	Mo-MLV	Rat T cell leukaemia
	Notch1	Mo-MLV	Mouse T cell lymphoma
G protein	*Hras1*	MAV-1	Chicken nephroblastoma
	Kras2	Fr-MLV	Mouse myeloid cell line
GDP–GTP regulation	*Tiam1*	Mo-MLV	Mouse T cell lymphoma cell line
	Nf1	BXH2-MLV	Mouse myeloid leukaemia
Non-receptor tyrosine kinase	*Lck*	Mo-MLV	Rat T cell lymphoma
Serine/threonine kinase	*Mos*	IAP	Mouse myeloma
	Pim1	Mo-MLV	Mouse T cell lymphoma
	Pim2	Mo-MLV	Mouse T cell lymphoma
	Tpl2	Mo-MLV	Rat T cell lymphoma
Transcription factor	*Bmi1*	Mo-MLV	Mouse B cell lymphoma
	Ets1	Mo-MLV	Rat T cell lymphoma
	Evi1	Fr-MLV	Mouse myeloblastic leukaemia
	Fli1	FR-MLV	Mouse erythroleukaemia
	c-fos	RAV-1	Chicken nephroblastoma
	Hox2.4	IAP	Mouse myeloid leukaemia cell line
	Hoxa9	BXH-2 MLV	Mouse myeloid leukaemia
	c-myb	ALV	Chicken B cell lymphoma
	c-myc	RAV-1/RAV-2	Chicken B cell lymphoma
	N-myc	Mo-MLV	Mouse T cell lymphoma
	c-rel	ALV	Chicken lymphoma cell line
	Scl	IAP	Mouse myeloid cell line
	Spi1	SFFV	Mouse erythroleukaemia
	p53	F-MLV/SFFV	Mouse erythroleukaemia

[a] In the interests of space, only those genes with known or predicted function have been included. Many other genes targeted by retroviral insertion have been identified. See for example Suzuki et al. (2002).
[b] Only one virus type is given for each gene as an example.

DNA from such foci was usually subjected to several cycles of transfection to sequentially reduce the amount of donor DNA retained (via selection), and ultimately examined to identify the active donor DNA sequence. Other means of selection of altered cells were also used. This included ability to form colonies in suspension in soft agar, a phenotype exhibited by many transformed cells, and ability to form tumours in animals. In practice, most users preferred the focus assay because of the ease with which foci could be scored against the uniform background of the confluent, contact inhibited monolayer of immortal mouse cells and the relative speed with which multiple assays could be carried out. Human sequences could be identified due to the presence of human specific repeat sequences

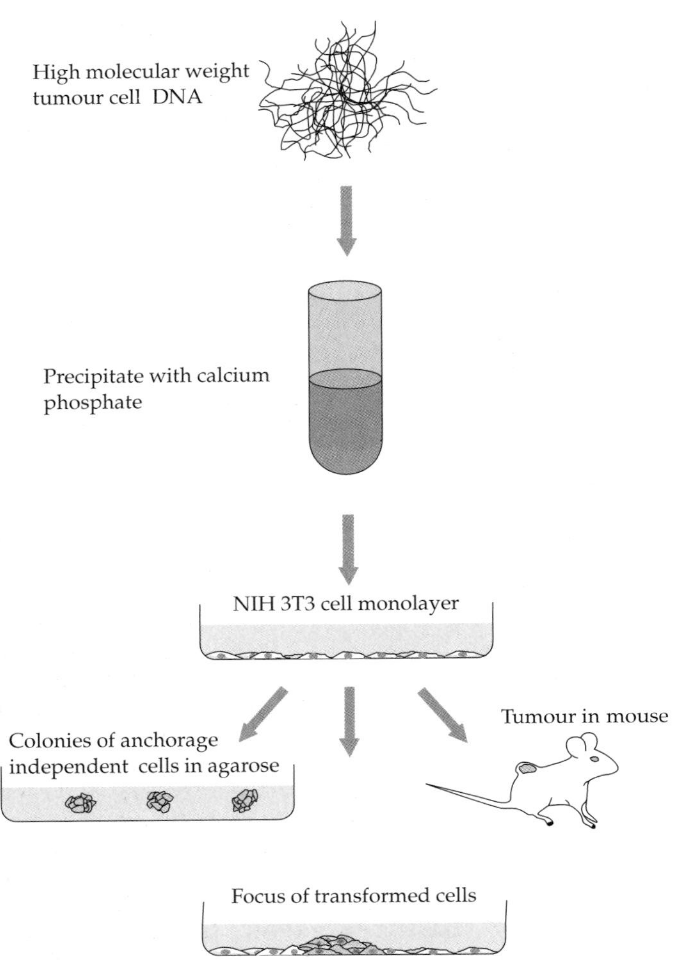

Figure 7.2 The NIH 3T3 transformation assay. High molecular weight DNA extracted from tumour cells is precipitated with calcium phosphate and added to a monolayer of NIH 3T3 cells which take up the precipitate. Some of this DNA becomes integrated into the cellular genome and if this contains an activated oncogene can induce phenotypic alterations in the transfected cells, including ability to form colonies in soft agarose, formation of piled up foci in the monolayer or tumour formation in mice. Cells with altered phenotype can be isolated for identification of transfected sequences.

(commonly Alu sequences), which facilitated downstream analysis of the transfected genes.

These functional analyses commonly identified members of the Ras gene family, already identified in retroviruses. In 1982 a human oncogene derived from the bladder tumour cell line EJ was shown to be homologous to the oncogene of Harvey murine sarcoma virus (Parada et al., 1982) and the cellular proto-oncogene was designated *HRAS*. Also identified by the assay was a homologue of the Kirsten murine sarcoma virus (*KRAS2*) and a new member of the ras gene family *NRAS*, that has no viral counterpart.

The mechanism of activation of these cellular genes was the subject of intense investigation. Excitingly, it was found that a single base change in the coding sequence altered a single amino acid in the encoded protein from glycine to valine, and functional studies demonstrated that this single point mutation was sufficient to confer transforming ability on the HRAS protein (Reddy et al., 1982; Tabin et al., 1982). Although Ras oncogenes (*HRAS, KRAS2,* and *NRAS*) were by far the most commonly identified human transforming genes using the NIH-3T3 assay, several other genes were also identified. These include *RET* and *TRK*, both identified as re-arranged genes that encoded novel fusion proteins (see below). The rat homologue of *ERBB2*, *Neu*, was identified using the assay and found to contain an activating mutation in the transmembrane domain of the receptor.

It should be noted that only a small proportion of tumour DNAs (less than 15%) score positive in the

NIH-3T3 assay. Possible explanations for this are the relative insensitivity of the assay, including the requirement that the genomic sequence of any oncogene remains intact during DNA extraction, which precludes detection of very large genes, subjectivity of scoring and the probability that only a few genes can transform this single immortal cell type. This latter issue might severely restrict the possibilities, given that NIH-3T3 cells which require only one additional event for transformation to tumorigenicity, are derived from a mesenchymal cell precursor rather than an epithelial cell that might be more applicable for the identification of epithelial tumour oncogenes. Nevertheless, the use of this simple assay provided a great deal of new information on human tumour genes and provided the impetus for further searches for human transforming genes.

7.3 Mechanisms of oncogene activation

7.3.1 Mutation

As we have seen, a single point mutation in a Ras proto-oncogene can lead to altered gene function. The Ras proteins are small (~21 kDa) guanosine triphosphatases (GTPases) that cycle between the GTP (active) and GDP-bound (inactive) state. In the normal cell, this is regulated by two classes of protein, guanine nucleotide exchange factors (GEFs), which increase the amount of GTP-bound Ras and the GTPase activating proteins (GAPs), which drive the formation of GDP-bound Ras. Upstream of these regulators, a wide range of stimuli from cell surface receptors influence these processes and downstream of the Ras proteins a plethora of effectors has been identified (Malumbres and Barbacid, 2003), resulting in a range of biological effects including stimulation of cell proliferation, differentiation and apoptosis. A major consequence of Ras activation following growth factor signalling via receptor tyrosine kinases is activation of the MAPK pathway (see Chapter 11).

The Ras oncogenes *NRAS*, *HRAS*, and *KRAS2* are mutated in 30% of human cancers including a high proportion of the major solid tumour types, for example, colorectal and lung and several forms of leukaemia (Bos, 1989). The mutations found are confined to codons 12, 13, and 61 and all result in an increase of the GTP-bound form of the protein (i.e. constitutive activation).

The key importance of the Ras-MAPK pathway led to the recent initiation of a systematic screen for mutations in the coding region of members of this pathway in a panel of human tumour types (cancer genome project: www.sanger.ac.uk/CGP/). The first finding of this initiative has been the identification of mutations of the *BRAF* gene in 66% of malignant melanomas and less frequently in a range of other tumour types (Davies et al., 2002). The mutations found are in the kinase domain of the protein and result in increased kinase activity. This finding in melanomas, which also show mutation of *NRAS*, indicates a possible alternative means to activate this pathway and underscores the importance of the Ras-MAPK pathway in this cell type.

Several other genes are activated by point mutation in human cancer. Activating point mutations in codons 301 and 969 of the *FMS* gene have been identified in acute myeloblastic leukaemia (Ridge et al., 1990). More recently mutations have been found in the *FMS*-like tyrosine kinase 3 (*FLT3*) in patients with acute lymphoblastic leukaemis, myelodysplasia, and acute myeloid leukaemia, making this one of the most frequently mutated genes in haematological malignancies (Stirewalt and Radich, 2003). Also in haematological malignancies, mutations in the receptor tyrosine kinase *KIT* are found in mastocytosis, a malignant disease involving mast cells and in myeloproliferative syndromes (Scheijen and Griffin, 2002). The most common mutation of *KIT* is D816V, in the phosphotransferase domain. Mutations are also found in some germ cell tumours (Tian et al., 1999) and gastrointestinal stromal tumours (GISTs) (Hirota et al., 1998).

The fibroblast growth factor receptor 3 (*FGFR3*) is mutated in a large proportion of bladder tumours (Munro and Knowles, 2003). In this case the mutations found are identical to mutations that in the germline cause lethal forms of dwarfism through constitutive activation of the tyrosine kinase activity of the receptor. In the long bones, FGFR3 signalling has a negative effect on chondrocyte proliferation. In the epithelium of the bladder it seems that a positive regulatory role is likely. *FGFR3* mutation appears surprisingly specific, found only in bladder cancer and a small number of cases of multiple myeloma.

Three oncogenes have been identified as causative genes in familial cancer syndromes. These are *RET*, *MET*, and *CDK4* (Chapter 3).

7.3.2 Overexpression

Insertional activation of oncogenes in animal tumours indicated that overexpression of some cellular genes or in some cases low-level expression in an unusual cellular context could have a profound effect on cell phenotype. During the early 1980s, aberrant expression of cellular genes was therefore considered as potentially oncogenic and the search was on for examples of this in human tumours.

Two genetic mechanisms have been identified that lead to the overexpression of cellular proto-oncogenes; genomic amplification and translocation. Identification of genes activated by both mechanisms has yielded an enormous amount of information not only on the genes involved in neoplastic development but also the pathways in which they function.

Amplification of oncogenes

An increase in the number of copies of a gene within the cell represents a possible mechanism for increased expression. Many early cytogenetic studies of human tumours described the presence of so-called double minute chromosomes (DMs) and homogenously staining regions (HSRs) within chromosomes (see Chapter 6). These were found to be the visible hallmarks of high-level amplification of specific genomic regions.

When tumour-derived cells containing DMs or HSRs were studied by Southern blotting or *in situ* hybridization using probes for known oncogenes, it was found that many amplified regions contained *MYC*-related sequences. Amplification of *MYC* (8q24) was identified in the acute lymphocytic leukaemia cell line HL-60 (Collins and Groudine, 1982) and a related sequence, *MYCN* (2p24), was amplified in many neuroblastomas (Schwab et al., 1983). A third myc family member, *MYCL1* (1p34), is amplified in cases of small cell lung carcinoma (SCCL) (Nau et al., 1985).

In breast and other epithelial malignancies, amplification of *ERBB2* (also known as *HER2*), a receptor tyrosine kinase with significant homology to *ERBB1* (previously identified as a retroviral oncogene) was found (Slamon et al., 1989). The rat homologue of *ERBB2*, *Neu*, had previously been identified as an oncogene by the NIH-3T3 assay. In the *Neu* oncogene, an activating mutation in the transmembrane domain of the protein was found to give rise to constitutive activation of the tyrosine kinase. In the case of human *ERBB2* (17q21), no activating mutations have been found in tumours and the gene has not been identified by functional screening in NIH-3T3 cells. More recently, other members of this protein family, *ERBB3* and *ERBB4* have been found to be overexpressed in breast and other cancers. In neither case does this appear to be the result of gene amplification but it has been shown that these two receptors can heterodimerize with ERBB2, allowing binding of the ligand heregulin, which does not bind to ERBB2 homodimers.

Initial identification of these amplified genes relied heavily on pre-existing knowledge of retroviral oncogenes and some inspired guesswork. With the vast amount of information now available on the human and other genomes, together with the development of some powerful molecular cytogenetic techniques, the localization of novel amplicons and the rapid identification of candidate genes within them has become almost routine. In recent years therefore, the catalogue of amplified genes found in human tumours has enlarged considerably. The methodology currently applied to map amplicons has been discussed in more detail in Chapter 6. For example, a whole genome comparison of DNA copy number changes by classical or microarray CGH can detect regions of high-level amplification with ease. With accurate mapping in the case of array CGH, where sequenced clones are used in the array, identification of candidate genes is simply achieved by reference to the current build of the human genome.

Many amplicons contain several genes. Final confirmation of the critical target(s) within such amplicons requires functional studies and for many candidate genes this has not yet been obtained. A comprehensive listing of these amplified genes is beyond the scope of this chapter but Table 7.3 lists examples of amplicons described in solid cancers together with some candidate genes identified within them.

As the numbers of amplicons and candidate oncogenes expand, it is becoming clear that validation of candidates is not always straightforward and much attention is currently focussed on the development of robust methods for this. Two regions of amplification that have received much recent attention are those on 17q and 20q that are amplified in many cancers. These are commonly large amplicons and fine mapping and measurement of copy number across the regions has revealed more than one peak of amplification in each (Monni et al., 2001;

Table 7.3 Amplified genes in human solid tumours

Genomic region	Candidate gene(s)	Tumour types with amplification
1p34	*MYCL1*	Lung, ovary
1q21–24	*COAS2, PRUNE, KIA1096*	Sarcoma, liver, breast, bladder, and others
2p24	*MYCN*	Neuroblastoma, retinoblastoma, medulloblastoma
2p15	*MEIS1*	Neuroblastoma
3q25–26	*PIK3CA, EIF-5A2*	Cervix, ovarian, prostate
6p22	*E2F3, CDKAL1*	Bladder
6q22–24	*MYB*	Hereditary breast (*BRCA1*), pancreatic
7p12	*EGFR*	Glioma, glioblastoma
7q31	*MET*	Colorectum
7q35–36	*EZH2*	Breast, colon, bladder larynx, gastric, lung, testis
8p12	*FGFR1, WHSC1L1*	Breast, bladder
8q21	*TCEB1, E2F5*	Breast
8q24	*MYC, KCNK9, RAD21, EIF3S3*	Many
9p23–24	*GASC1*	Oesophagus
10q24	*PLAU*	Prostate
10q26	*FGFR2*	Gastric, breast
11q13	*CCND1, EMS1, MYEOV*	Breast, bladder, liver, pancreas, oesophagus
11q22	*BIRC2, BIRC3*	Lung
12p12	*PTHLH, KRAS2*	Lung
12q14	*MDM2, GLI, CDK4, SAS,*	Sarcoma, bladder, glioma, salivary gland
15q26	*IQGAP1*	Gastric
17p12	*MAP2K4, ZNF18*	
17q12–23	*TERBB2, GRB7, MLN64, HSD17B1, TBX2, BIRC5, TOP2A, HOXB7, PAT1, RAD51C, SIGMA1B, BCAS3, and others*	Breast, pancreas, bladder, endometrium
19q13	*SEI1, AKT2, ZNF146, CCNE1*	Ovary, pancreas, bladder
20q11	*NCOA6*	
20q13	*CTSZ, ZNF217, CYP24, AURKA, BCAS1, BCAS4, NCOA3, MYBL2, and others*	Breast, ovary, pancreas, bladder

Hodgson et al., 2003). This implies that there may be more than one target gene that confers a selective advantage. On 17q for example there is one region at 17q13 that contains *ERBB2* and another at 17q23 that can be mapped separately in some tumours. Many breast tumours however contain a huge amplicon encompassing both regions. Expression analyses have generated a similarly complex picture. Consequently, there are several genes from each of these regions that show high level amplification, high levels of expression in the appropriate tumour samples and also show some characteristics expected of an oncogene in functional assays such as transforming ability *in vitro*. With these problems in mind it is worth noting that considerable luck was experienced during the early identification of *MYC* and *ERBB2* as functionally significant target genes within HSRs and DMs.

Current possibilities of combining both genome-wide assessment of copy number changes with expression profiling of the same tumour tissues are generating complex and exciting views of the molecular signatures of cancer cells. This approach potentially can lead to the direct identification of amplification targets. The reader is referred to two recent examples of studies of breast cancer in which, reassuringly this approach identified most of the previously identified amplicons in breast cancer together with many novel targets (Hyman et al., 2002; Pollack et al., 2002).

Potential mechanisms for the generation of high-level genomic amplification have now been proposed. Ultimately these will need to account for two distinct patterns of amplification, those that are high level but affect only a small region of DNA, for example, amplicons affecting *MYCN* in neuroblastomas and others such as those on 11q, 12p, 17q, and 20q that cover many megabases of DNA and contain variations in copy number across the amplicon. Drug-selected intrachromosomal gene amplification, for example that of *DHFR* amplification in the presence of methotrexate, can be explained by the chromatid breakage–fusion–bridge cycle (McClintock, 1941). Extra copies can also be acquired following unusual segregation at mitosis of extrachromosomal fragments (DMs or episomes) without centromeres (Windle et al., 1991). Amplicons are frequently found adjacent to fragile sites in the genome (Coquelle et al., 1997; Hellman et al., 2002) and hypoxia, commonly found in solid tumours, may be a potent trigger for expression of these sites providing breaks that can form the boundaries of new amplicons (Coquelle et al., 1998).

In practice, any overrepresentation of a gene can lead to a potentially pathogenic increase in expression levels and it is likely that for some genes, perhaps where levels of expression are normally very low, an increase in copy number by one or two may raise expression levels well above a critical normal threshold. In an aneuploid tumour cell, subtle imbalances may well lead to pathological changes in relative expression levels. The application of sensitive expression array analysis may allow any such changes to be identified in the future.

Chromosomal translocations and re-arrangements

Some of the most striking early observations made on the karyotypes of cells derived from tumours were of chromosomal translocations, often balanced translocations where two chromosomes appeared to have made a direct exchange of material. Chromosomal translocations are found in both chronic and acute haematopoetic malignancies and in some solid tumours of mesenchymal origin. In these contexts, striking specificity of translocation with tumour type or sub-type is observed. To date, despite rapid recent improvements in our ability to prepare and study chromosomes from the common epithelial malignancies, few balanced translocations have been identified. The reader is referred to excellent reviews (Rabbitts, 1994; Rowley, 1999; Bennicelli and Barr, 2002) and to Chapter 6 for more extensive descriptions of the range of translocations found in non-epithelial tumours.

Two consequences of chromosomal breakage and re-joining have been elucidated via the cloning and sequencing of translocation breakpoints from tumours. One consequence is that a gene close to the breakpoint on one derivative chromosome is not altered in its structure but its pattern of expression is altered. The second is that the structure of a gene (or genes) at the breakpoints is altered. Commonly this involves the fusion of exons from two different genes to give rise to a novel transcript and fusion protein product with altered or novel function.

Several examples of the first type of translocation involve the *MYC* gene (Kuppers and Dalla-Favera, 2001). These include three common translocations in Burkitt's lymphoma, t(8;14)(q24;q32), t(2;8)(p12; q24), and t(8;22)(q24;q11) in which the *MYC* gene is activated by translocation to the region of an immunoglobulin gene. Other lymphomas have different breakpoints and the orientation of the two genes can be head to head (5′ of *MYC* to 5′ of Ig) or head to tail (5′ of *MYC* to 3′ of Ig). Immunoglobulin and T-cell receptor genes are involved in many such translocations as they have a natural propensity to re-arrange in the generation of antibody diversity and errors in the process can occasionally lead to interchromosomal translocation.

An example of the second type of translocation is the 9;22 translocation in chronic myelogenous leukaemia that results in the fusion of the Abelson gene (*ABL*) on 9q34 with the 5′ region including the promoter of the *BCR* gene on chromosome 22. Both genes are broken in introns resulting in the formation of an in-frame fusion mRNA and protein that is unique to these tumour cells. Almost all CML patients show this translocation and express an abnormal 210 kDa protein (normal ABL protein 145 kDa). The derivative chromosome 22 is known as the Philadelphia (Ph) chromosome. A Ph chromosome is also found in some cases of acute lymphoid and myelogenous leukaemia and but here the breakpoint in the *BCR* gene is different and the fusion protein is 190 kDa. Functional assessment of these two fusions proteins *in vivo* indicates that the transforming ability of the 190 kDa protein is greater, which may explain its association with acute rather than chronic disease.

Most of the translocations identified in the myeloid leukaemias and in sarcomas are of this second type, resulting in the production of novel fusion proteins. It is difficult to give an accurate estimate of the number of translocation breakpoints that have been cloned as the number continues to increase but it is estimated to be well in excess of 100. Many of the fusion proteins encode transcription factors, suggesting that altered transcription, plays a key role in these tumour types, perhaps by altering the differentiation programme of the cell. Many fusion proteins have been tested for oncogenic function using a range of assays and several have been shown to be able to transform cultured cells. Some fusion proteins were in fact first identified in the NIH-3T3 assay. The NGF receptor *TRKA*, was identified as a fusion in which most of the extracellular part of the receptor was replaced by the coding sequence of a tropomyosin gene (Lamballe et al., 1991). *RET* was identified as a transforming gene in the DNA of a thyroid carcinoma. The cellular counterpart encodes a receptor for glial cell derived neurotrophic factor and oncogenic activation occurs by truncation of the tyrosine kinase domain and fusion to other genes, resulting in a product with constitutive tyrosine kinase activity (Nikiforov, 2002). As indicated above, *RET* can also be activated by point mutation and this represents one of only three familial cancer genes identified to date that is an oncogene rather than a tumour suppressor gene. *RET* is mutated in the MEN2A and MEN2B syndromes characterized by multiple endrocrine neoplasias and thyroid cancer.

These translocations are generally reciprocal and two chimaeric genes are produced, only one of which is usually considered essential in transformation. Sometimes, the second fusion does not produce a transcript. However, recent results indicate that some reciprocal products may have an effect on cell phenotype. For example, in acute myelogenous leukaemia with X-RARα translocations, where X-can be a range of partners including *PML, PLZF, NuMA*, or *STAT5B*, the reciprocal products are expressed and found to interfere by physical interaction with their respective X-pathways. In animal models at least, this appears to contribute to leukaemogenesis (Rego and Pandolfi, 2002).

7.4 Functions of proto-oncogenes

The enormous increase in knowledge of the past two decades has provided an insight into the complexity of cancer at the molecular level. Several principles have emerged; that multiple heritable changes are required to transform a cell, that several key cellular characteristics must be changed and that at least some of these characteristics are determined by a small number of critical pathways in the cell. Despite the complexity of detail that emerges from such a large human endeavour, already some simple concepts and rules that appear to apply to most cancer cells can be stated.

Hanahan and Weinberg (2000) summarize current understanding and provide a framework in which to consider novel findings. They list six essential alterations in cellular physiology that are required for malignant transformation and are shared by most, if not all cancer cells. These are self-sufficiency in growth signals, insensitivity to growth-inhibitory signals, evasion of programmed cell death (apoptosis), limitless replicative capacity, sustained angiogenesis and tissue invasion and metastasis. To describe the roles of oncogenes in the context of transformation of the cell, I will use these properties of transformed cells as a framework within which to give examples of the range of oncogene function.

7.4.1 Self-sufficiency in growth signals

Self-sufficiency in growth signals can arise via production of growth factors by the cancer cell, by alterations in expression of growth factor receptors or by changes in the levels of expression or activation status of signalling molecules and transcription factors (Hunter, 1997). Of the six characteristics, perhaps this is the characteristic of tumour cells to which dominant oncogenes contribute most frequently and dramatically to promote tumour cell proliferation. At the top of the growth signalling pathways, production of growth factors to which the cancer cell itself can respond (autocrine stimulation) is exemplified in several cases. The v-onc identified in simian sarcoma virus is the monkey homologue of *PDGFB* (Doolittle et al., 1983) and in human cancer, PDGFs are produced by glioblastomas (Lokker et al., 2002). In the skin tumour dermatofibrosarcoma protuberans (OMIM; 607907) PDGF is also produced. Here a reciprocal translocation, t(17;22) creates a fusion between *COL1A1* and *PDGFB* that is secreted and after proteolytic cleavage, produces excess PDGF-BB homodimers which act as an autocrine factor.

FGF4 is the product of an oncogene originally named HST, identified as amplified in gastric cancer, using the NIH-3T3 assay (Sakamoto et al., 1986). Homology was found with fibroblast growth factor and the *Int2* gene (≡ *Fgf3*) activated by insertion of MMTV in mouse mammary tumours. The same gene was also identified following transfection of DNA from Kaposi's sarcoma (Huebner et al., 1988) and designated K-FGF. *FGF4* is co-amplified with several other genes in the common 11q13 amplicon found in breast and other cancers and is overexpressed in many cancers.

Cell surface receptors, many with tyrosine kinase activity, have been identified as oncogenes in a wide range of cancers. The mechanisms of activation include mutations that activate the kinase, amplification, activation by the generation of fusion proteins and in many cases overexpression of the wild-type receptor has been recorded with no apparent genetic alteration. The epidermal growth factor receptor (*EGFR*) is amplified and/or overexpressed by stomach, brain and breast cancers and a truncated version that shows constitutive activation is found in glioblastomas with amplification of the gene (Ekstrand et al., 1994). The related receptor, *ERBB2*, is amplified and overexpressed in many breast, bladder, and other cancers. The fibroblast growth factor receptors are implicated in many cancers. *FGFR3* is mutated in bladder cancer and *FGFR2* is amplified in breast and gastric cancer. As this latter receptor binds FGF4, this may provide an alternative mechanism to activate the same signalling pathway as overexpression of FGF4. *FGFR4* is amplified in breast and gynaecological malignancies and a truncated version lacking the ligand-binding domain is found as an oncogenic variant in 40% of pituitary tumours. Mutational activation resulting in constitutive activation of the kinase activity of the receptor is also found for some other receptors, for example *CSF-1* receptor and *MET*. In addition to the growth factors themselves, some adaptor molecules are implicated for example CRK, an adaptor protein that is involved in signalling via several pathways (Feller et al., 1998).

Downstream of growth factors and their receptors signalling molecules in the same pathways are also implicated. Oncogenic Ras signalling has been studied extensively (McCormick, 1999). The *Ras* oncoproteins transduce signals from a range of growth factor receptors. Constitutive activation of their signalling activity via mutation thus renders the cell independent of both exogenous growth factors and cell surface receptors. Ras proteins activate several effector families, RAF, RALGDS, and PI3-kinase representing the most extensively studied to date. There is a complex literature describing the molecular mechanisms of effector activation, the identification of a range of novel effectors and the ways in which the downstream signalling pathways interact. This is discussed in more detail in Chapter 11. *Raf* has been identified as a retroviral oncogene and activation by Hras of Raf has been shown to be sufficient for malignant transformation in mice (Khosravi-Far et al., 1996). Several members of these pathways have transforming activity in *in vitro* assays, though they have not yet been identified as mutated in human tumours (e.g. RAC and RHO family members). Nevertheless there is evidence that some are overexpressed in cancer (e.g. RHOA, RHOC, and RAC1). Some GD/GTP exchange factors for these proteins are also implicated as oncogenes (e.g. TIAM1 which is mutated in renal cell carcinoma, DBL and VAV).

Finally, the transcription factors that are activated as the final targets in various signalling pathways are implicated. In the Ras-MAPK pathway, ETS (identified as a retroviral oncogene in the chicken virus E26-AMV) is activated downstream of RAF and this leads to transcription of a range of genes required for progression through the cell cycle, including cyclin D1 and FOS, both able to act as oncogenes themselves.

7.4.2 Insensitivity to negative signals and evasion of apoptosis

The normal cell possesses elegant control mechanisms that prevent acquisition of potentially damaging alterations and maintain quiescence and tissue homeostasis. These include soluble inhibitors such as transforming growth factor beta (TGFβ) that signal to maintain quiescence and cell cycle checkpoints that prevent damaged cells progressing through the cycle or prevent proliferation when environmental conditions are inappropriate. The major cell responses to negative signalling or to the activation of one of these checkpoints are cell cycle arrest (in G0 or G1) or programmed cell death, apoptosis. Cell cycle arrest provides time for necessary repair and apoptosis effectively removes damaged cells. The cellular proteins involved in monitoring the genome and cellular environment and eliciting these responses are for the most part tumour suppressor genes and it is loss of their function rather than gain of function that contributes to transformation. Examples include the various tumour suppressor genes involved in maintaining the all-important G1 checkpoint. These are members of the Rb and p53 pathways and regulators thereof (see Chapter 9). Nevertheless, some proteins involved in these pathways can contribute in a dominant manner. For example, cyclin D1, which as we have seen is overexpressed, often due to amplification, is implicated in many epithelial cancers. During G1, cyclin D1 activates CDKs 4 and 6, resulting in phosphorylation of Rb, which liberates bound E2Fs to initiate transcription of genes required for progression into S phase. Thus overexpression of cyclin D1 may phenocopy inactivation of Rb, p16 and/or p14^{ARF}. The cyclin dependent kinase CDK4 that is activated by cyclin D1 can itself act as an oncogene either by virtue of overexpression or by mutations that render the protein unable to bind to the negative regulator p16 (*CDKN2A*). This latter mechanism is responsible for some cases of familial melanoma (Zuo et al., 1996). E2Fs have also been implicated as oncogenes recently via overexpression or amplification in tumours (Table 7.3). In the p53 pathway, that provides the major DNA damage checkpoint, the MDM2 protein can provide an oncogenic stimulus when overexpressed by virtue of its function in targeting p53 for degradation via the ubiquitin pathway. Amplification of MDM2 has been found frequently in sarcomas and gliomas and less commonly in other tumour types. Overexpression has been described in many cancers.

The MYC transcription factor suppresses several negative regulatory functions that can act both to suppress differentiation and to stimulate cell proliferation and apoptosis. A comprehensive review of the role of MYC in cancer has been given by Pelengaris et al. (2002). Within the cell, MYC can complex with the factor MAX which in turn also complexes with MAD. MAD–MAX heterodimers provide differentiation-inducing signals. Overexpression of MYC swings the balance in favour of MYC–MAX heterodimers, activating transcription of many genes required for proliferation, including cyclin E-CDK2 and cyclin D-CDK4. Expression of cyclin D2 and CDK4 leads to sequestration of p27 (KIP1) and subsequent degradation, freeing cyclinE-CDK2 from complexes with p27 and allowing phosphorylation, which is required for subsequent phosphorylation of RB. MYC–MAX heterodimers also repress transcription via chromatin re-modelling induced by acetylation of histones and via binding to positively acting transcription factors such as MIZ1 which activates both p15 (*CDKN2B*) and p21 (WAF1). In this case MYC–MAX causes downregulation of the negative regulators p15 and p21. MYC also contributes to the increase in cell mass required during proliferation via induction of positive regulators of protein synthesis (e.g. eIF4).

Apoptosis is an effective means by which damaged cells are removed rapidly. It is also a likely mechanism for the removal of cells in which inappropriate oncogenic stimuli have been activated (e.g. a cell containing a mutated oncogene). In either case, survival might allow further changes to take place leading to the development of a fully transformed cell. The apoptotic machinery is therefore a vital defence against cancer development and detailed discussion of the mechanisms and control of apoptosis are given in Chapter 12.

Cell survival results from a balance in exposure to survival and death signals. This involves both sensors, for example, cell surface receptors that bind survival or death factors and effectors that initiate or participate in the apoptotic cascade. Examples of survival factors include insulin-like growth factors (IGFs) 1 and 2, which bind to IGF1-R. These can act as oncogenic stimuli. For example, overexpression of IGF-2 in pancreatic islet tumours provides a vital survival (rather than proliferative) signal (Christofori et al., 1994).

A range of factors and receptors transmit death signals. Examples include FAS ligand and FAS receptor and TNFα and TNFR1. Several so-called decoy receptors exist that lack a signalling domain and overexpression of these in tumours can sequester death factors and promote survival (Ashkenazi and Dixit, 1999). Intracellular monitors of DNA damage and environmental abnormalities can also trigger apoptosis. Some of the proteins that are involved in the control of the apoptotic process are implicated as oncogenes. BCL-2, an anti-apoptotic protein, is activated via translocation in follicular lymphomas (Korsmeyer, 1992) and in combination with *Myc*, *Bcl2* can elicit lymphomas in mice (Strasser et al., 1990). As MYC is a pro-apoptotic protein, activation of MYC in tumours is often (perhaps always) accompanied by overexpression of survival factors or disruption of death signalling (Pelengaris et al., 2002).

7.4.3 Acquisition of limitless proliferative capacity

Normal cells all have a finite ability to proliferate *in vitro* and *in vivo* this is likely to limit the ability of tumour cells to survive. A detailed discussion of the mechanisms by which tumour cells evade the senescence checkpoint and become immortal is given in Chapter 10. To date all evidence points to tumour suppressor genes as the major players in this process. The role of telomerase in immortalization is now well documented and in tumour cell this is clearly a dominant function that in the strict sense could merit its classification as an oncogene. However, as there is little evidence to date that up-regulation of telomerase activity dysregulates cellular processes, there has been some debate about the definition of telomerase as an oncogene (Kipling, 1995; Harley, 2002).

7.4.4 Angiogenesis

All tumours require the formation of a new blood supply if they are to grow to any significant size (Folkman, 1997). As described in Chapter 17, this is elicited by the tumour cells themselves via several mechanisms. Again there are counterbalancing positive and negative signals. VEGF and FGFs 1 and 2 are potent stimulatory molecules that signal via endothelial cell receptors and are potent mitogens for endothelial cells. These genes are not activated in tumours via any of the genetic mechanisms described above. However, the recent literature contains many references to known oncogenes and tumour suppressor genes that induce either directly or indirectly the expression of molecules including VEGF and FGFs that effect angiogenesis. An example is the induction of VEGF expression in ovarian carcinomas that have activation of the oncogene *PIK3CA* (Zhang et al., 2003). Similarly, the cellular response to hypoxia, a response that includes induction of VEGF expression, is affected by several oncoproteins including RAS, SRC, and ERBB2 (Rak et al., 1995).

7.4.5 Tissue invasion and metastasis

Much less is known about genes that determine invasion and metastasis than about those that contribute to the formation of primary tumours (Chapter 16 and Friedl and Wolf, 2003). These are complex processes and can only occur once a tumour has acquired all of the previous characteristics. The additional changes required involve alterations in the interaction of tumour cells with their neighbours and with the tissue micro-environment. Adhesion molecules are implicated, such as loss of expression of E-cadherin in many aggressive epithelial tumours. Interestingly in some cases of colorectal cancer, this can be linked to the presence of a truncated β-catenin, which disrupts the interaction between E-cadherin and α-catenin with consequent loss of cell adhesion. In this situation mutated β-catenin acts as a dominant oncogene.

Some secreted molecules, for example, matrix metalloproteinases (MMPs) contribute by proteolysis in the tumour stroma, leading to the degradation of matrix and the generation of promigratory, for example, chemotactic factors from precursors and the liberation of sequestered growth factors. There are several secreted factors that are promigratory in the tumour micro-environment (e.g. EGF, IGF1) that contribute to tumour invasion. Several known oncogenes including *RAS* and *MYC* can induce metastatic ability in model systems though complete information on the mechanisms is lacking. The interaction of the proto-oncogene tyrosine kinase receptor MET with hepatocyte growth factor/scatter factor induces cell scattering and increased motility in epithelial cells that is likely to contribute to invasion an/or metastasis in several tumour types. MET is activated by mutation, overexpression and HGF by overexpression in human cancers leading to autocrine stimulation (Birchmeier et al., 2003).

7.4.6 Determining mechanisms and facilitating the process

The ways in which each of the above six characteristics of tumour cells are acquired and the speed at which this occurs will be influenced by environmental factors such as the presence of various carcinogens, the tissue type involved and the ways in which different signalling pathways function to maintain tissue homeostasis. In one tissue for example, the pivotal importance of a particular pathway in a specific cell type or lineage may dictate the possible ways in which growth control is likely to be regulated in this context. This type of consideration may explain, at least in part, the tissue specific combinations of genetic alterations found in tumours. This is particularly apparent in the haematological malignancies as illustrated by some of the examples cited here.

It is also worth noting that a seventh characteristic of tumour cells, not absolutely necessary for tumour formation, but of great advantage in tumour progression and evolution is the propensity for genomic instability. This has been discussed in several excellent recent reviews (Feldser et al., 2003; Rajagopalan et al., 2003; Sieber et al., 2003).

One class of genes involved in this phenotype requires mention here as these genes clearly act as oncogenes in several types of cancer. These are genes that control chromosome segregation and when overexpressed lead to errors in segregation that lead to cellular aneuploidy. An example is aurora kinase A (*AURKA)* also known as STK15, a gene whose product associates with the centrosome in S phase and is involved in centrosome separation, duplication, and maturation. STK15 is amplified and overexpressed in several types of cancer and this is associated with the generation of aneuploidy (Dutertre et al., 2002).

7.5 Oncogenes as therapeutic targets

The dominant or gain of function effect of activated oncogenes makes these attractive targets for therapeutic intervention. The highly specific nature of many of the oncogenic events described above also raises the possibility of specific and targeted therapies. Although this possibility was recognized many years ago, until relatively recently success was limited and disappointment dominated the field. Rational drug design requires a thorough knowledge of the function of the target and of how this is altered in cancer cells and for several of the attractive targets (e.g. RAS, ERBB2) this information is available in large measure. Some specific examples and approaches are covered in Chapters 24 and 28 and only a few general comments will be made here.

A key consideration is whether the inactivation of a single oncogene in a cell with multiple other genetic changes will be sufficient to elicit a response. Transgenic models have recently provided evidence that inactivation of a single oncogene can provide specific and effective therapy. For example, inactivation of MYC in a range of tumour types in mice induces tumour regression with observation of cell cycle arrest, cell differentiation, and in some cases apoptosis. Similarly, RAS has been shown to be required for continued survival of melanoma and lung adenocarcinomas in mice and ABL is required in mouse lymphomas (Felsher, 2003). These promising results have led to the concept that cancers are 'addicted' to certain oncogenic stimuli involved in their induction. This is not surprising given that all subsequent genetic changes that are selected for in the tumour cell occurred against the background of changes in the signalling circuitry induced by the initiating oncogene and thus may be fine balanced to accommodate this. To date few oncogenes have been examined in this way, possibly these have been the most potent ones and in all cases the oncogenic activation was the initiating event in the tumour models. It remains to be seen what the outcome will be if an oncogene activated later in the transformation process is targeted.

Nevertheless, this evidence has been sufficient to stimulate renewed efforts to target oncogenes in human cancer. The best example to date is the treatment of patients with chronic myelogenous leukaemis (CML; Ph+ tumours) with the ABL kinase inhibitor Gleevec. Remarkable sustained remissions have been achieved in these and in gastrointestinalstromal-associated tumours (GISTs), which contain activated c-KIT. However, some of the early successes with the drug have already been tempered by examples of resistance mediated by novel BCR-ABL mutations and reduced effects in patients who following blast crisis develop an acute myeloid leukaemia (AML), presumably with additional genetic defects. This gives a hint that targeting more than one oncogene may be more effective.

BCR-ABL represents a protein unique to the tumour cells. RAS and other mutated oncogenes all differ from their wild-type counterparts and present the possibility of mutant-specific therapy. The prospect of inactivating oncogenes that are overexpressed wild-type proteins raises questions concerning possible serious systemic side effects. The MYC oncogene is a key example of this type. Interestingly, a recent study has provided tantalizing evidence that even very brief inactivation of the MYC in a transgenic model of osteosarcoma was sufficient not only to cause differentiation of the tumour cells but also to render them refractory to the effects of MYC re-activation, which surprisingly caused apoptosis (Jain et al., 2002). This has been interpreted as a differentiation context-specific effect, in which despite continued presence of other genetic changes, the state of the cell post-treatment was no longer permissive for MYC to contribute to transformation. This may result from epigenetic changes associated with the therapy-induced differentiation. Interestingly a similar effect had been reported decades ago when a temperature sensitive *Src* mutant in chick muscle induced cell death upon re-activation after a period at the non-permissive temperature. This additional layer of complexity, while difficult to dissect experimentally, may provide a valuable opportunity for therapy.

7.6 Conclusions

The identification and characterization of genes with dominant cellular effects has had enormous impact on our understanding of the molecular basis of neoplasia. Less than 30 years ago, despite the knowledge that viruses could cause cancer in animals, there was great scepticism in the human cancer research community about the relevance of these viruses and their transforming genes to human cancer. Fortunately, the persistence and curiosity of those working in that field provided the tools that have allowed the dramatic progress in understanding of the genes involved in human cancer that has been achieved since the 1980s. Within 20 years of the identification of the first human oncogenes, there have been direct applications of knowledge about these genes in the clinic. Examples range from the direct visualization of specific translocations for diagnosis of haematopoetic malignancies, through various molecular profiling applications for diagnosis and treatment planning in solid tumours to the use of oncogenes as therapeutic targets. These oncogene-based approaches to therapy have not yet met with widespread success but the promise offered by small molecules such as Gleevec coupled with current progress in solving the three-dimensional structure of many of the key targets and improved understanding of their function is likely to yield many potential drugs in the near future. Similarly, novel approaches to gene therapy such as the application of small interfering RNAs (siRNA) to knock down gene expression in mammalian cells show great promise. These are exciting times. Currently we have such a range of powerful technologies on hand to carry out profiling experiments on tumours and to manipulate the genome of model organisms and human cells that a deluge of new information is inevitable. So far it has proved difficult to interpret and use the vast array of information on gene expression that is coming from microarray experiments on tumours but current developments in methodology are already having great impact. In light of these changes in approach to biological questions, it is likely that the next decade will see a marked change, perhaps the most marked in the field to date, in the way we study oncogenes and the consequences of their alteration in human cancer.

References

Ashkenazi, A. and Dixit, V. M. (1999). Apoptosis control by death and decoy receptors. *Curr Opin Cell Biol*, **11**, 255–60.

Bennicelli, J. L. and Barr, F. G. (2002). Chromosomal translocations and sarcomas. *Curr Opin Oncol*, **14**, 412–9.

Birchmeier, C., Birchmeier, W., Gherardi, E., and Vande Woude, G. F. (2003). Met, metastasis, motility and more. *Nat Rev Mol Cell Biol*, **4**, 915–25.

Bos, J. L. (1989). ras oncogenes in human cancer: a review. *Cancer Res*, **49**, 4682–9.

Christofori, G., Naik, P., and Hanahan, D. (1994). A second signal supplied by insulin-like growth factor II in oncogene-induced tumorigenesis. *Nature*, **369**, 414–8.

Coffin, J. M., Hughes, S. H., and Varmus, H. E. (1997). *Retroviruses*, Cold Spring Harbor Laboratory Press.

Collins, S. and Groudine, M. (1982). Amplification of endogenous myc-related DNA sequences in a human myeloid leukaemia cell line. *Nature*, **298**, 679–81.

Coquelle, A., Pipiras, E., Toledo, F., Buttin, G., and Debatisse, M. (1997). Expression of fragile sites triggers intrachromosomal mammalian gene amplification and sets boundaries to early amplicons. *Cell*, **89**, 215–25.

Coquelle, A., Toledo, F., Stern, S., Bieth, A., and Debatisse, M. (1998). A new role for hypoxia in tumor progression: induction of fragile site triggering genomic rearrangements and formation of complex DMs and HSRs. *Mol Cell*, **2**, 259–65.

Davies, H., Bignell, G. R., Cox, C., Stephens, P., Edkins, S., Clegg, S. et al. (2002). Mutations of the BRAF gene in human cancer. *Nature*, **417**, 949–54.

Doolittle, R. F., Hunkapiller, M. W., Hood, L. E., Devare, S. G., Robbins, K. C., Aaronson, S. A. et al. (1983). Simian sarcoma virus onc gene, v-sis, is derived from the gene (or genes) encoding a platelet-derived growth factor. *Science*, **221**, 275–7.

Dutertre, S., Descamps, S., and Prigent, C. (2002). On the role of aurora-A in centrosome function. *Oncogene*, **21**, 6175–83.

Ekstrand, A. J., Longo, N., Hamid, M. L., Olson, J. J., Liu, L., Collins, V. P. et al. (1994). Functional characterization of an EGF receptor with a truncated extracellular domain expressed in glioblastomas with EGFR gene amplification. *Oncogene*, **9**, 2313–20.

Feldser, D. M., Hackett, J. A., and Greider, C. W. (2003). Telomere dysfunction and the initiation of genome instability. *Nat Rev Cancer*, **3**, 623–7.

Feller, S. M., Posern, G., Voss, J., Kardinal, C., Sakkab, D., Zheng, J. et al. (1998). Physiological signals and oncogenesis mediated through Crk family adapter proteins. *J Cell Physiol*, **177**, 535–52.

Felsher, D. W. (2003). Cancer revoked: oncogenes as therapeutic targets. *Nat Rev Cancer*, **3**, 375–80.

Folkman, J. (1997). Tumor angiogenesis In *Cancer Medicine* (eds. J. F. Holland, R. C. Bast, E. Morton, E. Frei, D. W., Kufe, and R. R. Weichselbaum) BC Decker, Hamilton Ontario.

Friedl, P. and Wolf, K. (2003). Tumour-cell invasion and migration: diversity and escape mechanisms. *Nat Rev Cancer*, **3**, 362–74.

Hanahan, D. and Weinberg, R. A. (2000). The hallmarks of cancer. *Cell*, **100**, 57–70.

Harley, C. B. (2002). Telomerase is not an oncogene. *Oncogene*, **21**, 494–502.

Hellman, A., Zlotorynski, E., Scherer, S. W., Cheung, J., Vincent, J. B., Smith, D. I. et al. (2002). A role for common fragile site induction in amplification of human oncogenes. *Cancer Cell*, **1**, 89–97.

Hirota, S., Isozaki, K., Moriyama, Y., Hashimoto, K., Nishida, T., Ishiguro, S. et al. (1998). Gain-of-function mutations of c-kit in human gastrointestinal stromal tumors. *Science*, **279**, 577–80.

Hodgson, J. G., Chin, K., Collins, C., and Gray, J. W. (2003). Genome amplification of chromosome 20 in breast cancer. *Breast Cancer Res Treat*, **78**, 337–45.

Huebner, K., Ferrari, A. C., Delli Bovi, P., Croce, C. M., and Basilico, C. (1988). The FGF-related oncogene, K-FGF, maps to human chromosome region 11q13, possibly near int-2. *Oncogene Res*, **3**, 263–70.

Hunter, T. (1997). Oncoprotein networks. *Cell*, **88**, 333–46.

Hyman, E., Kauraniemi, P., Hautaniemi, S., Wolf, M., Mousses, S., Rozenblum, E. et al. (2002). Impact of DNA amplification on gene expression patterns in breast cancer. *Cancer Res*, **62**, 6240–5.

Jain, M., Arvanitis, C., Chu, K., Dewey, W., Leonhardt, E., Trinh, M. et al. (2002). Sustained loss of a neoplastic phenotype by brief inactivation of MYC. *Science*, **297**, 102–4.

Khosravi-Far, R., White, M. A., Westwick, J. K., Solski, P. A., Chrzanowska-Wodnicka, M., Van Aelst, L. et al. (1996). Oncogenic Ras activation of Raf/mitogen-activated protein kinase-independent pathways is sufficient to cause tumorigenic transformation. *Mol Cell Biol*, **16**, 3923–33.

Kipling, D. (1995). Telomerase: immortality enzyme or oncogene?. *Nat Genet*, **9**, 104–6.

Korsmeyer, S. J. (1992). Chromosomal translocations in lymphoid malignancies reveal novel proto-oncogenes. *Annu Rev Immunol*, **10**, 785–807.

Kuppers, R. and Dalla-Favera, R. (2001). Mechanisms of chromosomal translocations in B cell lymphomas. *Oncogene*, **20**, 5580–94.

Lamballe, F., Klein, R., and Barbacid, M. (1991). The trk family of oncogenes and neurotrophin receptors. *Princess Takamatsu Symp*, **22**, 153–70.

Lokker, N. A., Sullivan, C. M., Hollenbach, S. J., Israel, M. A., and Giese, N. A. (2002). Platelet-derived growth factor (PDGF) autocrine signaling regulates survival and mitogenic pathways in glioblastoma cells: evidence that the novel PDGF-C and PDGF-D ligands may play a role in the development of brain tumors. *Cancer Res*, **62**, 3729–35.

Malumbres, M. and Barbacid, M. (2003). RAS oncogenes: the first 30 years. *Nat Rev Cancer*, **3**, 459–65.

McClintock, B. (1941). The stability of broken ends of chromosomes in *Zea mays*. *Genetica*, **41**, 234–82.

McCormick, F. (1999). Signalling networks that cause cancer. *Trends in Cell Biol*, **9**, M53–M56.

Monni, O., Barlund, M., Mousses, S., Kononen, J., Sauter, G., Heiskanen, M. et al. (2001). Comprehensive copy number and gene expression profiling of the 17q23 amplicon in human breast cancer. *Proc Natl Acad Sci USA*, **98**, 5711–6.

Munro, N. P. and Knowles, M. A. (2003). Fibroblast growth factors and their receptors in transitional cell carcinoma. *J Urol*, **169**, 675–82.

Nau, M. M., Brooks, B. J., Battey, J., Sausville, E., Gazdar, A. F., Kirsch, I. R. et al. (1985). L-myc, a new myc-related gene amplified and expressed in human small cell lung cancer. *Nature*, **318**, 69–73.

Nikiforov, Y. E. (2002). RET/PTC rearrangement in thyroid tumors. *Endocr Pathol*, **13**, 3–16.

Parada, L. F., Tabin, C. J., Shih, C., and Weinberg, R. A. (1982). Human EJ bladder carcinoma oncogene is homologue of Harvey sarcoma virus ras gene. *Nature*, **297**, 474–8.

Pelengaris, S., Khan, M., and Evan, G. (2002). c-MYC: more than just a matter of life and death. *Nat Rev Cancer*, **2**, 764–76.

Pollack, J. R., Sorlie, T., Perou, C. M., Rees, C. A., Jeffrey, S. S., Lonning, P. E. et al. (2002). Microarray analysis reveals a major direct role of DNA copy number alteration in the transcriptional program of human breast tumors. *Proc Natl Acad Sci USA*, **99**, 12963–8.

Rabbitts, T. H. (1994). Chromosomal translocations in human cancer. *Nature*, **372**, 143–9.

Rajagopalan, H., Nowak, M. A., Vogelstein, B., and Lengauer, C. (2003). The significance of unstable chromosomes in colorectal cancer. *Nat Rev Cancer*, **3**, 695–701.

Rak, J., Mitsuhashi, Y., Bayko, L., Filmus, J., Shirasawa, S., Sasazuki, T. et al. (1995). Mutant ras oncogenes upregulate VEGF/VPF expression: implications for induction and inhibition of tumor angiogenesis. *Cancer Res*, **55**, 4575–80.

Reddy, E. P., Reynolds, R. K., Santos, E., and Barbacid, M. (1982). A point mutation is responsible for the acquisition of transforming properties by the T24 human bladder carcinoma oncogene. *Nature*, **300**, 149–52.

Rego, E. M. and Pandolfi, P. P. (2002). Reciprocal products of chromosomal translocations in human cancer pathogenesis: key players or innocent bystanders?. *Trends Mol Med*, **8**, 396–405.

Ridge, S. A., Worwood, M., Oscier, D., Jacobs, A., and Padua, R. A. (1990). FMS mutations in myelodysplastic, leukemic, and normal subjects. *Proc Natl Acad Sci USA*, **87**, 1377–80.

Rowley, J. D. (1999). The role of chromosome translocations in leukemogenesis. *Semin Hematol*, **36**, 59–72.

Sakamoto, H., Mori, M., Taira, M., Yoshida, T., Matsukawa, S., Shimizu, K. et al. (1986). Transforming gene from human stomach cancers and a noncancerous portion of stomach mucosa. *Proc Natl Acad Sci USA*, **83**, 3997–4001.

Scheijen, B. and Griffin, J. D. (2002). Tyrosine kinase oncogenes in normal hematopoiesis and hematological disease. *Oncogene*, **21**, 3314–33.

Schwab, M., Alitalo, K., Klempnauer, K. H., Varmus, H. E., Bishop, J. M., Gilbert, F. et al. (1983). Amplified DNA with limited homology to myc cellular oncogene is shared by human neuroblastoma cell lines and a neuroblastoma tumour. *Nature*, **305**, 245–8.

Shih, C., Shilo, B. Z., Goldfarb, M. P., Dannenberg, A., and Weinberg, R. A. (1979). Passage of phenotypes of chemically transformed cells via transfection of DNA and chromatin. *Proc Natl Acad Sci USA*, **76**, 5714–8.

Sieber, O. M., Heinimann, K., and Tomlinson, I. P. (2003). Genomic instability—the engine of tumorigenesis?. *Nat Rev Cancer*, **3**, 701–8.

Slamon, D. J., Godolphin, W., Jones, L. A., Holt, J. A., Wong, S. G., Keith, D. E. et al. (1989). Studies of the HER-/neu proto-oncogene in human breast and ovarian cancer. *Science*, **244**, 707–12.

Stirewalt, D. L. and Radich, J. P. (2003). The role of FLT3 in haematopoietic malignancies. *Nat Rev Cancer*, **3**, 650–65.

Strasser, A., Harris, A. W., Bath, M. L., and Cory, S. (1990). Novel primitive lymphoid tumours induced in transgenic mice by cooperation between myc and bcl-2. *Nature*, **348**, 331–3.

Suzuki, T., Shen, H., Akagi, K., Morse, H. C., Malley, J. D., Naiman, D. Q. et al. (2002). New genes involved in cancer identified by retroviral tagging. *Nat Genet*, **32**, 166–74.

Tabin, C. J., Bradley, S. M., Bargmann, C. I., Weinberg, R. A., Papageorge, A. G., Scolnick, E. M. et al. (1982). Mechanism of activation of a human oncogene. *Nature*, **300**, 143–9.

Tian, Q., Frierson, H. F., Jr., Krystal, G. W., and Moskaluk, C. A. (1999). Activating c-kit gene mutations in human germ cell tumors. *Am J Pathol*, **154**, 1643–7.

Varmus, H. (1988). Retroviruses. *Science*, **240**, 1427–35.

Weinberg, R. A. (1981). Use of transfection to analyze genetic information and malignant transformation. *Biochim Biophys Acta*, **651**, 25–35.

Windle, B., Draper, B. W., Yin, Y. X., O'Gorman, S., and Wahl, G. M. (1991). A central role for chromosome breakage in gene amplification, deletion formation, and amplicon integration. *Genes Dev*, **5**, 160–74.

Zhang, L., Yang, N., Katsaros, D., Huang, W., Park, J. W., Fracchioli, S. et al. (2003). The oncogene phosphatidylinositol 3'-kinase catalytic subunit alpha promotes angiogenesis via vascular endothelial growth factor in ovarian carcinoma. *Cancer Res*, **63**, 4225–31.

Zuo, L., Weger, J., Yang, Q., Goldstein, A. M., Tucker, M. A., Walker, G. J. et al. (1996). Germline mutations in the p16INK4a binding domain of CDK4 in familial melanoma. *Nat Genet*, **12**, 97–9.

CHAPTER 8

Tumour suppressor genes

Sonia Laín and David P. Lane

8.1 Definition

Tumour suppressor genes (TSGs) encode proteins whose absence, repression, expression inactivation, or mutation promotes oncogenesis. In some instances, reactivation of the function of a TSG suppresses the malignant phenotype. This type of TSG is referred to as a gatekeeper gene. Inactivation of other TSGs (caretaker genes), leads instead to genomic instability and therefore to an increase in the mutation of other genes that may be gatekeeper genes or influence tumour development. Caretaker genes include genes involved in DNA repair and genes that maintain the integrity of chromosomes and their numbers. Unlike gatekeeper genes, reconstitution of caretaker genes fails to override these secondary effects and does not suppress malignancy. In many cases as described below, TSGs may be involved in both gatekeeping and in caretaking functions.

Tumour suppressor genes are altered via different mechanisms, including deletions and point mutations, which may result in an inactive or dominant negative product. Regions of chromosomes frequently deleted in tumour cells are thought to harbour TSGs. Often such deletions are easily detectable and provide a means to map the underlying mutant gene. Alternatively, methylation of the promoter of the TSG can down-regulate its expression. Dysregulation of genes encoding proteins that modulate tumour suppressors may also lead to a defect in a given tumour suppressive function. In other examples, chimaeric proteins formed by chromosomal translocations can produce dominant negative factors that can decrease expression, stability or function of TSGs.

This chapter describes the discovery of TSGs, their role in the transformation process and the mechanisms by which they are inactivated. We discuss several specific examples of TSGs and their function in more detail.

8.2 Discovery of tumour suppressor genes and Knudson's 'two hit' model

The existence of tumour suppressor functions was anticipated from the observation that fusion of a tumour cell with a non-tumorigenic cell, most frequently results in the inhibition of the tumorigenic phenotype. This, together with the finding that loss of specific chromosomes (chromosome 11 in early experiments), was associated with a tumorigenic phenotype and that the introduction of a normal chromosome 11 into a tumour cell restored the normal morphological phenotype, reinforced the idea that genes exist that are involved in preventing tumorigenicity.

The first TSG identified, *RB*, was found from studies on retinoblastoma, a rare inherited cancer syndrome occurring in children. Inheritance of this tumour predisposition was associated with the loss of the 13q14 chromosome region. As first suggested by Knudson, inactivation of the gene is a two hit phenomenon. One of the changes is inherited whereas the second occurs somatically during embryogenesis or early in life. More refined studies comparing restriction fragment length polymorphisms (RFLP) in DNA from retinoblastomas with DNA from normal tissue of the same patient, revealed loss of heterozygosity (LOH) of loci near 13q14. In 1986, Weinberg and colleagues identified *RB* as the critical gene in this chromosome region. Whereas expression of this gene was found to occur in normal retinal and other normal cells, it was absent in retinoblastomas. These observations and the observation of LOH in non-inherited cancers led to the conclusion that mutation (or other functional inactivation) of both copies of a TSG is required for tumour formation, implying that only complete loss of the gene product produces a cellular defect. This is known as Knudson's 'two hit' model (reviewed in Knudson, 2001). However, as discussed in the section on haploinsufficiency (8.5 below), mutation of a single copy of a TSG may also have important consequences. Since the first proposal that a TSG is involved in the formation of retinoblastomas, a growing number of genes with proven or suspected tumour suppressor activity have been discovered. Over the past 15 years there have been great advances in our understanding of the function of TSGs. These advances are critical for the elucidation of the tumorigenic process as well as for the development of novel anti-cancer therapies.

8.3 Multi-step tumorigenesis: the Vogelstein–Fearon model for colorectal cancer

It is widely accepted that a single mutation is not likely to lead to cancer. Our current concept is that a cell progresses towards malignancy by acquiring a series of mutations that allow it to evade the various controls that normally prevent malignant growth. According to epidemiological and experimental data, between four and eight rate-limiting mutations are predicted to occur during the development of human cancer. The mutations found are sometimes characteristic for particular tumour types, indicating that their relevance may be influenced by the type of tissue in which the tumour develops.

Colorectal cancer (CRC) is one of the most frequent causes of morbidity and mortality worldwide due to cancer. The average lifetime risk is 5%, and the incidence of CRC rises dramatically with age. The incidence varies up to 20-fold between different geographical areas. High-risk populations occur in developed countries and therefore there is a possible association with lifestyle and dietary habits (Chapter 2).

Mutation of the adenomatous polyposis coli (*APC*) gene is an early and frequent feature of CRC. Familial adenomatous polyposis (FAP), a hereditary predisposition to colorectal cancer, is associated with mutations in *APC* and most sporadic colorectal cancers have mutations in this gene. The appearance of characteristic mutations at each stage of malignant transformation in colon carcinoma progression suggested that there is selection for sequential premalignant stage genetic lesions. In 1990, Fearon and Vogelstein proposed a model in which successive genetic changes lead to CRC. Research over recent years has revealed further information on the function of key genes involved. These include *APC, KRAS2, SMAD2/SMAD4*, and *TP53*. The dominant or recessive nature of these genes implies that one mutation at *KRAS2* and six mutations to inactivate each allele of *APC, SMAD2–4*, and *TP53* may be required. For a detailed discussion and revision of this model and a detailed description of the functional relationships between each of the gene products involved see Knudson (2001) and Fodde and Smits (2001). In brief, the Vogelstein–Fearon model consists of the following successive steps:

Initiation. APC is involved in a wide variety of functions that control cell adhesion, migration, apoptosis, and chromosomal segregation at mitosis. Alteration of the Wnt signalling pathway due to *APC* mutation is considered to be the crucial initiating event leading to the appearance of non-dysplastic aberrant crypt foci (ACF). Upon binding of a Wnt peptide to its receptor, the glycogen synthase 3β (GSK-3β) is inactivated. This blocks phosphorylation of β-catenin, an event that is necessary for its binding to APC and for APC-mediated degradation of β-catenin. As a consequence, β-catenin accumulates and co-operates with the transcription factor Tcf-4. Mutated and truncated APC is unable to bind to β-catenin, and therefore, in cells bearing such mutations, this pathway is deregulated. Interestingly as a consequence of this alteration in Wnt signalling, c-Myc is inappropriately activated. c-Myc is a transcription factor that regulates a large set of genes including p53 and cTERT (the main component of the telomerase complex) and binds to important cell cycle regulatory proteins such as Rb and p107. In this way c-Myc exerts diverse overall effects, such as induction of proliferation, apoptosis, and inhibition of differentiation. As such, c-Myc is thought to be crucial in the balance between proliferation and apoptosis, and therefore, its abnormal expression may tip the balance in the wrong direction. Mutations in *APC* may therefore lead to inappropriate regulation and stimulate the oncogenic effects of c-Myc. In the minority of the CRCs without *APC* mutations, mutations in APC partners such as β-catenin or conductin may be expected. *KRAS2* mutations occur in most ACF but the frequency decreases during progression. The survival of cells with mutated *KRAS2* may be limited by the possible induction in human cells of p14ARF and therefore by the activation of p53 (see below). However, considering the known co-operation of K-ras and c-Myc in transformation, *KRAS2* mutation may confer an additional advantage to cells with a deregulated Wnt signalling pathway. APC also binds to and stabilizes microtubules and is an important regulator of cytoskeletal function. Accordingly, cells carrying a truncated APC gene have been shown to be defective in chromosome segregation which suggests that alterations in APC that eliminate microtubule binding may contribute to chromosomal instability in cancer cells. In summary, mutations in APC are involved in tumour initiation by constitutively activating the Wnt pathway and in favouring tumour promotion and progression by enhancing chromosomal instability.

Promotion. Defects in the TGF-β signalling pathway due to mutations of *SMAD2/SMAD4* may permit the small adenoma initiated by Wnt pathway defects to grow into a large adenoma. 18q deletions are known to be associated with poor prognosis for patients with colorectal cancer. SMAD-4, originally called DPC-4 (deleted in pancreatic cancer), one of the components of the TGF-β signalling pathway, is one of the genes affected by these deletions. *SMAD4* mutations occur in 6–30% of CRCs. Closely positioned to *SMAD4*, the *SMAD2* gene is another component of the TGF-β signalling pathway and may be deleted in a particular group of CRCs.

Progression. When a mutation is acquired in *TP53*, the 'guardian of the genome' (see below), apart from loss of cell cycle checkpoints and reduced apoptotic response, cells accumulate genetic alterations involving gross genomic aberrations and aneuploidy, allowing the progression of the adenoma into a carcinoma.

8.4 Mechanisms leading to tumour suppressor function loss

Knudson's 'two-hit' hypothesis that both alleles of a gene have to be inactivated to contribute to transformation, holds true for some TSGs. In fact, the genes for most dominantly inherited cancers, like retinoblastoma, show this relationship. Considering mutation hypothesis only, even supposing a high frequency of 6×10^{-6} mutations per locus, the probability of four mutations arising is remarkably low (roughly 10^{-21}) even in a human organism (approx. 10^{14} cells) with a long lifespan. Whatever the inaccuracy of this calculation, this probability is nowhere near the frequency at which humans develop cancer at some time in their life (1 in 3). To explain this discrepancy, factors other than simple mutation rate must contribute to the development of cancer. TSGs may be inactivated by mechanisms other than mutation, such as methylation and this may occur at higher frequency than mutations. Furthermore, if mutations occur in genes that control genetic stability (such as caretaker genes), this 'mutator phenotype' may contribute to the appearance of mutations and other genetic abnormalities. Finally, this discrepancy has led to a renewed interest in the concept of haploinsufficiency, a state in which loss of a single allele significantly impairs its function.

8.5 Haploinsufficiency

Recent data suggest that the function of some TSGs can be disrupted solely by haploinsufficiency; that is, alteration of one allele of a gene with the other allele remaining normal (Figure 8.1). If a single mutation confers a significant selective advantage, the resulting clonal expansion would increase the number of target cells susceptible to further alteration. Mutation of one allele of TSGs with strong haploinsufficiency allows clonal expansion of cells that are heterozygous for a TSG mutation and these cells are susceptible to further progression along a multi-step tumorigenesis pathway. For partially haploinsufficient TSGs, LOH (i.e. loss of the remaining TSG allele) is necessary to complete tumorigenesis. In the absence of haploinsufficiency, mutation of one allele of a given TSG does not lead to clonal expansion, and therefore, very few cells are available to complete the pathway. In this case, tumours occur very rarely. In familial cancers, all cells are heterozygous, and no clonal expansion is required to increase the population of susceptible cells. Therefore, tumours can arise even in the absence of haploinsufficiency. Quon and Berns (2001) propose that all TSGs that are frequently mutated in sporadic human cancers may show varying degrees of haploinsufficiency, with some genes showing strong effects and others showing partial or weak effects.

8.6 Retinoblastoma

Retinoblastomas are caused by a germline mutation of one *RB* allele and an acquired somatic mutation of the remaining allele of the *RB* gene. These findings led to the proposal for the 'two hit' model of carcinogenesis and the proposal of the existence of TSGs as described above. Supporting the role of *RB* in cancer development, several DNA tumour viruses encode proteins that directly bind to Rb

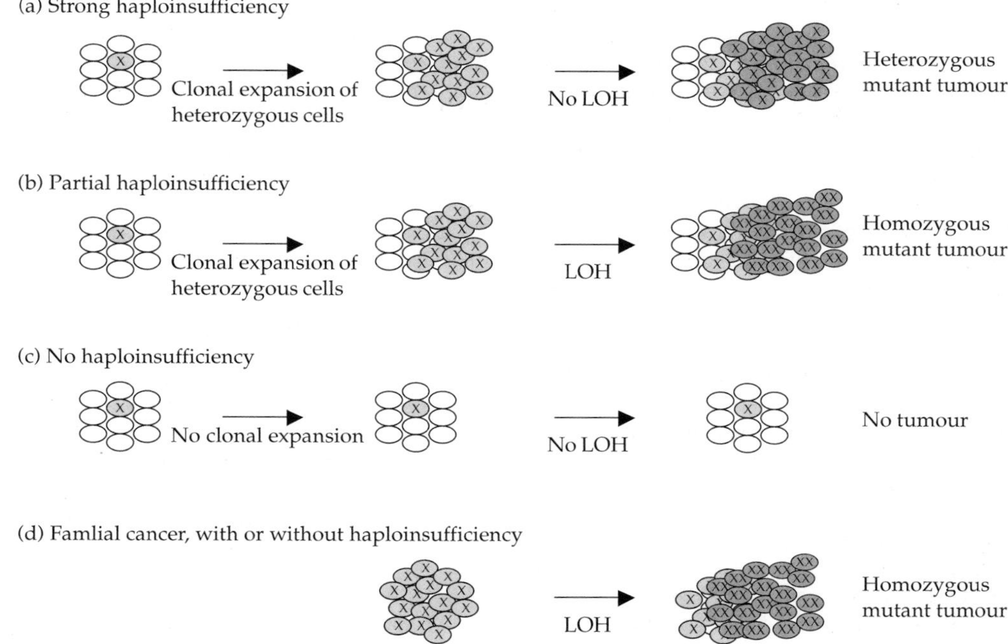

Figure 8.1 Strong haploinsufficiency increases the probability of completing a multi-step tumorigenesis pathway. Cells carrying two wild-type alleles of a TSG are shown in white. Heterozygous cells with one wild-type and one mutant (X) allele are shown in light grey. Tumour cells with one (X) or two (XX) mutant alleles are shown in dark grey. (Adapted from Quon and Berns, 2001)

(Chapter 13). The Rb family includes three members: Rb, p107, and p130. All of these proteins contain a protein interaction domain called the A/B pocket. This region binds proteins that contain the LXCXE motif in their sequence. Among these proteins are the SV40 large T antigen, adenovirus E1A protein and the human papillomavirus E7 proteins. Binding to the E2F family of transcription factors (see below) also involves the A/B pocket as well as the C-terminus of Rb and this is regulated by phosphorylation.

In addition to mutation in retinoblastoma, mutation of *RB* occurs in 80% of small cell lung cancers and 20–30% of non-small cell lung cancers as well as in osteosarcomas, sarcomas, breast, bladder and prostate carcinomas, myelomas, and leukaemias (reviewed in this book). The major effect of Rb expression is thought to occur during the G1 phase of the cell cycle (see below).

8.6.1 Rb mouse models

In 1992, three independent groups described the phenotype of the *Rb* knockout mouse. All three groups reported deficiencies in definitive erythropoiesis in homozygous *Rb* −/− embryos, finally leading to death of the embryos due to severe anaemia at day 15 post-conception. Surprisingly, heterozygous *Rb* +/− mice are not prone to retinoblastomas, but have a high incidence of pituitary adenocarcinomas. This result confirms the role of *Rb* mutation in tumorigenesis. In these pituitary tumours, the remaining *Rb* allele is lost, conforming to Knudson's 'two hit' hypothesis.

8.6.2 The G1/S checkpoint of the cell cycle

The cell cycle can be separated in four distinct phases: initial growth (G1), DNA replication (S), a gap (G2) and mitosis (M) (Chapter 9). The transitions between all of these phases are tightly regulated and involve the concerted action of cyclins and cyclin-dependent kinases (CDKs). This tight control of proteins involved in the regulation of the cell cycle is critical for an orderly cell division. A critical point in cell cycle control is the G1 to S transition. After passing this checkpoint, the cell is irreversibly committed to the next cell division. This has led to the proposal that alterations in this checkpoint are crucial for the development of cancer.

Key regulators of the G1 to S checkpoint are the cyclin D: CDK4/CDK6 and the cyclin E: CDK2 complexes. These complexes phosphorylate the retinoblastoma family proteins Rb, p107, and p130 (Figure 8.2). Hypophosphorylated proteins of the Rb family complex with the transcription factors of the E2F family. Five of the six members of the E2F family, E2F1-5, interact with Rb or other family members. These Rb family:E2F complexes inhibit the transcription of genes involved in S phase by several mechanisms: (1) They may act as active repressors on the promoters of the target genes, (2) they may recruit histone deacetylases (HDACs) to the target genes which cause nucleosome condensation, blocking access of transcription factors to the promoters, and (3) by sequestering E2Fs, the Rb family of proteins can prevent E2F transactivation of target genes. Upon phosphorylation of Rb by cyclin : CDK complexes, interaction with HDACs decreases and E2Fs are released and transactivate target genes involved in DNA synthesis. Additionally, CDK2 activity phosphorylates substrates that contribute to DNA synthesis.

Rb is not essential for cell cycle control and in normal fibroblasts, the G1/S checkpoint is mainly due to the activity of p107 and p130. Because mutations in p107 and p130 occur rarely, elucidating the differences between these two proteins and Rb may be crucial to understand the role of Rb as a tumour suppressor. One possibility is that Rb contributes to the regulation of gene expression only under particular circumstances, such as when cells differentiate or senesce.

The kinase activities of the cyclin D: CDK4/6 and cyclin E: CDK2 complexes are negatively regulated through two cyclin-dependent kinase inhibitor (CDKI) families: (1) The INK4 (inhibitor of CDK4) proteins: p16/INK4A/MTS1/ CDKN2A; p15/ INK4B/MTS2/CDKN2B; p18/INK4C/CDKN2C and p19/INK4D/CDKN2D. (2) The KIP (kinase inhibitor protein) molecules: p21/CIP1/CDKN1A/ WAF1; p27/KIP and p57/KIP2. The INK4 family of CDKIs are induced during cellular senescence and upon growth-inhibitory signals. They bind to CDK4 and CDK6, preventing the kinases from forming complexes with cyclin D.

Transcription of the *p21/CIP1* gene, a well-characterized KIP-family member, is activated by p53 upon DNA-damage and other stresses. p21/ CIP1 and p27KIP1 both inhibit the cyclinE : CDK2 activity, but *in vivo* they are less potent at inhibiting the activity of cyclinD:CDK4. Some authors even suggest that these inhibitors actually promote the assembly, stability, and nuclear retention of cyclin D: CDK4 complexes. These observations have led to the proposal that upon increase of cyclin D levels by mitogen stimulation, the levels of cyclin D: CDK4 complexes are increased and this leads to the sequestration of p27KIP1, preventing it from interacting with and inhibiting the activity of cyclinE : CDK2 complexes.

8.6.3 Inhibition of RNA pol I and III by Rb

Aside from its effects on E2F-induced RNA polymerase II transcription, Rb has also been shown to inhibit the function of RNA polymerases I and III, and may therefore have an important impact on

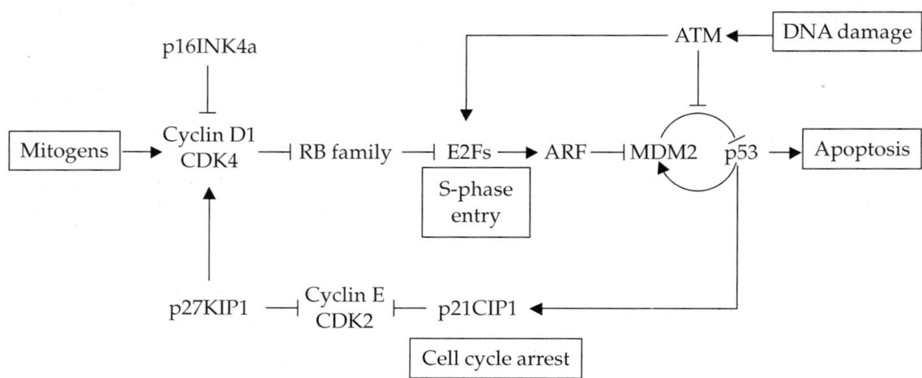

Figure 8.2 G1 to S transition of the cell cycle. See text for detailed description. Arrowheads represent stimulatory effects, and vertical black lines represent inhibitory effects. (Adapted from Sherr, 2001)

general protein expression. In particular, Rb binds to the UBF transcription factor, a component of the pol I machinery and blocks its binding to DNA. Rb is also able to inhibit the transcription of several pol III templates and Rb −/− mouse fibroblasts have higher levels of pol III transcription than their *Rb* positive counterparts. This inhibition of pol III activity may be due to the ability of Rb to bind to the TFIIIB component of the pol III complex.

By inhibiting the synthesis of ribosomal RNAs (dependent on pol I transcription) and tRNAs (dependent on pol III activity), Rb may limit cell growth. Deregulation of the synthesis of these RNAs may contribute to tumour development by providing large amounts of protein translation components sufficient to guarantee unrestrained cell growth.

8.6.4 Exploiting the Rb pathway in cancer therapy

Novel anti-tumour strategies, based on the manipulation of the Rb pathway in cancer cells, have been reviewed recently by Sherr and McCormick (2002). Disruption of the interaction between cyclins and CDKs is one obvious approach, although as noted by these authors, also a great challenge, because of the involvement of extensive interfaces in these interactions. Another approach is to interfere with the Ras-dependent signalling pathways which are required for the production of cyclin D1. Some selective small molecule inhibitors of kinases involved in these phosphorylation cascades (such as Raf, PI3K, and their corresponding downstream kinases) are now in clinical trials. Several CDK inhibitors, such as roscovitine, are also being tested in clinical trials. Although some of these studies are progressing favourably, determining specificity of these small molecules *in vivo* is a difficult task.

Adenoviruses that are deficient in E1A function, and therefore do not inhibit the activity of Rb have been tested for their ability to replicate selectively in and kill cells lacking functional Rb.

8.7 p53

8.7.1 p53 and cancer

In 1979 it was discovered that a host protein with an apparent molecular weight of 53/54 kDa binds to T antigen in SV40 transformed cells. Early studies suggested that the *TP53* gene acted as dominant oncogene and it was not until a decade later that *TP53* was found to be mutated in diverse human tumours. This important observation suggested that its real role is that of a tumour suppressor. At the same time, two labs reported that wild-type p53 protein can act as a suppressor of transformation by mutant p53 and oncogenes. Later, it was reported that *p53* knockout mice have a higher propensity to develop tumours spontaneously. This work firmly established the tumour suppressor function of p53. Supporting this evidence regarding the tumour suppressor role of p53 in humans, the Li–Fraumeni cancer predisposition syndrome was found to be associated with germline *TP53* mutations.

At least 50% (70–75% according to some estimations) of adult human tumours carry inactivating mutations in the *TP53* gene. The tumours in which *TP53* is most frequently mutated are CRC, breast cancer, and lung cancers. In many cases, loss of one allele and mutation of the other is detected. In carcinomas, most of the *TP53* alterations are due to missense point mutations. In sarcomas, deletions, insertions, and rearrangements are the most frequent events. Furthermore, in many of the tumours that encode wild-type p53, its levels and activity may be impaired due to alterations in other cellular factors or the expression of viral oncogenes (see below).

Tumours encoding wild-type p53 are thought to respond better to radiation and current chemotherapies than tumours lacking wild-type p53 and lose their responsiveness when *TP53* is mutated. A compelling demonstration of this comes from the observation that *TP53* mutations are associated with shorter survival of B-CLL patients, but also with selective resistance to alkylating agents. However, this is not a general rule, since in advanced breast cancers treated with epirubicin and cyclophosphamide and ovarian cancers treated with cisplatin and paclitaxel, a positive association between *TP53* mutation and success of the treatment has been reported. This difference in the influence of *TP53* status on the patient outcome may indicate that response is dependent on the type of tumour as well as on the characteristics (such as DNA-damaging activity) and dosage of the therapeutic drugs used.

8.7.2 p53 protein

p53 is a 393 amino acid protein that is highly conserved among mammals. The amino terminus of p53 contains its transactivation domain. This region is followed by a proline-rich segment that may be important for the stability of the protein. The central part of p53 contains its DNA binding domain. Downstream of the DNA binding region, there is a nuclear localization signal and an oligomerization domain that mediates the tetramerization of p53, which is necessary for its transcriptional activation function. Overexpression of the oligomerization domain of p53 in cells is an effective way to ablate full length p53 function. The C-terminus of p53 contains a negative regulatory domain as well as lysine residues that are susceptible to ubiquitination. This modification by ubiquitin, is involved in targeting the protein to degradation by the proteolytic activity of the proteasome. Supporting this, deletion of the 30 C-terminal amino acids of p53 results in an extremely stable form of the protein. Other modifications at the C- terminal domain that may affect p53 stability and activity include SUMO (small ubiquitin-like modifier) conjugation and acetylation. Phosphorylation, especially in the N-terminal and C-terminal domains can modulate protein stability and function.

In many tumours, DNA binding is impaired by mutations affecting specific aminoacids in the central hydrophobic domain which are necessary for direct binding to DNA and other protein factors. These mutants are still able to form tetramers, and therefore can have a dominant negative effect over wild-type protein. Other mutations alter the conformation of the protein. Thermosensitive conformational mutants of p53 have been of great use in functional studies. Aside from their loss of function and/or dominant negative effects over wild-type p53, mutated forms of p53 may also acquire the ability to perform new functions that are not carried out by wild-type p53 ('gain of function') as suggested by several authors.

8.7.3 p53 function

The tumour suppressor activity of wild-type p53 is mainly due to its ability to act as a transcription factor and induce the expression of a large number of proteins (Vousden and Lu, 2002). Accordingly, mice bearing a transcriptionally inactive mutant of p53 are prone to tumours, indicating that the transcription activation domain of p53 is necessary for its tumour suppressor function. Whether p53 can also specifically repress transcription in a direct way is still a matter of controversy.

Some p53 targets are involved in inhibition of cell proliferation by promoting cell cycle arrest (such as p21CIP1 and GADD45) and others can cause the induction of cell death by apoptosis (BAX, scottin, PIG3, etc.). Induction of other proteins induced by p53, such as histone H3, DNA polymerase-α and myb may have important effects in DNA replication.

The discovery of p53 alterations that promote selectivity on different promoters and the definition of cofactors that specifically promote p53-induced apoptosis suggest that the apoptotic and cell-cycle arrest activities of p53 can be separated. Supporting the view that c-Myc specifically modulates the effect of p53 on particular promoters, c-Myc expression specifically inhibits *p21/CIP1* transcription. This may explain why expression of c-Myc together with p53 leads to high levels of apoptosis.

8.7.4 Regulation of p53 levels

The primary function of p53 is to stop cell proliferation by halting the cell cycle or by inducing cell death by apoptosis. Therefore, its levels and activity must be tightly regulated. There are several reports on the mechanisms that control *p53* gene transcription. However, the current view is that p53 levels are mainly regulated at the post-transcriptional level.

In normal non-stressed cells, p53 has a very short half-life due to an autoregulatory feedback loop mechanism in which the MDM2 protein plays a key role (Figure 8.3). Wild-type p53 acts as a transcriptional activator of the *MDM2* gene (mouse double minute gene-2). In turn, MDM2, which itself has a very short half-life, interacts with p53 and functions as a ubiquitin E3 ligase that promotes the conjugation of p53 to ubiquitin. This conjugation to ubiquitin serves as a tag that effectively targets p53 for degradation by the proteasome. In this way, in normal non-stressed cells, p53 levels are kept low allowing cells to proliferate. Contributing to its 'anti-p53' function, MDM2 is also thought to impair the transcriptional activity of p53 by masking the transactivation domain of this tumour suppressor. Supporting the crucial role of MDM2 in the regulation of p53 activity, MDM2 knockout mice are rescued from embryonic lethality by deletion of p53. A similar requirement has also been observed when MDMX (MDM4) mice were developed, suggesting that MDMX is important in regulating the levels and activity of p53.

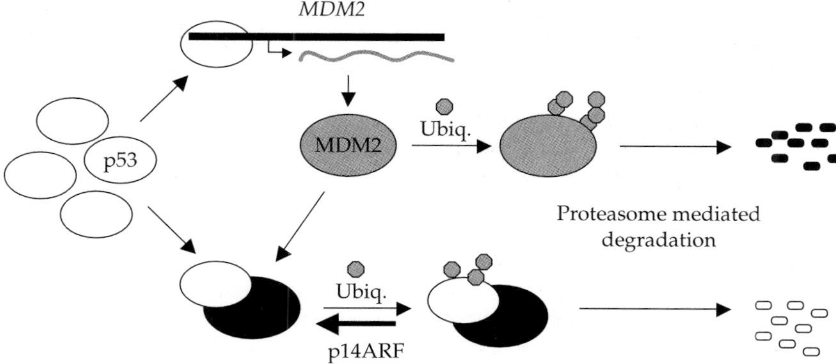

Figure 8.3 The p53/MDM2 autoregulatory feedback loop model.

In tumour cells that encode mutant p53, these forms are still susceptible to degradation by MDM2. However, the ability to act as a transcriptional activator is generally abolished, and therefore the levels of MDM2 are decreased, leading to the accumulation of p53 in the cells. This is why the detection of high levels of p53 in tumours can be used as an indicator (but not as full proof) for the existence of mutations in the *p53* gene.

8.7.5 Impairment of p53 function in tumours lacking p53 mutations

In cancers where the p53 gene is intact, its tumour suppressor function is thought to be blocked by the overexpression or inactivation of cellular factors that regulate the levels and activity of p53 or by the expression of certain oncoviral proteins. These include the overexpression of the MDM2 protein, defects in the expression of the p14ARF tumour suppressor (see below), mutations in kinases such as ATM or Chk2, chromosome translocations involving the PML or the nucleophosmin proteins or infection with certain viruses such as SV40, adenovirus, and human papillomavirus. The viruses encode proteins, like the SV40 large T-antigen, that interact with p53, or proteins that bind to p53 and target it for degradation. Important and well-studied examples of this are the malignant tumour-associated strains of the human papillomavirus (HPV). HPV protein E6 forms a complex with p53 and promotes its degradation through the ubiquitin pathway in a way that instead of involving MDM2, uses the ubiquitin E3 ligase activity of the celullar protein E6AP.

8.7.6 Activation of p53

It is well known that the levels of p53 and transcriptional activity increase in cells that are irradiated or treated with DNA damaging agents, including many of the currently used chemotherapeutic drugs. Additionally, p53 accumulates in the nucleus of human skin biopsies after exposure to UV light. Microinjection of cells with a restriction enzyme can induce the accumulation of p53, supporting the view that this activation is, at least in part, due to the appearance of DNA lesions. In at least some types of normal cells, p53 activation by DNA damage stops cell cycle progression, which is thought to be necessary to allow the cell to repair its damage. If the damage cannot be repaired, p53 triggers the apoptotic response. By allowing DNA repair in moderately damaged cells and promoting cell death of severely damaged cells, p53 ('the guardian of the genome') prevents the fixation of mutations in cell populations. Hence, loss of p53 function leads to genomic instability and the accumulation of cells with damaged DNA.

The elucidation of the mechanisms by which p53 is activated when cells are subjected to stress has been an area of intense research. In response to DNA damage, the activity of certain kinases (such as DNAPK, ATM, Chk2) may be increased and p53 and/or MDM2 may be modified by phosphorylation. In some cases, these phosphorylation events have been suggested to inhibit the ability of p53 and MDM2 to interact with each other or to inhibit the ability of MDM2 to carry out its functions.

p53 activity can also be increased by a variety of stresses that do not, at least not directly, involve DNA damage. These include hypoxia, serum starvation, heat, cold, pH changes, ribonucleotide depletion, glycerol, and inhibition of nuclear export. Oncogenic signals and certain viral oncoproteins can also increase the levels of p53. This activation, at least in some situations, is mediated by an increase in the levels of expression of the p14ARF tumour suppressor protein, an antagonist of MDM2 function (see below).

8.7.7 Mouse models

p53 double knockout mice are viable, suggesting that p53 function is not essential for normal development. However, after approximately six months of life, these mice spontaneously develop a variety of tumours at high frequency. One explanation for this delay is that sufficient DNA damage needs to accumulate before the absence of p53 is apparent. The phenotype of *p53* heterozygous mice is also of great interest, since they can be considered as a model of the Li–Fraumeni syndrome. These mice develop a slightly different variety of tumour types and as expected, with a longer latency period. The majority of these tumours show LOH of the *p53* genomic region, confirming that complete loss of p53 function contributes to tumorigenesis.

In a subset of human tumours with *p53* mutations and in over half of the tumours arising in *p53* +/− mice, LOH at the *p53* locus is not detected, suggesting that *p53* haploinsufficiency may promote tumour formation. However, as mentioned above, loss of both *p53* alleles is more tumorigenic than loss of one. Therefore, in the case of *p53*, haploinsufficiency is partial.

Donehower and colleagues have observed that a constitutive increase in p53 activity leads to the appearance of very clear symptoms of premature ageing in mice. In another study made in M. Serrano's lab, mice with an extra copy of the *p53* gene are protected from tumorigenesis but unlike the mice developed in the Donehower lab, do not show early ageing. This important difference between the phenotype observed by Donehower and colleagues and the phenotype of the mice with three copies of p53 is very likely to be due to the possibility that in the first case, p53 activity is constitutive, whereas in the latter case, p53 levels are properly regulated.

8.7.8 p53-based therapies

Selective killing of tumour cells lacking p53 or carrying inactivating mutations is a great challenge which has led to a variety of very exciting approaches (Woods and Lane, 2003). These include screening for drugs that bind to and reactivate mutant p53, using replication-defective adenoviral vectors expressing p53 or using viruses that selectively replicate in p53-deficient cells. Alternatively, the study of whether disruption of p53 function and/or accumulation of mutant p53 leads to the upregulation of specific activities in tumour cells may help to define new targets and preferably enzymatic activities that make tumour cells particularly susceptible to small molecule inhibitors.

Contrary to the findings in solid tumours occurring in adults, the rate of p53 mutations in haematological malignant diseases and childhood cancer is significantly lower. This may be the key to the much better prognosis of children with cancer. However, the DNA damaging effects of many current therapies is especially important to bear in mind when considering the treatment of young patients. Follow-up studies are showing that the damage induced by these treatments may lead to growth and development problems in children, infertility, and second malignant tumour induction later in life. Conceivably, these secondary tumours may derive from normal or tumour cells that were damaged during treatment. Supporting this, Sturm et al. (2003) have shown for the first time that treatment of B-CLL patients with DNA damaging alkylating agents correlates with the appearance of mutations in p53. As mentioned above, the appearance of these mutations is significantly associated with poor outcome and drug resistance. This is why the search for novel non-genotoxic activators of the p53 response is thought to be essential in improving the treatment of those cancers in which p53 function is not abolished by mutation.

If MDM2 is an important inhibitor of p53 function, a likely way to increase p53 levels in a non-genotoxic way is by impairing its function. We can decrease the effects of MDM2 on p53, by decreasing its expression with antisense RNAs and transcription inhibitors or by inhibiting the interaction between p53 and MDM2. Inhibiting the activity of the proteasome very effectively increases p53 levels. However, this increase is not associated with the activation of p53 transcriptional activity. Developing small molecules that inhibit ubiquitination of p53 by MDM2 or that mimic the function of the p14ARF tumour suppressor, a natural inhibitor of MDM2 (see below) may also be suitable approaches. A very effective alternative is to induce the accumulation of p53 in the nucleus, where it acts as a transcriptional activator. The nuclear export inhibitor leptomycin B (LMB) has been shown to be an extremely potent activator of p53 transcriptional activity.

When considering therapeutic strategies based on the activation of p53 activity an important question arises: are tumour cells significantly more susceptible to the killing effects of active p53? In tissue culture conditions, many tumour cells are very susceptible to apoptosis in response to activation of p53. This is probably due to defects in cell cycle checkpoints in these cells. Instead, certain types of normal cells, like fibroblasts, which tend to respond to stress by stopping their proliferation, are relatively resistant to the effects of some p53 activators. Furthermore, p53 can play a protective role against UV-induced apoptosis. Therefore, it is conceivable that chronic stress activation of p53 could protect cells from a subsequent stronger insult. In other normal cell types, such as T-lymphocytes, growth arrest is not the most likely response to p53 activation. Instead, these cells may elicit an apoptotic response as a consequence of p53 activity.

The induction of the p53 response in some normal tissues is thought to be at least partially responsible for many of the adverse side effects of current chemotherapeutic drugs, such as gastrointestinal dysfunction or hair loss. Therefore, one could think of taking a radically different approach and aim to decrease the devastating effects of p53 induction in normal tissues and in this way improve quality of life of patients during treatment. The use of drugs like the p53 inhibitor pifithrin α to protect normal cells from current therapies provide an example of this approach.

8.8 The INK4a/ARF locus

8.8.1 Rb and p53 pathways are connected

As described above, the INK4 proteins (p16INK4a, p155INK4b, p18INK4c, p19INK4d) inhibit the activity of cyclin-dependent kinases. This results in the inhibition of the phosphorylation of Rb family proteins and prevention of cell cycle progression. *INK4a* and *INK4b* are closely linked on chromosome 4 in mice and 9p in humans.

A striking finding was that the *INK4a* locus encodes a second gene product from an alternative reading frame (p14ARF in humans and p19ARF in mice) (Figure 8.4). Both proteins act as inhibitors of the G1 to S transition, even though they function in two different pathways: p16INK4A acts as an inhibitor of cyclin D:CDK4/6 complexes; and p14ARF protects p53 from MDM2-mediated degradation (Figures 8.2 and 8.4) and increases the transcriptional activity of p53 (Sherr, 2001; Sherr and McCormick, 2002).

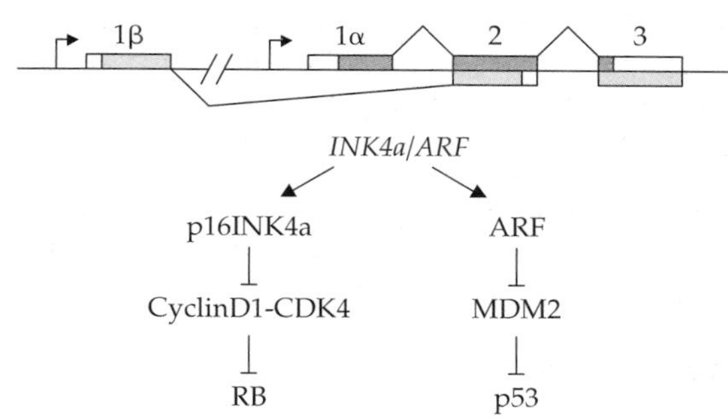

Figure 8.4 The *INK4a/ARF* locus and involvement of p16INK4a and p14ARF in the Rb and p53 tumour suppressor pathways, respectively.

p53 can modulate the Rb pathway through the induction of expression of the CDK inhibitor p21CIP1. Supporting this model, mice deficient in all three Rb family members (Rb, p107, and p130) are resistant to ARF-induced cell cycle arrest. However, mouse cells lacking *p21Cip1* are not immortal and undergo ARF-induced arrest, supporting the view that this activation is, at least in part, due to the appearance of DNA lesions. Reciprocally, E2F induces the expression of *ARF*. This, together with the overlap between the *ARF* and *p16INK4a* genes, provides another connection between the Rb and the p53 pathways.

8.8.2 p16INK4a function

One key observation indicating that p16INK4a acts primarily through the Rb pathway *in vivo* is that p16INK4a does not inhibit G1-phase progression in cells lacking Rb. p16INK4a directly inhibits the activities of cyclinD-dependent kinases CDK4 and 6. This inhibition is thought to occur by the interaction of p16INK4a with CDK4 in a way that prevents the formation of active cyclinD1/CDK4 complexes. This lack of interaction between cyclinD1/CDK4 may impair the interaction with CIP/KIP proteins. Therefore, an increase in the levels of p16INK4a may in turn indirectly impair the activity of CDK2 by increasing the levels of CIP/KIP proteins accessible to cyclinE : CDK2 complexes (Figure 8.2).

8.8.3 ARF function

The first studies on ARF function led to the suggestion that this small protein (132 residues in man) exerts its tumour suppressor function through its ability to potentiate p53 activity. However, p53-independent effects of ARF, and even MDM2-independent effects of ARF in cell culture and mouse models, have been documented. Even though the growth inhibitory and tumour suppressor effects of ARF may be potentiated by the presence of active p53 and MDM2 in cells, genetic studies indicate that the action of ARF on the p53 pathway may not be necessarily direct. Chuck Sherr's lab has recently shown that ARF can impair nucleolar function by inhibiting the processing of pre-ribosomal RNAs, supporting the idea that ARF may act through mechanisms other than binding to MDM2.

Whether through its binding to p53/MDM2 complexes and/or indirectly, it is clear that ARF protects p53 from MDM2-mediated degradation. However, it is also clear that p53 degradation is a multi-step process involving the interaction of p53 with MDM2, the ubiquitination of p53 by MDM2 and the MDM2-dependent interaction of p53 with the proteasome (Figure 8.3). Therefore, ARF could affect p53 degradation by MDM2 at different levels. This is now an area of intensive research.

8.8.4 Modulation of *INK4a/ARF* expression

ARF gene expression is induced by mitogenic signals in response to the overexpression of Myc, the adenovirus E1A, mutated Ras, v-Abl and β-catenin oncoproteins. Whereas Ras transforms established rodent cell lines lacking *ARF* or *p53*, ectopic expression of oncogenic Ras leads to growth arrest and the appearance of senescence-associated markers.

Mouse fibroblasts that overexpress Myc apoptose rapidly. In these cultures, cells that have lost either ARF or p53 function survive. A similar situation is found in mice bearing a Myc transgene under the control of a B-cell specific promoter (Eμ-Myc). In early stages, increased S-phase entry of B-cells in lymph nodes leads cells to apoptosis. Gradually, cells that have lost either p53 or ARF function are selected, giving rise to lymphomas in which one of these genes is frequently mutated. These effects of selective Myc expression are strongly enhanced in an *ARF* negative background but not in a *p16INK4a* negative background. However, a role for p16INK4a, but not for ARF, has been suggested in facilitating the curative response to cyclophosphamide in mice.

Neither p16INK4a or ARF is expressed at significant levels during development. This may be due to the transcriptional repressor Bmi-1 since the developmental anomalies observed in *Bmi-1* deficient mice are reversed in a *p16INK4a-ARF* negative background and Bmi-1 accelerates Eμ-Myc-induced lymphomagenesis. Other *ARF* repressors include Twist and TBX2. These factors are overexpressed in some cancers that retain wild-type p53.

8.8.5 *INK4a/ARF* genes and cancer

p16INK4a function is often deficient in cancer cells. In contrast, *p15INK4b* and *p18INK4c* are less frequently altered and the possible involvement of *p19INK4d* in cancer is not yet clear.

p16INK4a-ARF mutations have been detected in familial melanoma, and in some cases, the critical mutations affect only $p16^{INK4a}$ but not *ARF*. They are also present in other cancers such as small cell carcinomas of the lung. A mutation affecting exon 1β, and therefore, only the expression of p14ARF and not p16INK4a has been detected in a colon cancer and in familial melanoma.

The gene for p15INK4b is localized in close proximity to the INK4A locus on chromosome 9p21. All three genes (*p16INK4a, p15INK4b,* and *p14ARF*) are frequently altered in various haematological malignancies. Most alterations occur by inactivation of *p16INK4a* and *p15INK4b* due to hypermethylation of CpG islands in their promoters, or by deletions in the 9p21 region, frequently involving all three genes.

8.8.6 Knockout mouse models

Before *ARF* was discovered, the first *INK4a* knockout mice were described. These were shown to be tumour prone and develop various cancers early on in life. They were subsequently found to be deficient for the expression of both p16INK4a and ARF.

To unravel whether the observed effects were due to the lack of function of only one of these proteins, mice that were deficient in the expression of either gene were obtained. *p16INK4a* knockout mice are tumour-prone and develop a variety of cancers after exposure to carcinogens or radiation. Another important observation derived from experiments with mouse embryonic fibroblasts (MEFs) from the initial *INK4a/ARF* knockout mice was that these cells do not undergo senescence and they are susceptible to transformation by *Ras* in the absence of other immortalizing oncogenes. Later on it was shown that pure *INK4a*-null MEFs had normal growth properties and cannot be transformed by *Ras* alone. Like *p53* knockout mice, pure *ARF*-deficient mice, spontaneously develop tumours and die of cancer and primary MEFs cultured from these animals do not senesce in culture and give rise to immortal cell lines. However, in other mouse cell types, loss of *ARF* and silencing of *p16INK4a* are required for the establishment of cell lines.

In agreement with the fact that *INK4a* mutations are more frequent in human cancers than mutations of *INK4b*, *INK4b*-knockout mice do not spontaneously develop tumours, although they do show predisposition to extramedullary haematopoiesis (formation of blood outside the bone marrow) and lymphoid hyperplasia.

Unlike *p16INK4a* and *p15INK4b*, *p18INK4c*, and *p19INK4d* are ubiquitously expressed during mouse development and in a tissue-specific manner in adult mice. *INK4d*-null mice are not tumour prone and have a normal lifespan. Mice lacking both *INK4c* and *INK4d* are sterile. In contrast, *p18INK4c* null mice show spontaneous development of mid-lobe pituitary tumours and other endocrine neoplasias, indicating an important role for p18INK4c in these cell types.

8.9 von Hippel–Lindau syndrome

von Hippel–Lindau (VHL) is a rare inherited disease with an incidence of approximately 1 in 35,000. This syndrome is associated with a predisposition to develop retinal, spinal, and cerebellar haemangioblastomata, clear cell renal carcinoma, and phaeochromocytoma. Haemangiomas of the adrenals, lungs, and liver, and multiple cysts of the pancreas and kidneys are also observed. This disease is another example of Knudson's 'two hit' model. Affected individuals inherit one mutated *VHL* gene, and develop neoplastic disease in association with loss or inactivation of the remaining allele. Somatic inactivation of both *VHL* alleles is also common in non-familial clear cell renal carcinoma and CNS haemangioblastoma (Kaelin, 2002).

8.9.1 VHL function

The *VHL* gene contains an open reading frame encoding 213 aminoacids. An alternative translational initiation site at codon 54 encodes a truncated protein that retains tumour suppressor activity. Co-immunoprecipitation experiments suggested the association of VHL with elongins C and B, Cul-2, and Rbx-1. Subsequently, isolation of Rbx-1 as a common component of SCF (Skp-1-Cdc53/CUL 1-F-box) family of multi-component ubiquitin ligases and VHL-elongin B-elongin C-Cul 2 (VBCC) complexes provided further circumstantial evidence for a role in proteolysis.

The hypoxia-inducible factor subunit (HIF-1α) was shown to be a proteolytic target of the VBCC complex. This provided a direct link between the tumour suppressor function of VHL and tumour cell responses to hypoxia. HIF is a transcriptional regulator involved in the maintenance of cellular oxygen homeostasis through its effects on angiogenesis, vasomotor control, and regulation of energy metabolism. HIF is a heterodimer. The β-subunits of HIF are constitutive nuclear proteins and the α-subunits are the regulatory components. Under normoxic conditions, HIF-1α subunits are rapidly degraded by the proteasome. In hypoxia, this proteolysis is suppressed and high levels of HIF-1α are detected. Accordingly, there is an oxygen-dependent degradation domain (ODDD) that occupies a central position in HIF-1α and conveys proteolytic regulation by the ubiquitin proteasome pathway. VHL regulates HIF-1α proteolysis by interacting with the ODDD and VHL acts as the recognition component of an E3 ubiquitin ligase that targets HIF-1α subunits. The interaction of VHL with HIF-1α was shown to be dependent on hydroxylation of either of two critical prolyl residues lying in HIF-1α. *In vivo*, in *VHL*-associated renal carcinoma cells that lack functional VHL, expression of HIF target genes is upregulated.

8.9.2 Hypoxia in cancer

Upregulation of specific isoforms of glucose transporters and of glycolytic enzymes by HIF activation accounts at least in part for the enhanced rates of aerobic glycolysis observed in tumours. On the other hand, the HIF regulation of angiogenic growth factors such as vascular endothelial growth factor (VEGF), links HIF function to the enhanced angiogenic activity that is associated with aggressive tumour growth.

Interestingly, some upregulation of HIF has been observed following oncogenic activation or tumour suppressor inactivation in a wide variety of settings. Reciprocally, wild-type p53 and p14ARF can interact with HIF1-α. The interaction with p53 may be related to its ability to impair HIF1 stimulated transcription and promote the degradation of HIF1-α.

More hypoxic tumours generally have worse prognosis and are more resistant to current therapies. However, aggressive growth might itself promote hypoxic conditions in the tumour. Thus, a question that arises is whether HIF activation is causally implicated in cancer. Mouse models have not yet provided a clear answer. Another question is whether *VHL*-associated tumorigenesis is not due to HIF-independent effects of VHL. So far, no other ubiquitination substrate has been identified. Nevertheless, understanding the HIF/VHL pathway may possibly to identify molecular targets that can be used in rational drug design.

8.10 LKB1

8.10.1 Peutz–Jeghers Cancer Syndrome

Peutz–Jeghers Cancer Syndrome (PJS) is an autosomal-dominant inherited disorder that is characterized by multiple hamartomatous polyps in the gastrointestinal tract, pigmentation of the mucous membranes and an increased risk of cancer. Hamartomas are benign overgrowths of well-differentiated tissues. In PJS patients, the hamartomatous polyps are most common in the small intestine. The total numbers of polyps vary from a few to several hundreds. In addition to hamartomatous polyps, adenomatous and hyperplastic polyps can also be found. Histologically, the PJS polyps are characterized by proliferation of normal epithelium and smooth muscle. The branching of a well-defined smooth muscle bundle in the core of the polyp is a prominent feature of the hamartomatous polyp in PJS. The reported estimates of incidence of PJS vary significantly from 1:8300 to 1:120,000 live births. Although the majority of PJS patients have a family history, 10–20% of the cases are caused by *de novo* mutations in *LKB1* (Boudeau et al., 2003). The most common cancer types in PJS patients include colon, stomach, small intestinal, and pancreatic cancer. The relative risk for all cancers from this analysis was estimated to be 15.2-fold higher for PJS patients compared to the general population.

8.10.2 Identification of the PJS gene

Initial analysis of multiple hamartomas derived from a single PJS patient using comparative genomic hybridization revealed deletions of chromosome 19p, indicating that 19p was the locus for PJS. Further linkage analysis confirmed chromosome 19p13.3 as the PJS locus. In early 1998, two groups independently reported the identification of the same gene, a novel serine/threonine kinase, responsible for PJS. This kinase was named LKB1 by one group and serine threonine kinase-11 (STK11) by the other. This protein is ubiquitously expressed.

To date over 80 different germline and somatic mutations in *LKB1* have been identified from PJS patients. These include nonsense, small point mutations, deletions, insertions, splice site mutations, rearrangements, missense mutations, and promoter hypermethylation.

8.10.3 LKB1 function

Analysis of the *LKB1* primary sequence reveals that LKB1 has a core serine/threonine kinase domain (encompassing residues 44–309) and distinct N-terminal and C-terminal regulatory domains. LKB1 has been reported to possess autocatalytic activity but no physiological substrates have yet been identified. LKB1 is a target for PKA and RSK, which phosphorylate LKB1 at Ser431. Phosphorylation of LKB1 at Ser431 does not alter the LKB1 activity but mutation of this residue to Ala or Asp prevents LKB1 from suppressing cell growth. Interestingly, a similar result was obtained with the mutation of Thr336 to Glu but not to Ala.

IR induces the phosphorylation of LKB1 at Thr366, which lies in an optimal phosphorylation motif for the PI 3-kinase like kinases, DNA-PK, ATM, and ATR. These enzymes function as sensors for DNA damage in cells and mediate cellular responses to DNA damage. Both DNA-PK and ATM efficiently phosphorylate LKB1 at Thr366 *in vitro* and there is evidence that ATM mediates this phosphorylation *in vivo*.

LKB1 has been reported to be mainly nuclear, but some studies have reported cytosolic localization of a minor but significant proportion of LKB1. This may play an important role in regulating LKB1 growth inhibitory activity in cells. LKB1 associates with, and is functionally linked to, LKB1 Interacting Protein-1 (LIP1), which is suggested to regulate LKB1 by altering its cellular localization and anchoring it in the cytoplasm.

Overexpression of wild-type LKB1 in LKB1-deficient G361 or HeLa cells leads to suppression of cell proliferation caused by a G1-cell cycle block. Induction of proliferation suppression by LKB1 is associated with an increase in the levels of the $p21^{WAF1/CIP1}$ cell cycle inhibitor through a p53-dependent pathway. In these studies, it was suggested that LKB1 induced G361 growth arrest required LKB1 to translocate into the cytosol. Overexpression of several naturally occurring LKB1 mutations from PJS patients fail to cause G361 growth suppression, further suggesting that a functional LKB1 is required for the suppression of cell proliferation. The tumour suppressor protein p53 immunoprecipitates from cell lysates with endogenous LKB1 suggesting that p53 directly or indirectly associates with LKB1. Furthermore, it was shown that overexpression of LKB1 in HT1080 cells induced classical apoptosis via activation of caspases and DNA-fragmentation in a p53-dependent manner. LKB1 kinase activity was required for LKB1-induced cell death. In apoptotic cells, LKB1 translocated to mitochondria indicating that LKB1 could mediate the p53-dependent apoptosis by regulating a mitochondrial protein.

LKB1 association with Brahma-related gene-1 (Brg1) is required for Brg1-induced growth arrest. Brg1 possesses an ATP-dependent helicase activity that is necessary for chromatin remodelling. Brg1 also interacts with other proteins, including steroid hormone receptor, BRCA1 and cyclin E, stimulates the activity of several transcription factors and is necessary for retinoblastoma-dependent cell cycle arrest and senescence *in vivo*. Although the kinase activity of LKB1 is not required for its association with Brg1 or the activation of Brg1 *in vitro*, Brg1-induced cell cycle arrest requires LKB1 kinase activity.

8.10.4 LKB1 mouse models

Targeted disruption of the *LKB1* gene by homologous recombination in mouse embryonic stem cells has been reported by several groups. Analysis of LKB1 +/− heterozygous mice showed that by the age of 40–45 weeks all the mice developed polyps in the gastrointestinal tract which are histologically similar to PJS polyps. The location of polyp development predominantly in the glandular stomach in LKB1 +/− mice is distinct from PJS patients who develop polyps mainly in the small intestine. Many of these mice die before the onset of carcinomas and metastasis, as a result of intestinal obstruction and/or bleeding from polyps.

No *LKB1* mutations were identified in the polyps from *LKB1* +/− mice. These results indicate that *LKB1* +/− mice express wild type LKB1 in haploid amounts and that haploinsufficiency of LKB1 is enough to induce polyposis in *LKB1* +/− mice. However, a recent study reported that 3 of 12 polyps analysed from *LKB1* +/− mice showed clear loss of the wild-type *LKB1* allele. Moreover, no LKB1 protein was detectable in half of the polyps from *LKB1* +/− mice that retained wild type *LKB1* allele suggesting epigenetic gene inactivation.

Seventy per cent of the male and twenty per cent female *LKB1* +/− mice that survived beyond 50 weeks developed hepatocellular carcinoma, indicating that there could be a sex difference in cancer susceptibility. Interestingly, no expression of LKB1 mRNA and protein was observed in any of the hepatocellular carcinoma samples examined, indicating that the wild-type allele of *LKB1* in these tumours was lost or silenced. Therefore, it is currently thought that the initiation of polyp formation could result from reduction in the expression of LKB1. However, complete loss of LKB1 expression may be required for the development of hepatocellular carcinomas as well as progression of benign polyps into carcinomas.

8.11 Neurofibromatosis type 1

8.11.1 Neurofibromatosis type 1 or Recklinghausen's neurofibromatosis

Neurofibromatosis type 1 (NF1) is a neurocutaneous disorder and one of the most frequent human genetic diseases. The most common symptoms of NF1 are abnormal skin pigmentation, benign iris hamartomas, and cutaneous or subcutaneous neurofibromas. NF1 patients also suffer from distinctive skeletal lesions. Other frequent problems include macrocephaly and learning and behavioural problems. Individuals with NF1 are predisposed to the development of malignancies including peripheral nerve sheath tumours and astrocytomas. Peripheral nerve sheath tumours can be benign (neurofibromas) or malignant (MPNSTs). Most MPNSTs are thought to arise by malignant transformation of neurofibromas, an event occurs in about 2% of NF1 patients. The disruption of the p53 pathway is involved in this malignant progression. Neurofibromas, one of the most common manifestations of the disease, are unique among tumours with respect to their heterogeneity. They contain all of the cell types found in normal peripheral nerves (axonal processes of neurons, Schwann cells, perineural cells, fibroblasts, and mast cells).

8.11.2 *NF1* gene

The high frequency of NF1 worldwide is possibly related to the large size of the *NF1* gene (over 350 kb). This gene is mapped to chromosome 17q11.2 and consists of 57 constitutive and 3 alternatively spliced exons. The large size of *NF1* and the presence of several pseudogenes greatly complicate the search for mutations. The Human Gene mutation Database (http://archive.uwcm.ac.uk/uwcm/mg/hgmd0.html) lists more than 600 mutations. No clear genotype–phenotype correlations emerge from this mutation data except that patients with large deletions are more likely to exhibit more severe symptoms. Bone marrow cells from NF1 and myelogenous leukaemia showed homozygous inactivation of the *NF1* gene, providing support for a tumour suppressor role.

8.11.3 NF1 function

NF1 is expressed in many cell lines and is abundant during mouse foetal development. In adult rats Nf1 (neurofibromin) is most abundant in peripheral nervous system and CNS and in particular in neurons, oligodendrocytes, and non-myelinating Schwann cells. In several studies, NF1 has been suggested to be associated with mitochondria.

Neurofibromin is involved in the modulation of the Ras pathway. Ras GTPases (H-, K-, and N-Ras) have high affinity for both GTP and GDP and function as binary switches by cycling between inactive GDP- and active GTP-bound conformations. Upon growth factor receptor signalling, Ras is activated by at least four guanine nucleotide exchange factors that promote GTP for GDP exchange. Active Ras interacts with several effector proteins including Raf, PI3kinase, and Ral-GDS. Inactivation of Ras is mediated by exchange of GTP with GDP, a process mediated by several Ras-specific GTPase-activating proteins (RasGAP), including neurofibromin. The most common disruption of this pathway in human cancer is mutation of Ras, resulting in constitutively active, oncogenic Ras (Chapter 7). Another disruption of this pathway is by inactivation of neurofibromin, resulting in a higher proportion of active Ras. NF1-deficient neurons survive in the absence of neurotropic factors, supporting a role for neurofibromin in reducing cell growth.

8.11.4 *Nf1* mouse models: contribution of the surrounding somatic tissue to tumour formation

An excellent review on the observations from genetically engineered mice can be found in McLaughlin and Jacks (2002). *NF1* homozygous mice die during fetal development possibly due to a role for Nf1 in heart development. Mice heterozygous for a targeted disruption of the *Nf1* gene do not resemble the human phenotype with regard to either pigmentation abnormalities or neurofibromas, but they are susceptible to malignancies (pheochromocytoma and myeloid leukemia) as well as learning and memory defects. Therefore, although these mice do not provide a perfect model for all aspects of the human disease, the generation of *Nf1*-knockout mice has confirmed the role of neurofibromin as a tumour suppressor. This difficulty has been circumvented by the generation of chimeric mice partially composed of *Nf1* $-/-$ cells. Nearly all of these mice develop numerous neurofibromas that histologically resemble human plexiform neurofibromas. This confirms the hypothesis that somatic *Nf1* mutation is the rate-limiting step in neurofibroma formation. The chimeric mouse model, however, has its limitations; the cell type in which *Nf1* is deleted cannot be controlled and these animals cannot easily be crossed to other mutant mouse strains.

Using Cre-recombinase transgene technology in which this enzyme is under control of the Krox20 promoter and induces the ablation of a floxed *Nf1* gene, it has been possible to specifically abolish Nf1 function in Schwann cells. All progeny with the *Nf1flox/-;Krox20-cre* genotype developed neurofibromas, demonstrating that loss of Nf1 in the Schwann cell lineage is sufficient for this phenotype.

This is an important result, but not sufficient to explain the cellular heterogeneity in neurofibromas, nor does it address whether hetereozygous *Nf1* neighbouring cells may influence tumour development. To study this second issue, researchers compared the size and frequency of neurofibromas occurring in *Nf1flox/-;Krox20-cre* mice (in which all neighbouring cells are phenotypically heterozygous for *Nf1)* and *Nf1flox/flox;Krox20-cre* mice (in which all of the neighbouring cells are phenotypically wild type). In striking contrast to the widespread plexiform neurofibromas in the first case, the *Nf1flox/flox;Krox20-cre* mice only developed small, infrequent hyperplastic lesions in the cranial nerves. These observations provide genetic evidence that the haploinsufficient state of the somatic tissue surrounding tumour can contribute to tumour formation.

8.12 Wilms' tumour

8.12.1 *WT1* gene

Wilms' tumour is a paediatric kidney malignancy affecting 1/10,000 children making it the most common solid tumour in the young. Eighty per cent of the cases can be treated, but with increased survival rates, various side effects have become apparent. Therefore, unravelling the mechanism of the disease may help to refine therapeutic strategies.

Cytogenetic studies indicate that several chromosome regions are involved, but so far, only the *WT1* gene has been proven to play a role in the aetiology of this tumour (Scharnhorst et al., 2001). However, *WT1* mutations are found in only 5% of sporadic Wilms' tumours and *WT1* mutations appear to play a role only in a few familial cases. One possible reason for is that disruption of WT1 function may impair gonad development and hence the transmission of germinal *WT1* mutations. Therefore, only less disruptive alterations of WT1 may be transmitted. Alternatively, WT1 function may be altered by mutations affecting either regulators or effectors of WT1. Wilms' tumour also is associated with a group of rare syndromes (Denys–Drash syndrome, Frasier syndrome, and WAGR syndrome) and in the development of other tumours such as leukaemias, breast cancer, and mesothelioma.

8.12.2 WT1 function: importance of alternative splicing

There is little knowledge about the factors that regulate WT1 protein expression and function or about the downstream effectors of WT1. Analysis of the chromosomal regions related to the appearance of WT may help to reveal the identity of these regulatory factors. WT1 may function at three stages of kidney development. WT1 expression can be detected at the onset of nephrogenesis, is low in the developing blastema, increases as nephrogenesis progresses and upon further differentiation its expression is downregulated except in the podocytes, where it is maintained into adulthood. Consistent with its role in kidney development, inactivation of several WT1-target genes, such as *IGF-II, IGF-IR, Gαl-2, Pax-2,* or *Bcl-2,* results in reduced and abnormal nephrogenesis.

WT1 also plays a role in differentiation, proliferation and apoptosis in cell culture systems. Since *Wt1* knockout mice die early in development due to a failure in kidney development, and mice heterozygous for *Wt1* appear normal and do not develop tumours, the creation of conditional knockouts for *Wt1* may be required to evaluate the physiological function of Wt1.

WT1 initially was shown to be a transcription factor that is able to repress transcription of genes that are abnormally upregulated in Wilms' tumours, although more recent studies indicate that activation of transcription by WT1 is likely to be the critical function of this tumour suppressor. Nevertheless, discrepancies between the results obtained by different labs suggest that a specific cellular context may be required to manifest its function as a transcriptional activator. Consistent with this, some data suggest that WT1 splice variants may function as transcription factors with different transactivation activities on different target genes. These target genes include *IGF-II, PDGF-A,* amphiregulin, syndecan-2, *Bcl-2, p21CIP1,* and *hsp70.* WT1 may also affect promoter activity independently of DNA binding by binding other proteins such as the steroid binding factor 1 (SF1) or the hsp70 protein. Also, a conserved N-terminal RNA recognition motif is present in all known WT1 proteins. Therefore, WT1 proteins may also regulate gene expression at the post-transcriptional level through their ability to bind mRNA (e.g. the exon 2 region of IGF-II RNA) or by modulating RNA splicing as inferred by the localization of WT1 and snRNPs in the nucleus. A conserved N-terminal RNA recognition motif is present in all known WT-1 isoforms and the splicing factor U2AF65 may interact with WT1. The balance between the expression levels of WT1-induced genes may determine whether a cell will proliferate, differentiate or undergo apoptosis. Disruption of any of these three processes may result in tumour formation.

WT1 is subject to alternative splicing in two regions. The best characterized alternative splice variant involves the insertion of the three aminoacids, lysine–threonine–serine (KTS) between the third and fourth zinc fingers of the DNA-binding domain at the C-terminus of WT1. The inclusion of these aminoacids drastically reduces the affinity of WT1 for a specific DNA sequence, and instead this isoform binds preferentially to RNA. Moreover, the +KTS, but not the −KTS isoform of WT1, shows a speckled pattern by immunofluorescence analysis and colocalizes with splicing factors. Thus, it appears that WT1 may play a role in both transcription and RNA processing in a splice isoform-dependent manner.

Another alternative splice inserts 17 aminoacids (17AAs) between the WT1 transcriptional activation domain and the zinc finger region. Studies of the effect of the +17AA form of WT1 have shown variable effects on the transcriptional function of WT1. In some cell types, it augments the transcriptional activation domain, and in others it has been shown to constitute an independent transcriptional repression domain. The involvement of the Par4 protein, a coactivator of this splice variant, may help to explain these discrepancies. The 17AA insertion of WT1 also has been linked to both the regulation of the cell cycle and apoptosis, although the molecular mechanisms involved are not clear.

The relative level of the WT1 isoforms can vary during development and in disease. For example, Frasier syndrome results from an imbalance of the +KTS/−KTS ratio and the relative level of the WT1 + 17AA isoform can be elevated in Wilms' tumours and leukaemia. In addition, the +17AA variant is differentially expressed throughout development.

8.13 *PTEN*

8.13.1 *PTEN* gene

PTEN (phosphatase and tensin homologue deleted on chromosome ten), also known as *MMAC1* (mutated in multiple advanced cancers) and *TEP1* (TGF-regulated and epithelial cell-enriched phosphatase) was first identified as a tumour-suppressor gene localized on chromosome 10q23. *PTEN* mutations occur in many tumour types and are associated with different stages of tumorigenesis. Cowden disease (CD), an autosomal dominant familial cancer syndrome is characterized by multiple hamartomas of the skin, breast, thyroid and intestines, and increased risk of breast and thyroid malignancies. The phenotype of Bannayan–Zonana syndrome (BZS) patients partly overlaps CD, but these patients are not found to have an increased risk of malignancy. Germline mutations have been found in 81% of families with CD and 57% of BZS families. Somatic mutations of *PTEN* occur in high-grade gliomas, advanced stage prostate carcinomas, endometrial carcinomas and malignant melanomas. PTEN may exhibit differential roles in specific tumour types. In brain and prostate carcinomas, *PTEN* mutations probably occur late in tumorigenesis and in association with the metastatic phenotype. In endometrial carcinomas *PTEN* mutations may instead be initiating events. Germline mutations predispose CD patients to breast and thyroid cancers, supporting the role of PTEN as an inhibitor of transformation.

8.13.2 PTEN function

In response to mitogen or cytokine stimulation, phosphoinositide 3 kinase (PI3K) activation leads to the production of PtdIns(3,4,5)P_3 and subsequent recruitment of both PKB (Akt/RAC) and PDKs to the plasma membrane. The resulting colocalization of kinases facilitates PDK phosphorylation (activation) of PKB, which in turn phosphorylates substrates involved in cell growth and survival.

The *PTEN* gene encodes a dual-specificity phosphatase of the VHR family. These phosphatases dephosphorylate proteins and lipids by virtue of their HCXXGXXRS/T domain. PTEN has a phosphatase activity towards serine, threonine, and tyrosine phosphorylated residues in acidic regions. This preference for acidic substrates led to tests of its activity as a phospholipid phosphatase. PTEN specifically dephosphorylates the D3 position on the inositol ring of phosphatidyl inositol and inositol phosphates. This specificity for the 3 position suggested that PTEN acts as an antagonist of phosphoinositide PI3K signalling.

Loss of PTEN function was found to result in high levels of PtdIns(3,4,5)P_3 and elevated basal levels of the activated PKB. These data strongly suggested that PTEN functions downstream of PI3K and upstream of PKB in the PI3K–PKB signalling pathway. PTEN contains 403 aminoacid residues. Residues 10 to 353 constitute the minimal phosphatase domain and the C-terminal residues contain a PDZ binding site which may be involved in the assembly of multiprotein complexes at the cell membrane and regulation of the half life of the protein.

Particular mutations that retain protein phosphatase but not lipid phosphatase activity, have allowed it to be established that protein phosphatase activity is not sufficient for G1 arrest. Possibly, the protein phosphatase activity of PTEN may be important in other aspects of tumorigenesis related to cell spreading and motility. Overexpression of PTEN has been shown to inhibit cell migration while antisense PTEN enhances it. Accordingly, integrin-mediated cell spreading and the formation of focal adhesions are downregulated with wild-type PTEN but not a PTEN with an inactive phosphatase domain. These effects of PTEN may be mediated by its ability to dephosphorylate focal adhesion kinase (FAK). An excellent review of PTEN function is given by Yamada and Araki (2001).

8.13.3 *PTEN* mouse models

Numerous mouse transgenic studies support a role for PTEN in PKB-mediated tumorigenesis and disease. *Pten*-null mouse embryos exhibit a disruption in developmental patterning and regions of increased cellular proliferation that result in death before birth. Cells from *Pten*-null mice and PTEN-deficient human tumour cell lines both exhibit elevated levels of PtdIns(3,4,5)P_3 which correlates with increased PKB activity. Expression of wild-type Pten in these cells reduces PtdIns(3,4,5)P_3 levels and inhibits PKB and other targets of PI3K. Mice heterozygous for *Pten* are viable but develop spontaneous tumours, establishing the role of *Pten* as a TSG.

8.13.4 PTEN and the p53 pathway

Several elements in the *PTEN* promoter appear to regulate the level of protein expression, including binding sites for the tumour suppressor p53. On the other hand, recent observations show that PKB promotes the phosphorylation and possibly the movement of the MDM2 oncoprotein into the nucleus, where it downregulates the p53 tumour-suppressor protein. Through its ability to inhibit activation of PKB, PTEN could inactivate or restrict MDM2 to the cytoplasm, and therefore, induce the accumulation and promote p53 transcriptional function in the nucleus.

8.14 Breast cancer: BRCA1, BRCA2, and p53

After lung carcinoma, breast carcinoma is a leading cause of cancer mortality among women in the Western hemisphere. Current estimates suggest that one in eight American women will develop breast carcinoma. The molecular mechanisms and changes leading to the development and progression of breast carcinoma are extremely complex. Multiple factors contribute to its development and progression including certain steroid receptors (oestrogen receptor (ER), progesterone receptor (PR), and retinoic acid receptor), members of the HER/*ERBB* family, and several TSGs. Individuals with mutations of the *BRCA1*, *BRCA2*, or *TP53* TSGs are at a higher risk of developing breast carcinoma in their lifetime. Some of these mutations associate with early onset of disease, whereas others increase overall lifetime risk. Therefore, testing for mutations in these genes can contribute information regarding the risk of developing breast carcinoma, and also help to evaluate overall prognosis and response to specific therapy. The evaluation of certain molecular markers such as ER and PR expression in individual tumours may also contribute to the determination of prognosis in patients with breast carcinoma and be predictors of clinical outcome with current therapy. For example, the presence of ER and/or PR is reported to predict response to endocrine therapies.

Somatic cell mutation in *TP53* is observed in approximately 20–30% of primary breast carcinoma cases. Most of these mutations occur at the core DNA binding domain and result in decreased p53-dependent gene transactivation. In the majority of p53-negative tumours, a missense mutation of one allele is associated with deletion of the second allele. Tumours with *TP53* mutations are more likely to be highly invasive, poorly differentiated, high-grade breast tumours. It is hypothesized that

TP53 mutations may precede the development of tumours with fully malignant and invasive phenotypes. Therefore, mutant p53 has been suggested to be a biomarker predicting risk for subsequent breast carcinogenesis. However, the response to therapy may not always be related to *TP53* status. As recently described, in the case of advanced breast cancer tumours treated with epirubicin and cyclophosphamide, a positive association between p53 mutation and success of the treatment has been reported. Germline *TP53* mutation is also a risk factor for breast carcinoma. Although quite rare, Li–Fraumeni is a dominant inherited cancer syndrome that manifests itself with a high rate of early-onset breast carcinoma as well as multiple other tumour types.

The ER has been shown to associate physically with the aminoterminus of p53 to form complexes containing p53 and MDM2. It is interesting to note that ER protects p53 from MDM2-mediated degradation, suggesting that ER-signalling results in the up-regulation of p53 protein. However, overexpression of ER- has been reported to mediate the overexpression of MDM2 also and to decrease p53 transcriptional activity. This may be a potential mechanism leading to neoplastic transformation of the cell and suppression of p53 leading to increased cellular proliferation.

Hereditary breast carcinoma is reported to account for a small proportion (5–10%) of all breast carcinoma cases. Germline mutations in two breast carcinoma susceptibility genes, *BRCA1* and *BRCA2*, have been implicated in a fraction of these, and in particular those arising in young women, via an autosomal dominant inheritance mechanism. Patients carrying *BRCA1* mutations have up to a 94% risk of developing breast and/or ovarian cancer by the age of 70. These mutations also increase the risk of ovarian, colon, and prostate cancer.

Tumorigenesis in women with *BRCA1* or *BRCA2* mutations requires the loss or inactivation of the remaining wild-type allele, resulting in expression of a non-functional protein. Women with a mutation in one of these genes are reported to have an approximately 60–80% risk of developing breast carcinoma in their lifetime. Although these mutations are found scattered throughout the genes, some are more prevalent and have a higher penetrance than others. For example, three mutations (*BRCA1* 185delAG, *BRCA1* 5382insC, and *BRCA2* 6174delT) are found to have a high penetrance in the Ashkenazi Jewish population. *BRCA2* mutations account for approximately 40% of early breast cancers. Interestingly, almost all cell lines that show loss of *BRCA2* (at 13q12–q13) also show loss of *RB* (at 13q14). Screening for and detection of *BRCA1*/*BRCA2* mutations may be helpful in determining the overall risk for the development of breast carcinoma, especially in families with hereditary cases.

The observation that both BRCA1 and BRCA2 proteins form nuclear foci with Rad51 during S phase and after DNA damage led to the suggestion of their involvement in DNA repair. Accordingly, *BRCA1* and *BRCA2* mutant cells show defects in the repair of double-strand breaks (DSBs). Aside from this function, *BRCA1* has also been implicated in the regulation of gene transcription and ubiquitin ligase activity when dimerized to BARD1. The striking genetic instability observed in cells deficient in BRCA1 or BRCA2, which is greater than that observed in oncogene-induced tumours, suggests that chromosomal aberrations followed by gain or loss of function of other genes triggers BRCA-associated tumorigenesis. This model is strongly supported by experiments carried out by knocking out *BRCA1* or *BRCA2* functions in mice.

8.15 Concluding remarks

The identification of tumour suppressor genes has had enormous impact on our understanding of the neoplastic process and has already had a major impact in the clinic. Most directly the identification of the genetic basis of cancer family syndromes has allowed the unequivocal detection of which family members are at risk and has allowed that excess risk to be quantified. In many cases such at risk individuals can be offered enhanced screening access and even prophylactic surgery. Such populations of at risk individuals also provide ideal populations in which prevention trials can be conducted. Screening for *BRCA1* and *BRCA2* mutations in breast cancer families and for mismatch repair and *APC* gene mutations in colorectal cancer families is becoming more routine though it still faces technical, economic, and ethical challenges. As more TSG mutations are uncovered, the possibility of larger groups of the population being defined as 'genetically at enhanced risk' will pose great problems for health care but this does have the potential benefit of focusing screening and preventative strategies on those populations that will gain most benefit.

In the absence of a clear cancer family pedigree associated with a locus, TSGs have proven notoriously difficult to define. This situation is probably compounded by the level of haploinsufficiency of a TSG. Thus, in the case of TSGs with strong happloinsufficiency, mutations in the second allele may not be present. The realization of the importance of haploinsufficiency together with the use of mouse models with chromosomal deletions at defined loci, novel methods of gene knock down such as small interfering RNA techniques (siRNA), and the genome and proteome databases that are being developed should all help to resolve these problems rapidly.

Since TSG mutations classically represent loss of function, superficially they do not appear to be such good targets for the development of novel anti-cancer drugs as oncogenic gain of function mutations. However, an understanding of the pathways in which TSGs act can provide such 'druggable' targets. TSG reactivation is an attractive possibility in those cases where the TSG is inactivated by methylation or where the TSG gene product's function is blocked by the binding of overexpressed host or viral proteins. The critical roles of TSGs in regulating repair, cell cycle, and apoptotic decisions also suggest that they may act as key determinants of the tumour cell's relative sensitivity to existing therapeutic modalities such as ionizing radiation and chemotherapy. Thus the accurate individual profiling of the tumour may allow a more rational and effective selection of currently used therapies as well as the definition of new targets for therapy development. In the future one hopes to see cancer as a chronic disease controlled by accurately targeted and specific non-toxic therapies. The work on TSGs has a key role to play in realizing that vision.

References

Boudeau, J., Sapkota, G., and Alessi, D. R. (2003). LKB1, a protein kinase regulating cell proliferation and polarity. *FEBS Lett*, **546**, 159–65.

Fodde, R. and Smits, R. (2001). Disease model: familial adenomatous polyposis. *Trends Mol Med*, **7**, 369–73.

Kaelin, W. G., Jr. (2002). Molecular basis of the VHL hereditary cancer syndrome. *Nat Rev Cancer*, **2**, 673–82.

Knudson, A. G. (2001). Two genetic hits (more or less) to cancer. *Nat Rev Cancer*, **1**, 157–62.

McLaughlin, M. E. and Jacks, T. (2002). Thinking beyond the tumor cell: Nf1 haploinsufficiency in the tumor environment. *Cancer Cell*, **1**, 408–10.

Narod, S. A. (2002). Modifiers of risk of hereditary breast and ovarian cancer. *Nat Rev Cancer*, **2**, 113–23.

Quon, K. C. and Berns, A. (2001). Haplo-insufficiency? Let me count the ways. *Genes Dev*, **15**, 2917–21.

Scharnhorst, V., van der Eb, A. J., and Jochemsen, A. G. (2001). WT1 proteins: functions in growth and differentiation. *Gene*, **273**, 141–61.

Sherr, C. J. (2001). The INK4a/ARF network in tumour suppression. *Nat Rev Mol Cell Biol*, **2**, 731–7.

Sherr, C. J. and McCormick, F. (2002). The RB and p53 pathways in cancer. *Cancer Cell*, **2**, 103–12.

Sturm, I., Bosanquet, A. G., Hermann, S., Guner, D., Dorken, B., and Daniel, P. T. (2003). Mutation of p53 and consecutive selective drug resistance in B-CLL occurs as a consequence of prior DNA-damaging chemotherapy. *Cell Death Differ*, **10**, 477–84.

Vousden, K. H. and Lu, X. (2002). Live or let die: the cell's response to p53. *Nat Rev Cancer*, **2**, 594–604.

Woods, Y. L. and Lane, D. P. (2003). Exploiting the p53 pathway for cancer diagnosis and therapy. *Hematol J*, **4**, 233–47.

Yamada, K. M. and Araki, M. (2001). Tumor suppressor PTEN: modulator of cell signaling, growth, migration and apoptosis. *J Cell Sci*, **114**, 2375–82.

CHAPTER 9

The cancer cell cycle

Chris J. Norbury

9.1 Introduction: cell cycle events in normal and neoplastic cells

The relationship between cell cycle progression and tumour biology is both complex and fascinating. The major cell cycle events of chromosomal DNA replication in S (synthesis) phase and chromosome segregation in mitosis (M phase) must be orchestrated reasonably accurately if a neoplastic cell is to proliferate to an extent that is clinically significant. Disorderly DNA replication or uncontrolled progression through mitosis, if sufficiently extreme, would be incompatible with cell survival, and hence with tumour development. Like many other aspects of cell cycle regulation, this point is clearly illustrated by reference to model organisms such as yeasts. In these simple eukaryotes, cell cycle progression is governed by proteins that, in many cases, are highly conserved in human cells. Most loss-of-function mutations in yeast cell cycle genes cause cell cycle arrest and loss of viability. Indeed, it was through studies of such *cdc* (cell division cycle) mutants that many of the key components of the human cell cycle were indirectly identified. Most notable among these are the cyclin-dependent kinases (CDKs) that control both S phase and M phase entry (Figure 9.1).

Despite this requirement for retention of functional cell cycle apparatus, tumorigenesis is characterized by loss of controls that normally restrict cell growth and proliferation. Thus, one fundamental hallmark of neoplasia is persistent cell cycle progression in defiance of physiological cues that would normally signal cell cycle withdrawal. Much of this aberrant behaviour must be explicable in terms of the genetic lesions that drive tumour development. Indeed, it is increasingly possible to describe pathways that link oncoproteins and tumour suppressors with the core cell cycle machinery—the enzymatic apparatus that is directly responsible for DNA replication, chromosome segregation and the co-ordination of these processes. When considering such pathways it is important to distinguish between components that drive cell growth (hypertrophy) and those that promote cell cycle progression itself. This is fairly straightforward in model organisms such as yeast and *Drosophila*, where cell cycle progression is separable from, but dependent on, cell growth, (Fantes and Nurse, 1977; Prober and Edgar, 2001). The situation in human cells is less straightforward, however, and prominent oncoproteins such as MYC appear able to promote cell growth and cell cycle progression simultaneously via distinct pathways (Beier et al., 2000). Similarly, the tumour suppressor RB normally functions both to restrain cell cycle progression and, separately, to repress cell growth (White, 1997; Classon and Harlow, 2002).

Cytogenetic examination of cancer cells shows that they are often highly aneuploid, and this level

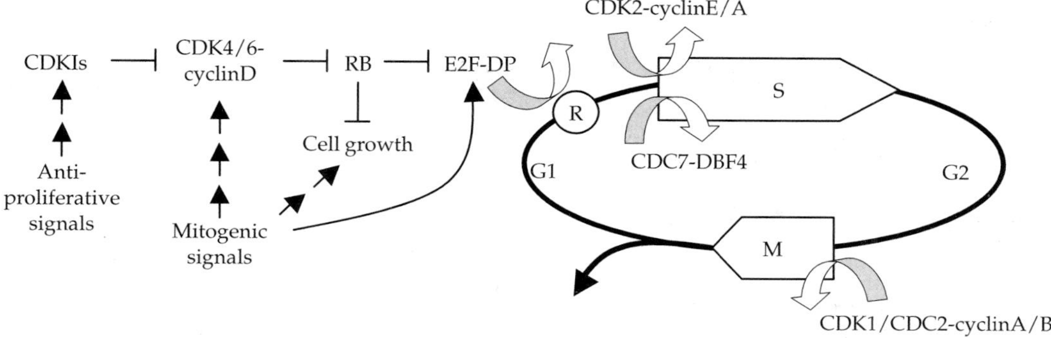

Figure 9.1 The interface between growth control and cell cycle control. Signal transduction pathways activated in response to diverse mitogens and anti-proliferative cues serve either to activate or, via CDK inhibitors (CDKIs), to inhibit CDK4/6-cyclinD, which in turn phosphorylates and inactivates RB. Hypophosphorylated RB represses transcription of genes required for R (restriction) point transit, in part through inhibition of E2F-DP transcription factors, and represses cell growth. Mitogenic signals can also activate cell growth and E2F activity independently of CDK4/6-cyclinD. Following cell cycle commitment, distinct heterodimeric protein kinases are required for successive cell cycle transitions as shown on the right hand side. Both CDK2-cyclinE (and to a lesser extent cyclin A) and CDC7-DBF4 are required for the initiation of DNA replication, while CDK1/CDC2-cyclinB (and to a lesser extent cyclin A) is responsible for M phase entry.

of genetic instability results in part from defects in 'checkpoint' mechanisms that normally govern cell cycle progression (Paulovich et al., 1997). Checkpoints can be defined as genetically determined signalling pathways that delay the execution of certain cell cycle events until earlier events are deemed to be complete. The mitotic spindle checkpoint, for example, serves to delay the onset of anaphase until the pair of kinetochores at each centromere has made balanced and bipolar connections to the spindle microtubules. Other checkpoint mechanisms operate to ensure that mitosis is not initiated until completion of DNA replication, to inhibit either mitosis or DNA replication in response to DNA damage, or to inhibit re-replication of DNA until mitosis has been completed. Defects in each of these checkpoint pathways could contribute to genomic instability, and many such checkpoint defects have been described in human cancers, as discussed below. It follows that, while many aspects of the cell cycle are normal in cancer cells, some aspects of its regulation are flawed, with disastrous consequences.

9.2 Restriction point control and its loss

Many of the controls that govern the transition between quiescence and active cell cycling in mammals operate in the G1 phase (Zetterberg et al., 1995; Blagosklonny and Pardee, 2002). This is particularly clear in the case of fibroblasts, which have been intensively studied in this respect. Such studies have identified a point of commitment in G1 beyond which cells lose their requirement for high levels of protein synthesis or exogenous growth factors. Progression beyond this 'restriction' (R) point commits a cell to enter and complete S phase and, in most cases, the subsequent mitosis. Cell types other than fibroblasts use closely analogous mechanisms to regulate cell cycle commitment. Over the past decade, the molecular details of R point control have started to become apparent. Broadly similar points of cell cycle commitment in G1 have been described in yeasts, but the molecular details of these controls are quite distinct, limiting the usefulness of the yeast model in this case. Loss of R point control appears to be a common, possibly even universal step in tumour development, and a number of genetic lesions that can contribute to this deregulation have been identified. Together with a wide variety of additional experimental data, these genetic studies have led to a fairly detailed understanding of how mitogenic signals are integrated during the process of cell cycle commitment.

RB, the product of the gene defective in familial retinoblastoma (see Chapter 8), plays a central role in R point control and is subject to regulatory phosphorylation events that determine its ability to interact with members of the E2F family of transcription factors (Classon and Harlow, 2002). In early G1, RB is hypophosphorylated and through its 'pocket' domain binds the transcriptional activation domain of E2F proteins. This interaction neutralizes the transcriptional activity of E2F, by preventing its interaction with general transcription factors, and tethers RB to the promoters of genes to which E2F can bind, along with its dimerization partner DP, in a sequence-specific manner. Known E2F/DP target genes encode a variety of proteins with roles in cell cycle progression, including CDK1 (otherwise known as CDC2) and cyclins A and E. Hypophosphorylated RB represses unscheduled expression of these cell cycle regulatory genes, in part through neutralization of E2F and in part through its capacity to act independently as a transcriptional repressor once recruited to a promoter. This repression depends partly on RB-mediated inhibition of protein kinase activity associated with the general transcription factor TFIID, and partly on the recruitment of histone deacetylases and interaction with SWI/SNF proteins, with subsequent chromatin modification (Dunaief et al., 1994; Brehm et al., 1998; Siegert and Robbins, 1999). Interpretation of the consequences of loss of RB function is further complicated by its repression of Pol I- and Pol III-dependent transcription (White, 1997). These polymerases, which are responsible for the synthesis of ribosomal and transfer RNAs, are frequently found to be hyperactive in experimental tumour models and their deregulation could play an important role in driving cancer cell growth.

Germline mutational loss of RB plays a clear causal role in familial retinoblastoma, and is associated with predisposition to other tumours such as osteosarcomas. Mutation of *RB* in sporadic tumours is also well documented, but other genetic lesions that have the effect of functionally inactivating wild-type RB through promoting its hyperphosphorylation are seen more frequently. Phosphorylation and inactivation of RB by heterodimeric CDK4/CDK6-cyclinD kinases is considered crucially important for R point transition (Classon and Harlow, 2002). As with other members of the CDK family, the activities of these kinases are limited by cyclin availability, and cyclin D1 overexpression helps to explain constitutive cell cycling in a number of tumour types. CDK inhibitor proteins including p16 and p27 also have the capacity to restrict the activities of R point-associated CDKs. Mutational inactivation of the *CDKN2A* gene leads to loss of p16 function in a wide variety of tumour types, though the interpretation of this observation is complicated by the fact that the same gene encodes the ARF protein, which serves to regulate the p53 tumour suppressor (see Chapter 8). Decreased levels of p27 have been associated with poor prognosis in a number of studies and result either from mutation or, more commonly, from the enhanced degradation of p27 by the ubiquitin-proteasome pathway (Slingerland and Pagano, 2000). Gain of function mutations in *CDK4*, which disrupt the interaction between the kinase and the CDK inhibitor p16, provide a further mechanism for loss of R point control, though such mutations are comparatively rare (Wolfel et al., 1995).

CDK4/CDK6-cyclinD kinases represent an important interface between growth factor signal transduction pathways and the cell cycle commitment machinery. Activation of RAS-regulated signalling results in transcriptional activation of cyclin D1, and through the RAF-MAPK pathway promotes assembly of cyclin D1 with its CDK partners (Cheng et al., 1998; Kerkhoff and Rapp, 1998). Conversely, inhibition of epithelial cell proliferation by transforming growth factor beta (TGFβ) is associated with its activation of the p27 CDK inhibitor and consequent inhibition of R point progression (Polyak et al., 1994).

9.3 Initiation of DNA replication

The initiation of DNA replication is biochemically distinct from R point transition and the two events can be separated by several hours. Current models of replication initiation in human cells are based largely on data from yeast, in which many of the key molecular components were first identified, though important contributions have come from *in vitro* DNA replication systems derived from human cells or *Xenopus* eggs. Detailed reviews of this area may be found elsewhere (Bell and Dutta, 2002; Blow and Hodgson, 2002).

Human S phase typically lasts just a few hours, and in cells such as activated T lymphocytes, DNA replication can be even faster. In order that the entire genome can be replicated within this time frame, a large number (perhaps tens of thousands) of bi-directional origins must be established and fired in an orderly fashion, such that each DNA sequence is normally copied once, but only once, per cell cycle. Origins of replication are defined by the primary DNA sequence in the budding yeast *Saccharomyces cerevisiae*, but this is not the case in metazoan cells where higher order structure such as chromatin looping is probably more important for determining origin position. Nonetheless, the events leading to origin firing follow a common pattern in yeast and human cells, and consist of the sequential assembly of a multi-protein pre-replication complex (PRC), its modification by regulatory protein kinases and the subsequent recruitment of the DNA replication machinery itself. Different parts of the genome are replicated at characteristic times during S phase, reflecting the sequential activation of defined sets of origins as replication proceeds.

Potential origins of replication are marked by a conserved hexameric origin recognition complex (ORC), to which the proteins CDC6 (an ATPase) and CDT1 are recruited. These then permit the ATP-dependent loading of a second hetero-hexameric complex consisting of proteins MCM2-7, completing the assembly of the PRC and establishing a state of replication competence or 'licensing'. It is likely that the MCM hexamer proteins together constitute the helicase activity required for origin unwinding. Activation of the PRC requires the activity of two heterodimeric protein kinases: the S-phase CDK (S-CDK) and CDC7/DBF4 (DBF4-dependent kinase or DDK). The B-type CDK Cdc28-Clb performs the S-CDK role in *S. cerevisiae*, whereas in metazoan cells S-phase promoting activity is provided by CDK2-cyclinE and CDK2-cyclinA. Both S-CDK and DDK promote origin unwinding, recruitment of replicative DNA polymerases and their accessory subunits, initiation of daughter strand synthesis and PRC disassembly. Important intermediate steps include the S-CDK/DDK-dependent recruitment of CDC45, a putative MCM2-7 cofactor that may be required for activation of their helicase activity. Efficient recruitment of CDC45 also depends on the MCM10 protein, which binds to the nascent origin in a CDK- and DDK-independent manner (Wohlschlegel et al., 2002). The key substrates of DDK in origin activation appear to be the MCM2-7 proteins, while those of S-CDK have yet to be clearly identified.

Licensing of origins must be tightly regulated if initiation from each is to be limited to once per cell cycle. The key to this aspect of cell cycle control lies in the dual action of CDKs, which both trigger replication and inhibit origin re-licensing (Blow and Hodgson, 2002). CDT1 levels, like those of many key regulatory proteins, are normally held in check by substrate-specific ubiquitin conjugation, which targets proteins for proteolysis by the proteasome, a large multi-catalytic protease complex. CDK-dependent phosphorylation promotes the CDC4-dependent ubiquitinylation of CDT1, and hence its degradation, as well as nuclear export of CDC6. Total CDK activity is normally dramatically reduced on exit from mitosis (see below) and it is only during the interval between mitotic exit and activation of G1- and S-CDKs that CDK activity is low enough to allow nuclear CDT1 and CDC6 to license origins. After the initiation of replication, competence at any given origin can therefore normally be re-established only following progression through mitosis. Metazoans, including humans, have a second, parallel mechanism of licensing control in which the geminin protein tightly binds and sequesters CDT1. During progression through mitosis, geminin is marked for proteolysis by a ubiquitin ligase termed the anaphase-promoting complex/cyclosome (APC/C), thus freeing CDT1 to perform its licensing role until geminin levels are restored. Origin licensing is generally limited to actively proliferating cells, and is not seen in quiescent populations. Recruitment of ORC components and other proteins of the PRC may therefore provide a biochemical distinction between G1 and G0, a term applied rather loosely to cells that have left the cycling compartment for a protracted period.

DNA replication can be deregulated during tumorigenesis through unscheduled expression of cyclinE-dependent CDK activity. Cyclin E overexpression in tumours or cancer cell lines can result from a variety of mechanisms, including mutation of the CDC4 protein that comprises part of the SCF ubiquitin ligase that targets cyclin E for proteolysis (Strohmaier et al., 2001). The consequent deregulation of CDK2-cyclinE activity could contribute to tumour development at two levels; first, precocious cell cycle commitment and origin firing (since experimental cyclin E overexpression can counteract RB-induced cell cycle arrest and drive cells into S phase) and secondly, induction of genomic instability (Spruck et al., 1999). The latter may reflect inappropriate partial inhibition of replication licensing, with chromosome breakage resulting as an indirect consequence of incomplete DNA replication, followed by progression into mitosis.

9.4 Completion of DNA replication

Following DNA replication, the newly generated sister chromatids remain associated in a pseudo-parallel fashion through the action of the multi-protein complex cohesin (Nasmyth et al., 2000). Cohesin includes among its constituents SMC1 and SMC3 (structural maintenance of chromosomes), which like other proteins of the SMC family are capable of forming extended coil structures with globular ATPase head domains. This cohesion between sisters is thought to be important for the provision of an undamaged template for homologous recombinational DNA repair (HRR). Recent studies of yeast cohesin have established that three of its subunits are capable of forming a ring structure that might physically encircle the two sisters, and through which the entire replication fork could conceivably pass. Such an arrangement would provide a ready explanation for the essential link between replication and the establishment of cohesion (Gruber et al., 2003). HRR provides the possibility of error-free repair of double-strand (ds) DNA breaks induced by ionizing radiation (IR), but is thought to be of equal or greater importance in the recovery of stalled replication forks. Data from a variety of experimental models suggest that DNA helicases of the RecQ family play a part in this aspect of S phase completion (Hickson, 2003). The importance of this process for the maintenance of genomic stability is underlined by the consequences of germ line mutation of the gene encoding the RecQ-like helicase BLM in Bloom's syndrome. This syndrome is characterized by growth retardation, increased incidence of a wide variety of cancers and, at the cellular level, increased levels of mitotic recombination between sister chromatids. Consistent with a role for BLM in the completion of DNA replication, cells from Bloom's syndrome patients have a characteristically extended S phase in culture.

9.5 Checkpoint responses to DNA damage in G1 and S phase

The presence of DNA lesions such as strand breaks, UV photoproducts and cross-links clearly complicates the mechanics of DNA replication and may result in replication-induced chromosomal damage and/or the irretrievable fixation of new mutations. For these reasons, checkpoint pathways have evolved that have the capacity to detect DNA lesions, to delay S phase entry or the firing of origins at which replication has not yet begun, or to stabilize stalled replication forks.

The p53 tumour suppressor is a key component of the pathway that operates in G1 cells to delay S phase entry in response to DNA damage (Kuerbitz et al., 1992). The abrupt increase in p53 level that normally results from DNA damage is largely attributable to the inhibition of p53 degradation by the ubiquitin-proteasome pathway. After induction of dsDNA breaks, p53 stabilization requires the activity of the ATM protein kinase, which is mutated in the cancer-prone disorder ataxia–telangiectasia (A-T) and which plays a pivotal role in several cellular responses to such damage (Lu and Lane, 1993; Shiloh, 2001). Once stabilized, tetrameric p53 is able to act as a transcription factor, and p53-driven transcription of the *CIP1/WAF1* gene encoding the p21 CDK inhibitor plays a major role in DNA damage-induced G1 arrest (Sherr and Roberts, 1999). In comparison with other CDK inhibitors, p21 has a broad specificity, such that it can suppress both R point transit and replication origin firing. It is difficult to assess the importance of loss of the G1 DNA damage checkpoint in tumorigenesis. Although germline defects in either p53 or ATM confer cancer predisposition, each of these proteins has additional roles outside the G1 checkpoint pathway. Similarly, cells from mice lacking p21 have a severe G1 checkpoint defect, but the fact that these animals are not inherently cancer prone could derive from a secondary function of p21 in inhibiting apoptosis.

Asynchronous populations of fibroblasts exposed to IR exhibit a characteristic rapid decrease in DNA synthesis. This decrease principally reflects the inhibition of further origin firing in cells that are already in S phase, with minor contributions coming from inhibition of the G1-S transition and, potentially, the slowing of active replication forks. Cells from patients with any one of several autosomal recessive genetic disorders characterized by radiosensitivity and/or cancer predisposition fail to reduce DNA replication after IR-induced damage and hence are said to exhibit 'radioresistant DNA synthesis' (RDS). These syndromes include A-T, Nijmegen breakage syndrome and an A-T-like disorder, which result from mutations in the *ATM*, *NBS1* and *MRE11* genes, respectively (Vessey et al., 1999). The corresponding proteins have been identified as components of 'intra-S phase' checkpoint signalling pathways, explaining the characteristic RDS phenotype. These data have been combined with information from the yeast models, in which many aspects of the cell cycle responses to DNA damage are conserved, to generate a detailed picture of the intra-S checkpoints that operate in human cells (Figure 9.2).

The ATM protein kinase is representative of a group of large (~350 kDa) PI3-kinase-like enzymes

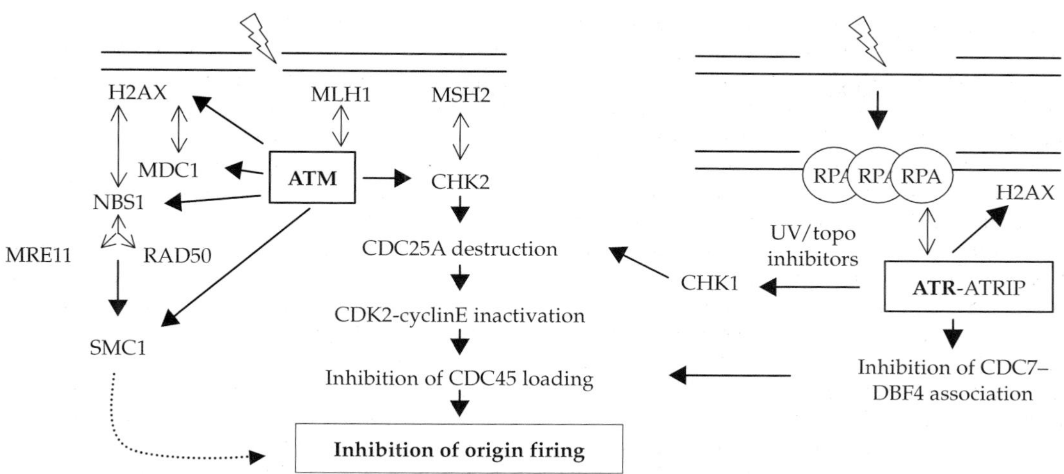

Figure 9.2 Intra-S phase checkpoint responses to DNA damage. ATM is central to the responses to dsDNA breaks (left). ATM interacts with MLH1, a MMR protein that may also serve to detect structures other than mismatched bases. At or near to the site of the DNA lesion, activated ATM phosphorylates the variant histone H2AX, which is then bound by MDC1 and NBS1. The NBS1–MRE11–RAD50 complex transmits a checkpoint signal via the cohesin protein SMC1, to inhibit origin firing by an as yet undetermined mechanism. NBS1 and SMC1 are also substrates of ATM. A parallel pathway downstream from ATM inhibits origin firing by promoting the inactivation of CDK2-cyclinE. This depends on the activation of CHK2, which may be brought into contact with ATM through its association with the MMR protein MSH2. Further substrates of ATM and protein–protein interactions (see Table 9.1) are omitted in the interests of clarity. Partially single stranded structures, including stalled replication forks and structures generated by nuclease-mediated processing of primary lesions, are coated in the single-strand binding protein RPA and then can activate ATR (right). ATR can phosphorylate H2AX, and inhibits CDC45 loading independently of CDK2-cyclinE by preventing the association between CDC7 and its activating subunit DBF4. In addition, activation of ATR by UV or topoisomerase (topo) inhibitors leads to CHK1 activation and suppression of CDC25A activity.

with central roles in checkpoint signalling in all eukaryotes. In this regard the other significant member of this family in human cells is ATR (ATM and Rad3-related), which acts independently of ATM to promote S phase delay after replication fork stalling or DNA damage (Shiloh, 2001). These kinases occupy apical positions in checkpoint pathways and presumably act either as damage sensors or in close association with such sensors. ATM and ATR are activated in response to different categories of DNA damage and inhibit origin firing via parallel pathways (Figure 9.2). Inactive ATM is largely sequestered in a pool of dimeric or multimeric protein; in response to dsDNA breaks this pool undergoes intermolecular autophosphorylation at Ser1981 prior to the release of active, monomeric ATM (Bakkenist and Kastan, 2003). Activation of ATR, which may involve analogous autophosphorylation, occurs specifically in response to DNA lesions of a partially single-stranded character and only after the single-stranded portions of such lesions have been coated by replication protein A (RPA), which performs a similar single-strand binding function during origin unwinding (Costanzo et al., 2003). Downstream from ATM, a relatively well-defined pathway culminates in the inhibition of CDK2-cyclinE activity and hence inhibition of origin firing (Costanzo et al., 2000). Understanding of this pathway was guided in part by the earlier description of S phase checkpoint pathways in fission yeast, where the ATM/ATR-like kinase Rad3 activates the downstream effector protein kinase Cds1. In human cells ATM activates the Cds1 homologue CHK2, which in turn phosphorylates the CDC25A phosphatase and targets it for degradation by the ubiquitin-proteasome pathway. Like other CDKs, CDK2 is subject to inhibitory phosphorylation at adjacent threonine and tyrosine residues in its ATP-binding cleft. Since CDC25A can reverse this inhibitory phosphorylation of CDK2, ATM activation promotes stabilization of CDK2 in its phosphorylated, inactive state and hence blocks origin firing at a point prior to CDC45 loading. Recent data suggest that, surprisingly, ionizing radiation-induced CHK2 activation is dependent on its association with the mismatch repair (MMR) protein MSH2, while ATM is activated in an MMR-independent fashion but binds to MLH1 (Brown et al., 2003). The implication is that, as well as being required for the repair of base mismatches, the MMR proteins perform further functions both in the recognition of dsDNA breaks and as a scaffold upon which ATM can be brought into contact with CHK2, one of its key substrates.

In fission yeast the 'checkpoint Rad' proteins Hus1 and Rad1, 3, 9, 17, and 26 are essential for all checkpoint responses to DNA damage and inhibition of DNA replication (Carr, 1997). In mammalian cells each of these proteins is conserved and is involved in checkpoint signalling, though the division of labour among them is more complex. Except for Rad3/ATM/ATR and the Rad3 accessory protein Rad26, which is conserved in human cells as ATRIP (Cortez et al., 2001), these checkpoint components are all structurally related to proteins involved in DNA replication. RAD1, RAD9, and HUS1 are related to the DNA polymerase sliding clamp proliferating cell nuclear antigen (PCNA), while RAD17 resembles subunits of replication factor C (RFC). These sequence similarities reflect physical associations, as RAD1, RAD9, and HUS1 are found together in a complex termed '9-1-1' (St. Onge et al., 1999), while RAD17 is associated with authentic RFC subunits on chromatin (Lindsey-Boltz et al., 2001). During DNA replication, RFC loads PCNA onto chromatin; similarly RAD17, in association with conventional RFC subunits, appears to load the 9-1-1 complex onto DNA in response to DNA damage (Roos-Mattjus et al., 2002; Zou et al., 2002). The 9-1-1 complex is thought to form a sliding clamp which has the dual purpose of checkpoint signalling and recruiting DNA repair enzymes. Localization of 9-1-1 to sites of DNA damage occurs independently of ATM/ATR, though both are required for normal levels of resistance to genotoxins. In mice, HUS1 (and, by implication, the 9-1-1 complex) is required for the intra-S phase response to bulky DNA adducts, but not to IR (Weiss et al., 2003). ATR and its downstream effector CHK1 play leading roles in checkpoints activated by UV, including the intra-S checkpoint (Heffernan et al., 2002). CHK1 has the capacity to inhibit CDC25 phosphatases directly by phosphorylation, or by promoting their cytoplasmic sequestration by 14-3-3 proteins, as well as by targeting them for ubiquitin-dependent degradation.

A number of additional mediators of DNA damage checkpoint signalling have been identified in recent years (Table 9.1). Several of these are relocalized in an ATM-dependent fashion to nuclear foci that probably represent sites of primary damage and also contain proteins such as RAD51 that are implicated in recombinational DNA repair. The details of this damage-dependent intranuclear redistribution of proteins are only beginning to emerge, but the process is clearly important for the appropriate orchestration of DNA repair and checkpoint responses. An early event appears to be phosphorylation of the histone variant H2AX by ATM and/or ATR at sites of damage, and the subsequent recruitment of NBS1 and MDC1 (mediator of damage checkpoint), which bind to H2AX via their forkhead-associated (FHA) domains. NBS1 and MRE11 are capable of stably associating with the SMC protein RAD50 and ATM specifically phosphorylates NBS1 after activation in response to dsDNA breaks. The NBS1–MRE11–RAD50 complex transduces the signal downstream to inhibit origin firing by a route that, in contrast to the CHK2 pathway, does not result in inhibition of CDC45 loading (Falck et al., 2002). The effector mechanism of this pathway is not yet clearly defined but intriguingly, one component appears to be the SMC1 cohesin subunit. SMC1 phosphorylation by ATM is required for intra-S checkpoint activation in response to IR and depends on prior phosphorylation of NBS1 (Kim et al., 2002; Yazdi et al., 2002). Yet another route to inhibition of origin firing operates downstream from ATR and culminates in the inhibition of association between CDC7 and DBF4 without inhibition of CDK2 (Costanzo et al., 2003).

Many of the components of the intra-S checkpoint pathway, including ATM, NBS1, MRE11, RAD50, MSH2, and MLH1, co-purify with the BRCA1 protein in what has been termed the BRCA1-associated genome surveillance complex (BASC) (Wang et al., 2000). BRCA1, first identified through its loss of function in familial breast and ovarian cancer, is also relocalized to nuclear foci after DNA damage, in a manner that depends on H2AX and the p53-interacting protein 53BP1. The latter is one of several checkpoint components that, like BRCA1, contain a protein–protein interaction motif called the BRCA1 carboxyl-terminal repeat (BRCT). SMC1 was not identified as a component of the BASC, but is also BRCA1-associated. It is tempting to speculate that the BASC, as its name suggests, represents a multifunctional

Table 9.1 Intra-S DNA damage checkpoint components acting downstream from ATM/ATR

Protein[a]	Associates with	Phosphorylation	Effect of loss of function	Structural motif(s)	References
H2AX	NBS1, MDC1	By ATM/ATR at Ser139	Genomic instability, radiation sensitivity	Variant histone	Ward and Chen (2001), Burma et al. (2001), Celeste et al. (2002), Kobayashi et al. (2002)
CHK2	MDC1, MSH2	By ATM at Thr68; MSH2/MLH1-and 53BP1-dependent	RDS, predisposition to osteosarcomas	Forkhead associated (FHA), protein kinase	Costanzo et al., 2000, Miller et al., 2002, Chaturvedi et al., 1999
MSH2	Other MMR proteins, CHK2	?	RDS; MMR deficiency; hereditary non-polyposis colorectal cancer (HNPCC)	MutS family	Brown et al., 2003
MLH1	Other MMR proteins, ATM	?	RDS; MMR deficiency; HNPCC	MutL family	Brown et al., 2003
NBS1	MRE11, RAD50, BRCA1, H2AX	By ATM at Ser343	Nijmegen breakage syndrome; RDS	BRCT, FHA	Falck et al., 2002, Lim et al., 2000
MRE11	NBS1, RAD50, BRCA1	NBS-dependent	AT-like disorder; RDS	-	Dong et al., 1999, Stewart et al., 1999
RAD50	NBS1, MRE11, BRCA1	?	Chromosomal instability, cancer predisposition (hypomorphic mouse mutant)	SMC	Bender et al., 2002
BRCA1	NBS1, MRE11, RAD50, ATM, SMC1, 53BP1, BRCA2	By ATM at Ser1423	Familial breast and ovarian cancer; RDS (hypomorphic mutant)	BRCT	Zhong et al., 1999, Cortez et al., 1999
53BP1	p53, CHK2, BRCA1	ATM-dependent	Partial RDS (siRNA); reduced phosphorylation of CHK2 and BRCA1	BRCT	Anderson et al., 2001, Ward et al., 2003
MDC1	CHK2 (phosphorylated at Thr68), NBS1, MRE11, RAD50, H2AX	ATM- and CHK2-dependent	RDS (siRNA)	BRCT, FHA	Lou et al., 2003, Goldberg et al., 2003, Stewart et al., 2003
SMC1	Other components of cohesin; BRCA1	By ATM at Ser957 and Ser966; NBS1-and BRCA1-dependent	RDS (phosphorylation site mutant)	SMC	Yazdi et al., 2002, Kim et al., 2002

[a] Mutations in genes encoding the components in bold type cause human cancer predisposition.

super-assembly of proteins capable of detecting DNA lesions and facilitating both checkpoint activation and DNA repair.

The replication factor RF-C and the BLM helicase are also BASC components, suggesting that the DNA structures sensed may extend to those generated at stalled replication forks. Consistent with this notion, after inhibition of DNA replication BRCA1, BLM, and the NBS1–MRE11–RAD50 complex are relocalized to foci containing PCNA (Wang et al., 2000). Partial inhibition of DNA replication results in the generation of fragile sites—gaps or breaks that appear at characteristic chromosomal positions in the subsequent mitotic metaphase. Recent findings suggest that ATR plays an important role in protection against the formation of these chromosome lesions, which probably contribute to chromosomal instability in tumorigenesis (Casper et al., 2002). Loss of ATR function results in the constitutive expression of fragile sites, even in the absence of replication inhibitors, suggesting that ATR (which is not a BASC component) may be targeted by RPA to stabilize stalled replication forks during normal S phase. Indeed, a function in replication fork stabilization has been directly demonstrated for the ATM/ATR homologue Mec1 in budding yeast (Tercero and Diffley, 2001). Yet another function of ATR is to transmit a mitosis-inhibitory checkpoint signal, which also requires BRCA1, when sister chromatid decatenation is prevented by inhibition of DNA topoisomerase II (Deming et al., 2001).

9.6 From G2 to mitotic metaphase

Several cell types can withdraw from the cycle for protracted periods between the S and M phases, while others proceed directly from S to M with no G2 lag (Norbury and Nurse, 1992). In most actively proliferating somatic cells, however, G2 is a period during which inactive CDK1/CDC2-cyclinA/B heterodimers are accumulated in preparation for their dramatic activation at the onset of mitosis. CDK1/CDC2 activation was recognized in the late 1980s as a universal, highly conserved and rate-limiting feature of entry into mitosis (Nurse, 1990). Cyclins B1 and B2 accumulate in somatic cells in G2 due to a combination of transcriptional activation and the inactivity of the APC/C ubiquitin ligase that targets B cyclins for destruction in other cell cycle phases. Though transcriptionally repressed in quiescence, the CDK1/CDC2 catalytic subunit is, by comparison, very long-lived and expressed at fairly constant levels in proliferating cells. CDK1/CDC2-cyclinA/B heterodimers are subject to constitutive activating phosphorylation by CDK-activating kinase at Thr161, and inhibitory phosphorylation at Thr14 and Tyr15 (Morgan, 1995). The inhibitory phosphorylation is carried out by the protein kinases WEE1, which is nuclear, and MYT1, which is predominantly associated with cytoplasmic membranes. Members of the CDC25 family of phosphatases remove the inhibitory phosphates from Thr14 and Tyr15. The abrupt activation of CDK1/CDC2-cyclin A/B is achieved by the concerted inhibition of WEE1 and MYT1 and activation of CDC25C and is responsible for initiating all of the major events of mitosis, including disassembly of the nuclear envelope and Golgi apparatus, chromosome condensation and spindle assembly (Nelson, 2000; Mitchison and Salmon, 2001; Gonczy, 2002). CDK1/CDC2-cyclinB heterodimers are assembled in the cytoplasm and are first activated at the centrosomes at the beginning of mitotic prophase. CDK1/CDC2-cyclinA activity appears slightly earlier and appears to play a priming role (Jackman and Pines, 1997; den Elzen and Pines, 2001; O'Farrell, 2001; Jackman et al., 2003). An emerging theme is that CDK-cyclin localization, rather than inherent substrate specificity, plays a primary role in determining the distinctive biological functions of these kinases. Thus cyclin B1 is capable of promoting S phase entry in experimental systems, but only if it is relocated from the cytoplasm to the nucleus (Moore et al., 2003). In line with the idea that reasonably orderly progression through mitosis is required for continued proliferation, there is so far no indication that mutations directly affecting CDK1/CDC2 regulation can play a part in tumorigenesis.

9.7 Checkpoints controlling mitotic entry

Since the consequences of CDK1/CDC2 activation are so dramatic, it is understandably the target of checkpoint pathways that prevent mitotic entry under inappropriate circumstances. Extensive overlap exists between the checkpoint pathways that inhibit mitotic entry and some of those that act within S phase. ATR and CHK1, for example, are essential for the S-M checkpoint that inhibits CDK1/CDC2 activation when DNA is incompletely replicated (Guo et al., 2000), while ATM and CHK2 contribute to the delay in mitotic entry that results from exposure to IR in G2. Here too there is an important role for BRCA1, which is required for CHK1 activation and G2 arrest after DNA damage (Yarden et al., 2002). CHK1 activation was also implicated in a checkpoint activated in response to CDC6 overexpression, and this mechanism may play a part in S-M checkpoint control under physiological conditions (Clay-Farrace et al., 2003). RAD17 is also required both for ATR-dependent checkpoint activation and for general chromosomal stability (Wang et al., 2003). The checkpoint pathways that delay origin firing and mitotic entry therefore share common lesion-sensing mechanisms and signal transducers and a major effector mechanism in each case is the inhibition of CDC25 activity. Notably excluded from this extensive overlap is the 9-1-1 complex, which does not seem to have a major role in inhibiting mitotic entry in mammalian cells (Weiss et al., 2003).

The duration of DNA damage-induced G2 delay is generally greater in the presence of functional p53. The effects of p53 on the G2 DNA damage checkpoint appear to operate in parallel with, and largely independently of, the ATM/ATR pathways. The relevant p53 effectors appear to be p21, which despite having a comparatively low affinity for CDK1/CDC2 can still inhibit its biological activity, and 14-3-3σ, which is also transcriptionally induced by p53 and serves to sequester CDK1/CDC2-cyclinB in the cytoplasm (Hermeking et al., 1997; Bunz et al., 1998; Winters et al., 1998).

9.8 Centrosome duplication and the maintenance of ploidy

Orderly duplication of the centrosome, which forms the basis for bipolar spindle formation in M phase, is fundamentally important for the maintenance of stable ploidy and is frequently deregulated in neoplasia, where multipolar mitoses are commonplace (Doxsey, 2002). An important advance in this area was the discovery that CDK2-cyclinE activity drives centrosome duplication through phosphorylation of nucleophosmin, a protein selectively associated with unduplicated centrosomes (Okuda et al., 2000). In this way, establishment of a bipolar spindle is normally linked to prior progression through S phase; promotion of multipolar mitoses could also help to explain the chromosomal instability seen following cyclin E deregulation (Spruck et al., 1999). An additional role for p53 in regulation of centrosome duplication has been described and this could involve p53-induced p21 expression with consequent downregulation of CDK2-cyclinE (Fukasawa et al., 1996). An alternative explanation is that centrosome amplification results indirectly from failure to complete mitosis and consequent tetraploidy (Meraldi et al., 2002), though it is not clear why such defects should be more frequent in the absence of functional p53. The normal regulation of human centrosome behaviour also requires the survivin protein, which has an additional function as an inhibitor of apoptosis (Li et al., 1999).

9.9 The metaphase–anaphase transition and exit from mitosis

The transition between metaphase and anaphase marks the point of no return in mitosis, and its accurate execution is fundamentally important for maintenance of diploidy. Anaphase separation of the chromosomes towards the spindle poles is normally only possible once each pair of sister centromeres, via the attached kinetochore complexes, has achieved bipolar attachment to spindle microtubules emanating from opposite poles. Loss of attachment of a single kinetochore is sufficient to block anaphase onset completely (Rieder et al., 1995). Evidence for the genetic control of this spindle checkpoint, and identification of some of the key players, came from studies of budding yeast *bub* (budding uninhibited by benomyl) and *mad* (mitotic arrest defective) mutants, which lack this checkpoint and hence fail to arrest mitotic progression in the presence of spindle poisons (Millband et al., 2002). Once again, the yeast model accurately predicted the overall organization of the corresponding mechanism in human cells. The ultimate target for this checkpoint is the APC/C ubiquitin ligase, which is responsible not only for targeting mitotic cyclins for destruction but also for initiating anaphase by indirectly promoting the proteolysis of the SCC1/RAD21 component of cohesin, thus allowing sister chromatid separation (Nasmyth et al., 2000). Cleavage of the cohesin subunit is performed by the protease separin and it is securin, a negative regulator of separin, that is subject to APC/C-dependent ubiquitinylation (Figure 9.3). The potential importance of this pathway in cancer was underscored by the finding that loss of securin caused deregulated separin activity and chromosomal instability in human cells (Jallepalli et al., 2001).

Heterodimeric complexes MAD1–MAD2, BUB1–BUB3, and BUBR1–BUB3 are recruited independently to kinetochores. In the absence of spindle tension and/or kinetochore–spindle attachment, the BUB3 and MAD1 proteins interact and generate a rapidly diffusible anaphase inhibitory signal in the form of MAD2, BUB3, and BUBR1 themselves, which bind to the CDC20 component of the APC/C and inhibit its activity. Bipolar attachment of the last pair of kinetochores and establishment of spindle tension allow this signal to decay, relieving the inhibition of the APC/C and triggering both cyclin B destruction and anaphase onset. Early indications that mutations in spindle checkpoint genes might be frequent in human cancer have not been substantiated, suggesting that this is another area of cell cycle regulation that is usually stringently controlled, even in neoplastic cells. Poleward chromosome movement is driven by kinetochore- and spindle pole-associated kinesin-like ATPases and, once completed, this is usually followed by the actin-dependent constriction of the cell and cytokinesis (Glotzer, 2001). The residual spindle midbody probably determines the site of this constriction but the details of this process in human cells are currently unclear. General phosphatase activities reverse mitotic phosphorylation events, allowing the assembly of nuclear

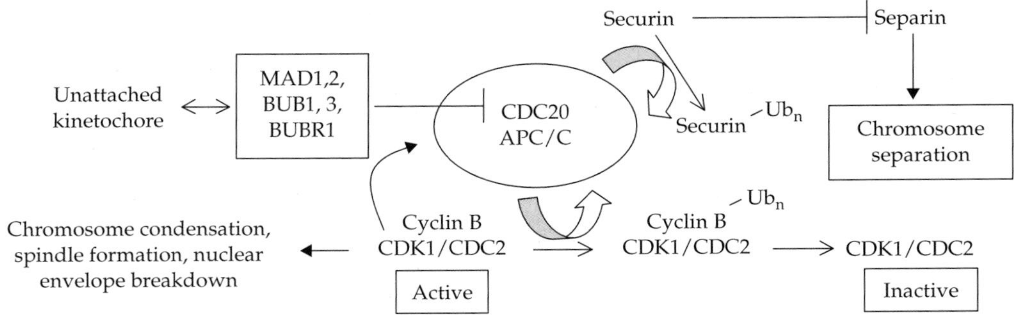

Figure 9.3 Regulation of anaphase onset and the exit from mitosis. Activation of CDK1/CDC2-cyclinB triggers all of the major events of mitosis, but also activates the multi-subunit APC/C ubiquitin ligase. Kinetochores that are not yet attached to the mitotic spindle, or at which spindle tension is not established, transmit APC/C inhibitory signals via the MAD and BUB/BUBR1 proteins indicated. Once all kinetochores are properly attached, this inhibition is lost, allowing the APC/C to catalyse polyubiquitin (Ub$_n$) transfer to key substrates including mitotic cyclins and securin; these proteins are then degraded by the proteasome. Securin maintains the separin protease in an inactive form; securin degradation releases active separin, which cleaves cohesin to allow the onset of anaphase.

envelopes around the new daughter nuclei and re-establishment of the interphase state.

9.10 Cell cycle proteins as prognostic markers and drug targets

The hope that a detailed understanding of the cell cycle might ultimately allow improvements in the management of cancer is gradually becoming more realistic. The studies reviewed in this chapter have identified a number of proteins that are expressed exclusively in proliferating cells. Several of these, including CDK1/CDC2, cyclin B, MCM2-7 and CDC6, may provide valuable proliferation markers with better discriminatory potential than, for example, Ki67, which is in widespread use although its biological function is unclear. Indeed, antibodies against CDC6 or MCM5 have been used for the sensitive detection of pre-malignant cells in cervical smears and for the detection of urothelial carcinoma cells in urine (Williams et al., 1998; Stoeber et al., 1999).

Might our understanding of cell cycle control also lead to the development of cytotoxic drugs with increased selectivity for neoplastic cells? Major efforts are currently being directed at the development of small molecule CDK inhibitors, even though it is not immediately apparent how these could selectively arrest cell cycle progression in cancer cells while sparing other proliferating populations. In fact, inhibitors targeting CDK2 have encouragingly selective cytotoxicity towards cancer cell lines, possibly because CDK2 inhibition in cells with deregulated R point control leads to the accumulation of active E2F transcription factors that can drive apoptotic death (Chen et al., 1999). Indeed, a more direct approach might be to target the most general distinctions between the cycles of cancer cells and their normal counterparts, namely R point deregulation and loss of p53 function. Inhibition of the residual G2 checkpoint function in p53-deficient cells, for example by inhibiting ATM/ATR or CHK1/CHK2 activities, can promote cell death following DNA damage, presumably as a result of mitotic entry in the presence of unrepaired strand breaks (Dixon and Norbury, 2002). Cells retaining p53-dependent G2 checkpoint pathways are comparatively resistant to the combination of limited DNA damage and inhibition of checkpoint kinases. This and related strategies look impressive on paper; it will be interesting to see how this promise holds up in the clinic.

References

Anderson, L., Henderson, C., and Adachi, Y. (2001). Phosphorylation and rapid relocalization of 53BP1 to nuclear foci upon DNA damage. *Mol Cell Biol*, **21**, 1719–29.

Bakkenist, C. J. and Kastan, M. B. (2003). DNA damage activates ATM through intermolecular autophosphorylation and dimer dissociation. *Nature*, **421**, 499–506.

Beier, R., Burgin, A., Kiermaier, A., Fero, M., Karsunky, H., Saffrich, R. et al. (2000). Induction of cyclin E-cdk2 kinase activity, E2F-dependent transcription and cell growth by Myc are genetically separable events. *EMBO J*, **19**, 5813–23.

Bell, S. P. and Dutta, A. (2002). DNA replication in eukaryotic cells. *Annu Rev Biochem*, **71**, 333–74.

Bender, C. F., Sikes, M. L., Sullivan, R., Huye, L. E., Le Beau, M. M., Roth, D. B. et al. (2002). Cancer predisposition and hematopoietic failure in Rad50(S/S) mice. *Genes Dev*, **16**, 2237–51.

Blagosklonny, M. V. and Pardee, A. B. (2002). The restriction point of the cell cycle. *Cell Cycle*, **1**, 103–10.

Blow, J. J. and Hodgson, B. (2002). Replication licensing—defining the proliferative state? *Trends Cell Biol*, **12**, 72–8.

Brehm, A., Miska, E. A., McCance, D. J., Reid, J. L., Bannister, A. J., and Kouzarides, T. (1998). Retinoblastoma protein recruits histone deacetylase to repress transcription. *Nature*, **391**, 597–601.

Brown, K. D., Rathi, A., Kamath, R., Beardsley, D. I., Zhan, Q., Mannino, J. L. et al. (2003). The mismatch repair system is required for S-phase checkpoint activation. *Nat Genet*, **33**, 80–4.

Bunz, F., Dutriaux, A., Lengauer, C., Waldman, T., Zhou, S., Brown, J. P. et al. (1998). Requirement for p53 and p21 to sustain G2 arrest after DNA damage. *Science*, **282**, 1497–501.

Burma, S., Chen, B. P., Murphy, M., Kurimasa, A., and Chen, D. J. (2001). ATM phosphorylates histone H2AX in response to DNA double-strand breaks. *J Biol Chem*, **276**, 42462–7.

Carr, A. M. (1997). Control of cell cycle arrest by the Mec1sc/Rad3sp DNA structure checkpoint pathway. *Curr Opin Genet Dev*, **7**, 93–8.

Casper, A. M., Nghiem, P., Arlt, M. F., and Glover, T. W. (2002). ATR regulates fragile site stability. *Cell*, **111**, 779–89.

Celeste, A., Petersen, S., Romanienko, P. J., Fernandez-Capetillo, O., Chen, H. T., Sedelnikova, O. A. et al. (2002). Genomic instability in mice lacking histone H2AX. *Science*, **296**, 922–7.

Chaturvedi, P., Eng, W. K., Zhu, Y., Mattern, M. R., Mishra, R., Hurle, M. R. et al. (1999). Mammalian Chk2 is a downstream effector of the ATM-dependent DNA damage checkpoint pathway. *Oncogene*, **18**, 4047–54.

Chen, Y. N., Sharma, S. K., Ramsey, T. M., Jiang, L., Martin, M. S., Baker, K. et al. (1999). Selective killing of transformed cells by cyclin/cyclin-dependent kinase 2 antagonists. *Proc Natl Acad Sci USA*, **96**, 4325–9.

Cheng, M., Sexl, V., Sherr, C. J., and Roussel, M. F. (1998). Assembly of cyclin D-dependent kinase and titration of p27Kip1 regulated by mitogen-activated protein kinase kinase (MEK1). *Proc Natl Acad Sci USA*, **95**, 1091–6.

Classon, M. and Harlow, E. (2002). The retinoblastoma tumour suppressor in development and cancer. *Nat Rev Cancer*, **2**, 910–7.

Clay-Farrace, L., Pelizon, C., Santamaria, D., Pines, J., and Laskey, R. A. (2003). Human replication protein Cdc6 prevents mitosis through a checkpoint mechanism that implicates Chk1. *EMBO J*, **22**, 704–12.

Cortez, D., Wang, Y., Qin, J., and Elledge, S. J. (1999). Requirement of ATM-dependent phosphorylation of brca1 in the DNA damage response to double-strand breaks. *Science*, **286**, 1162–6.

Cortez, D., Guntuku, S., Qin, J., and Elledge, S. J. (2001). ATR and ATRIP: partners in checkpoint signaling. *Science*, **294**, 1713–6.

Costanzo, V., Robertson, K., Ying, C. Y., Kim, E., Avvedimento, E., Gottesman, M. et al. (2000). Reconstitution of an ATM-dependent checkpoint that inhibits chromosomal DNA replication following DNA damage. *Mol Cell*, **6**, 649–59.

Costanzo, V., Shechter, D., Lupardus, P. J., Cimprich, K. A., Gottesman, M., and Gautier, J. (2003). An ATR- and Cdc7-dependent DNA damage checkpoint that inhibits initiation of DNA replication. *Mol Cell*, **11**, 203–13.

Deming, P. B., Cistulli, C. A., Zhao, H., Graves, P. R., Piwnica-Worms, H., Paules, R. S. et al. (2001). The human decatenation checkpoint. *Proc Natl Acad Sci USA*, **98**, 12044–9.

den Elzen, N. and Pines, J. (2001). Cyclin A is destroyed in prometaphase and can delay chromosome alignment and anaphase. *J Cell Biol*, **153**, 121–36.

Dixon, H. and Norbury, C. J. (2002). Therapeutic exploitation of checkpoint defects in cancer cells lacking p53 function. *Cell Cycle*, **1**, 362–8.

Dong, Z., Zhong, Q., and Chen, P. L. (1999). The Nijmegen breakage syndrome protein is essential for Mre11 phosphorylation upon DNA damage. *J Biol Chem*, **274**, 19513–6.

Doxsey, S. (2002). Duplicating dangerously: linking centrosome duplication and aneuploidy. *Mol Cell*, **10**, 439–40.

Dunaief, J. L., Strober, B. E., Guha, S., Khavari, P. A., Alin, K., Luban, J. et al. (1994). The retinoblastoma protein and BRG1 form a complex and cooperate to induce cell cycle arrest. *Cell*, **79**, 119–30.

Falck, J., Petrini, J. H., Williams, B. R., Lukas, J., and Bartek, J. (2002). The DNA damage-dependent intra-S phase checkpoint is regulated by parallel pathways. *Nat Genet*, **30**, 290–4.

Fantes, P. and Nurse, P. (1977). Control of cell size at division in fission yeast by a growth-modulated size control over nuclear division. *Exp Cell Res*, **107**, 377–86.

Fukasawa, K., Choi, T., Kuriyama, R., Rulong, S., and Vande Woude, G. F. (1996). Abnormal centrosome amplification in the absence of p53. *Science*, **271**, 1744–7.

Glotzer, M. (2001) Animal cell cytokinesis. *Annu Rev Cell Dev Biol*, **17**, 351–86.

Goldberg, M., Stucki, M., Falck, J., D'Amours, D., Rahman, D., Pappin, D. et al. (2003). MDC1 is required for the intra-S-phase DNA damage checkpoint. *Nature*, **421**, 952–6.

Gonczy, P. (2002). Nuclear envelope: torn apart at mitosis. *Curr Biol*, **12**, R242–4.

Gruber, S., Haering, C. H., and Nasmyth, K. (2003). Chromosomal cohesin forms a ring. *Cell*, **112**, 765–77.

Guo, Z., Kumagai, A., Wang, S. X., and Dunphy, W. G. (2000). Requirement for Atr in phosphorylation of

Chk1 and cell cycle regulation in response to DNA replication blocks and UV-damaged DNA in Xenopus egg extracts. *Genes Dev*, **14**, 2745–56.

Heffernan, T. P., Simpson, D. A., Frank, A. R., Heinloth, A. N., Paules, R. S., Cordeiro-Stone, M. et al. (2002). An ATR- and Chk1-dependent S checkpoint inhibits replicon initiation following UVC-induced DNA damage. *Mol Cell Biol*, **22**, 8552–61.

Hermeking, H., Lengauer, C., Polyak, K., He, T. C., Zhang, L., Thiagalingam, S. et al. (1997). 14-3-3 sigma is a p53-regulated inhibitor of G2/M progression. *Mol Cell*, **1**, 3–11.

Hickson, I. D. (2003). RecQ helicases: caretakers of the genome. *Nat Rev Cancer*, **3**, 169–78.

Jackman, M. R. and Pines, J. N. (1997). Cyclins and the G2/M transition. *Cancer Surv*, **29**, 47–73.

Jackman, M., Lindon, C., Nigg, E. A., and Pines, J. (2003). Active cyclin B1-Cdk1 first appears on centrosomes in prophase. *Nat Cell Biol*, **5**, 143–8.

Jallepalli, P. V., Waizenegger, I. C., Bunz, F., Langer, S., Speicher, M. R., Peters, J. M. et al. (2001). Securin is required for chromosomal stability in human cells. *Cell*, **105**, 445–57.

Kerkhoff, E. and Rapp, U. R. (1998). Cell cycle targets of Ras/Raf signalling. *Oncogene*, **17**, 1457–62.

Kim, S. T., Xu, B., and Kastan, M. B. (2002). Involvement of the cohesin protein, Smc1, in Atm-dependent and independent responses to DNA damage. *Genes Dev*, **16**, 560–70.

Kobayashi, J., Tauchi, H., Sakamoto, S., Nakamura, A., Morishima, K., Matsuura, S. et al. (2002). NBS1 localizes to gamma-H2AX foci through interaction with the FHA/BRCT domain. *Curr Biol*, **12**, 1846–51.

Kuerbitz, S. J., Plunkett, B. S., Walsh, W. V., and Kastan, M. B. (1992). Wild-type p53 is a cell cycle checkpoint determinant following irradiation. *Proc Natl Acad Sci USA*, **89**, 7491–5.

Li, F., Ackermann, E. J., Bennett, C. F., Rothermel, A. L., Plescia, J., Tognin, S. et al. (1999). Pleiotropic cell-division defects and apoptosis induced by interference with survivin function. *Nat Cell Biol*, **1**, 461–6.

Lim, D. S., Kim, S. T., Xu, B., Maser, R. S., Lin, J., Petrini, J. H. et al. (2000). ATM phosphorylates p95/nbs1 in an S-phase checkpoint pathway. *Nature*, **404**, 613–7.

Lindsey-Boltz, L. A., Bermudez, V. P., Hurwitz, J., and Sancar, A. (2001). Purification and characterization of human DNA damage checkpoint Rad complexes. *Proc Natl Acad Sci USA*, **98**, 11236–41.

Lou, Z., Minter-Dykhouse, K., Wu, X., and Chen, J. (2003). MDC1 is coupled to activated CHK2 in mammalian DNA damage response pathways. *Nature*, **421**, 957–61.

Lu, X. and Lane, D. P. (1993). Differential induction of transcriptionally active p53 following UV or ionizing radiation: defects in chromosome instability syndromes? *Cell*, **75**, 765–78.

Meraldi, P., Honda, R., and Nigg, E. A. (2002). Aurora-A overexpression reveals tetraploidization as a major route to centrosome amplification in p53-/- cells. *EMBO J*, **21**, 483–92.

Millband, D. N., Campbell, L., and Hardwick, K. G. (2002). The awesome power of multiple model systems: interpreting the complex nature of spindle checkpoint signaling. *Trends Cell Biol*, **12**, 205–9.

Miller, C. W., Ikezoe, T., Krug, U., Hofmann, W. K., Tavor, S., Vegesna, V. et al. (2002). Mutations of the CHK2 gene are found in some osteosarcomas, but are rare in breast, lung, and ovarian tumors. *Genes Chromosomes Cancer*, **33**, 17–21.

Mitchison, T. J. and Salmon, E. D. (2001). Mitosis: a history of division. *Nat Cell Biol*, **3**, E17–21.

Moore, J. D., Kirk, J. A., and Hunt, T. (2003). Unmasking the S-phase-promoting potential of cyclin B1. *Science*, **300**, 987–90.

Morgan, D. O. (1995). Principles of CDK regulation. *Nature*, **374**, 131–4.

Nasmyth, K., Peters, J. M., and Uhlmann, F. (2000). Splitting the chromosome: cutting the ties that bind sister chromatids. *Science*, **288**, 1379–85.

Nelson, W. J. (2000). W(h)ither the Golgi during mitosis? *J Cell Biol*, **149**, 243–8.

Norbury, C. and Nurse, P. (1992). Animal cell cycles and their control. *Annu Rev Biochem*, **61**, 441–70.

Nurse, P. (1990). Universal control mechanism regulating onset of M-phase. *Nature*, **344**, 503–8.

O'Farrell, P. H. (2001). Triggering the all-or-nothing switch into mitosis. *Trends Cell Biol*, **11**, 512–9.

Okuda, M., Horn, H. F., Tarapore, P., Tokuyama, Y., Smulian, A. G., Chan, P. K. et al. (2000). Nucleophosmin/B23 is a target of CDK2/cyclin E in centrosome duplication. *Cell*, **103**, 127–40.

Paulovich, A. G., Toczyski, D. P., and Hartwell, L. H. (1997). When checkpoints fail. *Cell*, **88**, 315–21.

Polyak, K., Kato, J. Y., Solomon, M. J., Sherr, C. J., Massague, J., Roberts, J. M. et al. (1994). p27Kip1, a cyclin-Cdk inhibitor, links transforming growth factor-beta and contact inhibition to cell cycle arrest. *Genes Dev*, **8**, 9–22.

Prober, D. A. and Edgar, B. A. (2001). Growth regulation by oncogenes—new insights from model organisms. *Curr Opin Genet Dev*, **11**, 19–26.

Rieder, C. L., Cole, R. W., Khodjakov, A., and Sluder, G. (1995). The checkpoint delaying anaphase in response to chromosome monoorientation is mediated by an inhibitory signal produced by unattached kinetochores. *J Cell Biol*, **130**, 941–8.

Roos-Mattjus, P., Vroman, B. T., Burtelow, M. A., Rauen, M., Eapen, A. K., and Karnitz, L. M. (2002). Genotoxin-induced Rad9-Hus1-Rad1 (9-1-1) chromatin association is an early checkpoint signaling event. *J Biol Chem*, **277**, 43809–12.

Sherr, C. J. and Roberts, J. M. (1999). CDK inhibitors: positive and negative regulators of G1-phase progression. *Genes Dev*, **13**, 1501–12.

Shiloh, Y. (2001). ATM and ATR: networking cellular responses to DNA damage. *Curr Opin Genet Dev*, **11**, 71–7.

Siegert, J. L. and Robbins, P. D. (1999). Rb inhibits the intrinsic kinase activity of TATA-binding protein-associated factor TAFII250. *Mol Cell Biol*, **19**, 846–54.

Slingerland, J. and Pagano, M. (2000). Regulation of the cdk inhibitor p27 and its deregulation in cancer. *J Cell Physiol*, **183**, 10–7.

Spruck, C. H., Won, K. A., and Reed, S. I. (1999). Deregulated cyclin E induces chromosome instability. *Nature*, **401**, 297–300.

St. Onge, R. P., Udell, C. M., Casselman, R., and Davey, S. (1999). The human G2 checkpoint control protein hRAD9 is a nuclear phosphoprotein that forms complexes with hRAD1 and hHUS1. *Mol Cell Biol*, **10**, 1985–95.

Stewart, G. S., Maser, R. S., Stankovic, T., Bressan, D. A., Kaplan, M. I., Jaspers, N. G. et al. (1999). The DNA double-strand break repair gene hMRE11 is mutated in individuals with an ataxia-telangiectasia-like disorder. *Cell*, **99**, 577–87.

Stewart, G. S., Wang, B., Bignell, C. R., Taylor, A. M., and Elledge, S. J. (2003). MDC1 is a mediator of the mammalian DNA damage checkpoint. *Nature*, **421**, 961–6.

Stoeber, K., Halsall, I., Freeman, A., Swinn, R., Doble, A., Morris, L. et al. (1999). Immunoassay for urothelial cancers that detects DNA replication protein Mcm5 in urine. *Lancet*, **354**, 1524–5.

Strohmaier, H., Spruck, C. H., Kaiser, P., Won, K. A., Sangfelt, O., and Reed, S. I. (2001). Human F-box protein hCdc4 targets cyclin E for proteolysis and is mutated in a breast cancer cell line. *Nature*, **413**, 316–22.

Tercero, J. A. and Diffley, J. F. (2001). Regulation of DNA replication fork progression through damaged DNA by the Mec1/Rad53 checkpoint. *Nature*, **412**, 553–7.

Vessey, C. J., Norbury, C. J., and Hickson, I. D. (1999). Genetic disorders associated with cancer predisposition and genomic instability. *Prog Nucleic Acid Res Mol Biol*, **63**, 189–221.

Wang, Y., Cortez, D., Yazdi, P., Neff, N., Elledge, S. J., and Qin, J. (2000). BASC, a super complex of BRCA1-associated proteins involved in the recognition and repair of aberrant DNA structures. *Genes Dev*, **14**, 927–39.

Wang, X., Zou, L., Zheng, H., Wei, Q., Elledge, S. J., and Li, L. (2003). Genomic instability and endoreduplication triggered by RAD17 deletion. *Genes Dev*, **17**, 965–70.

Ward, I. M. and Chen, J. (2001). Histone H2AX is phosphorylated in an ATR-dependent manner in response to replicational stress. *J Biol Chem*, **276**, 47759–62.

Ward, I. M., Minn, K., van Deursen, J., and Chen, J. (2003). p53 Binding protein 53BP1 is required for DNA damage responses and tumor suppression in mice. *Mol Cell Biol*, **23**, 2556–63.

Weiss, R. S., Leder, P., and Vaziri, C. (2003). Critical role for mouse Hus1 in an S-phase DNA damage cell cycle checkpoint. *Mol Cell Biol*, **23**, 791–803.

White, R. J. (1997). Regulation of RNA polymerases I and III by the retinoblastoma protein: a mechanism for growth control? *Trends Biochem Sci*, **22**, 77–80.

Williams, G. H., Romanowski, P., Morris, L., Madine, M., Mills, A. D., Stoeber, K. et al. (1998). Improved cervical smear assessment using antibodies against proteins that regulate DNA replication. *Proc Natl Acad Sci USA*, **95**, 14932–7.

Winters, Z. E., Ongkeko, W. M., Harris, A. L., and Norbury, C. J. (1998). p53 regulates Cdc2 independently of inhibitory phosphorylation to reinforce radiation-induced G2 arrest in human cells. *Oncogene*, **17**, 673–84.

Wohlschlegel, J. A., Dhar, S. K., Prokhorova, T. A., Dutta, A., and Walter, J. C. (2002). Xenopus Mcm10 binds to origins of DNA replication after Mcm2–7 and stimulates origin binding of Cdc45. *Mol Cell*, **9**, 233–40.

Wolfel, T., Hauer, M., Schneider, J., Serrano, M., Wolfel, C., Klehmann-Hieb, E. et al. (1995). A p16INK4a-insensitive CDK4 mutant targeted by cytolytic T lymphocytes in a human melanoma. *Science*, **269**, 1281–4.

Yarden, R. I., Pardo-Reoyo, S., Sgagias, M., Cowan, K. H., and Brody, L. C. (2002). BRCA1 regulates the G2/M checkpoint by activating Chk1 kinase upon DNA damage. *Nat Genet*, **30**, 285–9.

Yazdi, P. T., Wang, Y., Zhao, S., Patel, N., Lee, E. Y., and Qin, J. (2002). SMC1 is a downstream effector in the ATM/NBS1 branch of the human S-phase checkpoint. *Genes Dev*, **16**, 571–82.

Zetterberg, A., Larsson, O., and Wiman, K. G. (1995). What is the restriction point? *Curr Opin Cell Biol*, **7**, 835–42.

Zhong, Q., Chen, C. F., Li, S., Chen, Y., Wang, C. C., Xiao, J. et al. (1999). Association of BRCA1 with the hRad50-hMre11-p95 complex and the DNA damage response. *Science*, **285**, 747–50.

Zou, L., Cortez, D., and Elledge, S. J. (2002). Regulation of ATR substrate selection by Rad17-dependent loading of Rad9 complexes onto chromatin. *Genes Dev*, **16**, 198–208.

CHAPTER 10

Cellular immortalization and telomerase activation in cancer

Robert F. Newbold

10.1 Introduction

The development of cancer is a multi-step process, with the result that the cells of malignant tumours contain a number of superimposed heritable alterations that have accumulated in a neoplastic lineage over a protracted period of time (Newbold, 1985). The process by which this is thought to occur, known as 'clonal evolution', involves the repeated selection and succession, due to growth advantage, of variant cells that exhibit greater fitness to survive and proliferate in a particular environment (Figure 10.1). Malignant tumours are thus viewed as continually evolving populations of cells that can adapt to multiply in new sites distant from the primary growth. The life-threatening nature of cancer in humans, including the development of resistance to cytotoxic chemotherapy, is due almost entirely to this potential for unfettered somatic cell evolution.

For cancer to arise via clonal evolution, three basic requirements need to be met: (1) the initial step which sets in motion the whole train of events must allow a cell to compete effectively in terms of proliferation with its neighbours, (2) there must be a sufficiently high level of genetic (and possibly epigenetic) variability within the evolving lineage to permit rare variants to arise, and (3) the evolving clonal cell population must possess a very large reserve capacity for cell division, which means that in many instances the neoplastic clone will be immortal.

This chapter is concerned with what is currently known about the significance of cellular immortalization as a key event in carcinogenesis and will discuss several topics: the molecular mechanisms underlying cellular senescence; the importance of replicative senescence as a tumour suppressive mechanism in normal cells and how this is bypassed during immortalization/malignant transformation; and the role of telomerase in maintaining cellular immortality and the potential value of telomerase as an anti-cancer target.

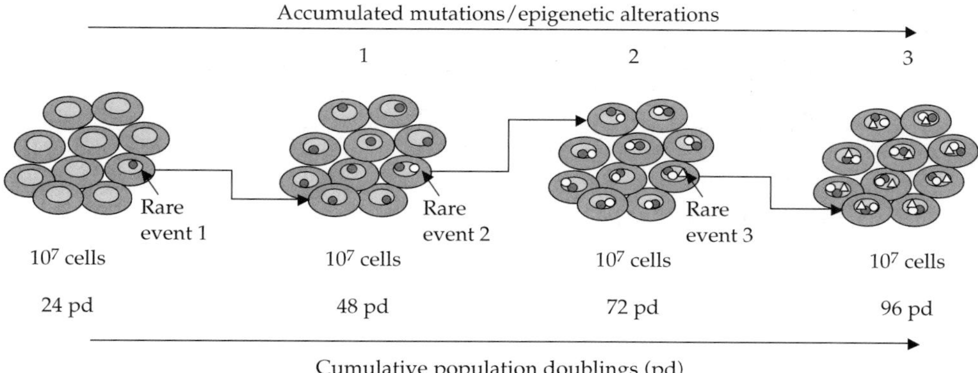

Figure 10.1 Clonal evolution lies at the heart of the process of cancer development in humans. Assuming a mutation (or epigenetic variant) frequency in a given cancer-related gene (e.g. tumour suppressor gene) of around 10^{-7}/cell division, the simplified model shown here indicates that a very large intrinsic cellular proliferative capacity is required to introduce more than a single mutation in an evolving clone of neoplastic cells. The model assumes that mutants/variants possess an increasing selective growth advantage over their counterparts. It is generally accepted that development of the common human carcinomas requires at least 5 or 6 of such rounds of mutation and clonal succession, and in many cases probably more. Therefore, an evolved mechanism limiting the proliferative capacity of somatic cells *in vivo* (e.g. via telomerase repression—see text) would be expected to provide us with a powerful protective barrier against cancer.

10.2 Historical perspective: early studies on the replicative lifespan of cells in culture

Observations made over 40 years ago (Hayflick and Moorhead, 1961) on the replicative potential of normal human cells (fibroblasts) explanted and grown as monolayers in tissue culture revealed that they possess an intrinsically programmed limit (now known as the 'Hayflick limit') to their capacity for proliferation that, even after a substantial healthy period of cell division, leads to permanent growth arrest (replicative senescence). In sharp contrast, cell cultures derived from the disaggregation of human cancer tissues, once successfully established *in vitro*, are often immortal. Before the advent of sophisticated molecular biological techniques it was not possible to demonstrate convincingly that cellular immortalization is associated with the development of human cancer, and it was often argued that the phenomenon represents a cell culture artefact. Furthermore, many human carcinomas (e.g. those developing from breast and prostate epithelia) were (and remain) very difficult to establish in culture, preventing any meaningful assessment of the proliferative potential of their constituent malignant cells. Tissue transplantation studies in inbred laboratory mouse strains, aimed at demonstrating limited proliferative capacity in serially transferred normal cells, proved inconclusive because of the ever-present possibility for cellular material to be damaged during transplantation.

In a series of important studies in the early 1980s with cultures of normal diploid rodent fibroblasts, experimental evidence was obtained that an immortal phenotype could actually be induced as a rare event following treatment with powerful chemical and physical carcinogens (Newbold, 2002). Only after immortalization were the cells, either spontaneously or after additional carcinogen treatment, able to undergo progression to a malignant phenotype. Moreover, immediately after the first human oncogenes (e.g. *Ha-rasV12*) had been cloned, it was found that such oncogenes could exert their powerful transforming effects only if transfected into cells that had previously been immortalized. Surprisingly, transfection of normal rodent cells with the *Ha-rasV12* oncogene induced premature senescence rather than malignant transformation, an observation that has been reproduced recently in primary human fibroblasts (Drayton and Peters, 2002). Independent studies performed at about the same time showed that rat fibroblasts could be fully transformed by co-transfection of *ras* with either a *myc* oncogene or the gene encoding the large-T antigen of simian virus (SV) 40, suggesting that combinations of oncogenes may be needed for immortalization and malignant transformation.

The susceptibility of human cells to immortalization, compared with that of rodent cells under similar conditions, was also comprehensively investigated at this time. Human cells usually proved refractory to immortalization by carcinogen treatment, even after repeated exposure to some of the most powerful known mammalian cell mutagens or clastogens. However, it was also demonstrated that variants displaying the anchorage-independent phenotype (a good marker for malignancy in fibroblasts) could be readily induced by exposure to such carcinogens. Transplanted into athymic mice, such variants produced small tumours whose growth was found to be limited by the finite intrinsic proliferative capacity retained by these cells, both in culture and in the tumorigenesis assays *in vivo*.

The above early observations on the cell biology of immortalization and malignant transformation were consistent with the idea that immortalization represents a prerequisite for the clonal evolution of neoplastic populations and in particular, the acquisition of advanced malignant (e.g. metastatic) properties. They also provided direct evidence for the multi-step nature of the transformation process and highlighted the exceptional refractoriness of human cells to immortalization, suggesting that replicative senescence in human cells may have evolved as a tumour suppressive mechanism (Reddel, 2000). However, the persuasiveness of such a hypothesis has, until relatively recently, been compromised by a lack of information concerning the molecular mechanisms of human cell senescence and immortalization.

The science of cell immortalization and its relationship to cancer was revolutionized in 1994 when a landmark paper appeared showing that the vast majority of human cancer tissues possess an enzyme activity, not present in normal human cells or tissues, that could account for the immortality of cancer cells (Kim et al., 1994). The enzyme, telomerase, was known to maintain the DNA of

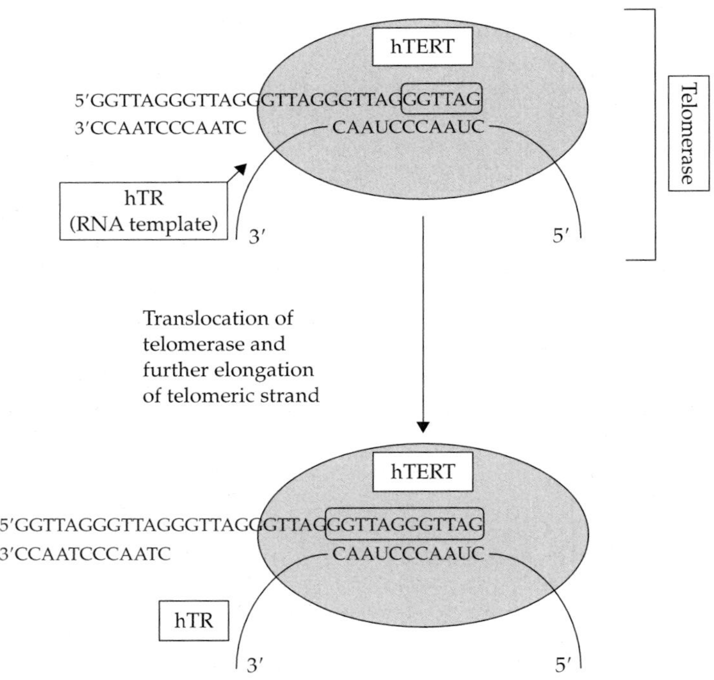

Figure 10.2 Telomerase is a ribonucleoprotein that synthesizes telomeric hexanucleotide repeats (TTAGGG in humans) to replace those lost during each round of the cell cycle, due to the inability of DNA polymerase to replicate completely both strands of a linear double DNA helix. The human telomerase complex consists of a protein catalytic sub-unit (hTERT—a type of reverse transcriptase) and an integral template RNA (hTR) for TTAGGG synthesis. Sensitive assays for human telomerase activity enabled it to be shown (Kim et al., 1994) that telomerase is constitutively active in around 90% of human cancers but is tightly down-regulated in normal cells and tissues.

structures at the ends of eukaryotic chromosomes, known as telomeres, through the synthesis of characteristic telomeric repeat sequences. Telomerase (telomere terminal transferase) had been described several years earlier in the ciliated single-celled protozoan Tetrahymena, and was subsequently shown to be present in human cancer cells (in which it synthesizes telomeric hexanucleotide, TTAGGG, repeats) (Figure 10.2). Following the observation that a mutant yeast strain est1 (ever shorter telomeres) underwent a kind of senescence after a certain number of divisions, several laboratories produced experimental evidence that the limited proliferative capacity of human cells may be due to the same mechanism. The definitive study in 1994, in which a large number of human cancer samples and cell lines, counterpart normal tissues, and *in vitro* transformed human cells were examined, was contingent on the development of a new, highly sensitive polymerase chain reaction (PCR)-based assay for functional telomerase known as telomere repeat amplification protocol (TRAP). The close association thereby obtained between telomerase activity, immortalization and cancer, provided the molecular underpinning required to launch an era of intensive investigation into the role of telomerase-mediated immortalization as a key event in human cancer.

10.3 Telomerase: the 'immortality enzyme'?

We now know that telomeres act as a mitotic clock in human cells, that is, as a specific timing mechanism to limit the division potential of human cells *in vitro* and presumably *in vivo*. This discovery involved the elaboration and experimental testing of a much earlier hypothesis (Olovnikov, 1973) in which it was proposed that the linear DNA of eukaryotic chromosomes would shorten with each round of DNA replication, and that this failure to maintain telomeric DNA might somehow trigger the phenomenon of replicative senescence that characterizes the Hayflick limit. An inevitable consequence of semi-conservative DNA replication in eukaryotic cells, known as the end-replication problem, is that the free DNA ends of each chromosome are not duplicated completely by DNA polymerase. Consequently, the ends of human chromosomes can lose up to 200 base pairs (bp) of DNA per cell division. Several reputable laboratories have now confirmed three basic observations: (1) that the vast majority of normal human tissues and primary cell lines lack telomerase activity, (2) that in the absence of telomerase, telomeres progressively shorten in normal human cells with each division cycle, culminating in replicative senescence, and (3) that the majority of human cancers have active telomerase and thereby maintain their telomeres. However, rigorous functional proof that telomerase is responsible for immortality of cancer cells and that lack of it triggers a cell division counting mechanism (namely telomere shortening) depended on the isolation of the genes encoding the elements of human telomerase.

Human telomerase is a ribonucleoprotein complex that is made up of two key components: (1) an RNA template molecule containing a sequence complementary to the telomeric TTAGGG repeat and (2) the catalytic component, known as hTERT, which is a type of reverse transcriptase able to synthesize TTAGGG repeats from the RNA template (Figure 10.2). The human genes encoding these components have been cloned and the availability of the two genes enabled it to be shown that the primary mode of regulation (i.e. repression) of telomerase in human cells is through silencing of the *hTERT* gene via transcriptional repression. Transfection of an *hTERT* cDNA expression vector into human fibroblasts leads to immortalization of the cells. Such cells have elongated telomeres, an apparently normal karyotype, and express none of the usual markers of malignancy. Telomerase-positive cells expressing a mutant telomerase enzyme fail to undergo immortalization, which has further strengthened the connection between telomere maintenance and immortalization. Furthermore, disruption of telomere maintenance by mutant forms of hTERT, acting in a dominant negative fashion, is known to restore limited lifespan in human cancer cells, resulting in loss of tumorigenicity.

The vast majority of studies carried out since these seminal observations have confirmed that the primary mode of repression and de-repression of telomerase in normal human cells and in cancers occurs at the level of transcription of *hTERT*. However, whether de-repression of the *hTERT* gene and telomerase activation is the sole requirement for immortalization in all human cell types has remained unresolved. Indeed, some investigators have questioned this premise and provided evidence that, in cultured primary human keratinocytes and breast epithelial cells, inactivation of a second tumour suppressive pathway in addition to telomerase reconstitution is necessary for immortalization (see Section 10.8).

10.4 Mortality barriers to human cell immortalization: the effectors of replicative cellular senescence in human cells

Prior to the discovery that telomere shortening and telomerase activation are the underlying primary causes of human cell replicative senescence and immortalization respectively, work with DNA tumour virus 'early' genes had shown that the senescence of human fibroblasts, which normally manifests itself as growth arrest of the cells after between 50 and 80 population doublings (pd) depending on donor age, can be blocked by transfection with viral early genes such as that encoding the SV40 large-T antigen (SV40-LT) or (co-transfer of) those encoding the HPV16 E6 and E7 transforming proteins (e.g. see Ozer, 2000). These viruses have evolved such genes to bypass negative host cell-cycle control mechanisms to enable them to replicate. We know that these viral transforming genes inactivate the p53 and pRB tumour suppressive proteins via sequestration and/or enhanced degradation. Human fibroblasts transfected with SV40-LT initially display a substantial increase (of around 20–30 pd) in their proliferative capacity rather than attaining immortality. The cells then enter a proliferative phase known as 'crisis' that is characterized by very slow cell turnover and cell death. Rare clones of rapidly dividing cells often emerge in these cultures at a frequency of around 10^{-6}, which thereafter remain immortal. T-antigen expression is therefore necessary, but not sufficient, for immortalization, pointing to a two-stage mechanism (Figure 10.3). The term M_1(Mortality 1) is now commonly used for the proliferative barrier (senescence) overcome by p53/pRB inactivation, and M_2 for the crisis restriction.

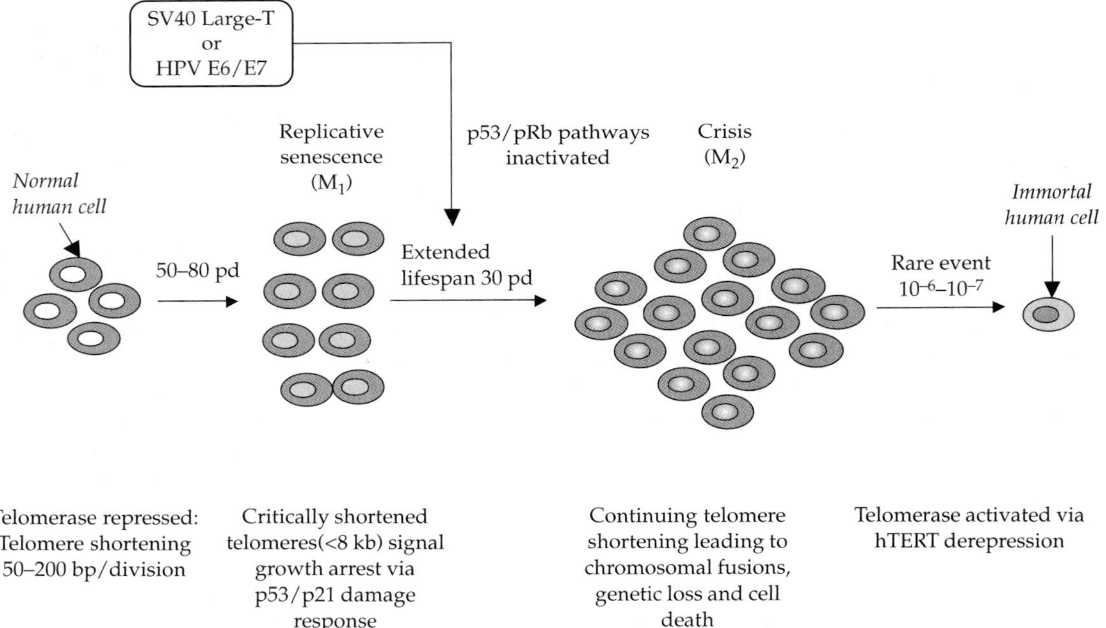

Figure 10.3 DNA tumour virus early genes, such as those encoding the SV40 Large T antigen or HPV E6/E7 proteins, bypass human fibroblast senescence (M_1) via inactivation of p53 and pRB cell growth suppressive proteins. Elimination of both suppressors appears to be necessary for human cell immortalization; together, they act as effectors of replicative cell senescence. The molecular mechanisms underlying the twin phenomena of cell senescence and immortalization can now be comprehensively explained in terms of: (i) progressive telomere shortening (leading to cell senescence), (ii) critically short telomeres (leading to chromosomal fusions, genetic instability and M_2 crisis), and, finally (iii) telomerase activation (a rare event involving hTERT de-repression) leading to cell immortalization.

An attractive explanation for the two stages observed in human fibroblast immortalization by DNA tumour virus early genes has emerged from our understanding of the role telomerase plays in the process. It is now thought that p53 acts as an *effector* of senescence by recognizing critically shortened telomeric DNA as a free end (i.e. as would be encountered following a double-strand break) and in this way inducing proliferative arrest via negative cell cycle control (i.e. by DNA damage recognition systems) through the p21 regulator, a key inhibitor of multiple cyclin/CDK complexes. The second target of Large-T and other viral early proteins, pRB, is also a negative cell cycle regulator acting in part via sequestration of the transcription factor E2F and family members. The latter proteins function as activators of cellular genes involved in DNA synthesis and are required for progression through the G1-S transition and S phase of the cell cycle. It is thought that M_1 occurs when telomeres become critically shortened, leading to destabilization of the protective 'cap' at the telomere formed by a foldback (lariat-type) structure known as a t-loop (Griffith et al., 1999). The critical event triggering DNA damage responses appears to be exposure and loss of the 3′ single-strand overhang sequence, due to t-loop disruption (rather than overall telomere length) and this may occur following critical telomere shortening or acute DNA damage (Li et al., 2003).

Inactivation of p53 and pRB by Large-T thus prevents the growth arrest signals mediated by these proteins, allowing transfected cells to continue to divide until M_2 (crisis) when telomeres become so short that chromosomal end–end fusions occur. The resulting dicentric chromosomes threaten cell viability either by blocking mitosis *per se* or via a fusion-breakage bridge-cycle that leads to the loss of essential chromosomal material. Rare immortal clones that emerge have usually (but not always, see Section 10.10 below) activated telomerase, probably through mutation/loss of *hTERT* transcriptional repressor genes during crisis. Human keratinocytes infected with SV40 emerge from M_2 crisis at a far greater frequency than their fibroblast counterparts, suggesting a non-mutational mechanism for the activation of telomerase in this cell type. The requirement for both p53 and pRB inactivation for the telomere-mediated M_1 proliferative restriction to be bypassed suggests that, in human cells, the two anti-proliferative pathways act in concert as effectors of replicative senescence.

The viral immortalization studies, when interpreted in the light of the telomere hypothesis of cellular senescence, suggest a possible model for the kinetics of cell immortalization in human cancer development (Figure 10.3). In such a model, immortalization is an important event in malignant transformation and the robust down-regulation of *hTERT* expression (and thereby telomerase) in human cells is assumed to have evolved as a protective mechanism against clonal evolution and neoplastic progression. Loss of p53 function (commonly observed in human carcinomas) would be expected to confer a selective advantage when proper telomere structure is disrupted at the M_1 restriction point in somatic cells. This would be expected to trigger lifespan extension, extensive chromosomal/genomic instability (a hallmark of cancer) and derepression of *hTERT* by genetic/epigenetic changes. The resulting telomerase-positive immortal lineage would then, having met all three requirements listed in Section 10.1, be primed to undergo further clonal evolution leading to the acquisition of malignant characteristics.

The *p16(INK4A)* gene is a third important tumour suppressor implicated as an effector (or in the maintenance) of cellular senescence and thus as a barrier to carcinogenesis. The encoded suppressor protein (and other related *INK4* family members) binds to cyclin-dependent kinases cdk-4 and cdk-6 and, by blocking their association with D-type cyclins, induces cell cycle arrest by preventing phosphorylation of pRB; p16 therefore lies upstream of pRB and loss of function of p16 is reported to be involved in immortalization as an alternative to inactivation of pRB. The *INK4A* (or *CDKN2A*) locus is unusual in that, through alternative splicing, it encodes two unrelated proteins in rodent and human cells by means of distinct but overlapping reading frames. One is p16, the other is the alternative reading frame (ARF)—also known as p14 in humans and p19 in mice. Both proteins appear to be involved in cell senescence: p16 activates pRB proteins through inhibition of their phosphorylation by cdk-4 and 6, while ARF activates p53. Thus, the *INK4A* locus regulates the two tumour suppressive pathways (Rb and p53) that are the most commonly disrupted in a wide range of human malignancies (Drayton and Peters, 2002) (Figure 10.4). The relative importance of the p16 and ARF proteins in the senescence process is becoming clearer. Their roles appear to differ substantially in different cell types and species. p16 is

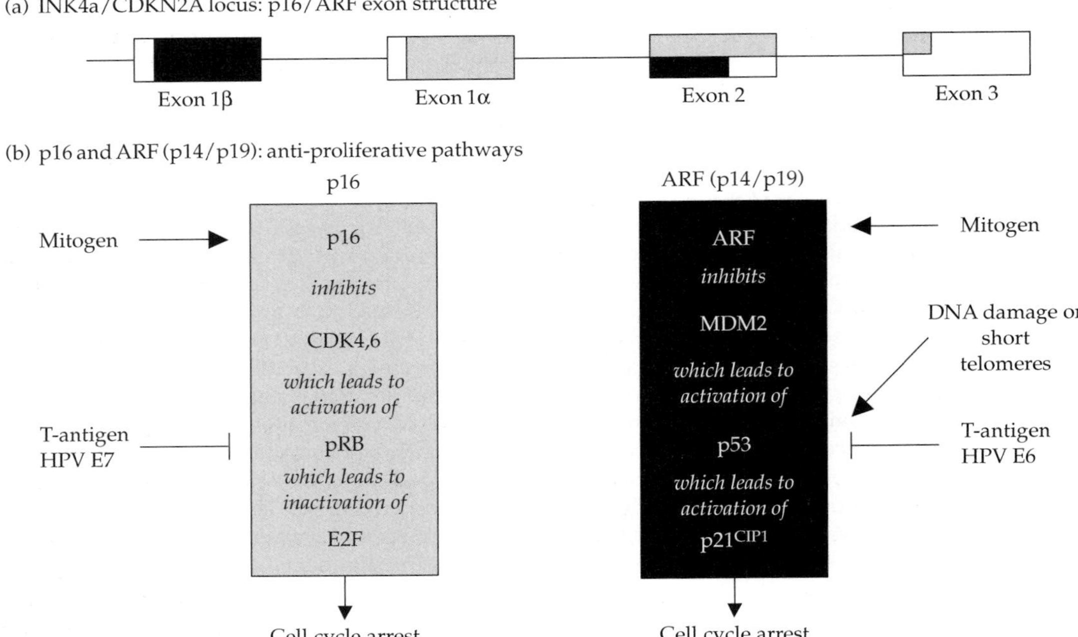

Figure 10.4 The *INK4a/CDKN2A* locus encodes two unrelated proteins: p16 and ARF (p14 in humans, p19 in mice) through the use of distinct but overlapping reading frames. (a) shows the exon structure of the complete *INK4a* locus indicating the p16 (grey) and ARF (black)-encoding regions. Both proteins are involved in replicative cell senescence (b) as upstream regulators of the RB (inhibited by p16) or p53 (inhibited by ARF) cell growth inhibitory pathways; MDM2 is a natural inhibitor of p53. *p16, RB,* and *TP53* are tumour suppressor genes disrupted in a wide range of human cancers. (Figure modified from Drayton and Peters (2002))

frequently silenced in a number of human cancers, often involving an epigenetic mechanism. In contrast, germline mutations in *p16* appear to predispose specifically to malignant melanoma (Bennett, 2003) leading to the proposal that *p16* silencing is central to melanocyte immortalization. ARF rather than p16 appears to be the key effector in rodent cell senescence. Recent studies have implicated several regulatory molecules (ETS, ID-1, BMI-1) as upstream transcriptional activators of p16 during senescence.

10.5 Recent progress in generating a malignant human cell *in vitro*

The availability of genetic reagents for manipulating each of the above tumour suppressive pathways and for reconstituting telomerase, opened the door to the experimental generation of malignant human cells from their normal counterparts in culture. Such work has helped pinpoint the key events required for human cell transformation. To investigate the role of hTERT in the transformation of human cells, combinations of hTERT, the SV40 large-T oncoprotein, and an oncogenic *Ha-ras* gene (*Ha-rasV12*) have been co-expressed in both human diploid fibroblasts and epithelial cells (the latter derived from normal kidney and breast epithelium) with the result that direct tumorigenic transformation of all the cell types could be achieved by these three genetic elements alone (Hahn et al., 1999). In human mammary epithelial cells transformed by the same three genetic elements, co-transfected cells form poorly differentiated carcinomas that infiltrate through adjacent tissue. Malignant transformation appears to be enhanced by the inclusion of the gene encoding the SV40 small-t antigen, that appears to act by perturbation of protein phosphatase 2A. While it is accepted that additional alterations are likely to be needed for tumour cells to metastasize, the observation that a defined set of genetic alterations can co-operate to achieve malignant transformation of human cells is a major advance in our understanding of the primary mechanisms operative in human cancer development.

The immortalization of human mammary epithelial cells (HMECs), potentially a clinically highly significant cell type in cancer research, has been characterized in some detail (Yaswen and Stampfer, 2002). HMEC cultures, commonly obtained from reduction mammoplasty tissue, normally proliferate for 15–30 population doublings (pd) in serum-containing medium, before undergoing a growth arrest (termed M_0) indistinguishable from replicative senescence. In a serum-free medium developed specifically for HMECs, culture lifespan is reduced to 10–20 pd. A cell population arises spontaneously in some cultures that is capable of long-term growth (up to 100 pd). This phenomenon, known as 'self-selection', generating longer lifespan cultures, is invariably associated with the epigenetic silencing of *p16* by promoter methylation. Post-selection cells, which have stable p53, hit the next replicative barrier (which has been termed 'agonescence', to distinguish it from the crisis that occurs in human fibroblasts immortalized with DNA tumour viruses) when their telomeres become critically shortened. At this point, such cells accumulate chromosome aberrations, particularly telomeric fusions. However, agonescence differs from fibroblast crisis in that most of the cells possess long-term viability, and immortal transformants have, in several independent studies, never been seen to arise spontaneously. Interestingly, spontaneous escape from M_0 senescence (but not immortalization) of HMECs eventually results in cells displaying the same types of chromosome aberrations seen in early breast cancers. Post-selection HMECs are readily immortalized by hTERT reconstitution, indicating that short telomeres are the main impediment to continuous growth in these cells. These stages in the immortalization process apply to other human epithelial cell types, such as keratinocytes.

The strict block to proliferation imposed by robust repression of the telomerase *hTERT* gene seems to be the primary barrier to clonal evolution of human breast epithelial and other human cells. If p53 is experimentally inactivated in post-selection breast cell cultures (e.g. by transfection of dominant negative *p53* mutant), activation of telomerase and conversion to an immortal phenotype is facilitated. From the information available, it appears that telomerase activation, at least in this particular model, could be a gradual process rather than an abrupt step-change typical of a mutation, raising the possibility that an epigenetic mechanism sometimes underlies derepression of the *hTERT* gene.

10.6 Regulation of telomerase in normal human cells and in cancer

We have seen that telomerase is necessary for the maintenance of telomeres because of the so-called end-replication problem (and possibly other assaults on telomeric integrity such as oxidative damage). Lack of telomerase characterizes the majority of normal human cells *in vivo*, while in cancers the gene encoding the telomerase reverse transcriptase subunit (hTERT) is de-repressed thereby permitting unlimited cell proliferation. How then is *hTERT* regulated in normal cells and by what mechanism is it reactivated during human carcinogenesis?

Of the two components of the core telomerase enzyme the catalytic sub-unit, hTERT, is limiting; consequently, a considerable amount of effort has been devoted to understanding the transcriptional regulation of *hTERT*. Most telomerase-negative normal human cells lack detectable *hTERT* transcripts, while in telomerase-positive tumour cells an average of 0.2–6 mRNA molecules/cell have been detected by using sensitive reverse transcription polymerase chain reaction (RT-PCR)-based techniques (Ducrest et al., 2002). The complete transcription unit of *hTERT* has been cloned and consists of 16 exons and 15 introns spanning around 37 kb of genomic sequence. The 5′ regulatory (promoter) sequences have been identified using reporter constructs. The promoter is inactive in normal human cells, but becomes active following immortalization, providing further evidence that transcriptional regulation of *hTERT* gene expression lies at the heart of replicative senescence and immortalization. Of the major factors binding to the core promoter, the c-Myc transcription factor (and oncoprotein) interacts with evolutionarily conserved E-boxes (CACGTG) and is able to stimulate *hTERT* transcription and telomerase activity in *hTERT*-silenced human cells (probably in conjunction with the transcription factor SP1, which also binds to a cognate GC-box within the core promoter). Overexpression of the Myc/Max dimer (again in conjunction with SP1 binding) leads to the activation of *hTERT* transcription, whereas Mad/Max acts as a repressor. The highly GC-rich content of the 5′ region extending into intron-1 constitutes a CpG island, again (see above) raising the possibility that epigenetic mechanisms may play a key role in silencing *hTERT* transcription in normal cells and possibly therefore also during its reactivation in carcinogenesis. This notion is supported by studies using the demethylating agent 5-azacytidine and the histone deactetylase inhibitor trichostatin A (TSA), both of which will activate *hTERT* in human fibroblasts and lymphocytes. Furthermore, *hTERT* chromatin (particularly that constituting the second intron) is invariably more condensed in telomerase-negative normal human cells compared with that in telomerase-positive human cancer cells (Szutorisz et al., 2003) indicating that chromatin remodelling to an 'open' transcriptionally active form is associated with telomerase activation during cancer development.

Controls working at the level of the 5′ core promoter appear to be concerned with regulating *hTERT* during differentiation, the cell cycle or quiescence. However, at least in normal somatic human cells, the presence is indicated of an additional, far more stringent process for permanently silencing *hTERT* transcription. Somatic cell genetic analysis, involving microcell-mediated monochromosome transfer (MMCT) has provided evidence for the existence of several genes that repress telomerase in normal human cells. Thus far, human chromosomes 3, 4, 6, 7, and 10 have been shown to suppress telomerase when transferred by MMCT into certain tumour cell lines (Newbold, 2002). For example, normal chromosome 3 induces senescence on transfer into a human renal cell carcinoma cell line, with growth arrest manifesting after 23–43 pd. This is associated with loss of telomerase activity as measured by TRAP (due to down-regulation of hTERT) and telomere shortening. Powerful repression of telomerase activity is also induced by chromosome 3 in early passage breast cancer cells. By fine-mapping deletions in the introduced chromosome in segregant hybrids the telomerase repressor gene has been localized to a region at 3p14–21. Similarly, chromosomes 4, 6, 7, and 10 repress telomerase activity in, respectively, HeLa cervical carcinoma cells, the HPV-16-containing cervical cancer cell line SiHa, a telomerase-positive human mesothelial cell line, MeT5A, and the hepatocellular carcinoma cell line, Li7HM. While the individual genes responsible for the repressive activity of these chromosomes remain to be identified, repression of telomerase in breast cancer cells by normal chromosome 3 is evidently due to a highly specific silencing effect on *hTERT* transcription by complex mechanisms involving regulatory elements distant from the 5′ regulatory region, and including alterations in *hTERT* chromatin structure (Szutorisz et al., 2003).

10.7 Origins of telomerase in cancer cells: two competing hypotheses

The suggestion from chromosome transfer studies that genes exist in normal human cells that repress telomerase activity in cancer cells, via a highly specific effect on *hTERT* transcriptional silencing, is consistent with the idea that the telomerase activity found in the vast majority of cancers arises from mutational or epigenetic disruption of such repressor genes. The kinetics of viral immortalization of human fibroblasts, that is, the emergence of a faster growing clone of cells as a rare event during M_2 crisis would be consistent with a step change in a single cell involving the mutational inactivation of a repressor. In addition, the fact that many human cancers, particularly carcinomas, have short dysfunctional telomeres maintained in steady state, often by relatively low levels of telomerase, would suggest that telomerase had been activated only after a considerable period of telomere shortening had taken place in the originating (telomerase-negative) target cell.

There is, however, a second possibility for the origin of telomerase in cancers that continues to warrant serious investigation. It is that the majority of human cancers arise from stem cells, or from transiently amplifying populations in renewing tissues, that already have active telomerase. We now know that the initial view that telomerase is present only in cancers and germ cells is too simplistic. Relatively low levels of activity are now known to be present in the proliferative cells of certain self-renewing tissues (e.g. the bone marrow), trachea and bronchi, skin (basal layer) and gut (lower crypt), and glandular prostate tissue (Forsyth et al., 2002). Moreover, very recently, Masutomi et al. (2003) have provided evidence (using immunoprecipitation techniques) that active telomerase is expressed at low levels during the S-phase of the cell cycle in proliferating normal human fibroblasts. It has been suggested that such levels of telomerase are sufficient to slow down, but certainly are not adequate to prevent telomere shortening during tissue renewal. The evidence for this comes from the observation that telomeres shorten in human skin and gut with increasing age, in spite of the presence of telomerase. Thus, although telomerase is silenced in almost all human organs at between 18 and 21 weeks of gestation, it is retained at low levels in rapidly dividing self-renewing tissues presumably to offset the effects that rapid telomere loss might have on chromosomal stability and the potential initiation of cancer. The consequences of inhibiting telomerase in these normal tissues (e.g. by anti-telomerase drugs used to control the proliferation of cancer cells) is unclear but needs further investigation.

The key question that remains unresolved is, therefore, whether the cells from which human cancers originate are in fact those cells that apparently have not robustly down-regulated hTERT or, alternatively, whether hTERT repressed cells undergo hTERT de-repression. If the former prevails, then the presence of telomerase in most cancers could be regarded as a process of 'selection' of pre-existing telomerase-positive cells with possible subsequent enhancement of activity (e.g. through further selection of clones with minor epigenetic changes) sufficient to maintain telomeres indefinitely. If the latter is true, telomerase activation would occur primarily through a process of 'induction' possibly resulting from a single or small number of genetic/epigenetic events inactivating *hTERT* repressor gene(s). Of course, the two models are not necessarily mutually exclusive.

10.8 Do telomere-independent senescence mechanisms exist in rodent and human cells?

As discussed in Section 10.2, the majority of early studies aimed at transforming normal diploid cells in culture (e.g. by carcinogens and cloned oncogenes) were carried out using freshly explanted diploid rodent cells. This was simply because, after many attempts, human cells proved virtually impossible to transform (except with DNA tumour viruses) due to the replicative senescence barrier and their intrinsic resistance to immortalization. How then does our contemporary understanding of telomerase regulation help us explain the increased transformability of rodent cells?

Mouse, rat, and Syrian hamster cells from trypsinized embryos, neonatal dermis or other tissues undergo a process that closely resembles replicative senescence in human cells. Fibroblasts normally dominate such cultures and terminal division generally occurs earlier with these cells (after around 10–25 pd) than with human fibroblasts (40–70 pd). In sharp contrast to human cells, rodent cells show a greater propensity to undergo immortalization in culture either spontaneously or following a single exposure to a carcinogen. Mouse cells appear to be more susceptible than rat cells in this respect, almost invariably immortalizing spontaneously, whereas in hamster cell cultures spontaneous immortalization is rare but can be readily induced by carcinogen treatment. The reason for the increased susceptibility of rodent cells to immortalization is explained by the fact that, unlike their human counterparts, primary rodent cell cultures possess high levels of active telomerase and maintain it throughout their culture lifespan (Newbold, 2002). As a result, the chromosomes of these cells have long telomeres that do not shorten with time in culture. Tissues taken from rodents also have active telomerase and show much less evidence of the stringent controls on *hTERT* expression found in their human equivalents. Telomere-mediated senescence does not therefore appear to exist as a barrier to immortalization and malignant transformation in rodent cells. Rodents, being physically much smaller and shorter-lived, may not have needed to evolve the protection of a powerful telomerase repressive mechanism to prevent cancer. However, the fact that primary rodent cells still undergo a senescence-like process *in vitro*, raises the question of the existence of telomere-independent 'clocks' that limit the proliferative capacity of somatic cells.

It has recently been argued (Ramirez et al., 2001) that the loss of division potential of rodent cells *in vitro* is a cell culture artefact, which implies that the immortalization of these cells in culture models does not reflect a genuine event that must occur in rodent carcinogenesis *in vivo*. It is suggested that the cause of the 'senescence' seen in these cells is in fact inadequate culture conditions leading to 'stress' and DNA damage. The primary effector of growth arrest in cultured mouse fibroblasts appears to be the ARF/p53 pathway, inactivation of which seems to be sufficient for immortalization whereas specific silencing of p16 leaving ARF intact indicates that p16 is not involved. Indeed, the p16/pRb response to telomere dysfunction appears not to operate in mouse cells (Smogorzewska and de Lange, 2002). 'Stress' and resulting DNA damage may, it is speculated, be the consequence of free radicals produced by amine oxidase in serum, since the immortal growth of diploid mouse cells in a serum-free medium has been demonstrated and also of rat oligodendrocyte precursor cells cultured under conditions that inhibit differentiation.

An analogous phenomenon of telomere-independent growth arrest is also encountered in the immortalization of human epithelial cells, as discussed earlier in this chapter. For example, the initial proliferative potential of HMECs in chemically defined media is approximately 20 pd. This mortality barrier (M_0; see above) is mediated by p16 rather than ARF as the effector, and raises the possibility of the existence of additional tumour suppressive mechanisms for counting cell divisions. However, experimental evidence has been produced against this explanation (Ramirez et al., 2001) showing that the proliferative capacity of cultured HMECs can be extended all the way to the telomere-dependent M_1 barrier, merely by growing the cells on feeder layers. Under these conditions, HMECs could be immortalized directly by *hTERT* without the need to inactivate the p16/pRB pathway. In this model, the telomere-dependent barrier limiting division potential is seen as the only true mechanism of replicative senescence, with all other limits to mammalian cell proliferative capacity in culture being artefacts. However, it should be pointed out that the interpretation of the above feeder layer study is, at the time of writing, controversial. For example, in a variety of human keratinocyte cell types, Rheinwald et al. (2002) were able to show comprehensively that such cells possess a telomere-independent replicative senescence mechanism (mediated by p16 and p53) that functions as an immortalization barrier, irrespective of culture conditions.

An alternative view is therefore persuasive. Dividing cells in differentiating tissues are naturally programmed, as part of a commitment process, to enter terminal division. The process of differentiation can be assumed to be highly complex, depending on signalling either through contact with other cell types in the tissue 'niche' or through humoral factors that orchestrate unfolding programmes of gene expression and repression, culminating in the ultimately specialized (usually post-mitotic) terminally differentiated cell. This kind of process does in essence incorporate a cell counting mechanism that imparts a limit to the division capacity of the differentiating cell lineage. It is reasonable to suppose that such programmes would need to be bypassed in both rodent and humans during carcinogenesis and would therefore represent important tumour suppressive mechanisms.

In any event, M_0 senescence in the absence of feeder cells does not necessarily indicate an artefact, but rather may reflect a natural response of cells to being removed from their tissue niche (and as such could still be regarded as a kind of stress). This type of response would represent a genuine safeguard against cancer because, by definition, clonally evolving neoplastic cell lineages ultimately need to escape from niche constraints (e.g. by removal of the p16/pRB negative cell cycle regulator pathway) to undergo malignant transformation. Such populations would then come up against the telomere-mediated M_1 replicative block as a second-line safeguard. The fact that the p16/pRB pathway has been shown to be functionally inactivated in many human cancers would tend to support the view that its loss of function represents an early and important event in tumour development. Furthermore, there are other well-characterized examples of telomere-independent replicative senescence in specific cultured human cell types, including thyroid epithelial cells and melanocytes, where germline p16 loss of function is associated with high melanoma incidence and an abnormally large number of precursor lesions (naevi or moles). The potential for exploiting such telomere-independent senescence mechanisms in cancer treatment has been comprehensively reviewed (Roninson, 2003).

Somatic cell genetics has also provided evidence for the presence of genes that induce telomere-independent senescence in immortal human cells derived from cancers or viral transformation (Tominaga et al., 2002). Somatic cell fusion has demonstrated that senescence is dominant over immortality; four senescence-inducing complementation groups have been identified. Microcell-mediated monochromosome transfer has pinpointed the location of several genes that induce senescence in the absence of telomerase repression. One gene, *MORF4* (on chromosome 4) associated with one of the complementation groups has been cloned. As yet the precise significance of the majority of these genes as *bona fide* tumour suppressors remains to be determined.

10.9 Does inactivation of telomerase protect against immortalization and cancer: evidence from the telomerase 'knockout' mouse

Work with rodent cell cultures and from observations that telomerase is expressed in many rodent tissues, strongly points towards major differences between humans and rodents with respect to telomerase regulation in the soma. However, despite this fact, genetically engineered rodents have proved to be extremely valuable in studying both the consequences for the whole organism of telomere attrition due to lack of telomerase, and also the modulating effects of telomerase inactivation and, conversely, its overexpression on tumour suppression and carcinogenesis respectively.

Blasco et al. (1997) were first to construct a telomerase 'knockout' mouse strain by deleting the gene encoding the telomerase RNA component (mTR) from the germline. Such mice possess no detectable telomerase in any tissue but are viable for six generations, presumably reflecting the fact that the original mouse strain had long telomeres. Cells isolated from animals at the fourth generation onwards have no detectable telomeric repeats and display severe chromosomal abnormalities. Do cells from such mice display total resistance to immortalization? The answer is surprisingly that they do not. Telomerase-deficient cells can be immortalized in culture (albeit at a lower frequency than telomerase-positive cells) and transformed by viral oncogenes to the point that they produce tumours in athymic mice following subcutaneous injection.

The acquisition of immortality by telomerase-deficient mouse cells confounds expectations and also raises concerns about the prevailing notion that telomerase repression in human cells represents an evolutionary anti-cancer strategy. Some light has been shed on this conundrum by work showing that, in immortal cells from telomerase-null mice, telomere length becomes stabilized in a chromosome-specific manner, indicating that a telomerase-independent telomere maintenance mechanism can be activated in mouse cells.

Collectively, results to date from telomerase 'knockout' mouse studies provide evidence that lack of telomerase protects against cancer whilst its expression promotes carcinogenesis. However, very short telomeres, in certain circumstances (e.g. in the absence of p53) increase the propensity for chromosomal instability and this may, paradoxically, promote cancer induction. Telomerase repression probably exerts its maximum effect during normal reproductive age when telomeres are long (i.e. when evolutionary selective pressures for survival are at their highest). As telomeres shorten with age, or when unusual demands are placed on renewing tissues, lack of telomerase may, particularly in abnormal clones in which p53 and/or p16 have been functionally inactivated, have the opposite effect and increase the probability of crisis, telomerase reactivation, immortalization, clonal evolution, and cancer.

10.10 Alternative mechanisms of telomere maintenance

From the results of the telomerase mTR knockout studies, it is clear that mouse cells are able to activate an alternative mechanism for telomere maintenance under the selective pressure that results from the absence of telomerase. Moreover, the fact that not all human tumour cells and *in vitro* immortalized (e.g. with SV40) cell lines have detectable telomerase activity (Kim et al. 1994) points to the existence of similar mechanisms in humans. Some of these telomerase-negative cancers may genuinely not be immortalized, particularly those localized focal growths that have not undergone much in the way of clonal evolution. However, the majority have been shown to maintain the length of their telomeres by a mechanism that has become known as Alternative Lengthening of Telomeres (ALT).

Studies in various eukaryotes have revealed the existence of telomerase-independent telomere maintenance pathways. Mutational inactivation of telomerase in the yeast *Saccharomyces cerevisiae* results in senescence of the majority of the population (Lundblad and Blackburn, 1993). Clones of immortal cells emerge, however, that are able to maintain their telomeres via a RAD52-dependent recombination pathway that involves amplification of sub-telomeric elements. It now appears that there are two different classes of telomerase-negative survivors: those that possess amplified subtelomeric sequences and short telomeric elements, and those that have much longer telomeres made up of amplified telomeric (TTAGGG) repeats. Analysis of telomere restriction fragments from human cells that rely on ALT for telomere maintenance has revealed that they possess telomeric tracts that are extremely heterogeneous in length, ranging from undetectable to abnormally long which would also point towards a recombinational origin.

The incidence of ALT in human cancer cells and in *in vitro*-immortalized human cell lines has been studied in some detail (Newbold, 2002). In SV40-immortalized fibroblasts up to 50% utilize an ALT mechanism rather than telomerase. However, the available evidence indicates that epithelial and mesothelial cells lines are predominantly telomerase-positive. In human tumours and tumour-derived cell lines, ALT has been identified in around 7% of samples assayed in each case. Intriguingly, the majority of ALT-positive cell lines are sarcomas.

There is intense interest in the ALT pathway because it represents a potential stumbling-block to the application of anti-telomerase approaches to cancer therapy. The key question still requiring resolution is whether and at what frequency ALT variants arise when telomerase-positive human cancer cells are challenged with telomerase inhibitors. Some clues can already be gained from *in vitro* experiments, which indicate that the appearance of ALT variants in telomerase-inhibited human cancer cell populations is extremely rare. Furthermore, it also appears that even if ALT is activated it does not fully substitute for telomerase in malignant transformation. It is now believed that telomerase has an additional function that acts independently of telomere maintenance to promote tumorigenesis (Stewart et al., 2002). This is probably why ALT is rarely seen as the sole telomere-maintenance mechanism in human cancers, because ALT cannot adequately replace telomerase function during the process of tumour progression.

10.11 Telomerase and cellular immortality as anti-cancer targets

Because telomerase is dysregulated in around 90% of human cancers and is essential for the continued proliferation (and clonal evolution) of cancer cells, it represents arguably one of the most exciting anti-cancer targets thus far discovered. The telomerase ribonucleoprotein complex is biochemically unique, since it possesses a functional RNA component as well as a catalytic protein sub-unit, and therefore would, *a priori*, be expected to be well suited to highly specific functional inhibition by small molecules. Telomerase inhibition has to date been accomplished in the laboratory by a range of experimental procedures (White et al., 2001) including the use of: (1) antisense oligonucleotides or hammerhead ribozymes directed against the RNA (hTR) component of telomerase, (2) dominant-negative mutant *hTERT* constructs, (3) reverse transcriptase inhibitors aimed at blocking the catalytic function of hTERT, (4) agents that stabilize and/or encourage the formation of four-stranded G-quadruplex structures by telomeric DNA (which inhibit telomerase function), (5) other small molecule inhibitors targeted at a variety of processes involved in telomere maintenance, and (6) the use of hTERT as a cancer-specific antigen in immunotherapy. As might be expected there has been a large number of studies using these specific approaches. However, only a few of them have been shown to generate a response consistent with a highly specific effect on telomere dynamics (i.e. reduced telomerase activity, progressive telomere shortening, absence of non-specific toxicity, and phenotypic lag followed by replicative senescence, or apoptosis, after a period of time that reflected initial mean telomere length).

Small molecule inhibitors of telomerase thus far described include compounds that inhibit the action of telomerase at the telomere through the stabilization of G-quadruplex structures. Such tetraplex DNA conformations have been shown to form, thus far only *in vitro*, from the G-rich regions that exist in the 3′ telomere single-stranded overhang. A wide variety of agents has been discovered that stabilize such structures and exert cytotoxic effects on cells in culture. The main problem with such studies is that telomere shortening has not been demonstrated and cytotoxic effects could be interpreted as being non-specific. However, recently a 'second generation' of quinoline-based G-quadruplex stabilizing molecules has been described that induce telomere shortening and delayed growth arrest in cancer cells, in the absence of rapid cytotoxicity. A second class of G-quadruplex-active compound (a trisubstituted acridine) that is an extremely potent telomerase inhibitor at nanomolar concentrations has also been characterized; again this agent did not show the non-specific toxicity to human cancer cells that was an undesirable feature of previous inhibitors. These latest advances have improved the prospects for G-quadruplex stabilization as an effective strategy on which to base new anti-cancer drugs.

Other classes of small molecule inhibitors identified to date include reverse transcriptase inhibitors, nucleoside analogues and cisplatin derivatives. However, such drugs often inhibit the proliferation of telomerase-negative as well as telomerase-positive cells, again indicating a lack of specificity for the chosen target and therefore the potential for side effects *in vivo*. One recently discovered compound BIBR1532 (a synthetic non-nucleosidic telomerase inhibitor) developed by researchers at Boehringer Ingelheim Pharma (Damm et al., 2001) was found to possess the degree of selectivity to justify further investigation as a promising drug candidate. The compound was shown to disrupt telomere maintenance in tumour cells by inhibition of the processivity of telomerase through a non-competitive mechanism, similar to that mediated by inhibitors of HIV1 reverse transcriptase.

10.12 Conclusions

Cell culture models of cancer have, in conjunction with genetic 'knockout' and transgenic strains of mice, permitted considerable advances to be made in understanding the specific cellular and molecular events required to generate a malignant cell. The discovery of telomerase, its role in maintaining the immortality of the mammalian germline and cancer cells, coupled with its critical importance in human somatic cell immortalization *in vitro*, have over the past decade provided strong molecular underpinning for the hypothesis that cell immortalization is a critically important event in human carcinogenesis. Somatic cell genetic studies, involving the reconstitution of active telomerase, have shown that the reason that human cells are so difficult to immortalize is because telomerase is stringently repressed. With the availability of hTERT cDNA vectors this can now be readily achieved and malignant human cells can be created from normal cells purely in culture. At the very least, it is now widely accepted that neoplastic cells must be immortal (through the presence of telomerase, or rarely via ALT) for *repeated* clonal evolution and advanced malignant progression to occur. Evidence demonstrating the presence in human tissues of clonally expanded cell populations (e.g. with compromised p16 or p53) that have undergone replicative senescence *in vivo* can now be expected to emerge.

This does not always mean, however, that all human cancers are immortal, particularly carcinomas *in situ* that have not undergone widespread dissemination. Indeed, work on the molecular characterization of stages in the development of human head and neck carcinomas (which, unlike breast or prostate cancers, can be readily established in tissue culture) (Gordon et al., 2003) indicates that a significant proportion senesce in culture, even in the best known culture conditions, while others possess only low levels of telomerase apparently insufficient to maintain telomeric integrity. Short telomeres maintained by relatively low levels of active telomerase are also a characteristic of other primary carcinomas (e.g. those of the breast and prostate). Thus, many carcinomas appear to exist on a knife-edge of survival in a state that equates to M_2 crisis characterized by extensive telomere dysfunction (which can be detected cytogenetically, for example, by quantifying anaphase bridges). This property would seem to make such cancers excellent candidates for curative anti-telomerase drug therapy.

The advances outlined above strongly suggest that most carcinomas arise from telomerase-deficient cells following the sequential bypass of the M_0 and M_1 senescence checkpoints. Firm evidence for an induction mechanism should emerge from establishing the identity of putative telomerase repressor genes identified by monochromosome transfer and studying their structural integrity in human cancer tissues. The consistent presence of mutations, methylated promoters and/or silenced chromatin in such genes would furnish the required unequivocal support for an induction mechanism.

The other important issue relates to the precise function of telomerase in telomerase-positive cells found in the dividing layers of normal human tissues, and thereby to a prediction of the likely effects on normal tissues of anti-telomerase cancer therapies. Since telomerase-deficient mice do not display pathological phenotypes until the sixth generation, absence of the enzyme seems not to be particularly harmful to cells except when telomeres are critically short. As discussed above, a large proportion of human cancers are made up of cells with very short telomeres (ca. 5 kbp or less). From the *in vitro* evidence obtained to date, if telomerase function were abrogated in such cells, they would be expected to revert to an M_2 crisis state relatively quickly leading to cell death from apoptosis. There is reason to believe (Newbold, 2002) that drug-induced telomere attrition would be reversible in normal human tissues where cells have considerable reserves of telomeric repeats. Furthermore, patients with the human disorder dyskeratosis congenita, which affects telomerase function either through a mutation in the *hTR* gene or in dyskerin, do not display severe phenotypes (pancytopenia and early cancers) until many years after birth, providing further evidence that lack of telomerase, even in renewing tissues, may well be tolerated for some considerable time.

Telomerase, and the immortal phenotype it maintains, remains one of the most attractive anti-cancer targets yet discovered. Since most primates, and possibly other large long-lived animals, appear to control rigorously the expression of telomerase in somatic tissues, this tumour suppressive mechanism is likely to have appeared relatively early in mammalian evolution (Steinert et al., 2002). What better route to adopt for the treatment of cancer than that chosen, by chance and necessity, as a preventative strategy over millions of years of natural selection?

Acknowledgements

The author is indebted to Ken Parkinson and Dorothy Bennett for helpful advice and discussion.

References*

Bennett, D. C. (2003). Human melanocyte senescence and melanoma susceptibility genes. *Oncogene*, **22**, 3063–9.

Blasco, M. A., Lee, H. W., Hande, M. P., Samper, E., Lansdorp, P. M., DePinho, R. A. et al. (1997). Telomere shortening and tumor formation by mouse cells lacking telomerase RNA. *Cell*, **91**, 25–34.

Damm, K., Hemmann, U., Garin-Chesa, P., Hauel, N., Kauffmann, I., Priepke, H. et al. (2001). A highly selective telomerase inhibitor limiting human cancer cell proliferation. *Embo J*, **20**, 6958–68.

Drayton, S. and Peters, G. (2002). Immortalisation and transformation revisited. *Curr Opin Genet Dev*, **12**, 98–104.

Ducrest, A. L., Szutorisz, H., Lingner, J., and Nabholz, M. (2002). Regulation of the human telomerase reverse transcriptase gene. *Oncogene*, **21**, 541–52.

Forsyth, N. R., Wright, W. E., and Shay, J. W. (2002). Telomerase and differentiation in multicellular organisms: turn it off, turn it on, and turn it off again. *Differentiation*, **69**, 188–97.

Gordon, K. E., Ireland, H., Roberts, M., Steeghs, K., McCaul, J. A., MacDonald, D. G. et al. (2003). High levels of telomere dysfunction bestow a selective disadvantage during the progression of human oral squamous cell carcinoma. *Cancer Res*, **63**, 458–67.

Griffith, J. D., Comeau, L., Rosenfield, S., Stansel, R. M., Bianchi, A., Moss, H. et al. (1999). Mammalian telomeres end in a large duplex loop. *Cell*, **97**, 503–14.

Hahn, W. C., Counter, C. M., Lundberg, A. S., Beijersbergen, R. L., Brooks, M. W., and Weinberg, R. A. (1999). Creation of human tumour cells with defined genetic elements. *Nature*, **400**, 464–8.

Hayflick, L. and Moorhead, P. S. (1961). The serial cultivation of human diploid cell strains. *Exp Cell Res*, **25**, 585–621.

Kim, N. W., Piatyszek, M. A., Prowse, K. R., Harley, C. B., West, M. D., Ho, P. L. et al. (1994). Specific association of human telomerase activity with immortal cells and cancer. *Science*, **266**, 2011–5.

Li, G. Z., Eller, M. S., Firoozabadi, R., and Gilchrest, B. A. (2003). Evidence that exposure of the telomere 3′ overhang sequence induces senescence. *Proc Natl Acad Sci U S A*, **100**, 527–31.

Lundblad, V. and Blackburn, E. H. (1993). An alternative pathway for yeast telomere maintenance rescues est1-senescence. *Cell*, **73**, 347–60.

Masutomi, K., Yu, E.Y., Khurts, S., Ben-Porath, I., Currier, J., Metz, G.B. et al. (2003). Telomerase maintains telomere structure in normal human cells. *Cell*, **114**, 241–253.

Newbold, R. F. (1985). Multistep malignant transformation of mammalian cells by carcinogens: induction of immortality as a key event. *Carcinog Compr Surv*, **9**, 17–28.

Newbold, R. F. (2002). The significance of telomerase activation and cellular immortalization in human cancer. *Mutagenesis*, **17**, 539–50.

Olovnikov, A. M. (1973). A theory of marginotomy. The incomplete copying of template margin in enzymic synthesis of polynucleotides and biological significance of the phenomenon. *J Theor Biol*, **41**, 181–90.

Ozer, H. L. (2000). SV40-mediated immortalization. In *Cell Immortalization* (Ed., A. Macieira-Coelho) Springer, Berlin, pp. 121–54.

Ramirez, R. D., Morales, C. P., Herbert, B. S., Rohde, J. M., Passons, C., Shay, J. W. et al. (2001). Putative telomere-independent mechanisms of replicative aging reflect inadequate growth conditions. *Genes Dev*, **15**, 398–403.

Reddel, R. R. (2000). The role of senescence and immortalization in carcinogenesis. *Carcinogenesis*, **21**, 477–84.

Rheinwald, J. G., Hahn, W. C., Ramsey, M. R., Wu, J. Y., Guo, Z., Tsao, H. et al. (2002). A two-stage, p16(INK4A)- and p53-dependent keratinocyte senescence mechanism that limits replicative potential independent of telomere status. *Mol Cell Biol*, **22**, 5157–72.

Roninson, I. B. (2003). Tumor cell senescence in cancer treatment. *Cancer Res*, **63**, 2705–15.

Smogorzewska, A. and de Lange, T. (2002). Different telomere damage signaling pathways in human and mouse cells. *Embo J*, **21**, 4338–48.

Steinert, S., White, D. M., Zou, Y., Shay, J. W., and Wright, W. E. (2002). Telomere biology and cellular aging in nonhuman primate cells. *Exp Cell Res*, **272,** 146–52.

Stewart, S. A., Hahn, W. C., O'Connor, B. F., Banner, E. N., Lundberg, A. S., Modha, P. et al. (2002). Telomerase contributes to tumorigenesis by a telomere length-independent mechanism. *Proc Natl Acad Sci USA*, **99,** 12606–11.

Szutorisz, H., Lingner, J., Cuthbert, A. P., Trott, D. A., Newbold, R. F., and Nabholz, M. (2003). A chromosome 3-encoded repressor of the human telomerase reverse transcriptase (hTERT) gene controls the state of hTERT chromatin. *Cancer Res*, **63,** 689–95.

Tominaga, K., Olgun, A., Smith, J. R., and Pereira-Smith, O. M. (2002). Genetics of cellular senescence. *Mech Ageing Dev*, **123,** 927–36.

White, L. K., Wright, W. E., and Shay, J. W. (2001). Telomerase inhibitors. *Trends Biotechnol*, **19,** 114–20.

Yaswen, P. and Stampfer, M. R. (2002). Molecular changes accompanying senescence and immortalization of cultured human mammary epithelial cells. *Int J Biochem Cell Biol*, **1300,** 1–13.

*The reader is directed to a recent review by the author (Newbold, 2002) for a comprehensive list of references underpinning the various topics covered in this chapter.

CHAPTER 11

Growth factors and their signalling pathways in cancer

Sally A. Prigent

11.1 Introduction

The organization of cells into multicellular organisms depends upon sophisticated communication systems. During development, and in the mature organism, cells need to be able to sense the appropriate time to grow, divide, migrate, differentiate, survive, or die. These processes are all controlled by families of growth factors, which bind to specific receptors on the surface of their target cells. Once activated, these receptors initiate signalling pathways, which determine the response of the cells. Aberrant activation of one or more of these pathways can lead to unregulated cell division, and the formation of a tumour.

While there are many kinds of growth factor receptors, two families have emerged as promising therapeutic targets in the treatment of cancer; the epidermal growth factor receptor (EGFR) family, and the vascular endothelial growth factor (VEGF) receptors. While EGFR and its relatives are expressed on epithelial cell-derived tumour cells and contribute directly to tumour cell growth, VEGF receptors are expressed on the endothelial cells lining blood vessels, which are normal, untransformed cells. VEGF receptors contribute to tumour growth by triggering vessel growth which is essential to supply nutrients to a growing tumour. This chapter will consider the signalling pathways initiated by EGFR and VEGF receptors, their respective roles in normal growth and development, and the mechanisms by which signalling can become deregulated in cancer.

11.2 The EGF/ErbB family of growth factors and receptors

11.2.1 Epidermal growth factor receptors

The EGF family of growth factor receptors comprises four family members: EGF receptor (ErbB1/HER1), ErbB2 (HER2/neu), ErbB3 (HER3), and ErbB4 (HER4) (Jorissen et al., 2003). These receptors share a similar domain structure, as illustrated in Figure 11.1. The extracellular domain of each consists of four subdomains: ligand-binding domains L1 and L2, and two cysteine-rich domains C1 and C2. L1 and L2 fold to form a ligand-binding pocket, whereas the C1 and C2 domains contain disulphide bonded modules and support the structure of the ligand-binding regions (Garrett et al., 2002; Ogiso et al., 2002). The C2 domain appears to be involved in ensuring that the receptors are targeted to the lipid raft sub-domains of the cell membrane, which are regions rich in signalling molecules. Parts of the C1 domain are also involved in interactions between two receptors present in a dimer. The receptors are anchored in the membrane by means of a single membrane-spanning region consisting of around 22 hydrophobic residues forming an α-helix. The cytoplasmic domain of the receptors contains the highly conserved kinase domain, which is responsible for binding ATP and transferring phosphate groups onto tyrosine residues of other receptors and signalling molecules. In the case of ErbB3, the kinase is inactive due to the substitution of critical residues within the catalytic domain (Guy et al., 1994). The juxtamembrane region is responsible for binding proteins involved in receptor internalization and sorting, and recruitment of some proteins involved in downstream signalling (see below). The C-terminal tail differs between each of the receptors and is the main region responsible for recruitment of signalling molecules.

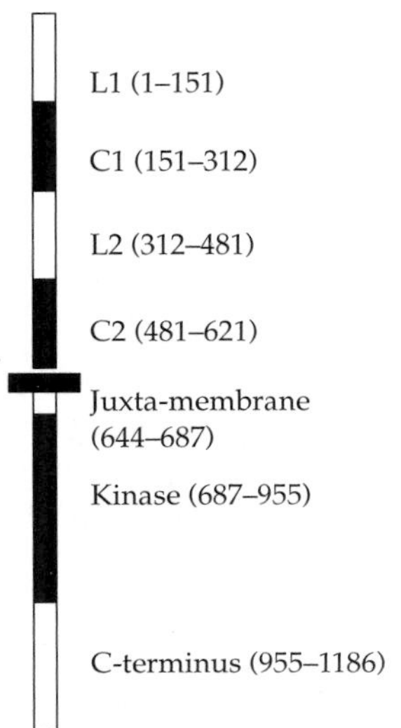

Figure 11.1 Domain structure of the EGF receptor. L1 and L2 refer to ligand-binding domains, C1 and C2 indicate cysteine-rich domains. Aminoacid residues are indicated in parentheses.

11.2.2 Ligands

Eleven related ligands have been identified for ErbB receptors, each containing an EGF-like domain (Harris et al., 2003). These can be divided into three categories on the basis of their receptor binding specificity (Table 11.1). The first group includes EGF, transforming growth factor alpha (TGFα), epigen and amphiregulin, and bind selectively to EGFR. The second group comprising betacellulin, heparin-binding EGF and epiregulin also bind EGFR, but in addition can bind to ErbB4. The third group, the neuregulins, do not bind EGFR, but have different binding specificities for ErbB3 and ErbB4. These can be divided into two sub-groups; NRG-1 and NRG-2 bind ErbB3 and ErbB4, whereas NRG-3 and NRG-4 bind exclusively to ErbB4. ErbB2 does not bind directly to any ligand.

Table 11.1 EGF-related growth factors and their receptors

Receptor	Ligand
EGFR/ErbB1	EGF TGFα
	Amphiregulin
	Betacellulin
	HB-EGF
	Epiregulin
ErbB2	No ligand
ErbB3	NRG-1
	NRG-2
ErbB4	Betacellulin
	HB-EGF
	Epiregulin
	NRG-1
	NRG-2
	NRG-3
	NRG-4

EGFR binding ligands are all synthesized as precursors which are transmembrane proteins with a single membrane spanning segment. The mature peptide is in each case cleaved from the extracellular domain of the precursor by the action of proteases, to release a soluble growth factor. In the case of TGFα, the metalloprotease, tumour necrosis factor alpha converting enzyme, (TACE or ADAM17) has been shown by knock-out studies to be involved in its processing (Sunnarborg et al., 2002). This enzyme is most likely involved in the processing of other EGF-like ligands. While TGFα is rapidly cleaved at the membrane to produce a soluble growth factor, one of the EGF-like ligands, HB-EGF remains at the membrane in its precursor form (pro-HB-EGF) for a longer time, such that the majority of the protein remains at the cell surface (Nanba and Higashiyama, 2004). All of the mature, soluble EGF-like growth factors are characterized by the presence of six conserved cysteine residues in the consensus (CX7 CX4-5 CX10-13 CXCX8 C). The cysteine residues form three disulfide bonds, critical for function such that Cys1 forms a bond with Cys3; Cys2 with Cys4, and Cys5 with Cys6. The disulfide-bonded region is termed the EGF-like motif. Of the EGF-like ligands, TGFα has most frequently been the ligand implicated in cancer.

The neuregulins (NRGs) represent perhaps the most complex family of all growth factors (Falls, 2003). Of this family, NRG-1 is the best characterized. NRG-1 is encoded by an enormous gene, some 1.4 megabases long. Through alternative splicing and the use of more than one promoter at least 15 distinct protein products are produced from this gene. NRGs can most simply be divided into two groups depending on the presence of an immunoglobulin-like domain in addition to the EGF-like domain (Ig-NRGs), or the presence of an additional cysteine-rich domain (CRD-NRGs). Of the 11 Ig-NRGs, 7 are produced as type I transmembrane proteins (in common with the EGFR ligands described above). Similarly the bioactive peptide is shed by protein cleavage possibly involving the metalloproteases ADAM17 and ADAM19 (Montero et al., 2000; Shirakabe et al., 2001). One Ig-NRG splice variant is produced as a secreted form, the remaining forms are unlikely to be released from the cell, or to be bioactive. The distinguishing feature of the CRD-NRGs, is the presence of a second membrane localization sequence, such that the protein spans the membrane twice, with both N- and C-termini being cytoplasmic. While the EGF-like domain is exposed, very little peptide is shed by proteolytic cleavage such that the majority of the peptide remains membrane-bound (Wang et al., 2001). The presentation of these splice variants of NRG-1 has important bearing on their biological properties. While the majority of the Ig-NRGs are produced as soluble peptides that can diffuse short distances and can act either on the same cell or cell type (i.e. in an autocrine fashion), or a different cell type (paracrine signalling), CRD-NRGs can only signal efficiently by direct cell–cell contact with the receptor (juxtacrine signalling). Thus CRD-NRGs perform an analagous role to proHB-EGF of the EGFR binding ligands.

11.3 Receptor activation

It is generally accepted that ligand binding to a receptor tyrosine kinase (RTK) leads to dimerization, or oligomerization, resulting in a conformational change in the receptor which leads to activation of the tyrosine kinase. In some cases, the ligand itself is a dimer, as is the case for VEGF, and it is easy to understand how ligand binding could promote dimerization. In the case of EGF, and its related growth factors, these are monomers, and it is only recently that the crystal structure of ligand-bound EGF receptor extracellular domains has shed light on the mechanism by which dimerization is enhanced upon ligand binding (Garrett et al., 2002; Ogiso et al., 2002) (Figure 11.2). In the absence of ligand, EGFR exists in an equilibrium between a low-affinity monomer, and a high-affinity monomer. In the low-affinity form, intramolecular interactions occur between the C1 and C2 domains, whereas in the high-affinity form, these interactions are absent. Dimerization can occur between these monomers in the absence of ligand, driven by interactions between the kinase or transmembrane domains. These dimers are not however activated until a ligand binds. In the ligand-bound form, a loop from one C1 ectodomain interlocks with a pocket in the adjacent receptor C1 domain, thereby stabilizing the dimeric form. This interaction is necessary to promote a conformational change required for activation of the RTK (Walker et al., 2004). Some RTKs, such as the insulin receptor, require phosphorylation of a critical tyrosine residue with the activation loop of the kinase for optimal kinase activity (Hubbard et al., 1998), however this does not appear to be the case for EGF receptor. Once activated, adjacent receptors

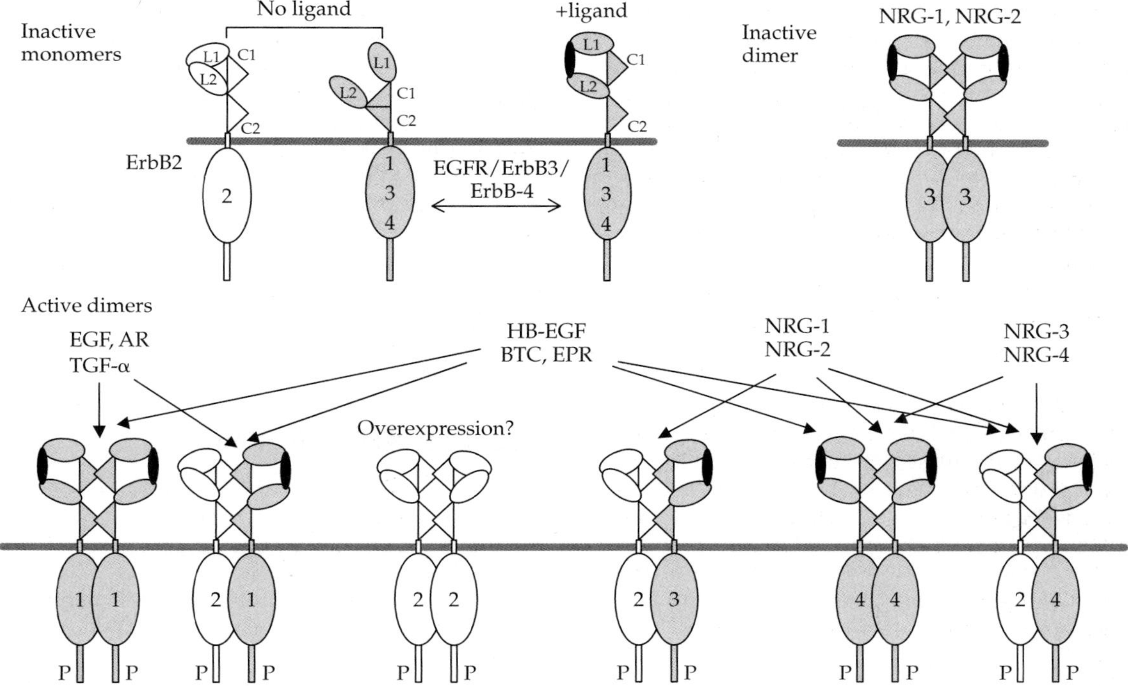

Figure 11.2 Ligand-induced dimerization and activation of ErbB receptors. In the absence of ligand, intramolecular interactions between the C1 and C2 domains of EGFR, ErbB3 and ErbB4 prevent exposure of dimerization loops, and maintain the receptors in an inactive state. Upon ligand binding, dimerization loops within the C1 and C2 domains (represented by triangles) become exposed, facilitating either homo-, or heterodimerization as indicated. In the case of ErbB2, dimerisation loops are exposed in the absence of ligand, enabling it to form dimers with ligand-bound EGFR, ErbB3, and ErbB4. Overexpression of ErbB2 may facilitate spontaneous homodimerization and activation.

cross-phosphorylate each other at distinct tyrosine residues thereby initiating signalling pathways.

11.4 Heterodimerization

Dimerization between identical receptors is referred to as homodimerization. In addition to promoting homodimer formation, all ErbB ligands are able to promote heterodimerization between different receptors of the ErbB family. ErbB2 is the preferred heterodimerization partner for all ErbB receptors. In fact the most potent signalling dimer is that containing ErbB2 and ErbB3. This is remarkable as ErbB2 has no ligand and ErbB3 has no catalytic activity. The reason that ErbB2 makes such a good dimerization partner is that the 'dimerization loop' that protrudes from the C1 extracellular domain in a ligand-dependent fashion in the case of EGFR, is permanently extended in the case of ErbB2 (Garrett et al., 2003). Thus ErbB2 is able to dimerize with any ligand-bound monomeric ErbB receptor. When ErbB2 is overexpressed, as occurs in certain tumours (see below) it is able to spontaneously dimerize and become activated in a ligand-independent fashion.

11.5 The role of tyrosine phosphorylation

A major breakthrough in understanding how RTKs signal was made in the early 1990s with the discovery of structural modules termed SH2 (Src-homology-2) domains. SH2 domains are found in a wide variety of proteins involved in signalling and selectively bind to phosphorylated tyrosine residues. The specificity of binding of distinct SH2 domains is determined by the sequence of amino-acids surrounding the phosphotyrosine residue. Generally it is the three residues C-terminal to the phosphorylated tyrosine which determine binding specificity. This discovery led to the conceptual breakthrough that the subset of pathways activated by a receptor can be determined by its primary aminoacid sequence. Subsequently the phosphotyrosine binding (PTB) domain was identified as a phosphotyrosine interaction domain of quite different structure. In this case binding specificity is determined by residues N-terminal to the phosphorylated tyrosine. The domain structure of various signalling proteins is illustrated in Figure 11.3.

In the case of EGFR, five major autophosphorylation sites have been reported at tyrosines 992, 1068, 1086, 1148, and 1173. These act as docking sites for a variety of signalling molecules illustrated in Figure 11.4. Additional sites have been shown to be phosphorylated by Src (Y891, Y920) (Stover et al., 1995), and phosphorylation of Y1068 by Jak2 has been shown to provide a cross-talk mechanism for signalling via growth hormone (Yamauchi et al., 1997). Of the proteins recruited to activated EGFR, some are adaptor proteins, or scaffolds, which assemble complexes of other active molecules on the receptor. These include Grb2, Shc, Crk, Nck, and Dok-R (Okutani et al., 1994; Hashimoto et al., 1998; McCarty, 1998; Okabayashi et al., 1994; Jones et al., 1999). Others possess enzymatic activity and include non-RTKs such as Src and Abl (Zhu et al., 1994; Stover et al., 1995); tyrosine phosphatases PTB-1B and SHP-1 (Milarski et al., 1993; Keilhack et al., 1998), Phospholipase C-γ (Chattopadhyay et al., 1999) and the GTPase activating protein for Ras, p120 RasGAP (Serth et al., 1992). Once bound to the activated receptor, some of the proteins are themselves phosphorylated with a resulting increase in enzymatic activity (e.g. PLCγ), or phosphorylation of the bound protein creates a further docking site for another protein (e.g. phosphorylation of Shc creates a docking site for Grb2). The major pathways initiated by interactions with EGFR will be considered below, and are reviewed in detail elsewhere (Jorissen et al., 2003).

11.5.1 Ras-Raf-MAP kinase pathway

One of the major mitogenic signalling pathways initiated by RTKs in the mitogen-activated protein

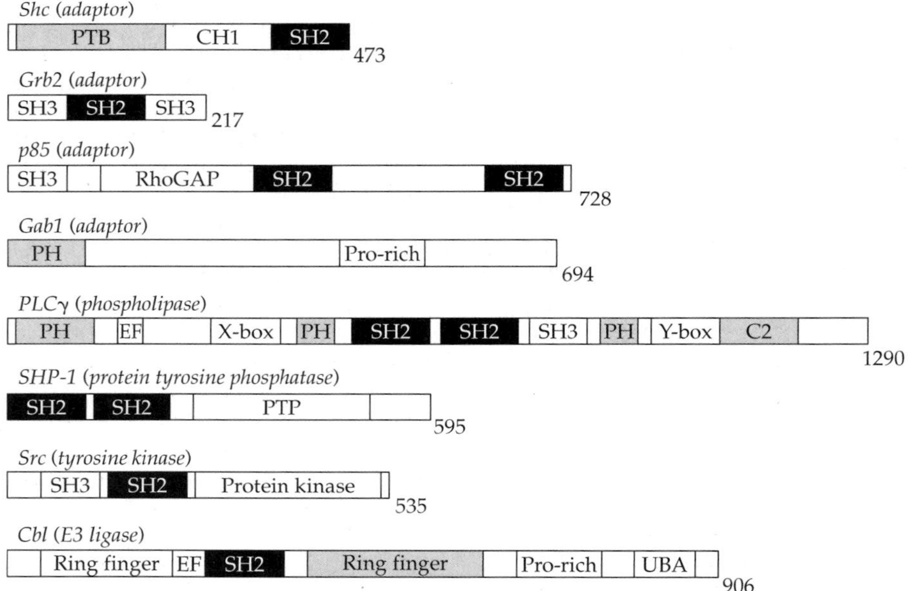

Figure 11.3 Domain structure of selected signalling proteins. Proteins involved in cell signaling comprise various functional domains which either possess catalytic activity (e.g. protein kinase; protein tyrosine phosphatase (PTP); X- and Y-box of phospholipase C) or are involved in interactions with other proteins, lipids or ions. Src homology 2 (SH2) and phosphotyrosine binding (PTB) domains recognize motifs containing phosphotyrosine; Pleckstrin homology (PH) domains are involved in protein–protein and protein–lipid interactions; SH3 domains recognize proline-rich motifs RXLPPLPXX or XXXPPLPXR (where X is any aminoacid); EF-hand (EF) and C2 domains bind calcium ions; ring-finger domains bind zinc ions; 4H domains contain four helices; RhoGAP domain has homology to Rho GTPase activating protein (GAP).

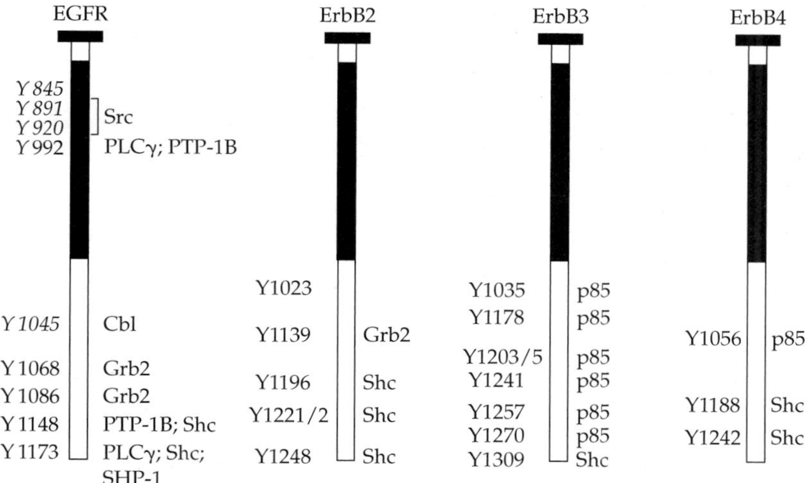

Figure 11.4 Binding of signalling proteins to phosphorylation sites on ErbB receptors. Some of the signalling proteins that have been shown to bind specific phosphorylation sites of ErbB receptors are indicated. In the case of EGFR and ErbB2, autophosphorylation sites have been mapped directly by *in vivo* labelling studies, whereas sites on ErbB3 and ErbB4 have been inferred by phosphopeptide competition studies. Sites indicated in italics are phosphorylated by Src.

(MAP) kinase pathway (Figure 11.5(a)). This pathway is initiated by binding of either Grb2 or Shc to the activated EGFR. Both Grb2 and Shc are modular proteins comprising of protein–protein interaction domains. Grb2 contains one SH2 domain which binds either phosphorylated Y1068 or Y1086 of the EGFR, and two SH3 domains. Shc contains one SH2, one PTB and a collagen homology domain which can be phosphorylated by the EGFR at three distinct sites Y239, Y240, and Y317. Phosphorylation of these sites creates two potential p-YXN motifs which can bind the SH2 domain of Grb2. Shc interacts predominantly with Y1173 and Y1148 of EGFR through its PTB domain. Thus Grb2 can bind either directly to the EGFR or indirectly through Shc. The N-terminal SH3 domain of Grb2 constitutively associates with a proline-rich sequence on the nucleotide exchange factor, SOS, which regulates the activity of Ras proteins. Thus when Grb2 associates with the EGFR it brings with it the key regulator of the Ras-Raf-MAP kinase pathway. Ras is a guanosine triphosphate (GTP) binding protein, which is localized to the plasma membrane by virtue of a fatty acid, farnesyl chain modification. In fact there are three Ras genes *KRAS*, *NRAS*, and *HRAS*, which are commonly mutated in cancer. In its inactive form, Ras is bound to guanosine diphosphate (GDP). Recruitment of SOS to activated EGFR places it in close proximity to Ras, enabling it to catalyse the exchange of GTP for GDP, converting Ras into the GTP-bound active form. When Ras is in its GTP-bound state, it is able to associate with the serine-threonine kinase Raf-1. All three Ras proteins (H-Ras, K-Ras, and N-Ras) are able to bind Raf-1 and will be referred to collectively as Ras. Binding of Raf-1 to Ras leads to direct activation of Raf-1, but also leads to changes in its phosphorylation state regulated by other kinases and phosphatases. It has been reported that in its inactive form Raf-1 is phosphorylated at two serine residues (259 and 621) which enable it to bind to 14-3-3 proteins which sequester it in its inactive form. Displacement of 14-3-3 upon Ras binding permits dephosphorylation of these residues. Additional phosphorylation events have been reported which lead to further activation of Raf-1, including phosphorylation of serine 338, and tyrosine phosphorylation of residue 341 (Mason et al., 1999; Sun et al., 2000). The best characterized targets for phosphorylation by activated Raf-1 are the dual specificity kinases MEK1 and MEK2. Both kinases contain a proline-rich region which is thought to be responsible for recognition by Raf proteins. MEK1 is activated by phosphorylation at two serine residues (S218 and S222) (Alessi et al., 1994). The dual specificity kinases MEK1 and MEK2 in turn phosphorylate and activate the MAP kinases, ERK1 and ERK2, at threonine and tyrosine residues with a conserved TEY motif in the activation loop. ERK1

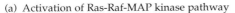

(a) Activation of Ras-Raf-MAP kinase pathway

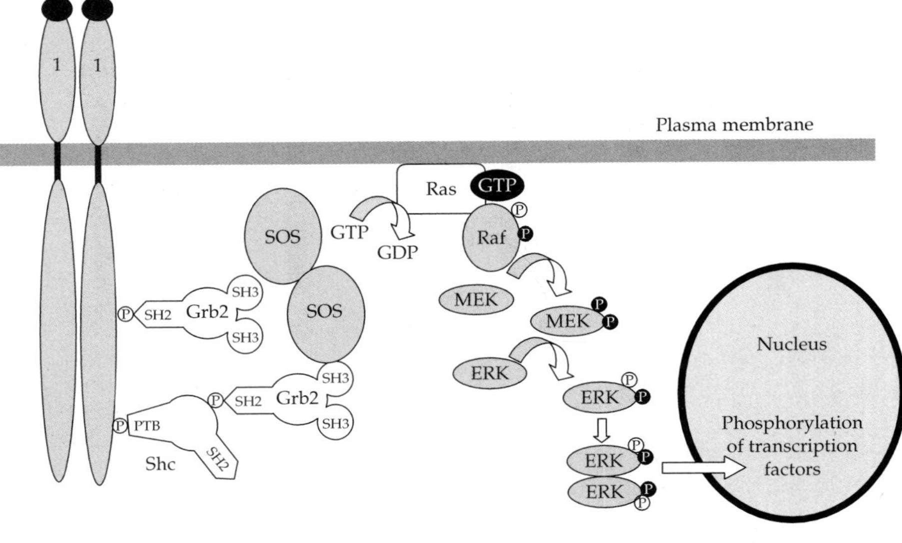

(b) Lipid signalling

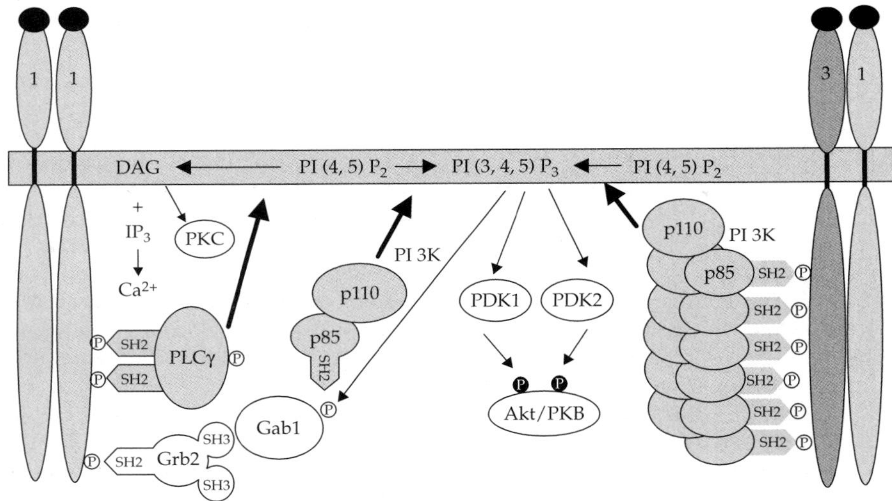

Figure 11.5 Major EGF-regulated signalling pathways. (a) Adaptor proteins Grb2 and Shc are recruited to phosphtyrosine residues on activated EGF receptor (1). Shc is phosphorylated by EGFR creating two further docking sites for Grb2. Grb2 is constitutively bound to the nucleotide exchange factor SOS, thus recruitment of Grb2 to activated receptors brings SOS close to the membrane where it catalyses the guanine nucleotide exchange on Ras. Activated Ras associates with Raf serine/threonine kinases, which require phosphorylation on tyrosine and serine residues for optimal activity. Raf phosphorylates and activates the dual specificity kinases MEK1 and MEK2, which in turn phosphorylate, and activate ERK1 and ERK2 on both a tyrosine and threonine residue. Active ERK undergoes dimerization and translocation to the nucleus where it phosphorylates and activates transcription factors. (b) Activated EGFR (1) directly binds PLCγ through either its N- or C-terminal SH2 domain, and itself becomes phosphorylated on tyrosine. PLCγ catalyses the conversion of phosphatidylinositol (PI) 4,5 bisphosphate to inositol trisphospate (IP_3) and diacylglycerol (DAG). DAG is an activator of protein kinase C (PKC), whereas IP_3 stimulates the release of calcium ions from intracellular stores thereby activating calcium-regulated enzymes. Phosphoinositide 3-kinase (PI 3K) is comprised of two subunits, an inactive adaptor subunit, p85, and a catalytic subunit p110. PI 3K does not efficiently bind directly to EGFR. It is recruited indirectly via the adaptor protein Gab1, which interacts with the SH3 domain of Grb2, or by binding to ErbB3 (3), which is a heterodimerization partner for EGFR. Both Gab1 and ErbB3 contain multiple YXXM motifs which, when phosphorylated bind p85. PI 3K phosphorylates the 3-OH position of the inositol ring of phosphatidlyinositol lipids, generating lipids that bind PH-domains. PDK-1 and PDK-2 are serine/threonine kinases activated by PI (3,4,5) P3, which in turn phosphorylate, and activate the serine/threonine kinase Akt/PKB.

and ERK2 translocate to the nucleus where they catalyse the phosphorylation of nuclear transcription factors such as AP1, Sp1, E2F, Myc, and Elk-1 leading to increased transcription. ERK1 and 2 also phosphorylate SOS leading to the dissociation of the Grb2-SOS complex, thereby inactivating the initial signal (Langlois et al., 1995).

Although Raf-1 was originally identified as the major effector of Ras, partly due to the fact that it is the most abundant, ubiquitously expressed form, and partly due to experiments using dominant-negative Raf-1 constructs to inhibit signalling induced by active forms of Ras, there is increasing evidence to suggest that the related B-Raf protein may be the most important physiological regulator of the Ras-Raf-MAP kinase pathway. Although B-Raf is expressed at very low levels in many tissues, its activity is disproportionately high. For example, in mouse embryo fibroblasts where Raf-1 is expressed at high levels and B-raf protein is barely detectable, B-Raf displays a much higher level of biochemical activity (Huser et al., 2001). Results from knock-out studies in mice suggest that Raf-1 does not play a major role in normal cell proliferation, but may be involved in protecting cells from apoptosis, whereas B-Raf appears to be the major regulator of ERK activity and associated cell proliferation.

11.5.2 Phospholipid metabolism

Phospholipase C-γ binds directly to activated EGFR at tyrosine residues Y1173 and Y993, and is itself a substrate for phosphorylation at Y771 and Y1254. Once activated, PLCγ catalyses the conversion of PtdIns (4,5)-P2 to inositol (1,3,5) trisphosphate (IP3) and diacylglycerol (DAG) (Figure 11.5(b)). DAG is an activator of the serine-threonine kinase, protein kinase C (PKC). PKC activates a number of signalling pathways, including the MAP kinase pathway through direct activation of Raf-1. IP3 induces the mobilization of Ca^{2+} from intracellular stores, resulting in the activation of Ca^{2+}/calmodulin dependent-enzymes.

A second phospholipase, phospholipase D2 (PLD2) has also been shown to directly associate with, and be activated by EGFR, although the mechanism for association and activation remains less clear. PLD2 catalyses the conversion of phosphatidylcholine into choline and phosphatidic acid (PA). PA, and its metabolic product are important second messengers (Houle and Bourgoin, 1999).

One of the most important phospholipid modifying enzymes in signal transduction downstream of RTKs is phosphatidyl inositol 3′ kinase Ia. Other classes of phosphatidyl inositol 3′ kinase exist with different subunit composition and substrate specificity, but as they are not activated by RTKs, they will not be discussed here. Phosphatidyl inositol 3′ kinase Ia (hereafter referred to as PI3 kinase) phosphorylates the 3′ position of phosphatidyl inositols to create phospholipids capable of binding protein domains. Specifically, PI3 kinase catalyses the conversion of phosphatidylinositol (4,5) bisphosphate to phosphatidylinositol (3,4,5) trisphosphate (Figure 11.5(b)). The 5′-phosphate group is then hydrolysed through the action of 5′-inositol phosphatases to generate PtdIns (3,4) P2. Both of these lipid products bind PH domains. One of the most important biological consequences of this reaction is that it promotes the relocalization of specific proteins containing PH domains to various membrane compartments, most notably, the plasma membrane. EGF is an important activator of PI3 kinase in cells, but in contrast to other receptors, it does not associate directly with PI3 kinase. PI3 kinase consists of an adaptor subunit, p85, and a catalytic subunit, p110 with lipid kinase activity. It is the p85 subunit which contains an SH2 domain able to interact with phosphotyrosines in the consensus sequence pYXXM. Following p85 binding to a phosphorylated receptor, or docking protein, the p110 subunit is activated by an allosteric mechanism.

EGFR utilizes two main indirect mechanisms for activating PI3 kinase. The first of these mechanisms involves an additional scaffold protein, Gab1 (Gu and Neel, 2003), which is able to bind to the C-terminal SH3 domain of Grb2. Gab1 is termed a scaffold as it is able to recruit multiple signalling proteins but has no enzymatic activity itself. Gab1 contains a PH domain which binds to 3′ phosphoinositides, multiple phosphorylation sites which interact with SH2-domain containing proteins and three prolyl-rich domains which interact with SH3 domain-containing proteins. Following recruitment to activated EGFR through Grb2, Gab1 becomes phosphorylated by the EGFR. Phosphorylation permits the binding of PI3 kinase to phosphorylated YXXM motifs on Gab1. PtdIns (3,4,5)P3 at the membrane is then able to bind the PH domain of Gab1, thereby promoting a more sustained signalling event. Thus utilization of Gab1 permits the activation of additional signalling pathways by increasing the number of available effector docking sites.

The second mechanism through which EGF promotes activation of PI3 kinase is through heterodimerization with the related erbB3 receptor. In contrast to EGFR, erbB3 contains six potential p85 binding motifs, and is the major p85 binding receptor (Prigent and Gullick, 1994).

The best characterized downstream mediator of PI3 kinase activity is the serine/threonine kinase Akt/PKB (Vanhaesebroeck and Alessi, 2000). This kinase contains a PH domain and is recruited to the membrane upon PI3 kinase activation where it is phosphorylated and activated by another PH-domain-containing kinase, PDK1. Akt is involved in inhibiting the activity of proapoptosis proteins such as BAD, Glycogen synthase kinase 3 and the forkhead transcription factor FKHR-L1, thereby promoting cell survival. Another effect of Akt activation is the downregulation of the cell-cycle inhibitor p27, thereby promoting cell-cycle progression and proliferation.

11.5.3 Other pathways

Although the precise details of activation are unclear, there is abundant evidence in the literature that non-RTKs such as Src are involved in EGFR signalling and consequent induction of cell proliferation (Leu and Maa, 2003). The physiological binding site for Src on EGFR has not been defined. However Src is able to phosphorylate EGFR at two sites (Y891 and Y920), both of which are capable of binding the Src SH2 domain. One of these sites is also able to bind p85, but this does not appear to be the main mechanism for activation of PI3 kinase by EGFR. Another class of signalling molecule involved in EGFR signalling are the STAT transcription factors (David et al., 1996). These transcription factors have a major role in cytokine signalling where they are classically activated by Janus kinases (JAKs). JAKs bind constitutively to receptors such as growth hormone receptor, which has no kinase activity of its own, and are activated upon ligand binding to promote phosphorylation of the receptor. STATs are then recruited to the receptor through their SH2 domain, phosphorylated by JAK enabling them to homo- or heterodimerize and translocate to the nucleus where they initiate transcription. GH activation of JAK2 has been shown to lead to phosphorylation of EGFR such that it is able to recruit Grb2 and initiate the MAP kinase pathway, an example of transactivation of an EGFR-mediated pathway by a distinct ligand/receptor family. Activation of STATs by EGFR does not involve JAKs, and there are reports which suggest that STATs are constitutively bound to EGFR (Olayioye et al., 1999). It is not clear whether they are phosphorylated and activated by the EGFR itself, or Src kinase.

11.6 Signalling through ErbB2, ErbB3

As already mentioned, ErbB2 has no ligand and therefore cannot signal on its own, unless expressed at such high levels that it spontaneously dimerizes. ErbB3 has no catalytic activity and therefore requires a kinase-competent dimerization partner to signal. Together, ErbB2/ErbB3 heterodimers make a highly effective signalling dimer (Citri et al., 2003). Transphosphorylation of ErbB3 by ErbB2 creates six binding sites for PI3 kinase and potently activates this survival pathway, whereas ErbB2 itself is not able to interact directly with p85. ErbB2 on the other hand is able to potently activate the Ras-MAP kinase pathway as it possesses several Grb2 and Shc binding sites. ErbB3 can similarly activate MAP kinase by interaction with the Shc adaptor. The major downstream target of signalling via ErbB2 is cyclin D1, which is critically involved in progression through the G1/S phase of cell cycle by activation of cyclin-dependent kinases CDK4 and CDK6. Cyclin D1 is transcriptionally upregulated by E2F, Myc, and Sp1 transcription factors, substrates of Erk1/2 MAP kinases. Thus the heterodimer of ErbB2/ErbB3 drives cell proliferation though activation of the MAP kinase pathway, and promotes cell survival and resistance to apoptosis through very efficient activation of PI3 kinase. PLCγ is also activated by the heterodimer, by recruitment of the enzyme to ErbB2.

As well as promoting optimal activation of all major signalling pathways, an additional property of ErbB2-containing heterodimers is their relatively long half-life at the cell surface. This is a consequence of a very slow rate of internalization following ligand binding, resulting in more sustained signalling (see below). An additional means by which ErbB2 promotes optimal sustained signalling is by increasing the affinity of its dimerization partner for ligand, again resulting in more sustained signalling.

An 85 kDa secreted ErbB3 ectodomain has recently been described which is able to attenuate signalling via ErbB2, ErbB3, and ErbB4 by sequestration of ligands (Lee et al., 2001).

11.7 ErbB4

ErbB4 is perhaps the least well characterized of the ErbB receptors, and no unique signalling pathways have been shown to be associated with this receptor (Carpenter, 2003*a*). It possesses binding sites for Shc and Grb2 suggesting that it signals through the Ras/MAP kinase pathways and a single binding site for p85, enabling it to activate PI3 kinase, albeit less potently than ErbB3. A splice variant of ErbB4 lacks this p85 binding site, and presumably does not signal though PI3 kinase. The JAK/STAT pathway has also been shown to be activated down stream of ErbB4. A unique feature of this receptor is the regulation of its activity though proteolytic cleavage of the extracellular domain (see below).

11.8 Switching off the signal

Following activation of ErbB kinases by ligand binding, various mechanisms exist to terminate the signals induced. One of the earliest feedback mechanisms identified was the phosphorylation of EGFR by PKC resulting in a reduced kinase activity (Cochet et al., 1984). A more significant mechanism for downregulation of EGFR activity is through ligand-induced internalization, and subsequent degradation (Lipkowitz, 2003). Although ErbB2, ErbB3, and ErbB4 display a basal level of internalization, this is not enhanced by the presence of ligand. In contrast, binding of ligand to EGFR results in rapid internalization followed, in general, by degradation of the receptor and ligand. One of the major proteins involved in this ligand-stimulated degradation is the ubiquitin ligase Cbl, which contains a PTB domain and binds to a subset of RTKs including EGFR (Levkowitz et al., 1996). Ubiquitin ligases catalyse the covalent attachment of ubiquitin, a 76 aminoacid peptide, to specific lysine residues on substrate proteins. Ubiquitin molecules can be added individually resulting in monoubiquitination, or as a chain of ubiquitin molecules resulting in polyubiquitination. Classically polyubiquitination has been linked to protein degradation via the proteasome. Monoubiquitination of EGFR has been shown to be sufficient for internalization and degradation of the EGFR via the lysosome (Haglund et al., 2003) (Figure 11.6). Following ligand-induced autophosphorylation of EGFR, Cbl is recruited to Y1045 via its PTB domain, or it binds indirectly via Grb2. Once bound, Cbl is phosphorylated by Src kinases which enhances its binding to Grb2, and facilitates association with the protein CIN85 and its constitutively bound partner endophilin. Endophilins in turn have been shown to bind a number of proteins involved in clathrin-mediated endocytosis, including the GTPase dynamin. Thus the Cbl initiated multi-protein complex targets the EGFR to the machinery controlling clathrin-mediated endocytois. Cbl catalyses the ubiquitination of EGFR providing interaction sites for two protein adaptors, Epsin and Eps15, which contain ubiquitin-interaction motifs (UIMs). Evidence suggests that these proteins have a role in directing the EGFR to clathrin-coated pits. Internalized EGFR passes through three distinct endocytic compartments: the early endosome, the late endosome, and finally the lysosome. Cbl association is required throughout the endocytic pathway in order to target the receptor for degradation by the hydrolytic enzymes in the lysosome. Interestingly, the acid conditions within the early endocytic vesicles result in the dissociation of the low-affinity ligand TGFα from the EGFR, the release of Cbl, and the subsequent recycling of EGFR instead of degradation. Thus the ligand can influence the fate of the receptor. Consequently, TGFα-induced signalling is more sustained than that induced by other EGF-like ligands, which may be the reason this growth factor is most commonly overexpressed in tumours. Receptors can also be 'diverted' to the recycling pathway by PKC-induced threonine phosphorylation. The reason that ErbB2, ErbB3, and ErbB4 do not undergo ligand-induced internalization and degradation is that they do not couple efficiently to Cbl.

Although ErbB4 does not undergo rapid ligand-induced internalization, it displays a different, very effective mechanism for terminating signals. The 120 kDa extracellular domain is shed from the cell surface following stimulation with NRG-1, by a mechanism involving the metalloproteinase, TACE (also involved in the processing of EGF-like ligands), leaving an 80 kDa, membrane-associated cytoplasmic domain. A second protease γ-secretin cleaves the 80 kDa truncated receptor within the membrane, releasing it into the cytosol. This soluble ErbB4 cytoplasmic domain has been shown to

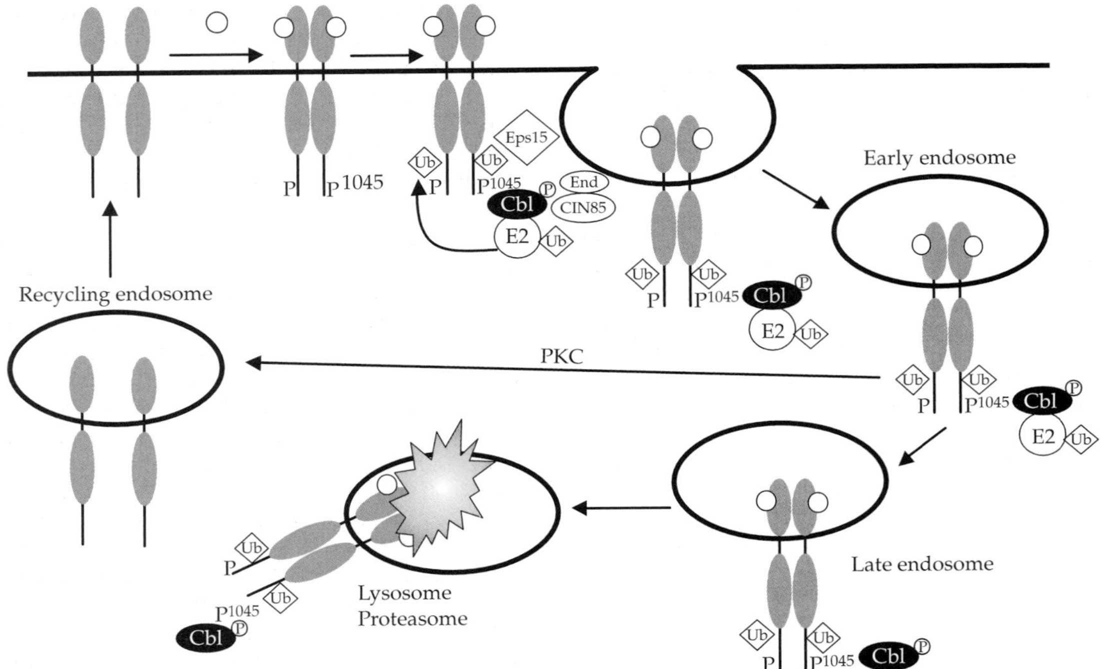

Figure 11.6 Ligand-induced EGFR downregulation. Following ligand binding, the E3 ubiquitin ligase, Cbl, is recruited to Y1045 of the EGFR, and in association with the E2 conjugating enzyme, catalyses the ubiquitination of the EGFR, and subsequent internalization and degradation. CIN85 and its associated endophilins, and Eps15 are involved in growth factor receptor internalization, the former through interaction with Cbl, the latter through interaction with ubiquitin. Phosphorylation by protein kinase C (PKC), stimulates recycling of EGFR from the early endosome.

translocate to the nucleus, though its function there is unclear (Carpenter, 2003*b*).

Tyrosine phosphatases associated directly with EGFR (SHP-1, PTP1B) or indirectly via the adaptor Gab1 (SHP-2), might be expected to have a role in dephosphorylation and switching off receptor signalling. While there is some evidence that SHP-1 negatively regulates EGFR signalling (Keilhack et al., 1998), most of the evidence for SHP-2 suggests that it is a positive effector of EGF signalling and enhances MAP kinase activation. The mechanism by which SHP-2 increases MAP kinase activation has recently been shown to involve the dephosphorylation of Y992 of EGFR, the binding site for RasGAP, a negative regulator of Ras activity (Agazie and Hayman, 2003). Failure to recruit RasGAP results in an increase in Ras activity and activation of the MAP kinase pathway.

An important enzyme involved in termination of signalling via the PI3 kinase pathway is the tumour suppressor PTEN (phosphatase and tensin homologue deleted on chromosome 10). PTEN is a lipid phosphatase that dephosphorylates the 3′ phosphate of PtdIns (3,4,5) P3 and PtdIns (3,4) P2. Effectively this protein switches off the PI3 kinase pathway.

11.9 Activation of ErbB receptors in cancer

The observation that altered signalling through EGF receptors is involved in cancer progression was first suspected when v-erbB, one of the oncogenes carried by the avian erythroblastosis virus was shown to encode a homologue of the human EGFR (Downward et al., 1984). Shortly thereafter an oncogenic form of rat ErbB2 (NeuT), which contained a point mutation within the transmembrane domain, was identified in animals treated with a carcinogen (Bargmann et al., 1986). Although mutations corresponding to either of the mutations in v-erbB, or NeuT do not exist in human cancers, activation of signalling pathways downstream of ErbB receptors has been linked to many different tumours. Of the ErbB receptors, evidence is most compelling for a role for EGFR and ErbB2 in cancer progression (Holbro et al., 2003). In addition to promoting tumour cell growth and inhibiting apoptosis, activation of ErbB-induced signalling pathways has been shown to result in an upregulation of matrix metalloproteases MMP2 and MMP9 involved in proteolysis of the extracellular matrix and invasion (O-charoenrat et al., 2000), and in the induction of expression of angiogenic growth factors such as VEGF-A (Petit et al., 1997). Various mechanisms exist for upregulation of ErbB-controlled pathways including receptor overexpression, often together with ligand; activating mutations of the receptor or downstream effector; or an inactivating mutation affecting a negative regulatory pathway.

The most common mechanism by which EGFR contributes to cancer is through overexpression, frequently along with one of its ligands, TGFα or EGF. Overexpression of EGFR is found in a proportion of tumours, particularly those of the breast, head and neck, and lung, either as a consequence of gene amplification, or more commonly due to increased mRNA production. Co-expression of TGFα and EGFR is associated with poor patient prognosis in invasive breast carcinomas. Several different mutant EGFRs have been identified in human tumours, the most common of which involves deletion of exons 2–7 from the extracellular domain (Kuan et al., 2001). This results in the deletion of residues 6–273 of the mature polypeptide, and the expression of an EGFR mutant (EGFRvIII) that cannot bind ligand, but is constitutively active due to a presumed conformational change. EGFRvIII was first identified in human glioblastomas, where it is observed in about 40–50% of advanced cases, but has since been described in cancers of the breast, lung and ovary, albeit at lower frequency. Expression of the EGFRvIII in cultured fibroblasts leads to cell transformation that is dependent upon PI3 kinase activity, but independent of ERK activity. Interestingly, the ERK-related stress-activated kinase, Jun N-terminal kinase, is constitutively activated in EGFRvIII transformed fibroblasts. In addition to being constitutively active, the mutant receptor has a reduced ability to recruit Cbl, and CIN85, and does not undergo ubiquitination or internalization (Schmidt et al., 2003). Escape from Cbl-mediated downregulation is an emerging theme for oncogenic deregulation of other receptor tyosine kinases (Peschard and Park, 2003).

ErbB2 is dramatically overexpressed in 20–25% of breast cancers as a result of gene amplification. This overexpresion correlates with poor tumour prognosis and resistance to chemotherapeutic agents. Overexpression is also observed in cancers of the ovary, bladder and stomach. Overexpression most likely leads to transformation by spontaneous formation of receptor homodimers with elevated kinase activity. In addition ErbB2-induced transformation probably results from signalling through ligand-dependent heterodimerization with EGFR, ErbB3, or ErbB4. Heterodimer formation with EGFR results in prolonged signalling as the heterodimer displays a slower rate of internalization, and diversion of EGFR to the recycling pathway rather than the degradation pathways.

ErbB3 and ErbB4 are expressed in a range of cancers including those of the breast, ovary, lung, skin, and gastrointestinal tract. ErbB3 shows enhanced tyrosine phosphorylation in tumours co-expressing ErbB2, and it is tempting to speculate that activation of ErbB3 via ErbB2 contributes to the transformation. The role of ErbB4 in cancer is the least well defined. Of particular interest is its role in paediatric brain tumours, where it is frequently co-expressed with ErbB2 (Gilbertson et al., 1997). Co-expression of the two receptors correlates with enhanced tumour proliferation and reduced patient survival.

Mutations in various signalling proteins downstream of the ErbB receptors contribute to tumorigenesis independently, or in co-operation with active ErbB signalling pathways. Mutations can activate components of the Ras/Raf/MAP kinase pathway leading to enhanced cell proliferation, or affect the regulation of the PI3 kinase/Akt pathway resulting in enhanced survival and resistance to apoptosis. Mutations in one of the three Ras genes *HRAS*, *NRAS*, or *KRAS* have been identified in around 30% of human tumours. *KRAS* mutations are the most common and are found in 70–90% of pancreatic adenocarcinomas, 50% of colon carcinomas and 25–50% of lung adenocarcinomas. Three codons (codons 12, 12, and 61) are affected by missense mutation, all of which result in the expression of mutant Ras proteins with increased levels of bound GTP, which are able to constitutively activate downstream signalling pathways. Downstream of Ras, activating mutations of the B-Raf kinase have been identified in a high percentage of malignant melanomas, and a proportion of colorectal cancers. Similar mutations in Raf-1 have yet to be identified. The predominant mutation involves the replacement of a glutamate residue for a valine residue within the activation segment of the kinase. This aminoacid substitution introduces a negative charge which is thought to mimic the activated form of B-Raf when it is phosphorylated on threonine 598 and serine 601 (Mercer and Pritchard, 1993).

Defects in the lipid phosphatase, PTEN, result in unchecked signalling via Akt and PDK1, as a result of an accumulation of PtdIns (3,4,5) P3. PTEN is a tumour suppressor protein located on chromosome 10q23.3. Somatic mutations in *PTEN* occur in a wide variety of sporadic tumours, most commonly in endometrial carcinomas and glioblastomas. Germline mutations in PTEN give rise to a variety of syndromes. Of particular note is Cowden disease, in which patients display an increased susceptibility to various cancers, including breast, thyroid, and endometrial carcinomas (Eng, 2003).

11.10 VEGF and its receptors

It has been accepted since the 1970s that tumour growth is dependent upon vascularization to supply oxygen and nutrients to the growing tumour (Folkman, 1990). For vascularization to occur, the nearest vessel or capillary needs to become destabilized so that the endothelial cells lining the vessel can loosen from their neighbours, migrate through the extracellular matrix towards the tumour, and redifferentiate into mature vessels. This process is termed angiogenesis and is described in more detail in Chapter 17. In this chapter we will focus on the key signalling events involved, and how interference with this signalling process can provide an attractive target for anti-cancer therapy.

Possibly the most important regulator of angiogenesis is VEGF (Ferrara et al., 2003; Cross et al., 2003). VEGF was first identified as a vascular permeability factor which promotes the leakage of plasma proteins, such as fibrinogen, into the extracellular spaces. It is proposed that this provides a provisional matrix that promotes the migration of endothelial cells. Since the identification of a number of related factors, VEGF is now commonly referred to as VEGF-A. VEGF-A binds to two related RTKs, VEGFR-1 (also known as Flt-1), and VEGFR-2 (also known as KDR, kinase domain-containing receptor, in humans, and Flk-1, fms-like kinase 1, in mice). VEGFR-1 is also a receptor for two related growth factors, VEGF-B and placental growth factor (PlGF, or sometimes called PGF). VEGFR-2 is a receptor for VEGF-C and VEGF-D (at least in humans, but not mice). VEGFR-1 and VEGFR-2 are expressed almost exclusively in endothelial cells lining blood vessels. A third VEGF receptor, VEGFR-3 (or Flt-3), binds VEGF-C and VEGF-D, and has been predominantly implicated in the process of lymphangiogenesis. This complex series of receptor–ligand interactions is illustrated in Figure 11.7. A soluble, secreted VEGFR-1 protein has also been described. A number of other co-receptors have been reported to modulate signalling through VEGFR-2 including VE-cadherin, $\alpha v\beta 3$ integrin, and neuropilin-1 and -2 (Soker et al., 1998; Rahimi et al.,1999; Borges et al., 2000). VE-cadherin is a cell–cell adhesion molecule which may negatively regulate the activity of VEGFR-2 in densely growing cells in culture. $\alpha v\beta 3$ integrin binds components of the extracellular matrix and is upregulated in endothelial cells undergoing angiogenesis. $\alpha v\beta 3$ integrin has been detected in complexes with VEGFR-2, and been shown to potentiate VEGFR-2 signalling. Neuropilin-1 and -2 are transmembrane proteins with short cytoplasmic tails, and no catalytic activity. They bind several VEGF-like ligands and are thought to enhance VEGFR signalling by presenting the ligand to the receptor in an efficient way. Neuropilins are able to bind PDZ-domain-containing proteins, and may have an independent signalling role, though this has yet to be defined.

Of the VEGFs, VEGF-A is still thought to be the most important regulator of angiogenesis. This information is partly due to the results of gene knock-out studies, where even the heterozygous mouse dies from severe vascular abnormalities, providing a rare example of a half-dosage effect (haploinsufficiency) causing embryonic lethality (Ferrara et al., 1996). In contrast, mice containing a targeted deletion of VEGF-B or PlGF (ligands for VEGFR-1) have very modest defects. The VEGF-B knock-out mice have small hearts, suggesting a possible role in cardiac angiogenesis, while the PlGF knock-out mice are overtly normal. Interestingly, while embryonic development is normal in mice

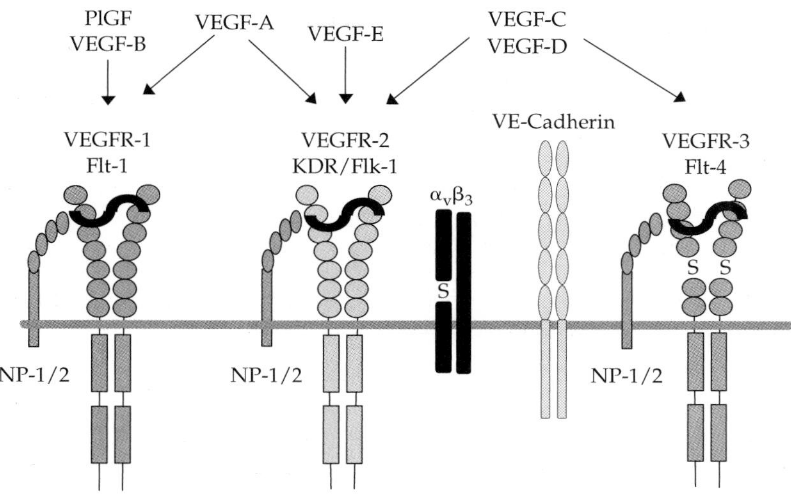

Figure 11.7 VEGF ligands and receptors. The binding-specificty of six VEGF receptor ligands (VEGF-A-E, PlGF) is indicated. Neuopilin-1 and -2 (NP1/2) are co-receptors which bind selectively to certain VEGF isoforms and potentiate signalling through VEGF receptors. $\alpha_v\beta_3$ integrin and VE-cadherin have been reported to associate with VEGFR-2 and enhance signalling through this receptor.

lacking PlGF, they do display defects in pathological angiogenesis in the adult mouse, for example having an impaired angiogeneic response to ischaemia (Carmeliet et al., 2001). This suggests that signalling through VEGFR-1 may be more important during pathological angiogenesis. Overexpression of VEGF-C in transgenic mice results in lymphatic hyperplasia, consistent with the fact that this ligand binds VEGFR-3, the expression of which is predominantly restricted to lymphatic endothelial cells.

VEGF-A expression is predominantly regulated at the transcriptional level through the transcription factor hypoxia inducible factor (HIF-1) (Safran and Kaelin, 2003). HIF-1 is composed of two subunits, α and β, both of which are required for its function. While the β-subunit is a stable protein, the α-subunit is rapidly degraded under normoxic cellular conditions. The oxygen-sensing mechanism controlling HIF-1α expression and activity has recently been shown to involve two oxygen-sensitive enzymes, a prolyl hydroxylase of the EGLN family, which hydroxylates two proline residues at positions 402 and 564 within the oxygen destruction domain; and an asparaginyl hyroxylase (FIH1) which hyroxylates HIF-1α at position 803 within the C-terminal transactivation domain. The hydroxylation reaction performed by both enzymes involves the splitting of molecular oxygen, thus both are highly sensitive to oxygen concentration. Hydroxylation of prolines 402 and 564 results in the binding of the Von Hippel Lindau (VHL) protein, a ubiquitin ligase, which polyubiquitinates HIF-1α and targets it for degradation via the proteasome. Thus under normoxic conditions HIF-1α is rapidly destroyed. Under hypoxic conditions, such as those that occur in the centre of a growing tumour more than 1 mm away from a blood vessel, prolyl hydroxylase activity is switched off, HIF-1α is no longer able to bind VHL and therefore accumulates within the cell. Translocation to the nucleus results in transcriptional activation via complex formation with HIF-1β (Figure 11.8). While prolyl hydroxylation regulates HIF-1α expression, activity of HIF-1α is controlled by aspariginyl hydroxylation of the C-terminal transactivation domain, as transcriptional co-activators such as p300 and CBP, are unable to bind to hydroxylated HIF-1α.

In addition to VEGF-A mRNA being transcriptionally upregulated by hypoxia, there is evidence that VEGF-A mRNA stability is also enhanced under hypoxic conditions, although the RNA-binding proteins involved have not been fully characterized (Levy et al., 1996). Expression of VEGF-A at the protein level also requires an additional level of complexity, as normal CAP-dependent translation mechanisms are switched off under hypoxic conditions. Translation of VEGF-A is made possible under these conditions as the

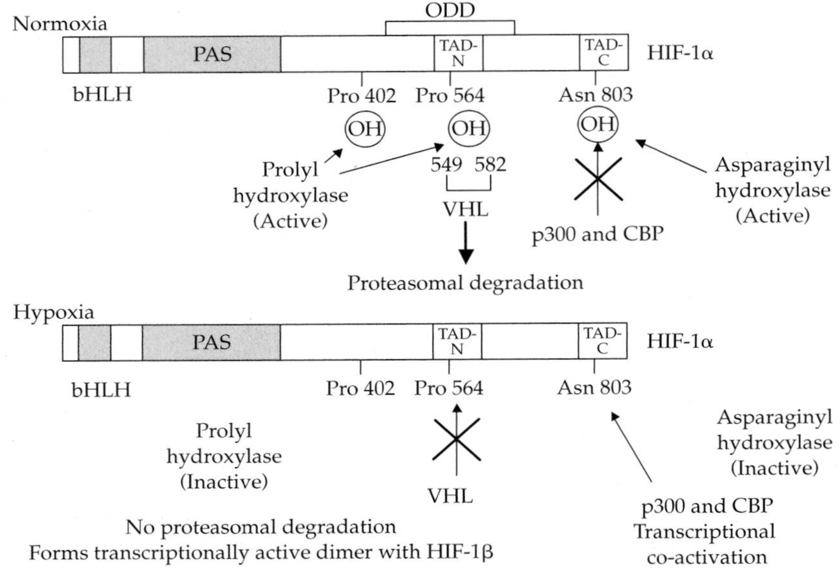

Figure 11.8 Regulation of HIF-1α by hypoxia. Under normoxic conditions prolyl and asparaginyl hydroxylases catalyse the hydroxylation of prolines 402/564 and asparagine 803. Hydroxylation of Pro 402 and Pro 564 facilitates the binding of von Hippel Lindau (VHL) protein, a component of a ubiquitin ligase complex targetting HIF-1α for proeasomal degradation. Hydroxylation of Asn 803 inhibits binding of the transcriptional coactivators p300 and Creb binding protein (CBP). Thus under normoxic condition the HIF-1α protein is both unstable and transcriptionally inactive. Under hypoxic conditions, the hydroxylases are inactive, allowing HIF-1α protein to accumulate and form a nuclear complex with HIF-1β. In the absence of Asn 803 hydroxylation, p300 and CBP are able to bind HIF-1α and stimulate the transcription of hypoxia-responsive genes such as VEGF-A.

VEGF-A mRNA has a long, GC-rich structured 5′UTR, containing an internal ribosome entry segment (IRES) which permits translation even under conditions where CAP-dependent translation is switched off (Lang et al., 2002).

11.10.1 VEGF-A signalling

VEGF-A signals through two related RTKs: VEGFR-1 and VEGFR-2. Both receptors are characterized by their possession of seven immunoglobulin-like domains in the extracellular region, a single membrane-spanning domain and a cytoplasmic region containing the tyrosine kinase domain. The kinase domain contains an insert region, in common with members of the platelet-derived growth factor (PDGF) receptor family. VEGFR-1 has a 10-fold higher affinity for VEGF-A than VEGFR-2, but a 10-fold lower catalytic activity. Knock-out studies in mice have established that both receptors are essential for embryonic development, the absence of either receptor resulting in embryonic lethally due to vascular defects (Shalaby et al., 1995; Fong et al., 1995). The role of each receptor during development appears to be distinct since in mice lacking VEGFR-1, endothelial cells are produced, but overproliferate and fail to organize themselves into vessels, whereas in the VEGFR-2 knock-out mouse, endothelial cell precursors fail to form altogether. Interestingly, a transgenic mouse which expresses only the extracellular and transmembrane domain of VEGFR-1, and lacks the catalytic domain, shows no striking defects in vascularization, the mice are healthy, and show only a subtle defect in monocyte migration. This observation has led to the notion that VEGFR-1 may not have a classical signalling role during embryonic angiogenesis, but may instead regulate the activity of VEGFR-2, for example by regulating the availability of VEGF-A. Deletion of the VEGFR-1 kinase domain (Hiratsuka et al., 2001), or inhibition of ligand binding using antagonists (Luttun et al., 2002) result in impaired pathological angiogenesis suggesting a signalling role in the adult.

11.10.2 VEGFR signalling pathways

As already discussed, signalling downstream of RTKs involves ligand binding, dimerization, autophosphorylation and the recruitment of signalling molecules containing SH2 or PTB domains. Various approaches have been used to identify proteins interacting with the cytoplasmic domain of VEGFRs that may be involved in signalling. These include the use of synthetic phosphopeptides corresponding to potential autophosphorylation sites to purify proteins from cell extracts and the use of the cytoplasmic domain of VEGFR-1 or VEGFR-2 as bait proteins to screen yeast two-hybrid libraries. Several potential effectors have been identified in this way as illustrated in Figure 11.9, though their biological relevance is not clear in all cases (Cunningham et al., 1997; Igarashi et al., 1998*a*, *b*; Ito et al., 1998; Warner et al., 2000; Wu et al., 2000).

Investigators have used many different cell models to delineate the pathways downstream of VEGFR-1 and VEGFR-2, sometimes yielding conflicting results. These include the use of primary endothelial cells, fibroblasts or porcine aortic endothelial cells transfected individually with VEGFR-1, or VEGFR-2, and engineered chimeric VEGFRs that can be regulated in a VEGF-independent fashion. Early results suggested that VEGFRs may signal differently in fibroblasts and endothelial cells suggesting the existence of endothelial cell-specific effectors. Despite extensive efforts, such endothelial-cell selective proteins have remained elusive, and it appears that the major pathways used by other RTKs, such as EGFR, are the ones utilized by VEGFRs, though their mechanisms of activation differ in detail (Figure 11.10). VEGF-induced PI3 kinase activation is essential for survival and migration of endothelial cells (Qi et al., 1999). The p85 subunit of PI3 kinase is phosphorylated in response to VEGF (Thakker et al., 1999) and activation of the enzyme has been identified in many endothelial cells of different origin. Activation has generally been attributed to VEGFR-2, and indeed a repressor segment has been reported in the juxtamembrane domain of VEGFR-1 which may negatively regulate its activity towards PI3 kinase (Gille et al., 2000). Interestingly however, VEGFR-2 does not possess a p85 interaction motif, and it is not clear how it is recruited, or activated by the receptor. In analogy with the ErbB receptors, when co-expressed, VEGFR-1 could act as a dimerization partner and, once phosphorylated by VEGFR-2, provide the docking site for p85. Indeed, VEGFR-1 has been shown to bind p85 in yeast (Igarashi et al., 1998*a*), and to activate the downstream kinase, Akt, using chimeric cytoplasmic receptors activated by dimerization (Knight et al., 2000). Deletion of the cytoplasmic domain of VE-cadherin has been shown to result in impaired VEGF-induced PI3 kinase activation and cell survival (Carmeliet et al., 1999), and complex formation between focal adhesion kinase and PI3 kinase in response to VEGF has also been reported (Qi and Claesson-Welsh., 2001). Whatever the initial mechanism of activation, the downstream effects of PI3 kinase activation are similar to those described for EGFR signalling.

Many studies have shown phosphorylation and activation of PLCγ in response to VEGF in

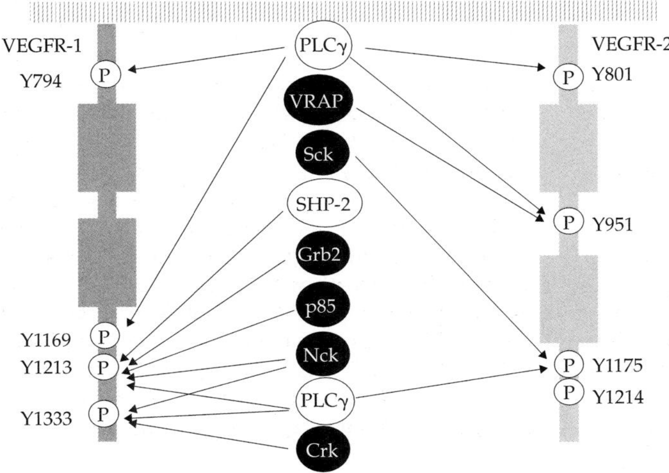

Figure 11.9 Binding of SH2-domain proteins to VEGFR-1 and VEGFR-2. Binding sites for various adaptor proteins (black circles), and enzymes involved in cell signalling (white circles) are indicated. Many of these interactions have been reported in yeast two-hybrid studies, or through binding to phosphopeptides, and consequently their significance *in vivo* is not completely established.

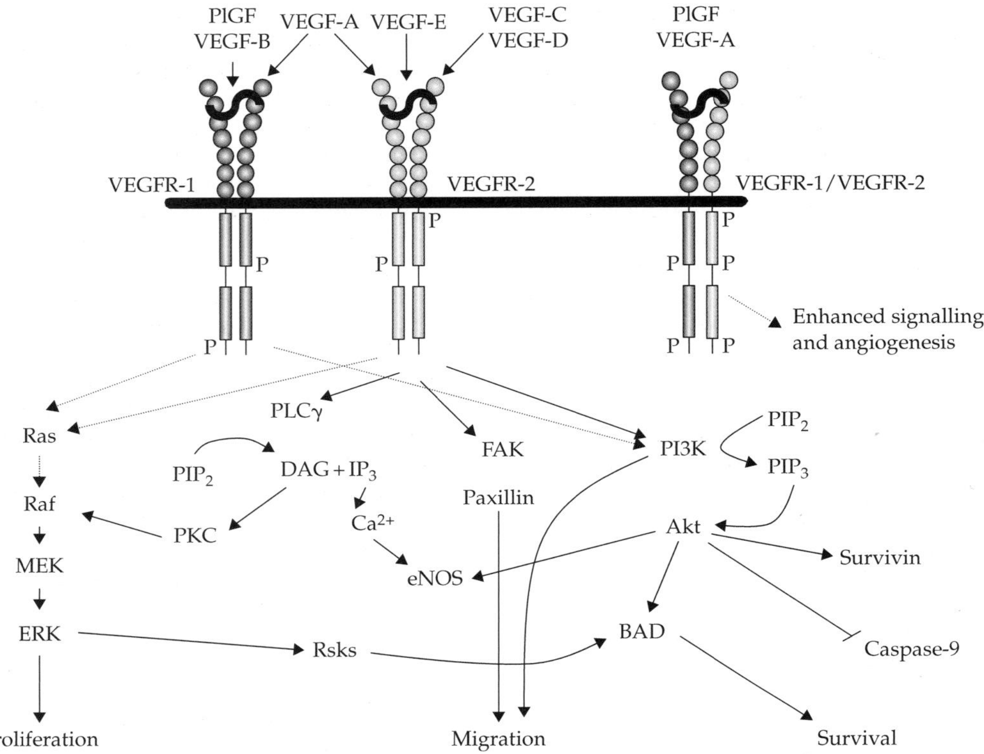

Figure 11.10 VEGF receptor signalling pathways in vascular endothelial cells. VEGFR-2 is activated more potently upon ligand binding than VEGFR-1. PLCγ has been shown to bind directly to VEGFR-2 and catalyses the conversion of phosphatidylinositol 4,5, bisphosphate (PIP_2) to inositol trisphosphate (IP_3) and diacylglycerol (DAG). PLCγ does not appear to be activated efficiently by VEGFR-1. Both phosphoinositide 3-kinase (PI 3K) and the Raf-MEK-ERK pathway are activated by VEGFR-2, however the mechanism by which these are initiated is unclear, as direct recruitment of Grb2, Shc, and p85 to VEGFR-2 has been difficult to demonstrate *in vivo*. Protein kinase C (PKC) activated downstream of PLCγ has been shown to activate the Raf-MEK-ERK pathway directly. Phosphorylation of focal adhesion kinase (FAK) and paxillin have been linked to the pro-migratory action of VEGF-A. Activation of Akt downsteam of PI 3K is involved in survival signalling through phosphorylation and inactivation of the proapoptosis proteins BAD and caspase-9, and upregulation of the anti-apoptotic protein survivin. Ribosomal subunit kinases (Rsks) activated downstream of ERK also promote cell survival through phosphorylation of BAD. Akt also phosphorylates endothelial nitric oxide synthase (eNOS), an enzyme involved in the production of nitric oxide, which has a role in regulating vascular tone and angiogenesis. VEGFR-1 has been shown to activate the Raf-MEK-ERK pathway and PI 3K, and recent evidence suggests that VEGFR-1 and VEGFR-2 may co-operate through an ill-defined mechanism to promote optimal angiogenesis.

endothelial cells. While this enzyme can bind both VEGFR-1 and VEGFR-2 in yeast, VEGFR-2 appears to be the physiological regulator. Recruitment of PLCγ to VEGFR-2 initiates the classical signalling pathway described for EGFR. A potentially novel mechanism by which VEGFR-2 has been reported to activate PLCγ is through phosphorylation of the intermediate VEGF-associated protein, VRAP (Wu et al., 2000). The role of VRAP in VEGF-A signalling is poorly defined, but is analagous to that of Gab1 in EGFR signalling.

Activation of the MAP kinase pathway is required for proliferation in response to most growth factors. Indeed the Raf-MEK-ERK pathway is activated downstream of VEGFRs, but, as is the case for PI3 kinase, the mechanism by which the pathway is initiated is incompletely defined. The majority of evidence suggests that activation is downstream of PKC, as inhibitors of PKC block VEGF-A-induced ERK activation, DNA synthesis and proliferation (Takahashi et al., 1999). Shc can be phosphorylated to a limited extent in cells engineered to overexpress

VEGFR-2, and under these conditions Shc forms complexes with Grb2. There is however no direct evidence that the Shc-Grb2 complex is involved in the activation of Ras in endothelial cells. The related Shc-like adaptor, Sck, has been shown to bind VEGFR-2 more efficiently than Shc in yeast. Mutation of its binding site on VEGFR-2 does not inhibit ERK activation suggesting that this adaptor does not have a primary role in regulating ERK activity (Knight et al., 2000). In addition to ERK, the related stress-activated MAP kinase p38 is activated by VEGF, probably through VEGFR-2, and is involved in endothelial cell motility. This effect probably involves the downstream effector of p38, HSP27, which is an actin-polymerizing factor.

While VEGFR-1 has the potential to associate with many signalling proteins *in vitro*, or in yeast two-hybrid assays, the signalling role of this receptor in intact endothelial cells has proved difficult to define. A recent report suggests that VEGFR-1 may have an important role in transactivation of VEGFR-2 by enhancing its phosphorylation and angiogenic activity (Autiero et al., 2003). This cross-talk can be mediated by VEGFR-1 homodimers when activated by PlGF, or by VEGFR-1 present within VEGFR-1/VEGFR-2 heterodimers, activated by VEGF/PlGF dimers. Interestingly these investigators demonstrated that PlGF and VEGF induce phosphorylation of distinct sites within VEGFR-1 suggesting that different ligands can activate distinct signalling pathways through the same receptor, possibly having quite different consequences.

The downregulation of VEGFR signalling is less well characterized than for ErbB receptors, however there is evidence that the ubiquitin ligase Cbl is involved in the degradation of both VEGFR-1 and VEGFR-2 (Duval et al., 2003).

11.10.3 VEGF and its receptors in cancer

VEGF receptors are expressed in normal endothelial cells in the blood vessels supplying the tumour. No naturally occurring VEGF receptor mutations have been identified predisposing individuals to cancer. VEGF-A is upregulated as a consequence of the low oxygen tension within tumours, providing a sensitive mechanism for ensuring blood vessel growth when vascularization is deficient. The VEGFR-1 promoter (but not that of VEGFR-2) also possesses a binding site for HIF-1 and is upregulated by hypoxia (Gerber et al., 1997). Thus upregulation of VEGFR-1 within the hypoxic tumour vasculature may potentiate signalling through VEGFR-2, and angiogenesis. Certain tumours, such as hypervascular renal cell carcinomas also express high levels of the VEGFR-1 selective ligand PlGF, though upregulation in this case is independent of hypoxia (Takahashi et al., 1994). Signalling via many growth factors, including EGF and TGFα, leads to an induction of VEGF-A mRNA. Thus hyperactivation of ErbB pathways in many tumours will lead to increased VEGF-A expression and angiogenesis. Oncogenic mutation, or amplification of components of the EGFR signalling pathway, such as Ras, also leads to increased VEGF-A expression (Kranenburg et al., 2004).

One cancer syndrome associated with high levels of VEGF expression is VHL disease. This syndrome is the result of germline mutations in the *VHL* gene predisposing patients to a variety of benign and malignant tumours of the CNS, kidneys, adrenal glands, pancreas, and reproductive adnexal organs (Lonser et al., 2003). These tumours are characterized by their highly vascular properties. Defects in the VHL protein most likely result in an inability to ubiquitinate HIF-1α, thus rendering it insensitive to degradation under normoxic conditions. Unregulated expression of active HIF-1 permits sustained expression of VEGF-A and enhanced angiogenesis.

11.11 Targeting RTKs as a therapeutic strategy for the treatment of cancer

The overwhelming evidence that EGFR and ErbB2 contribute to the growth and survival of tumours has led to intensive efforts to develop inhibitors of these kinases for therapeutic use. This approach is possible as the function of both receptors is dispensible in normal adult tissues. An obvious limitation is that such inhibitors will, at best, only be effective in those cancers where abnormalities in ErbB signalling have an essential role in the growth and survival of the tumour cells. The VEGFRs on the other hand contribute to the growth of virtually all tumours, as their action is necessary for promoting angiogenesis and essential for tumour expansion and metastasis. Moreover, in normal healthy adults, the process of angiogenesis is limited to wound healing, and the female reproductive cycle, thus it should, at least in theory, be possible to inhibit tumour angiogenesis without affecting normal tissues. The identification of VEGFR-2 as a pivotal regulator of angiogenesis has prompted extensive efforts to develop therapeutic agents able to interfere with its signalling ability.

11.12 Approaches targeting EGFR and ErbB2

Many agents are currently in clinical trials, the most promising of these being antibodies directed towards the extracellular domain of the RTKs, or small molecule inhibitors of tyrosine kinase activity (see Table 11.2) (Grunwald and Hidalgo, 2003; Bennasroune et al., 2004; Dancey, 2004). Cetuximab (C225) and ABX-EGF are both humanized monoclonal antibodies (mAbs) directed towards the extracellular domain of EGFR. C225 and ABX-EGF both inhibit binding of EGF and TGFα to EGFR, and stimulate its dimerization and downregulation. Several studies using cultured tumour cells, have demonstrated that these antibodies inhibit EGFR signalling causing an induction of the cell cycle inhibitor p27, inhibition of Cdk2, and arrest in the G1 phase of the cell cycle. The binding of antibodies to tumour cells *in vivo*, may also facilitate recruitment of immune effector cells and subsequent tumour cell destruction. Herceptin (Trastuzumab), an antibody targeting the extracellular domain of ErbB2, has already been approved for treatment of breast cancer. As observed for the anti-EGFR mAbs, Herceptin functions by inducing endocytic downregulation of ErbB2 by a process that may involve Cbl, and induces the expression of p27 and consequent cell cycle arrest. Another anti-ErbB2 antibody, Pertuzamab (Omnitarg, 2C4), which targets a different region of the extracellular domain, sterically blocks dimerization of ErbB2 with EGFR and ErbB3 and blocks signalling from these heterodimers. Studies in cultured cells suggest that Herceptin and Pertuzamab may act in synergy to inhibit the survival of breast cancer cells (Nahta et al., 2004). An interesting possibility for the treatment of cancers expressing the EGFRvIII mutant involves the generation of antibodies specifically recognizing the novel epitope sequence produced by the deletion of aminoacids 6–273. Preclinical studies using such an antibody, mAb-806, have shown promise in reducing the growth of tumour xenographs expressing the mutant receptor (Luwor et al., 2001).

Small molecule inhibitors of EGFR and ErbB2 are also being developed and evaluated in clinical trials. This strategy exploits subtle differences in the structure of ATP-binding sites of different RTKs, and aims to develop receptor-specific competitive or irreversible inhibitors of ATP binding. The most promising inhibitor of EGFR, Iressa (ZD1839), has been approved in Japan for treatment of non-small cell lung cancer. Inhibition of EGFR with Iressa induces apoptosis of mammary epithelial cells by inhibiting phosphorylation of the proapoptosis mediator BAD. Interestingly, low doses of Iressa also inhibit phosphorylation of ErbB2 in breast cancer cells overexpressing this receptor. This inhibitory effect occurs at doses which do not affect the ErbB2 kinase directly, suggesting that it is the transactivation of ErbB2 by EGFR that is inhibited. An irreversible inhibitor of ErbB2, CI-1033, displays an interesting mechanism of action, in that it modifies a cysteine residue in ErbB2 thereby disrupting association with the chaperone Hsp90 leading to ErbB2 degradation (Citri et al., 2002).

11.13 Approaches targeting VEGFR-2

VEGFR-2 is generally considered to be the most important receptor for mediating proliferation and

Table 11.2 Drugs targeting EGFR, ErbB2, and VEGFR-2

Target	Drug	Mode of action	Company	Stage of development
EGFR	ABX-EGF	mAb against EGFR	Abgenix	Phase II
EGFR	Cetuximab (C225)	mAb against EGFR	ImClone systems	Phase III
EGFR	Iressa (ZD1839)	Inhibitor of EGFR kinase	AstraZeneca	Approved in Japan for some cancers
EGFRvIII	mAb-806	mAb against mutant EGFR	LICR	pre-clinical
ErbB-2	Herceptin (Trastuzumab)	mAb against ErbB-2	Genentech	Approved for breast cancer
ErbB-2	Pertuzumab	mAb against ErbB-2	Genentech	Phase I
VEGF	Bevacizumab (Avastin)	mAb against VEGF-A	Genentech	Phase III
VEGFR-2	SU5416	Inhibitor VEGFR-2 kinase	SUGEN	Phase II
VEGFR-2	SU6668	Inhibitor VEGFR-2 kinase	SUGEN	Phase I
VEGFR-2	ZD6474	Inhibitor VEGFR-2 kinase	AstraZeneca	Phase II

migration of endothelial cells. Studies in the early 1990s provided the first direct evidence that inhibition of VEGFR-2 action could interfere with tumour growth in mice, by inhibition of angiogenesis. In these studies the action of VEGF was prevented through use of VEGF sequestering antibodies, or viruses encoding dominant-negative VEGFR-2 proteins to block the activation of VEGFR-2 (Kim et al., 1993; Millauer et al., 1994). As for the ErbB receptors, current strategies under development for cancer therapy involve monoclonal antibodies and tyrosine kinase inhibitors (Sridhar and Shepherd, 2003). Bevacizumab (Avastin), is an antibody against VEGF-A that inhibits its binding to VEGFR-2, and subsequent signalling. In clinical trials, this antibody has been shown to reduce serum VEGF levels to undetectable levels. It is currently under evaluation for the treatment of lung, breast, prostate, colorectal, and renal cancers. A number of small molecule VEGFR-2 kinase inhibitors are also undergoing clinical evaluation. These differ with respect to their inhibitory activity towards other RTKs. SU5416, a relatively selective inhibitor of VEGFR-2 that also inhibits the c-kit tyrosine kinase, showed great promise in pre-clinical studies demonstrating broad anti-tumour activity. Unfortunately, clinical trials revealed a rather severe toxicity profile for this compound, which, coupled with its requirement for intravenous administration have limited its development. SU6668 inhibits VEGFR-2 in addition to PDGF receptor (PDGFR) and fibroblast growth factor receptor (FGFR). This compound has the advantage that it can be orally administered, but also has rather toxic side effects. Another promising VEGFR-2 inhibitor, which has some inhibitory action on EGFR, is ZD6474. Initial trials suggest that this compound is well tolerated by patients. Other agents are under investigation.

Our knowledge of signalling pathways involved in cancer has permitted the rational design of promising agents targeting RTKs. Further knowledge is required to optimize treatment regimens, and improve drug design. In the case of inhibitors targeting ErbB family members, a key issue is identifying those patients most likely to respond. In this regard we need to understand the details of receptor cross-talk and identify markers predicting likely success. Overexpression of certain combinations of ErbB receptors may suggest a more favourable outcome of therapy. For example, tumours overexpressing ErbB3 in addition to ErbB2 may transduce a more potent survival signal through PI3 kinase than those expressing ErbB2 in isolation. Such tumours may be more sensitive to ErbB2 targeted therapy. Inhibitors of VEGFR-2 kinase activity have shown potent anti-angiogenic, and anti-tumour activity in pre-clinical models, but some have caused unacceptable toxic side effects in clinical trials. This may be due in part to their inhibition of other tyrosine kinases. Although endothelial cells generally proliferate very slowly in healthy adults, and with a few physiological exceptions are not involved in angiogenesis, they may be dependent on VEGFR-induced signalling events for their survival. The challenge in this area is to develop an inhibitor with the optimal receptor cross-specificity and activity to selectively inhibit signalling pathways in actively proliferating, migratory endothelial cells.

References

Agazie, Y. M. and Hayman, M. J. (2003). Molecular mechanism for a role of SHP2 in epidermal growth factor receptor signaling. *Mol Cell Biol*, **23**, 7875–86.

Alessi, D. R., Saito, Y., Campbell, D. G., Cohen, P., Sithanandam, G., Rapp, U. et al. (1994). Identification of the sites in MAP kinase kinase-1 phosphorylated by p74raf-1. *EMBO J*, **13**, 1610–9.

Autiero, M., Waltenberger, J., Communi, D., Kranz, A., Moons, L., Lambrechts D. et al. (2003). Role of PlGF in the intra- and intermolecular cross talk between the VEGF receptors Flt1 and Flk1. *Nat Med*, **9**, 936–43.

Bargmann, C. I., Hung, M. C., and Weinberg, R. A. (1986). Multiple independent activations of the neu oncogene by a point mutation altering the transmembrane domain of p185. *Cell*, **45**, 649–57.

Bennasroune, A., Gardin, A., Aunis, D., Cremel, G., and Hubert, P. (2004). Tyrosine kinase receptors as attractive targets of cancer therapy. *Crit Rev Oncol Hematol*, **50**, 23–38.

Borges, E., Jan, Y., and Ruoslahti, E.(2000). Platelet-derived growth factor receptor beta and vascular endothelial growth factor receptor 2 bind to the beta 3 integrin through its extracellular domain. *J Biol Chem*, **275**, 39867–73.

Carmeliet, P., Moons, L, Luttun, A, Vincenti, V., Compernolle, V., De Mol, M. et al. (2001). Synergism between vascular endothelial growth factor and placental growth factor contributes to angiogenesis and plasma extravasation in pathological conditions. *Nat Med*, **7**, 575–83.

Carmeliet, P., Lampugnani, M. G., Moons, L., Breviario, F. et al. (1999). Targeted deficiency or cytosolic truncation of the VE-cadherin gene in mice impairs VEGF-mediated endothelial survival and angiogenesis. *Cell*, **98**, 147–57.

Carpenter, G. (2003*a*). ErbB-4: mechanism of action and biology. *Exp Cell Res* **284**, 66–77.

Carpenter, G. (2003*b*). Nuclear localization and possible functions of receptor tyrosine kinases. *Curr Opin Cell Biol*, 15, 143–8.

Chattopadhyay, A., Vecchi, M., Ji, Q., Mernaugh, R., and Carpenter, G. (1999). The role of individual SH2 domains in mediating association of phospholipase C-gamma1 with the activated EGF receptor. *J Biol Chem*, **274**, 26091–7.

Citri, A., Alroy, I., Lavi, S., Rubin, C., Xu, W., Grammatikakis, N. C. et al. (2002). Drug-induced ubiquitylation and degradation of ErbB receptor tyrosine kinases: implications for cancer therapy. *EMBO J*, **21**, 2407–17.

Citri, A., Skaria, K. B., and Yarden, Y. (2003). The deaf and the dumb: the biology of ErbB-2 and ErbB-3. *Exp Cell Res*, **284**, 54–65.

Cochet, C., Gill, G. N., Meisenhelder, J., Cooper, J. A., and Hunter, T. (1984). C-kinase phosphorylates the epidermal growth factor receptor and reduces its epidermal growth factor-stimulated tyrosine protein kinase activity. J *Biol Chem*, **259**, 2553–8.

Cross, M. J., Dixelius, J., Matsumoto, T., and Claesson-Welsh, L. (2003). VEGF-receptor signal transduction. *Trends Biochem Sci*, **28**, 488–94.

Cunningham. S. A., Arrate, M. P., Brock, T. A., and Waxham, M. N. (1997). Interactions of FLT-1 and KDR with phospholipase C gamma: identification of the phosphotyrosine binding sites. *Biochem Biophys Res Commun*, **240**, 635–9.

Dancey, J. (2004). Epidermal growth factor receptor inhibitors in clinical development. *Int J Radiat Oncol Biol Phys*, **58**, 1003–7.

David, M., Wong, L, Flavell, R., Thompson, S. A., Wells, A., Larner, A. C. et al. (1996). STAT activation by epidermal growth factor (EGF) and amphiregulin. Requirement for the EGF receptor kinase but not for tyrosine phosphorylation sites or JAK1. *J Biol Chem*, **271**, 9185–8.

Downward, J., Yarden, Y., Mayes, E., Scrace, G., Totty, N., Stockwell, P. et al. (1984). Close similarity of epidermal growth factor receptor and v-erb-B oncogene protein sequences. *Nature*, **307**, 521–7.

Duval, M., Bedard-Goulet, S., Delisle, C., and Gratton, J. P. (2003). Vascular endothelial growth factor-dependent down-regulation of Flk-1/KDR involves Cbl-mediated ubiquitination. Consequences on nitric oxide production from endothelial cells. *J Biol Chem*, **278**, 20091–7.

Eng, C. (2003). PTEN: one gene, many syndromes. *Hum Mutat*, **22**, 183–98.

Falls, D. L. (2003). Neuregulins: functions, forms, and signaling strategies. *Exp Cell Res*, **284**, 14–30.

Ferrara, N., Carver-Moore, K., Chen, H., Dowd, M., Lu, L., O'Shea, K. S. et al. (1996). Heterozygous embryonic lethality induced by targeted inactivation of the VEGF gene. *Nature*, **380**, 439–42.

Ferrara, N., Gerber, H. P. and LeCouter, J. (2003). The biology of VEGF and its receptors. *Nat Med*, **9**, 669–76.

Folkman, J. (1990). What is the evidence that tumors are angiogenesis dependent? *J Natl Cancer Inst*, **82**, 4–6.

Fong, G. H., Rossant, J., Gertsenstein, M. and Breitman, M.L. (1995). Role of the Flt-1 receptor tyrosine kinase in regulating the assembly of vascular endothelium. *Nature*, **376**, 66–70.

Garrett, T. P., McKern, N. M,, Lou, M., Elleman, T, C., Adams, T, E., Lovrecz, G. O. et al. (2002). Crystal structure of a truncated epidermal growth factor receptor extracellular domain bound to transforming growth factor alpha. *Cell*, **110**, 763–73

Garrett, T. P., McKern, N. M,, Lou, M., Elleman, T, C., Adams, T, E., Lovrecz, G. O. et al. (2003). The crystal structure of a truncated ErbB2 ectodomain reveals an active conformation, poised to interact with other ErbB receptors. *Mol Cell*, **11**, 495–505.

Gerber, H. P., Condorelli, F. Park, J., and Ferrara, N. (1997). Differential transcriptional regulation of the two vascular endothelial growth factor receptor genes. Flt-1, but not Flk-1/KDR, is up-regulated by hypoxia. *J Biol Chem*, **272**, 23659–67.

Gilbertson, R. J., Perry, R. H., Kelly, P. J., Pearson, A. D., and Lunec, J. (1997). Prognostic significance of HER2 and HER4 coexpression in childhood medulloblastoma. *Cancer Res*, **57**, 3272–80.

Gille, H., Kowalski, J. Yu, L., Chen, H., Pisabarro, M. T. Davis-Smyth, T. et al. (2000). A repressor sequence in the juxtamembrane domain of Flt-1 (VEGFR-1) constitutively inhibits vascular endothelial growth factor-dependent phosphatidylinositol 3′-kinase activation and endothelial cell migration. *EMBO J*, **19**, 4064–73.

Grunwald, V. and Hidalgo, M. (2003). Developing inhibitors of the epidermal growth factor receptor for cancer treatment. *J Natl Cancer Inst*, **95**, 851–67.

Gu, H. and Neel, B. G. (2003). The 'Gab' in Signal Transduction. *Trends Cell Biol*, **13**, 122–130.

Guy, P. M., Platko, J. V., Cantley, L. C., Cerione, R. A., and Carraway, K. L. 3rd. (1994). Insect cell-expressed p180erbB3 possesses an impaired tyrosine kinase activity. *Proc Natl Acad Sci USA*, **91**, 8132–6.

Haglund, K, Sigismund, S. Polo, S., Szymkiewicz, I., Di Fiore, P. P., and Dikic, I. (2003). Multiple monoubiquitination of RTKs is sufficient for their endocytosis and degradation. *Nat Cell Biol*, **5**, 461–6.

Harris, R. C., Chung, E., and Coffey, R. J. (2003). EGF receptor ligands. *Exp Cell Res*, **284**, 2–13.

Hashimoto, Y., Katayama, H., Kiyokawa, E. Ota, S., Kurata, T., Gotoh, N. et al. (1998). Phosphorylation of CrkII adaptor protein at tyrosine 221 by epidermal growth factor receptor. *J Biol Chem*, **273**, 17186–91.

Hiratsuka, S., Maru, Y., Okada, A., Seiki, M., Noda, T., and Shibuya, M. (2001). Involvement of Flt-1 tyrosine kinase (vascular endothelial growth factor receptor-1) in pathological angiogenesis. *Cancer Res*, **61**, 1207–13.

Holbro, T. Civenni, G., and Hynes, N. E. (2003). The ErbB receptors and their role in cancer progression. *Exp Cell Res*, **284**, 99–110.

Houle, M. G. and Bourgoin, S. (1999). Regulation of phospholipase D by phosphorylation-dependent mechanisms. *Biochim Biophys Acta*, **1439**, 135–49.

Hubbard, S. R., Mohammadi, M., and Schlessinger, J. (1998). Autoregulatory mechanisms in protein-tyrosine kinases. *J Biol Chem*, **273**, 11987–90.

Huser, M., Luckett, J., Chiloeches, A., Mercer, K., Iwobi, M., Giblett, S. et al. (2001). MEK kinase activity is not necessary for Raf-1 function. *EMBO J*, **20**, 1940–51.

Igarashi, K., Isohara, T., Kato, T., Shigeta, K., Yamano, T., and Uno, I. (1998*a*). Tyrosine 1213 of Flt-1 is a major binding site of Nck and SHP-2. *Biochem Biophys Res Commun*, **246**, 95–9.

Igarashi, K., Shigeta, K., Isohara, T., Yamano, T., and Uno, I. (1998*b*). Sck interacts with KDR and Flt-1 via its SH2 domain. *Biochem Biophys Res Commun*, **251**, 77–82.

Ito, N., Wernstedt, C., Engstrom, U., and Claesson-Welsh, L. (1998). Identification of vascular endothelial growth factor receptor-1 tyrosine phosphorylation sites and binding of SH2 domain-containing molecules. *J Biol Chem*, **273**, 23410–8.

Jones, N. and Dumont, D. J. (1999). Recruitment of Dok-R to the EGF receptor through its PTB domain is required for attenuation of Erk MAP kinase activation. *Curr Biol*, **9**, 1057–60.

Jorissen, R. N., Walker, F., Pouliot, N., Garrett, T. P, Ward, C. W., and Burgess, A. (2003). Epidermal growth factor receptor: mechanisms of activation and signalling. *Exp Cell Res*, **284**, 31–53.

Keilhack, H., Tenev, T., Nyakatura, E., Godovac-Zimmermann, J., Nielsen, L., Seedorf, K. et al. (1998). Phosphotyrosine 1173 mediates binding of the protein-tyrosine phosphatase SHP-1 to the epidermal growth factor receptor and attenuation of receptor signaling. *J Biol Chem*, **273**, 24839–46.

Kim et al. (1993). Inhibition of VEGF induced angiogenesis suppresses tumour growth in vivo. *Nature*, **362**, 841–44.

Knight, E. L., Warner, A. J., Maxwell, A., and Prigent, S.A. (2000). Chimeric VEGFRs are activated by a small-molecule dimerizer and mediate downstream signalling cascades in endothelial cells. *Oncogene*, **19**, 5398–405.

Kobayashi, S., Sawano, A., Nojima, Y., Shibuya, M., and Maru Y. (2004). The c-Cbl/CD2AP complex regulates VEGF-induced endocytosis and degradation of Flt-1 (VEGFR-1). *FASEB J*. **18**, 929–931.

Kranenburg, O., Gebbink, M. F., and Voest, E. E. (2004). Stimulation of angiogenesis by Ras proteins. *Biochim Biophys Acta*, **1654**, 23–37.

Kuan, C. T., Wikstrand, C. J., and Bigner, D. D. (2001). EGF mutant receptor vIII as a molecular target in cancer therapy. *Endocr Relat Cancer*, **8**, 83–96.

Lang, K. J., Kappel, A., and Goodall, G. J. (2002). Hypoxia-inducible factor-1alpha mRNA contains an internal ribosome entry site that allows efficient translation during normoxia and hypoxia. *Mol Biol Cell*, **13**, 1792–801.

Langlois, W. J., Sasaoka, T., Saltiel, A. R., and Olefsky, J. M. (1995). Negative feedback regulation and desensitization of insulin- and epidermal growth factor-stimulated p21ras activation. *J Biol Chem*, **270**, 25320–3.

Lee, H., Akita, R. W., Sliwkowski, M. X., and Maihle, N. J. (2001). A naturally occurring secreted human ErbB3 receptor isoform inhibits heregulin-stimulated activation of ErbB2, ErbB3, and ErbB4. *Cancer Res*, **61**, 4467–73

Leu, T. H. and Maa, M. C.(2003). Functional implication of the interaction between EGF receptor and c-Src. *Front Biosci*, **8**, s28–38.

Levkowitz, G. Klapper, L. N., Tzahar, E., Freywald, A., Sela, M., and Yarden, Y. (1996). Coupling of the c-Cbl protooncogene product to ErbB-1/EGF-receptor but not to other ErbB proteins. *Oncogene*, **12**, 1117–25.

Levy, A. P., Levy, N. S., and Goldberg, M. A. (1996). Post-transcriptional regulation of vascular endothelial growth factor by hypoxia. *J Biol Chem*, **271**, 2746–53.

Lipkowitz, S.(2003). The role of the ubiquitination-proteasome pathway in breast cancer: ubiquitin mediated degradation of growth factor receptors in the pathogenesis and treatment of cancer. *Breast Cancer Res*, **5**, 8–15.

Lonser, R. R., Glenn, G. M., Walther, M. C, E. Y., Libutti, S. K., Linehan, W. M. et al. (2003). von Hippel-Lindau disease. *Lancet*, **361**, 2059–67.

Luttun, A., Tjwa, M., Moons, L., Wu, Y., Angelillo-Scherrer, A., Liao, F. et al. (2002). Revascularization of ischemic tissues by PlGF treatment, and inhibition of tumor angiogenesis, arthritis and atherosclerosis by anti-Flt1. *Nat Med*, **8**, 831–40.

Luwor, R. B., Johns, T. G., Murone, C., Huang, H. J., Cavenee, W. K., Ritter, G., Old, L. J., Burgess, A. W., and Scott, A. M. (2001). Monoclonal antibody 806 inhibits the growth of tumor xenografts expressing either the de2-7 or amplified epidermal growth factor receptor (EGFR) but not wild-type EGFR. *Cancer Res*, **61**, 5355–61.

Mason, C. S., Springer, C. J., Cooper, R. G., Superti-Furga, G., Marshall, C. J., and Marais, R. (1999). Serine and tyrosine phosphorylations cooperate in Raf-1, but not B-Raf activation. *EMBO J*, **18**, 2137–48.

McCarty, J. H. (1998). The Nck SH2/SH3 adaptor protein: a regulator of multiple intracellular signal transduction events. *Bioessays*, **20**, 913–21.

Mercer, K. E. and Pritchard, C. A. (1993). Raf proteins and cancer: B-Raf is identified as a mutational target. *Biochim Biophys Acta*, **1653**, 25–40.

Milarski, K. L., Zhu, G., Pearl, C. G., McNamara, D. J., Dobrusin, E. M., MacLean, D. et al. (1993). Sequence specificity in recognition of the epidermal growth factor receptor by protein tyrosine phosphatase 1B. *J Biol Chem*, **268**, 23634–9.

Millauer et al. (1994). Glioblastoma growth inhibited in vivo by dominant negative Flk-1 mutant. *Nature*, **367**, 576–9.

Montero, J. C., Yuste, L., Diaz-Rodriguez, E., Esparis-Ogando, A., and Pandiella, A. (2000). Differential shedding of transmembrane neuregulin isoforms by the tumor necrosis factor-alpha-converting enzyme. *Mol Cell Neurosci*, **16**, 631–48.

Nahta, R., Hung, M.-C., and Esteva, F. J. (2004). The HER-2 targeting antibodies Trastuzumab and Pertuzumab synergistically inhibit survival of breast cancer cells. *Cancer Res* **64**, 2343–6.

Nanba, D. and Higashiyama, S. (2004). Dual intracellular signaling by proteolytic cleavage of membrane-anchored heparin-binding EGF-like growth factor. *Cytokine Growth Factor Rev*, **15**, 13–19.

O-charoenrat., P, Modjtahedi, H., Rhys-Evans, P., Court, W. J., Box, G. M., and Eccles, S. A. (2000). Epidermal growth factor-like ligands differentially up-regulate matrix metalloproteinase 9 in head and neck squamous carcinoma cells. *Cancer Res*, **60**, 1121–8.

Ogiso, H., Ishitani, R., Nureki, O., Fukai, S., Yamanaka, M., Kim, J. H. et al. (2002). Crystal structure of the complex of human epidermal growth factor and receptor extracellular domains. *Cell*, **110**, 775–87.

Okabayashi, Y., Kido, Y., Okutani, T., Sugimoto, Y., Sakaguchi, K., and Kasuga, M. (1994). Tyrosines 1148 and 1173 of activated human epidermal growth factor receptors are binding sites of Shc in intact cells. *J Biol Chem*, **269**, 18674–8

Okutani, T., Okabayashi, Y., Kido, Y., Sugimoto, Y., Sakaguchi, K., Matuoka, K. et al. (1994). Grb2/Ash binds directly to tyrosines 1068 and 1086 and indirectly to tyrosine 1148 of activated human epidermal growth factor receptors in intact cells. *J Biol Chem*. **269**, 31310–4.

Olayioye, M. A., Beuvink, I., Horsch, K., Daly, J. M., and Hynes, N. E. (1999). ErbB receptor-induced activation of stat transcription factors is mediated by Src tyrosine kinases. *J Biol Chem*, **274**, 17209–18.

Peschard, P. and Park, M. (2003). Escape from Cbl-mediated downregulation: A recurrent theme for oncogenic deregulation of receptor tyrosine kinases. *Cancer Cell*, **3**, 519–23.

Petit, A. M., Rak, J., Hung, M. C., Rockwell, P., Goldstein, N., Fendly, B. et al. (1997). Neutralizing antibodies against epidermal growth factor and ErbB-2/neu receptor tyrosine kinases down-regulate vascular endothelial growth factor production by tumor cells in vitro and in vivo: angiogenic implications for signal transduction therapy of solid tumors. *Am J Pathol*, **151**, 1523–30.

Prigent, S. A. and Gullick, W. J.(1994). Identification of c-erbB-3 binding sites for phosphatidylinositol 3′-kinase and SHC using an EGF receptor/c-erbB-3 chimera. *EMBO J*, **13**, 2831–41.

Qi, J. H., Matsumoto, T., Huang, K, Olausson, K. Christofferson, R., and Claesson-Welsh, L. (1999). Phosphoinositide 3 kinase is critical for survival, mitogenesis and migration but not for differentiation of endothelial cells. *Angiogenesis*, **3**, 371–80.

Qi, J. H. and Claesson-Welsh, L. (2001). VEGF-induced activation of phosphoinositide 3-kinase is dependent on focal adhesion kinase. *Exp Cell Res*, **263**, 173–82.

Rahimi, N. and Kazlauskas, A.(1999). A role for cadherin-5 in regulation of vascular endothelial growth factor receptor 2 activity in endothelial cells. *Mol Biol Cell*, **10**, 3401–7.

Safran, M. and Kaelin, W. G., Jr. (2003). HIF hydroxylation and the mammalian oxygen-sensing pathway. *J Clin Invest*, **111**, 779–83.

Schmidt, M. H., Furnari, F. B., Cavenee, W. K., and Bogler O. (2003). Epidermal growth factor receptor signaling intensity determines intracellular protein interactions, ubiquitination, and internalization. *Proc Natl Acad Sci USA*, **100**, 6505–10.

Serth, J., Weber, W., Frech, M., Wittinghofer, A., and Pingoud, A. (1992). Binding of the H-ras p21 GTPase activating protein by the activated epidermal growth factor receptor leads to inhibition of the p21 GTPase activity in vitro. *Biochemistry*, **31**, 6361–5.

Shalaby, F., Rossant, J., Yamaguchi, T. P., Gertsenstein, M., Wu, X. F., Breitman, M. L. et al. (1995). Failure of blood-island formation and vasculogenesis in Flk-1-deficient mice. *Nature*, **376**, 62–6.

Shirakabe, K., Wakatsuki, S., Kurisaki, T., and Fujisawa-Sehara, A. (2001). Roles of Meltrin beta/ADAM19 in the processing of neuregulin. *J Biol Chem*, **276**, 9352–8.

Soker, S., Takashima, S., Miao, H. Q., Neufeld, G., and Klagsbrun, M. (1998). Neuropilin-1 is expressed by endothelial and tumor cells as an isoform-specific receptor for vascular endothelial growth factor. *Cell*, **92**, 735–45.

Sridhar, S. S. and Shepherd, F. A. (2003). Targeting angiogenesis: a review of angiogenesis inhibitors in the treatment of lung cancer. *Lung Cancer*, **42**, 581–91.

Stover, D. R., Becker, M., Liebetanz, J., and Lydon, N. B. (1995). Src phosphorylation of the epidermal growth factor receptor at novel sites mediates receptor interaction with Src and P85 alpha. *J Biol Chem*, **270**, 15591–7.

Sun, H., King, A. J., Diaz, H. B., and Marshall, M. S. (2000). Regulation of the protein kinase Raf-1 by oncogenic Ras through phosphatidylinositol 3-kinase, Cdc42/Rac and Pak. *Curr Biol*, **10**, 281–4.

Sunnarborg, S. W., Hinkle, C. L., Stevenson, M., Russell, W. E., Raska, C. S., Peschon, J. J. et al. (2002). Tumor necrosis factor-alpha converting enzyme (TACE) regulates epidermal growth factor receptor ligand availability. *J Biol Chem*, **277**, 12838–45.

Takahashi, A., Sasaki, H., Kim, S. J., Tobisu, K., Kakizoe, T., Tsukamoto, T. et al. (1994). Markedly increased amounts of messenger RNAs for vascular endothelial growth factor and placenta growth factor in renal cell carcinoma associated with angiogenesis. *Cancer Res*, **54**, 4233–7.

Takahashi, T., Ueno, H., and Shibuya, M.(1999). VEGF activates protein kinase C-dependent, but Ras-independent Raf-MEK-MAP kinase pathway for DNA synthesis in primary endothelial cells. *Oncogene*, **18**, 2221–30.

Thakker, G. D., Hajjar, D. P., Muller, W. A., and Rosengart, T. K. (1999). The role of phosphatidylinositol 3-kinase in vascular endothelial growth factor signalling. *J Biol Chem*, **274**, 10002–7.

Vanhaesebroeck, B. and Alessi, D. R.(2000). The PI3K-PDK1 connection: more than just a road to PKB. *Biochem J*, **346**, 561–76.

Walker, F., Orchard, S. G., Jorissen, R. N., Hall, N. E., Zhang, H. H., Hoyne, P. A. et al. (2004). CR1/CR2 interactions modulate the functions of the cell-surface epidermal growth factor receptor. *J Biol Chem*, **279**, 22387–398.

Wang, J. Y., Miller, S. J., and Falls, D. L.(2001). The N-terminal region of neuregulin isoforms determines the accumulation of cell surface and released neuregulin ectodomain. *J Biol Chem*, **276**, 2841–51.

Warner, A. J., Lopez-Dee, J., Knight, E. L., Feramisco, J. R., and Prigent, S. A. (2000). The Shc-related adaptor protein, Sck, forms a complex with the vascular-endothelial-growth-factor receptor KDR in transfected cells. *Biochem J*, **347**, 501–9.

Wu, L. W., Mayo, L. D., Dunbar, J. D., Kessler, K. M., Ozes, O. N., Warren, R. S. et al. (2000). VRAP is an adaptor protein that binds KDR, a receptor for vascular endothelial cell growth factor. *J Biol Chem*, **275**, 6059–62.

Yamauchi, T., Ueki, K., Tobe, K., Tamemoto, H., Sekine, N., Wada, M. et al. (1997). Tyrosine phosphorylation of the EGF receptor by the kinase Jak2 is induced by growth hormone. *Nature*, **390**, 91–6.

Zhu, G., Decker, S. J., Maclean, D., McNamara, D. J., Singh, J., Sawyer, T. K. et al. (1994). Sequence specificity in the recognition of the epidermal growth factor receptor by the abl Src homology 2 domain. *Oncogene*, **9**, 1379–85.

CHAPTER 12

Apoptosis: molecular physiology and significance for cancer therapeutics

Dean A. Fennell

Apoptosis, also referred to as programmed cell death, is a highly regulated, evolutionarily conserved, and biochemically stereotyped process with tremendous relevance to cancer therapeutics. Understanding the molecular basis of apoptosis regulation in cancer is a prerequisite for the development of new effective medicines. This chapter will broadly overview current knowledge of core apoptosis mechanisms, with a focus on the mammalian cell. Novel approaches for overcoming defects in apoptosis signalling have opened up an active and exciting area of drug discovery relevant to cancer, and will be highlighted.

12.1 Apoptosis as a morphological phenomenon

The term *apoptosis* first appeared in the literature in 1972 (Kerr et al., 1972), and was termed *programmed cell death* by Lockshin in 1974 (Lockshin and Beaulaton, 1974). Glücksmann recognized more than two decades earlier in 1951, that cell death could occur during a developmental programme. Cells begin to show features of apoptosis by losing specialized membrane structures such as microvilli and desmosomes, involved in cell–cell contact. As a result, there is separation of neighbouring cells. The plasma–lipid bilayer undergoes a period of blebbing involving organelle-free extensions of membrane-enveloped cytosol that undergo reversible extrusion and resorption. Rapid and irreversible condensation of cytoplasm follows and this is accompanied by an increase in cell density, compaction of cytoplasmic organelles, and condensation of the nuclear chromatin to form dense granular caps or toroidal structures underlying the nuclear membrane. The nuclear pores disappear from the membrane adjacent to the chromatin condensations, and within the nucleus, the nucleolus separates. The nucleus shrinks (pyknosis), and this is followed by nuclear fragmentation (karyorhexis). During these latter changes, the cell splits into a cluster of membrane-bound bodies, each containing a variety of organelles that are largely conserved. Aminophospholipids including phosphotidylserine are normally asymmetrically distributed in the inner plasma membrane, but undergo symmetricalization and outer membrane exposure enabling phagocytes to recognize and ingest the apoptotic cell without evoking an inflammatory response.

These features contrast with necrosis in which dying cells swell, and cytosolic as well as nuclear structures alter, but the nuclear pores are maintained, as are the hetero- and euchromatin. The integrity of the plasma membrane is lost leading to dispersal of the cytoplasmic contents into the extracellular space, a process that triggers an inflammatory reaction.

The last decade of the twentieth century saw an explosive growth in understanding of the underlying molecular physiology of programmed cell death in eukaryotic cells, its fundamental role in development and tissue homeostasis, and its critical involvement in the mode of action of a wide range of cytotoxicity inducers. Phylogenetic conservation of this pathway has enabled investigators to identify human apoptosis proteins that share homology in lower eukaryotes such as *Caenorhabditis elegans*.

12.2 Apoptosis is a process in three phases: a synopsis

The mitochondrion plays a critical role in the induction of apoptosis, acting as an integrator of diverse biochemical signals within the cell. Studies in the early 1990s from Martin Raff's Laboratory at University College London provided early evidence for the cytoplasmic control of apoptosis in cytoplasts devoid of a nucleus (Jacobson et al., 1994). Since those seminal experiments, the mitochondrion has become established as the principle integrating centre for death stimuli within the cell.

The process of apoptosis may be simplified into three discrete phases (shown in Figure 12.1). The *stimulus* or *initiation phase* activates the apoptotic pathway, either via an environmental toxic stimulus (intrinsic pathway), or via a physiological death-inducing stimulus such as ligation of cell surface death receptors (extrinsic pathway). Withdrawal of survival factors may also initiate apoptosis. The *regulatory phase* involves the cellular decision to undergo irreversible commitment to cell death. Mitochondria play a critical role in integrating apoptotic signals, as well as amplifying death signals originating via death receptor signalling. The *execution phase* represents the final common pathway of cell death and involves proteolytic cleavage, nuclear degradation, and plasma membrane changes mediated by enzymes, termed caspases. Activation of this phase is essentially irreversible and results in the display of apoptotic morphology, and stereotyped biochemical changes.

Many aspects of the intrinsic signalling pathway remain to be elucidated. Death is not an inevitability following cell damage; cell cycle arrest and

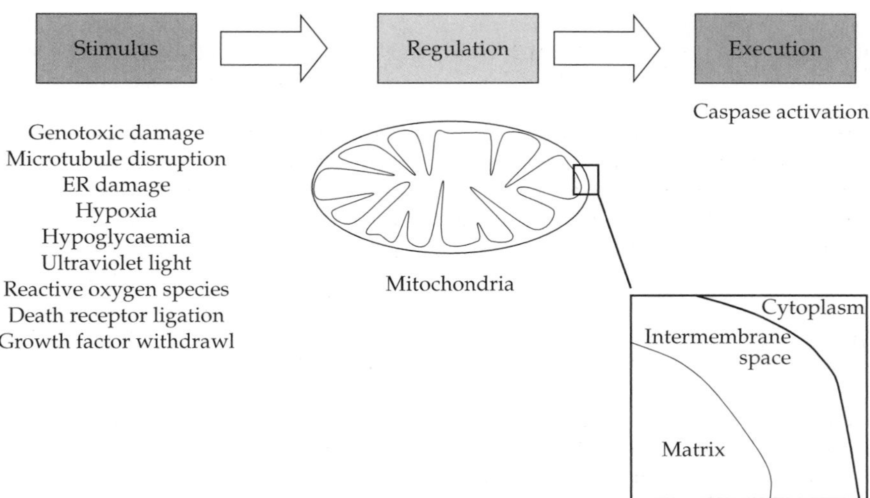

Figure 12.1 Apoptosis as a process in three phases. Mitochondria integrate a diverse range of toxic stimuli, ultimately signalling to cytosol to launch the execution phase involving caspase activation. Breeching of the outer mitochondrial membrane is a critical event, leading to the release of apoptogenic factors that initiate the caspase-dependent effector phase of apoptosis, and caspase-independent cell death.

DNA repair are decisions available to the cell under control by p53. Under conditions when a cell is overwhelmed by the degree of damage (dosage), the signalling of this damage is directed into the apoptosis pathway.

Transduction of a death stimulus involves the translocation of death agonist proteins from the cytoplasm to the outer mitochondrial membrane. Docking of death agonists induces permeabilization of both the outer and the inner mitochondrial membranes. This is accompanied by the release of proapoptotic proteins localized to the intermembrane space that induces caspase dependent and independent apoptosis. Permeabilization of the inner mitochondrial membrane by death agonist proteins results in cessation of respiration and can evoke release of proapoptotic proteins across the outer mitochondrial membrane.

12.2.1 The execution phase of apoptosis

Cellular demolition during apoptosis is an active phenomenon and is achieved by *caspases*, a highly conserved family of aspartate-specific cysteine proteases. Caspases are unique among mammalian cysteine proteases, as they specifically cleave proteins after an aspartate residue. The origin of the term caspase derives from the Cysteine, and *ASP*artate enzyme (*ASE*) specificity. The phylogenetic subdivision *paracaspase* has been applied to metazoans and dictyostelium, while *metacaspase* is applied to caspases in fungi and protozoa. Caspases exhibit specificity for consensus sequences QAC(R/Q)G.

Caspases are synthesized as inactive precursors

Pro-caspases are inactive polypeptides (zymogens), and are constitutively expressed. They comprise an N-terminal prodomain fused to large and small catalytic domains. During activation, the prodomain is cleaved at internal aspartate residues, enabling the catalytic domains to assemble into an active tetrameric enzyme, comprising two large and two small subunits (Figure 12.2).

The prodomain harbours a consensus sequence termed the caspase activation and recruitment domain or CARD. This domain consists of 6–7 antiparallel alpha helices that are involved in homophilic protein–protein interactions. CARDs are present in all caspases and other adaptor proteins that recruit caspase prodomains to cell surface death inducing signalling complex or DISC (Figure 12.3).

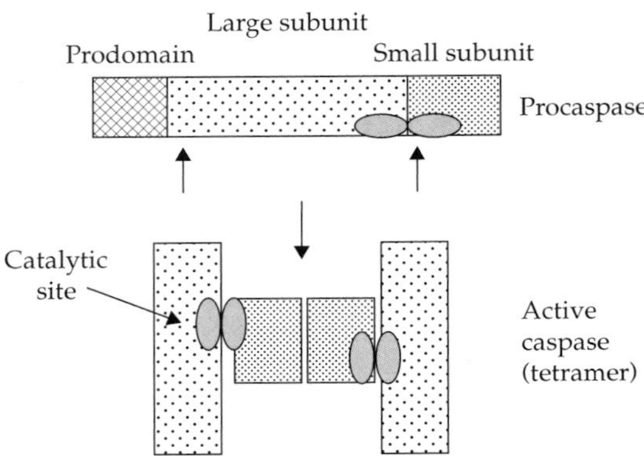

Figure 12.2 Caspase activation. Proteolytic cleavage of the caspase prodomain, results in domain rearrangement and assembly of an active tetramer with two active sites. Caspases are activated in a ballistic manner and target specific.

Caspase 9 is the apical caspase in the intrinsic pathway

Caspase 9 (CASP9) plays a critical role in initiating the caspase cascade and resides in the cytoplasm. Activation of CASP9 involves the assembly of a heterotrimeric complex with cytochrome *c* and the CARD containing protein, APAF-1 (apoptosis protease activating factor 1) (Li et al., 1997; Zou et al., 1997). In the presence of dATP, the prodomain of CASP9 is cleaved resulting in its activation and cleavage of other family members. A splice variant of CASP9 called CASP9S, has been identified in normal liver. It has an intact prodomain and small catalytic subunit, but no large catalytic subunit. CASP9S can inhibit CASP9, and blocks apoptosis mediated by a wide range of stimuli.

APAF-1 comprises three domains; an N-terminal CARD, a middle region with CED4 homology involved in self-assembly (homo-oligomerization), and a C-terminal region comprising WD40 repeats (Figure 12.4). APAF-1 does not normally interact with CASP9 as the CARD is masked by the WD40 repeats. However, in the presence of cytoplasmic cytochrome *c* and dATP, APAF-1 undergoes unfolding, and the CARD and CED4 regions are exposed, resulting in APAF-1 oligomerization, and homophilic CARD interaction with CASP9. The resulting heterotrimeric complex is called the *apoptosome* (Figure 12.5).

Mitochondria harbour and release several apoptogenic factors

Cytochrome *c* is only one of a number of apoptogenic factors that are localized to the mitochondrial

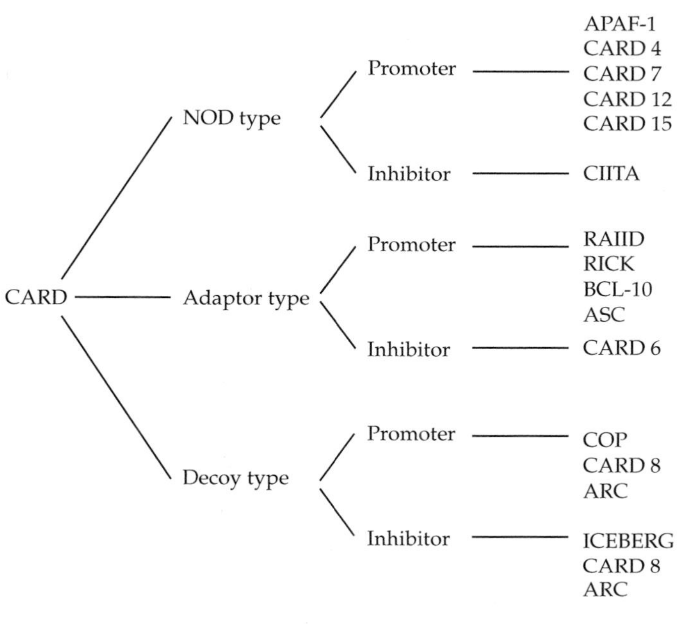

Figure 12.3 Proteins possessing the CARD domain, involved in apoptosis regulation. These proteins possess a consensus domain involved in homophilic protein–protein interactions. A simple classification of CARD proteins is shown.

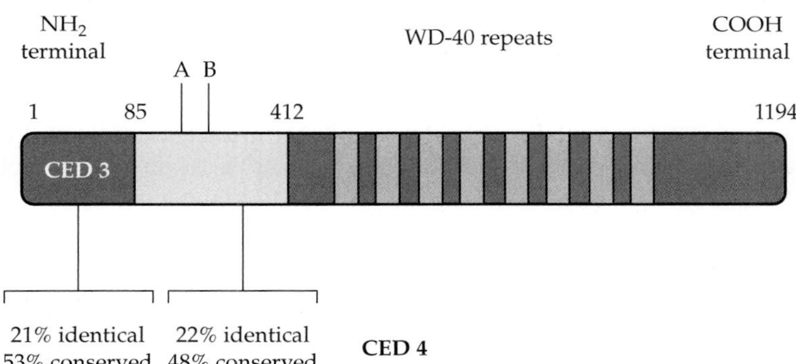

Figure 12.4 APAF-1 is a CARD domain-containing protein that acts as a scaffold with cytochrome *c*, within the pro-CASP9 activating apoptosome. This heterotrimeric structure activates the caspase pathway via prodomain cleavage and activation of the apical CASP9, resulting in the activation of downstream effector caspases.

intermembrane space. During apoptosis, these factors may be selectively or non-specifically released into the cytoplasm. In some models of cell death, proteomic analysis of mitochondrial cytosols has demonstrated a release of up to 200 proteins (Patterson et al., 2000).

Mitochondrial release of cytochrome *c* occurs transiently, and is kinetically invariant (Goldstein et al., 2000). The molecular mechanism underlying its release has not been fully elucidated, but may involve non-specific outer membrane rupture, exit through the voltage-dependent anion channel, or via a specific cytochrome *c* conducting channel.

Executioner caspases and their substrates

Once activated, CASP9 binds to CASP3 and CASP7 (executioner caspases) via homophilic CARD interactions, resulting in cleavage of their prodomains, and activation. CASP3 and CASP7, then cleave downstream caspases. The organized destruction of the cell involves targeting of several intracellular substrates by the activated caspases. DNA

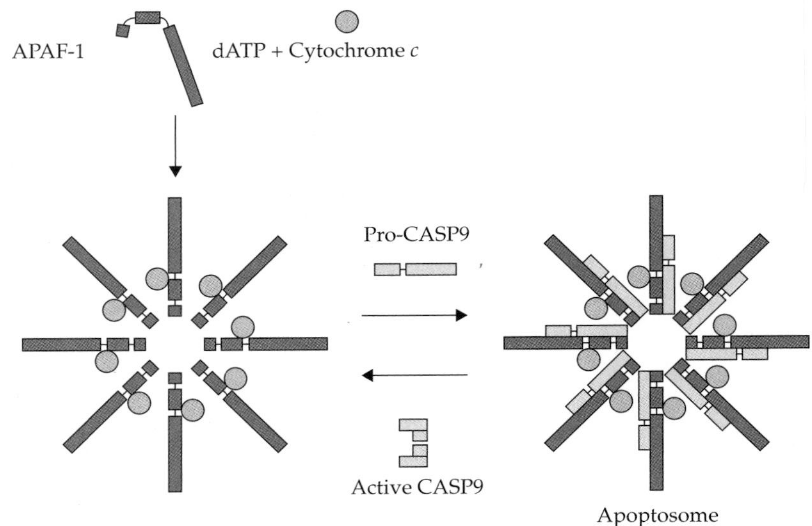

Figure 12.5 Assembly of the CASP9-activating apoptosome, follows cytochrome *c* release in the presence of dATP. APAF-1 recruits pro-CASP9 via a CARD domain interaction. The molecular details involved in the release of cytochrome *c* have not been elucidated but may involve more than one mechanism. Assembly of the APAF-1 apoptosome is one of several pro-apoptotic events resulting from outer mitochondrial membrane permeabilization.

fragmentation factor (DFF) is a substrate for CASP3, which mediates both nuclear condensation and DNA fragmentation (Enari et al., 1998). It is a heterodimeric protein composed of 40 kDa (DFF-40) and 45 kDa (DFF-45) subunits. CASP3 cleaves DFF-45 into two subunits that dissociate from DFF-40. The magnesium-ion-dependent endonuclease activity of DFF is associated with the smaller subunit, DFF-40. The larger 45 kDa subunit (DFF-45) has a regulatory function, and inhibits cell death inducing DFF-45-like effectors, CIDE-A and CIDE-B.

Lamin A is a protein component of the nuclear lamina, a structure that lies beneath the nuclear envelope, maintains its integrity, and organizes interphase chromatin. Lamins are a phylogenetically conserved family of proteins. During apoptosis, CASP6 degrades lamin A, and this occurs during chromatin condensation. Neither CASP3 nor CASP7 exhibit apoptotic laminase activity. CASP6 is required for chromatin condensation and the formation of apoptotic bodies. Other important substrates for caspases include gelsolin, and PARP.

CASP2 is an initiator caspase that targets mitochondria

CASP2 is a stress-induced initiator of downstream effector caspase activation. CASP2 mediates permeabilization of the mitochondrial membrane resulting in apoptogenic factor release, APAF-1/cytochrome *c*/apoptosome. CASP2 is co-released from mitochondria with CASP9 (Susin et al., 1999), and also mediates cell death by promoting translocation of the death agonist protein, BAX from the cytoplasm to the mitochondria.

CASP12 mediates endoplasmic reticulum stress-induced apoptosis

Procaspase 12 is localized to the endoplasmic reticulum (ER), and is activated by CASP7, TRAF-2 (tumour necrosis receptor associated factor 2), and calpain. In addition, glucose starvation, hypoxia, and ER-targeting poisons such as thapsigargin or brefeldin-A activate CASP12. Gene knockout of CASP12 prevents ER stress-induced apoptosis, indicating a critical role for this protein in mediating apoptosis secondary to ER damage (Nakagawa et al., 2000).

Caspase-independent effectors of apoptosis

A number of proteins have been identified that can mediate cell death in the absence of caspases. These proteins include apoptosis-inducing factor (AIF), and endonuclease G (endo G). They function in parallel with caspases, to effect the morphological and biochemical phenomena that constitute apoptosis. They share the common property of being constitutively localized to the mitochondrial intermembrane space, and undergo release upon induction of apoptosis.

Apoptosis inducing factor (PDCD-8)
This 57-kDa protein, was discovered by Guido Kroemer's group. It is localized to the mitochondrial intermembrane space, and undergoes release during initiation of apoptosis (Joza et al., 2001). It is not solubilized in the intermembrane space, but is probably an integral membrane protein in the inner mitochondrial membrane. Human AIF is encoded by a single gene that maps to the X-chromosome, at Xq25–26. It is phylogenetically conserved with a homologue in *C. elegans*, termed WAH-1. Strongest structural homology of AIF with other eukaryotic proteins is shared with the plant flavoproteins, semi-dihydroascorbate, and ascorbate reductase. AIF also shares homology with bacterial NADH (nicotinamide adenine dinucleotide) oxidoreductases. Upon release from mitochondria, AIF translocates to the nucleus where it is able to induce chromatin condensation and internucleosomal DNA fragmentation. AIF does not require the apoptosome or activated caspases to induce nuclear apoptosis. However, recent evidence from Jean-Claude Martinou's group suggests that release of AIF following BAX, occurs downstream of cytochrome *c* release and requires caspase activation.

Endo G
This mitochondrial intermembrane space protein is a mammalian homologue of the *C. elegans* protein, CPS-6. It is an endonuclease that cleaves GC-rich stretches of DNA. During apoptosis, endo G is released from the mitochondrial intermembrane space, and translocates to the nucleus, where it mediates DNA fragmentation independently of DFF45. Unlike DFF45, activation of caspases is not a prerequisite for function of endo G.

12.2.2 Initiation of apoptosis via the intrinsic pathway

During transduction of a toxic environmental signal, or activation of physiological death receptors, a common pathway leading to apoptosome assembly and activation of caspases has been defined that involves mitochondrial membrane permeabilization. The control of mitochondrial permeabilization is a critical event that is both positively and negatively regulated by specific proteins within cells. The balance of pro- versus anti-apoptotic protein activity is a major determinant of cellular apoptotic threshold. In recent years, a considerable growth in knowledge has been achieved with regard to understanding the important controlling checkpoints that regulate mitochondrial permeabilization. However, the precise molecular mechanisms have yet to be fully elucidated.

Death agonist proteins: effectors of mitochondrial permeabilization
BAX and BAK are homologous, multidomain death agonist proteins, that are structurally related to the anti-apoptosis protein BCL-2. These proteins play an essential role in mediating apoptotic signals from a diverse range of stimuli. Enforced overexpression of *BAX,BAK* induces cell death by apoptosis, through a process that involves permeabilization of the outer and inner mitochondrial membranes.

BAX (BCL-2 associated X protein) is a 21 kDa protein that is encoded by a gene located on chromosome 19 (19q13.4–13.5), and contains six exons. Several splice isoforms of BAX have been described. BAX was originally identified from a screen of BCL-2 interacting proteins, and possesses three BCL-2 homology (BH) domains, BH1, BH2, and BH3. The BH3 domain is a nine-amino acid α-helical domain required for apoptosis, and its deletion suppresses BAX,BAK apoptosis-inducing activity. The C-terminal transmembrane domain is involved in mitochondrial localization. These BH domains are involved in homo-dimerization. BAX also heterodimerizes with the anti-apoptotic protein BCL-2. This interaction involves the BH3 domain of BAX, and the BH1–3 domains of BCL-2. Multidomain proapoptotic proteins of the BCL-2 family contrast with shorter BH3-only domain containing proteins, which integrate a diversity of death signalling pathways, through BAX,BAK (Figure 12.6).

In the non-apoptotic setting, BAX resides in the cytoplasm in a folded conformation that brings the C-terminus into proximity with the N-terminus. The mitochondrial localizing transmembrane domain is essentially hidden, and BAX is inactive. During a death stimulus, BAX unfolds, exposing the N-terminal. Monomeric BAX then translocates to the mitochondrial outer membrane, where it undergoes multimerization, assembling into large clusters containing up to several hundred monomeric forms (Wolter et al., 1997; De Giorgi et al.,

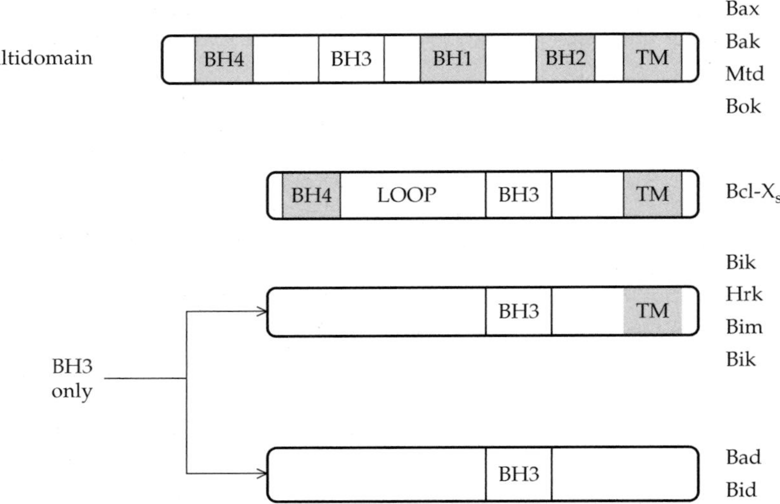

Figure 12.6 Pro-apoptotic (death agonist) proteins of the BCL-2 family can be subdivided into multidomain, and BH3 domain-only subgroups. The BH3 domain is a prequisite for pro-apoptotic function. BH3 proteins mediate mitochondrial permeabilization in association with multidomain pro-apoptotic proteins BAX, BAK. Multidomain domain homologues can oligomerize; this has been shown to occur prior to mitochondrial permeabilization.

2002). BAX-clusters can be visualized by immunofluorescence microscopy. Multimerization is a prerequisite for mitochondrial permeabilization, and is prevented by enforced expression of *BCL-2*. *BAX* is both transcriptionally and directly activated by cytoplasmic p53 (Miyashita and Reed, 1995; Chipuk et al., 2004).

BAK (BCL-2 antagonist killer) is structurally and functionally similar to BAX, undergoing conformation change in the outer mitochondrial membrane during apoptosis. It is encoded by a gene on chromosome 6 (6p21.3), which contains six exons. The splice variant N-BAK is expressed exclusively in neurons, however, the unspliced form is expressed in a wide variety of tissues including terminally differentiated cells.

Mechanism of BAX,BAK at the mitochondrial outer membrane

BAX and BAK have been shown to localize to areas of contact between the inner and outer mitochondrial membrane (De Giorgi et al., 2002). These regions are highly organized *contact sites*, that possess junctional complexes comprising inner/outer membrane, and intermembrane space proteins. These complexes are implicated in the control of mitochondrial permeabilization. Monomeric BAX and BAK bind to the outer membrane protein, VDAC (voltage-dependent anion channel) (Shimizu et al., 1999). This is an abundant outer mitochondrial membrane protein that normally conducts anionic solutes including pyridine nucleotides. VDAC has been shown to exhibit BAX,BAK-inducible conductance of cytochrome *c* by Tsujimoto's group. It has been postulated that this may represent one mechanism of cytochrome *c* release (Shimizu et al., 1999). This model contrasts with the recent work of Colombini and colleagues who have shown that closure of VDAC and antagonism of pyridine nucleotide exchange during apoptosis may be a critical proapoptotic event. The true role of VDAC during apoptosis remains to be elucidated.

Recent work from Korsmeyer's group has shown that a specific isoform of VDAC is important in mediating BAX,BAK-induced outer membrane permeabilization. VDAC1 is proapoptotic while VDAC2 binds BAK, sequestering it in an inactive form, effectively blocking apoptosis (Cheng et al., 2003).

Electrophysiological studies by Kinnally's group have suggested that a novel conductance is established by BAX in the outer mitochondrial membrane, and has been termed the mitochondrial apoptosis channel or MAC (Pavlov et al., 2001). The molecular composition of the MAC is not known. Electrophysiological studies have demonstrated that BAX and BAK have ion channel activity with cationic specificity; a property common to homologous BCL-2 family members, and may contribute electrophysiologically.

Mechanism of BAX,BAK at the mitochondrial inner membrane

BAX,BAK have also been shown to mediate permeabilization of the inner mitochondrial membrane. This results in dissipation of the transmembrane potential gradient ($\Delta\Psi_m$) established during electron transport by the export of protons out of the matrix, into the intermembrane space. Potential energy associated with $\Delta\Psi_m$, is utilized by complex V of the respiratory chain (F_1F_0ATPase), to synthesize ATP. $\Delta\Psi_m$ collapse results in cessation of ATP synthesis, and reversal of the F_1F_0ATPase leading to ATP hydrolysis. Respiration ceases due to failure of electron transport, and cellular ATP levels fall, leading to cell death.

$\Delta\Psi_m$ collapse is accompanied by a non-specific permeability of the inner mitochondrial membrane to solutes below 1500 Da molecular weight. This process is associated with the formation of a novel conductance, and is termed permeability transition or PT (Haworth and Hunter, 1979). Induction of PT involves a pore structure in the inner mitochondrial membrane, the permeability transition pore (PTP) which is part of a multimeric structure comprising junctional complex proteins, implicated in localization of BAX,BAK and cytochrome *c* release (Shimizu et al., 1999; De Giorgi et al., 2002) (Figure 12.7). The inner membrane adenine nucleotide translocator (ANT), normally exchanges newly synthesized ATP within the mitochondrial matrix with ADP. ANT regulates the PTP, although it is not the pore per se (Kokoszka et al., 2004). Three isoforms of ANT are encoded by individual genes. Overexpression of ANT1 induces apoptosis, however, ANT2 overexpression does not. ANT1-mediated PT is promoted by the viral proapoptotic protein Vpr, whereas vMIA expressed by cytomegalovirus, inhibits ANT1-induced PT. BAX and BAK directly interact with the ANT to mediate PT, however, the physical nature of this interaction has not been fully elucidated. BAX inhibits translocase activity of ANT (Marzo et al., 1998).

Evidence suggests that PT can precede or follow cytochrome *c* release, and determines the mode of cell death; this may be dependent upon the nature of the toxic stimulus. Irreversible opening of the PTP results in an influx of water along a gradient of osmolarity, into the mitochondrial matrix resulting in matrix swelling. The inner mitochondrial membrane is folded into cristae and has a high surface area compared to the outer membrane. The swelling therefore results in rupture of the outer but not the inner membrane. Outer membrane rupture releases cytochrome *c* to mediate caspase activation in the presence of dATP.

The BH3-only proteins PUMA and NOXA mediate p53-associated apoptosis

The tumour suppressor protein p53 mediates cell death or cell cycle arrest following genotoxic stress.

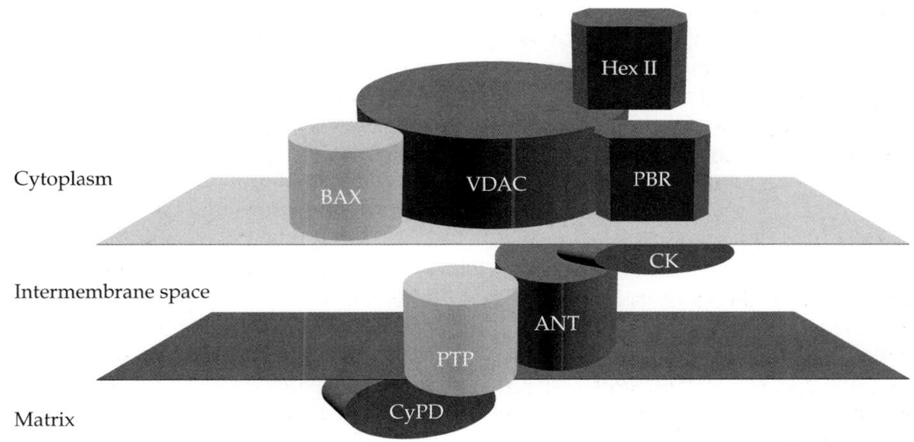

Figure 12.7 The PT pore complex. This multimeric structure comprises nucleated BCL-2 family proteins. In the outer mitochondrial membrane it comprises VDAC, peripheral benzodiazepine receptors (PBRs), hexokinase II; in the intermembrane space, creatinine kinase (CK); in the inner mitochondrial membrane, the ANT, cyclophillin D. The PTP itself has not yet been identified.

NOXA and PUMA are proapoptotic BH3-only proteins that are expressed in a p53-dependent manner, and are involved in mediating apoptosis by p53. During genotoxic stress, NOXA and PUMA mobilize to the mitochondrial outer membrane, where they interact with the anti-apoptotic BCL-2 family members, BCL-2 and BCL-X_L via the BH3 domain to mediate outer mitochondrial membrane permeabilization and apoptosome-dependent apoptosis. Downregulation of PUMA by antisense RNA, suppresses induction of apoptosis by p53, reflecting the important role of this protein in regulation of *p53*-induced cell death. The gene encoding NOXA is responsive to phorbol 12 myristate 13-actetate (PMA) and is rapidly expressed upon exposure. Recent evidence suggests that NOXA can mediate mitochondrial permeabilization via a mechanism that does not involve BAK oligomerization, but may involve direct induction of PT.

Granzyme B induces apoptosis in a BAX,BAK-independent manner

Granzyme B is one of a number of serine proteases that are localized to the cytotoxic granules of cytotoxic T lymphocytes (CTLs) and natural killer (NK) cells. It is released following their activation and induces apoptosis in the target cell. The mechanism leading to apoptosis has been shown to involve two independent pathways. Granzyme B mediates direct intracellular cleavage of BID, resulting in BAX,BAK-dependent mitochondrial permeabilization and cytochrome *c* release. Granzyme B is also able to induce mitochondrial inner membrane depolarization in *bax/bak* double knockout cells, independently from cytochrome *c* release and caspase activation, and this appears to occur via a novel pathway that does not involve PT. It has been postulated that granzyme B may require a novel cofactor to mediate mitochondrial depolarization.

Direct mitochondrial permeabilization by reactive oxygen intermediates

Superoxide directly induces apoptosis by opening of VDAC and releases cytochrome *c* (Madesh and Hajnoczky, 2001). Oxidative stress can directly induce PT. This is mediated by oxidation of a critical vicinal thiol, localized to the matrix facing side of the ANT at cysteine 56 (cys^{56}). Pro-oxidants capable of oxidizing cys^{56} can directly induce apoptosis following induction of PT (Costantini et al., 2000). This is due to osmotic swelling of mitochondria, and outer mitochondrial membrane rupture. Pro-oxidants sensitize cells to other apoptosis inducers, and this property is inhibited by antioxidants such as *N*-acetylcysteine or glutathione.

12.2.3 Initiation of apoptosis via the extrinsic pathway

The extrinsic apoptosis pathway rapidly transduces physiological apoptotic signals mediated at the cell surface, following engagement of a death receptor with its endogenous ligand. Apoptosis mediated by the extrinsic pathway involves caspase activation, and may occur independently from, or in association with the apoptosome which provides a parallel amplificatory pathway. The growing family of death receptors are transmembrane proteins that ligate specific death-inducing ligands, resulting in recruitment of adaptor proteins. The major death ligands are FAS ligand, (tumour necrosis factor) TNF-α, TNF-β, TRAIL, and Apo 3 ligand.

Death domains help assemble the DISC

Death receptors possess a homologous death domain (DD) that mediates protein–protein interaction resulting in either self-association or association with heterologous proteins with DD motifs. A wide variety of adaptor proteins that transduce death signals possess DD motifs. These include FADD, CRADD, and CASP8.

Following engagement of the receptor/adaptor protein via DD interaction, CASP8 and CASP10 are recruited. This occurs via homologous interaction of death effector domains or DEDs (Figure 12.8). The DED is required for death signal transduction through the DISC, and interacts with the prodomain of the apical caspase. Non-caspase proteins containing DEDs, also interact with adaptor proteins and include DEDAF, which facilitates interaction between CD95, FADD, and CASP8. Some DED-containing proteins can activate apical caspases independently of death receptor crosslinking. The DED-containing proteins form cytoplasmic death effector filaments, that recruit and activate apical pro-caspases.

BID: a link between death receptors and the mitochondrial pathway

Upon recruitment of pro-caspase 8 to the DED of the DISC, it is cleaved and activated, resulting in downstream activation of effector caspases. This pathway

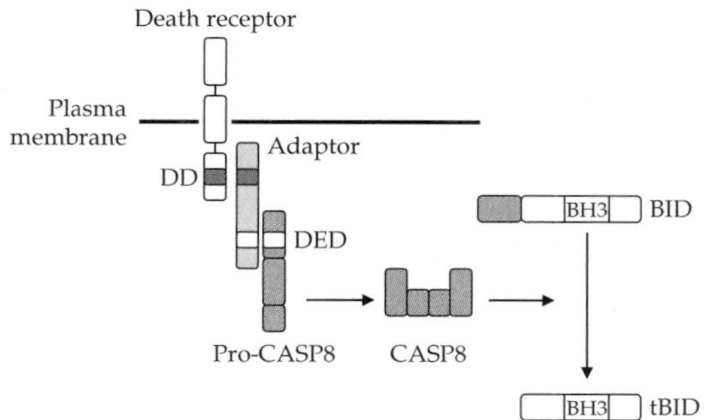

Figure 12.8 The Extrinsic death pathway. Activation of CASP8 and the BH3 domain-only pro-apoptotic protein BID following ligation of death receptor. BID is cleaved resulting in its translocation to the mitochondrial outer membrane. BID directly activates the caspase pathway independent of mitochondrial permeabilization. However, it also facilitates oligomerization of multidomain death agonists and promotes mitochondrial permeabilization. Cells preferentially signalling via direct CASP8 activation following engagement of CD95 receptors have been termed type I cells, whereas preferential use of the mitochondrial pathway is seen in type II cells.

therefore mediates apoptosome-independent caspase activation and cell death. However, the BH3-only protein BID (BH3-interacting domain death agonist) is a substrate for CASP8, which mediates its cleavage as shown in Figure 12.8 (Wang et al., 1996). The C-terminal of BID is a 15 kDa truncated protein (tBID), and translocates to the mitochondrial outer membrane following post-translational *N*-myristolylation (Zha et al., 2000). It has been shown that cardiolipin provides the specificity for targeting of tBID to mitochondria, via a novel three-helix domain. Following transmembrane insertion, tBID oligomerizes and mediates membrane insertion/oligomerization of BAX, through which it is able to effect mitochondrial outer and inner membrane permeabilization. Interaction of tBID with a multidomain death agonist is a prerequisite for its proapoptotic action. Ultrastructural studies have shown that tBID remodels mitochondrial cristae, in a VDAC-dependent manner, resulting in the release of cytochrome *c*.

Type I and type II apoptosis
Krammer's group have identified two types of CD95 pathway. One involves predominant signalling via the DISC, resulting in CASP3 cleavage and apoptosis in type I cells. Type II cells rely upon mitochondrial permeabilization to undergo apoptosis. Apoptosis can therefore be suppressed in type II but not in type I cells by membrane stabilizing anti-apoptotic proteins such as BCL-2 (Scaffidi et al., 1999).

Death receptors and the ceramide pathway
Sphingomyelin is a phospholipid component of the plasma membrane. Ceramide, derived from hydrolysis of sphingomyelin is a proapoptotic signalling molecule, which also regulates cellular proliferation and differentiation. The DD-containing proteins FADD and TRADD activate acid sphingomyelinase (A-Smase), resulting in ceramide synthesis. A-Smase is also activated by a wide range of cell-damaging stimuli including radiation. Ceramide induces apoptosis via activation of MEKK1/MEK4/JNK pathway, by activation of BAX-mediated mitochondrial permeabilization, and via activation of protein kinase C ξ. Ceramide forms large stable channels in the mitochondrial outer membrane capable of conducting cytochrome *c* and could form a release pathway for apoptogenic proteins (Siskind et al., 2002).

12.2.4 Physiological suppression of apoptosis

The mammalian genome encodes many proteins that antagonize the core apoptosis machinery. Overexpression of such genes may confer survival advantage with implications for cancer pathogenesis and treatment. Cells have evolved further levels of regulatory complexity through the expression of proapoptotic genes that antagonize endogenous apoptosis inhibitors, and this may be exploited as a therapeutic strategy to reverse apoptosis resistance.

Apoptosis inhibitors of the BCL-2 family
BCL-2 was originally cloned from the t(14;18) translocation in B-cell non-Hodgkin's lymphoma. Its discovery in the late 1980s arguably heralded the era of rapid growth in apoptosis biology. BCL-2 is encoded on 18q21, and is expressed as a 26 kDa protein comprising BH1, BH2, and BH3 domains. BCL-2 is related to several anti-apoptotic homologues including BCL-X_L, BCL-W, BCL-B, MCL-1, and A1 as shown in Figure 12.9. Overexpression of BCL-2 inhibits apoptosis by a wide variety of inducers including chemicals, irradiation, ultraviolet light, engagement of death receptors, and growth factor withdrawal (Reed et al., 1988). BCL-2 plays an important role during development. Knockout of the *BCL-2* gene results in growth retardation and massive splenic involution due to excessive apoptosis. Conversely, mice

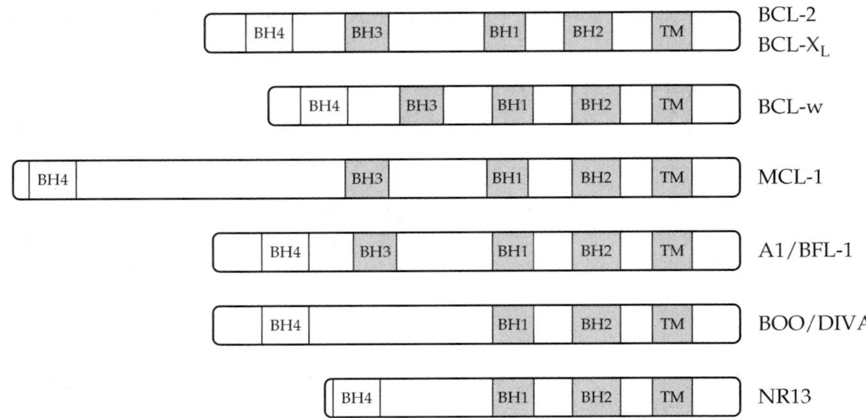

Figure 12.9 BCL-2 family death antagonist proteins. The BH4 domain confers anti-apoptotic activity. This domain is associated with regulation of VDAC permeability and antagonizes multidomain pro-apoptotic activity, however, the precise mechanism of anti-apoptotic action has not been elucidated.

overexpressing *BCL-2* exhibit increased lifespan of memory B cells, and persistence of immunoglobulin secreting cells.

BAX,BAK interacts with BCL-2 and are antagonistic to its activity (Oltvai et al., 1993). The structural basis of this interaction has been elucidated, and reveals a receptor/ligand-like docking in which the BH3 domain of BAX,BAK engages with a cleft formed from BH1, BH2, and BH3 domains. Thus, the BH1 and BH2 domains are required to inhibit apoptosis (Yin et al., 1994). The ratio of anti-apoptotic BCL-2 to proapoptotic BAX has been likened to a rheostat that governs the cellular apoptosis threshold (Korsmeyer et al., 1993). Thus, overexpression of BCL-2 confers an increased apoptosis threshold, whereas overexpression of BAX/BAK increases apoptosis sensitivity.

BCL-2 protein exhibits cationic ion-channel properties and localizes to the mitochondrial outer membrane, ER, and nucleus. BCL-2 also acts independently as an efficient inhibitor of mitochondrial permeabilization, blocking both the release of apoptogenic factors, and preventing PT. It has been shown that during apoptosis BCL-2 antagonizes BAX-mediated opening of VDAC, effectively preventing cytochrome c conductance. The binding site of BCL-2 on VDAC has been shown to be synoptic with BAX. The BH4 domain of BCL-2 is required for anti-apoptotic activity, and this domain has been shown to be sufficient to prevent VDAC opening. Deletion of BH4 does not prevent homo- nor heterodimerization, however.

BCL-2 functionally interacts with the ANT to maintain its translocase activity, and thus prevents formation of the PTP. BCL-2 can be inhibited by the thiol oxidant diamide, and this activity is due to oxidation of ANT (cys^{56}), which overcomes BCL-2-mediated suppression of PT. The small molecule, PK11195 directly interacts with the PTP complex via the peripheral benzodiazepine receptor, and can also inhibit BCL-2. However, this activity may depend upon its ability to generate oxidative stress (Fennell et al., 2001). Recent evidence suggests that BCL-2 can act upstream of mitochondria to prevent caspase activation (Marsden et al., 2002). The molecular basis for this action has not been elucidated.

Tumour hypoxia upregulates anti-apoptotic proteins

As tumours increase in dimension, they acquire regions of low oxygenation (hypoxia). Cancer cells respond to this environmental stress by increasing expression of hypoxia-activated transcription factor, a heterodimeric protein which in turn transcriptionally activates genes involved in anti-apoptosis, glycolytic energy metabolism, and tumour progression.

BCL-X$_L$: anti-apoptotic homologue of BCL-2

The BCL-2 homologue BCL-X$_L$ is a 233-amino acid splice variant of the *BCL-X* gene that is a multidomain apoptosis repressor (Boise et al., 1993). Deletion of BCL-X$_L$ is lethal, owing to massive apoptosis in the haematopoietic and nervous systems during embryogenesis. Transgenic mice overexpressing BCL-X_L develop bone marrow expansion of pro-B cells with aberrant immunoglobulin gene rearrangements. The 170-amino acid splice variant, BCL-X_s lacks the BH1 and BH2 domains, and is proapoptotic. BCL-X_L promotes cell survival in the absence of an apoptotic stimulus, with greater potency than BCL-2, and has been shown to involve maintenance of ADP/ATP exchange through stabilization of a pyridine nucleotide conducting conformation of VDAC. This activity contrasts with the anti-apoptotic action of BCL-X_L, whereby BAX-induced cytochrome *c* release through VDAC is inhibited (Shimizu et al., 1999).

Inhibitors of BAX translocation

BAX activity may be regulated by proteins which directly prevent translocation. Proteins identified with this activity include humanin, 14-3-3 isoforms σ and τ, Ku70, ARC, and hexokinase II. Humanin is a 24-amino acid secreted peptide that is not expressed in the immune system, but exhibits high levels in the liver, skeletal muscle, and heart. Expression is significant also in the brain and gut. Humanin blocks beta-amyloid peptide or serum withdrawal-induced apoptosis. The mechanism of anti-apoptotic action by humanin has been shown to involve sequestration of BAX, and prevention of translocation from cytosol to mitochondria. Downregulation of humanin derepresses BAX, and facilitates cell death (Guo et al., 2003).

The cytoskeletal protein 14-3-3σ, is involved in regulating cell cycle arrest by the tumour suppressor p53 during genotoxic stress, and suppresses apoptosis by preventing BAX translocation. The identification of a trimeric complex comprising 14-3-3σ BAX, and cyclin-dependent kinase 1 (CDK-1) has been postulated to mediate BAX suppression, possibly via sequestration. The isoform 14-3-3τ sequesters BAX, effectively suppressing apoptosis. Ku70 was recently identified as a BAX-suppressing protein that also acts via sequestration of BAX. Disruption of the Ku70–BAX interaction by small peptides is sufficient to facilitate BAX translocation and apoptosis in cells overexpressing Ku70 (Sawada et al., 2003).

Bax inhibitor 1 (BI-1) is a non-BCL-2 family protein, that is bound to intracellular membranes and interacts with BAX, BCL-2, and BCL-X_L. Its overexpression prevents BAX-induced apoptosis, but does not inhibit apoptosis induced via ligation of the FAS receptor. Downregulation of BI-1 expression by antisense oligonucleotides induces cell death. The gene is also termed testis-enhanced gene transcript (TEGT), and mediates cell survival in a developmentally regulated manner, and is expressed in testis and perinatal lung tissue.

The glycolytic enzyme hexokinase II interacts with VDAC and exploits its proximity to newly synthesized ATP, exported through this channel. Hexokinase II has been shown to inhibit BAX-mediated apoptosis, and this activity is related to suppression of BAX translocation.

BAG-1

Human BAG-1 is a protein with four isoforms, that does not exhibit structural homology to BCL-2, but augments its anti-apoptotic activity when co-expressed (Takayama et al., 1995). It functions by interacting with the activated steroid hormone receptors via interaction with heat shock protein 90 (Hsp90), a molecular chaperone required for steroid receptor activation. BAG-1 promotes ATP hydrolysis in the presence of Hsp40 and Hsp70. BAG-1 also interacts with the intracellular domain of platelet-derived growth factor.

FLICE inhibitory proteins (FLIPs) inhibits the DISC

FLIPs are proteins with viral homologues expressed by bovine Herpesvirus 4, Herpesvirus 8 associated with Kaposi's sarcoma, herpesvirus saimiri, and human molloscipoxvirus. FLIPs interact with the adaptor FADD and CASP8, and effectively block death receptor signal transduction. However, FLIPs do not block apoptosis mediated via the intrinsic pathway, nor granzyme B. Two forms (cellular FLIP or c-FLIP), have been identified, and are predominantly expressed in lymphoid tissue and muscle. The long isoform of FLIP (FLIP-L) possesses homology to caspases, but lacks proteolytic activity. FLIP-S, the short form is characterized by two DEDs and has structural homology to viral FLIPs.

The inhibitor of apoptosis protein family

Endogenous caspase inhibitors have been identified, that can antagonize both intrinsic and extrinsic apoptosis pathways. The inhibitor of apoptosis protein (IAP) family, comprises phylogenetically conserved homologues of an anti-apoptotic protein encoded by the baculovirus (polyhydrosis virus) genome. These proteins, collectively termed BIR-containing proteins or BIRCs, are characterized by a baculoviral internal repeat, or BIR domain, comprising histidine- and cysteine-rich motifs. The

BIR domain is essential for function, and interaction with other apoptosis-regulating proteins, including caspases and APAF-1. The structural detail of the binding interaction between the BIR-3 domain of XIAP (X-linked inhibitor of apoptosis protein) has been determined (Huang et al., 2001).

The C-terminal domain is characterized by a cysteine and histidine containing ring finger, which can coordinate two zinc atoms. This domain has ubiquitin ligase protease activity, and mediates degradation upon auto-ubiquitination during an apoptotic stimulus. XIAP sequesters CASP3 in the apoptosome complex with processed CASP9 and oligomerized APAF-1. This effectively prevents release of activated CASP3.

Survivin is a 16 kDa protein which contains a single BIR domain, and lacks the C-terminal ring finger (Ambrosini et al., 1997). Structurally, survivin resembles the *C. elegans* protein BIR-1. Expression of survivin is turned off in normally differentiated adult tissues. Survivin binds to CASP3 and CASP7, but not to the initiator CASP8, and thus inhibits apoptosis (Tamm et al., 1998). Expression of survivin is also increased in the G2/M-phase of the cell cycle, and it associates with the mitotic spindle at the beginning of mitosis. This interaction is essential for anti-apoptotic function.

The XIAP is expressed in all foetal and adult tissues, except for peripheral blood leucocytes (Deveraux et al., 1997). Like survivin, XIAP directly interacts with and inhibits CASP3 and CASP7. In addition, it interacts with the CASP9–APAF1 apoptosome via the small p12 subunit of processed CASP9. This interaction is required for XIAP function. Mutational analysis has shown that the inhibitory effect on CASP3 can be separated from inhibition of CASP9. The ring finger domain of XIAP interacts with ubiquitin, and during an apoptotic stimulus in T cells, is degraded by the proteosome. As XIAP possesses ubiquitin protein ligase (E3) activity, it is able to undergo auto-ubiquitination.

The proteins c-IAP1 and c-IAP2 bind and directly inactivate CASP3 and CASP7 in a BIR domain-dependent manner (Roy et al., 1997). Both of these proteins possess C-terminal ring finger domains and possess ubiquitin protein ligase (E3) activity. An increasing number of IAP proteins have been identified including NAIP, livin, and apollon.

Mitochondria release inhibitors of IAPs

Harboured within the intermembrane space of mitochondria, are proteins which specifically derepress caspases, by inhibiting IAPs. During apoptosis, the proteins SMAC (second mitochondria derived activator of caspases), and OMI (serine protease 25) or HtrA2 are released from the mitochondria. SMAC was the first mitochondrial IAP inhibitor to be discovered, and is co-released with cytochrome *c* (Du et al., 2000). OMI is a mitochondrial intermembrane space protein that has close structural resemblance to the bacterial hsp HtrA, a protein involved in the endoproteolytic degradation of denatured proteins, involved in allowing survival of the bacterial cell in high temperature environments. The C-terminus of OMI bears structural resemblance to human HtrA (L56), a secreted protein. During apoptosis, OMI is released from the mitochondrial intermembrane space into the cytoplasm in a processed form, binds to XIAP (but not survivin), and inhibits its caspase-inhibitor activity. The interaction between OMI and XIAP involves a reaper-like domain. The full-length (unprocessed) precursor of OMI does not bind XIAP.

Apoptosis suppression mediated by growth factor pathways

The core apoptosis machinery is regulated by survival signals originating from growth factor receptors at the cell surface. The erbB family of growth factor receptors is a structurally related family of transmembrane proteins with intrinsic tyrosine kinase activity. They include ERBB1 (epidermal growth factor receptor, EGFR), ERBB2 (Her2), ERBB3, and ERBB4. Natural ligands are EGF amphiregulin, (transforming growth factor) TGF-alpha, and epiregulin. Upon ligation, the receptors heterodimerize and undergo tyrosine autophosphorylation of the intracellular domain. This results in the recruitment of phosphoinositide 3 kinase, which in turn is phosphorylated, mediating downstream phosphorylation and activation of AKT (Figure 12.10). Phosphorylated AKT (p-AKT) mediates anti-apoptosis by promoting glycolysis via recruitment of hexokinase II to the outer mitochondrial membrane, adjacent to VDAC. CASP9, an AKT substrate is inhibited by phosphorylation (Cardone et al., 1998).

BAD: a link between survival pathways and cell death

The BH3 domain-only protein BAD is inactivated by AKT, by phosphorylation of serine 136 (ser^{136}) (Zha et al., 1996). BAD is an endogenous inhibitor of BCL-X_L and antagonizes its interaction with BAK, BAX (Yang et al., 1995; Kelekar et al., 1997).

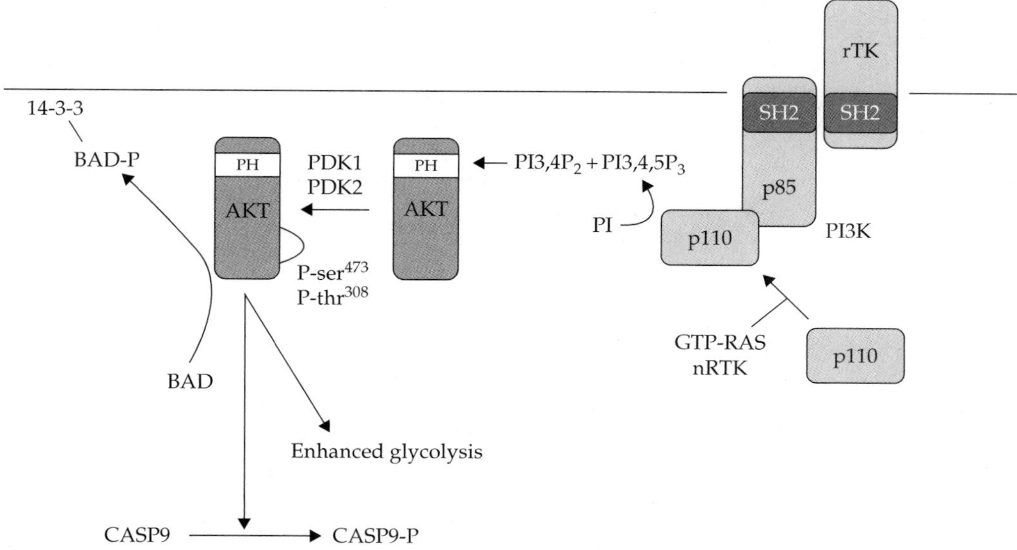

Figure 12.10 BAD inactivation by growth factor receptor signalling. Phosphoinositide 3 kinase is activated upon growth factor receptor ligation. The active enzyme possesses two subunits (p85 and p110). Phosphorylation of phosphoinositide (PtdIns), yields PtdIns 1,4,5P$_3$, which binds the pleckstrin homology domain of AKT leading to its activation via phosphorylation by PDK1/2. AKT phosphorylates BAD, leading to 14-3-3 sequestration.

This results in sequestration to the scaffold protein 14-3-3. BAD is also inactivated by phosphorylation associated with activation of the mitogen-activated protein kinase (MAPK) pathway, on ser^{115} and ser^{155}. Inhibition of PI3K by the inhibitor LY294002, or the MAPK pathway by PD98059, promotes apoptosis by enabling BAD to be released from 14-3-3 and in turn dissociates BAK, BAX, and BCL-X$_L$.

12.3 Exploiting apoptosis biology for effective cancer therapy

The effectiveness of radiotherapy- or drug-based cytotoxic therapy for cancer relies primarily on the ability to kill the cancer cell, a process that is achieved via induction of apoptosis. Success in achieving this is associated with cytoreduction to undetectable levels, termed complete remission (CR). Some cancers are curable, and attainment of CR is a prerequisite. Metastatic disease does not preclude curative systemic therapy. Hodgkin and non-Hodgkin lymphomas, and germ cell cancers such as seminoma, are rapidly proliferating and metastasizing tumours, yet their sensitivity to chemotherapy and radiotherapy underlies their curability in the majority of patients.

Unfortunately, the majority of solid cancers have considerably higher tolerance to cytotoxic therapy. A spectrum of tolerance to chemotherapy-induced cell death can be defined in which certain metastatic cancers, including advanced non-small cell lung cancer (non-SCLC), mesothelioma, pancreatic cancer, cholangiocarcinoma, and renal cell cancer, constitute a group that exhibit major apoptosis resistance. Conversely, germ cell cancers and haematological malignancies reside at the most chemosensitive and potentially curable end of the spectrum. The impact of chemotherapy alone displays dramatically different effects on natural history for diseases at either end of the spectrum, and this is manifest in median survival as illustrated in Figure 12.11.

Acquisition of resistance to therapy is a commonly observed phenomenon in many malignancies. The most striking examples of this include SCLC and follicular lymphoma (FL). SCLC is exquisitely sensitive to chemotherapy, and will respond with tumour shrinkage in the majority of patients. A significant proportion of tumours may indeed exhibit CR. However, some tumours exhibit early recurrence with a resistant phenotype (variant SCLC, v-SCLC) that is unresponsive to therapy. The genetic basis of this phenotype is not understood.

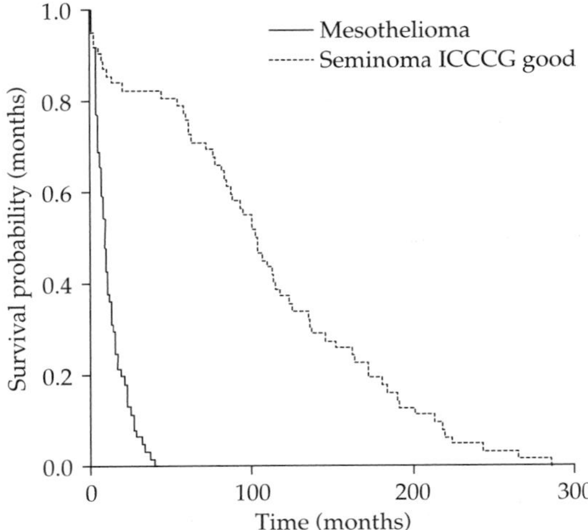

Figure 12.11 Kaplan–Meier survival curves comparing the relative survival of patients with malignant pleural mesothelioma, compared with seminoma.

Failure of therapy results in uncontrolled progression of the disease. FL exhibits relatively long-term sensitivity to treatment, and will respond, often for years. The disease undergoes *transformation* associated with a change in phenotype to diffuse large B-cell lymphoma. This form is aggressive, and exhibits significantly lower tolerance to cytotoxic therapy compared with FL. Genetic analysis has shown that apoptosis regulation may determine outcome in large B-cell lymphoma.

Apoptosis resistance is a major factor involved in failure of systemic cytotoxic therapy. This phenomenon is multifactorial. Local factors within a tumour such as pH, and perfusion may be poor, limiting drug bioavailability. Mutations leading to upregulation of drug efflux pumps such as multidrug resistance proteins (MDR-1, MRP, LRP), may significantly affect intracellular bioavailability. Chemotherapeutic drugs typically effect cell death via damage sensors associated with DNA, cellular metabolism, or microtubule stabilization, and specific mutations may be sufficient to attenuate apoptosis induction.

Common patterns of dysregulation of the core apoptosis pathway have been identified recently. Mutations leading to inhibition of the final common pathway to apoptosis will effectively suppress cell death induced by most cytotoxic stimuli. Overcoming this problem requires functional dissection of the core death apparatus in specific cancers, to increase understanding of how such processes can be reversed. Some of the major lesions in core apoptosis signalling and their potential for therapeutic reversal are outlined below, and summarized in Figure 12.12.

12.3.1 Apoptosome and caspase suppression in cancer

Some cancers have been shown to exhibit reduced expression of CASP9, resulting in reduced caspase activation potential. Approximately 15% of non-Hodgkin lymphomas have inactivating mutations of CASP10, attenuating death signalling via the extrinsic death pathway.

Expression of IAPs appears to be widespread in several malignancies, such as non-SCLC, which expresses survivin, and XIAP. Downregulation of these proteins using antisense oligonucleotides confers apoptosis sensitivity. The interaction between IAPs and the endogenous IAP inhibitor SMAC has been elucidated, with potential for drug discovery. SMAC peptides can sensitize several tumour models to chemotherapy *in vivo*, suggesting utility of this approach in the clinic. Small molecule SMAC mimetics discovered by combinatorial library screening exhibit chemosensitizing efficacy, and are an exciting development. The lack of expression of survivin in differentiated adult tissue, suggests that its targeting may exhibit tumour selectively, and thus minimize systemic toxicity of chemosensitization strategies.

12.3.2 Regulation of BCL-2 family death agonist proteins in cancer

Testicular cancer cells are highly susceptible to apoptosis induction, and have been shown to exhibit a high BAX : BCL-2 ratio. The tumour suppressor *TP53* is mutated in several cancers, resulting in failure of stabilization and accumulation following sensing of DNA damage. The BH3-only death agonists PUMA and NOXA are mediated by p53 expression, and are potentially attenuated in cancer due to defective p53.

12.3.3 BCL-2 and its homologues in cancer: novel therapeutic targets

Several cancers overexpress BCL-2 and BCL-X_L, with the potential to suppress mitochondrial

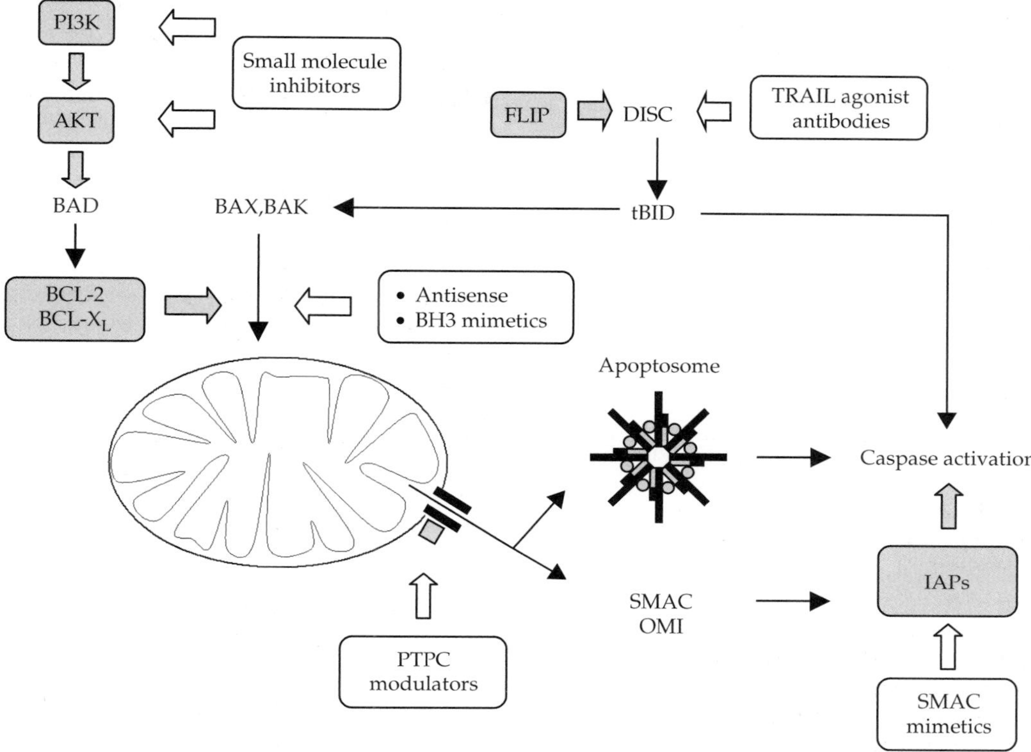

Figure 12.12 Molecular targets with a potential to reverse apoptosis resistance in cancer.

permeabilization. Downregulation of *BCL-2* or *BCL-X$_L$* using antisense oligonucleotides has been reported in patients with Non-Hodgkin's lymphoma and melanoma, validating this approach as a novel therapeutic strategy. Antisense BCL-2 facilitates apoptosis induced by chemotherapeutic drugs, and represents a novel strategy for chemosensitization (Webb et al., 1997; Jansen et al., 1998; Waters et al., 2000). This approach is currently being evaluated in clinical trials in a range of solid and haematological malignancies. Suppression of RNA translation by antisense oligonucleotides requires a time lag to allow for endogenous proteolysis of the target in order to achieve protein downregulation. Anti-tumour properties of the phosphorothioate backbone of antisense oligonucleotides may exhibit additional desirable properties such as reduced cellular proliferation in addition to target downregulation, due to binding of growth factor receptors. Development of novel bi-specific antisense oligonucleotides targeting *BCL-2* and *BCL-X$_L$* simultaneously, have been shown to overcome the potential problem of redundant expression.

The *BAX* gene exhibits frameshift mutations in gastrointestinal cancer, with the potential to inhibit core apoptosis signalling (Rampino et al., 1997). Reduced expression of *BAX* in breast cancer is associated with poor response rates to chemotherapy and worse survival (Krajewski et al., 1995). Knowledge of the structural basis underlying heterodimerization between BCL-2/BCL-X$_L$ and BAX/BAK is currently being exploited to develop small molecule antagonists of this interaction. The BH3 domain of BAK can be mimicked by small molecules, selected by random screening of a large combinatorial library of small compounds, or via theoretical determination of optimal pharmacophore structure to enable high-affinity binding. First-generation small molecule BAK BH3 peptide mimetics (BBPMs) have been discovered with micromolar binding affinity (Wang et al., 2000; Enyedy et al., 2001; Tzung et al., 2001). Second-generation nanomolar affinity ('drugable')

BBPMs have been identified, and will soon enter clinical evaluation.

12.3.4 Exploiting the extrinsic apoptosis pathway in cancer

TRAIL receptors have been shown to be functionally active in several cancers and are a target for therapeutic drug development. Agonist monoclonal antibodies to TRAIL receptors DR1 and DR2 are currently undergoing early clinical evaluation. Furthermore, activation of caspases via this pathway has been shown to exhibit low systemic toxicity, although potential for hepatotoxicity has been suggested from studies in mice. The FADD/CASP8 inhibitor FLIP-L is expressed at high levels in melanoma, and effectively suppresses apoptosis signalling via the DISC. FAS ligand exhibits significant hepatotoxicity in preclinical models, and is therefore not a valid target for anticancer drug development.

12.3.5 Survival pathways as targets for therapeutic intervention in cancer

Several cancers express EGFR, and this is a poor prognostic factor for survival. Constitutive EGFR activation effects PI3K-dependent phosphorylation and activation of AKT, with concomitant inactivation of BAD. The EGFR is a target for therapy. Several strategies for inhibiting EGFR are being evaluated in the clinic, and include monoclonal antibodies such as cetuximab, and small molecule receptor tyrosine kinases such as ZD1839 and OSI774. These molecules rely for their activity on suppressing all downstream events from the receptor within the PI3K pathway. Her2 (ERBB2) is a prognostic factor in breast cancer, and a humanized monoclonal antibody to this receptor, termed Herceptin, has been validated as an effective therapy in the management of breast cancer. There is evidence however, that crosstalk between the PI3K and MAPK pathways may promote constitutive activation of PI3K and AKT, and that this may not be prevented by specific inhibition of the ERBB receptors alone. For example, constitutive Ras activation may promote phosphorylation of MAPK and therefore lead to phosphorylation of BAD even in the presence of blocked EGFR. This mechanism could account for the failure of response to EGFR inhibitors in some patients.

Phosphorylated AKT can be measured *in vivo* in cancers, and represents a potent anti-apoptotic protein and putative therapeutic target. The small molecule SRI13368 is a specific AKT inhibitor, and more novel small molecules are in development.

The receptor tyrosine kinase c-kit is constitutively activated in gastrointestinal stromal tumours (GISTs), and mediates intracellular survival signals via the PI3K pathway. GISTs exhibit significant chemoresistance with short median survival. Recent clinical evidence has demonstrated the dramatic antitumour activity of a small molecule c-kit tyrosine kinase inhibitor, imatinib mesylate (Gleevec/STI571). This agent has demonstrated efficacy in chronic lymphocytic leukaemia (CML), with the translocation t(9,22) bcr-abl expressed in over 90% of cells. This results in the constitutive activation of the tyrosine kinase abl, which exhibits anti-apoptotic function. Imatinib has been rapidly established as a new standard therapy in the management of chronic phase CML and GISTs, and represents a paradigm shift in cancer therapeutics.

12.4 Concluding remarks

The last decade has witnessed extensive growth of knowledge relating to mammalian apoptosis. Application of this knowledge is helping to define the important pathways that determine the apoptosis-resistant phenotype of the most common but difficult to treat cancers. Despite the complexity of regulation of apoptosis pathways, functional genomics, and target validation using small molecules, are identifying new potentially therapeutic molecules at an advancing rate. This will inevitably increase the number of new agents entering clinical trial, and thus the likelihood of effective drug discovery.

References

Ambrosini, G., Adida, C., and Altieri, D. C. (1997). A novel anti-apoptosis gene, survivin, expressed in cancer and lymphoma. *Nat Med*, **3**, 917–21.

Boise, L. H., Gonzalez-Garcia, M., Postema C. E., Ding, L., Lindsten, T., Turka, L. A. et al. (1993). Bcl-X, a Bcl-2 related gene that functions as a dominant regulator of apoptotic cell death. *Cell*, **74**, 597–608.

Cardone, M. H., Roy, N., Stennicke, H. R., Salvesen, G. S., Franke, T. F., Stanbridge, E. et al. (1998). Regulation of cell death protease caspase-9 by phosphorylation. *Science*, **282**, 1318–21.

Cheng, E. H., Sheiko, T. V., Fisher, J. K., Craigen, W. J., and Korsmeyer, S. J. (2003). VDAC2 inhibits BAK activation and mitochondrial apoptosis. *Science*, **301**, 513–7.

Chipuk, J. E., Kuwana, T., Bouchier-Hayes, L., Droin, N. M., Newmeyer, D. D., Schuler, M. et al. (2004). Direct activation of Bax by p53 mediates mitochondrial membrane permeabilization and apoptosis. *Science*, **303**, 1010–4.

Costantini, P., Belzacq, A. S., Vieira, H. L., Larochette, N., de Pablo, M. A., Zamzami, N. et al. (2000). Oxidation of a critical thiol residue of the adenine nucleotide translocator enforces bcl-2-independent permeability transition pore opening and apoptosis (in process citation). *Oncogene*, **19**, 307–14.

De Giorgi, F., Lartigue, L., Bauer, M. K., Schubert, A., Grimm, S., Hanson, G. T. et al. (2002). The permeability transition pore signals apoptosis by directing Bax translocation and multimerization. *Faseb J*, **16**, 607–9.

Deveraux, Q. L., Takahashi, R., Salvesen, G. S., and Reed, J. C. (1997). X-linked IAP is a direct inhibitor of cell-death proteases. *Nature*, **388**, 300–4.

Du, C., Fang, M., Li, Y., Li, L., and Wang, X. (2000). Smac, a mitochondrial protein that promotes cytochrome c-dependent caspase activation by eliminating IAP inhibition. *Cell*, **102**, 33–42.

Enari, M., Sakahira, H., Yokoyama, H., Okawa, K., Iwamatsu, A. and Nagata, S. (1998). A caspase-activated DNase that degrades DNA during apoptosis, and its inhibitor ICAD (see comments) (published erratum appears in Nature 1998 May 28;393(6683):396). *Nature*, **391**, 96–9.

Enyedy, I. J., Ling, Y., Nacro, K., Tomita, Y., Wu, X., Cao, Y. et al. (2001). Discovery of small-molecule inhibitors of Bcl-2 through structure-based computer screening. *J Med Chem*, **44**, 4313–24.

Fennell, D. A., Corbo, M., Pallaska, A., and Cotter, F. E. (2001). Bcl-2 resistant mitochondrial toxicity mediated by the isoquinoline carboxamide PK11195 involves de novo generation of reactive oxygen species. *Br J Cancer*, **84**, 1397–404.

Goldstein, J. C., Waterhouse, N. J., Juin, P., Evan, G. I., and Green, D. R. (2000). The coordinate release of cytochrome *c* during apoptosis is rapid, complete and kinetically invariant (In Process Citation). *Nat Cell Biol*, **2**, 156–62.

Guo, B., Zhai, D., Cabezas, E., Welsh, K., Nouraini, S., Satterthwait, A. C. et al. (2003). Humanin peptide suppresses apoptosis by interfering with Bax activation. *Nature*, **423**, 456–61.

Haworth, R. A. and Hunter, D. R. (1979). The Ca2+-induced membrane transition in mitochondria. II. Nature of the Ca2+ trigger site. *Arch Biochem Biophys*, **195**, 460–7.

Huang, Y., Park, Y. C., Rich, R. L., Segal, D., Myszka, D. G., and Wu, H. (2001). Structural basis of caspase inhibition by XIAP: differential roles of the linker versus the BIR domain. *Cell*, **104**, 781–90.

Jacobson, M. D., Burne, J. F., and Raff, M. C. (1994). Programmed cell death and Bcl-2 protection in the absence of a nucleus. *Embo J*, **13**, 1899–910.

Jansen, B., Schlagbauer-Wadl, H., Brown, B. D., Bryan, R. N., van Elsas, A., Muller, M. et al. (1998). bcl-2 antisense therapy chemosensitizes human melanoma in SCID mice. *Nat Med*, **4**, 232–4.

Joza, N., Susin, S. A., Daugas, E., Stanford, W. L., Cho, S. K., Li, C. Y. et al. (2001). Essential role of the mitochondrial apoptosis-inducing factor in programmed cell death. *Nature*, **410**, 549–54.

Kelekar, A., Chang, B. S., Harlan, J. E., Fesik, S. W., and Thompson, C. B. (1997). Bad is a BH3 domain-containing protein that forms an inactivating dimer with Bcl-XL. *Mol Cell Biol*, **17**, 7040–6.

Kerr, J. F., Wyllie, A. H., and Currie, A. R. (1972). Apoptosis: a basic biological phenomenon with wide-ranging implications in tissue kinetics. *Br J Cancer*, **26**, 239–57.

Kokoszka, J. E., Waymire, K. G., Levy, S. E., Sligh, J. E., Cai, J., Jones, D. P. et al. (2004). The ADP/ATP translocator is not essential for the mitochondrial permeability transition pore. *Nature*, **427**, 461–5.

Korsmeyer, S. J., Shutter, J. R., Veis, D. J., Merry, D. E., and Oltvai, Z. N. (1993). Bcl-2/Bax: a rheostat that regulates an anti-oxidant pathway and cell death. *Semin Cancer Biol*, **4**, 327–32.

Krajewski, S., Blomqvist, C., Franssila, K., Krajewska, M., Wasenius, V. M., Niskanen, E. et al. (1995). Reduced expression of proapoptotic gene BAX is associated with poor response rates to combination chemotherapy and shorter survival in women with metastatic breast adenocarcinoma. *Cancer Res*, **55**, 4471–8.

Li, P., Nijhawan, D., Budlhardjo, I., Srinivasula, S. M., Ahmad, M., Alnemri, E. S. et al. (1997). Cytochrome c and dATP-dependent formation of Apaf-1/caspase-9 complex initiates an apoptotic protease cascade. *Cell*, **91**, 479–89.

Lockshin, R. A. and Beaulaton, J. (1974). Programmed cell death. *Life Sci*, **15**, 1549–65.

Madesh, M. and Hajnoczky, G. (2001). VDAC-dependent permeabilization of the outer mitochondrial membrane by superoxide induces rapid and massive cytochrome *c* release. *J Cell Biol*, **155**, 1003–15.

Marsden, V. S., O'Connor, L., O'Reilly, L. A., Silke, J., Metcalf, D., Ekert, P. G. et al. (2002). Apoptosis initiated by Bcl-2-regulated caspase activation independently of the cytochrome c/Apaf-1/caspase-9 apoptosome. *Nature*, **419**, 634–7.

Marzo, I., Brenner, C., Zamzami, N., Jurgensmeier, J. M., Susin, S. A., Vieira, H. L. A. et al. (1998). Bax and adenine nucleotide translocator cooperate in the mitochondrial control of apoptosis. *Science*, **281**, 2027–31.

Miyashita, T. and Reed, J. C. (1995). Tumor suppressor p53 is a direct transcriptional activator of the human bax gene. *Cell*, **80**, 293–9.

Nakagawa, T., Zhu, H., Morishima, N., Li, E., Xu, J., Yankner, B. A. et al. (2000). Caspase-12 mediates endoplasmic-reticulum-specific apoptosis and cytotoxicity by amyloid-beta. *FEBS Lett*, **472**, 39–44.

Oltvai, Z. N., Milliman, C. L., and Korsmeyer, S. J. (1993). Bcl-2 heterodimerizes in vivo with a conserved homolog, Bax, that accelerates programmed cell death. *Cell*, **74**, 609–19.

Patterson, S. D., Spahr, C. S., Daugas, E., Susin, S. A., Irinopoulou, T., Koehler, C. et al. (2000). Mass spectrometric identification of proteins released from mitochondria undergoing permeability transition (in process citation). *Cell Death Differ*, **7**, 137–44.

Pavlov, E. V., Priault, M., Pietkiewicz, D., Cheng, E. H., Antonsson, B., Manon, S. et al. (2001). A novel, high conductance channel of mitochondria linked to apoptosis in mammalian cells and Bax expression in yeast. *J Cell Biol*, **155**, 725–31.

Rampino, N., Yamamoto, H., Ionov, Y., Li, Y., Sawai, H., Reed, J. C. et al. (1997). Somatic frameshift mutations in the BAX gene in colon cancers of the microsatellite mutator phenotype. *Science*, **275**, 967–9.

Reed, J. C., Cuddy, M., Slabiak, T., Croce, C. M., and Nowell, P.C. (1988). Oncogenic potential of bcl-2 demonstrated by gene transfer. *Nature*, **336**, 259–61.

Roy, N., Deveraux, Q. L., Takahashi, R., Salvesen, G. S., and Reed, J. C. (1997). The c-IAP-1 and c-IAP-2 proteins are direct inhibitors of specific caspases. *Embo J*, **16**, 6914–25.

Sawada, M., Hayes, P., and Matsuyama, S. (2003). Cytoprotective membrane-permeable peptides designed from the Bax- binding domain of Ku70. *Nat Cell Biol*, **5**, 352–7.

Scaffidi, C., Schmitz, I., Zha, J., Korsmeyer, S. J., Krammer, P. H., and Peter, M. E. (1999). Differential modulation of apoptosis sensitivity in CD95 type I and type II cells. *J Biol Chem*, **274**, 22532–8.

Shimizu, S., Narita, M., and Tsujimoto, Y. (1999). Bcl-2 family proteins regulate the release of apoptogenic cytochrome *c* by the mitochondrial channel VDAC. *Nature*, **399**, 483–7.

Siskind, L. J., Kolesnick, R. N., and Colombini, M. (2002). Ceramide channels increase the permeability of the mitochondrial outer membrane to small proteins. *J Biol Chem*, **277**, 26796–803.

Susin, S. A., Lorenzo, H. K., Zamzami, N., Marzo, I., Brenner, C., Larochette, N. et al. (1999). Mitochondrial release of caspase-2 and -9 during the apoptotic process. *J Exp Med*, **189**, 381–94.

Takayama, S., Sato, T., Krajewski, S., Kochel, K., Irie, S., Millan, J. A. et al. (1995). Cloning and functional analysis of BAG-1: a novel Bcl-2-binding protein with anti-cell death activity. *Cell*, **80**, 279–84.

Tamm, I., Wang, Y., Sausville, E., Scudiero, D. A., Vigna, N., Oltersdorf, T. et al. (1998). IAP-family protein survivin inhibits caspase activity and apoptosis induced by Fas (CD95), Bax, caspases, and anticancer drugs. *Cancer Res*, **58**, 5315–20.

Tzung, S. P., Kim, K. M., Basanez, G., Giedt, C. D., Simon, J., Zimmerberg, J. et al. (2001). Antimycin A mimics a cell-death-inducing Bcl-2 homology domain 3. *Nat Cell Biol*, **3**, 183–91.

Wang, J. L., Liu, D., Zhang, Z. J., Shan, S., Han, X., Srinivasula, S. M. et al. (2000). Structure-based discovery of an organic compound that binds Bcl-2 protein and induces apoptosis of tumor cells. *Proc Natl Acad Sci USA*, **97**, 7124–9.

Wang, K., Yin, X. M., Chao, D. T., Milliman, C. L., and Korsmeyer, S. J. (1996). BID: a novel BH3 domain-only death agonist. *Genes Dev*, **10**, 2859–69.

Waters, J. S., Webb, A., Cunningham, D., Clarke, P. A., Raynaud, F., di Stefano, F. et al. (2000). Phase I clinical and pharmacokinetic study of bcl-2 antisense oligonucleotide therapy in patients with non-Hodgkin's lymphoma (see comments). *J Clin Oncol*, **18**, 1812–23.

Webb, A., Cunningham, D., Cotter, F., Clarke, P. A., di Stefano, F., Ross, P. et al. (1997). BCL-2 antisense therapy in patients with non-Hodgkin lymphoma. *Lancet*, **349**, 1137–41.

Wolter, K. G., Hsu, Y. T., Smith, C. L., Nechushtan, A., Xi, X. G., and Youle, R. J. (1997). Movement of Bax from the cytosol to mitochondria during apoptosis. *J Cell Biol*, **139**, 1281–92.

Yang, E., Zha, J., Jockel, J., Boise, L. H., Thompson, C. B., and Korsmeyer, S. J. (1995). Bad, a heterodimeric partner for Bcl-x(L), and Bcl-2, displaces Bax and promotes cell death. *Cell*, **80**, 285–91.

Yin, X. M., Oltvai, Z. N., and Korsmeyer, S. J. (1994). BH1 and BH2 domains of Bcl-2 are required for inhibition of apoptosis and heterodimerization with Bax. *Nature*, **369**, 321–3.

Zha, J., Harada, H., Yang, E., Jockel, J., and Korsmeyer, S.J. (1996). Serine phosphorylation of death agonist BAD in response to survival factor results in binding to 14–3–3 not BCL-X(L) (see comments). *Cell*, **87**, 619–28.

Zha, J., Weiler, S., Oh, K. J., Wei, M. C., and Korsmeyer, S. J. (2000). Posttranslational N-myristoylation of BID as a molecular switch for targeting mitochondria and apoptosis. *Science*, **290**, 1761–5.

Zou, H., Henzel, W. J., Liu, X., Lutschg, A., and Wang, X. (1997). Apaf-1, a human protein homologous to *C. elegans* CED-4, participates in cytochrome c-dependent activation of caspase-3. *Cell*, **90**, 405–13.

CHAPTER 13

Mechanisms of viral carcinogenesis

Paul Farrell

There are many controls on proliferation and survival of cells. These prevent development of cancer unless multiple genetic or epigenetic changes accumulate in the cells. As part of their normal growth strategy, certain viruses happen to cause changes in infected cells that are equivalent to some of the changes required to make a cancer cell. In this way these viruses make an important contribution to certain types of cancer, to the extent that prevention of the virus infection may effectively prevent the cancer. About 14% of all human cancer worldwide has this type of viral component to its aetiology (Stewart and Kleihues, 2003). Studies on viruses associated with cancer have been central to the discovery of the mechanisms of cancer development and may provide novel approaches to prevention or treatment of cancers.

The long time taken to accumulate the genetic or epigenetic changes that cause cancer generally requires persistence of a virus if it is to contribute to the disease. Some viruses involved in cancer normally persist in their hosts long-term (e.g. the herpesviruses EBV, Epstein–Barr viruses and KSHV, Kaposi's sarcoma herpesvirus), or cancer may be associated with aberrant chronic persistence of a normally acute virus infection. There is not much evidence for a third theoretical possibility (sometimes called 'hit and run') that the virus contributes a key step in carcinogenesis but is then lost.

The purpose of this chapter is to provide an integrated overview of the mechanisms by which viruses contribute to cancer. More detail about all of the individual viruses discussed here can be found in the relevant chapters of Fields Virology (Knipe and Howley, 2001).

13.1 Tumour viruses in animals

Experimental systems for studying virus-associated cancer in animals have been very important in understanding the mechanism of cancer but the viruses are generally different from the viruses that are associated with human cancer (considered separately below).

13.1.1 Early history

The idea that viruses could be involved in causing cancer in animals received direct experimental support from several discoveries in the first half of the twentieth century. In 1908 Ellerman and Bangerman described a form of infectious leukaemia in chickens and in 1911 Rous showed that a virus could induce sarcomas (Rous sarcoma virus, RSV). In 1930, Shope demonstrated that papillomas (warts) could be caused in cottontail rabbits by a virus (the Shope papilloma virus) and that these warts had a propensity to become malignant. In 1936 Bittner discovered the transmission of a virus (mouse mammary tumour virus, MMTV) that could cause mammary cancer in mice and later, in 1951, Gross reported the first mouse leukaemia virus. This was followed rapidly in 1953 by his discovery of polyoma virus, which causes many types of tumour in mice. Most of these discoveries of animal cancer viruses subsequently proved not to have direct equivalents in human cancer but they were pivotal in providing experimental systems in which the mechanism of cell transformation to the malignant state became understood. They also illustrate mechanisms that are important in human cancer.

13.1.2 Animal retroviruses and cancer

Over many years, selective breeding of animals, either for agriculture or for laboratory purposes, revealed strains with a high incidence of cancer. In a few cases, particularly in birds and in mice, this has lead to the isolation of viruses that caused the disease. The first of these to be isolated were retroviruses of the oncovirus group. These viruses (Figure 13.1) have a simple structure comprising three genes called *gag*, *pol*, and *env* positioned between the long terminal repeat region, which contains a strong transcription promoter and enhancer. There are two ways in which these viruses can cause cancer.

(1) The normal life cycle of the retrovirus involves reverse transcription of its RNA genome into DNA, integration of the DNA into the host cell genome and subsequent transcription of viral mRNAs and new viral genomic RNA from that integrated DNA. The position of integration of viral genomes in infected cells is largely random. Occasionally a viral genome may happen to integrate close to a cellular gene that can cause cell proliferation. In this case the viral LTR (long terminal repeat) sequence can induce expression of the cellular gene and promote tumour formation. Well-known examples of this include integration of chicken, cat, or mouse retroviruses near the *c-myc* gene to cause leukaemia and integration of the MMTV near the *int-1* and *int-2* genes to cause mammary tumours. Although the virus integrated at random, identification of the integration site in cells that grow out as a tumour shows that these integration sites have been selected and this can be used as a method to identify cell genes that contribute to cancer formation.

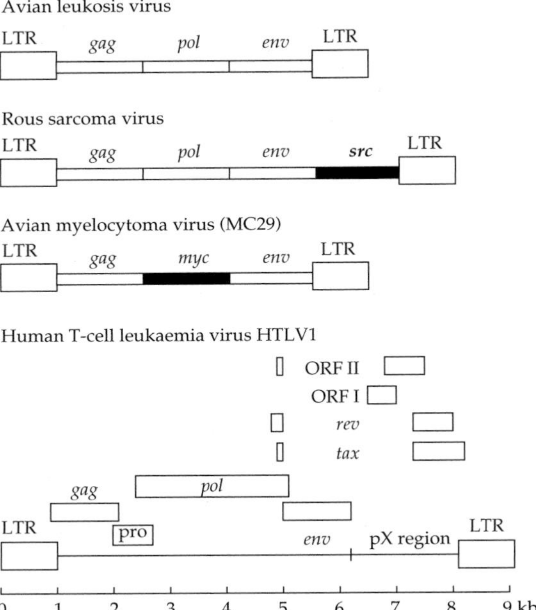

Figure 13.1 Retrovirus structures. Avian leukaemia virus is an example of a wild type retrovirus of the oncovirus family. Acutely transforming retroviruses are derived from such viruses by rare recombination events that include a cell gene whose normal function is in cell proliferation into the viral genome. RSV and Avian Myelocytoma virus are examples of this. The cellular proto-oncogene (in these cases *c-src* or *c-myc*) is converted to a viral oncogene, *v-src* or *v-myc*. Often the viral oncogene is altered to some extent, truncated, or mutated so that it has lost some of the normal constraints on its activity. The viruses containing the oncogene are frequently defective and require complementation by a wild type virus to permit their replication. HTLV1 is also a retrovirus but naturally includes extra viral genes additional to *gag*, *pol*, and *env*. The HTLV1 *Tax* gene is important for cell proliferation caused by HTLV1.

(2) Very rarely, an error in the retrovirus replication strategy can result in a modified retrovirus that has acquired an extra gene by insertion of cell

DNA. This usually involves loss of some of the viral genetic material so these viruses are generally dependent on complementing wild type virus to permit their replication. If the cell DNA inserted into the virus happens to encode a gene that promotes cell proliferation or cancer, then this acutely transforming retrovirus (Figure 13.1) can cause cancer with very high frequency in infected animals. Many examples of this have been studied and they are described in more detail in Chapter 7. The realization that the viral oncogenes present in acutely transforming retroviruses are derived from cell genes involved in growth control was a key step in identifying some of the genes involved in cancer.

Two common examples of retroviral-mediated cancers in animals are the leukaemia caused by bovine leukosis virus in cattle and a variety of tumours caused by feline leukaemia virus in cats. FeLV is the most common cause of non-traumatic death in domestic cats in western countries and cats are now generally required to be vaccinated against FeLV before boarding in catteries. Both of these viruses cause tumours by the mechanism 1 described above.

13.1.3 SV40 and polyoma

These small DNA viruses (now described as the polyoma virus family) rely on the host cell DNA polymerase to replicate their DNA so that they have evolved mechanisms to cause the infected cell to move into the late G1 and S phases of the cell cycle (Figure 13. 2). This is a feature of many cancer-associated viruses. SV40 (a monkey virus) causes tumours in rodents, that is, not in its natural host, where the replication cycle can be incomplete and there is continued expression of the viral early genes. These viruses also neutralize some of the apoptosis and cell cycle checkpoint mechanisms that normally protect against malignant transformation. All of these properties favour production of cancer cells. SV40 large T-antigen binds the Rb and p53 tumour suppressor proteins and prevents their function. SV40 small T inhibits protein phosphatase 2A, another regulator of cell cycle progression. The binding of the p53 protein to SV40 large T was one of the ways in which the significance of p53 was discovered.

There was a large-scale exposure of humans to SV40 in the 1950s because it was an unknown contaminant of the Salk polio vaccine (which had been

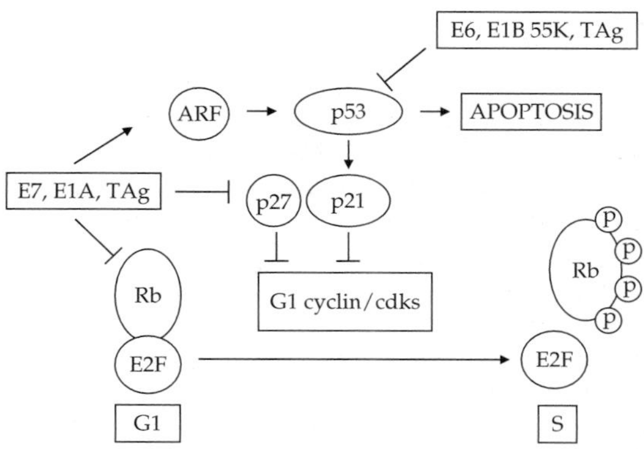

Figure 13.2 Transforming proteins of the SV40, papillomaviruses, and adenoviruses all regulate the G1 to S cell cycle transition in analogous ways. E2F transcription factor activity required for the G1 to S cell cycle transition is regulated by Rb family proteins. In normal cell proliferation, cyclin dependent kinases that have been activated in response to growth factors or similar signals phosphorylate Rb, causing it to unmask E2F activity and allow cell cycle progression. SV40 large T antigen, papillomavirus E7, and adenovirus E1A can all bind Rb and cause it to dissociate from E2F without G1 cyclin dependent kinase activity. The same proteins also prevent that activity of the p21 and p27 inhibitors of cyclin dependent kinase. Activation of p53 dependent apoptosis or cell cycle arrest is prevented by the SV40 large T antigen, papillomavirus E6, and adenovirus E1B proteins. SV40 large T and adenovirus E1B bind to p53 to inactivate it but papillomavirus E6 causes p53 degradation, with the same functional outcome.

grown in monkey cells that carried SV40). Fortunately this did not result in any obvious pathogenic effect but there is a suspicion that the virus might play a role in some human mesothelioma; SV40 DNA has been detected in biopsies of this tumour type in several studies but there is no direct evidence that it caused the disease.

Polyoma virus can also cause tumours in mice in cell types where its infection is non-productive. The ability of polyoma large T-antigen to bind pRb, although essential for cell-cycle activation and immortalization of cells in culture, is not essential for virus replication or tumour induction in the mouse. Tumour induction by polyoma virus varies according to mouse strain; this effect is partly reflected in the expression of the mouse p150 Sal2 protein, which binds to polyoma large T (Li et al., 2001). The Sal2 protein is a transcription factor that can act as a tumour suppressor and is inactivated by large T-antigen. For polyoma virus, most of the transforming action is exerted by the middle T-antigen, which has the ability to convert established cell lines to an oncogenic state. Middle T is a membrane bound polypeptide that interacts with several of the proteins used by tyrosine kinase associated receptors to stimulate cell proliferation. Middle T assembles a large multi-protein complex at the cell membrane, comprising MT, the core dimer of protein phosphatase 2A, a src-family tyrosine kinase, ShcA, phosphatidylinositol (3′) kinase (PI3 K), and phospholipase Cγ-1 (PLCγ). Tyrosine phosphorylation stimulates PI3 K and PLCγ enzymatic activity, and on ShcA creates binding sites for Grb2 with its associated Sos1 and Gab1. This activates p21(ras) and hence the MAP kinase cascade. Other studies have shown that the ability of the virus to induce tumours is not strictly dependent on its transforming functions as defined *in vitro*. No inactivation of p53 has yet been described for polyoma virus but there is evidence that the polyoma early proteins disrupt $P14^{ARF}$ activation of p53 (Lomax and Fried, 2001) and might thus avoid p53 dependent cell cycle checkpoints or apoptosis.

13.1.4 Adenovirus

In humans, adenoviruses generally cause severe cold-like symptoms but in some animal cells where replication of the virus is incomplete, cell transformation can occur. Certain adenovirus DNA fragments can also cause cell transformation when transfected. The fragments containing the viral *E1A* and *E1B* genes are required for this. E1A binds to and inactivates pRb and the E1B proteins (56k and 19k) bind and inactivate p53 and bax, suppressing apoptosis, so that the virus is able to overcome the check point associated with G1 and promote cell proliferation and survival. Purification and sequencing of the cell proteins that bind to adenovirus E1A led to the identification of the pRb protein and other members of the Rb protein family.

13.1.5 Marek's Disease Virus and other animal herpesviruses

Marek's Disease Virus (MDV) is a herpesvirus that causes a commercially significant disease of chickens. The disease became prevalent in commercial flocks during the mid part of the twentieth century but is now largely controlled by vaccination. Before vaccination was introduced, outbreaks would typically involve up to 20% of a flock, with a substantial proportion developing T-cell lymphomas (the virus also affects the nervous system). The vaccines are now made from a mixture of related non-oncogenic herpesviruses of turkeys and chickens.

The most important viral gene of MDV for transformation appears to be the *Meq* gene. Virus strains that are attenuated in transformation have mutations in *Meq* and *Meq* can transform rat cells in culture when transfected. The Meq protein is a transcription factor of the b-ZIP family that is able to dimerize with c-jun and various other cell bZIP proteins (Liu et al., 1997). It has also been reported to associate with complexes of cell proteins that can include CDK2 (Liu et al., 1999), pRb, and p53. The detailed mechanism of action of Meq is not yet understood but it evidently can interact with several factors involved in cell proliferation and death. Recently, oncogenic strains of MDV have been found to encode a functional viral homologue of the RNA component of telomerase, which may also help survival of cells infected with this virus (Fragnet et al., 2003).

Several other animal herpesviruses have been shown to cause tumours. The Lucké frog herpesvirus (RaHV-1) causes renal adenocarcinoma in the northern leopard frog, *Rana pipiens*. Interestingly, metastasis of this tumour occurs as a function of ambient temperature; frogs kept at 28° develop many metastases whereas those kept at 7° do not. The mechanism by which the virus contributes to tumour development is as yet unknown.

In monkeys, herpesvirus ateles and herpesvirus saimiri (HVS) can cause T-cell lymphomas. HVS has been studied in some detail (Fickenscher and Fleckenstein, 2001). In its natural host, the squirrel monkey, HVS infects and persists without any signs of disease. In contrast, the virus causes acute peripheral T-cell lymphoma after experimental infection of several other types of monkey. HVS strains have been assigned to three subgroups (A, B, and C). The transformation-associated genes in subgroup C viruses, stpC (saimiri transformation-associated protein) and tip (tyrosine kinase-interacting protein), are adjacent in the viral genome. Both stpC and tip are necessary for the transforming activity of HVS. StpC was shown to directly associate with cellular Ras, leading to activation of the Ras pathway and it also binds to TRAFs and causes activation of NF-kB. The other transformation-associated protein, tip, associates with the Src family tyrosine kinase p56lck, an mRNA export factor Tap. Phosphorylated Tip also binds to and activates STAT transcription factors. All the HVS strains also have the viral FLIP, cyclin D, and LANA equivalents, discussed below under KSHV, a human virus with some similarity to HVS.

13.1.6 Papillomaviruses in animals

The papillomaviruses will be discussed in more detail below in the human cancer virus section but Shope PV in cotton-tailed rabbits and BPV in cattle are examples of PVs that have been studied in animals.

Bovine papillomavirus (BPV)-induced papillomas in cattle are benign tumours of cutaneous or mucosal epithelia and generally regress. Occasionally, the papillomas persist and undergo malignant transformation to squamous cell carcinoma, particularly in the presence of co-carcinogens from the environment. This occurs with BPV-2 and cancer of the urinary bladder, and BPV-4 and cancer of the upper alimentary canal in cattle feeding on bracken fern. Quercetin appears to be the active co-carcinogen in the bracken fern. In cell culture transformation systems with PV DNA, the E5, E6, and E7 proteins all play a role. E7 protein binds to pRb and inactivates p21 and p27, overcoming the G1 cell cycle checkpoint mediated by those proteins. E6 binds to p53 and causes its degradation. These activities are analogous to the mechanisms described above for SV40 and adenovirus. The E5 protein is a small membrane protein that can stabilize other membrane proteins, for example, the epidermal growth factor receptor (EGFR) and thus enhances cell proliferation by increasing signal transduction through EGFR.

13.2 Tumour viruses in humans

13.2.1 Papillomaviruses

There are many different subtypes of the herpesvirus (HPVs) (subtypes are distinguished by lack of cross hybridization or percentage sequence dissimilarity). The disease associations of papillomaviruses are highly specific to subtypes.

Squamous carcinoma of the cervix is one of the major cancers in women worldwide and most cases are now thought to involve infection by one of the high risk types 16, 18, 31, or 33 of HPV. Of these, HPV16 accounts for about 65% and HPV18 about 20% of cases. Cervical carcinoma accounts for the great majority of HPV-associated cancers but many other anogenital cancers also involve the same HPV types. Up to 20% of oropharyngeal carcinomas have also been reported to contain the high risk types of HPV. Cervical intraepithelial neoplasia (CIN) is the precursor lesion to cervical carcinoma that contains proliferating cells. These cells can be detected in cervical smears, which are currently used to screen for women at risk of developing cervical cancer. CIN also very frequently contains HPV so the virus infection is thought to be a relatively early event in the development of disease; some investigators consider that the CIN I stage is equivalent to infection of the cervical epithelium by a high risk HPV type. In Western countries about 10% of normal women have been infected with HPV high risk types. There has recently been progress in developing a vaccine that is highly effective in preventing infection by the high risk HPV types, as assessed by serum antibodies. This vaccine uses virus-like particles (VLPs) that assemble spontaneously when the virus capsid proteins are expressed artificially and these VLPs are immunogenic (Koutsky et al., 2002). There are preliminary indications that the vaccine prevents CIN (Koutsky et al., 2002) and large-scale trials are now underway to determine whether the apparent prevention of infection ultimately results in prevention of cervical cancer. If effective, this vaccine approach could also be applied to other HPV associated cancers in immunocompetent people.

The main transforming activity of HPV16 is associated with the E6 and E7 proteins (Figure 13.2); as in BPV there is also some evidence for a contribution from E5. In cancers, some or all of the HPV genomes are frequently found to have become integrated at random locations in the cell chromosomes. The linearization of the HPV genome that is required for this frequently interrupts the *E2* gene and thus prevents the E2 protein from repressing the viral promoter that expresses *E6* and *E7*. This favours increased expression of E6 and E7 and continued expression of these proteins has been shown to be required for continued growth of cervical carcinoma cells in culture. Disruption of *E4*, which overlaps *E2*, also evades negative effects of E4 on cyclin B activity and evades a G2 checkpoint.

The E7 protein from high risk HPV types binds the pRb protein and prevents its checkpoint function in the G1 phase of the cell cycle, favouring cell proliferation. The E7 proteins of high risk types are much more effective at this than those of low risk

HPV types. E7 also inactivates the cdk inhibitors p27 and p21, which normally also act as brakes on cell proliferation. E7 has also been reported to affect pyruvate kinase activity, perhaps suggesting an additional modulation of carbohydrate metabolism in infected cells.

The E6 protein binds p53 and overcomes the tumour suppressor and apoptotic function of p53. E6 promotes the ubiquitination of p53 and its subsequent degradation by interaction with the E6-AP ubiquitin ligase enzyme. E6 can also block induction of beta-interferon in papillomavirus infected cells through an effect on interferon regulatory factor 3 (IRF-3) and associates with the focal adhesion plaque protein paxillin. E6 can additionally bind to the proapoptotic Bak protein (Jackson et al., 2000) and to E6TP1, a GAP protein regulating transduction of mitogenic signals. The C-terminus of E6 can also bind to some cell proteins containing the PDZ domain (e.g. Dlg and various other signalling proteins) and cause their degradation. The relative importance of these interactions is still being investigated but both E6 and E7 are clearly multifunctional proteins that can increase cell proliferation and survival by several mechanisms.

The E5 protein of HPV has been shown to act in a similar way to that of BPV and may thus also contribute to cell transformation. Early data favoured stabilization of EGFR on the cell surface as a mechanism by which E5 contributes to cell transformation but more recent studies in human keratinocytes suggest that EGFR may not be the key component that is affected, since the effects of E5 were independent of the addition of EGF.

In addition to the consequences of HPV gene expression, it is clear that other genetic or epigenetic changes in the cell are involved in cervical cancer. In this context, the ability of HPV *E6* and *E7* to promote genome instability is likely to be important. Expression of *E6* and *E7* can permit accumulation of many different types of abnormalities in chromosome number and structure.

Although the long-term hope for the major cancers associated with HPVs is that a vaccine will prevent the disease, this is still uncertain and there is also a very large cohort of people currently infected who presumably would not benefit from a vaccine. There is thus great interest also in developing therapeutic drugs or vaccines that might target HPV gene expression in human disease.

Since HPVs are clearly important in squamous carcinoma of the cervix, there has also been extensive investigation of whether HPVs might be involved more generally in skin cancers. Although various HPV types can often be detected by PCR (polymerase chain reaction) in normal skin, there is no substantial evidence for a general involvement of HPVs in skin cancer. The exception to this is a very rare inherited condition called epidermodysplasia verruciformis (EV). The *EV* gene has not yet been identified but two genetic loci have been linked to the disease. HPV type 5 is found in the EV cutaneous lesions and the lesions are susceptible to malignant transformation, particularly at sites exposed to sunlight. It is thus suggested that the HPV might play a role in the carcinomas that can develop in EV patients.

13.2.2 Epstein-Barr virus

EBV is the clearest example of a human virus that directly causes cell proliferation and it is also involved in several types of human cancer. EBV infects B lymphocytes and causes resting B cells to proliferate; immortalized cell lines (lymphoblastoid cell lines, LCLs) are readily obtained. EBV can also infect epithelial cells and this is reflected in its association with most undifferentiated nasopharyngeal carcinoma and a small proportion of gastric carcinomas. Other cancers associated with EBV are Burkitt's lymphoma (a B-cell lymphoma), some cases of Hodgkin's disease and, in immunosuppressed people, immunoblastic lymphomas, or post-transplant lymphoproliferative disease. A small number of leiomyosarcomas and certain T-cell lymphomas are also EBV associated.

The great majority of people in the world (90%) are thought to be infected with EBV and carry the virus for life, so epidemiological evidence linking the virus to cancer at the population level is generally weak. Serological studies in Africa have linked an enhanced EBV antibody titre to incidence of Burkitt's lymphoma (BL) and rising titres of certain EBV antibodies are strong predictors of nasopharyngeal carcinoma in China. However, the number of B cells infected in a normal carrier is very low (about 1 in 100,000 peripheral B cells) (Thorley-Lawson, 2001) so the presence of EBV in almost every tumour cell in Burkitt's lymphoma or naso pharyngeal carcinoma (NPC) is an impressive degree of association. The fraction of normal lymphocytes infected by EBV is somewhat higher in people suffering from malaria, one of the cofactors for BL in Africa but the proportion is still low. Infection usually occurs asymptomatically in early childhood but in Western countries infection is sometimes delayed until adolescence or adulthood. Primary infection at this stage often causes infectious mononucleosis (glandular fever). Here EBV infection and replication causes an initial proliferation of EBV infected B cells followed by a massive immune response to those cells and replicating virus. Up to 25% of the cytotoxic T-lymphocyte population can be directed against single EBV antigens in this situation (Callan et al., 1996). The symptoms of IM (infectious mononucleosis) are essentially a consequence of the immune response, so the illness resolves as the immune response subsides to that in a normal virus carrier. A few rare families have an inherited X-linked mutation that prevents an effective immune response to EBV (the mutation is in the *SAP* gene, also called *SH2D1A*). Boys affected by this mutation (Duncan's syndrome, X-linked lymphoproliferative disease) can suffer severe lymphomas after primary EBV infection, which are frequently fatal.

The genes of EBV whose expression causes proliferation of normal cells have been identified and are summarized in Figure 13.3. Their functions are consistent with EBV constitutively subverting growth pathways of the B cell that would be normally used in the response to antigen. LMP1 can mimic the cell survival effects of CD40 signalling, inducing the bcl-2 and A20 proteins that can protect against apoptosis. The EBNA-2 transcription factor induces *c-myc* and *Runx3* expression (Spender et al., 2002), causing cell proliferation. EBNA-2 has a strong transcription activation domain but does not bind DNA directly, instead associating with specific DNA binding cellular proteins such as the PU.1 transcription factor and the RBP-Jk component of the Notch signal transduction pathway. RBP-Jk also binds to the EBNA-3 family of proteins. EBNA-3A and EBNA-3C can additionally bind to the CtBP repressor in the polycomb complex (Touitou et al., 2001; Hickabottom et al., 2002) and overcome cell cycle checkpoints (Parker et al., 2000; O'nions and Allday, 2003), perhaps also allowing chromosomal instability that can be associated with cancer. Lymphomas similar to LCLs also occur in patients immunosuppressed after transplants. The EBNA and LMP proteins described above cause cell proliferation and survival in these tumours but

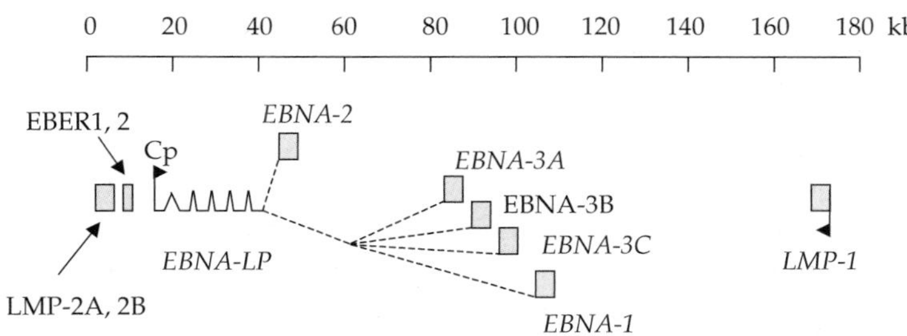

EBV proteins essential for B cell immortalization

Nuclear proteins	
EBNA-1	Plasmid maintenance in latent replication
EBNA-2	Transcription factor–induces Myc, Runx-3
EBNA-LP	Cooperates with EBNA-2
EBNA-3A and 3C	Overcome cell cycle checkpoints, bind CtBP
Cytoplasmic membrane protein	
LMP-1	partly mimics CD40, activates NF-kB, JNK, Tpl2

Figure 13.3 EBV latent cycle gene expression EBV latent cycle gene positions in the viral genome are shown relative to a scale in kb. The *EBNA* genes are transcribed from a common promoter in LCLs (Cp) and the mRNAs are made by alternative splicing of a repetitive leader section onto the coding portions of the RNAs. Additional alternative splicing at the 5′ end can create an initiator met residue to allow expression of EBNA-LP from the repetitive leader section.

All the genes shown are expressed in EBV immortalized B lymphocytes (latency III). Those labelled in italics and listed in the table below are essential for efficient B-cell immortalization. In latency I in BL cells, only *EBNA-1* and *EBER RNAs* are expressed. Latency II, found in NPC is intermediate with no EBNA-2. *In vivo*, latent persistence in memory B cells may involve only EBER RNA and residual stable EBNA-1 protein with some cells also containing LMP2A.

the cells have also acquired additional mutations that make the lymphoma cells more tumorigenic than simple EBV LCLs. Although it is not essential for immortalization, LMP2A plays an important role in latent B-cell infections, blocking signalling through the B-cell receptor and consequently preventing induction of the virus lytic cycle.

The role of EBV in cancers of people who are not immunosuppressed is more difficult to interpret because the genes that are clearly involved in causing proliferation in LCLs are frequently not expressed in those cancer cells. The most striking example is in EBV positive Burkitt's lymphomas, where there seems to be a selection against expression of *EBNA-2* (Kelly et al., 2002), in contrast to the LCLs, where continued expression of *EBNA-2* is required for proliferation. BL cells characteristically have a translocation of *MYC* to one of the immunoglobulin loci, which de-regulates MYC expression and the *MYC* gene is also sometimes mutated (Gu et al., 1994) so that the MYC protein is stabilized. Defects in proteasome-mediated protein degradation also contribute to the stabilization of MYC protein in BL cells. EBNA1, the EBER RNAs, and a very low level of BART/CST RNAs are the EBV transcripts detected in most BL cells of the group I type that retain the correct BL phenotype. Cloning EBV positive and negative cells from BL cell lines that have a tendency to lose their EBV genomes in culture indicates that the EBV positive lines are more tumorigenic. The EBER RNAs have been reported to mediate this contribution to tumorigenicity (Nanbo et al., 2002) but the mechanism by which this may work remains to be fully established.

There is a low background of sporadic BL worldwide in which the tumour cells do not contain EBV, but a 10-fold higher incidence of endemic BL in parts of the world where malaria is hyperendemic. These cases usually have EBV in the tumour cells and the mechanism by which the tumours develop is slightly different since they are derived from subtly different stages of B-cell development. The role of EBV in BL might include:

(1) The *EBNA* and *LMP* genes involved in LCL immortalization enhance survival or proliferation of an early stage of the disease followed by selection of cells which have down-regulated the immunogenic EBNAs and LMPs.

(2) The tumorigenic contribution of EBV in BL might differ from LCL immortalization, implied by the EBER results described above.

The mechanism remains to be established but it is clear from clonality of the BL cells and the EBV present in them that the virus was present in the tumour cells at the beginning of tumour development. Because of the low frequency of EBV positive normal B cells, there is thus a much greater chance of BL developing in an EBV positive B cell than an EBV negative one. There is also an interesting difference in the positions of the *MYC* translocations between the EBV positive and negative tumours. In EBV negative tumours the breakpoints relative to *MYC* are always very close to the *MYC* gene, usually just upstream of the start or in the first exon. In the EBV positive BLs, the breakpoints can be spread over a long distance either up or downstream of the *MYC* gene. If the errors leading to translocation are random, this implies that only a very restricted subset of translocation events go on to cause BL in EBV negative cells. The broader range of *c-MYC* translocation points found in the endemic (EBV positive) BL cells suggests that more of the translocation events were able to cause BL in EBV positive cells. The mechanism by which this effect of EBV might occur is unknown.

In Hodgkin's disease the tumour mass comprises mainly non-malignant reactive B cells, which are usually EBV negative but there is also a characteristic tumour cell type, the Reed-Sternberg cell, originally also derived from the B lineage. These Reed Sternberg cells carry EBV in about 30% of cases and there is high expression of *LMP1* and *LMP2* in them. It seems likely that this contributes to the survival of these cells.

The link between EBV and NPC was initially discovered serologically (Old et al., 1966) but EBV DNA was soon demonstrated in the tumour cells (zur Hausen et al., 1970). The disease has a much higher incidence in Chinese people in the South of China and in Singapore than in Western countries. Some North African and Inuit populations have an intermediate incidence. NPC patients characteristically have high titres of antibodies to EBV lytic cycle antigens (a puzzle since the EBV infection of the tumour cells is almost completely latent). Rising titres of antibodies to some early lytic cycle EBV antigens have been used in population screening in Southern China to identify people at risk of NPC, which can be treated effectively by radiotherapy if it is identified early. The NPC tumour is a mixture of lymphoid and epithelial cells but it is the malignant epithelial cells that virtually contain EBV. The EBV LMP-2 protein is transcribed in NPC tumour cells and about half of the cells also express variable levels of LMP-1. The contribution of EBV to the transformation of the cells is poorly understood—changes in several cell genes have been reported in a proportion of NPC tumours, including loss of p16 / P14^{ARF} expression (Lo and Huang, 2002). NPC is thought to result from a combination of inherited susceptibility in the populations at risk (Feng et al., 2002), EBV and chemical carcinogenesis from ethnic foodstuffs or environmental carcinogens. Recent data indicating that relevant genetic and epigenetic changes can be detected in normal oropharyngeal epithelium in susceptible populations in South East Asia has lead to the suggestion that EBV infection may not be an initiating event in the epithelial cells but contribute to the later stages of tumour development. LMP-2A has been shown to cause hyperplasia in epithelial cell raft cultures (Scholle et al., 2000) so this might be a mechanism for an EBV contribution.

13.2.3 Kaposi's sarcoma herpesvirus

Discovery of DNA from this virus (systematically named human herpesvirus 8 (HHV-8)) was reported in 1994 in a biopsy of Kaposi's sarcoma (KS) and the complete virus was then characterized very rapidly. Like EBV, it is a member of the herpesvirus family but it is only present in about 5% of the population and incidence of the virus infection can be related epidemiologically to disease (Boshoff and Weiss, 2001). KS occurs classically in the absence of HIV in southern European, and Mediterranean Arab and Jewish populations. A much higher incidence has appeared as a result of the AIDS epidemic in many parts of the world so that, for example, KS now comprises 10% of malignancies in Uganda. Some rare lymphomas in AIDS patients known as multicentric Castleman's Disease and plasmablast variant primary effusion lymphomas also contain KSHV.

The tumours contain a latent viral infection and the virus expresses several genes that can affect cell proliferation and prevent cell death. Some of these are adjacent on the viral genome and are transcribed together. Two of the viral genes are clearly able to affect cell proliferation and promote cell transformation. Like adenovirus E1A, KSHV LANA is reported to bind pRb and to cooperate with an activated *Ras* oncogene to transform cells in culture, suggesting that it has an ability to overcome a cell cycle checkpoint. In addition, LANA also includes a replication/plasmid maintenance function similar to EBV EBNA-1. KSHV also encodes a cyclin, which is expressed in the tumour cells. This viral cyclin combines properties of the cell cyclins E and D, so that it is very effective at promoting cell cycle progression and has been shown to be much more tumorigenic in the absence of the cellular p53 function in a transgenic mouse model (Verschuren et al., 2002). Both LANA and the product of orf K10 are reported to bind p53 and reduce its ability to cause transcriptional activation and this may expose the proliferative activity of the KSHV cyclin.

A protein known as vFLIP (FLICE inhibitory protein) is expressed during latency by KSHV and is effective at preventing apoptosis of cells through inhibition of signal transduction from, for example, the Fas receptor or TNF receptor. The virus also encodes an analogue of the cell bcl-2 apoptosis inhibitor. There is clearly an overall similarity to the cell proliferative and apoptotic cell pathways affected by several other tumour viruses but the detailed mechanism that has evolved in KSHV is slightly different. The greatly enhanced incidence of KS in AIDS patients (who also have a higher rate of KSHV infection) might be explained by reduced immune surveillance but there is also evidence for a direct contribution from HIV, perhaps through the HIV-1 Tat protein. Tat is able to induce cell angiogenic and proliferative pathways and to directly activate the NF–kB pathway and thus may cooperate with KSHV to cause KS.

The KSHV infection in tumours is mainly latent but there are a few lytically infected cells and these may produce growth factors such as viral IL6 and cellular VEGF that are involved in the KSHV-mediated disease pathogenesis. The action of the KSHV G protein coupled receptor protein (vGPCR) that signals constitutively to the JNK and p38 MAP kinases, PI3 kinase, and to the NF-kB transcription factor is thought to mediate expression of these soluble factors.

13.2.4 Human T-cell leukaemia/lymphoma virus

This virus is endemic in the south-west part of Japan, parts of West Africa, and in the Caribbean. It is also found in the peoples of some Pacific islands and in Australian aborigines. It can infect many cell types *in vitro* but *in vivo* infection is almost totally confined to T-lymphocytes. HTLV-1 causes adult T-cell leukaemia (ATL) in a small proportion of infected people. Although ATL is generally a rare disease, there are about 800 new cases per annum in Japan. HTLV-1 also causes (probably indirectly) a condition known as HTLV-1 associated myelopathy or tropical spastic paraparesis (HAM/TSP), that was recognized initially in a Caribbean population infected with HTLV-1 but is also present in Japanese people infected with the virus.

HTLV1 is a retrovirus of the oncovirus sub-family but contains extra genes in addition to the basic *gag*, *pol*, and *env* (Figure 13.1). Of these, the *Tax* gene appears to be the most important for the ability of HTLV1 to cause cell proliferation. *Tax* induces cell and viral gene expression by activating other DNA-binding transcription factors. It binds to IkB to cause the activation of NF-kB and activates the HTLV-1 transcription from the LTR. Via NFkB, *Tax* also induces IL-2 and the IL2 receptor. It can thus stimulate T-cell growth through an autocrine IL-2 mechanism. Tax can additionally bind and inactivate cell cycle checkpoint proteins p16 and MAD1 (a mitotic checkpoint protein) so there are several ways in which it can contribute to cell proliferation and transformation, particularly in CD4+ T cells. There also appears to be an inactivation of p53 function, possibly involving phosphorylation of serine 15 of p53 in cell lines transformed by HTLV-1. The position at which the HTLV-1 provirus is integrated in the cell chromosome appears to be random but the cell populations in ATL are normally clonal with respect to the integration site.

The long-term persistence of HTLV-1 involves the virus causing T-cell proliferation and can involve a much higher viral load than, for example, EBV. Immune surveillance maintains a balance of virus-infected cells and CTL-mediated killing that can persist life-long without significant disease. If ATL develops, this will normally be many years after primary infection (up to 50 years later) and there will have been progressive accumulation of changes in tumour suppressor genes and oncogenes in the HTLV-1 infected cells as the tumorigenic ATL cell population eventually emerges. These associated changes in cellular tumour suppressor genes and oncogenes have not been fully characterized but examples of deletion or mutation of *CDKN2A*(p16) and *TP53* have been reported. The smouldering ATL that can be present in intervening years involves proliferation of T-cells that appears to be dependent on *Tax* expression. Mature ATL cells were originally reported not to express *Tax* but with improved methods it can now sometimes be detected at low levels in ATL.

Tax protein is a major target for the Cytotoxic T lymphocytes (CTL)-mediated immune surveillance that operates in HTLV-1 infected people. The CTLs are constantly killing HTLV-1 infected cells. There can be large differences between individuals in the virus load at which the balance between virus replication and CTL mediated killing of infected cells becomes established. The virus load can differ between individuals by more than 10,000-fold but in each individual the virus load reaches a stable 'fixed point', which appears to represent a balance between virus replication and CTL-mediated killing of infected cells. There is evidence for an effect of major histocompatability complex (MHC) type in determining the proviral load, which in turn affects the risk of HAM/TSP disease that is associated with HTLV-1.

13.2.5 Hepatitis viruses and cancer

Chronic infection with hepatitis B virus (HBV) or hepatitis C virus (HCV) is a major cause of primary liver cancer (hepatocellular carcinoma, HCC), one of the major cancers in South East Asia and in Africa. HCC accounts for about 4% of all cancer worldwide; HCC and cervical cancer are the virus associated cancers with much the highest incidence in humans. Classic epidemiological studies in Taiwan showed that chronic infection with HBV conferred a very high-risk factor for development of HCC. In high-risk areas most of the population was infected with HBV in early childhood and many years of chronic carriage of HBV are normally required for tumour development of HCC. The development of a vaccine for HBV in the 1980s has permitted mass vaccination of populations but it takes many years for the young cohort who avoid infection as a result of vaccination to reach the typical age for development of HCC. Nevertheless, initial results are very encouraging and there are signs that vaccination may play a major role in preventing liver cancer caused by HBV (Kao and Chen, 2002).

HBV and HCV are completely different viruses, merely connected by their ability to infect the liver and cause hepatitis. There has been a long debate as to whether these viruses encode proteins with direct oncogenic functions or whether the cancer is a result of chronic damage caused to the liver because of the hepatitis. The liver is able to regenerate after cell death of part of the liver and this proliferation could provide the opportunity for accumulation of the genetic errors that can lead to cancer, particularly if carcinogenic chemicals are also present. Cirrhosis caused by alcohol abuse also involves death of liver cells and their replacement and is an independent risk factor for liver cancer by such a chronic damage mechanism.

HBV is a hepadnavirus and thus has a small ds DNA genome. Integration of the viral DNA into the host cell chromosomes can occur but is not a normal part of the viral life cycle. Although there are examples of integration events at genes relevant to cell growth control (cyclin A, thyroid hormone receptor), in animal model systems, these do not reflect the human situation, where HBV integration events appear to be random. The *X* gene of HBV is a transactivator of transcription, can cause transformation of cells in culture and may block the function of p53 by binding to it. Some strains of transgenic mice expressing the *X* gene are prone to liver cancer and have enhanced sensitivity to chemical carcinogenesis. X protein has also been reported to bind to XAP-1, a protein involved in repair of DNA damage, suggesting an additional mechanism by which it could contribute to cancer development.

Repeated exposure to aflatoxin B1, which can be produced by Aspergillus fungus contaminating food, is another major risk factor for HCC. Aflatoxin induces a specific mutation in amino acid 249 of p53, the clearest example of a targeted mutation of p53. There are thus several direct and indirect routes for HBV to contribute to HCC development. It is likely that all of these are important to some degree.

HCV is a flavivirus (RNA genome). The existence of non-A, non-B hepatitis viruses was inferred from cases of transfusion hepatitis that were not explained by the A or B viruses but HCV was not identified until 1989. Patients with HCV-related HCC tend to be older than HBV related cases and the HCV cancers are linked more frequently to alcohol-induced cirrhosis. There is little evidence for a direct oncogenic effect of HCV, so liver cell damage and repair in response to viral infection seems to be the most likely mechanism by which it contributes to liver cancer. In some European countries where HBV related HCC is relatively rare, HCV can account for up to 80% of primary liver cancers. No vaccine is yet available for HCV. In some parts of Africa, it seems likely that HCV was unwittingly transmitted widely by the re-use of syringes and needles during early mass vaccination programmes for other diseases. For example, in Egypt 20% of the population is now infected with HCV.

13.2.6 HIV and AIDS

Although HIV is not thought to be directly oncogenic, the loss of immune surveillance and enhanced cell proliferation in the immune response provide a mechanism for cancer development. KS was an obscure disease until the AIDS epidemic, when it was soon recognized as a sign of advancing disease in AIDS patients. With improved therapies for HIV in Western countries patients are surviving longer, resulting in an increase in numbers of lymphomas, although with the latest triple drug therapies survival is further extended without additional incidence of lymphoma. Some of these lymphomas are linked to EBV but the majority are not. There is thus an increase in cancers as a result of HIV and the huge scale of the AIDS pandemic will make this increasingly numerically important.

13.3 Other infectious agents and cancer

Although it is not a virus, for completeness it is useful to note the important role of the bacterium *Helicobacter pylori* in gastric carcinoma. *H. pylori* infects up to 50% of the world's population and is the leading cause of chronic gastritis, which is known to precede gastric cancer. Current ideas on the mechanism by which *H. pylori* might contribute to gastric carcinoma focus on the inflammation produced by the bacterium and the reduction in acid secretion it causes. Inflammation can result in reactive oxygen species and reduced acid in the stomach, which is associated with increased levels of mutagenic nitrosamines and increased secretion of gastrin (which promotes epithelial cell growth). It therefore appears to be an indirect mechanism by which *H. pylori* contributes to gastric cancer. Antibiotic treatment is clearly beneficial for peptic ulcers caused by *H. pylori* but it remains to be determined whether use of antibiotics to prevent gastric carcinoma will be pursued because the bacterial infection is also associated with reduced levels of certain other diseases.

Several other human viruses have been considered as possibly being involved in human cancer. Herpes simplex virus type 2 was studied for many years in connection with cervical cancer prior to the discovery of HPV16. Since HSV2 and HPV16 are both transmitted through sexual contact, HSV2 infection is now thought to be frequently co-incidental with HPV16 rather than causative of cervical cancer. Another herpesvirus, cytomegalovirus has also been studied in connection with cancer because certain fragments of CMV DNA were found to cause transformation of human cells when transfected. There is, however, no substantial evidence for CMV causing any human cancer.

Human viruses of the polyoma family have also been studied for cancer connections. BK virus has been detected in pancreatic adenomas and various types of brain tumour but it can also be present in normal tissue of these types. BKV is oncogenic in rodents but there is no other evidence that it contributes to human cancer. Similarly JC virus has been reported in tumours of the brain, colon, and in some leukamias but there is no evidence for a causative role.

13.4 Therapeutic implications—vaccination and targeting therapy to cancer cells

If a virus causes cancer, the obvious approach is to vaccinate against the virus infection. This has been implemented for HBV and there are some preliminary indications that this may be effective in reducing HCC. Early trials of the HPV vaccine also look promising and this is being tested for its ability to prevent cervical carcinoma. Vaccines for the other human viruses discussed here are still a long way in the future.

Even when vaccines are available, there is a large burden of disease in people already infected by the viruses in whom vaccines will have no effect. In these cases it will be interesting to consider the possiblity of novel therapeutic approaches based on the presence of the virus in the tumour cells. The fundamental problem in cancer therapy is how to distinguish cancer cells from normal cells and then kill the cancer cells. The differences between cancer cells and normal cells are frequently very subtle but in the case of the virus associated cancers the presence of the virus provides an obvious opportunity for development of novel therapeutic agents that could be selective for virus infected cells.

References

Primary literature references can be found generally in Knipe and Howley (2001).

Boshoff, C. and Weiss, R. A. (2001). Epidemiology and pathogenesis of Kaposi's sarcoma-associated herpesvirus. *Philos Trans R Soc Lond B Biol Sci*, **356**, 517–34.

Callan, M. F., Steven, N., Krausa, P., Wilson, J. D., Moss, P. A., Gillespie, G. M. et al. (1996). Large clonal expansions of CD8+ T cells in acute infectious mononucleosis. *Nat Med*, **2**, 906–11.

Feng, B. J., Huang, W., Shugart, Y. Y., Lee, M. K., Zhang, F., Xia, J. C. et al. (2002). Genomewide scan for familial nasopharyngeal carcinoma reveals evidence of linkage to chromosome 4. *Nat Genet*, **31**, 395–9.

Fickenscher, H. and Fleckenstein, B. (2001). Herpesvirus saimiri. *Philos Trans R Soc Lond B Biol Sci*, **356**, 545–67.

Fragnet, L., Blasco, M. A., Klapper, W., and Rasschaert, D. (2003). The RNA subunit of telomerase is encoded by Marek's disease virus. *J Virol*, **77**, 5985–96.

Gu, W., Bhatia, K., Magrath, I. T., Dang, C. V., and Dalla-Favera, R. (1994). Binding and Suppression of the Myc Transcriptional Activation Domain by p107. *Science*, **264**, 251–4.

Hickabottom, M., Parker, G. A., Freemont, P., Crook, T., and Allday, M. J. (2002). Two nonconsensus sites in the Epstein-Barr virus oncoprotein EBNA3A cooperate to bind the co-repressor carboxyl-terminal-binding protein (CtBP). *J Biol Chem*, **277**, 47197–204.

Jackson, S., Harwood, C., Thomas, M., Banks, L., and Storey, A. (2000). Role of Bak in UV-induced apoptosis in skin cancer and abrogation by HPV E6 proteins. *Genes Dev*, **14**, 3065–73.

Kao, J. H. and Chen, D. S. (2002) Global control of hepatitis B virus infection *Lancet Infect Dis*, **2**, 395–403.

Kelly, G., Bell, A., and Rickinson, A. (2002) Epstein-Barr virus-associated Burkitt lymphomagenesis selects for downregulation of the nuclear antigen EBNA2 *Nat Med*, **8**, 1098–1104.

Knipe, D. and Howley, P. (2001) *Fields Virology*. Lippincott Williams and Wilkins, Philadelphia.

Koutsky, L. A., Ault, K. A., Wheeler, C. M., Brown, D. R., Barr, E., Alvarez, F. B. et al. (2002). A controlled trial of a human papillomavirus type 16 vaccine. *N Engl J Med*, **347**, 1645–51.

Li, D., Dower, K., Ma, Y., Tian, Y., and Benjamin, T. L. (2001). A tumor host range selection procedure identifies p150(sal2) as a target of polyoma virus large T antigen. *Proc Natl Acad Sci USA*, **98**, 14619–24.

Liu, J. L., Lee, L. F., Ye, Y., Qian, Z., and Kung, H. J. (1997). Nucleolar and nuclear localization properties of a herpesvirus bZIP oncoprotein, MEQ. *J Virol*, **71**, 3188–96.

Liu, J. L., Ye, Y., Qian, Z., Qian, Y., Templeton, D. J., Lee, L. F. et al. (1999). Functional interactions between herpesvirus oncoprotein MEQ and cell cycle regulator CDK2. *J Virol*, **73**, 4208–19.

Lo, K. W. and Huang, D. P. (2002). Genetic and epigenetic changes in nasopharyngeal carcinoma. *Semin Cancer Biol*, **12**, 451–62.

Lomax, M. and Fried, M. (2001). Polyoma virus disrupts ARF signaling to p53. *Oncogene*, **20**, 4951–60.

Nanbo, A., Inoue, K., Adachi-Takasawa, K., and Takada, K. (2002). Epstein-Barr virus RNA confers resistance to interferon-alpha-induced apoptosis in Burkitt's lymphoma. *Embo J*, **21**, 954–65.

O'nions, J. and Allday, M. (2003). Epstein-Barr virus can inhibit genotoxin-induced G1 arrest downstream of p53 by preventing the inactivation of CDK2. *Oncogene*, **22**, 7181–91.

Old, L., Clifford, P., Boyse, E., de Harven, E., Geering, G., Oettgen, H. et al.(1966). Precipitating antibody in human serum to an antigen present in cultured Burkitt lymphoma cells. *Proc Natl Acad Sci USA*, **56**, 1699–704.

Parker, G. A., Touitou, R., and Allday, M. J. (2000). Epstein-Barr virus EBNA3C can disrupt multiple cell cycle checkpoints and induce nuclear division divorced from cytokinesis. *Oncogene*, **19**, 700–9.

Scholle, F., Bendt, K. M., and Raab-Traub, N. (2000). Epstein-Barr virus LMP2A transforms epithelial cells, inhibits cell differentiation, and activates Akt. *J Virol*, **74**, 10681–9.

Spender, L. C., Cornish, G. H., Sullivan, A., and Farrell, P. J. (2002). Expression of transcription factor AML-2 (RUNX3, CBF(alpha)-3) is induced by Epstein-Barr virus EBNA-2 and correlates with the B-cell activation phenotype. *J Virol*, **76**, 4919–27.

Stewart, B. and Kleihues, P. (2003). *WHO World Cancer Report*. IARC Press, Lyon.

Thorley-Lawson, D. (2001). Epstein-Barr virus: exploiting the immune system. *Nature Rev Immunol*, **1**, 75–82.

Touitou, R., Hickabottom, M., Parker, G., Crook, T., and Allday, M. J. (2001). Physical and functional interactions between the corepressor CtBP and the Epstein-Barr virus nuclear antigen EBNA3C. *J Virol*, **75**, 7749–55.

Verschuren, E. W., Klefstrom, J., Evan, G. I., and Jones, N. (2002). The oncogenic potential of Kaposi's sarcoma-associated herpesvirus cyclin is exposed by p53 loss *in vitro* and *in vivo*. *Cancer Cell*, **2**, 229–41.

zur Hausen, H., Schulte-Holthausen, H., Klein, G., Henle, W., Henle, G., Clifford, P. et al. (1970). EBV DNA in biopsies of Burkitt tumours and anaplastic carcinomas of the nasopharynx. *Nature*, **228**, 1056–8.

CHAPTER 14

Cytokines and cancer

Peter W. Szlosarek and Frances R. Balkwill

14.1 Introduction

Complex multicellular organisms maintain cellular homeostasis at the local tissue level via a diverse array of secreted low-molecular weight mediators collectively called cytokines. These include tumour necrosis factor-α (TNF-α), interleukins (ILs), interferons (IFNs), colony-stimulating factors, chemokines, angiogenic factors, and growth factors. Unlike classical endocrine hormones, these proteins act in an autocrine, paracrine, and/or juxtacrine fashion on a variety of cells, ranging from stem cells to those that are fully differentiated. Cytokines act within an informational network consisting of ligands and their respective cell-surface receptors and downstream intracellular signalling pathways, enabling cells to participate in a range of processes including cell activation (survival, growth, and differentiation), cell death (apoptosis), cell motility, inflammation, and immunity (see Table 14.1). Since cancer is intimately linked with aberrations in these pathways (reviewed in Hanahan and Weinberg, 2000) either at a genetic or epigenetic level, disturbances in the 'cytokine network' may promote the malignant phenotype. Evidence in recent years has documented that this is undoubtedly the case, and that cytokines often display seemingly paradoxical roles in tumorigenesis.

The factors determining the 'double-edged' nature of cytokines in relation to cancer are poorly understood; however, dose, timing (e.g. proliferative state), cell type, and the effect of other cytokines, nutritional factors, and local mediators are all important (see also Ardestani et al., 1999; Mocellin et al., 2001). For example, transforming growth factor-β (TGF-β) is considered a tumour suppressor early on in mammary oncogenesis, and assumes a tumour-promoting role with more advanced breast tumours. Thus, modulation of the cytokine network and, in turn, the tumour–stroma landscape, whether with cytokine ligands or antagonists provides a rationale for cancer therapy. Here, following a review of the tumour microenvironment, we discuss the roles of several cytokines in cancer emphasizing their clinical use and areas currently under development (i.e. cytokine antagonists).

Table 14.1 The role of endogenous cytokines in the tumour microenvironment

Tumour/stromal cell proliferation
Tumour cell apoptosis
Tumour cell motility and invasion
Tumour cell surface antigen expression
Angiogenesis
ECM formation
Immune responses
Nutritional/hormonal balance
Modulators of cancer therapy

14.2 The tumour microenvironment

Cancer comprises both a neoplastic clonal cell population in a continuous state of evolution and stromal cells which provide sustenance and facilitate the metastatic process of the malignant cell. The stromal cell component varies between and within tumour types and consists of fibroblasts (myofibroblasts, carcinoma-associated fibroblasts), endothelial cells and pericytes, and cells of the innate (macrophages, eosinophils, and natural killer (NK) cells) and adaptive immune system (B and T lymphocytes). The extracellular matrix (ECM) with its proteases and scaffolding proteins, constitutes the final element of the tumour microenvironment. Thus, the tumour mass has been likened to an 'outlaw organ' which has co-opted normal cells and reprogrammed their biology at the service of the cancer cell. Attempts made by the immune system to inhibit tumour progression, including the release of various cytokines, are often inadequate and instead provide a means for the cancer cell to further adapt to its host (reviewed in Szlosarek and Dalgleish, 2002).

The critical importance of stroma in tumorigenesis has been confirmed by a series of experiments that, by modulating the stromal cell and/or ECM composition, have demonstrated either an inhibitory or enhanced effect on cancer growth.

A striking feature of many epithelial cancers is an underlying inflammation, which often predates the disease, functioning both as a tumour promoter and as a key determinant of tumour stroma (see Table 14.2). Dvorak compared tumours to 'wounds that do not heal' and several recent reviews have revisited and expanded upon these observations (see O'Byrne et al., 2000; Balkwill and Mantovani, 2001; Coussens and Werb, 2002; Bogenrieder and Herlyn, 2003; Dranoff, 2004). Since biological reactions display a finite number of possible outcomes, it is unsurprising that on a pathophysiological level many conditions share similar processes. For instance, rheumatoid arthritis, which is characterized by an inflammatory stromal tissue or 'pannus' invading synovial joints exhibits hyperproliferation, angiogenesis, and leucocyte infiltration, all of which are features of a developing tumour. Moreover, TNF-α (tumour necrosis factor-α) is both a molecule of fundamental importance to rheumatoid arthritis and a critical player in the evolution of certain haematological and epithelial tumours (see below). In the following discussion of several classical cytokines, their dual function in cancer is a recurring theme. Thus, opposing treatment strategies may be envisaged not only in different tumours but also at different stages in the history of the same tumour.

Table 14.2 Cancer and inflammation

Malignancy	Inflammatory stimulus
Bladder	Schistosomiasis
Bronchial	Asbestos, smoking
Breast	Chronic mastitis[a]
Cervical	Human papillomavirus[a]
Colorectal	Inflammatory bowel disease
Gastric	*Helicobacter pylori*-induced gastritis
Hepatocellular	Hepatitis B/C
Kaposi's sarcoma	Human herpes virus 8
Lymphoma	HIV, EBV ?
Mesothelioma	Asbestos
Oesophageal	Barrett's metaplasia
Ovarian	Pelvic inflammatory disease, talc, tissue remodelling[a]
Pancreatic	Chronic pancreatitis
Prostatic	Chronic prostatitis[a]

[a] Additional hormonal modulation.

14.3 Tumour necrosis factor-α

Isolated in 1975, following almost a century of investigation with inactivated bacterial filtrates for the treatment of cancer, TNF-α has remained an important cytokine in cancer research. It exists as a 50 kDa homotrimeric molecule with each polypeptide containing 157 amino acids (cleaved from a larger 233 amino acid pro-TNF-α molecule), and binds two alternative homotrimeric receptors, TNFRI and TNFRII. Although TNF-α is licensed for the locoregional treatment of sarcoma (i.e. isolated

Table 14.3 Tumour promoting effects of TNF-α

Production of NO (DNA/enzyme damage, cyclic guanosine monophosphate (cGMP)-mediated tumour promotion)
Autocrine growth and survival factor for malignant cells
Activation of E6/E7 mRNA in HPV-infected cells
Tissue remodelling via induction of MMPs
Control of leucocyte infiltration in tumours via modulation of chemokines and their receptors
Downregulation of E-cadherin, increased nuclear pool of β-catenin
Enhance tumour cell motility and invasion
Induction of angiogenic factors
Loss of androgen responsiveness
Resistance to cytotoxic drugs

limb perfusion), experimental data over the last decade has paradoxically suggested a significant tumour-promoting role for this cytokine (see Tsimberidou and Giles, 2002; Szlosarek and Balkwill, 2003 for reviews). In contrast to the underlying anti-angiogenic and immunostimulatory mechanism of high-dose TNF-α in sarcoma therapy, low-dose TNF-α positively regulates tumour growth, invasion, angiogenesis, and metastasis (Table 14.3).

Several TNF-α/TNFR knockout mouse models have emphasized a central role for this cytokine in both solid tumours and lymphoproliferative disease. A study by Moore et al. (1999) documented a tenfold decrease in skin tumours in TNF-$\alpha^{-/-}$ mice compared with wild-type mice exposed to skin carcinogens. Recent analysis indicates that the difference during tumour promotion is due, in part, to a temporal delay in the activation of protein kinase Cα (PKCα) and AP-1, key carcinogen-responsive signalling molecules. This modulates the transcription of several genes involved in tumour development (GM-CSF (granulocyte-macrophage colony-stimulating factor), MMP-3, (matrix metalloproteinase-3) and MMP-9), which are suppressed in the TNF-$\alpha^{-/-}$ mice compared to wild-type animals exposed to carcinogen. Furthermore, both TNFRI$^{-/-}$ and TNFRII$^{-/-}$ mice have also confirmed a requirement for TNF-α in promoting skin carcinogenesis. Similarly, TNFRI$^{-/-}$mice have proven useful in elucidating the mechanisms involved in liver carcinogenesis. TNFRI$^{-/-}$ mice displayed reduced oval cell (hepatic stem cell) proliferation during the preneoplastic phase of liver carcinogenesis, resulting in fewer tumours. A more recent study by Kitakata et al. (2002) has used TNFRI$^{-/-}$ mice to show that endogenous TNF-α is critical in promoting liver metastasis following intrasplenic administration of a colonic adenocarcinoma cell line. The fatal lymphoproliferative disorder that develops in Fas ligand-deficient mice was attenuated by crossing these animals with TNF-$\alpha^{-/-}$ mice. Here, TNF-α may have induced the expression of chemokines (see below), which regulate trafficking and accumulation of tumour cells into lymph nodes.

Transgenic mice overexpressing TNF-α are poor models for investigating the effects of TNF-α in tumour promotion, since they succumb early on to severe inflammatory pathologies. However, both the administration of exogenous TNF-α and tumour cells containing a TNF-α transgene have revealed enhanced tumorigenesis in several studies. In human xenograft models of ovarian cancer, TNF-α injected intraperitoneally converts malignant ascites into solid tumour deposits, reflecting modulation of both tumour stroma and metastasis. Alternative approaches employing TNF-α overexpression have also demonstrated enhanced invasive properties in xenograft tumours.

In direct contrast, studies in TNF-$\alpha^{-/-}$ mice have confirmed important roles of TNF-α in tumour immunity. Both CD8+ T cells, lymphokine activated killer (LAK) cells, and NK cells displayed impaired cytotoxicity against an immunogenic syngeneic tumour in TNF-$\alpha^{-/-}$ mice which was reversible with the injection of recombinant TNF-α. Similarly, rejection of sarcomas using near lethal doses of TNF-α was abrogated in T-cell deficient mice; both the haemorrhagic necrosis and eventual tumour regression was dependent upon T-cell activity.

Evidence for involvement of TNF-α in human cancer is derived from several sources. First, expression studies using immunohistochemistry and *in situ* hybridization to mRNA have shown that TNF-α is present in a variety of tumours. This is supported by an increasing amount of *in vitro* data defining TNF-α's role within the cytokine network. Ovarian cancer, a tumour rich in cytokines, has been the focus of several studies. The autocrine regulation of TNF-α mRNA expression differs markedly between normal and malignant ovarian epithelium emphasizing that malignant transformation is accompanied by deregulated TNF-α activity. Both IL-1 and CXCL12 (see below) are known inducers of TNF-α in ovarian cancer but the initial trigger for deregulated TNF-α activity remains elusive. TNF-α activation results in the following: upregulation of several autocrine and paracrine loops including TNF-α itself, IL-6, IL-8, M-CSF, and the IL-1 family (IL-1α, IL-1β and IL1RA); invasion (MMP-9); leucocyte recruitment via chemokines (MCP-1 (monocyte chemotactic protein-1), IL-8); and an array of local mediators (prostaglandins, free radicals, e.g. nitric oxide (NO)), which fuel further mutations and clonal expansion. More recently in the case of glioma, TNF-α mRNA stabilization has been characterized as a factor in the downstream activation of key angiogenic molecules, VEGF (vascular endothelial growth factor) and IL-8 (Nabors et al., 2003). The paradoxical effects of TNF-α on tumour vasculature may reflect the difference in chronic synthesis, which may favour angiogenesis, while acute high-dose local administration triggers vascular collapse.

Several *in vitro* studies have explored the mechanisms underlying tumour cell resistance to TNF-α cytotoxicity. These include downregulation of TNFRs, the gain of a TNF-α autocrine/paracrine loop, and the activation of free radical scavenging pathways (e.g. manganese superoxide dismutase). TNF-α resistance is associated with loss of p53 in breast cancer and upregulation of E6/E7 in human papillomavirus (HPV)-induced cervical carcinogenesis. TNF-α is implicated in anthracyline chemoresistance and induces androgen independence via repression of the androgen receptor in prostate cancer. Signalling via TNFRI also provides a vital level of control, with a cell's fate (i.e. apoptosis or survival) determined by the balance between two opposing complexes: complex I (membrane-associated) regulates activation of NF-κB1 (nuclear factor-κB1) and cell survival; and complex II (cytoplasmic) signals apoptosis via caspase-8. A checkpoint is maintained by this arrangement, as complex II harbours an inhibitor of caspase-8 upon activation of complex I. Apoptosis will therefore occur in the presence of incomplete NF-κB1 activation by complex I (reviewed in Micheau and Tschopp, 2003).

Paraneoplastic syndromes that accompany cancer may also be orchestrated to varying degrees by TNF-α. Cachexia, or the progressive weight loss associated with muscle and lipid wasting, appears to be driven by several tumour-and/or host-derived factors including cytokines, such as TNF-α, IL-1, IL-6, and IFN-γ. Here, animal data is more convincing for the involvement of TNF-α, with clinical studies evaluating the cytokine in human cachexia being less consistent. However, pancreatic carcinoma is an exception with recent studies in patients with cachexia confirming both increased TNF-α mRNA and protein in blood cells and plasma, respectively. TNF-α has also been characterized as an endogenous pyrogen, osteoclast-activating factor facilitating skeletal metastases (reviewed in Roodman, 2003), and as an inhibitor of erythropoietin production linking the cytokine to typical tumour presentations of fever, hypercalcaemia, anaemia, and fatigue.

Lastly, if TNF-α is an endogenous tumour promoter, it is possible that functional single nucleotide polymorphisms (SNPs) in the genes for TNF-α, TNFRs, or events downstream in the TNF-α signalling pathway may be associated with cancer severity and susceptibility. A number of recent studies have associated TNF-α SNPs with cancer development. However, the small numbers of patients in these studies have been insufficient to draw any firm conclusions, and further work is required.

There have been two decades of clinical research with TNF-α. First, TNF-α isolation led quickly to a large number of clinical trials in the mid-to-late 1980s, documenting both high toxicity and a disappointing (<10%) response rate with no discernible impact on patient survival. Various alternative strategies are currently in development including modification of the TNF-α molecule (so-called TNF-α muteins), the use of hyperthermia in conjunction with locoregional TNF-α, and radiation-inducible TNF-α in an attempt to eliminate side effects while preserving cytotoxicity. The latter approach employs an adenoviral vector containing an epidermal growth receptor 1 (EGR1) promoter (with radiation-sensitive *CArG* elements) upstream of cDNA encoding TNF-α. Preliminary clinical studies with intratumoural *Ad.EGR-TNF* (TNFerade) in combination with ionizing radiation have yielded some complete and partial responses of accessible lesions in patients with breast, lung, pancreas, and rectal tumours.

Second, in view of the data concerning TNF-α as a tumour promoter, the pendulum has presently swung in the opposite direction and TNF-α antagonists, such as infliximab (a humanized murine immunoglobulin G1 (IgG1) monoclonal antibody) and etanercept (a dimeric molecule consisting of two molecules of the extracellular portion of the human TNFRII fused to the Fc portion of human IgG) are currently the focus of several phase I/II clinical trials. Other specific TNF-α antagonists in development include a human IgG1 antibody, a pegylated truncated form of TNFRI, and antisense; a TNF 'Trap' molecule based on a fusion molecule of the extracellular domains of TNFRI and TNFRII (i.e. similar to the VEGF 'Trap' currently in clinical trials) is another possibility. Some reports of beneficial activity are emerging in myelodysplatic disease and graft-versus-host disease with biological indices of cytokine activation being affected in patients with breast and ovarian cancer. Other studies are in progress in patients with non-small cell lung cancer (in combination with docetaxel), pancreatic cancer (in combination with gemcitabine), and palliative care studies examining the role of TNF-α in cancer cachexia. It is noteworthy that several broad-spectrum anti-inflammatory/anti-angiogenic drugs, such as dexamethasone, thalidomide, aspirin, and cyclo-oxygenase inhibitors (especially targeting COX2) as well as naturally occurring compounds found in green tea, black raspberry, and turmeric (i.e. curcumin) are also inhibitors of TNF-α activity and may partly account for their chemopreventative and/or therapeutic properties in cancer. Lastly, TNF-α antagonists may also have a role to play in limiting the nephrotoxicity of cisplatin and the pulmonary toxicity of bleomycin.

The cytokine release syndrome, distinguished by fever and rigors with abdominal pain, hypotension, and orthopnoea present in more severe reactions, is a common event following treatment with rituximab (>50% of first treatment episodes) and is associated with high circulating levels of TNF-α. The mechanism underlying the TNF-α-induced cardiopulmonary toxicity is unclear but is thought to include the release of NO and leukostasis in pulmonary vasculature. Drugs such as oxaliplatin and irinotecan also produce fevers occasionally (without infection) associated with increased plasma levels of TNF-α.

In summary, research into TNF-α and cancer has aptly illustrated the complexity of cytokine tumour biology. Indeed members of the TNF superfamily, with some further 20 ligands and receptors, all have in common the ability to activate NFκB and c-Jun and hence regulate apoptosis, cell survival, and the immune system (reviewed in Younes and Kadin, 2003). Some TNF superfamily members, such as CD30L, CD40L, RANKL, and TRAIL implicated in a number of haematological cancers and therapies based on their biology are in development.

14.4 Interferons

14.4.1 Interferon-α

Although first noted for their antiviral effect over four decades ago, it is only recently that the IFN family, consisting of type I (IFN-α, β, τ, ω) and type II (IFN-γ) IFNs, has emerged as a central mediator in tumour immunity and immunosurveillance. Previously, the use of IFN-α as an antitumour agent has been explained mainly in terms of its direct antiproliferative activity (on both tumour and endothelial cells). However, key animal experiments have now revealed important immune mechanisms at play, ranging from dendritic cell (DC) activation to enhanced humoral and cellular immunity with considerable uncertainty about the relative contributions of direct or indirect mechanisms for anti-cancer effects. Much less is known regarding IFN-τ and ω, although recent work with the latter IFN in human tumour xenograft models indicates, as with IFN-α, that it also has significant direct antiproliferative activity when injected intratumorally or systemically. Since no murine IFN-ω gene has been isolated, an assessment of any immunomodulatory properties will require study within the patient population.

IFN-α has a role in the therapy of a variety of tumours including, chronic myeloid leukaemia (CML) (although this is now superseded by imatinib), hairy cell leukaemia, renal cell carcinoma, melanoma, Kaposi's sarcoma, and some B- and T-cell lymphomas. The type I IFNs all bind to a dimer of two receptors, IFNARI and IFNAR2. Upon binding IFN-α the receptor dimer undergoes phosphorylation, triggering subsequent phosphorylation of JAK (Janus Kinases) and STAT (signal transducers and activators of transcription) proteins, which then proceed to modulate a wide array of IFN-α inducible genes. Direct effects on tumour cells include downregulation of oncogene expression (e.g. BCR/ABL) and induction of tumour suppressor genes (e.g. p53) thereby promoting a growth inhibitory response. IFN-α also inhibits tumour angiogenesis and induces haemorrhagic necrosis by interrupting the tumour endothelium. The immunomodulatory action of IFN-α was initially observed in studies of mice transplanted with IFN-resistant cells. Here, mice transplanted with a syngeneic IFN-α-resistant clone of Friend leukaemia cells (FLC) mounted an effective antitumour response upon injection of IFN-α, similar to that observed in mice injected with IFN-α-sensitive cells. The intrinsic IFN-α resistance of the cells remained unaffected, as demonstrated by an absence of H-2 class I antigen expression and the failure to induce an antiviral state. Instead, an analysis of the antitumour mechanism revealed immunopotentiation of several parameters, including the presence of FLC gp70 cytotoxic antibodies (IgG2a isotype) and CD4+ T cells. Other models have illustrated a requirement for the codelivery of tumour-antigen primed T cells (either CD4+ or CD8+) and IFN-α for effective inhibition of visceral metastases.

In contrast, the role of endogenous IFN-α, normally expressed at very low levels by liver and spleen cells, has been addressed with neutralizing antibodies. Using IFN-α-resistant tumour cells, (thereby limiting the analysis to IFN-α-mediated immune events), these antibody experiments revealed enhanced tumorigenicity of IFN-α-resistant tumour cells in syngeneic mice. Clearly, endogenous IFN-α was important in suppressing tumour development in this model, but via an indirect mechanism. A major source for the endogenous IFN-α, mediating the immunological rejection of the tumour cells, is now attributed to a rare blood cell population—the so-called plamacytoid DC or 'natural IFN-producing cell'. These cells are CD4+ CD11c- type 2 DC precursors (pDC2s) and are capable of a 200–1000-fold greater IFN-α production compared with other blood cells. As such they provide a bridge between the innate and adaptive immune system and emphasize the importance of adjuvant IFN-α. Apart from DC activation, IFN-α enhances the following parameters: NK cell, macrophage, and (cytotoxic T lymphocyte) CTL activity; expression of (major histocompatibility complex) MHC class I antigen; differentiation of the Th1 subset; the *in vivo* proliferation, expansion, and long-term survival of CD8+ cells; and the effect of CpG DNA administration on T cells. Moreover, certain chemo/adoptive cell therapy approaches (e.g. cyclophosphamide in combination with tumour-sensitized lymphocytes) stimulate an IFN-α immunomodulatory effect, since IFN-α antibodies abrogate the antitumour response in mice.

Gene transfer has also been employed in an attempt to both limit the adverse effects of systemically delivered cytokine and generate a more focussed immune response. Several different tumour models, including syngeneic (FLC, TS/A mammary adenocarcinoma, murine colon carcinoma, B16 melanoma, and ESb lymphoma) and human xenograft mouse experiments have confirmed that IFN-α-producing cells provoke a specific antitumour response in established parental tumours (CD4+, CD8+, and DCs) and confer protection against subsequent rechallenge, indicating an effect on memory T cells. Furthermore, several points need to be emphasized regarding IFN-α biotherapy. First, IFN-α-transduced normal cells (e.g. fibroblasts) and intramuscular delivery of IFN-α-expressing plasmid DNA (CD8+ response) have also proven to be effective in inhibiting the growth of established murine tumours. Second, a synergistic effect with chemotherapy has been demonstrated in several murine and human tumour models. IFN-α potentiated the apoptosis induced by cisplatin, 5-fluorouracil, and enzyme-prodrug gene therapy (i.e. thymidine kinase/ganciclovir), concurrently triggering antitumour immune responses.

The clinical application of systemic IFN-α, although of value in several of the cancers outlined above, continues to be problematic particularly due to dose-limiting side effects (e.g. fever, myalgia, general malaise). In addition, for tumours such as melanoma and renal cell cancer the overall response rates are low, in the order of 4–26%. A recent meta-analysis of adjuvant IFN-α (i.e. no evidence of metastatic disease) for the treatment of melanoma has shown that while IFN-α has improved the relapse-free interval, the question of survival benefit remains unanswered (Wheatley et al., 2003). However, the most convincing evidence to date for the antitumour immune-mediated activity of IFN-α stems from studies in patients with CML. Here, IFN-α can induce a 60–80% haematological remission rate, with an albeit much lower level of complete cytological remission. A strong correlation exists between CML antigen-specific T cells and antibodies and a clinical response to IFN-α. Moreover, analysis of DCs obtained from patients with CML suggests that the mechanism involves IFN-α-mediated differentiation and maturation of these cells. A pegylated version of IFN-α, allowing once weekly dosing and improved compliance, has recently become available. The immunomodulatory data on IFN-α that has emerged should hopefully facilitate further development.

14.4.2 Interferon-γ

IFN-γ is produced mainly by T cells, NK T cells, and NK cells following challenge with non-viral immune and inflammatory stimuli. It exists as a 50 kDa homodimeric molecule, with each glycosylated polypeptide consisting of 134 amino acids arranged in an antiparallel fashion, thereby revealing two identical receptor-binding sites. Signalling is achieved by binding to a high-affinity heterodimeric receptor found on most cell types: IFNGR1 (also known as IFN-γRI, IFN-γ α chain, CDw119) which binds IFN-γ; and IFNGR2 (also known as IFN-γRII, IFN-γ β chain, or accessory factor 1) which facilitates transmission of the IFN-γ signal. The latter depends on a functional JAK–STAT pathway, with initial activation of JAKs involving auto- and *trans*-phosphorylation. Subsequently, a signalling cascade leading to activation and nuclear translocation of a Stat1 homodimer results in the activation of IFN-γ-dependent genes. Several studies with mutant or null members of this pathway have concluded the obligatory role of Jak1, Jak2, and Stat1 for effective IFN-γ signalling.

Experiments with methylcholanthrene (MCA)-induced sarcomas in mice provided evidence for a role of IFN-γ in immune-mediated tumour rejection. Mice treated with sublethal doses of lipopolysaccharide (LPS) normally rejected transplantable tumours. Antibodies to IFN-γ not only abrogated the effect of LPS, but also facilitated tumour growth. The importance of endogenous IFN-γ was resolved once mice with aberrant IFN-γ signalling (i.e. IFN-γ-insensitive mice: IFN-γ−/−, IFN-γR−/−, or Stat1−/−) were exposed to MCA: a 16-fold increase in tumorigenicity was observed in IFN-γ-insensitive mice compared with wild-type mice. More striking results were obtained when IFN-γ-insensitive mice were bred onto p53−/− backgrounds. Whereas all the p53−/− and IFN-γ-sensitive mice developed exclusively lymphoid tumours, over a third of the p53−/− and IFN-γ-insensitive mice developed a variety of non-lymphoid tumours (e.g. teratomas, haemangiomas, and chondrosarcomas), with a comparably earlier time of onset. Further work in this area revealed an interdependence between IFN-γ and lymphocytes. By deleting a gene critical for lymphocyte development (*RAG2*), an increase was observed in the spontaneous appearance of breast and intestinal adenocarcinomas. Moreover, the antitumour effects of IL-12 (see below) were abolished following administration of neutralizing IFN-γ antibodies. Studies of IFN-γ-resistant tumours with a non-functional IFNGR1, demonstrated increased growth in naïve syngeneic mice compared with IFN-γ-sensitive tumours. On the other hand, these same IFNGRI-defective tumours and their wild-type counterparts grew equally well in severe combined immunodeficiency (SCID) mice, again indicating the close relationship between IFN-γ and the immune system. Therefore, a tumour escape mechanism can be envisaged which is driven by the immune system itself. Indeed, about 25% of certain human tumour cell lines contain aberrations in IFN-γ signalling, such as mutations in IFNGR1 and JAKs. Moreover, recent experiments using short-term primary ovarian carcinoma cells treated with IFN-γ and co-cultured with allospecific CD8+ T cells have produced surprising results. Here, IFN-γ neutralized antitumour CTL activity due to the concomitant upregulation of an inhibitory CD94/NKG2A-dependent pathway in the effector cells, associated with the expression of HLA-E (human leucocyte antigen-E) and G on the tumour cells (see Lukacher, 2002). Thus, evidence suggesting a central role for IFN-γ in modulating the innate and adaptive immune system in respect of tumours, has given rise to the concept of 'immunoediting' in preference to 'immunosurveillance' (see Sporn and Vilcek, 2002; Dunn et al., 2002).

Experimental data also supports a significant direct antitumour effect for IFN-γ, inhibiting both tumour cell proliferation and metabolism. STAT1-deficient tumour cells, for instance, are insensitive to the growth inhibitory effects of IFN-γ *in vitro*, which proceed via upregulation of the cell cycle inhibitors, $p21^{WAF1/CIP1}$ and $p27^{Kip1}$. These bind to the cyclin-dependent kinases, CDK-2 and CDK-4 respectively, and prevent their activation by CDK-activating kinase—an effect observed in a variety of cancer cell types from epidermoid cells to rhabdomyosarcoma. The apoptotic activity of IFN-γ is also mediated by STAT-1, via activation of caspase-1 or Fas/Fas ligand. This pathway is in addition to the basal levels of apoptotic proteins (e.g. caspase-1, Cpp32, and Ich-1) maintained by STAT1. In contrast, STAT3 activation can directly transform immortalized fibroblasts *in vitro*. Both STAT3 and the related STAT5 are linked to growth factor receptor pathways and are activated in a variety of tumours (breast, ovary, prostate, lung, kidney, head, and neck), promoting cell survival via induction of Bcl-2 and Bcl-X_L. Lastly, an anti-angiogenic mechanism has been proposed with the following features: the upregulation of several IFN-γ-dependent CXC non-ELR chemokines acting via CXCR3 (see below), including CXCL10 (IP-10), CXCL9 (MIG), and I-TAC, all with an inhibitory effect on neovascularization. This pathway appears to be a feature of IL-12-directed angiogenesis, as CXCL10 antibodies antagonize the phenomenon.

Early clinical investigation with IFN-γ proved disappointing, with the majority of trials in a variety of advanced tumours showing no effect. To date, some of the more encouraging data for IFN-γ comes from studies with ovarian carcinoma (Pujade-Lauraine et al., 1996 Windbichler et al., 2000). A large global randomized phase-III trial called GRACES (Gamma Interferon and Chemotherapy Efficacy Study) is currently assessing the activity of IFN-γ in combination with carboplatin and paclitaxel. A recent clinical study has assessed the mechanism of action of intraperitoneal IFN-γ on primary ovarian tumour cells and has provided evidence of apoptosis in 6/6 patients with clinical response in 2/6 patients (Wall et al., 2003).

14.5 Interleukins

Our knowledge of the IL family has increased substantially in the last few years with the total now at around 30 members. IL-1, 6, 8, and 10, are implicated in tumour promotion, whereas others including IL-2, 12, and 24 possess antitumour activity, or in the case of IL-11 may be used clinically as a thrombopoietin during chemotherapy (reviewed in Brown and Demetri, 2002). Moreover, IL-8 has recently been reclassified as a CXC chemokine (see CXCL8 below and Xie, 2001 for a review), and a whole new family of IL-10 cytokines has been identified. The following section briefly reviews the spectrum of activity of several ILs in tumorigenesis, particularly IL-1, IL-6, and the IL-10 cytokine family, as well as the current status of IL-2 and IL-12 in tumour immunotherapy.

14.5.1 Interleukin-1 and -6

Both IL-1 and IL-6 are associated with enhanced growth of haematological and solid cancers, in addition to influencing paraneoplastic phenomena, such as cancer cachexia, fatigue, and fever. Since these cytokines are involved in autocrine/paracrine loops, in some cases driven by activating oncogenic mutations (e.g. RAS activation of IL-1β in leukaemia), this may provoke yet further deregulation of the cytokine network. The IL-1(α/β)/IL-1Ra (IL-1 receptor antagonist) family provides a unique insight into the complexity involved in cytokine cancer biology (see Arend, 2002 and Kurzrock, 2001 for reviews). The two IL-1 isoforms activate the 80 kDa type 1 receptor (IL-1RI), whereas IL-1RII functions as a decoy receptor. In contrast, IL-1Ra which attenuates IL-1 signalling by inhibiting the interaction of IL-1RI with its accessory protein (IL-1R AcP), has at least three isoforms: the soluble IL-1Ra (sIL-1Ra) present in monocytes/macrophages, neutrophils, and other cells; and two characterized intracellular forms (icIL–1Ra), with icIL–1Ra1 expressed by various cell types (epithelial and endothelial cells, fibroblasts, and monocytes/macrophages) and icIL–1Ra3 found in monocytes/macrophages and hepatocytes. Although icIL-1Ra2 has been cloned from lymphocytes, its 25 kDa protein remains putative.

Several organ systems, which undergo cellular remodelling, appear to have a cycling IL-1 system. For instance, ovulation is characterized by peak levels of IL-1Ra, with both IL-1 and IL-1RI also being expressed in ovarian tissue. Furthermore, for IL-1Ra to downregulate IL-1 activity the former needs to be produced in relative excess due to the so-called spare receptor effect. This phenomenon of unoccupied receptors is observed when agonists with high efficacy (i.e. IL-1) produce maximal responses with activation of relatively few receptors. Thus, the biological response can only be inactivated once all the spare receptors are occupied by a non-competitive antagonist (i.e. IL-1Ra).

Clinically, a high IL-1 : IL-1Ra ratio is observed in several proinflammatory conditions, such as inflammatory bowel disease and rheumatoid arthritis. Similarly, in malignancy an imbalance of IL-1 and IL-1Ra may be present favouring the protumorigenic effects of the former. Studies of patients with CML and acute myeloid leukaemia (AML), for instance, have indicated an inverse relationship between IL-1 levels and the low levels of its endogenous inhibitor, IL-1Ra. Indeed, proliferation of both cell types may be inhibited *in vitro* by the addition of IL-1Ra into the culture medium. A similar anticancer role of IL-1Ra has been observed in B16 melanoma, with a reduction in the size and number of hepatic metastases, but the story changes with respect to several other tumour types. Thus, IL-1Ra is involved in murine hepatic carcinogenesis and supports the metastatic growth of glioblastoma by downregulating an inhibitory autocrine IL-1 loop. The data in ovarian cancer remains unclear with ovarian cancer cell lines spontaneously expressing both IL-1Ra and IL-1. The SNP for allele 2 of IL-1Ra (IL-1RN*2) is linked to a proinflammatory state, with increased IL-1β and/or decreased icIL–1Ra1 production and may be involved in ovarian cancer.

A high serum IL-6 level has proven a robust independent prognostic factor with worse survival in diffuse large cell lymphoma, renal cell, and ovarian carcinoma. A pathogenic role for IL-6 in lymphoma has been derived from several different studies: overexpression of IL-6 is pro-tumorigenic; transfection of IL-6 into Epstein-Barr virus (EBV)-transformed B lymphocytes confers tumorigenicity in nude mice; IL-6 acts as a growth factor for certain lymphoma cell lines; and high IL-6 levels correlate with a greater risk of lymphoma in AIDS and renal transplant patients. Antagonists, whether in the form of endogenous antagonists (e.g. IL-1Ra), soluble receptors, or converting enzyme inhibitors, are currently being evaluated to determine the role of these cytokines in cancer therapy.

14.5.2 Interleukin-10 family

Identification of the IL-10-related cytokines, consisting of IL-19, 20, 22 (IL-10-related T-cell-derived inducible factor, IL-TIF) IL-24 (melanoma differentiation–associated antigen 7, MDA-7), and IL-26 (AK155) has also opened up several new avenues of research (reviewed in Fickenscher et al., 2002). These cytokines have 20–83% sequence identity with IL-10 and are all homodimeric molecules that interact with specific heterodimers of different type-2 cytokine receptors (i.e. IFN receptor and IL-10 receptor family) leading to a diverse array of biological effects via the STAT pathway. Furthermore, a family of viral homologues of IL-10 have been identified, such as EBV IL-10 (BCRF1) and human cytomegalovirus (HCMV) IL-10; these seem to share the same receptor as cellular IL-10. Since IL-10 (produced by Th2 cells, B cells, monocytes, and macrophages) is a known immunomodulatory cytokine, with inhibitory effects on the Th1 response and stimulatory effects on B cells, viral IL-10 may be critical in facilitating autocrine cellular transformation. High levels of viral IL-10, for example, correlate with a poor prognosis in patients with non-Hodgkin's lymphoma (NHL) and chronic lymphocytic leukaemia (CLL). Moreover, IL-10 overexpression stimulates B-cell proliferation and rituximab, an anti-CD20 antibody, abrogates the autocrine/paracrine IL-10 loop, sensitizing malignant B cells to cytotoxic drugs. This effect is achieved via downregulation of STAT3 (and bcl-2), whose activation is IL-10-dependent. Thus, specific IL-10 antagonists raise the possibility of overcoming NHL chemoresistance. Other effects of IL-10 include suppression of Th1 cytokines (IL-2 and IFN-γ) and human T-cell proliferation, enhanced production of IL-1Ra, and downregulation of MHC class-II expression on monocytes. In direct contrast to the IL-10 members discussed so far, IL-24/MDA-7, which was identified from cultured human melanoma cells treated with a differentiation protocol (IFN-β and a PKC activator), resembles a classical tumour suppressor gene (reviewed in Sauane et al., 2003). It can be proapoptotic in tumour cell lines, an effect that is dependent upon caspases and a STAT3 pathway, but independent of p53. Moreover, recent work shows that IL-24 can inhibit endothelial cell differentiation and migration induced by VEGF and bFGF. IFN-γ and IP10 *in vitro*, and intravenous (i.v.) administration of IL-24 in xenograft tumour models reveals a decrease in tumour size with a corresponding reduction in microvessel density and haemoglobin content. Certain IL-24-resistant tumours, such as pancreatic carcinoma, have responded to IL-24 after pretreatment with K-*ras* antisense. Normal cells on the other hand remain resistant to the proapoptotic effects of IL-24, and the basis of this selectivity is unknown. Recent phase-I trials in patients with advanced cancer employing an adenoviral vector expressing IL-24 (Ad. *mda-7*) revealed substantial levels of apoptosis in injected tumours.

14.5.3 Interleukin-2, -12, and -15

IL-12 is an essential cytokine in coordinating the innate and adaptive immune responses (reviewed in Trinchieri, 2003). Released by phagocytes, B cells, and DCs, IL-12 functions in a positive feedback loop via IFN-γ derived from T and NK cells to generate potent immunity. The active form of IL-12 is composed of a heterodimeric glycoprotein (p35, p40) linked by a disulfide bridge, which binds to a heterodimeric receptor (IL-12Rβ1 and IL-12Rβ2) found mainly on activated T and NK cells. The signalling cascade downstream of the IL-12R involves phosphorylation of JAK2 and STAT4 resulting in the production of IFN-γ. Although IFN-γ is a critical mediator of IL-12 activity, it is not the only explanation of its antitumour effect. Furthermore, dissection of the antitumour immune response has demonstrated paradoxically a temporary period of immunosuppression associated with IL-12. This is mediated by a hyperinduction of IFN-γ and a concomitant increase in NO which induces apoptotic deletion of antigen-specific T cells during priming. Administration of IL-12 with a nitric oxide synthase (NOS) inhibitor during vaccination studies with irradiated tumours in mice results in enhanced tumour immunity compared with IL-12 alone.

Additional non-immune (i.e. anti-angiogenic) mechanisms also account for IL-12 antitumour activity. It is now clear that IL-12 induces a cytokine/chemokine cascade involving IFN-γ, CXCL10, and CXCL9, with direct inhibitory effects on the endothelium, with an additional mechanism employing the recruitment of NK and T cells. To date, clinical trials employing IL-12 have confirmed both modest clinical efficacy and significant toxicity (fever/chills, fatigue, nausea, vomiting, headache, mental depression, oral mucositis, anaemia, leukopenia, and elevated liver function tests). Phase I/II studies have demonstrated IL-12 activity in a range of tumours including melanoma, renal cell carcinoma, ovarian carcinoma, mesothelioma, and cutaneous T-cell lymphoma. In view of the toxicity observed with high i.v. proinflammatory doses of IL-12, the field has in recent years shifted towards an adjuvant role for IL-12, using lower immunostimulatory doses via the subcutaneous (s.c.) route.

IL-2 or T-cell growth factor mainly regulates the adaptive immune system, activating T-cell subsets (helper, suppressor, and cytotoxic cells) and promoting B-cell proliferation and differentiation. Deficiencies in the IL-2/IL-2 receptor system are associated with SCID in humans, whereas human T-cell leukaemia virus 1(HTLV1)-associated leukaemia is characterized by an early IL-2-dependent growth phase. However, there is a degree of redundancy in the system (reviewed in Ozaki and Leonard, 2002) at least early on in development, since IL-2$^{-/-}$ mice are essentially normal at birth (see IL-15 below). IL-2R$^{-/-}$ mice on the other hand demonstrate major T-cell abnormalities. More recently, IL-2 has been shown to modulate NK cell and macrophage activity, influence non-immune cells (neuronal and glial cells) and the cytokine network (an inducer of IL-1, TNF-α, and IFN-γ).

Cloned in 1983, the 15 kDa molecule was soon introduced as an immunostimulant in cancer protocols and, despite many years of investigation, clinical use of IL-2 remains restricted to patients with renal cell carcinoma and melanoma. However, the past decade has shed new light on the complex biology of IL-2 paving the way for more sophisticated applications, such as vaccine strategies and expanding antigen-specific T cells *in vitro*. Several forms of the IL-2 receptor have been identified, each with characteristic signalling properties, involving: Src; MAPK cascade, PI-3K, and Akt; and JAK (1/3) and STAT (3/5). These range from a low-affinity receptor (IL-2Rα, K_d 10^{-8}M) which has no downstream signal, to an intermediate (IL-2R, K_d 10^{-9}M) and high-affinity receptor (IL-2R$\alpha\beta\gamma$, K 10^{-11}M). Numerous immune cells express components of the IL-2 receptor including NK cells and CD4+ and CD8+ cells, with different doses of IL-2 impacting on these receptors in a variety of ways. Thus, high dose bolus IL-2 therapy correlating with nanomolar concentrations of IL-2 in the serum, activates several immune cells expressing IL-2R (NK cells, activated T cells, monocyte/macrophages, and activated B cells), simultaneously triggering a generalized proinflammatory state with hypotension and capillary leak syndrome. In contrast, low-dose therapy typical of s.c. or continuous infusion IL-2 regimens, stimulates IL-2R$\alpha\beta\gamma$, avoiding systemic toxicity with picomolar levels, yet producing immunologically relevant antitumour responses (i.e. the selective expansion of NK cells).

Application of high-dose therapy in renal cell cancer and melanoma has produced responses in some 20% of patients with some durable remissions. The low-dose regimens may be equally effective. A recent trial by Yang et al. (2003) in patients with renal cell cancer showed that despite a higher response rate with high-dose i.v. IL-2 (21%) there was no difference in overall survival between low-dose i.v. (13% response rate) or low-dose s.c. IL-2 (10% response rate). Several small phase-III studies in advanced melanoma have recently reported a lack of survival benefit on the question of biochemotherapy compared to biotherapy or chemotherapy alone, and the results from several larger studies are awaited (reviewed in Keilholz and Gore, 2002).

Studies employing IL-2 in combination with tumour-specific antigen from melanoma (e.g. IL-2 and gp100) remains a credible approach but, as with conventional chemotherapy, this may be limited by the emergence of resistant clones (immunological escape). However, several recent studies indicate that tolerance to tumour antigen, in particular, may be amenable to manipulation. Thus, patients with metastatic melanoma, who were pretreated with a non-myeloablative conditioning regimen (cyclophosphamide and fludaribine), responded to adoptive T-cell transfer in combination with high-dose IL-2. Patients with significant tumour regression also exhibited antimelanocyte autoimmunity with the onset of vitiligo and anterior uveitis (Dudley et al., 2002). Additional approaches include the following: combination treatments of low-dose/bolus IL-2 with monoclonal antitumour antibodies seeking to expand antibody-dependent cellular cytotoxicity (ADCC)-effector NK cells (e.g. IL-2 + trastuzumab/rituximab); and cytokine-coupled tumour-specific antibodies.

Finally, IL-15 is a cytokine that displays much of the biology of IL-2 *in vitro*, sharing, for example, the same intermediate affinity receptor, and in recent years has been shown to be an important lymphocyte activator. In particular, it is viewed as a 'second-generation' cytokine with an enhanced ability to promote NK cell differentiation and the survival of memory CD8 + T cells. Devoid of IL-2 properties such as activation-induced cell death (AICD) of T cells, IL-15 may be explored as a potential therapeutic in cancer immunotherapy.

14.6 Colony stimulating factors

Although originally defined as haematopoietic growth factors, the CSFs are now recognized as a family of molecules with diverse properties. Thus, CSFs have roles in the following: stem cell mobilization and the treatment of chemotherapy-induced neutropenia (granulocyte or G-CSF); as immune adjuvants (GM-CSF); and, in contrast, facilitate tumorigenesis by modulating the number of tumour-associated macrophages (macrophage or M-CSF).

14.6.1 Granulocyte-colony-stimulating factor

G-CSF obtained a licence in 1991 for the prevention and treatment of febrile neutropenia secondary to cytotoxic administration. Pegylated versions have recently become available resulting in weekly dosing and more stable pharmacokinetics, with an equivalent reduction in febrile neutropenia (i.e. pegfilgrastim). However, despite the documented benefits of reduced hospitalization, antibiotic use, and neutropenic complications, in general, the use of G-CSF has not translated into an increased overall survival for patients. Hence, current clinical guidelines recommend confining the use of these products to situations in which the expected incidence of febrile neutropenia exceeds 40% (see Dale, 2003 and Lyman, 2003 for reviews). Dose-dense or accelerated chemotherapy, whereby treatment is delivered in a shorter time frame (e.g. a cycle of chemotherapy being delivered every two instead of every three weeks), is dependent upon G-CSF-maintained neutrophil counts, and is a notable exception. Recent studies in patients with early breast cancer have revealed a survival benefit with dose-dense chemotherapy regimens (Citron et al., 2003), and this principle may apply to a range of other tumours currently under study (see also Bohlius et al., 2003).

14.6.2 Granulocyte-macrophage colony-stimulating factor

GM-CSF has gained prominence as an immunomodulatory cytokine, being incorporated into cancer vaccines protocols either in the form of GM-CSF-transduced tumour cells or as a DC maturation factor, along with TNF-α and IL-4 (see Dranoff, 2002 and Villinger, 2003 for reviews). Early vaccination trials using GM-CSF-secreting autologous and allogeneic tumour cells have documented encouraging responses, even in heavily pretreated patients. Simplification of vaccine delivery along with better characterization of immune responses is a prerequisite for effective future development of GM-CSF-based cancer therapies.

14.6.3 Macrophage-colony-stimulating factors

M-CSF (CSF-1) is a haematopoietic growth factor with an important role in macrophage activation, and more recently evidence has accumulated implicating the cytokine in tumorigenesis (reviewed in Kascinski, 2002). For example, levels of CSF-1 and its receptor (CSF-1R, encoded by the *c-fms* proto-oncogene) correlate with tumour cell invasiveness and an adverse prognosis in patients with ovarian carcinoma. The mechanism for enhanced invasiveness involves an increase in urokinase-type plasminogen activator (uPA) activity in tumour cells and macrophages, a feature common to several tumours. CSF-1 also promotes angiogenesis by stimulating VEGF release from monocytes.

The development of novel therapeutics based on modulation of the CSF-1/CSF-1R axis is currently an area of active research. M-CSF has also been studied as an immune adjuvant (mirimostim) in patients with cancer receiving chemotherapy, with reported improvements in several parameters including NK cell activity and the Th1/Th2 balance; however, further studies addressing relapse-free and overall survival are needed.

14.7 Chemokines

The discovery in recent years of a family of small (8–11 kDa) chemoattractant cytokines or chemokines and their respective receptors has provided new insights into several aspects of tumorigenesis. Chemokines were initially characterized as leukocyte trafficking molecules, facilitating, for instance, the homing of a neutrophil to a site of injury (i.e. CXCL8). There are currently about 50 identified ligands (subclassified according to the position of the first two cysteines: C–C, C–X–C, C and C–X_3–C), operating via half as many G-protein-coupled (GPCRs) seven-transmembrane-domain (7TM) receptors. It is now evident that apart from cell recruitment in inflammation, chemokines have additional roles in immunity and several developmental processes including angiogenesis and haematopoiesis (reviewed in Wilson and Balkwill, 2002). Moreover, cancer has usurped many elements of the chemokine system to enhance tumour cell growth, invasion, and metastasis. Indeed, the latter phenomenon, namely the non-random migration of cancer cells and their colonization of distant organs, has been reassessed in light of new data showing that cancer cells express a specific and restricted range of chemokine receptors. Breast cancer, for example, is differentiated into two common patterns of spread: cutaneous/bone and a visceral presentation affecting liver, lung, brain (and bone). CXCL12–CXCR4 chemokine interactions are central to metastasis in a murine model of breast cancer. Signalling through CXCR4 mediated actin polymerization and pseudopodia formation stimulating tumour cell invasion and migration towards a gradient of CXCL12. With high levels of CXCL12 expression in lymph nodes and lungs, CXCR4 antagonism significantly impaired spread to these tissues. This proof of principle indicates that chemokine antagonists may be considered as inhibitors of metastasis (reviewed in Homey et al., 2002). Work in our laboratory has also provided evidence for this chemokine pairing in human ovarian cancer metastasis (Scotton et al., 2001) with other groups implicating CXCL12-CXCR4 in haematological malignancies, glioma, and pancreatic cancer. Table 14.4 summarizes data relating to known chemokine ligand–receptor pairings in cancer metastasis.

Table 14.4 Involvement of chemokine ligand/receptor pairs in cancer

	Chemokine Receptor on tumour cell	Stromal Chemokines	
Breast	CXCR4	CXCL12	Lung and lymph nodes
	CCR7	CCL21	
Ovary	CXCR4	CXCL12	
Prostate	CXCR4	CXCL12	Osteoblasts
Melanoma	CXCR4	CXCL12	Lung, lymph nodes, and bone
	CCR7	CCL21	
	CCR10	CCL27	
Oesophageal	CCR7	CCL21	Lymph nodes
Intraocular	CXCR4	CXCL12	Retinal pigment, epithelium
Lymphoma	CXCR5	BLA1	

The leucocyte infiltrate as indicated in previous sections appears to play a critical role in cancer invasion and dissemination, yet our current understanding of the relationship between the leucocyte and the tumour cell remains at a rudimentary level. Nevertheless, the explosion of knowledge in the chemokine field is redressing the balance and a major effort is now in place to dissect out the leucocyte content of tumours in terms of the prevailing chemokine ligands and receptors.

Ascites formation is a common occurrence in human epithelial ovarian cancer. mRNA and pico to nanomolar levels of protein for CCL2, CCL3, CCL4, CCL5, CCL8 (MCP-2), and CCL22 were found in the cellular and fluid. Ascitic fluid contained variable numbers of tumour cells, macrophages, and CD3+ T lymphocytes that were predominantly CD4+. A direct correlation was found between CCL5 concentration in ascitic fluid and CD3+ T cell infiltrate. Infiltrating leucocytes may not only contribute to tumour progression by producing MMPs and growth, angiogenic, and immunosuppressive factors, but the profile of the cells attracted by chemokines to the tumour may contribute to an immunosuppressive environment. There is often a prevalence of Th2 cells in tumours and this polarization may be a general strategy to subvert immune responses against tumours. Hodgkin's disease, for instance, is characterized by constitutive activation of NFκB and overproduction of Th2 cytokines and chemokines into the tumour, causing an influx of Th2 cells and eosinophils (reviewed in Skinnider and Mak, 2002).

Chronic exposure to high chemokine concentrations in the tumour microenvironment may encourage activated type-II macrophages that release immunosuppressive IL-10 and TGF-β. These macrophages may also release CCL2, which could contribute to a Th2 polarized immunity and stimulate a type-II inflammatory response. Tumours are also known to inhibit DC1 migration and function, thus suppressing any specific immune response.

In ovarian cancer, there is evidence that tumour cell production of CXCL12 weakens immunity by attracting and protecting CXCR4-expressing preDC2 cells, and altering preDC1 distribution, immunity, and stimulation of fibrosis. Another example of a strategy to encourage a Th2 environment in tumours comes from Kaposi's sarcoma. The viral genome encodes three chemokines (vMIPI, II, and III) that are selective attractants for polarized Th2 cells.

Angiogenesis is regulated by two types of chemokines: pro-angiogenic CXC chemokines possess a Glu–Leu–Arg at the immediate amino-end to the CXC motif (ELR+); and chemokines without this triplet (ELR-) are angiostatic. However, CXCL12 (an ELR- chemokine) by upregulating VEGF in a synergistic fashion, is an exception that breaks the rule. CXCL8 (IL-8) release is stimulated by TNF-α, IL-1, acidosis, and hypoxia and in addition to its potent angiogenic effects, has important mitogenic and motogenic properties. IL-8 antagonism is effective in reducing angiogenesis and growth in a range of tumour models including lung, ovarian and prostate cancer, and melanoma. ELR- chemokines with angiostatic properties include CXCL9 in Burkitt's lymphoma (BL) and CXCL10 in BL and lung carcinoma; CCL21 also inhibited the latter in SCID mice.

Finally, deregulated chemokines may contribute directly to transformation of tumour cells by acting as growth and survival factors, generally in an autocrine manner. This action of chemokines has been extensively characterized in malignant melanoma. CXCL1 and CXCL8 are constitutively produced by melanoma cells, but not by untransformed melanocytes. Melanoma cells also show elevated levels of the CXCR2 receptor for these chemokines, and autocrine chemokine stimulation enhances survival, proliferation, and tumour cell migration. In addition, CXCL8, CXCL1, as well as the CC chemokine CCL20, all stimulate growth of pancreatic tumour cell lines.

In epithelial ovarian cancer, tumour cells express CXCR4 and its ligand CXCL12 enhances tumour cell proliferation in conditions of suboptimal growth. This autocrine chemokine stimulation may also have paracrine implications because CXCL12 stimulated the production of TNF-α by ovarian tumour cells. Production of TNF-α in the tumour microenvironment has been implicated in tumour progression. The ability of tumour cells to proliferate in response to chemokines appears to have been exploited by the human Kaposi's sarcoma herpes virus, KSHV. The KSHV genome encodes a GPCR that signals constitutively and is structurally similar to CXCR2. Expression of this receptor is associated with cellular transformation. Cells transfected with a constitutively signalling mutated CXCR2 are similarly transformed. Transgenic mice overexpressing the KSHV-GPCR under the control of the CD2 promoter develop lesions with remarkable similarity to Kaposi's sarcoma.

To conclude, the importance of understanding the function of the chemokine network within a given tumour is underscored by recent experiments manipulating the levels of chemokines to induce tumour rejection. Thus, CCL20 (MIP-3α) overexpression in a transplantable murine tumour induced a DC-rich tumour infiltrate activating CTLs to suppress tumour growth; CCL19 (MIP-3β) and CCL21 (6Ckine) triggered NK and CD4+ T cell antitumour activity in a murine breast and colon cancer model, respectively; and CXCL10 reduced tumour growth via a thymus-dependent pathway.

14.8 Summary and conclusions

Cancer as a biological process is intricately linked to a deregulated cytokine network with inflammation directing many aspects of tumour promotion and stromal reorganization. The current emphasis on microarray and RNA interference technology should enable the characterization of pathways central to cytokine cancer biology and their modulation will provide novel therapeutic opportunities. The complexity of the tumour microenvironment will necessitate the use of both cytokines and their antagonists at different stages

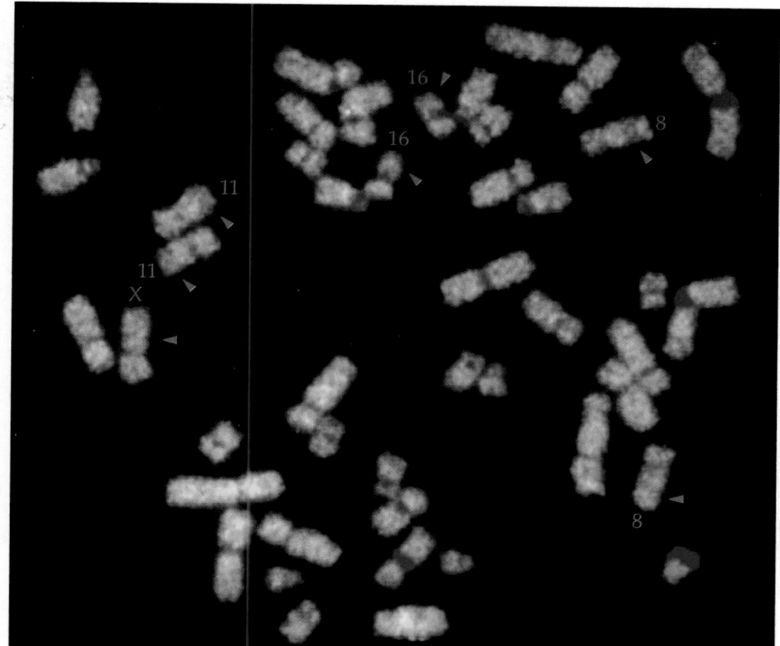

Plate 1 Comparative genomic hybridization experiment to determine genomic copy number changes in a primitive neuroectodermal tumour from a two-year old boy. Tumour and female control DNA were labelled with fluorescein isothiocyanate (FITC) and Texas red, respectively. Regions of deletion are visualized in red (arrowed). The X-chromosome acts as an internal control as it appears red when male DNA (green) and female DNA (red) are co-hybridized to male metaphase chromosomes.

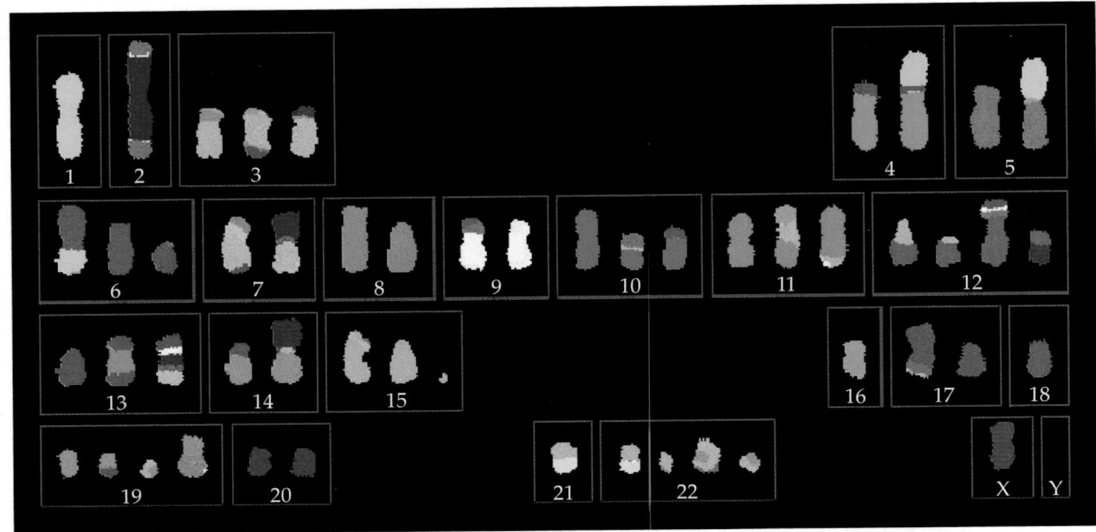

Plate 2 Spectral karyotype (SKY) from breast carcinoma cell line showing multiple chromosome rearrangements (Courtesy: Mira Grigorova and Paul Edwards).

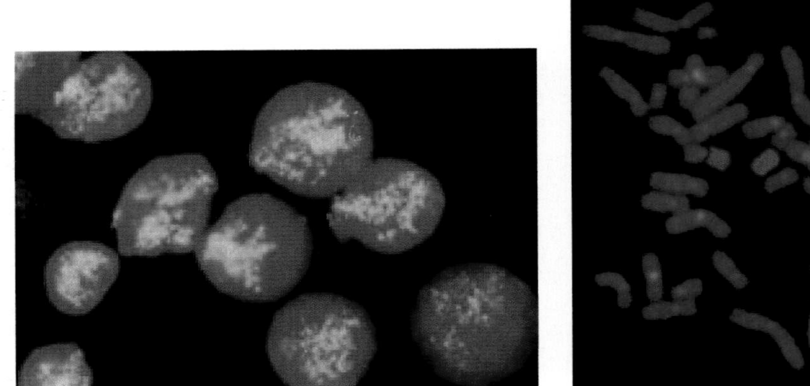

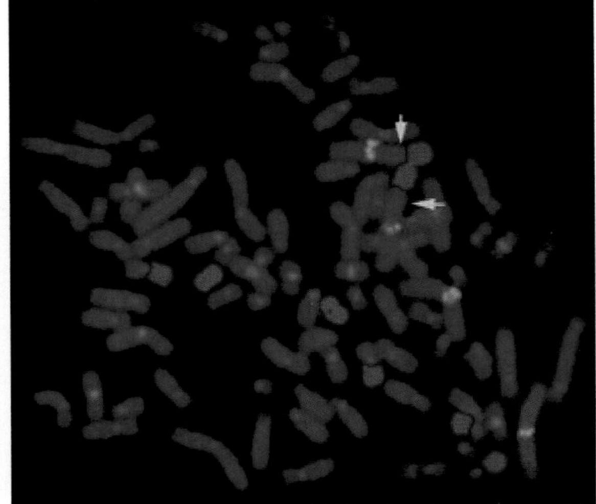

Plate 3 Detection by fluorescence *in situ* hybridization (FISH) of prognostic markers in neuroblastoma. Left: Interphase FISH on nuclei showing multiple copies of *MYCN* labelled yellow. Right: Metaphase spread from neuroblastoma cell line with deleted 1p (arrowed), and additional copies of 17q labelled red. Centromeres of chromosome 1 are labelled green.

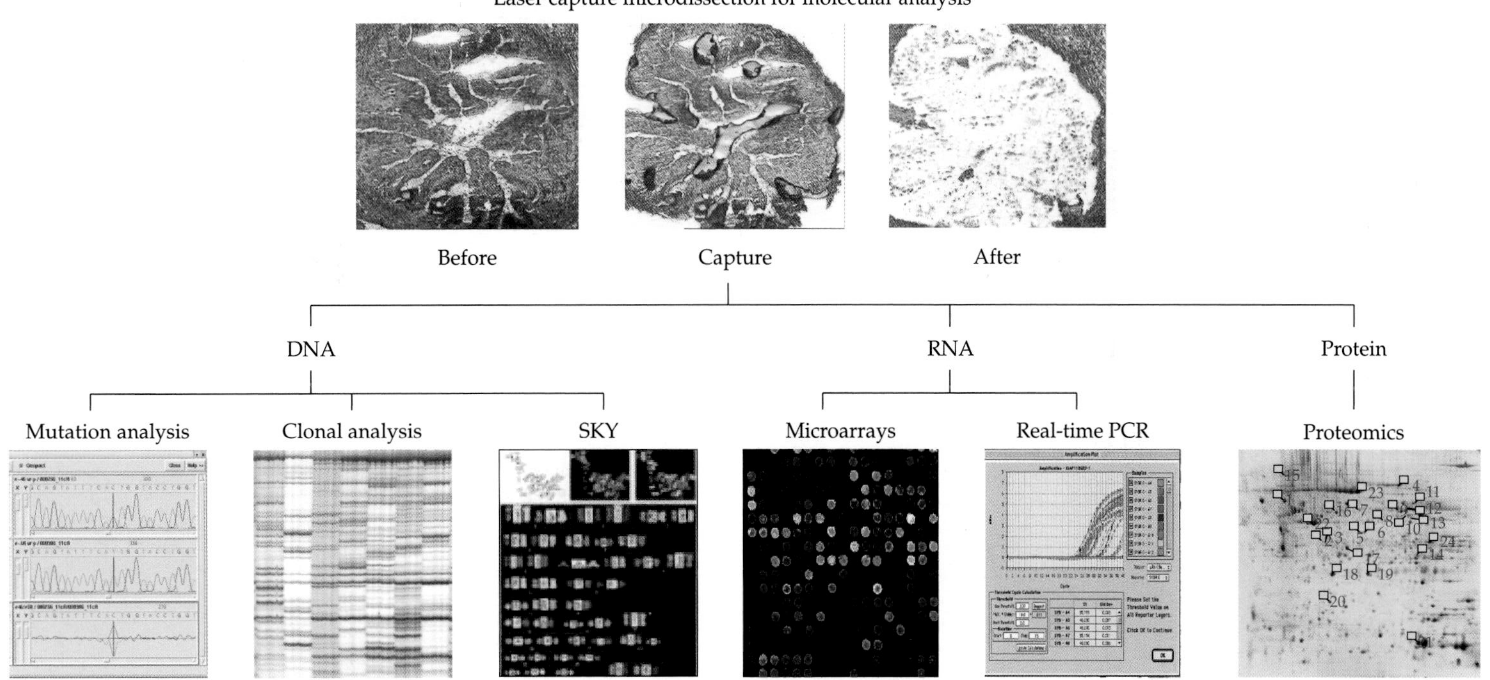

Plate 4 Illustration of laser capture microdissection and the utility of subsequently isolated material in molecular analysis.

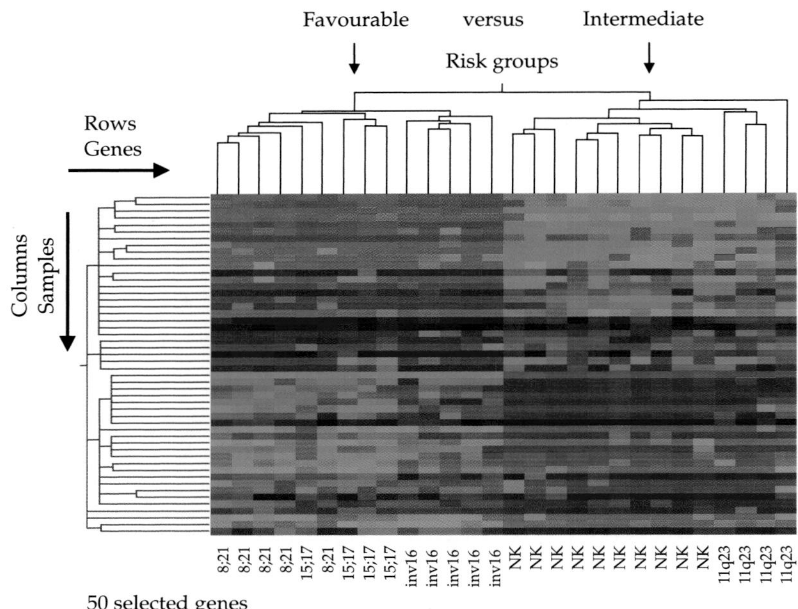

Plate 5 Cytogenetic risk groups in AML: favourable versus intermediate risk groups hierarchical cluster of the 50 genes selected to be the more predictive in the two class comparison performed. Each column represents a sample, and each row represents a single gene. Expression levels are normalized for each gene, where the mean is 1. Expression levels greater than the mean are shown in red and levels less than the mean are in green.

of cancer progression. Integration with conventional therapies and vaccines will provide yet further challenges.

References

Ardestani, S. K., Inserra, P., Solkoff, D., and Watson, R. R. (1999). The role of cytokines and chemokines on tumour progression: a review. *Cancer Detect Prevent*, **23**, 215–25.

Arend, W. P. (2002). The balance between IL-1 and IL-1Ra in disease. *Cytokine Growth Factor Rev*, **13**, 323–40.

Balkwill, F. R. and Mantovani A. (2001). Inflammation and cancer: back to Virchow? *Lancet*, **357**, 539–45.

Bogenrieder, T. and Herlyn, M. (2003). Axis of evil: molecular mechanisms of cancer metastasis. *Oncogene*, **22**, 6524–36.

Bohlius, J., Reiser M., Schwarzer G., and Engert A. (2003). Impact of granulocyte colony-stimulating factor (CSF) and granulocyte-macrophage CSF in patients with malignant lymphoma: a systematic review. *Br J Haematol*, **122**, 413–23.

Brown, J. R. and Demetri, G. D. (2002). Challenges in the development of platelet growth factors: low expectations for low counts. *Curr Hematol Rep*, **1**, 110–8.

Citron, M. L., Berry, D. A, Cirrincione C., Hudis, C., Winer, E. P., Gradishar, W. J. et al. (2003). Randomized trial of dose-dense versus conventionally scheduled and sequential versus concurrent combination chemotherapy as postoperative adjuvant treatment of node-positive primary breast cancer: first report of intergroup trial C9741/cancer and leukaemia group B trial 9741. *J Clin Oncol*, **21**,1431–9.

Coussens, L. M. and Werb, Z. (2002). Inflammation and cancer. *Nature*, **420**, 860–7.

Dale, D. (2003). Current management of chemotherapy-induced neutropenia: the role of colony stimulating factors. *Semin Oncol*, **30**, 3–9.

Dranoff, G. (2002). GM-CSF-based cancer vaccines. *Immunol Rev*, **188**, 147–54.

Dranoff, G. (2004). Cytokines in cancer pathogenesis and cancer therapy. *Nat Rev Cancer*, **4**, 11–22.

Dudley, M. E., Wunderlich, J. R., Robbins, P. F., Yang J. C., Hwu, P., Schwartzentruber, D. J. et al. (2002). Cancer regression and autoimmunity in patients after clonal repopulation with antitumor lymphocytes. *Science*, **298**, 850–4.

Dunn, G. P., Bruce, A. T, Ikeda, H., Old, L. J., and Schreiber, R. D. (2002). Cancer immunoediting: from immunosurveillance to tumor escape. *Nat Immunol*, **11**, 991–8.

Fickenscher, H., Hör, S., Küpers, Knappe, A., Wittmann, S., and Sticht, H. (2002). The interleukin-10 family of cytokines. *Trends Immunol*, **23**, 89–96.

Hanahan, D. and Weinberg, R. A. (2000). The hallmarks of cancer. *Cell*, **100**, 57–70.

Homey, B., Müller, A., and Zlotnik, A. (2002). Chemokines: agents for the immunotherapy of cancer? *Nat Rev Immunol*, **2**, 175–84.

Kascinski, B. (2002). Expression of CSF-1 and its receptor CSF-1R in non-hematopoietic neoplasms. *Cancer Treat Res*, **107**, 285–92.

Keilholz, U. and Gore, ME., (2002). Biochemotherapy for advanced melanoma. *Semin Oncol*, **29**, 456–61.

Kitakata, H., Nemoto-Sasaki, Y., Takahashi Y., Kondo, T., Mai, M., and Mukaida, N. (2002). Essential roles of tumor necrosis factor receptor p55 in liver metastasis of intrasplenic administration of colon 26 cells. *Cancer Res*, **62**, 6682–7.

Kurzrock, R. (2001). Cytokine deregulation in cancer. *Biomed Pharmacother*, **55**, 543–7.

Lukacher, A. E. (2002). IFN-γ suspends the killing licence of antitumor CTLs. *J Clin Invest*, **110**, 1407–9.

Lyman, G. H. (2003). Balancing the benefits and costs of colony stimulating factors: a current perspective. *Semin Oncol*, **30**, 10–17.

Micheau, O., and Tschopp, J., (2003). Induction of TNF receptor I-mediated apoptosis via two sequential signaling complexes. *Cell*, **114**, 181–90.

Mocellin, S., Wang, E., and Marincola, F. M. (2001). Cytokines and immune response in the tumor microenvironment. *J Immunotherapy*, **24**, 392–407.

Moore, R. J., Owens, D. M, Stamp, G., Arnott, C., Burke, F., East, N. et al. (1999). Mice deficient in tumor necrosis factor-alpha are resistant to skin carcinogenesis. *Nat Med*, **5**, 828–31.

Nabors, L. B., Suswam, E., Huang, Y., Yang, X., Johnson, M. J., and King, P. H. (2003). Tumor necrosis factor α induces angiogenic factor upregulation in malignant glioma cells: a role for RNA stabilization and HuR. *Cancer Res*, **63**, 4181–7.

O'Byrne, K. J., Dalgleish, A. G., Browning, M. J., Steward, W. P., and Harris, A. L. (2000). The relationship between angiogenesis and the immune response in carcinogenesis and the progression of malignant disease. *Eur J Cancer*, **36**, 151–69.

Ozaki, K. and Leonard, W. J. (2002). Cytokine and cytokine receptor pleiotropy and redundancy. *J Biol Chem*, **277**, 29355–8.

Pujade-Lauraine, E., Guastalla, J. P., Colombo, N., Devillier, P., Francois, E., Fumoleau, P. et al. (1996). Intraperitoneal recombinant interferon γ in ovarian cancer patients with residual disease at second-look laparotomy. *J Clin Oncol*, **14**, 343–50.

Roodman, G. D. (2003). Role of stromal-derived cytokines and growth factors in bone metastasis. *Cancer*, **97**, 733–8.

Sauane, M., Gopalkrishnan, R. V., Lebedeva, I., Mei, M. X., Sarkar, D., Su, Z. Z. et al. (2003). MDA-7/IL-24: a novel cancer growth suppressing and apoptosis inducing cytokine. *Cytokine Growth Factor Rev*, **14**, 35–51.

Scotton, C. J., Wilson, J.L., Milliken, D., Stamp, G., and Balkwill, F. R. (2001). Epithelial cancer cell migration: a role for chemokine recptors? *Cancer Res*, **61**, 4961–5.

Skinnider, B. F. and Mak, T. W. (2002). The role of cytokines in classical Hodgkin lymphoma. *Blood*, **99**, 4283–97.

Sporn, M. B. and Vilcek, J. T. (2002). Cytokines in tumor immunity and immunotherapy. *Cytokine Growth Factor Rev*, **13**, 93–193.

Szlosarek, P. W., and Balkwill, F. R. (2003). Tumour necrosis factor-α: a potential target for the therapy of solid tumours. *Lancet Oncol*, **4**, 565–73.

Szlosarek, P. W., and Dalgleish, A. G. (2002). Anticancer mechanisms involving the immune system. In *The Psychoimmunology of Cancer*. (Eds C. E. Lewis, R. M. O'Brien, and J. Barraclough) Oxford University Press, Oxford, pp. 100–45.

Trinchieri, G. (2003). Interleukin-12 and the regulation of innate resistance and adaptive immunity. *Nat Rev Immunol*, **3**, 133–46.

Tsimberidou, A. M. and Giles, F. J. (2002). TNF-α targeted therapeutic approaches in patients with hematologic malignancies. *Expert Rev Anticancer Ther*, **2**, 277–86.

Villinger, F. (2003). Cytokines as clinical adjuvants: how far are we ? *Expert Rev Vaccines*, **2**, 317–26.

Wall, L., Burke, F., Barton, C., Smyth, J., and Balkwill, F. (2003). IFN-γ induces apoptosis in ovarian cancer cells *in vivo* and *in vitro*. *Clin Cancer Res*, **9**, 2487–96.

Wheatley, K., Ives, N., Hancock, B., Gore, M., Eggermont, A., and Suciu, S. (2003). Does adjuvant interferon-α for high risk melanoma provide a worthwhile benefit? A meta-analysis of the randomised trials. *Cancer Treatment Rev*, **29**, 241–52.

Wilson, J. and Balkwill, F. (2002). The role of cytokines in the epithelial cancer microenvironment. *Semin Cancer Biol*, **12**, 113–20.

Windbichler, G. H., Hausmaninger, H., Stummvoll, W., Graf, A. H. , Kainz, C., Lahodny, J. et al. (2000). Interferon-γ in the first line therapy of ovarian cancer: a randomized phase III trial. *Br J Cancer* **82**, 1138–44.

Xie, K. (2001). Interleukin-8 and cancer biology. *Cytokine Growth Factor Rev*, **12**, 375–91

Yang, J. C., Sherry, R. M., Steinberg, S. M., Topalian, S. L., Schwartzentruber ,D. J., Hwu, P., et al. (2003). Randomized study of high-dose and low-dose interleukin-2 in patients with metastatic renal cancer. *J Clin Oncol*, **21**, 3127–32.

Younes, A. and Kadin, M. E. (2003). Emerging applications of the tumor necrosis factor family of ligands and receptors in cancer therapy. *J Clin Oncol*, **21**, 3526–34.

CHAPTER 15

Hormones and cancer

Charlotte L. Bevan

15.1 Introduction

Hormone-dependent cancer is increasingly a major concern. In the United Kingdom, breast and prostate cancer are the commonest cancer and the second leading cause of cancer death in women and men respectively, and their incidence is increasing (Cancer Research UK, 2003). They are also both tumours which arise in hormone-responsive tissues and which themselves require steroid hormones for growth, at least in the initial stages. Thus, the study of hormone action in cancer is of utmost importance.

The fact that these tumours depend on hormones also means that manipulation of the hormonal environment should allow control of tumour growth. The first documented use of hormone therapy for cancer was towards the end of the nineteenth century, when Beatson reported regression of breast cancer in some patients after ovariectomy, and Rann and White also noted remission in prostate cancer patients after castration. In both cases, removal of gonads removed the primary source of sex steroids—oestrogens in the breast cancer patients, androgens in the prostate cancer patients—which were causing the tumour to grow. Gonadectomy is still a primary treatment for such tumours today, although it is likely to be chemical rather than surgical. In this chapter, we will consider the action of hormones and their role in carcinogenesis and cancer progression, but also their role in cancer therapy. Much of the discussion will focus on breast and prostate cancer as these together make up 24% of newly diagnosed cancers each year in the United Kingdom, as well as being the best characterized hormone-dependent cancers.

15.2 Endocrinology

15.2.1 Types of hormone action

The classical definition of a hormone is a substance secreted by one organ (an endocrine gland) that increases the activity of distant organs. This is still a useful definition for endocrine effects of hormones—where hormones secreted by an endocrine gland are carried by the blood to distant target organs, for instance testicular androgens act on the hair follicles to promote beard growth. However, we should also consider paracrine and autocrine effects of hormones. Paracrine effects, where hormones produced by one organ act on adjacent tissue directly, are seen for example during Wolffian duct development when testicular androgens are taken up by the adjacent Wolffian duct by pinocytosis and cause its differentiation into seminal vesicles. Autocrine effects are less well characterized during normal development but may have a role in cancer progression. They occur when a cell or tissue is acted upon by hormones it has secreted, and in cancer this could cause auto-induced growth of malignant cells. The term 'intracrine' has been used to describe the action of hormones within the cells in which they are synthesized, without secretion. For instance breast, endometrial, and ovarian cancers may convert androgens to oestrogens which then act in an intracrine manner.

15.2.2 Hormones involved in carcinogenesis

This chapter will consider the action of several steroid hormones and peptide hormones in cancer. There are also many other signalling molecules with hormone-like effects, such as growth factors and cytokines, which are discussed elsewhere (Chapters 11 and 14).

Steroid hormones and related hydrophilic ligands
Steroid hormones, which are synthesized from cholesterol and share the same characteristic 4-ring structure, are lipid-soluble and so are able to enter cells via passive diffusion. They are produced in specific steroidogenic organs—the gonads and adrenal glands. This class of hormones includes mineralocorticoids, glucocorticoids, progestins, oestrogens, and androgens. Only the latter two appear to be involved in carcinogenesis as they are strongly mitogenic in several organs, while glucocorticoids and progestins generally inhibit mitosis and so are potential anti-cancer agents. Synthesis often involves conversion of one steroid to another, for instance the major gonadal androgen, testosterone, can be converted to the more potent androgen 5α-dihydrotestosterone (DHT) by the action of the enzyme 5α-reductase and this occurs in the androgen target tissue, such as prostate (Figure 15.1). It can also be converted to 17β-oestradiol (E2), the most abundant circulating form of oestrogen, by the action of aromatase. This occurs in adipose tissue and in the ovaries and is one major route of E2 synthesis in males and females (Johnson and Everitt, 1995). Steroid hormone receptors, the androgen receptor (AR), progesterone receptor (PR), glucocorticoid receptor (GR), mineralocorticoid receptor (MR), and oestrogen receptor (ER), form a subfamily of the nuclear hormone receptor superfamily. This consists of 48 currently characterized proteins, all transcription factors and many of them, like the steroid receptors, ligand-activated (Tsai and O'Malley, 1994; Escriva et al., 2000). Nuclear receptors consist of a central DNA-binding domain (DBD), which shows high amino acid conservation between all members and especially between steroid receptors, a moderately conserved ligand-binding domain (LBD) at the C-terminal end, and an N-terminal domain that is divergent and often houses activation functions and protein–protein interaction domains (Figure 15.2). These receptors are discussed in detail in Section 15.4. The thyroid-secreted hormones thyroxine (T4) and triiodothyroxine (T3) are not structurally

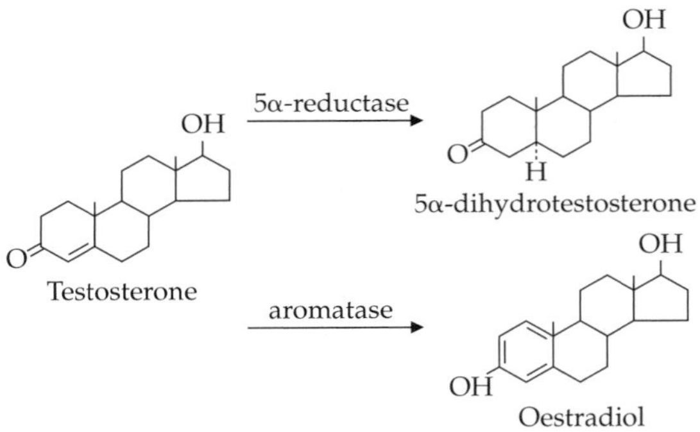

Figure 15.1 Interconversion of steroid hormones. Steroid hormones share a characteristic carbon ring structure (3 benzene rings and a pentane ring), exemplified here by testosterone. Testosterone can be converted to DHT, a more potent androgen with a higher binding affinity for the AR, in androgen target tissues by the action of 5α-reductase. Testosterone is also converted to 17β-oestradiol (E2) in the ovaries and peripheral tissues by the enzyme aromatase.

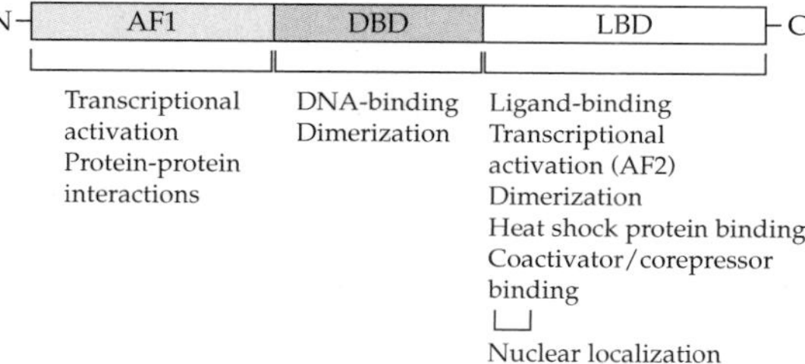

Figure 15.2 Nuclear receptor functional domains. The N-terminus is the most variable domain and generally contains an activation function, AF1, which is inhibited in the absence of ligand by the LBD. The highly conserved DBD contains 2 zinc-finger-like structures that interact with DNA, and is also important for dimerization. LBD interacts with ligand and with other proteins, including cofactors. It contains a ligand-dependent activation function, AF2. Between the DBD and LBD is a charged conserved sequence required for nuclear localization.

similar to steroid hormones, but have highly related nuclear receptors. These hormones affect many target tissues, influencing cell metabolism and growth widely as evidenced by mental and physical retardation in individuals with a deficiency in these hormones. Another substance (not strictly a hormone at all) that has a receptor of the same family is retinoic acid, a derivative of vitamin A. This does not promote tumour growth but does induce differentiation in many tissues and will be discussed in terms of therapy. The thyroid hormone receptor (THR) and retinoic acid receptor (RAR) belong to a different subfamily of nuclear receptors than steroid receptors, termed type I nuclear receptors. There are 3 THR isoforms ($\alpha1$, $\alpha2$ and β) generated by alternate splicing. The RAR, which binds *all-trans* retinoic acid and RXR, which binds *9-cis* retinoic acid, are each transcribed from 3 genes generating forms α, β, and γ, which then undergo differential splicing to generate further isoforms, differing in the N-terminal region. Until recently it was believed that there was only one gene for each steroid receptor, until a second form of ER was discovered. This was termed ERβ and differs from the previously identified receptor (now renamed ERα) in the N-terminus. Although this may have a role in breast and prostate cancer, its physiological role is only just becoming characterized, and in this review 'ER' will refer to the ERα form unless otherwise stated.

Peptide hormones

The other class of hormones is peptide or protein hormones and several of these are also implicated in cancer or its treatment, either in their own right or due to their roles in control of steroid production (see later). Since many tumours also aberrantly produce peptide hormones they are also used as diagnostic markers of particular types of tumours.

The hypothalamus secretes the small peptide hormones gonadotrophin-releasing hormone (GnRH) and TSH-releasing hormone (TRH). GnRH consists of only 10 amino acids and alterations in the N-terminal residues can be used to engineer antagonists or superactive forms.

The gonadotrophins, follicle-stimulating hormone (FSH) and luteinising hormone (LH), which control sex steroid production and the related thyroid-stimulating hormone (TSH) are glycoprotein hormones produced by the pituitary gland. They consist of two glycosylated polypeptides one of which, the alpha chain, is common to all, while the beta chain is unique for each and confers specific activity. The stability of these hormones is controlled by oligosaccharide side-arm structures on each polypeptide.

The anterior pituitary also secretes two other peptide hormones that may be influential in cancer: somatotropin and prolactin. Somatotropin may have a general role in carcinogenesis since it promotes the growth and division of many cell types. Prolactin, a single-chain polypeptide hormone, was originally identified as an inducer of lactation. It promotes cellular growth as well as differentiation in the breast and prostate, and its receptor is expressed in 80–90% of breast cancers. However, it can also be classified as a local growth factor or cytokine and its role in cancer may reflect these types of action, with locally produced rather than pituitary-produced prolactin being important in breast and prostate growth and function (Ben-Jonathan et al., 2002).

The majority of peptide hormones are not able to pass through the cell membrane and signal via membrane-bound receptors on the surface of target cells that share many of the characteristics of growth factor and cytokine receptors, discussed in Chapter 11. These respond to external stimuli by activating second messenger pathways, inside the cell. This cascade can efficiently amplify the initial signal so that a very few molecules of peptide hormone can have a strong effect in the cell. For instance, receptors for gonadotrophins and GnRH are G protein-coupled, 7-span transmembrane proteins that exert their effects mainly via cyclic AMP and phospholipase C signalling pathways, respectively. Paradoxically, overstimulation of the GnRH receptor with continuous high doses of agonists or 'superactive' analogues leads to downregulation of the receptor protein and loss of sensitivity, and this is exploited in chemical methods of gonadectomy.

15.2.3 Control of hormone production

The endocrine glands under consideration here include the gonads—the ovaries and testes—which secrete E2 and testosterone; the thyroid, which secretes thyroxine; and the adrenal gland, which secretes glucocorticoids and also testosterone and other weaker androgens. The secreted hormones are carried by the bloodstream to their distant sites of action, the hormone-responsive tissues. This hormone production (summarized in Figure 15.3) is under the control of the pituitary gland, which communicates with the endocrine glands by means of peptide hormones known as trophins, each secreted by specialized cells in the anterior pituitary. The gonadotrophins trigger steroid secretion from the ovary and testis while ACTH (adrenocorticotrophic hormone) prompts their secretion from adrenal glands. TSH signals the thyroid gland to secrete thyroxine. The secretion of these trophins by the anterior pituitary into the bloodstream is controlled, in turn, by the hypothalamus. Neuroendocrine cells in the hypothalamus secrete peptide hormones: GnRH triggers LH and FSH production, TRH prompts secretion of TSH and corticotrophin-releasing hormone (CRH) targets different cells to release ACTH. In this case the effect of the releasing hormones could be described as paracrine, since they are released from the hypothalamus directly into veins that drain into the anterior pituitary. Finally, feedback at each step of the pathway regulates hormone production. For instance, the hypothalamus and anterior pituitary, which both contain AR, respond to high levels of testosterone in the blood by downregulating GnRH and LH production, respectively, thus preventing excess circulating testosterone. Feedback by E2 is more complex: E2 initially downregulates LH and FSH but after 2–3 days it upregulates LH production, as well as enhancing the responsiveness of the GnRH receptor, in synergy with progesterone (Marshall, 2001). This biphasic feedback presumably reflects and regulates the variations in these hormones associated with the menstrual cycle.

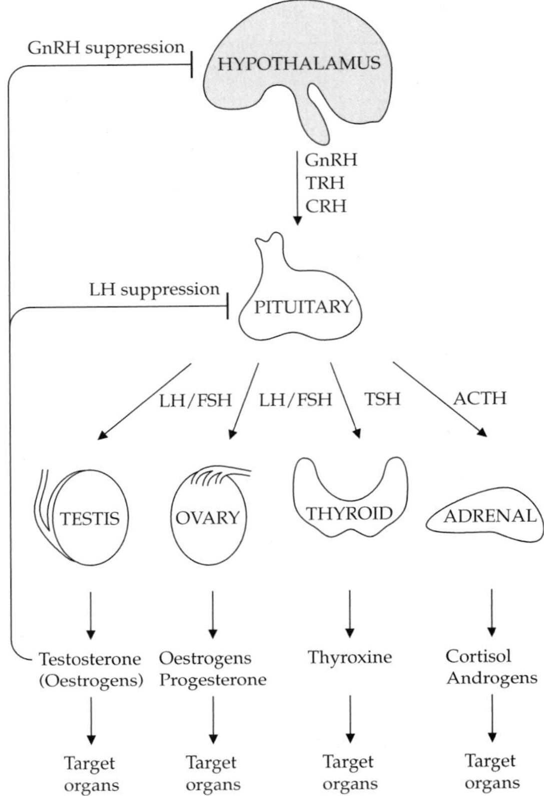

Figure 15.3 Control of hormone secretion by the hypothalamic-pituitary axis. The hypothalamus controls pituitary secretion of gonadotrophins, TSH and ACTH, which in turn control production of steroid hormones and thyroxine from the endocrine glands. Feedback loops operate to prevent excess production, for instance as shown here high levels of testosterone prevent further GnRH and LH release. For abbreviations see text.

Another level of control is provided by the fact that the majority (97–99%) of sex steroids in the blood are bound to sex hormone binding globulin (SHBG). The ratio of free to bound steroid is critical in determining effective steroid concentrations since SHBG-bound steroids may not be available to freely enter the target tissues, although a role for SHBG in promoting membrane transport has been postulated (Selby, 1990).

15.2.4 Hormone-responsive tissues and tumours

Target tissues of androgens and oestrogens include the internal and external genitalia, bone, brain, cardiovascular system, and tissues displaying secondary sexual characteristics, such as hair follicles. Steroid action on these target organs can result in mitosis and growth or differentiation, and it is sometimes difficult to determine which effects are due to androgens and which to oestrogens. For instance in bone, the pubertal growth spurt occurs in response to adrenarche (the pubertal rise in androgen levels) in both males and females thus androgens were believed to be the major hormone for bone growth. It is now thought that it is actually oestrogen (once thought to be a bone growth inhibitor), derived from aromatization of testosterone, that drives this growth. Oestrogens then ultimately drive fusion of the end plates and cessation of growth as well as maintenance of bone density. This was illustrated most dramatically in a man with no functional ERα, who due to incomplete closure of the epiphyses kept growing after puberty to reach a height of over 2 m and was found to have decreased bone density (Smith et al., 1994). Testosterone also has a role in bone since androgen insensitive patients, with no functional AR, also have decreased bone density. It seems intuitive that, at least in tissues showing sexual differentiation, androgens and oestrogens would have opposing effects and this also seems to occur—for instance in breast, which atrophies in females taking exogenous androgens.

The two target tissues that are most prone to malignancy, breast and prostate, are exocrine glands (Figure 15.4). These consist of ducts lined by luminal epithelial cells, which secrete substances into the lumen of the gland for dispersal outside the body—components of the seminal fluid in the case of the prostate, milk in the case of the breast. The luminal cell layer is surrounded by a second layer of epithelial cells, known as basal epithelial or myoepithelial cells, which contact the basement membrane. The ducts are then surrounded by a mixture of stromal cells (mainly smooth muscle cells in the prostate), blood vessels, neuroendocrine cells and, in the breast, adipose tissue. The gland—prostate or mammary—consists of many such ducts, which form a branching network eventually joining together to exit the body via the urethra or the nipple respectively. Over 90% of breast, and prostate cancers are adenocarcinomas arising in the luminal epithelial cells, and histological examination reveals that the basal epithelial cell layer is absent in most tumours.

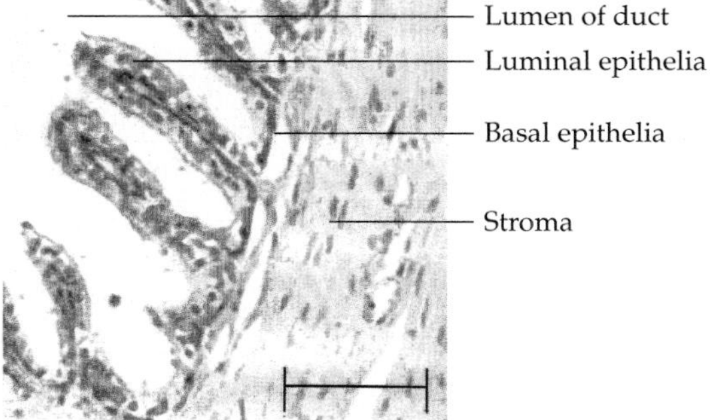

Figure 15.4 A prostatic duct. Cuboidal, luminal epithelial cells line the lumen of the duct and are surrounded by a layer of flatter basal epithelial cells. Mammary gland ducts show similar cellular arrangements. Cells have been stained to visualize the nuclei. Bar represents 100 μm.

Rudimentary prostate and mammary glands are formed in response to hormones during foetal development, and remain unchanged until the rise in hormones at puberty, when they again undergo cell division and grow to mature size. In the case of the prostate, although high levels of testosterone are maintained, the prostate ceases growth and instead requires androgens to become differentiated and begin secretory function. The breast, however, undergoes growth and subsequent involution during each menstrual cycle, in response to the fluctuating levels of E2 and progesterone. It is the luminal epithelial cells that divide in response to steroid hormones but this growth is probably not a direct response. During growth of the prostate, the epithelial cells do not express AR protein. The stromal cells do, and it is likely that they respond to the androgen signal by secreting paracrine factors causing proliferation of the epithelial cells (Thompson, 2001). In the mature prostate, epithelial cells themselves express AR, which is believed to mediate the secretory response. In the breast, only 15–25% of epithelial cells express ER but this fraction is largely non-dividing and it is the ER-negative cells surrounding them that divide in response to oestrogens. Again, this is believed to be due to paracrine secreted factors from the ER-positive cells. Candidates for the paracrine factors responsible include members of the fibroblast growth factor family. However, in both breast and prostate, when malignant growth occurs in receptor-positive epithelial cells, it appears to be directly regulated by the steroid hormone and so the patterns of hormone-responsive growth are different from those seen in normal tissue.

The endometrium of the uterus is another hormone-responsive tissue prone to cancer. The pre-malignant stages of hyperplasia, preneoplasia, and the neoplastic phase itself are all promoted by oestrogens and opposed by progestins. Thus oral contraceptives or hormone replacement therapy containing high doses of oestrogens are associated with a slight increase in uterine cancer risk, while high-dose, long-term progestin therapy appears to be protective.

15.2.5 Hormone-producing tumours

Tumours in hormone-producing organs are likely to disrupt hormone production and, while impairment of hormone production is a possibility, since tumours involve hyperproliferation they often result in excess hormone production which may cause problematic symptoms. For example, Cushing's syndrome results from overexposure to cortisol and includes obesity, hirsutism, weakened bones and decreased fertility. More helpfully, the 'signature' of hormones produced by a particular type of tumour can be used in diagnosis.

The adrenal cortex produces glucocorticoids, mineralocorticoids, androgens, and oestrogens, and tumours in this area are usually benign adenomas, treated by adrenalectomy. Carcinomas are rare and are usually fatal because of metastasis to vital organs rather than hormonal disturbance. That said, overproduction of mineralocorticoids and glucocorticoids from adrenal tumours can result in hypertension and Cushing's syndrome. Adrenal adenomas are more common in women and the associated overproduction of androgens can lead to extensive virilization, including hirsutism. This hyperandrogenic phenotype is also observed with ovarian tumours, which can produce androgens as well as oestrogens when the tumour arises in the stromal sex cord cells that normally produce steroids. However, the frequency of these is rare since most ovarian tumours arise in the surface epithelium or germ cells (Keeney, 2001). This is also the case in testicular cancer—tumours rarely arise in the steroid-secreting interstitial and Sertoli cells, but when they do an increase in androgens or oestrogens may result. Excess oestrogen production in males leads to feminization including gynaecomastia.

Peptide hormone production can also be affected by tumours. The production of ACTH, TSH, LH and FSH by the pituitary can be affected by pituitary tumours, with knock-on consequences for cortisol, sex steroid and thyroxine production. Pituitary adenomas are the most common cause of Cushing's syndrome due to increased ACTH production driving high cortisol levels. Cushing's syndrome can also be caused by ectopic secretion of ACTH by some types of gonadal tumours. Thyroid tumours (one cause of which is constitutively activating mutations in the TSH receptor) alter thyroxine levels, with increased production as a consequence of constitutive activation of malignant cells or increased malignant tissue mass. Ectopic hormone production may involve the secretion of an altered spectrum of hormones, such as germ cell tumours in the gonads secreting gonadotrophins. Even organs that do not normally secrete hormones may acquire the ability to do so ectopically when malignantly transformed. For instance, some small-cell lung cancers acquire the ability to secrete ACTH and so can lead to Cushing's syndrome (Terzolo et al., 2001).

15.3 The role of hormones in carcinogenesis

Steroid hormones are powerful mitogens and appear to affect the rate of mitosis by acting in the G1 phase of the cell cycle—shortening G1 length and promoting entry into S phase. It is to be expected then that steroid target genes include those involved in regulation of the G1 phase or those controlling entry into S phase. The gene targets of steroid hormones are not well characterized currently, but those that are known include several potential cell-cycle control genes, for instance D-type cyclins promote S-phase entry and are upregulated by E2. This mitotic action could have two roles in carcinogenesis, both of which are likely to be important. First, by increasing the number of dividing cells in target organs that can be at risk from carcinogens, steroids can act as sensitizing agents. Second, they can increase the number of malignant cells by clonal expansion, resulting in increased tumour mass. It is towards this second action that hormonal therapies are aimed.

It is unlikely that hormones are *bona fide* carcinogens. The proven carcinogens, such as chemicals, ionizing radiation, and viruses, are usually powerful mutagens. Hormones are not mutagenic and it seems that their role in carcinogenesis is more likely to be that of a promoting factor rather than an initiator. That said, initiation of cancer by hormones can occur and has been demonstrated in animal models. For instance oestrogens can promote mammary tumours in male mice, and kidney tumours in hamsters (but not other species). This species specificity is often seen in research involving hormones and reminds us that results of experiments in laboratory animals are not necessarily applicable to the human situation, especially where sex steroids are concerned as these can have quite different effects on different species. In humans, perhaps the only known case of hormones acting as bone fide carcinogens is the small increase in risk of vaginal adenocarcinoma and invasive cervical cancer in females whose mothers were given diethylstilboestrol during pregnancy (Emens, 1999). It now seems incredible that powerful hormone analogues were once used during pregnancy but this potent oestrogen analogue was used between the 1950s and 1970s to prevent miscarriage. The most obvious place to seek hormone-initiated cancer would be the mammary gland and prostate, asking whether oestrogens and androgens, respectively, are responsible for driving carcinogenesis in these tissues. Experiments in animals are inconclusive. To take the prostate: dogs (the only species apart from man known to suffer from prostate cancer) treated with potent androgens for long periods have been reported to develop prostate tumours. In a rat model engineered to develop spontaneous prostate tumours, exogenous androgens increased tumour frequency. So does exposure to androgens cause prostate cancer in men? The negative control experiment has been performed in history and there are no recorded cases of prostate cancer in eunuchs or castrati (male singers castrated to prevent their voices breaking), unsurprising as eunuchs are recorded as having nonpalpable prostates in the majority of cases studied. The positive control is more problematic, as until now human males have not been given potent androgens, although the recent trend for 'testosterone therapy' may provide more data in the long term. However, the fact that prostate cancer incidence increases with age, but testosterone (and, most importantly, free testosterone) decreases with age suggests that androgens do not drive initiation of prostate cancer but drive its progression.

In the female, there is more evidence for a role of oestrogen as a carcinogen, if only because women not only undergo natural variations in hormone levels during menstruation but are also more likely to take exogenous hormones. The best-known risk factors for breast cancer, apart from genetic factors, include young age at menarche, late menopause, and late first pregnancy. All of these have the effect of exposing the body to more uninterrupted menstrual cycles, and thus surges of oestrogen. Pregnancy, during which progesterone levels increase, is protective for breast cancer in humans. The use of oral contraceptives containing high doses of oestrogens have been shown to increase the risk of breast and uterine cancer slightly, while those containing progesterone only or very low oestrogen do not (and may even decrease risk of breast, ovarian, and uterine cancer). In these preparations, the progesterone is believed to be 'antioestrogenic' and protective against cancer of the breast and uterus. For this reason, progestins are now included in hormone replacement therapy treatments for postmenopausal women.

Dietary factors are an issue when studying the epidemiology of hormone-dependent cancers. Both breast and prostate cancer have their highest incidence in the west, especially the United States, and are less common in Asian countries such as China and Japan. However, when their incidence is measured in migrants from eastern countries to the United States it is nearer to the western level. This is believed to be due at least in part to the adoption of a more western diet, higher in unsaturated fats (meat and dairy products). Since steroid hormones are derived from cholesterol, and oestrogen is synthesized in fat cells, this could be altering the hormonal milieu and promoting cancer. A more direct link may be the relative reduction in the diet of substances derived from soy, which is a major component of the eastern diet. Phytoestrogens derived from soy may be protective against prostate and breast cancer.

Carcinogenic effects of oestrogens may be via non receptor-mediated effects. Both steroidal oestrogens and nonsteroidal pharmacological oestrogens such as diethylstilbestrol can be converted to catecholestrogens, potentially mutagenic substances due to their ability to promote formation of DNA adducts and also the generation of free radicals during the conversion (Liehr, 2000). Such global effects could potentially cause tumours in any tissue, but the higher levels of oestrogen-metabolizing enzymes in breast and uterus might explain the higher rates of malignancy in these tissues.

15.4 Steroid/nuclear hormone receptors

15.4.1 Receptor action

Binding of ligand (hormone) to a nuclear hormone receptor can occur in the cytoplasm or the nucleus. It appears that some steroid receptors, for example, the AR and GR, exist mainly in the cytoplasm in the absence of ligand, while the ER and PR are mainly nuclear. In the presence of ligand all receptors are nuclear. In fact, it is likely that receptors continually shuttle back and forth between the nucleus and cytoplasm, and the presence of ligand forces this equilibrium towards nuclear localization, while in the absence of ligand the equilibrium varies depending on receptor type. Unbound steroid receptors are complexed with heat shock proteins (hsps), which may be required to maintain the receptor in a ligand-binding-competent state and/or to prevent ligand-independent receptor activity by blocking nuclear translocation or DNA-binding. Upon ligand-binding hsps dissociate from the complex, the receptor dimerizes, in the case of cytoplasmic receptors it moves into the nucleus, and it binds to sequence-specific response elements in the promoter of target genes (Figure 15.5 (a)). The hormone response elements are 2 repeats of short sequences. The DBD of the receptor consists of two zinc finger-like structures that interact with the major groove of DNA. The ER homodimer binds to an imperfect inverted repeat of A/GGTCA separated by 3 nucleotides (ERE). The other steroid receptors all bind to a similar inverted repeat but the sequence of the half-site differs. Thus a glucocorticoid response element (GRE) is also responsive to activated PR, MR, or AR. Recently, more specific androgen response elements (AREs) have been characterized in androgen responsive gene promoters and enhancers, which look more like imperfect direct repeats (Claessens et al., 2001). From the response element, the receptor dimer promotes transcription via co-activator proteins as described below. The response elements for type I nuclear receptors such as THR and RAR are generally imperfect direct repeats of an ERE half-site, with variable spacing between. These bind as heterodimers with the ubiquitously expressed RXR (Figure 15.5(b)). Like steroid receptors, in the presence of ligand they recruit co-activators and promote transcription. However, they differ in the absence of ligand in that they do not bind hsps and instead bind to DNA in a repressive manner.

It should be remembered that nuclear receptors do not generally bind to a promoter in isolation, there are binding sites for other transcription factors nearby and the different transcription factors are likely to influence DNA binding activity. They can also affect each other's activity in a non-DNA-binding dependent manner. For instance, glucocorticoids have an anti-inflammatory effect partly because activated GR can repress transcription of the collagenase gene, which is activated by

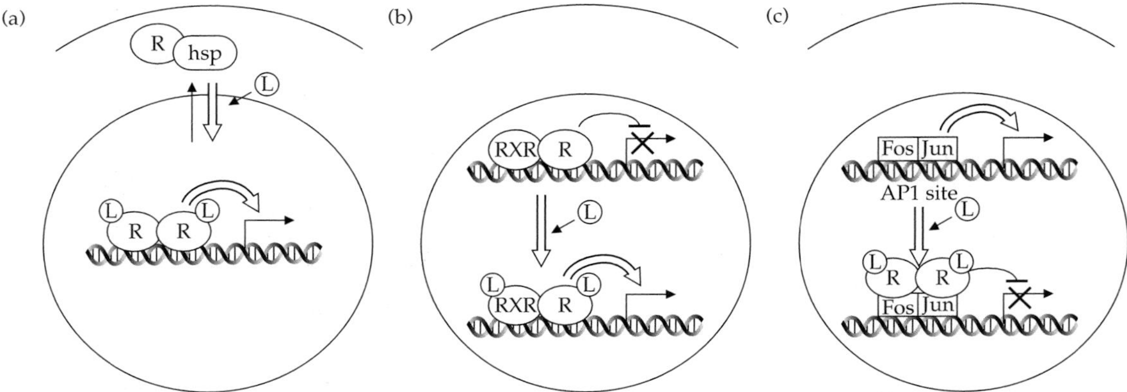

Figure 15.5 Modes of action of nuclear receptors (R). (a) Steroid receptors are complexed with heat shock proteins in the absence of ligand; they may be cytoplasmic as shown here or nuclear. On ligand binding they move into the nucleus and bind to response elements in the promoters of target genes to activate transcription. (b) Type I nuclear receptors are bound to response elements in the absence of ligand and repress transcription, as a heterodimer with RXR. When ligand binds, they switch to activating transcription from the promoter. (c) Receptors can also modulate the activity of AP1 transcription factors, positively or negatively depending on the composition of the AP1 dimer, probably via direct interaction with the AP1 dimer. hsp = heat shock protein complex.

AP1 binding to the promoter. This does not require DNA-binding of the GR but appears to be via direct protein–protein interaction between the GR and DNA-bound AP1 (Figure 15.5(c)).

The next step is activation of transcription of the target gene, achieved via the activation functions AF1 and AF2. AF1 in the N-terminus is intrinsically ligand-independent, but is inhibited by the LBD in the absence of ligand. It can also be activated in certain receptors by phosphorylation, induced by growth factors. AF2 is a ligand-dependent activation function in the LBD itself. Crystallographic studies have shown that the LBDs of all nuclear receptors modelled to date consist of 12 α-helices (Wurtz et al., 1996). When ligand enters the ligand-binding pocket (consisting of residues from helices 1, 3, 5, and 11), the domain undergoes a conformational change as helix 12 flips to lie over the pocket, stabilizing ligand binding and forming a new surface to which co-activator proteins can bind (Figure 15.6). This co-activator-binding surface, which forms the core of AF2, consists of residues from helices 3, 4, 5, and 12. The relative contributions of AF1 and AF2 to receptor activity depend on the receptor in question, with AF1 being stronger for the AR and AF2 for the ER. However, even for a given receptor, circumstances such as the cell type or target promoter can affect the relative importance of the two domains. For instance, the ER activates mainly via AF2 in breast issue, but in the uterine endometrium AF1 has been shown to be more important. This is presumably due to the different cofactors, growth factors, etc. present in the different cell types.

15.4.2 Coactivators and corepressors

Reporter assays using overexpressed receptor proteins in mammalian cells showed that one activated steroid receptor is able to inhibit activity of another in the presence of its cognate ligand, implying that there is a limiting cofactor common to activation by the two receptors. Many such co-activators have been identified in recent years by virtue of their ability to interact with nuclear receptors in a ligand-dependent manner and to potentiate activity of receptors in *in vitro* assays (Bevan and Parker, 1999). Some are common to all the receptors examined to date, such as the co-integrator CREB binding protein (CBP), while others may be more restricted to certain receptors. Transcription involves chromatin remodelling prior to recruitment of the basal transcriptional machinery, the assembly of the pre-initiation complex on the promoter, and the movement of the

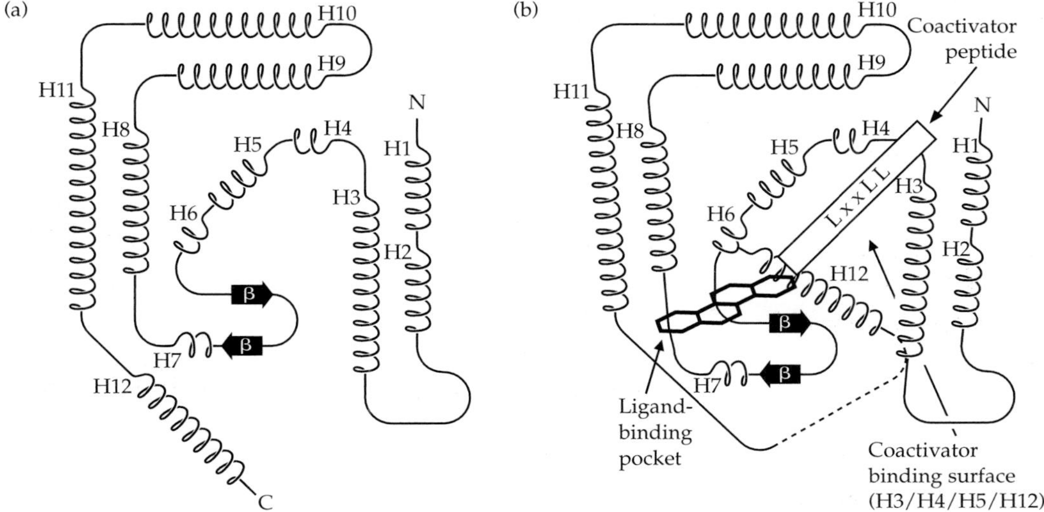

Figure 15.6 LBD structure. This consists of 12 α-helices and a β-sheet. (a) In the absence of ligand, helix 12 lies at an angle away from the main body of the LBD. (b) In the presence of ligand, it is folded back over the ligand-binding pocket to form a 'lid'. This conformational change results in a coactivator-binding surface being formed consisting of residues in helices 3,4,5, and 12. LxxLL = the receptor-interaction motif of the coactivator.

polymerase along the gene. Proteins that enhance transcription could do so by promoting one or more of these steps. Initially, it was hypothesized that coactivators act as bridging factors between transcription factors and the transcription machinery, stabilizing the formation of the pre-initiation complex. The TRAP (thyroid receptor associated proteins) complex appears to have such a role. This large, multiprotein complex was first identified as binding to the THR via a single protein termed TRAP220. Parallel work led to the characterization of related complexes binding other type I and steroid receptors. It has emerged that these complexes, containing at least 12 polypeptides, are almost identical to one another and about half the peptides are similar to those found in the yeast mediator complex. The mediator complex may serve several functions but importantly it recruits RNA polymerase II to target genes by its association with the C-terminal repeat domain of the large subunit. The TRAP complex is also believed to phosphorylate the C-terminus of RNA polymerase II, enabling it to move along the coding strand thus promoting elongation as well as initiation of transcription (Figure 15.7b).

Other coactivators promote transcription by altering the organization of DNA at the promoter. Chromatin structure consists of histone protein complexes associated with DNA in units known as nucleosomes, which generally repress transcription from adjacent promoters, presumably by preventing access of transcription factors and the pre-initiation complex (Kadanoga, 1998). This restrictive heterochromatin structure can be 'loosened' by destabilizing histone-DNA contacts by post-translational modification, including acetylation of the histone tails. Enzymes with this capability are called histone acetyltransferases (HATs). Two major classes of coactivators have been identified which possess HAT activity: the related 300 kDa proteins CBP and p300, and the p160 co-activator family. The p160 family consists of 3 co-activators: SRC1 (the first identified coactivator, also known as NCoA1 (Oñate et al., 1995)), TIF2 (also known as GRIP1 or NCoA2), and AIB1 (also known as pCIP, ACTR, RAC3, or NCoA3). The confusing collection of different names for these proteins is the result of different labs cloning them at different times or from different organisms and renaming them each time. The p160s may have some weak HAT activity but appear to function primarily by recruiting CBP/p300 and another HAT, pCAF, to the receptor. Thus a complex of HAT coactivators may build on a DNA-bound receptor to promote transcription from that promoter by remodelling chromatin structure (Figure 15.7a). How these complexes disassociate is likely to involve modification of the coactivators themselves by other components of the complex—for instance, acetylation of AIB1 by p300 has been shown to promote dissociation of the HAT complex bound to ER (Liao et al., 2002). The interaction of coactivators with receptors is primarily via a receptor-binding motif that consists of LxxLL, where L is leucine and x is any amino acid. This motif, one or more copies of which are found in most coactivators studied to date, forms an α-helix that binds in the co-activator-binding surface of the active LBD (Figure 15.6).

The repression of basal transcription of target genes by type I nuclear receptors also requires cofactors, known as corepressors, which bind to the receptor only in the absence of ligand

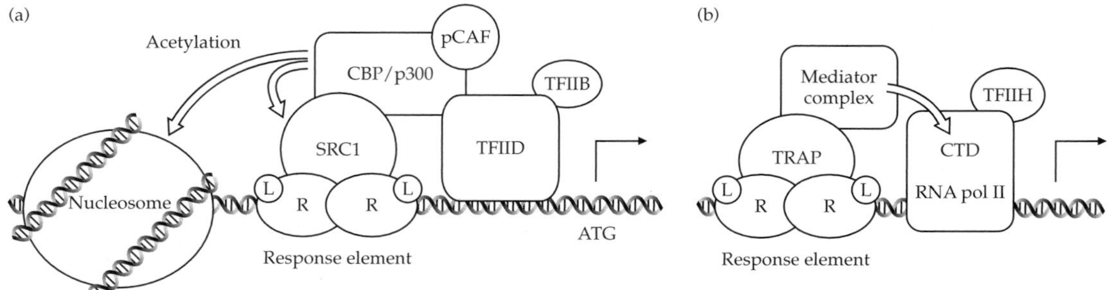

Figure 15.7 Coactivator recruitment to DNA-bound nuclear receptors. (a) A complex of HAT coactivators can build that remodel chromatin structure by acetylation of histones and also acetylate each other, promoting dissociation of the complex. (b) Coactivator complexes can also promote initiation of transcription by forming contacts with the basal transcriptional machinery, and promote elongation by phosphorylation of the C-terminus of RNA polymerase II.

(Hu and Lazar, 2000). The best-characterized corepressors are the related proteins NCoR and SMRT. Their action opposes that of HAT coactivators as they recruit proteins with histone deacetylase (HDAC) activity, promoting the formation of heterochromatin at the promoter, thus restricting the access of transcription factors and the pre-initiation complex and inhibiting transcription. The corepressor interaction site in receptors overlaps with the coactivator interaction site and when ligand binds the receptor, the conformational change results in co-repressors being released and coactivators recruited (Figure 15.8). Until recently it was thought that nuclear corepressors had no role in steroid hormone action, since steroid receptors are not thought to bind DNA or repress basal transcription in the absence of hormones. Although unliganded steroid receptors do not bind to corepressors in interaction assays, several groups have found that NCoR and SMRT associate with the ER and PR in the presence of certain antagonists (see later). Therefore, co-repressors may also be required for any DNA-bound nuclear receptor to inhibit transcriptional activity. This is of interest in the context of cancer since antagonists are the most common therapies for breast and prostate cancer.

15.4.3 Hormone receptors as oncogenes

The physiological importance of the basal repression of target genes by type I receptors is illustrated by the case of acute promyelocytic leukaemia (APL), caused by a block of differentiation of primary bone marrow cells into mature granulocytes. This is a retinoic acid-dependent process and in most cases high-dose retinoic acid therapy overcomes the block and results in disease remission. In many patients, APL is associated with a reciprocal translocation between chromosomes 15 and 17. The breakpoint occurs in the coding sequence of a gene called *PML* (for promyelocytic leukaemia) on chromosome 15, function unknown, and the retinoic acid receptor α gene *(RARα)* on chromosome 17. Of the two resulting fusion genes, the one that is associated with the disease in patients, *PML–RARα*, encodes a fusion protein containing the DBD and LBD domains of RARα (Figure 15.9). The PML–RARα fusion protein binds to retinoic acid response elements and inhibits their transcription through recruitment of corepressors to the RARα C-terminus. However, it is impaired in its ability to release corepressors, possibly due to interference from the PML part, and higher pharmacological doses of retinoic acid are required to release corepressors and relieve this repression. Unfortunately, some APL patients do not respond to retinoic acid treatment. Most of these carry a different chromosomal translocation resulting in a gene rearrangement between *RARα* and the promyelocytic zinc finger (*PLZF*) gene. The PLZF protein itself is able to recruit the corepressors NCoR and SMRT, and this ability is retained in the fusion protein, PLZF–RARα (Zelent et al., 2001). While retinoic acid treatment results in the dissociation of corepressors bound to the RARα part, those bound to the PLZF part remain and prevent activation of target genes, thus inhibiting differentiation of

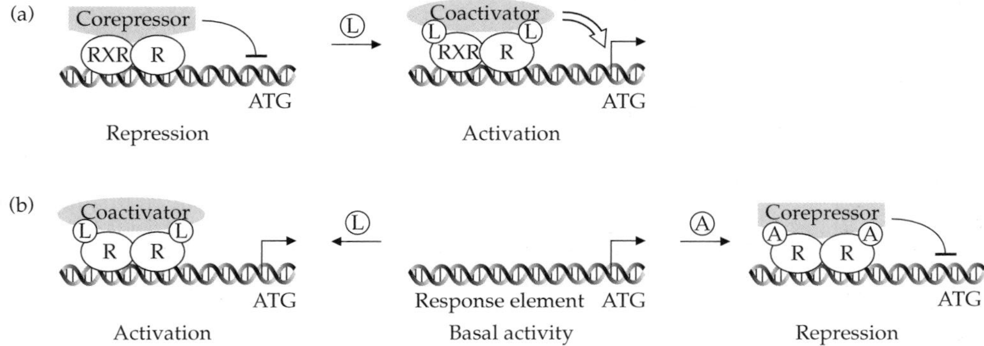

Figure 15.8 Role of corepressors. (a) Corepressors are required for repression of basal transcription by type I receptors in the absence of ligand. When ligand (L) binds, corepressors are released, coactivators recruited and transcription is activated. (b) Steroid receptors are not thought to bind DNA in the absence of ligand. However, some antagonists (A) promote DNA-binding and it is postulated that these may function by causing the recruitment of corepressors.

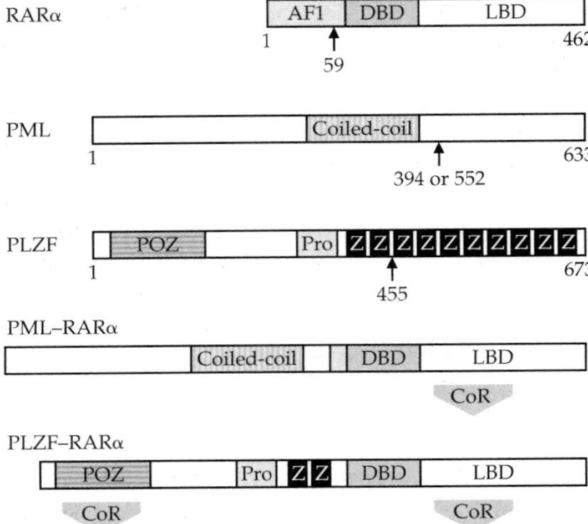

Figure 15.9 Schematic representation of APL fusion proteins and their component proteins. Breakpoints are indicated by arrows. Both PML–RARα and PLZF–RARα contain the RARα LBD, which binds corepressors (CoR) in the absence of retinoic acid. However, PLZF–RARα also binds corepressors via the POZ domain of the PLZF part in a retinoic acid-insensitive manner, thus patients with this fusion protein do not respond to high-dose retinoic acid therapy. Z = zinc finger, Pro = proline-rich region.

granulocytes. Since repression by corepressors is mediated at least partly through histone deacetylation, inhibitors of histone deacetylation such as trichostatin A (TSA) may be effective treatments for retinoic acid-resistant APL.

In chicks, erythroblastosis can be caused by a virus encoding a mutant, oncogenic form of *THRα*, *v-ErbA*. This arrests differentiation of erythroblasts by repressing target gene transcription and enhances the proliferative effects of a second oncoprotein *v-ErbB*, a truncated form of the EGF receptor. A similar role of THR has not yet been seen in human erythroleukaemias.

15.5 Hormone therapy for cancer

While organ-confined cancers can be treated effectively by surgical removal, in the United Kingdom over 60% of men presenting with prostate cancer have disease that has spread, either locally to the seminal vesicles and bladder, or metastatically to the bone (Foster et al., 1999). In such cases, and when disease recurs after surgery, hormone therapy is most often used. Breast cancer patients usually present with localized disease—however,

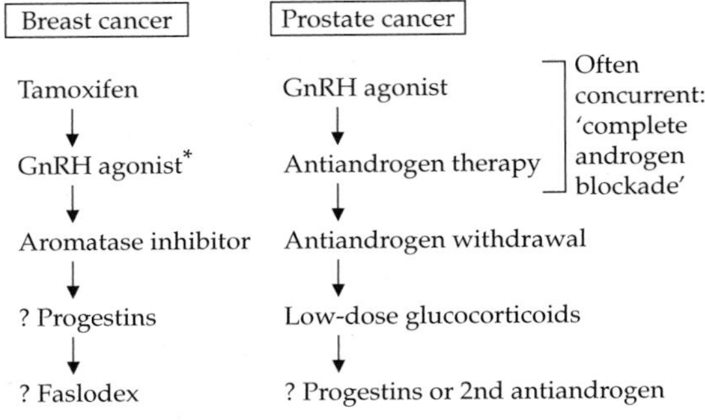

Figure 15.10 Hormone therapy regimes. This is not a blueprint for order of therapies but rather an overview of how the therapies discussed might be applied in clinic. After surgery, if appropriate, gonadal ablation and/or antihormone treatment are generally the first treatments used, and second-line therapies used after relapse will vary. In breast cancer, aromatase inhibitors are only useful after GnRH agonist treatment or menopause has removed ovarian E2.

despite surgery, over half will eventually relapse presumably due to undetectable 'micrometastases'. They are therefore treated with hormone therapy for at least 5 years to reduce this risk (Ali and Coombes, 2002). The aim of hormone therapy is to prevent steroid-mediated growth of the tumour and/or metastases, by removing gonadal steroid hormones from the patient and opposing the action of remaining steroids (produced by the adrenal, tumour, or peripheral tissues) using antagonists. An example of a possible sequence of therapies for both breast and prostate cancer is given in Figure 15.10.

15.5.1 Gonadectomy

Since 1786 when the surgeon John Hunter noted that 'the prostate gland ... of the perfect male (is) large and pulpy, while in the castrated animal (it is) ... small, flabby tough and filamentous and has little secretion', it has been known that prostate relies on testicular secretions, later identified as androgens, for growth and function. It was logical, then, for Huggins and Hodges to try treating prostate cancer patients with castration in the 1940s and indeed the experiment had a fair degree of success. Similarly, the ovaries produce the majority of oestrogen in women, and in 1900 Boyd and Beatson used ovariectomy to treat women with metastatic breast cancer, successfully in 30% of cases. These days, rather than surgical gonadectomy, testicular or ovarian 'ablation' is performed by treating patients with 'super' analogues of GnRH such as goserelin, buserelin, or leuprolide acetate. Paradoxically, these ultimately reduce the levels of LH and testosterone or oestradiol down to levels similar to those seen in surgically gonadectomized patients. This is because GnRH works by promoting the release of stored LH and FSH after which it downregulates GnRH receptors to inhibit further release (a negative feedback mechanism). Normally, GnRH production is also inhibited and the stores of gonadotrophins can be replenished, but continuous goserelin therapy results in continued receptor downregulation so that there is no response even to endogenous GnRH. Antagonists of GnRH are currently in trials with the same aim of preventing LH/FSH release. While gonadectomy or gonadal ablation effectively removes the majority of circulating androgens or oestrogens, there are still hormones secreted by the adrenal or synthesized in peripheral tissue. For instance, while 90% of the circulating androgens in an adult male are gonadal in origin, androgens synthesized by the adrenal gland can be converted to testosterone and thence to DHT, which promotes prostate growth. The unimpaired activity of 5α-reductase in prostate acting on adrenally derived testosterone means that tissue concentrations of DHT are only reduced by approximately 40%. For this reason, prostate cancer is often treated with a combination of gonadectomy and antiandrogen therapy (see further), termed 'total androgen blockade'. In breast cancer, gonadectomy and antioestrogen therapy are more often used sequentially.

15.5.2 Inhibition of peripheral and intracrine steroid synthesis

As DHT is the most important androgen in the prostate, inhibiting the enzyme responsible for its synthesis should effectively reduce prostate growth. This is illustrated by a tribe in the Dominican Republic with a high frequency of 5α-reductase I inactivating mutations. A number of the outwardly female children of this tribe develop into fully fledged males at puberty—those affected are given the name 'guevedoces' which translates as 'penis at 12'. These children lack DHT but have normal levels of testosterone, which is sufficient to virilize the internal genitalia. The external genitalia are normally virilized by the more potent DHT, but at puberty the increase in testosterone levels is sufficient to cause penile growth and development of male secondary sexual characteristics. The one organ that does not fully develop is the prostate, which remains small, as DHT is absolutely required for its growth. (In fact, these children are likely to have some low levels of DHT since there is a second 5α-reductase gene in which they do not carry mutations.) Study of this tribe led to the development of finasteride, a 5α-reductase inhibitor used to treat patients with prostate cancer or, more commonly, benign prostatic hyperplasia with some success in slowing and even reversing prostatic growth.

Peripheral synthesis of E2 from testosterone occurs principally in fat cells, also skin, muscle, and bone, and requires the cytochrome p450 enzyme complex aromatase. This normally contributes less than 30% of circulating levels of E2 in premenopausal women but is likely to be more significant in breast cancer, as *in situ* production of oestrogens appears to drive tumour growth and 60–70% of breast cancers contain the aromatase enzyme. The ability of such cells to produce their own oestrogen is presumably selected for during ovarian oestrogen depletion. Aromatase inhibitors such as exemestane (a 'suicide substrate') and anastrazole (a competitive inhibitor) effectively prevent this synthesis, in both peripheral tissues and tumour cells, and have recently been licensed for use in breast cancer patients. They are used for patients who have developed hormone-independent disease and are postmenopausal or have undergone ovarian ablation (Dowsett, 1997).

15.5.3 Steroid receptor antagonists: antioestrogens and antiandrogens

Hormone antagonists, the best-known of which is the antioestrogen tamoxifen, repress receptor-mediated signalling at the level of the receptor itself. Antagonists are molecules, often bearing structural similarities to the ligand, that bind to the receptor in the ligand-binding pocket but do not cause it to become active. The mechanism by which they prevent activity is not absolutely clear (see Figure 15.11). They may function simply by competition. However, antagonists generally have a much lower binding affinity for receptors than the cognate ligand so competitive inhibition is unlikely to be the whole story. They may prevent nuclear

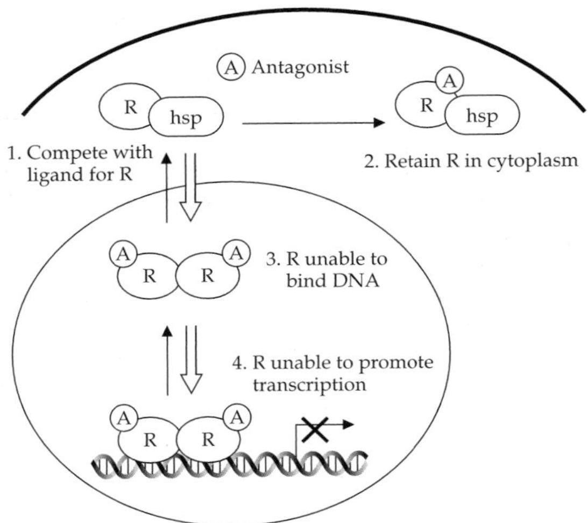

Figure 15.11 Mechanisms of antagonist action. Possible steps in the steroid receptor pathway at which antagonists might act are indicated. A combination of these is likely: for instance faslodex promotes cytoplasmic retention and degradation but may also inhibit ER dimerization thus DNA-binding.

translocation of the receptor, keeping it in the cytoplasmic compartment, perhaps complexed with inactivating hsps. This was found to be a likely explanation for the action of the antioestrogen faslodex, recently introduced as a breast cancer treatment. Faslodex alters the equilibrium of nucleo-cytoplasmic shuttling of the ER such that it becomes mainly cytoplasmic—further, it is degraded more rapidly (Dauvois et al., 1993). However, other ER and AR antagonists, such as flutamide (an antiandrogen) and tamoxifen, are known to promote receptor movement into the nucleus. Later steps that could be inhibited by such antagonists include dimerization, DNA-binding or coactivator binding. Co-crystallization of receptor LBDs with the receptor-interacting regions of coactivator proteins in the presence of ligand showed that coactivators bound to a surface formed by helix 12 in the 'active' conformation, and helices 3, 4, and 5. When LBDs were crystallized in the presence of antagonists, however, helix 12 adopted an alternative orientation. This time, it occupied the coactivator-binding surface itself, presumably preventing coactivators from binding (Brzozowski et al., 1997). Thus, the presence of an antagonist in the ligand-binding pocket would, by virtue of its shape difference from the agonist, prevent helix 12 adopting the 'active' conformation and instead promote an inactive conformation unable to bind coactivators. Research is currently underway to determine whether these inactive conformations are actually able to bind to corepressor proteins instead, and so actively repress transcription.

While some of the antagonists used in clinics will repress receptor activity under any circumstances, most are more complex and in some circumstances can actually activate the receptor. These are termed partial or mixed antagonists and examples include the antioestrogens tamoxifen and raloxifene, and the antiandrogens flutamide and cyproterone acetate. In cell culture experiments using reporter assays, tamoxifen is able to activate ER in certain cell types but represses it in others. The promoter sequence used also determines the outcome. In the body, the same phenomenon is seen—tamoxifen is an effective repressor of ER activity in breast, but it activates ER in the uterine endometrium and in bone. This is believed to explain the slight increase in uterine cancer risk in women treated with tamoxifen. The explanation of this dual role of tamoxifen is that it inhibits AF2, but not AF1 activity, and AF1 is the dominant activation function in uterine and bone cells. Another, not incompatible, explanation of how partial antagonists can have different effects in different tissues was suggested by structural studies of mutant ER crystallized in the presence of a partial antioestrogen (Gangloff et al., 2001). Helix 12 was found to 'flip-flop' between the active and inactive positions and it is hypothesized that the local concentration of cofactors might affect which position it preferentially adopts when bound to a partial antagonist. Hence in different tissues, with a different milieu of cofactors, either the active or the repressed state will predominate. It might seem odd that such a drug would continue to be used, but in fact the dual actions of these drugs in promoting ER action in certain tissues but repressing it in breast are being exploited to develop the next generation of agents for hormone therapy.

Finally, it should be noted that not all of the inhibitory effects of hormone antagonists may be due to their antagonism of hormone action. Tamoxifen can sometimes cause regression even of tumours that are classed as ER–negative. This could be due to very low levels of ERα, or the presence of the second ER, ERβ, which is not yet routinely tested for in breast tumour samples due to the lack of a specific antibody. However, tamoxifen also appears to reduce the free radical generation due to conversion of oestrogens to catecholestrogens and thus may prevent cancer initiation (Liehr, 2000). Antioestrogens can also block growth factor-mediated mitogenic effects by mechanisms unknown.

15.5.4 Other hormone therapies

By their very nature, oestrogen and androgen can oppose each other's effects in certain tissues. Thus, the first 'antiandrogen' used in prostate cancer therapy was actually oestrogen, and the non-steroidal oestrogen analogue diethylstilboestrol is still sometimes used today. This opposition could come about by feedback, with high levels of oestrogens preventing gonadotrophin release and hence blocking testosterone production, but more direct effects must also occur. The prostate contains ER and the mouse model lacking functional ERβ showed hyperproliferation of the prostate, suggesting that oestrogens act via ERβ to inhibit prostate cell proliferation (Weihua et al., 2001). In cell culture, testosterone inhibits the growth of breast cancer cell lines in the presence or absence of oestradiol. Also, approximately 50% of human breast cancers express AR and androgen therapy for breast cancer has been shown to be effective. Androgens act additively when used in combination with antioestrogens, confirming that they are not acting via the ER pathway (Labrie et al., 2003). A protective role of androgens against breast cancer is also indicated by the very low rate of breast cancer in men and the fact that in more than one case, familial male breast cancer was found to be associated with AR mutations. In general however, androgens and oestrogens are not often used as first- or second-line therapy, due to the side-effects engendered by using such powerful agents.

15.5.5 Development of hormone resistance

While hormone therapy for breast and prostate cancer is initially extremely successful, it almost inevitably eventually fails. Tamoxifen therapy causes tumour regression in 50% of patients with ER-positive tumours and 10% of patients with ER-negative tumours but after a median of 20 months, many of these relapse and show further tumour growth. In prostate cancer, antiandrogen therapy has an even higher success rate (75%), but almost all patients will relapse after an even shorter period. The growth of tumours in such a steroid-depleted environment, despite the use of antagonists, is often termed 'hormone-independent'. As we shall see, this term may be misleading.

Hormonal therapy imposes harsh, growth inhibitory conditions on the tumour cells and any individual cells with a growth advantage over the others will be selected and clonally expanded, resulting in a cluster of tumour cells able to grow in spite of hormonal therapy. Many theories for how cells adapt to be able to grow under these conditions have been put forward and it is likely that there is no unifying explanation and each of the theories may account for resistance in a proportion of patients. Most of the putative pathways, however, still rely on continued expression and activation of the hormone receptor, unsurprising in light of the fact that almost all 'hormone-independent' prostate tumours and 70% of advanced breast tumours remain receptor positive. The possible pathways by which hormone resistance may develop are described below. See also Jenster, 1999; Feldman and Feldman, 2001; Sommer and Fuqua, 2001.

Receptor amplification

As discussed, no therapy is able to completely eliminate all steroid hormones from the body. Residual oestrogens and androgens still circulate in patients treated by gonadectomy and/or antagonist therapy. An amplification of the response to these low levels, or weaker steroids, could explain how tumours can grow under these conditions, and the simplest way to achieve this would be by increasing the number of molecules of receptor proteins. Indeed, this is seen in up to 30% of cases of prostate and breast cancer. Increase in receptor protein can be achieved via an increase in transcription of the gene (overexpression) or an increase in copy number of the gene (amplification) and both of these mechanisms have been observed.

Cofactor changes

A second way of amplifying the response to residual steroids might be to increase the number of coactivator proteins. Coactivators seem to be limiting, hence not every ligand-bound steroid receptor will be able to activate transcription to the maximum extent. Increasing coactivator proteins until they are present in excess would allow the maximum activity to be extracted from each receptor molecule, as is seen in cell culture experiments where activity of a reporter gene in the presence of a fixed amount of receptor can be increased by co-transfecting increasing amounts of coactivator until a saturating concentration is reached.

One coactivator, AIB1 (which stands for Amplified In Breast Cancer 1), was as its name suggests identified as a gene amplified in breast cancer (Liao et al., 2002). Several studies since have confirmed that a subset of breast cancers (5–10%) have amplification of the *AIB1* gene and a higher percentage show increased levels of the protein, but this does not always correlate with ER expression. Thus the role of AIB1 in breast cancer may not be limited to its effect on ER activity. Further, mice lacking *AIB1* were less susceptible than wild-type mice to oncogene-induced mammary gland tumorigenesis, suggesting a possible role in tumour initiation. A recent study of a small cohort of prostate cancer patients has also shown that levels of *AIB1* are increased in prostate tumours as compared to benign prostate.

Conversely, if hormone antagonists require corepressors to achieve repression of hormone-responsive genes, then a shortage of corepressors would prevent antagonists working to their full extent. If the loss of corepressors allows coactivator binding, due to lack of competitive inhibition, it could even switch partial antagonists to agonists, contributing to hormone-independent activation and growth. Although there is a lack of direct evidence that corepressors are required for antagonist action, a mouse model of breast cancer showed a decrease in the corepressor NCoR correlating with progression to tamoxifen resistance (Lavinsky et al., 1998).

Studies measuring expression of individual coactivator and corepressor proteins in both breast and prostate cancer have so far failed to show convincing changes in expression levels correlating with progression to hormone independence. However, this could be a consequence of the fact that only small subsets of cofactors are being investigated. Over 200 potential cofactors have been identified so far, most of these are ubiquitously expressed and many appear to operate as part of large, multiprotein complexes (McKenna et al., 1999). Thus if changes in coactivator and corepressors do contribute to hormone resistance, it is likely to be more subtle changes in the milieu and ratios between various types of cofactor. A more global approach, such as microarray analysis, may eventually allow the identification of signature cofactor changes associated with disease progression.

Crosstalk with growth factor/receptor tyrosine kinase-activated pathways

In the absence of ligand, other pathways may be able to activate steroid receptors and promote tumour growth. Hormone receptors are phosphoproteins, with both the liganded and unliganded forms being phosphorylated. This has been best characterized for the ER in which several phosphorylation sites have been mapped corresponding to target sites for known kinases (Figure 15.12). Phosphorylation of the ER by growth factors such as EGF, protein kinase A, TFIIH, mitogen-activated protein kinases (MAPKs) and the serine/threonine protein kinase AKT can activate the receptor, in some cases acting synergistically with E2 and so amplifying the hormone response, but in others activating the receptor in a completely ligand-independent manner (Ali and Coombes, 2002). Overexpression or constitutive activation of any of the components of growth factor signalling pathways, including the growth factor ligands, the membrane-associated receptors, or downstream kinases, could result in activation of the ER in breast cancer. The target of TFIIH and ERK1 and 2 is serine 118, phosphorylation of which can result in ligand-independent activation of the ER. Overexpression of the TFIIH-associated kinase CDK7 in cell culture experiments reduces the ability of tamoxifen to repress ER activity, and ERK1/2 expression or activity has been found to be increased in several hormone-resistant breast cancer cell

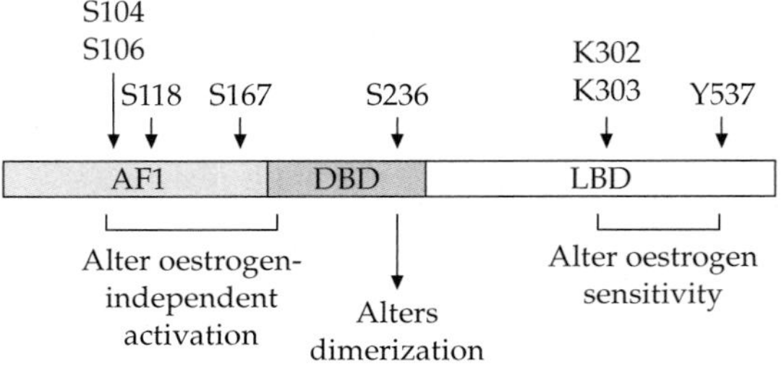

Figure 15.12 Post-translational modifications of the ER. Serine residues as indicated are targets for phosphorylation by growth factor pathways, including EGF, insulin, IGF-1, and TGFα. These can increase ER activity, sometimes in the absence of ligand, by increasing AF1 activity or promoting dimerization. In the LBD, acetylation of K302 and K303 by CBP increases sensitivity to ligand while phosphorylation of Y537 causes ligand-independent activity.

lines. *PTEN*, a tumour suppressor gene that is frequently inactivated in both breast and prostate cancer, is a repressor of AKT activity, and AKT proteins are often increased in breast cancer, suggesting that the ligand-independent ER activity induced by phosphorylation by AKT can also occur *in vivo*. At the growth factor receptor level, the EGF receptor and the related membrane-associated tyrosine kinase ERB-B2/HER-2/NEU are both often overexpressed in breast tumours, often correlating with hormone independence (Pietras et al., 1995). Both of these are targets for new therapies for breast cancer, Iressa™ and Herceptin™ respectively, which inhibit their kinase activity.

The AR has likewise been shown to be activated in a ligand-independent manner by certain growth factors including IGF-1, KGF, and EGF, but a direct effect on phosphorylation of the AR has not been shown (Culig et al., 1994). Notwithstanding, it is possible that the targets of these growth factor pathways could be other proteins in the AR-signalling pathway—coactivators, for instance. ERB-B2 can activate the AR in the absence of ligand as well as amplify its response to low levels of androgens, while overexpression of *ERB-B2* in androgen-dependent prostate cell lines allowed them to grow in the absence of androgens *in vitro* and as xenografts in castrated mice (Craft et al., 1999). Some studies have found overexpression or amplification of *ERB-B2* DNA in between 16 and 69% of patients, while in patients with advanced androgen-independent disease serum levels of the extracellular domain of ERB-B2 are often elevated (Daliani and Papandreou, 1999). Thus *ERB-B2* overexpression may be a mechanism of escape from androgen independence in prostate cancer and Herceptin™ could be a possible future therapy for advanced disease. ERB-B2 is known to activate the PI3K/AKT and MAPK signalling pathways but how exactly it promotes prostate cancer cell growth is not clear—both MAPK and AKT can phosphorylate the AR and cause it to become active. Involvement of the AKT pathway with prostate and possibly breast cancer progression also occurs at the level of PTEN.

Nuclear receptors may also affect response to growth factors by interference with growth factor targets such as AP1. Direct protein–protein interactions between nuclear receptors and AP1 can either increase or decrease its activity, as discussed. In the breast cancer cell line MCF7, oestrogens increase growth factor-induced AP1 activity and antioestrogens inhibit it, while also inhibiting their growth. Changes in growth factor pathways could alter this response.

Receptor mutation

In prostate cancer, while mutation of the AR is rare in primary and hormone-dependent tumours, in screens of patients with advanced metastatic hormone-independent disease the frequency of mutation rises to 30–40%, evidence in itself that these mutations are likely to contribute to the progression to hormone independence (Gottlieb et al., 1999). Around 75 different mutations have been identified to date, most of them being point mutations leading to single amino acid substitutions, and they are found in all of the functional domains of the AR. Of the missense mutations that have been studied by *in vitro* mutagenesis and functional studies, several increase the spectrum of activation of the AR. They allow it to become activated by alternative ligands such as E2, progesterone, glucocorticoids and the antiandrogens hydroxyflutamide and cyproterone acetate, and/or increase its activation by weak androgens such as androstenediol. As many of these hormones are present in the patients, either naturally (e.g. E2) or administered (e.g. antiandrogens), such aberrant receptor activation could contribute to tumour growth. Further, the activation of such mutant receptors by antiandrogens has been suggested as an explanation for the 'antiandrogen withdrawal syndrome'. This describes the situation where a patient shows symptomatic improvement for a few weeks after antiandrogen therapy is stopped. If antiandrogens are actually contributing to tumour growth by activating the AR, this is understandable. One argument against this explanation is that the antiandrogen withdrawal syndrome occurs with higher frequency than do AR mutations. However, advanced, metastatic tumours are not routinely sampled and are likely to be heterogeneous, so it is possible that the frequency of mutation is underestimated.

Missense mutation of the ER in breast cancer is not so common, with less than 1% of primary tumours carrying coding mutations although the percentage appears to be higher in metastatic tumours (Sommer and Fuqua, 2001). One mutation has been reported, of the tyrosine residue at 357 to asparagine, that results in a constitutively active receptor, not repressed by tamoxifen. Tyrosine 537 is a possible phosphorylation target of src kinases and thus the mutation may mimic some of the effects of phosphorylation. Another point mutation at a site of receptor modification was found in 4% of pre-malignant hyperplastic lesions in one study. This resulted in a lysine to arginine substitution at residue 303. Residue 303 is the site of acetylation of ER by CBP and mutation of this site *in vitro* was shown to increase the sensitivity of ER to E2, which could result in increased response to low levels of E2 after gonadectomy (Figure 15.12). Much has been published on the significance or otherwise of a splice variant of ERα, termed ERΔ5, lacking the LBD. This mutant form is unable to bind ligands, including tamoxifen, but can still bind to DNA and activate target genes in cell culture assay systems. However, its role *in vivo* is uncertain, as while the variant mRNA is common in most oestrogen target tissues, the protein is not often detected. Even if it were, the expression of the mutant form does not appear to be increased in hormone-independent tumours, so would not be able to explain the disease progression.

Non receptor-dependent pathways

All of the mechanisms for progression to hormone-independence require mutation of a tumour cell and subsequent selection and clonal expansion. While the mutations, understandably, occur most often in genes linked to the hormone response pathway, it is feasible that certain mutations could allow another growth pathway to take over completely, bypassing the requirement for hormone receptor involvement. For instance, autocrine growth control is a possible mechanism for continued growth of tumour cells. Breast and prostate epithelial cells are believed to divide in response to growth factors secreted by neighbouring cells (stromal or epithelial) in a paracrine fashion. If the growing cells themselves secreted these growth factors as well as responding to them, an autocrine, self-serving growth loop would be set up resulting in hyperproliferation. For example, primary androgen-sensitive prostate cells show high levels of the growth factor TGFα only in the stromal cells and high levels of its receptor, EGFR, only in the epithelial cells. However, metastatic androgen-independent prostate epithelial cells express high levels of both TGFα and EGFR, suggesting a switch from paracrine to autocrine growth control (Daliani and Papandreou, 1999). An autocrine loop could also involve steroid receptors—for instance oestrogens increase expression of TGFα and EGFR, thus oestrogens could be functioning indirectly to promote cell growth by increasing sensitivity to autocrine and paracrine-acting growth factors.

Anti-apoptotic pathways are also likely candidates for driving truly hormone-independent tumour growth, since tumour regression due to hormone withdrawal occurs via apoptosis. While the kinase AKT is anti-apoptotic, inactivating pro-apoptotic proteins by phosphorylation, PTEN is a phosphatase that blocks AKT effects so allows apoptosis. Thus loss of functional PTEN, frequently seen in breast and prostate cancer, is transforming in that it decreases the ability of a cell to undergo apoptosis, as well as in the ways previously described. BCL2 is a survival or anti-apoptotic factor that is not normally expressed in prostate epithelial cells, but is frequently expressed in hormone-independent prostate cancer. Selecting for androgen-independent prostate cells by growing BCL2-negative cells as xenografts in castrated mice resulted in emergence of BCL2 expression in the xenografts that grew under these conditions. Thus BCL2 overexpression is one pathway by which AR can be bypassed entirely, but others are likely to exist including those involving oncogenes and tumour suppressor genes. For instance, a few studies report a correlation between prostate cancer progression and mutant forms of p53, but the significance of this is controversial.

Finally, it is inescapable that the majority of cancer deaths are caused by metastasis. One of the reasons that patients with ER-negative breast cancers have a poorer prognosis is that these tumours are more likely to metastasize. If we can understand what enables a cancer cell to metastasize, it should be possible to develop therapies aimed at preventing this. Possible targets are the metastasis-associated genes (MTAs), identified based on their differential expression between metastasizing and non-metastasising tumour cells. They appear to indirectly regulate expression of E-cadherin, a cell adhesion protein, loss of which leads to increased metastasis. Further, this regulation appears to involve ER itself, so loss of ER results in loss of E-cadherin, promoting invasive behaviour. This also raises the possibility that in ER-positive tumours, alterations in MTA proteins could lead to invasive behaviour (Kumar, 2003).

15.6 New developments/prospects

It seems clear that hormone-dependent cancers are initiated largely by the same types of carcinogens as other types of cancer and thus therapies such as chemotherapy and radiotherapy can be used with a fair degree of success. However, since the tumours retain hormone responsiveness at least initially, we are also able to manipulate the tumour by manipulating the hormonal environment. The recent huge increase in hormone receptor research has led to many exciting developments, such as the elucidation of the crystal structure of the LBD and the discovery of coactivators and corepressors, which are accelerating the development of new therapies.

15.6.1 Endocrine therapies

It has been mentioned that many of the so-called antagonists used in therapy today are actually partial or mixed antagonists, which under certain circumstances inhibit and under others activate the receptor. Far from being undesirable this is being exploited to develop new hormonal therapies, termed SERMs or SARMs (selective ER/AR modulators). The effects of steroids on different target tissues include protective effects, which physicians would like to preserve in cancer patients. For instance, oestrogens appear to protect against heart disease in women—the risk of heart disease is lower in women then in men until the menopause, when oestrogen levels naturally decline and the risk becomes equal. In pre-menopausal women with breast cancer, pure antioestrogens would have the same effect and effectively increase the risk of heart disease. A SERM which is antioestrogenic in breast and uterus, but oestrogenic in heart tissue and bone, would act as therapy for breast cancer while protecting against uterine cancer, heart disease, and osteoporosis. Pharmaceutical companies are thus making concerted efforts to develop new SERMS with similar activation profiles. SARMs are also a major target of drugs companies, as antiandrogens that reduce AR activity in prostate but not in other target tissues such as erectile tissue and breast adipose tissue would avert side-effects such as impotence and gynaecomastia. Another advantage of having a wide range of hormone antagonists licensed for use in cancer therapy is that when a patient relapses on treatment with one antiandrogen or antioestrogen, switching to another type known to act via different mechanisms may be effective. While this is not yet routinely tried in prostate cancer therapy, two-thirds of women with breast cancer who developed resistance to tamoxifen showed improvement on treatment with the pure antioestrogen faslodex. An important implication of this is that the ER signalling pathway is still driving tumour growth in these women.

15.6.2 Non-endocrine therapies

Novel therapeutic targets for hormone-dependent cancers have been identified as a result of the research on steroid mechanisms of action. For instance, a peptide containing an LxxLL motif could act as a competitive inhibitor to prevent coactivators binding to the AF2 of hormone receptors and would have application in any hormone-driven pathway. The problem here may be in refining the system to prevent global inhibition of hormone pathways, either by targeting or by increasing our knowledge of receptor specificity for different motifs. If corepressors prove to be bona fide essential proteins for antagonist function, a targeted local increase in corepressors could be used to improve the response to antagonist therapy.

The discovery that in a subset of breast cancers, HAT coactivators are increased has led to the development of HAT inhibitors as possible future therapies for hormone-resistant cancer. Conversely, it might be expected that increasing HDAC activity would be beneficial, by increasing repression of target genes, but in fact the opposite appears to be true. Breast cancer cell lines are growth-inhibited by the HDAC inhibitor trichostatin A (TSA) and rodent models of breast cancer have shown tumour regression and differentiation in the presence of HDAC inhibitors, which have the advantage of low toxicity. HDAC inhibitors are thus currently in clinical trials for use in breast cancer patients and the results are encouraging. Their efficacy presumably is not linked to suppression of corepressor activity, but to lifting inappropriate repression of genes and promoting differentiation, as suspected in the case of acute promyelocytic leukaemia (Vigushin and Coombes, 2002). The fact is that it is not at all clear by what mechanisms HDAC inhibitors are inhibiting APL or breast cancer, but it is not unusual for therapies to be used successfully for many years before how they are working becomes clear, if indeed it ever does—tamoxifen being a case in point.

15.6.3 Cancer prevention

As one in nine women in the United States and United Kingdom are likely to suffer from breast cancer during their lifetime, prevention is a major issue. As tamoxifen has been so effective as a therapy for metastatic breast cancer and in prolonging the relapse-free period, presumably by inhibiting development of micrometastases, several clinical trials have been initiated to evaluate its effectiveness as a preventative agent. A trial in the United States appeared to show a high success rate, but was stopped early due to premature disclosure of the results, while trials in the United Kingdom and Italy showed little benefit (Ali and Coombes, 2002). The antioestrogen raloxifene is now being tested with more encouraging results, and has the added benefit of being an inhibitor of ER activity in endometrium thus it should not increase risk of endometrial tumours.

Currently, the major challenge in treatment of hormone-dependent cancers is to exploit their hormone-responsiveness for as long as possible, to prolong the relapse-free period. This may involve combinations of therapies, such as gonadal ablation plus antihormone therapy. It may involve swapping therapies as soon as one fails—this is becoming more effective as new second-line therapies are being developed, such as aromatase inhibitors for breast cancer which may even be more effective than tamoxifen treatment for postmenopausal women. However, the ultimate goal will be to develop effective therapies for the truly hormone-independent stage of the disease, therapies aimed at the new targets constantly being identified by the research surrounding these cancers.

References

Ali, S. and Coombes, R. C. C. (2002). Endocrine-responsive breast cancer and strategies for combating resistance. *Nat Rev Cancer*, **2**, 101–12.

Ben-Jonathan, N., Liby, K., McFarland, M., and Zinger, M. (2002). Prolactin as an autocrine/paracrine growth factor in human cancer. *TEM*, **13**, 245–50.

Bevan, C. L. and Parker, M. G. (1999). The role of coactivators in steroid hormone action. *Exp Cell Res*, **253**, 349–56.

Brzozowski, A. M., Pike, A. C. W., Dauter, Z., Hubbard, R. E., Bonn, T., Engstrsm, O. et al. (1997). Molecular basis of agonism and antagonism in the oestrogen receptor. *Nature*, **389**, 753–8.

Cancer Research UK (2003). CancerStats: Incidence-UK, London.

Claessens, F., Verrijdt, G., Schoenmakers, E., Haelens, A., Peeters, B., Verhoeven, G. et al. (2001). Selective DNA binding by the androgen receptor as a mechanism for hormone-specific gene regulation. *J Steroid Biochem Mol Biol*, **76**, 23–30.

Craft, N., Shostak, Y., Carey, M., and Sawyers, C. L. (1999). A mechanism for hormone-independent prostate cancer through modulation of androgen receptor signaling by the HER-2/neu tyrosine kinase. *Nat Med*, **5**, 280–5.

Culig, Z., Hobisch, A., Cronauer, M. V., Radmayr, C., Trapman, J., Hittmair, A. et al. (1994). Androgen receptor activation in prostatic tumor cell lines by insulin-like growth factor-I, keratinocyte growth factor, and epidermal growth factor. *Cancer Res.*, **54**, 5474–8.

Daliani, D. and Papandreou, C. N. (1999). Markers of androgen-independent progression of prostatic carcinoma. *Semin Oncol*, **26**, 399–406.

Dauvois, S., White, R., and Parker, M. G. (1993). The antiestrogen ICI 182780 disrupts estrogen receptor nucleocytoplasmic shuttling. *J Cell Sci*, **106**, 1377–88.

Dowsett, M. (1997). Aromatase inhibitors come of age. *Annal Oncol*, **8**, 631–2.

Emens, J. M. (1999). Hormones (including diethylstilboestrol) and vaginal and vulval cancer. In *Hormones and Cancer* (Eds., P.M.S. O'Brien, and A. B. MacLean,) RCOG Press, London, pp. 124–135.

Escriva, H., Delaunay, F. and Laudet, V. (2000). Ligand binding and nuclear receptor evolution. *Bioessays*, **22**, 717–27.

Feldman, B. J. and Feldman, D. (2001). The development of androgen-independent prostate cancer. *Nat Rev Cancer*, **1**, 34–45.

Foster, C. S., Cornford, P., Forsyth, L., Djamgoz, M. B., and Ke, Y. (1999). The cellular and molecular basis of prostate cancer. *BJU Int*, **83**, 171–94.

Gangloff, M., Ruff, M., Eiler, S., Duclaud, S., Wurtz, J. M., and Moras, D. (2001). Crystal structure of a mutant hERa ligand-binding domain reveals key structural features for the mechanism of partial agonism. *J Biol Chem*, **276**, 15059–65.

Gottlieb, B., Beitel, L. K., Lumbroso, R., Pinsky, L., and Trifiro, M. (1999). Update of the androgen receptor gene mutations database. *Hum Mut.*, **14**, 103–14.

Hu, X. and Lazar, M. A. (2000). Transcriptional repression by nuclear hormone receptors. *Trends Endocrinol Metab*, **11**, 6–10.

Jenster, G. (1999). The role of the androgen receptor in the development and progression of prostate cancer. *Semin Oncol*, **26**, 407–21.

Johnson, M. H. and Everitt, B. J. (1995). *Chapter 2: Reproductive Messengers*,. Blackwell Science, Oxford.

Kadanoga, J. T. (1998). Eukaryotic transcription: an interlaced network of transcription factors and chromatin-modifying machines. *Cell*, **92**, 307–13.

Keeney, G. L. (2001). Ovarian tumours with endocrine manifestations. In *Endocrinology*, Vol. 3 (Eds., L. J. DeGroot, and J. L. Jameson,) W. B. Saunders Co., Philadelphia, pp. 2172–9.

Kumar, R. (2003). Another tie that binds the MTA family to breast cancer. *Cell*, **113**, 142–3.

Labrie, F., Luu-The, V., Labrie, C., Bélanger, A., Simard, J., Lin, S. X. et al. (2003). Endocrine and intracrine sources of androgens in women: inhibition of breast cancer and other roles of androgens and their precursor dehydroepiandrosterone. *Endocr Rev*, **24**, 152–182.

Lavinsky, R. M., Jepsen, K., Heinzel, T., Torchia, J., Mullen, T.-M., Schiff, R. et al. (1998). Diverse signalling pathways modulate nuclear receptor recruitment of N-CoR and SMRT complexes. *Proc Natl Acad Sci USA*, **95**, 2920–5.

Liao, L., Kuang, S. Q., Yuan, Y., Gonzalez, S. M., O'Malley, B. W., and Xu, J. (2002). Molecular structure and biological function of the cancer-amplified nuclear receptor coactivator SRC-3/AIB1. *J Steroid Biochem Mol Biol*, **83**, 3–14.

Liehr, J. G. (2000). Is estradiol a genotoxic mutagenic carcinogen? *Endocr Rev*, **21**, 40–54.

Marshall, J. C. (2001). Regulation of gonadotropin synthesis and secretion. In *Endocrinology*, Vol. 3 (Eds., L. J. DeGroot, and J. L. Jameson) W. B. Saunders Co., Philadelphia, pp. 1916–25.

McKenna, N. J., Lanz, R. B., and O'Malley, B. W. (1999). Nuclear receptor coregulators: cellular and molecular biology. *Endocrine Rev*, **20**, 321–344.

Oñate, S. A., Tsai, S. Y., Tsai, M.-J., and O'Malley, B. W. (1995). Sequence and characterization of a coactivator for the steroid hormone receptor superfamily. *Science*, **270**, 1354–7.

Pietras, R. J., Arboleda, J., Reese, D. M., Wongvipat, N., Pegram, M. D., Ramos, L. et al. (1995). HER-2 tyrosine kinase pathway targets estrogen receptor and promotes hormone-independent growth in human breast cancer cells. *Oncogene*, **10**, 2435–46.

Selby, C. (1990). Sex hormone binding globulin: origin function and clinical significance. *Ann Clin Biochem*, **27**, 532–41.

Smith, E. P., Boyd, J., Frank, G. R., Takahashi, H., Cohen, R. M., Specker, B. et al. (1994). Estrogen resistance caused by a mutation in the estrogen-receptor gene in a man. *N Engl J Med*, **331**, 1056–61.

Sommer, S. and Fuqua, S. A. W. (2001). Estrogen receptor and breast cancer. *Semin Cancer Biol*, **11**, 339–52.

Terzolo, M., Reimondo, G., Ali, A., Bovio, S., Daffara, F., Paccotti, P. et al.(2001). Ectopic ACTH syndrome: molecular bases and clinical heterogeneity. *Ann Oncol*, **12 (Suppl)**, 83–7.

Thompson, A. (2001). Role of androgens and fibroblast growth factors in prostatic development. *Reproduction*, **121**, 187–95.

Tsai, M.-J. and O'Malley, B. (1994). Molecular mechanisms of action of steroid/thyroid receptor superfamily members. *Annu. Rev. Biochem*, **63**, 451–86.

Vigushin, D. M. and Coombes, R. C. (2002). Histone deacetylase inhibitors in cancer treatment. *Anticancer Drugs*, **13**, 1–13.

Weihua, Z., Makela, S., Andersson, L. C., Salmi, S., Saji, S., Webster, J. I. et al. (2001). A role for estrogen receptor beta in the regulation of growth of the ventral prostate. *Proc Natl Acad Sci USA*, **98**, 6330–5.

Wurtz, J.-M., Bourguet, W., Renaud, J. P., Vivat, V., Chambon, P., Moras, D. et al. (1996). A canonical structure for the ligand-binding domain of nuclear receptors. *Nature Struct Biol*, **3**, 87–94.

Zelent, A., Guidez, F., Melnick, A., Waxman, S., and Licht, J. D. (2001). Translocations of the RARalpha gene in acute promyelocytic leukaemia. *Oncogene*, **20**, 7186–203.

CHAPTER 16

The spread of tumours

Ian Hart

16.1 Introduction

Metastasis is 'the transfer of disease from one organ or part to another not directly connected with it. It may be due to the transfer of pathogenic organisms or to the transfer of cells, as in malignant tumours'. This transfer of cancer cells, which underlies the metastasis of malignant tumours, is perhaps the fundamental problem in oncology. Surgical removal, often combined with irradiation and chemotherapy, frequently is successful in the treatment of primary tumours (particularly when initiated early in tumour development) but widespread dissemination of the cancer cells often defeats this approach to treatment. Neoplastic cell spread is responsible for the major portion of cancer deaths, while the relentless and seemingly intractable movement of a cancer from a primary site to distant organs is a major factor in people's fear of neoplastic disease.

16.1.1 Pathogenesis of the process

Tumour spread is a complex process where the eventual outcome, in terms of secondary tumour development, depends on the result of a number of interactions between the disseminating tumour cell and the cells and tissues of the host. There are five major steps involved in metastasis, though it should be realized that the process, which is a dynamic one, passes from one step to another without interruption while a number of steps will be operating concurrently. Breaking the steps into a neat sequential series of events therefore gives a sense that there is more apparent order to the phenomenon than may actually be the case.

Following tumour initiation and growth of the primary tumour mass (dealt with elsewhere in this volume) there must be:-

(1) invasion and infiltration of cancer cells into surrounding normal host tissue with penetration of small vascular channels or lymphatics;
(2) release of tumour cells, either as individual cells or as small clumps, into the lumen of the penetrated vessels;
(3) survival of the tumour cells in the circulation;
(4) arrest of the surviving cancer cells in the capillary beds of distant organs; and
(5) extravasation (or movement out of the lumen of the arresting lymphatic or blood vessel), followed by growth, of the disseminating tumour cells at the distant site (see Figure 16.1).

If all these steps are completed the result will be the formation of a secondary tumour in a distant organ.

As mentioned in Chapter 1 tumours typically have been thought not to come into existence with all their characteristics pre-developed. This view of cancer as being one of static populations of cells which merely grow has been replaced by one in which they are seen as dynamic entities where there is a gradual acquisition of new characteristics

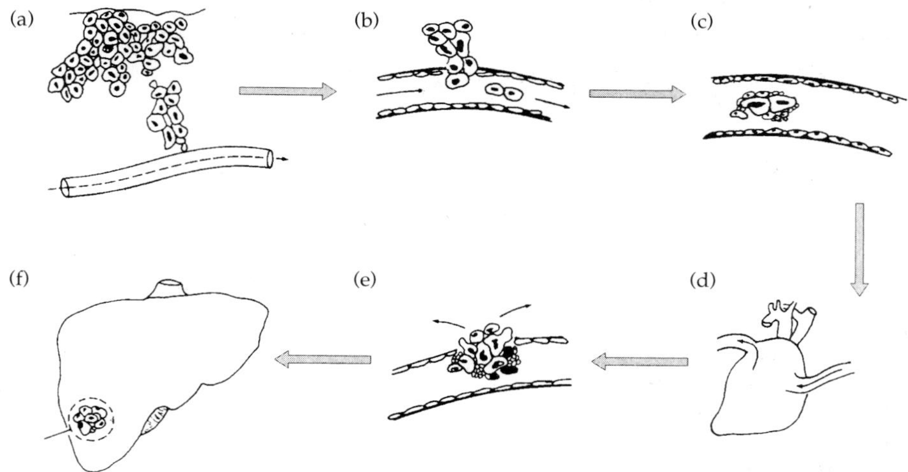

Figure 16.1 The spread of malignant tumours, (a) Primary tumour invades and spreads into adjacent normal tissue, eventually coming into contact with small blood vessels or lymphatics. (b) These small vessels are penetrated by tumour cells which are releazed into the circulation. (c) In the circulation a number of interactions occur between the releazed tumour cells and circulating host cells, such as platelets, lymphocytes, and monocytes. (d) The passage of individual neoplastic cells or small emboli throughout the body is made possible by a number of junctions between the lymphatics and blood vessels; few tumour cells survive this passage. (e) Those tumour cells that survive must arrest in distant organs, possibly in mixed clumps containing both neoplastic cells and platelets or lymphocytes, breach the integrity of the vessel wall, and move out into the surrounding normal tissues. (f) Growth of such extravasating tumour cells give rise to secondary tumour deposits (here shown growing in the liver) and the process may be repeated.

as the tumour develops. This process has been termed 'tumour progression' and, in general, the trend is for tumours to go from 'bad to worse'. Thus, with tumour progression, there is a movement towards a more aggressive behavioural pattern and it has been considered that the ability to invade and to metastasize may not be manifested until relatively late in the course of neoplastic development. Some of the possible difficulties and contradictions in this view of the process of evolution and progression are discussed later in this chapter. However, for the present, it should be considered that the fully malignant tumour cell, that is, one which is able to invade and metastasize, might differ considerably in its characteristics from a cancer cell in its early stages of the transformation process. Modern techniques, such as microarray analysis of gene expression, have been able to shed considerable light on which genes need to be expressed in order to render tumour cells metastatic and, as a consequence of this knowledge, the encoded proteins provide targets, which might be exploited to prevent the process from occurring. Since, for the vast majority (about 80%) of tumours, the likelihood of metastasis occurring is in direct proportion to the size of the primary tumour mass it may be that the propensity to spread is a consequence of the gradual step-wise acquisition of these characteristics or, alternatively, that the stochastic nature of the process simply dictates that the larger the number of cancer cells the greater the random possibility that some will spread and survive to establish distant growths. We will examine evidence for and against these possibilities at the end of this chapter.

16.1.2 Loss of cell–cell cohesion

About 90–95% of human cancers are carcinomas, that is, epithelial in origin (see Chapter 2), and thus a loss of normal epithelial tissue cohesion, which depends on cell–cell adhesion, is a pre-requisite of cancer cell spread. To a large extent this cell–cell cohesion of normal epithelial cells is mediated via members of the cadherin superfamily and, in particular, by E-(for epithelial) cadherin, which is a so-called 'classical cadherin'. Cadherins represent a family of transmembrane, cell–cell adhesion molecules which mediate predominantly homotypic cell–cell (i.e. between cells of the same type) interactions in a calcium-dependent fashion. The highly conserved cytoplasmic tails of the cadherins interact via a series of linking intracellular proteins (α-, β-, and γ-catenin in the case of the classical cadherins) with the cytoskeleton (the actin filaments in classical cadherins) thereby providing a link from the exterior of the cell to the cellular machinery responsible for changes in cell shape and migratory activity. Many investigations into clinical cancer have indicated that loss of E-cadherin protein, primarily as detected by immunohistochemistry, is a common finding in more aggressive/advanced carcinomas. The conclusion is that movement of transformed epithelial cells requires down-regulation of E-cadherin levels or function to permit the occurrence of the initial events in tumour cell spread. This loss of cell surface-located cadherin may arise through a variety of mechanisms. Thus it may relate to inactivation, via mutations in the gene, as occurs in invasive lobular carcinoma of the breast, or to silencing at the transcriptional level via a mechanism such as methylation of the promoter region (see Chapter 5) of the E-cadherin gene, as occurs in colorectal cancer. Recently the transcription factors *Snail* and *Slug*, identified originally as playing a role in the development of lower organisms, have been identified as direct transcriptional repressors of E-cadherin expression; raising the possibility that increased expression of these transcription factors in cancer may be associated with the loss of differentiation and acquisition of metastatic activity that follows the loss of normal epithelial architecture. At the time of writing an extremely exciting report has just been published which links control of the *Snail* transcription factor to oestrogen receptor (ER) signalling. The report suggests that the loss of ER, and ER-negative breast carcinomas generally have a poor prognosis, is associated with increased *Snail* levels and concomitant down-regulation of E-cadherin, providing a logical basis for the increased invasion and metastasis associated with this poorer prognosis subset of breast cancers (Fujita et al., 2003).

16.2 Mechanisms of tumour invasion

Of the five steps outlined above as being essential for the pathogenesis of cancer spread, two depend on the ability of tumour cells to invade or infiltrate into areas of normal tissue. The process of tumour invasion has been defined as 'a derangement in the proper sorting of cell populations, causing a violation of normal tissue boundaries'. In recent years there has been considerable investigation of two of the three proposed mechanisms of tumour cell invasion and we now understand much regarding the molecular basis of steps 2 and 3 below. The three general mechanisms are

(1) mechanical pressure;
(2) release of lytic enzymes; and
(3) the increased motility of tumour cells either as individual cells or as small clumps.

Interestingly, while it has been steps 2 and 3 that have received the most experimental investigation it quite probably is mechanism 1, which accounts for a large amount of the observed invasion by carcinomas. Process 1 though is difficult to analyse in the reductionist way that forms the backbone of most experimental investigations. The absence of appropriate and well-defined model systems with which to interrogate this possibility has inevitably led to a shift in the focus of researchers which does not necessarily reflect the primacy of the mechanism in the tumours which matter, that is, those which arise spontaneously in man.

Obviously these mechanisms are not mutually exclusive and it is possible that in any given tumour a combination of all three processes may be involved in mediating invasion with the relative importance of each process varying both according to tumour type and to the anatomical location in the tumour-bearing host where the invasion is occurring.

As covered elsewhere in this volume (Chapter 1) neoplastic cells are characterized by their unregulated proliferation and this proliferation within a confined tumour mass may build up pressure which forces sheets, or fingers, of tumour cells along lines of least mechanical resistance in the surrounding tissue. This process may be analogous to the way that plants force their roots through the soil. According to this hypothesis invasion simply is a direct consequence of uncontrolled growth causing pressure from the growing tumour mass. The fact that the expansion of the tumour blocks or occludes local blood vessels and lymphatics and leads to local normal tissue death, with a concomitant reduction in mechanical resistance, further facilitates the process. It certainly is true that the gross appearance of many malignant tumours conforms to this concept, with finger-like projections of contiguous cords of tumour cells emanating from the main cancer mass. It also is true, however, that there are many observations, both experimental and clinical, which cannot be explained solely by this hypothesis. For example, some highly invasive tumours grow more slowly than their benign counterparts; this would not be expected were pressure building up from increased individual cell proliferation the sole requisite for invasive behaviour. Equally, serial histological sections, which take in isolated individual tumour cells or small clumps of invading cells and then track back to the main tumour mass, often reveal no connection of these isolated neoplastic cells with the main neoplasm; it is difficult to explain how such cells could have got to such a position without the involvement of active amoeboid movement on their part. Finally, cancer cells can often invade and penetrate loose tissue, or even infiltrate from the surface of the tissue, where it would not seem possible to build up any pressure effect. Thus mechanisms 2 and 3 have to be invoked to explain how many invading cancer cells have accomplished this infiltrative process.

As stated above there has been considerable work on these possible driving forces behind tumour cell invasion and the rather basic summary given here is expanded on by some excellent reviews listed in the references and further reading section at the end of this chapter. Normal host tissue adjacent to areas of tumour invasion frequently is severely disrupted and shows considerable amounts of lytic damage. Since many animal and human tumours have higher levels of proteases and collagenases (enzymes capable of digesting proteins and extracellular matrix components such as the collagens) than do their normal counterpart tissues, the concept has arisen that malignant tumours produce and secrete lytic enzymes capable of degrading normal tissue. Even now, after years of investigation, there are difficulties involved in establishing the precise molecular mechanisms that lie behind such correlations between malignant behaviour and increased proteolytic enzyme activity, which have been established by biochemical analysis. Direct sampling of tissue (biopsy) actually can induce damage in the sampled tissue which in itself may give rise to the observed elevated levels of enzyme activity. Moreover, tumours are not composed solely of neoplastic cells but instead contain both neoplastic cells and infiltrating normal stromal cells (indeed some tumours apparently may contain more normal cells and normal tissue than they contain neoplastic cells). Many of these infiltrating cells, such as the monocytes and polymorphonuclear leucocytes, contain high levels of exactly those enzymes thought to be involved in tissue degradation (they may well use these enzymes to facilitate their own invasive abilities) such that it is their presence which contributes to the lytic activity determined by direct sampling. Using combinations of *in situ* hybridization, to determine mRNA production, and immunohistochemistry, to localize protein, it has become apparent that the tumour cells themselves may have a direct influence on surrounding or juxtaposed normal cells, causing them to elaborate the tissue-degrading enzymes which cause tissue damage and promote tumour cell invasion. Thus the majority of the proteases which complex at the invasive front of a tumour may not be contributed by the invading carcinoma cells themselves but are contributed by the stromal cells, such as fibroblasts, inflammatory cells, and endothelial cells, whose production of these enzymes is under the control of various soluble mediators produced by the carcinoma cells themselves. Interestingly some of these matrix-degrading enzymes may not only play a role in breaking down the proteins of the extracellular matrix, thereby allowing the penetration of invading cancer cells, but they also can influence tumour cell proliferation. They do this by releasing growth factors, which have been sequestered within the extracellular matrix (ECM), which can then act in a paracrine fashion on those tumour cells which express the cognate receptor for such growth-stimulating molecules.

There are numerous reports in the clinical literature where correlations have been established between the amounts of proteolytic enzymes detected in cancer samples and increased tumour progression, that is, those cancers where the highest levels of enzymatic activity have been determined frequently have the worst prognosis or outlook. However, the central portions of many large tumours often are necrotic and it may be that the death of cells in these areas releases enzymes; these show up in the measurements made but they may have no direct involvement in determining the actual invasive behaviour which occurs in the viable, peripheral rim of the tumour. For these reasons perhaps the most compelling evidence on the role of proteolytic enzymes in tumour invasion has come from experimental studies. Here it has proved possible to modulate enzyme production by tumour cells grown in tissue culture, either up- or down-regulated, and to correlate this capacity with the subsequent invasive behaviour of the cells in *in vitro* analyses or *in vivo* after transplantation into animals. However, the problem with such analyses is, as discussed above, that in the natural situation the tumour cells may not be the source of these enzymes and that the model systems are simplified to such an extent that they fail to take into account the complex cellular interactions that inevitably occur in a growing tumour mass. Thus these enzymes play a fundamental role in the process of angiogenesis (covered in Chapter 17), in part by facilitating the invasion and penetration of endothelial cells (a process very analogous to tumour cell invasion) and in part by causing the liberation of pro-angiogenic molecules which have been sequestered by the ECM. It may be that their role in facilitating tumour neovascularization through empowering normal endothelial cells to invade is what may enhance metastatic spread and not through a direct tumour-mediated effect that would be detected by the *in vitro* cell based approaches. For these reasons the supplementary information which has been derived from 'knock-out' mice (see Chapter 19) has been particularly useful. In general tumours growing in mice where the individual genes for members of the various protease families have been knocked out or eliminated are less aggressive than those growing in the control, wild-type mice. Such tumours in the knockout mice seem to have a reduced capacity to invade and metastasize. Again though caution should be exercised in the interpretation of such results which, at face value, appear to support an unequivocal role for proteases in mediating tumour invasion. This is because, as already emphasized, the proteases may have multiple roles to play in the pathogenesis of tumour growth as well as in regulating invasive behaviour. Reduced invasive and metastatic capacity may just be a reflection of reduced tumour size.

Notwithstanding these reservations the case for the involvement of proteolytic enzymes in tumour invasion is a compelling one and considerable effort has been made to develop synthetic enzyme inhibitors, which can block this enzymatic activity and thereby block the invasive behaviour of tumour cells. That clinical studies using such inhibitors have met with such limited success should not be taken as evidence that the postulated involvement of the targeted enzymes in invasion is incorrect. The proteases are not released diffusely into the extracellular milieu but, instead, may be focused at sites of tumour cell-extracellular matrix attachment, often by an interaction with members of the integrin family of adhesion receptors (see later), and getting the inhibitors to such protected sites of activity may be a particularly difficult proposition.

It is apparent that tissues vary considerably in their ability to withstand tumour invasion. Thus tumours rarely penetrate the walls of arteries, arterioles, or even the larger veins while they readily invade the walls of capillaries and lymphatics. Such resistance is thought to be due, in part, to greater mechanical strength of the larger vessels but there also is the suggestion that certain of those tissues which are resistant to invasion, such as cartilage or the elastic fibres surrounding the larger blood vessels, do so as a consequence of the release of cell-produced factors that inhibit proteases. These factors bind, in a one to one stoichiometric fashion, to both inactive and active proteolytic enzymes and thereby inhibit their capacity to initiate proteolytic degradation.

The probable involvement of active tumour cell motility in the process of cancer invasion seems equally likely at an intuitive level yet has proven just as difficult to establish unequivocally. Thus the finding of individual tumour cells, or small clumps of tumour cells, which are separate from and have no obvious connection with the main tumour mass, has been taken as a certain indication of individual tumour cell motility. Cinematography has been used to show that cancer cells in the body are, as they are in tissue culture, capable of active movement and migration. Moreover blocking the cells' motility machinery (either by controlled regulation of gene expression or by pharmacological inhibition) in experimental systems can lead to the inhibition of tumour spread. It seems highly likely therefore that the ability of neoplastic cells to move through normal tissues involves at least some component of active locomotion. A possible criticism of the data in the literature is that most of the studies which have been conducted on the active motility of tumour cells have been undertaken within the 2D constraints of the tissue culture dish. However, recently more relevant 3D models have become available which also have shown that cancer cells manifest a number of migratory and invasive mechanisms and, moreover, that they can shift from one to another of these mechanisms during the process of invasion should specific pathways be blocked. How tumour cells interact with the extracellular matrix largely is through the members of the integrin family of cell surface receptors. These heterodimeric glycoproteins, composed of non-covalently associated α and β subunits, not only mediate attachment to the various extracellular matrix component ligands but also serve as transducing molecules, capable of evoking changes in gene expression as a consequence of such attachment; so-called 'outside-in' signalling. Conversely, by activating or de-activating these molecules ('inside-out' signalling), the integrin-expressing cell is able to rapidly modulate and control adhesive and de-adhesive activity which is such an important component of cellular motility. While the situation is far from clear-cut there is a suggestion that, in carcinomas, there is a general down-regulation of integrin levels with increasing malignancy though there is considerable evidence that an increase in one particular integrin heterodimer, $\alpha6\beta4$, may be associated with an increased migratory activity in a range of tumour types.

16.3 Dissemination of tumour cells via the lymphatics or the blood vessels

Once a tumour cell enters the lumen of a lymphatic or a blood vessel it can either remain there, at the site of penetration, and grow with the consequent occlusion of that vessel or individual cancer cells or small clumps (emboli) of cells may be released and carried away in the lymph or the blood. The release of individual cells or small emboli within the circulation may be attributable to the less strong cohesion that malignant cancer cells exhibit to each other (see earlier in this chapter).

It is a common clinical observation that carcinomas, which are epithelial in origin, generally spread initially via the lymphatic system while the sarcomas, which are of mesenchymal origin, appear to spread via the haematogenous route. This may be an arbitrary division. There are connections between the lymphatics and the blood vessels and experimental analyses, using radio-labelled circulating tumour cells, have shown that such cancer cells are capable of moving between these two systems. This is either through direct veno-lymphatic communications (anastomoses) or from the lymphatics through the thoracic duct, which then empties into the jugular vein and the venous circulation.

It is known that the newly developed blood vessels which form during the process of tumour angiogenesis are irregular and chaotic in their structure and have vessel walls which contain widened interendothelial junctions and defective basement membranes that permit the easier access of tumour cells into the circulation. Once entered into the vessel lumen the disseminating cancer cell encounters sluggish, non-laminar blood flow, which is conducive to tumour cell survival. All these features might explain why the numbers of new blood vessels within a tumour frequently have been shown to serve as prognostic indicators, that is, the greater the number of new blood vessels within or adjacent to a tumour the more likely it is that metastasis will occur.

The situation with regard to the penetration of lymphatic vessels (probably easier to access because apart from the lack of a continuous basement membrane, poor interendothelial junctions and frequent gaps which they share with new tumour capillaries, they also lack a surrounding layer of pericytes), is much less clear-cut. For many carcinomas the patterns of metastatic spread follow natural drainage routes of afferent lymphatics with sentinel lymph nodes, which are the first to receive drainage, often being preferentially colonized by malignant cells. What is still not clear is whether this represents invasion into a pre-existent lymphatic system, which may be more dense in epithelial tissues, or whether it is the consequence of *de novo* formation of lymphatic capillaries (lymphangiogenesis). A few years ago most pathologists would have said that lymphatics did not occur within tumour tissue and this, in part, was one contributing reason for the increased hydrostatic pressure observed within many tumour masses. In part this failure to identify lymphatic vessels within tumours might be attributable to a lack of specific immuno-histochemical markers (a similar situation had existed with regard to tumour blood vessels up to the early 1990s). Recently though the development of reagents which recognize specific markers of lymphatic endothelium has facilitated the detection of lymphatic vessels both around and within the periphery of tumours. Early results using these reagents appear to be indicative of the occurrence of lymphangiogenesis in a range of cancer types. These dilated and engorged lymphatics, which often are observed around the tumour/stroma interface and which may occasionally penetrate the tumour rim, appear to be a consequence of expression of a specific lymphangiogenic factor (a particular member of the VEGF family which has been known to be the major growth factor family involved in stimulating angiogenic development). Enhanced expression of this VEGF member (VEGF-C) has been associated with increased tumour spread in both experimental studies and clinical analyses.

Also from both clinical observations and experimental studies it is known that the mere presence of neoplastic cells within either circulatory system (i.e. blood or lymph) does not necessarily constitute metastasis. Cells in these fluids may not survive to establish a distant tumour. Refinements in molecular biology and immunohistochemistry have been able to demonstrate that blood and bone marrow samples taken from cancer patients often contain disseminating cancer cells. However, the process of metastasis is an inefficient one with most of the cells which are released into the circulation dying without forming a metastatic deposit. Much of this death may be attributable to non-specific factors, such as turbulence, or it may be a consequence of specific immuno-mediated destruction of the circulating cancer cells. As will be discussed below, the way the body potentially reacts to tumour cells in the circulation may be 'double-edged'. Thus aggregation, either with other tumour cells or with host cells such as lymphocytes and platelets, may result in the formation of larger heterotypic emboli, which are more easily filtered out in arresting capillary beds. Moreover this aggregation into clumps with non-neoplastic cells may provide a protective outer layer, which prevents damage to the central tumour cells and thereby protects them from both turbulence and immune attack.

In order to leave the circulation tumour cells must be arrested and must implant in the capillary bed of a distant organ or lymph node. Generally circulating tumour cells do not adhere to the walls of the large vessels where, presumably, blood flow is sufficiently vigorous to sweep them away but instead attach to the walls of the narrower capillaries in the capillary bed. This arrest may be non-specific, as in the case of the large emboli, or it may represent an active process. It has been shown experimentally that tumour cells, like platelets, generally do not adhere to intact non-activated endothelium but rather they attach preferentially to exposed basement membrane. Tissue culture studies have suggested that the tumour cells themselves stimulate endothelial cell retraction and loss (though the shedding of endothelial cells from blood vessel walls is a normal physiological process) and cause exposure of the underlying basement membrane. This endothelial damage leads to tumour cell and platelet adherence and tumour cell/platelet clumps may attach passively to such areas of endothelial retraction. Equally it also has become apparent that there are selective interactions between endothelial cells and tumour cells which are regulated by specific receptor/ligand interactions and which, if appropriate changes occur in the endothelial cells, can lead to the direct interaction of tumour cells with intact endothelium.

For example, it is known that leucocyte extravasation at sites of inflammation is controlled by upregulation of adhesion receptors on activated endothelium in response to inflammatory cytokines. These receptors bind specific molecules, members of the selectin and integrin family of attachment proteins, expressed by the leucocytes and mediate trans-endothelial movement. Interestingly many tumour cells express and secrete precisely the inflammatory cytokines known to activate endothelium and they already express the specific receptors for the up-regulated molecules at their cell surface. The possibility exists, therefore, that the tumour cells simply mimic the mechanisms used by normal cells to extravasate at distant sites and utilize most of the same molecules to achieve these ends.

16.4 Patterns of metastatic spread

Certain tumours frequently metastasize to particular organs. Thus, for example, neuroblastomas most commonly spread to the liver whereas osteosarcomas normally give rise to pulmonary metastases. The reasons for this organ selectivity of colonization are unknown but three general hypotheses have been proposed to explain the phenomenon. In the first hypothesis, the so-called mechanistic theory, the eventual site of metasatic development is held to be a consequence solely of the anatomical location of the primary tumour. In other words the number of viable tumour cells delivered to the capillary bed of the first organ encountered is due simply to the pattern of blood flow. Thus venous blood flow from the large bowel goes to the liver through the portal veins and, probably as a consequence of this, the liver therefore is the commonest site for secondary deposits from bowel tumours. Although this frequently invoked explanation undoubtedly is true for many tumours it does not explain all patterns of cancer spread. For example, muscle is well vascularized and the kidney receives up to 25% of cardiac blood output yet both these organs are involved infrequently in metastasis formation. The second hypothesis or concept which has gained much currency in recent years has been based to a large extent upon particularly clever experiments using Phage display peptide libraries injected intravenously into mouse and human recipients. These studies have revealed that the endothelium of blood vessels in specific tissue or organs is able to recognize specific peptide sequences expressed by particular phage. The obvious inference is that the endothelial cells express specific receptors which bind to specific ligands (represented by the peptide sequences expressed by the phage) and that there are, therefore, potential differences between organ endothelia in their capacity to bind circulating agents. While this phenomenon is now being examined as a means of exploiting selective organ delivery of drugs it also is possible that these characteristics could play a role in determining the arrest of circulating tumour cells in specific sites. There has been further support for such a possibility from recent related observations. Like many leucocytes which are involved in selective targeting to particular organs some tumour cells express at their cell surface so-called 'chemokine receptors' which respond to cytokines responsible for stimulating directional motility (chemokines) of target leucocytes. It is believed that an increased expression of these chemokines in particular organs may lead to the selective extravasation of arrested tumour cells, expressing the appropriate chemokine receptor, at those sites and work has established a correlation between those organs which produce the appropriate chemokine and their propensity to be involved with metastatic deposits.

The third hypothesis, suggested approximately 150 years ago by Stephen Paget, is the so-called 'seed and soil' hypothesis. Here it was held that the provision of a fertile environment (the soil) in which compatible tumour cells (the seed) could grow was the determining factor in deciding patterns of metastatic spread. Failure of an organ to support metastatic growth was not a consequence of the failure of disseminating cells to reach that site but was a reflection of the inability of that organ to provide a favourable environment for growth; a situation akin to 'seed falling on stony ground'. There is a remarkable clinical study which supports this contention. Some patients with ovarian cancer have extensive accumulation of fluid in the peritoneal cavity (ascites). To relieve this considerable volume of fluid, which causes marked distress and discomfort, it is necessary to withdraw this fluid. However, repeated withdrawal is an unpleasant procedure and it has proved possible in such patients to insert an artificial shunt from the abdomen directly into the jugular vein. Fluid is thus returned continuously to the venous circulation and the uncomfortable build up of ascites is avoided. It was shown that huge numbers of viable tumour cells were contained within this ascitic fluid and returning them to the jugular veins meant that the first capillary bed encountered was that located in the lungs. In spite of this many patients, who survived this treatment for a number of weeks or more, showed no evidence of pulmonary metastasis; even though many millions of viable tumour cells must have passed into their lungs. According to the mechanistic theory of metastasis development circulating tumour cells should have been filtered out in the lung capillary bed. There has to be some factor which has contributed to this lack of pulmonary metastasis. It could be that the lung lacks the requisite chemokine to stimulate chemokine receptor-mediated motility, that local growth factor production was insufficient or inadequate to support ovarian cancer growth or any other of a number of factors. What it does demonstrate though is that simple tumour cell delivery cannot, on its own, account for all selective patterns of metastatic development.

16.5 The role of the immune system in modulating metastasis

It must be that any influence of the immune system on cancer metastasis occurs after there has been the existence of potentially immunogenic material, in the form of the primary tumour growth, which might be expected to prime the host. Therefore it might be thought that if the immune response against human cancer was in any way to be effective it would particularly be so in determining the elimination of individual cells or small clumps of circulating cancer cells. The role of the immune system in cancer is dealt with in detail elsewhere in this volume (Chapter 20) and it is not the purpose of this section to review this facet of tumour biology. Paradoxically though the immune system does not always exert an inhibitory effect on metastatic development but may act as a 'double edged sword'. Thus the aggregation of lymphocytes with circulating tumour cells may increase the size of emboli, thereby assisting their arrest and lodgement in capillary beds as already discussed. Moreover lymphocytes are capable of inducing angiogenesis, which may actually facilitate the provision of nutrients and allow the proliferation of such arrested tumour cells. The issue of the role of the immune system in modulating metastatic spread is complicated by the fact that the majority of direct investigations into this topic have, of necessity, utilized rodent tumour lines. The relevance of these systems to the human situation is questionable and even though our molecular understanding of the basis of tumour cell/T-cell interactions has been made much clearer at the molecular level in the past decade the way that this actually impinges on the spread of naturally occurring tumours still remains largely unknown.

16.6 Tumour cell heterogeneity and the search for metastasis genes

All neoplastic cells in a single tumour are not identical. Instead they exhibit a range of different characters (phenotype) among which may be the capacity to invade and metastasize. It has been widely accepted, until now, that this acquisition of metastatic ability is a late event in the course of tumour progression. Indeed it was just this view that gave rise to the single most important experiment to have been conducted in metastasis research in the last century. Pondering on the possibility that, since metastasis is an inefficient process, the few cells which do survive to establish metastatic foci do so because they possess characteristics which are different from those of the majority of cancer cells, Fidler and Kripke set out in the mid-1970s to determine if there was a pre-existent metastatic subpopulation of tumour cells. They adapted the Luria–Delbruck fluctuation analysis, used to demonstrate the pre-existence rather than adaptation of resistant bacteria, to investigate metastatic potential of murine tumour cells. Thus an heterogeneous population of tumour cells was split into two; one half was used to derive a series of clones, each derived from a single cell, while the other half was divided into a series of aliquots representing fractions of the bulk population. Matched numbers of cells from the single-cell-derived clones or the multi-cell-derived aliquots were then injected intravenously into cohorts of identical (syngeneic) mice. At a set time after tumour cell injection the groups of mice were killed and the numbers of tumour nodules in the lung were enumerated. This simple experimental model of metastasis showed that the different groups of mice injected with the multi-cell-derived aliquots all had very comparable numbers of lung tumour growths. In marked contrast the lung tumour burden of the groups of mice injected with identical numbers of cells from the single-cell-derived clones varied enormously. Whereas some clones gave rise to only one or two lung nodules other clones gave rise to literally hundreds for the input of the same number of cells. Subcloning experiments showed that the clones 'bred true'; that is low metastatic potential clones remained low and high metastatic potential clones remained high, indicating a heritable basis to this ability to develop into secondary tumours. This classic experiment produced a paradigm-shift in the way that cancer researchers thought about the process of metastasis and set up the search for genes specifically involved in regulating the process of metastasis. To do this they were, for the first time, able to compare matched populations of high- and low-metastatic capacity tumour cells without resorting to the difficulty of comparing unrelated tumour types.

With the advent of microarray technology this approach has proven possible to apply to clinical samples and it is the results from these microarray studies that have engendered renewed debate about the established view of tumour progression. Thus microarrays, with their capacity to interrogate changes in the expression of large numbers of genes in a single experiment, have shown that the gene-expression patterns of metastases may be markedly similar to the primary tumour from which they were derived. This suggests that the major cell population in the primary tumour is almost identical to the cells in the metastases; not what would be expected if metastatic ability had been acquired late in the course of tumour progression and then by only a few cancer cells. Second, using this technology, it has proved possible to determine, with a high degree of accuracy, whether clinical tumours will remain localized or whether they will spread simply by profiling the primary tumour mass; a result which suggests that the characteristics which determine metastatic spread are acquired relatively early in tumorigenesis. A major practical consideration of these studies is that they 'support the emerging notion that the clinical outcome of individuals with cancer can be predicted using the gene-expression profiles of primary tumours at diagnosis'; a possibility which could revolutionize the individual approach to cancer therapy.

The implication of these and other results then is threefold:

(1) That the tendency of a tumour to metastasize is pre-determined by a spectrum of mutations which is acquired relatively early in the course of tumorigenesis; that is, that particular mechanisms of transformation confer the ability to form distant metastases as opposed to a selection process per se allowing the emergence of minor populations.

(2) That, in general, the genes which are changed are those which already are suspected of having a role in tumorigenesis; that is, the known oncogenes and tumour suppressor genes. The implication being that genes which are involved specifically and exclusively in orchestrating metastasis do not exist or are few.

(3) That even relatively small primary tumours may have the capacity to metastasize because of this early acquisition of regulating genetic events; a concept which, as discussed, holds considerable implications for future therapy.

Certainly there are additional elements, apart from just the microarray data, which support this revised view of tumour progression. For example, the ability of primary tumours to spread early is exemplified by primary tumours of unknown origin. This is where the presenting tumour is a secondary deposit and the primary mass is so small that nothing short of a complete histological analysis of the entire body can reveal its location. It does, however, tend to ignore other features/results which do not necessarily sit entirely comfortably with this revised view of tumour progression. Thus the search for genes which are involved in regulating metastasis, sought as a consequence of the Fidler and Kripke experiment, has been successful and has thrown up genes whose differential expression, originally determined in selected rodent tumours, has stood the test of transition to the clinical situation. Metastasis-associated genes (MTAs) constitute a novel gene family, the founding member of which, *MTA1*, originally was identified as a differentially expressed gene in metastatic rat tumours, which seem to function as part of a complex which forms a repressive chromatin state. One of the downstream targets of the MTAs is the transcription factor *Snail* whose effect on the cell–cell adhesion molecule E-cadherin, and thus its effect on tumour dissemination, already has been discussed. Interestingly this family of genes does not occur in the relatively small number of genes characterized as representing the molecular signature of metastasis in the tumours thus far characterized. Was it just that the sub-group of tumours in which these genes play an important role in determining metastasis were not included in the analysis? It seems likely that further and more extensive microarray experiments will clarify these and other points and will enhance our understanding of the nature of metastatic spread. Irrespective of whether the ability to metastasize is a characteristic of only a small sub-set of cells or whether it is inherent in major cellular constituents of small primary tumours is clear that variations in gene expression lie at the heart of the ability of a malignant tumour to spread. Functional analyses of the signature genes identified by microarray analysis should determine what, if any, role they play in the metastatic cascade and could lead eventually to targeting novel therapeutic targets aimed at preventing this most devastating aspect of oncological disease.

References and further reading

Bernards, R. and Weinberg, R. A. (2002). A progression puzzle. *Nature*, **418**, 823.

Chang, C. and Werb, Z. (2001). The many faces of metalloproteases: cell growth, invasion, angiogenesis and metastasis. *Trends Cell Biol*, **11**, S37–S43.

Fidler, J. and Kripke, M. L. (1977). Metastasis results from pre-existent variant cells within a malignant tumor. *Science*, **197**, 893–5.

Fidler, I. J. and Kripke, M. L. (2003). Genomic analysis of primary tumours does not address the prevalence of metastatic cells in the population. *Nature Genet*, **34**, 23.

Friedl, P. and Wolf, K. (2003). Tumour-cell invasion and migration: diversity and escape mechanisms *Nature Rev Cancer*, **3**, 362–74.

Fujita, N., Jaye, D. L., Kajita, M., Geigerman, C., Moreno, C. S., and Wade, P. A. (2003). MTA3, a Mi-2/NuRD complex subunit, regulates an invasive growth pathway in breast cancer. *Cell*, **113**, 207–19.

Jackson, D. G., Prevo, R., Clasper, S., and Banerji, S. (2001). LYVE-1, the lymphatic system and tumour lymphangiogenesis. *Trends Immun*, **22**, 317–21.

Liotta, L. A. and Kohn, E. C. (2001). The microenvironment of the tumour-host interface. *Nature*, **411**, 375–79.

Muller, A., Homey, B., Soto, H., Ge, N., Catron, D., Buchanan, M. E. et al. (2001). Involvement of chemokine receptors in breast cancer metastasis. *Nature*, **410**, 50–6.

Pepper, M. S. (2001). Lymphangiogenesis and tumor metastasis: Myth or reality? *Clin Cancer Res*, **7**, 462–8.

Ramaswamy, S., Ross, K. N., Lander, E. S., and Gloub, T. R. (2003). A molecular signature of metastasis in primary solid tumors. *Nature Genet*, **33**, 49–54.

Theiry, J. P. (2002). Epithelial-mesenchymal transitions in tumour progression *Nature Rev Cancer*, **2**, 442–54.

van de Vijver, M. J., He, Y. D., van't Veer, I. J., Dai, H., Hart, A. A., Voskuil, D. W. et al. (2002). A gene expression signature as a predictor of survival in breast cancer. *N Eng J Med*, **19**, 1999–209.

CHAPTER 17

Tumour angiogenesis

Kiki Tahtis and Roy Bicknell

17.1 Introduction

It is now some 20 years since it became widely appreciated that the growth of solid tumours requires a functional vasculature and that disruption of this functional vasculature could lead to novel anti-cancer therapies. This has led to the development of many anti-angiogenic drugs, the first of which are now completing clinical trial. The purpose of this chapter is to review our current understanding of tumour angiogenesis and what the prospects are for anti-angiogenic therapies.

17.1.1 Angiogenesis

Solid neoplasms, including epithelial cancers, require the formation of a supporting stroma and vascular supply if they are to grow beyond the size of 1–2 mm (Figure 17.1). Epithelial cancers induce the formation of stroma, which is a complex extracellular matrix (ECM) rich tissue that comprises three main components. These include newly formed blood vessels (which supply the tumour with nutrients and also provide a means for gas exchange and waste disposal), activated fibroblasts, and inflammatory infiltrates such as lymphocytes and macrophages, and a complex network of matrix proteins (Figure 17.1) (Dvorak, 1986).

Angiogenesis involves the formation of new capillary microvessels from pre-existing parent vessels. This process is extensive during embryonic development, but restricted in normal adults, occurring only during the female reproductive cycle, wound healing, and in certain disease states such as psoriasis, diabetic retinopathy, and cancer (Gerwins et al., 2000). In the developing embryo, two distinct processes give rise to the embryonic vascular network: vasculogenesis and angiogenesis. Vasculogenesis gives rise to the embryonic blood vessels such as the heart and the first primitive vascular plexus, while angiogenesis is responsible for subsequent remodelling and expansion of the network (Asahara et al., 1997; Patan, 2000). Under normal conditions, endothelial cells (ECs)

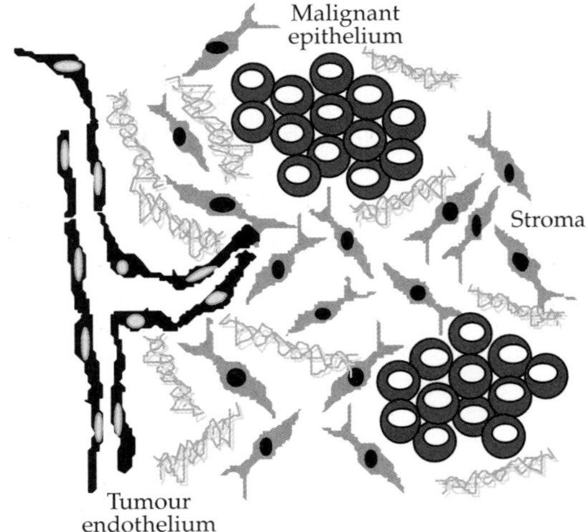

Figure 17.1 Epithelial tumours are comprised of malignant epithelium and stroma. The stroma includes tumour endothelium, activated fibroblasts, inflammatory infiltrates, and matrix proteins.

seldom divide. However, during angiogenesis, quiescent ECs of the post-capillary and small terminal venules are stimulated by a variety of cytokines and growth factors to begin a cascade of events leading to the formation of new vessels. These include proteolytic degradation of the basement membrane, an event closely followed by EC proliferation, directed migration, and differentiation, giving rise to the formation of a lumen or sprout. Newly formed sprouts anastomose with one another, as well as with pre-existing vessels to form a hollow tube through which blood flow starts (Yancopoulos et al., 2000). The newly formed endothelial vessels have been shown to lack cellular differentiation and to have a markedly different morphology from normal vessels. They acquire support from pericytes and a basement membrane, although this is often incomplete, resulting in leaky blood vessels from which protein macromolecules extravasate into the surrounding stroma (Molema et al., 1998). They also undergo alterations in their cell surface expression of adhesion molecules, receptors, and other proteins, characteristically expressing unique antigenic markers such as the VEGF (vascular endothelial growth factor receptor) receptors, integrins such as $\alpha_v\beta_3$ (Hynes, 2002), Delta-4 (Shima and Mailhos, 2000), and the recently discovered EC-specific magic roundabout protein (Huminiecki and Bicknell, 2000; Huminiecki et al., 2002; Suchting et al., 2005).

While angiogenesis is believed to result exclusively from the proliferation, migration, and remodelling of fully differentiated ECs, vasculogenesis refers to the formation of embryonic blood vessels from EC progenitors or angioblasts (Yancopoulos et al., 1998). However, in a study by Asahara et al. (1997) isolated human EC progenitors from peripheral blood, were capable of differentiating into mature ECs both in *in vitro* and *in vivo* experiments, incorporating into sites of active angiogenesis. Later studies showed that circulating EC progenitors were mobilized in response to tissue ischaemia or cytokine therapy, thereby augmenting neovascularization of ischaemic tissues (Takahashi et al., 1999). These findings imply that post-natal vascularization (angiogenesis) does not rely exclusively on sprouting from pre-existing blood vessels. Instead bone marrow derived EC progenitors may also contribute to angiogenesis (Asahara et al., 1997; Asahara et al., 1999; Takahashi et al., 1999). Studies by Lyden et al. (2001), have also confirmed that endothelial progenitor cells arising in the bone marrow are active in tumour angiogenesis and are significant contributors to tumour vasculature. These findings arose from work in which it was found that adult mice that expressed reduced levels of the transcription factor Id were unable to support tumour angiogenesis (Lyden et al., 1999). The Id proteins interact with other transcription factors to modulate cellular differentiation in early foetal development. It was subsequently shown that transplantation of β-galactosidase expressing wild type bone marrow into lethally irradiated *Id*-mutant mice was sufficient to restore vascularization of implanted tumours (Lyden et al., 2001). If tumours are achieving substantial vascularization by recruitment of circulating endothelial progenitors this has profound implications for the development of new strategies to block tumour angiogenesis.

17.1.2 The tumour stromal compartment

Neovascularization is accompanied by the formation of a supporting stromal network in tumour lesions, which often makes up between 20 and 50% of the mass of a solid tumour (Figure 17.1). Depending on the type of neoplasm, the amount and composition of the stroma varies and in some cancers may contribute to more than 90% of the mass of the tumour (Niedermeyer et al., 1997). The

ECM of tumour stroma comprises fibres including collagen and elastin, a fibrin gel matrix, and glycoproteins such as fibronectin. Activated fibroblasts synthesize and secrete many of these ECM proteins, in addition to a variety of proteolytic enzymes and their inhibitors, which exert control over the composition and renewal of the ECM. The formation of the tumour stromal compartment closely resembles that of granulation tissue in wound healing (Pupa et al., 2002). Stromal breakdown has been associated with malignant growth, with metastasis resulting from the degradation of basement membranes, and the ECM of tumours by proteolytic enzymes such as collagenases, and other metallo- and serine-proteases. Fibroblasts, in addition to macrophages and mast cells, appear to be involved in the synthesis and regulation of these enzymes. Studies indicate that malignant tumour cells release factors that stimulate fibroblasts to synthesize enzymes, suggesting a close cooperation between the tumour and stromal cells in the regulation of proteolysis (Liotta and Kohn, 2001).

Activated stromal fibroblasts are involved in a number of physiological processes, including desmoplastic reactions during neoplasia, fibromatoses (non-malignant fibroblastic transformations), wound healing (e.g. burns, scleroderma), and cirrhosis (Dvorak, 1986). In these situations, active fibroblasts grow abnormally but are not transformed, showing characteristic patterns of gene expression not observed in resting fibrocytes (Liotta and Kohn, 2001). They also characteristically induce the formation of fibroblast activation protein (FAP), a cell surface bound member of the serine protease gene family. The FAP antigen is an attractive antigenic target because it has broad applicability to several common and as yet poorly-treatable cancer types, and it also displays a restricted expression in normal tissue, shown by detailed immunohistochemical analyses (Garin-Chesa et al., 1990; Tahtis et al., 2003).

17.2 Factors affecting growth of new vessels

Angiogenesis is under stringent control and appears to occur as a result of the complex interplay of a myriad of soluble and insoluble factors that regulate the growth and differentiation of ECs (Bikfalvi and Bicknell, 2002). Some of the most well recognized soluble stimulatory factors include VEGF and family members, acidic fibroblast growth factor (aFGF), basic fibroblast growth factor (bFGF), platelet derived growth factor (PDGF), thymidine phosphorylase (TP), transforming growth factor β (TGFβ), tumour necrosis factor α (TNFα), IL-4 and IL-8. These molecules are secreted by ECs, tumour cells, or by other cell types that have been mobilized and recruited to the site of angiogenesis, such as pericytes, macrophages, mast cells, and platelets (Ellis et al., 2001). Formation of a mature vascular system also requires the coordinated signalling of various insoluble mediators. The VEGF family stimulate the most well-characterised angiogenic signal transduction pathway. However, other families of integrins and growth factors have emerged, which also exhibit high specificity for the vascular endothelium. These act independently or in concert with the VEGF family of proteins and receptors to influence vascular development. The time of release and molecular mechanism of action, and whether there is any synergy between these molecules, still require further investigation, as does the impact of other stimulatory forces such as hypoxia and oxidative stress (Bikfalvi and Bicknell, 2002).

Recently, intriguing structural parallels have been made between the vascular and nervous systems, with an increasing collection of molecules showing involvement in the development of both organ systems. Two of the best examples are the Eph/ephrin signalling pathway (discussed in Section 17.2.3) and the Neuropilin-1 receptor (NRP1)/Semophorin-3 ligand (Sem-3) pathway (Figure 17.2). NRP1/Sem-3 are critical during embryonic development, providing guidance signals for growing axons and migrating neural crest cells (Wilkinson, 2000). The pair also integrate into the VEGF signalling pathway, where they appear to modulate blood vessel development (Shima and Mailhos, 2000). NRP1 is a high affinity co-receptor for VEGF-165 with simultaneous binding of VEGF-165 to NRP1 and VEGFR-2 augmenting the migratory and proliferative effects observed through VEGFR-2 signalling alone (Soker et al., 1998; Gagnon et al., 2000) (Figure 17.2). Similarly, results suggest that members of the Eph/ephrin family have identical roles in the vascular and nervous systems of the developing embryo, where they provide guidance signals which help define organ boundaries (Wilkinson, 2000). For example, inactivation of the EphB4 receptor or its ligand, ephrinB2, results in loss of angiogenic

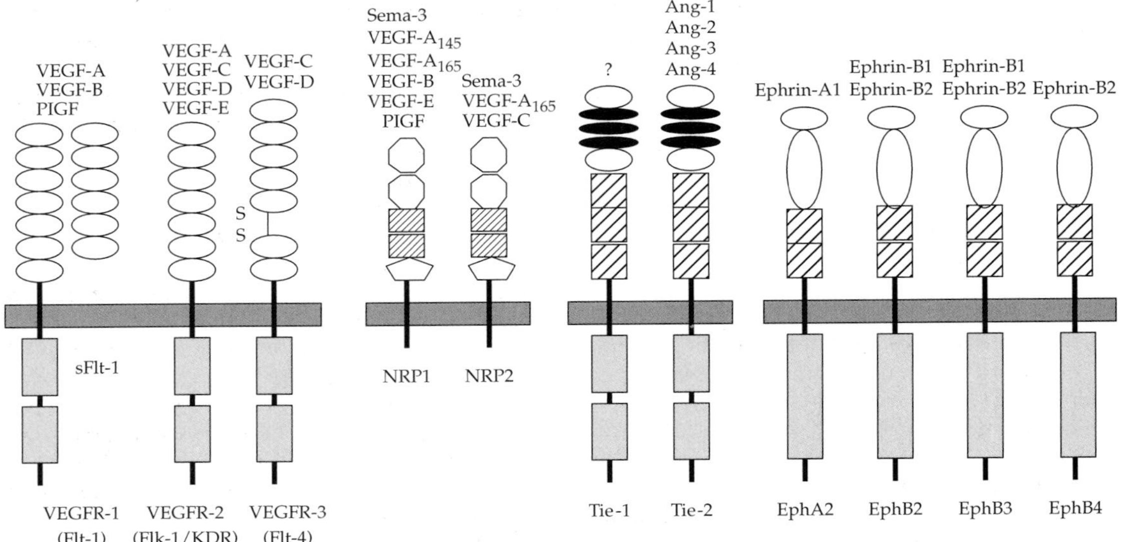

Figure 17.2 Endothelial signalling systems. Receptor tyrosine kinases of the vascular endothelial growth factor receptor (VEGFR) family bind different members of the VEGF family of growth factors. A secreted, soluble splice variant of Flt-1/VEGFR-1 (sFlt-1) is known. Neuropilin-1, and -2, previously identified as receptors for samaphorins, also specifically bind members of the VEGF family of growth factors. Angiopoietins-1 to -4 are the ligands of the Tie-2 receptor tyrosine kinase. Tie-1 is an orphan receptor. Certain members of the large Eph receptor tyrosine kinases and their counterpart Ephrin ligands have been implicated in vascular development. Modified from Breier, G (2000) and Yancopoulos, G.D (2000).

remodelling of the primary capillary beds and as a consequence, early embryonic death (Figure 17.2) (Wang et al., 1998).

Finally, other signaling pathways such as the Notch/Delta, hedgehog, sprouty, and slit/roundabout families have recently been implicated in angiogenesis. The interested reader is referred to Sullivan and Bicknell (2003).

17.2.1 The VEGF family of proteins and receptors

The VEGF family of proteins and receptors are the most well described pro-angiogenic molecules and are critical mediators of vasculogenesis and physiologic and pathogenic angiogenesis, intimately associated with the growth of solid tumours and the formation of metastases (Nicosia, 1998; Bikfalvi and Bicknell, 2002). The VEGF family comprises VEGF-A, VEGF-B, VEGF-C, VEGF-D, VEGF-E, and placental growth factor (PIGF). All of these molecules share amino acid sequence homology, including eight cysteine residue motifs, and bind to the same class of tyrosine kinase receptors (Breier, 2000).

VEGF-A

VEGF-A is a 34–42 kDa homodimeric glycoprotein that is considered as a prime regulator of angiogenesis. By alternative splicing of VEGF-A mRNA five main isoforms of 121, 145, 165, 189, or 206 amino acids arise; VEGF-A_{121}, VEGF-A_{145}, VEGF-A_{165}, VEGF-A_{189}, and VEGF-A_{206}, respectively (Breier, 2000). VEGF-A is mitogenic for ECs, is a potent inducer of vasodilation, and is responsible for generation of blood vessels in the developing embryo. VEGF-A mRNA is highly upregulated in most human tumours, with tumour cells representing the main source of VEGF-A. Its expression has been found in carcinoma of the lung, thyroid, gastric tract, colon, kidney, bladder, ovary, and cervix. Immunoreactivity has also been observed in angiosarcomas, germ cell tumours, and neoplasms of the central nervous system. However, tumour-associated stroma is also an important site of VEGF-A production (Ferrara and Alitalo, 1999). VEGF potentiates its effect by binding to VEGF receptor-1 (VEGFR-1) and VEGFR-2 tyrosine kinases and is reportedly capable of inducing heterodimer formation between the two (Figure 17.2) (Yancopoulos et al., 2000). VEGF-A is upregulated by a variety of factors such as the Ras oncogene, hypoxia, and the mutant form of p53 (Harris, 2002). Embryos that are defective in either one (VEGF-A +/−) or both (VEGF-A −/−) *VEGF-A* alleles are unable to undergo vasculogenesis, leading to *in utero* death of the embryo by day 10–12. The fact that heterozygous embryos (VEGF-A +/−) also display a vasculogenic defect, illustrates that there is a threshold level of VEGF-A expression below which new blood vessels are unable to form (Neufeld et al., 1999).

VEGF-B

VEGF-B is the most stable of the VEGF family members and has two alternatively spliced isoforms, VEGF-B_{167} and VEGF-B_{186}, which share 46% amino acid identity with VEGF-A. VEGF-B is a highly basic heparin binding protein that is not readily secreted unless it is in a heterodimeric form with VEGF-A (Olofsson et al., 1996a, b). VEGF-B is mitogenic for ECs with evidence that it mediates its effect through VEGFR-1 (Figure 17.2). However, the factors that regulate VEGF-B remain undetermined (Nicosia, 1998). The protein is expressed in over 90% of tumours and in a variety of normal organs, with most prolific expression observed in skeletal muscle and in the heart, suggesting that it may be involved in the angiogenesis of these tissues (Olofsson et al., 1996b).

VEGF-C

VEGF-C was initially isolated as a high affinity ligand for VEGFR-3, but has also been shown to exert its effect via VEGFR-2 (Figure 17.2). VEGF-C is produced as a propeptide that is proteolytically processed into a mature 21 kDa form that shares approximately 30% homology with VEGF-A. VEGF-C enhances vessel hyperpermeability and induces migration and proliferation of ECs (Nicosia, 1998). The high expression of *VEGF-C* in lymphatic vessels of the developing mouse embryo and studies with avian chorioallantoic membrane and transgenic mice suggests a specific role in lymphangiogenesis. In non-neoplastic adult tissue, restricted VEGF-C expression has been observed, while 50% of tumours show elevated levels of VEGF-C, including a number of prostatic, lung, and renal cell carcinomas (Kukk et al., 1996).

VEGF-D

VEGF-D is a recently identified member of the VEGF family, signalling via VEGFR-2 and VEGFR-3 (Figure 17.2). The primary structure of VEGF-D most closely resembles VEGF-C, the two molecules sharing 48% amino acid homology (Achen et al., 1998). VEGF-D stimulates EC proliferation following induction by the transcriptional regulator FOS. Prolific expression of VEGF-D is observed during foetal lung development, and in adults its expression is restricted to the heart, lung, intestine, and skeletal muscle (Nicosia, 1998).

VEGF Receptors

Three receptors for the VEGF family proteins have been characterized; VEGFR-1 (Flt-1), VEGFR-2 (KDR/Flk-1), and VEGFR-3 (Flt-4) (Figure 17.2). Binding of the VEGF family of ligands to these receptor tyrosine kinases induces receptor dimerization, followed by autophosphorylation and signal transduction (Neufeld et al., 1999). The receptors may also signal via several secondary pathways, for example, MAP kinase and AKT. VEGFR-1 is a high affinity VEGF receptor and has a naturally occurring splice variant, which encodes only the extracellular domain (Figure 17.2). When this domain is secreted as a soluble protein (sFlt-1), it is a potent antagonist of VEGF-A by binding VEGF-A with high affinity and reducing its interactions with its receptors. In VEGFR-1 knockout mice, EC differentiation still occurs but there is disorganized assembly of the developing vessel network and embryos die *in utero* by day 8.5–10 (Fong et al., 1995). VEGFR-2 is considered to be the main receptor mediating proliferation of ECs after stimulation by VEGF-A. In VEGFR-2 knockout embryos, inactivation of the receptor results in failure of vasculogenesis and an inability to form blood islands and to generate hemopoietic precursors, and hence ECs. Because the vascular abnormalities are so severe, VEGFR-2 knockout embryos die *in utero* by day 10.0 (Shalaby et al., 1995). VEGFR-3 is necessary for embryonic blood vessel development. In the adult, VEGFR-3 is associated with lymphatics and is also expressed in the abnormal blood vessels in pathological conditions including inflammation and malignancy. A recent study by Matsumura et al. (2003), demonstrated that targeted disruption of the *VEGFR-3* gene suggested that the receptor may be involved in the maintenance of vascular integrity through modulation of VEGFR-2 signals. Neuropilins are extracellular receptors for two different secreted protein families, VEGF and semaphorin (Neufeld et al., 2002) (Figure 17.2). Binding to NRP1 (by VEGF-A_{145}, VEGF-A_{165}, or VEGF-B) enhances signalling several fold through VEGFR-2. However, a naturally occurring extracellular form of NRP1 is an antagonist of VEGF signalling and SEMA3A antagonises VEGF signalling by interacting with NRP1 (Gagnon et al., 2000). Tumour cells overexpressing NRP1 have enhanced *in vivo* growth with increased angiogenesis. A second NRP, NRP2, is less well defined but is also important for yolk sac and embryonic angiogenesis. NRP2 is a receptor for VEGF-A_{165} and VEGF-C (Neufeld et al., 2002).

17.2.2 Angiopoietins and Tie receptors

The angiopoietins comprise a unique family of ligands that appear to bind exclusively to the Tek/Tie-2 receptor tyrosine kinase. There are four currently known angiopoietins Angiopoietin-1 (Ang-1)–Ang-4, with Ang-1 and Ang-2 the most well characterized—exerting their effect via the Tie-2 receptor (Figure 17.2) (Jones and Dumont, 2000). The angiopoietin/Tie-2 system is very tightly regulated, showing restricted expression at sites of active vessel remodelling and stabilization, which follow on from the initial angiogenic effects of VEGFR-1 and VEGFR-2 (Jones et al., 2001). Ang-1 and Ang-2 appear to have opposing actions on ECs at these sites, stimulating or inhibiting tyrosine phosphorylation of the Tie-2 receptor, respectively. In contrast to Tie-2, Tie-1 is an orphan receptor whose ligand or ligands remain to be identified (Figure 17.2) (Jones and Dumont, 2000).

The role of Ang-1 in EC biology has not been completely determined. However, Ang-1 has been implicated in EC migration and sprouting and also in promoting EC survival *in vitro*. Survival of ECs is encouraged in response to Ang-1, which acts independently or in synergy with VEGF, by the apparent inhibition of apoptosis and the recruitment of pericytes and other periendothelial support cells, which stabilize the newly forming vascular network (Gale et al., 2002). Investigations performed in Ang-1 deficient mice, demonstrated that embryos were still able to undergo VEGF-dependant angiogenesis, but displayed angiogenic defects resulting in an inability to interact with periendothelial cells, leading to severe vascular regression by embryonic day 11 (E11) and death by E12.5. Ang-1 and Tie-2 knockouts display comparable phenotypes, characterized by an abnormally developed primary capillary plexus, including a reduction in blood vessel integrity, decreased vessel sprouting, and remodelling as a consequence of migratory defects, and a general loss of ECs (Suri et al., 1996). In contrast, Ang-2 is the natural antagonist for Tie-2, and with the support of VEGF, appears to block the stabilizing effects of Ang-1. However, the interaction fails to induce phosphorylation of Tie-2, leading to EC destabilization and the subsequent induction of angiogenesis, providing further evidence for the precise regulation of the angiopoietin/Tie-2 system (Jones and Dumont, 2000).

In vivo tumour xenograft studies have been performed with cell lines stably transfected with full-length cDNA constructs for Ang-1 or Ang-2. The stable clones were subcutaneously injected into immunocompromised mice and tumour growth rate was monitored. Tumour weight was significantly lower in the Ang-1 group, compared with Ang-2 overexpressing tumours where tumour weight increased. The results corresponded with vessel density, which decreased in tumours grown from Ang-1 overexpressing cells, but increased in tumour cells overexpressing Ang-2. The data suggests that overexpression of Ang-1 may stabilize ECs, so that they are not released from pericytes and the basement membrane to initiate EC proliferation and ultimately angiogenesis (Liu et al., 2002). More comprehensive studies are required to understand further the importance of angiopoietins in cancer and evaluate their usefulness as anti-angiogenic targets.

17.2.3 Eph receptor/ephrin signalling

The ephrins are the largest known family of signalling molecules, with 14 Eph receptors and 8 ephrin ligands described to date. The ephrins can be divided into two subclasses, ephrin-A and ephrin-B, depending on their mechanism of cell surface attachment and their preference for Eph receptors (Figure 17.2) (Klein, 2001). Unlike most other ligands, ephrins must be anchored to the cell surface and do not function in a soluble form. A characteristic of the Eph/ephrin system is bidirectional signalling, where the ligand activates its receptor and is in turn activated. This reciprocal signalling may provide guidance cues in cell-to-cell interactions (Yancopoulos et al., 1998). The ephrins have traditionally been studied for their role in the nervous system in axon guidance, where they play a critical role in the formation of tissue and organ interfaces in the developing embryo.

However, they have also now been identified at the boundaries of arteries and veins in the developing embryonic vasculature (Wang et al., 1998), with results indicating that the early embryonic arterial and venous endothelium have distinct patterns of Eph and ephrin cell surface expression (Wang et al., 1998). This was illustrated in the study by Wang et al. (1998), where it was reported that during the establishment of the primary capillary plexus, ephrin-B2 marks ECs of developing arteries, while EphB4 (one of the receptors for ephrin-B2) marks the venous endothelium. In addition, homozygous ephrin-B2 knockout mice exhibited growth retardation at E10 and lethality at E11, with multiple vascular anomalies including an enlarged yolk sac and an abnormal vascular network of the head and cardiovascular system (Wang et al., 1998). Importantly, expression of Eph / ephrins has also been observed in the vascular ECs of surrounding tissues, implying that Eph / ephrin interactions are not restricted to vascular boundaries, but may also occur between the endothelium and mesenchyme (Klein, 2001).

Expression of ephrin A1 and its EphA2 receptor have been demonstrated in tumour angiogenesis (Ogawa et al., 2000). Double immunostaining of endothelial cells for CD34 showed ephrin A1 and its EphA2 receptor to be expressed throughout the endothelium in mouse xenografts of human MDA435 and K1767 Kaposi's sarcoma cells and in the vasculature of human cancers. A dominant-negative EphA2 receptor blocked formation of capillary endothelial tubes *in vitro*. Further studies have shown that soluble EphA2-Fc and EphA3-Fc receptor constructs inhibit tumour angiogenesis and growth *in vivo*, providing the first functional evidence for EphA receptor regulation in tumour angiogenesis (Brantley et al., 2002). Recent mechanistic studies have shown that blockade of the EphA receptor specifically inhibits VEGF-induced angiogenesis (Cheng et al., 2002). This activity is not restricted to members of the A subclass, as similar effects have been reported with the soluble extracellular domains of the EphB2 and EphB4 receptors. This is an expanding area of research, but it appears that abrogation of the function of both he A and B class ephrins may provide novel anti-ngiogenic and anti-tumour activities.

7.2.4 Integrins

he integrins are a large family of heterodimeric cell ırface adhesion molecules, whose transmembrane receptor complexes comprise non-covalently bound α and β chains. Ligands for the integrins include fibronectin, laminin, collagen, and vitronectin as components of the ECM; certain integrins can also bind soluble ligands such as fibrinogen (Hynes, 2002). The primary function of integrins is in mediating cellular adhesion interactions to ECM proteins and adjacent cells but they also appear to be involved in intracellular signalling pathways that contribute to EC survival, migration, and proliferation. For EC survival, integrin $\alpha_v\beta_3$, $\alpha_v\beta_5$, and some β1-integrin complexes appear to be predominantly involved. The interaction of $\alpha_v\beta_3$ and the ECM has been identified as a critical event for EC survival in nascent vessels. They are also believed to enhance the mitogenic potential of VEGFR-2, following binding of the VEGF-A_{165} ligand (Liu et al., 2002). Integrins are minimally expressed in quiescent blood vessels, but their expression is significantly upregulated and fundamental during angiogenesis *in vivo*, particularly that of $\alpha_v\beta_3$ and $\alpha_v\beta_5$, with the interaction between $\alpha_v\beta_3$ and the ECM identified as a critical event for EC survival in angiogenic blood vessels. Furthermore, the examination of clinical breast cancer specimens indicates that $\alpha_v\beta_3$ expression correlates with the extent of disease (Gasparini et al., 1998), implying that $\alpha_v\beta_3$ is potentially a valuable prognostic marker and therapeutic target. This is exemplified by studies showing that integrin inhibitors, especially against $\alpha_v\beta_3$, induce selective apoptosis of proliferating vascular ECs (Walton et al., 2000).

17.2.5 Hypoxia and oxidative stress

Hypoxia

Hypoxia and oxidative stress often occur concurrently within tumours and both act as strong angiogenic stimulators. Hypoxia is a decline in oxygen below the normal levels found in a tissue (~5%), manifesting itself in acute and chronic vascular disease, pulmonary disease, and cancer. During neoplasia intratumoral hypoxia is associated with a poor clinical outcome, and resistance to conventional treatment modalities such as radiotherapy. This is primarily because neoplastic cells adapt to hypoxic environments and subsequently survive and even proliferate under these conditions, resulting in aggressive tumour behaviour (Harris, 2002). Growing tumours develop hypoxic regions because the new blood vessels form an aberrant vascular network, have poor blood flow, and the stores of oxygen and glucose are rapidly metabolized, so that the tumour effectively outgrows its blood supply (Bikfalvi and Bicknell, 2002). The irregularity of these vessels and their inability to provide oxygen and nutrients to the surrounding tissue stimulates the release of growth factors, which induce tumour angiogenesis and contribute to the malignant phenotype. Endothelial cells are critical in the maintenance of vascular homeostasis and are directly affected by hypoxia, because they must specifically cope with the variations in oxygen tension that occur in the blood. The vascular endothelium undergoes molecular modifications in response to reduced oxygen levels, which impact significantly on EC function, and may result in changes to cell–cell interactions (Michiels et al., 2000). Exposure to hypoxia activates ECs in one of two ways. Acute hypoxia promotes the recruitment, adherence, and activation of neutrophils to blood vessels by the release of inflammatory mediators and growth factors. While in chronic hypoxia there is elevated expression of specific genes, which encode various cytokines and growth factors involved in angiogenesis, including PDGF and VEGF (Harris, 2002).

As tumours outgrow angiogenesis or are deprived of oxygen, a gene expression response to hypoxia is initiated. These genes regulate several biological pathways, including cell proliferation, apoptosis, and angiogenesis. Although several transcription factor pathways are involved in hypoxia regulation, most attention has focused on hypoxia inducible factors (HIFs). These are heterodimeric transcription elements of which HIF-1 is the best described. HIF-1 comprises the HIF-1α and HIF-1β sub-units with HIF-1α being the key transcription factor. HIF-1 regulates DNA response elements, in turn controlling the expression of more than 40 target genes (Semenza, 2002). In response to low cellular oxygen levels, HIF-1 binds to hypoxia response elements, which activate the expression of numerous hypoxia response genes such as *VEGF*, PDGF, endothelin, insulin-like growth factor-II (IGF-II), adrenomedullin, and endothelial growth factor (EGF), which have pro-angiogenic effects (Goonewardene et al., 2002). The intrinsic role that HIF plays in angiogenesis has been examined using both *in vitro* and *in vivo* studies, with investigators showing that loss of HIF-1 activity impacts negatively on tumour growth and vascularization (Semenza, 2002). Analyses using embryonic stem cells lacking the *HIF-1α* gene showed reduced levels of VEGF *in vitro* and *in vivo* tumour xenografts derived from this cell line had fewer vessels and significantly impaired vessel function (Carmeliet et al., 1998). In addition, HIF-1α knockout mice display inefficient angiogenesis and are characterized by a complete lack of cephalic vascularization (Ryan et al., 1998). In the last two years, the pathways mediating the hypoxia signal have been elucidated; HIF-1α is post-translationally modified on two prolyl residues by prolyl hydroxylases that require oxygen as a cofactor as well as ferrous iron, vitamin C and 2-oxoglutarate (Jaakkola et al., 2001). There are three well-characterized enzymes that have prolyl hydroxylase domains (PHDs 1, 2, and 3) (Epstein et al., 2001). PHD-2 is hypoxia inducible and the most widely expressed. The consequence of hydroxylation is that HIF-1α is then recognized by the Von Hippel–Lindau protein, which is a ubiquitin ligase that targets HIF-1α for destruction in the proteosome (Ivan et al., 2001). Clearly as oxygen becomes less available, there is less modification and therefore HIF-1α is stabilized.

Oxidative stress

Reactive oxygen species (ROS) naturally occur in many biological systems and are prevented from damaging molecules such as DNA, proteins, and lipids by the cell's antioxidant defenses, which supposedly scavenge free radicals and subsequently prevent DNA damage. During oxidative stress, the balance between ROS and antioxidants is disrupted in favour of ROS, which subsequently become toxic to the cell. It is unclear if this is due to excessive ROS production or loss of antioxidant defenses (Kang, 2002). It has been established that oxidative stress induces mutations in tumour suppressor genes and causes DNA damage, including base modifications, frame-shift mutations, and DNA strand breaks, critical molecular events in the initial stages of neoplasia (Kang, 2002). An imbalance in ROS also stimulates tumour cells to release stress-induced angiogenic factors such as VEGF, IL-8, and the matrix metalloproteinase-1 (MMP-1). Release of these molecules also occurs in the presence of thymidine phosphorylase (TP), a stimulator of angiogenesis and oxidative stress in tumour lesions, whose expression correlates with poor clinical outcome (Brown et al., 2000; Brown and Bicknell, 2001). Increased TP activity promotes angiogenesis in a range of pathologies and TP over-expression correlates with altered vascular density and poor prognosis in many human tumour types. Despite the wealth of data linking TP and angiogenesis, the molecular mechanisms underlying this link remain unclear. Site-directed mutagenesis and antibody studies have proved that promotion of vessel growth by TP is dependent on its enzyme activity which catabolizes thymidine to thymine and 2-dideoxyribose-1-phosphate. This reaction induces carcinoma cell oxidative stress, causing tumour cells to secrete stress-induced angiogenic factors (VEGF, IL-8, and MMP-1), which promote angiogenesis (Brown et al., 2000; Brown and Bicknell, 2001).

17.3 Approaches to anti-angiogenic therapy

Strategies designed at crippling a tumour by targeting the vascular supply were first proposed over 30 years ago by Folkman (1972), and since then a large amount of research has been carried out in this field to determine the role of angiogenesis in promoting tumour growth and metastasis, and to develop new treatment modalities. Approaches currently under evaluation for inhibiting angiogenesis may either be direct (targeting cell surface bound proteins/receptors) or indirect (targeting growth factor molecules). Although the EC is the prime target, because angiogenesis is a complex process with multiple, sequential, and interdependent steps, this complexity creates many potential targets for inhibition. Therefore, an anti-angiogenic effect can be achieved by targeting angiogenic stimulators, angiogenic receptors, ECM proteins, ECM proteolysis, control mechanisms of angiogenesis, or the ECs directly. Therapeutic approaches that specifically target the ECs, rather than indirectly inhibiting specific angiogenic factors appear to be the most practical, since the plasticity of most tumour cell populations would allow them to circumvent or become resistant to a treatment approach that interferes with a single pathway or blocks an individual stimulatory molecule. This point will be resolved over the coming years, as anti-angiogenesis immunotherapeutics are evaluated in the clinic.

17.3.1 Advantages of vascular targeting

The targeting of antigens selectively expressed on the surface of tumour capillary ECs or tumour stromal fibroblasts is currently being explored for the immunotherapy of cancer. By targeting or preventing the generation of angiogenic blood vessels or tumour stroma, tumour lesions may be deprived of the essential support functions or nutrients required for survival and growth (Dvorak, 1986). This targeting approach may also be applicable to many tumour types because it is not dependant on a specific tumour cell type. The theoretical advantages that anti-angiogenic therapeutics may have in the treatment of cancer are several-fold. First, ECs involved in angiogenesis show several fundamental differences compared with quiescent ECs, primarily their proliferation rate and antigen expression, which can be exploited so that anti-angiogenic therapeutics specifically target tumour ECs and not normal endothelium. Tumour blood vessels are also highly irregular (varying diameters), tortuous, have arterio-venous shunts, blind ends, lack smooth muscle, or enervation and have incomplete endothelial linings and basement membranes (Molema et al., 1998). As a result, blood flow is often slow or highly irregular, and the vessels are much 'leakier' than those in normal tissues, enabling the passage of large macromolecules. Second, anti-angiogenic therapy may circumvent insufficient drug penetration into the interior of a tumour mass due to high interstitial pressure gradients within tumours because ECs are highly accessible to circulating drugs. Third, unlike targeting of tumour cells where failure to destroy a proportion of the cells results in those cells proliferating and subsequent regrowth of the tumour, successful targeting of a few ECs within a growing vessel may be sufficient to completely destroy that vessel. Consequently, disruption of a small percentage of the angiogenic vasculature may result in ischaemic necrosis of a substantial volume of tumour. Fourth, in contrast to the malignant epithelial cells of carcinomas, ECs are not genetically transformed, and also do not display the genetic and phenotypic heterogeneity observed in malignant cells (such as gene amplification, chromosomal translocations, chromosome loss, and simple point mutations) and hence the outgrowth of antigen-loss variants or mutants is less likely to occur (Brown and Giaccia, 1998).

17.3.2 Natural inhibitors of angiogenesis

Tumour cells appear to produce both stimulators and inhibitors of angiogenesis and the balance of these dictates the degree of angiogenesis both locally and at distal sites. A large and structurally diverse family of endogenous protein inhibitors of angiogenesis have now been discovered including Thrombospondin-1 (TSP-1), angiostatin, endostatin, INF-α/β, vascular endothelial cell growth inhibitor, vasostatin, and metalloproteinase inhibitors among others. Angiostatin, endostatin, and TSP-1 are selective and potent endogenous inhibitors of neovascularization and show promise as future therapeutic agents as they begin to enter the clinic.

Angiostatin

Angiostatin was the first molecule specifically isolated as a potential tumour-derived angiogenesis inhibitor. Angiostatin is a 38 kDa fragment of the clotting cascade protease precursor plasminogen (which does not itself have anti-angiogenic properties). It is believed that tumours can produce or activate proteases capable of generating angiostatin from circulating plasminogen (Zetter, 1998). Angiostatin appears to inhibit both EC proliferation and migration, and can act as a circulating angiogenesis inhibitor that suppresses angiogenesis at downstream sites distant from the primary tumour. Treatment of tumour-bearing mice with angiostatin causes regression of the primary tumour and prevents vascularization and growth of metastatic colonies (Burke and DeNardo, 2001).

Endostatin

Endostatin, like angiostatin, is a fragment (20 kDa) of a larger precursor molecule, in this case collagen XVIII, a novel collagen frequently found near blood vessels which itself is not anti-angiogenic (Burke and DeNardo, 2001). Endostatin appears to be a highly active endothelial-specific inhibitor of microvascular EC proliferation, and inhibits primary tumour growth as well as establishment and growth of metastases (Ellis et al., 2001). Combinations of endostatin and angiostatin act synergistically and can result in complete tumour regression with no tumour regrowth after treatment is terminated in mice-bearing B16F10 melanoma and L1210 leukemia tumour xenografts (Scappaticci, 2002). Endostatin is the first endogenous angiogenesis inhibitor to enter clinical trials, with recombinant human endostatin currently in Phase I and Phase II/III clinical trials.

Thrombospondin-1

It has been demonstrated that TSP-1 is an inhibitor of EC proliferation, adhesion, migration, and morphogenesis, and its anti-angiogenic activity is derived from its interaction with the microvascular EC receptor CD36 (Lawler, 2000). Expression and secretion of TSP1 by epithelial and mesenchymal cells is modulated by hypoxia and by genes such as p53. In several tumour types (thyroid, colon, and bladder carcinoma) TSP1 expression is inversely correlated with tumour grade and survival rate, but interestingly in others (e.g. breast carcinomas), it is correlated with stromal response and is of little prognostic value. TSP-1 is an important inhibitor of angiogenesis and its anti-tumour potential has been investigated in several tumour xenograft models. Studies involving transfection of glioblastoma, fibrosarcoma, breast carcinoma, and cutaneous carcinoma cells with plasmids expressing the TSP-1 protein reported reduced tumour xenograft growth rate in immunocompromised mice compared with controls. Because of their large size (>450 kDa) TSP-1 and -2 have yet to enter the clinic, but peptides derived from TSP1 might have promising clinical applications. Methods for stabilizing these peptides *in vivo* and delivering them to tumour sites are currently being researched and will be essential in the development of treatments based on TSP-1 (de Fraipont et al., 2001).

17.3.3 Direct targeting of endothelial cells (anti-vascular strategies)

One of the most promising angiogenesis targeting approaches is to use molecules or design strategies against antigens that are selectively upregulated on tumour ECs, that may potentially lead to tumour blood vessel occlusion. Some of these approaches will be discussed here.

Anti-angiogenic monoclonal antibodies (mAbs) are being rigorously investigated in pre-clinical animal models (DC101 against Flk-1 and C-p1c11 against KDR) and in the clinic, with most success observed with agents that inhibit integrin activation. Anti-integrin mAbs or peptides may interfere with neovascular EC adhesion through inhibition of normal ligand binding and cell signalling, or induce vascular permeability. One such mAb has been evaluated for safety and pharmacokinetics in patients with advanced cancer. A phase I dose escalation study involving 17 patients with late stage metastatic disease, evaluated a humanized mAb generated against the $\alpha_v\beta_3$ integrin (Vitaxin), which is capable of inducing apoptosis in ECs of newly forming capillary blood vessel. In the 14 patients that were evaluable, the antibody was well tolerated with minimal toxicity, and demonstrated a terminal half-title of 120 h at high doses. In addition, a partial response was observed in one patient and seven others demonstrated stable disease, with three patients continuing on to further treatment cycles (Gutheil et al., 2000). However, a disadvantage of this system and others that specifically target angiogenic vessels, is that it has no effect on quiescent tumour vessels, which constitute a large proportion of the tumour endothelium. This type of treatment strategy will therefore probably have greatest potential in adjuvant settings where it could be used to prevent the growth of micrometastases, where angiogenesis is likely to be at its most intense (Eatock et al., 2000). Consequently, some mAbs may be more useful when conjugated to cytotoxic compounds such as radioactive isotopes. This approach has already been used with $\alpha_v\beta_3$, anti-endoglin, and anti-thrombomodulin antibodies with promising pre-clinical results. Anti-angiogenic radioconjugates may inhibit tumours by killing ECs directly and thereby indirectly killing tumour cells, so the effect is two-fold. This, however, depends on the path length of the radioisotope, and on the intrinsic radiosensitivity of the tumour cell.

Novel inhibitors of VEGF receptor tyrosine kinases and their downstream effects are attractive anti-angiogenic agents, that could also potentially inhibit EC activation, proliferation, and invasion (Eatock et al., 2000). SU5416 is a small, membrane permeable tyrosine kinase inhibitor for VEGFR-2, which is currently being assessed in phase I/II and III clinical trials. SU5416 has been shown to successfully inhibit VEGF-driven EC proliferation of cultured cells and also growth of a number of tumour types *in vivo* (Burke and DeNardo, 2001). Another related small molecule tyrosine kinase inhibitor (SU6668) is currently in Phase I clinical trials. SU6668 also inhibits tumour EC proliferation and decreases tumour vascularization and appears to be the superior molecule because it can also inhibit bFGF and PDGF in addition to VEGFR-2. Furthermore, it has been shown to have significantly greater effect on EC apoptosis and on mouse tumour xenografts than SU5416 (Burke and DeNardo, 2001).

Vaccines to VEGF receptors are also under development. Expression of vascular EGF receptors is known to be upregulated on tumour compared to normal vasculature. Recently two animal studies have demonstrated that active immunization against Flk-1 (Li et al., 2002) or use of cytotoxic T lymphocytes engineered to express *VEGF* (and so target VEGF receptor-expressing cells) (Niederman et al., 2002) were shown to elicit significant anti-tumour activities. In the first of these studies an immune response to Flk-1 was elicited by immunization with dendritic cells pulsed with a soluble Flk-1 protein. The immunization generated Flk-1 specific neutralizing antibodies and CD8+ cytotoxic T-cell responses, breaking tolerance to self-Flk-1 antigen. Both tumour-induced angiogenesis in an alginate bead assay and pulmonary metastases from B16 or Lewis lung carcinomas were strongly suppressed in the immunized mice. In the second approach, recombinant retroviral vectors were generated that encoded a chimeric T-cell receptor comprising VEGF sequences linked to intracellular signalling sequences derived from the zeta chain of the T-cell receptor. Transduced murine CD8 cells effectively killed Flk-1 expressing cells *in vitro*. Adoptive transfer into tumour-bearing mice strongly inhibited the growth of a range of syngeneic murine tumours and human tumour xenografts.

Another EC-specific targeting strategy is to selectively disrupt rapidly proliferating and immature tumour ECs using tubulin binding agents which are intrinsically anti-angiogenic. The use of these agents is based on the reliance of ECs for a tubulin cytoskeleton to maintain their architecture, and results in inhibition of spindle formation (mitotic arrest) and reduced tumour blood flow (Eatock et al., 2000). Examples of such agents include colchicines, vinblastine, and combretastatins. ZD6126 is a novel vascular targeting agent that was developed for its tubulin-binding properties and its ability to induce vascular damage in tumours. In a range of experimental tumour models, ZD6126 demonstrated selective disruption of tumour vasculature, which resulted in loss of tumour blood vessel integrity, vessel shutdown, and extensive tumour necrosis (Micheletti et al., 2003).

17.3.4 Targeting control of angiogenesis (anti-angiogenic strategies)

Angiogenesis is a complicated process regulated by numerous pro- and anti-angiogenic factors in a coordinated fashion. These play a fundamental role in regulating the proliferation of cancer cells and supporting tumour endothelium, and are consequently attractive anti-angiogenic therapeutics. One of the considerations with this therapeutic approach is that by blocking a particular tumour cell property, such as VEGF production, this may be subject to inactivation over time by classic acquired resistance mechanisms since, for example, tumour cells can produce a number of different pro-angiogenic growth factors. Furthermore, VEGF is produced by many different cell types and may also be sequestered in the ECM and the interstitial spaces between tissues. However, because angiogenesis is dependent on an appropriate growth factor environment, and VEGF is the most important of these growth factors, the use of blocking molecules to VEGF is keenly investigated. The most successful of these has been Avastin™ (bevacizumab), being the first targeted angiogenesis inhibitor to receive U.S. Food and Drug Administration Approval (February 2004). Avastin is an antibody that works by blocking VEGF and therefore preventing the formation of new blood vessels. It was approved for the treatment of colon cancer in combination with 5-fluorouracil (5-FU) based chemotherapy, following the results of a large, placebo controlled, randomised Phase III study demonstrating prolongation in the median survival of study patients. However five months after its approval, safety concerns about Avastin have been highlighted by the company, which discovered a twofold increase in serious arterial thromboembolic events in certain patients who received the combination treatment. Another example of an antibody inhibitor is rhuMabVEGF, which was initially pre-clinically assessed in cynomolgus monkeys (Ryan et al., 1999). In a phase Ib trial, the antibody was administered in combination with one of three chemotherapy regimens. Responses were observed in three patients, who continued on to further treatment cycles. The study demonstrated the safety and potential clinical activity of the combined treatment (Margolin et al., 2001). The antibody has now completed Phase I and II clinical studies and is currently undergoing Phase III investigation for breast and colorectal cancers. The 'VEGF trap' is another interesting VEGF inhibitor currently in clinical trials. It combines portions of human VEGF and VEGF receptor, and literally 'traps' the VEGF being made by the tumour, again precluding further tumour blood vessel formation.

Matrix inhibitors provide the best examples of anti-angiogenic therapeutics that prevent EC invasion. During angiogenesis proteolytic enzymes are released by ECs and are involved in basement membrane and matrix degradation (Eatock et al., 2000). Molecules that inhibit ECM proteolysis act to block the activity of two types of proteolytic enzymes, urokinase-plasminogen activator (uPA) and the matrix metalloproteinases (MMPs). Increased expression of MMPs correlates with invasive behaviour and metastatic potential and has been documented in a number of human cancers. Several inhibitors are now in advanced clinical trials, including marimastat (phase I/II/III) and AG3340 (phase II/III). MMPs have also been assessed in clinical trials in combination with other angiogenesis inhibitors. Interestingly, the combination of captopril, heparin, and marimastat resulted in either a partial response or stable disease in 3 of 6 patients with renal carcinoma in a study of 27 patients with a variety of malignancies. This finding may warrant further investigation (Pegram and Reese, 2002).

Other strategies for targeting control of angiogenesis include interference with oncogenes and hypoxia response pathways. Farnesyltransferase inhibitors block the activity of oncogenic-*ras* and antibodies against the epidermal growth factor receptor suppress angiogenesis and tumour proliferation in xenograft experiments. Hypoxia response pathways are also promising anti-angiogenic targets, particularly because hypoxic cells release many anti-angiogenic factors and are also often resistant to radiotherapy and chemotherapy. Experiments using knockouts of HIF-1α, dominant negative constructs, peptide mimetics, antisense techniques, or mutations in HIF-1α suggest that therapeutics targeting the HIF pathway should be further evaluated for their anti-tumour potential (Pegram and Reese, 2002).

17.3.5 Clinical considerations

Much has already been discussed concerning anti-angiogenic approaches to cancer but a few additional points are worthy of mention. There are now more anti-angiogenics in anti-cancer clinical trials than drugs that fit into any other mechanistic category (around a third of all drugs). This is indeed a large number, reflecting a huge financial investment and the intense interest in this approach to cancer treatment that has been apparent in recent years. Current anti-angiogenic clinical trial activity can be assessed at www.cancer.gov at the 'Angiogenesis Inhibitors in Clinical Trials' page. The most promising of these has been Avastin™ (Genentech) and hence it is worth considering this drug further. It had long been thought that anti-angiogenics would not be effective anti-cancer agents when administered alone but would need to be given in combination with cytotoxic drugs. While this has been questioned by some, it is generally accepted by those in the field. Another point concerns the recent discovery of VEGF isoforms, such as $VEGF_{165b}$, that are actually competitive inhibitors of VEGF and block angiogenesis themselves (Bates et al., 2002). The antibodies were raised to the N-terminus of the molecule and thus will recognize both the pro- and anti-angiogenic forms of VEGF. As such, it is difficult to predict *ab initio* whether anti-VEGF administration will be beneficial or otherwise to the patient. This illustrates the complexity of developing such novel approaches to cancer therapy. A final clinical consideration concerns the difficulty in assessing the efficacy of an anti-angiogenic drug that produces disease stabilization rather than tumour regression. One possibility is to use surrogate markers released by damaged endothelium, which are expected to be gene products restricted to endothelium. There have been several studies that have met with some success. For example, the soluble Tie-2 and Flt-1 domains have been shown to be elevated in the serum of patients receiving anti-angiogenic therapy (Harris et al., 2001).

17.4 Conclusions

Angiogenesis research is clearly at an exciting time. The next few years will show whether the first anti-angiogenics such as VEGF blockers have sustained clinical efficacy. Blood vessel growth has turned out to be complex, with many factors playing a role in the process. This complexity in itself, however, leads to many opportunities for therapeutic targeting that will test the ingenuity of cancer biologists and clinicians over the next decade.

References and further reading

Achen, M. G., Jeltsch, M., Kukk, E., Makinen, T., Vitali, A., Wilks, A. F. et al. (1998). Vascular endothelial growth factor D (VEGF-D) is a ligand for the tyrosine kinases VEGF receptor 2 (Flk1) and VEGF receptor 3 (Flt4). *Proc Natl Acad Sci USA*, **95**, 548–53.

Asahara, T., Murohara, T., Sullivan, A., Silver, M., van der Zee, R., Li, T. et al. (1997). Isolation of putative progenitor endothelial cells for angiogenesis. *Science*, **275**, 964–7.

Asahara, T., Masuda, H., Takahashi, T., Kalka, C., Pastore, C., Silver, M. et al. (1999). Bone marrow origin of endothelial progenitor cells responsible for postnatal vasculogenesis in physiological and pathological neovascularization. *Circ Res*, **85**, 221–8.

Bates, D. O., Cui, T. G., Doughty, J. M., Winkler, M., Sugiono, M., Shields, J. D. (2002). VEGF165b, an inhibitory splice variant of vascular endothelial growth factor, is down-regulated in renal cell carcinoma. *Cancer Res*, **62**, 4123–31.

Bikfalvi, A. and Bicknell, R. (2002). Recent advances in angiogenesis, anti-angiogenesis and vascular targeting. *Trends Pharmacol Sci*, **23**, 576–82.

Brantley, D. M., Cheng, N., Thompson, E. J., Lin, Q., Brekken, R. A., Thorpe, P. E. et al. (2002). Soluble Eph A receptors inhibit tumor angiogenesis and progression in vivo. *Oncogene*, **21**, 7011–26.

Breier, G. (2000). Angiogenesis in embryonic development–a review. *Placenta*, **21** (Suppl A.), S11–5.

Brown, J. M. and Giaccia, A. J. (1998). The unique physiology of solid tumors: opportunities (and problems) for cancer therapy. *Cancer Res*, **58**, 1408–16.

Brown, N. S. and Bicknell, R. (2001). Hypoxia and oxidative stress in breast cancer. Oxidative stress: its effects on the growth, metastatic potential and response to therapy of breast cancer. *Breast Cancer Res*, **3**, 323–7.

Brown, N. S., Jones, A., Fujiyama, C., Harris, A. L., and Bicknell, R. (2000). Thymidine phosphorylase induces carcinoma cell oxidative stress and promotes secretion of angiogenic factors. *Cancer Res*, **60**, 6298–302.

Burke, P. A. and DeNardo, S. J. (2001). Antiangiogenic agents and their promising potential in combined therapy. *Crit Rev Oncol Hematol*, **39**, 155–71.

Carmeliet, P., Dor, Y., Herbert, J. M., Fukumura, D., Brusselmans, K., Dewerchin, M. et al. (1998). Role of HIF-1alpha in hypoxia-mediated apoptosis, cell proliferation and tumour angiogenesis. *Nature*, **394**, 485–90.

Cheng, N., Brantley, D. M., Liu, H., Lin, Q., Enriquez, M., Gale, N. et al. (2002). Blockade of EphA Receptor Tyrosine Kinase Activation Inhibits Vascular Endothelial Cell Growth Factor-Induced Angiogenesis. *Mol Cancer Res*, **1**, 2–11.

de Fraipont, F., Nicholson, A. C., Feige, J. J., and Van Meir, E. G. (2001). Thrombospondins and tumor angiogenesis. *Trends Mol Med*, **7**, 401–7.

Dvorak, H. F. (1986). Tumors: wounds that do not heal. Similarities between tumor stroma generation and wound healing. *N Engl J Med*, **315**, 1650–9.

Eatock, M. M., Schatzlein, A., and Kaye, S. B. (2000). Tumour vasculature as a target for anticancer therapy. *Cancer Treat Rev*, **26**, 191–204.

Ellis, L. M., Liu, W., Ahmad, S. A., Fan, F., Jung, Y. D., Shaheen, R. M. et al., (2001). Overview of angiogenesis: Biologic implications for antiangiogenic therapy. *Semin Oncol*, **28**, 94–104.

Epstein, A. C., Gleadle, J. M., McNeill, L. A., Hewitson, K. S., O'Rourke, J., Mole, D. R. et al. (2001). C. elegans EGL-9 and mammalian homologs define a family of dioxygenases that regulate HIF by prolyl hydroxylation. *Cell*, **107**, 43–54.

Ferrara, N. and Alitalo, K. (1999). Clinical applications of angiogenic growth factors and their inhibitors. *Nat Med*, **5**, 1359–64.

Folkman, J. (1972). Anti-angiogenesis: new concept for therapy of solid tumors. *Ann Surg*, **175**, 409–16.

Fong, G. H., Rossant, J., Gertsenstein, M., and Breitman, M. L. (1995). Role of the Flt-1 receptor tyrosine kinase in regulating the assembly of vascular endothelium. *Nature*, **376**, 66–70.

Gagnon, M. L., Bielenberg, D. R., Gechtman, Z., Miao, H. Q., Takashima, S., Soker, S. et al. (2000). Identification of a natural soluble neuropilin-1 that binds vascular endothelial growth factor: In vivo expression and antitumor activity. *Proc Natl Acad Sci USA*, **97**, 2573–8.

Gale, N. W., Thurston, G., Hackett, S. F., Renard, R., Wang, Q., McClain, J. et al. (2002). Angiopoietin-2 is required for postnatal angiogenesis and lymphatic patterning, and only the latter role is rescued by Angiopoietin-1. *Dev Cell*, **3**, 411–23.

Garin-Chesa, P., Old, L. J., and Rettig, W. J. (1990). Cell surface glycoprotein of reactive stromal fibroblasts as a potential antibody target in human epithelial cancers. *Proc Natl Acad Sci USA*, **87**, 7235–9.

Gasparini, G., Brooks, P. C., Biganzoli, E., Vermeulen, P. B., Bonoldi, E., Dirix, L. Y. et al. (1998). Vascular integrin alpha(v)beta3: a new prognostic indicator in breast cancer. *Clin Cancer Res*, **4**, 2625–34.

Gerwins, P., Skoldenberg, E., and Claesson-Welsh, L. (2000). Function of fibroblast growth factors and vascular endothelial growth factors and their receptors in angiogenesis. *Crit Rev Oncol Hematol*, **34**, 185–94.

Goonewardene, T. I., Sowter, H. M., and Harris, A. L. (2002). Hypoxia-induced pathways in breast cancer. *Microsc Res Tech*, **59**, 41–8.

Gutheil, J. C., Campbell, T. N., Pierce, P. R., Watkins, J. D., Huse, W. D., Bodkin, D. J. et al. (2000). Targeted antiangiogenic therapy for cancer using Vitaxin: a humanized monoclonal antibody to the integrin alphavbeta3. *Clin Cancer Res*, **6**, 3056–61.

Harris, A. L. (2002). Hypoxia–a key regulatory factor in tumour growth. *Nat Rev Cancer*, **2**, 38–47.

Harris, A. L., Reusch, P., Barleon, B., Hang, C., Dobbs, N., and Marme, D. (2001). Soluble Tie2 and Flt1 extracellular domains in serum of patients with renal cancer and response to antiangiogenic therapy. *Clin Cancer Res*, **7**, 1992–7.

Huminiecki, L. and Bicknell, R. (2000). In silico cloning of novel endothelial-specific genes. *Genome Res*, **10**, 1796–806.

Huminiecki, L., Gorn, M., Suchting, S., Poulsom, R., and Bicknell, R. (2002). Magic roundabout is a new member of the roundabout receptor family that is endothelial specific and expressed at sites of active angiogenesis. *Genomics*, **79**, 547–52.

Hynes, R. O. (2002). A reevaluation of integrins as regulators of angiogenesis. *Nat Med*, **8**, 918–21.

Ivan, M., Kondo, K., Yang, H., Kim, W., Valiando, J., Ohh, M., et al. (2001). HIFalpha targeted for VHL-mediated destruction by proline hydroxylation: implications for O2 sensing. *Science*, **292**, 464–8.

Jaakkola, P., Mole, D. R., Tian, Y. M., Wilson, M. I., Gielbert, J., Gaskell, S. J. et al. (2001). Targeting of HIF-alpha to the von Hippel-Lindau ubiquitylation complex by O2-regulated prolyl hydroxylation. *Science*, **292**, 468–72.

Jones, N. and Dumont, D. J. (2000). Tek/Tie2 signaling: new and old partners. *Cancer Metastasis Rev*, **19**, 13–17.

Jones, N., Iljin, K., Dumont, D. J., and Alitalo, K. (2001). Tie receptors: new modulators of angiogenic and lymphangiogenic, responses. *Nat Rev Mol Cell Biol*, **2**, 257–67.

Kang, D. H. (2002). Oxidative stress, DNA damage, and breast cancer. *AACN Clin Issues*, **13**, 540–9.

Klein, R. (2001). Excitatory Eph receptors and adhesive ephrin ligands. *Curr Opin Cell Biol*, **13**, 196–203.

Kukk, E., Lymboussaki, A., Taira, S., Kaipainen, A., Jeltsch, M., Joukov, V. et al. (1996). VEGF-C receptor binding and pattern of expression with VEGFR-3 suggests a role in lymphatic vascular development. *Development*, **122**, 3829–37.

Lawler, J. (2000). The functions of thrombospondin-1 and-2. *Curr Opin Cell Biol*, **12**, 634–40.

Li, Y., Wang, M. N., Li, H., King, K. D., Bassi, R., Sun, H. et al. (2002). Active immunization against the vascular endothelial growth factor receptor flk1 inhibits tumor angiogenesis and metastasis. *J Exp Med*, **195**, 1575–84.

Liotta, L. A. and Kohn, E. C. (2001). The microenvironment of the tumour-host interface. *Nature*, **411**, 375–9.

Liu, W., Reinmuth, N., Stoeltzing, O., Parikh, A. A., Fan, F., Ahmad, S. A. et al. (2002). Antiangiogenic therapy targeting factors that enhance endothelial cell survival. *Semin Oncol*, **29**, 96–103.

Lyden, D., Young, A. Z., Zagzag, D., Yan, W., Gerald, W., O'Reilly, R. et al. (1999). Id1 and Id3 are required for neurogenesis, angiogenesis and vascularization of tumour xenografts. *Nature*, **401**, 670–7.

Lyden, D., Hattori, K., Dias, S., Costa, C., Blaikie, P., Butros, L. et al. (2001). Impaired recruitment of bone-marrow-derived endothelial and hematopoietic precursor cells blocks tumor angiogenesis and growth. *Nat Med*, **7**, 1194–201.

Margolin, K., Gordon, M. S., Holmgren, E., Gaudreault, J., Novotny, W., Fyfe, G. et al. (2001). Phase Ib trial of intravenous recombinant humanized monoclonal antibody to vascular endothelial growth factor in combination with chemotherapy in patients with advanced cancer: pharmacologic and long-term safety data. *J Clin Oncol*, **19**, 851–6.

Matsumura, K., Hirashima, M., Ogawa, M., Kubo, H., Hisatsune, H., Kondo, et al. (2003). Modulation of VEGFR-2-mediated endothelial-cell activity by VEGF-C/VEGFR-3. *Blood*, **101**, 1367–74.

Micheletti, G., Poli, M., Borsotti, P., Martinelli, M., Imberti, B., Taraboletti, G. et al. (2003). Vascular-targeting activity of ZD6126, a novel tubulin-binding agent. *Cancer Res*, **63**, 1534–7.

Michiels, C., Arnould, T., and Remacle, J. (2000). Endothelial cell responses to hypoxia: initiation of a cascade of cellular interactions. *Biochim Biophys Acta*, **1497**, 1–10.

Molema, G., Meijer, D. K., and de Leij, L. F. (1998). Tumor vasculature targeted therapies: getting the players organized. *Biochem Pharmacol*, **55**, 1939–45.

Neufeld, G., Cohen, T., Gengrinovitch, S., and Poltorak, Z. (1999). Vascular endothelial growth factor (VEGF) and its receptors. *Faseb J*, **13**, 9–22.

Neufeld, G., Cohen, T., Shraga, N., Lange, T., Kessler, O., and Herzog, Y. (2002). The neuropilins: multifunctional semaphorin and VEGF receptors that modulate axon guidance and angiogenesis. *Trends Cardiovasc Med*, **12**, 13–9.

Nicosia, R. F. (1998). What is the role of vascular endothelial growth factor-related molecules in tumor angiogenesis? *Am J Pathol*, **153**, 11–6.

Niederman, T. M., Ghogawala, Z., Carter, B. S., Tompkins, H. S., Russell, M. M., and Mulligan, R. C. (2002). Antitumor activity of cytotoxic T lymphocytes engineered to target vascular endothelial growth factor receptors. *Proc Natl Acad Sci USA*, **99**, 7009–14.

Niedermeyer, J., Scanlan, M. J., Garin-Chesa, P., Daiber, C., Fiebig, H. H., Old, L. J. et al. (1997). Mouse fibroblast activation protein: molecular cloning, alternative splicing and expression in the reactive stroma of epithelial cancers. *Int J Cancer*, **71**, 383–9.

Ogawa, K., Pasqualini, R., Lindberg, R. A., Kain, R., Freeman, A. L., and Pasquale, E. B. (2000). The ephrin-A1 ligand and its receptor, EphA2, are expressed during tumor neovascularization. *Oncogene*, **19**, 6043–52.

Olofsson, B., Pajusola, K., Kaipainen, A., von Euler, G., Joukov, V., Saksela, O. et al. (1996a). Vascular endothelial growth factor B, a novel growth factor for endothelial cells. *Proc Natl Acad Sci USA*, **93**, 2576–81.

Olofsson, B., Pajusola, K., von Euler, G., Chilov, D., Alitalo, K., and Eriksson, U. (1996b). Genomic organization of the mouse and human genes for vascular endothelial growth factor B (VEGF-B) and characterization of a second splice isoform. *J Biol Chem*, **271**, 19310–7.

Patan, S. (2000). Vasculogenesis and angiogenesis as mechanisms of vascular network formation, growth and remodeling. *J Neurooncol*, **50**, 1–15.

Pegram, M. D. and Reese, D. M. (2002). Combined biological therapy of breast cancer using monoclonal antibodies directed against HER2/neu protein and vascular endothelial growth factor. *Semin Oncol*, **29**, 29–37.

Pupa, S. M., Menard, S., Forti, S., and Tagliabue, E. (2002). New insights into the role of extracellular matrix during tumor onset and progression. *J Cell Physiol*, **192**, 259–67.

Ryan, A. M., Eppler, D. B., Hagler, K. E., Bruner, R. H., Thomford, P. J., Hall, R. L. et al. (1999). Preclinical safety evaluation of rhuMAbVEGF, an antiangiogenic humanized monoclonal antibody. *Toxicol Pathol*, **27**, 78–86.

Ryan, H. E., Lo, J., and Johnson, R. S. (1998). HIF-1 alpha is required for solid tumor formation and embryonic vascularization. *Embo J*, **17**, 3005–15.

Scappaticci, F. A. (2002). Mechanisms and future directions for angiogenesis-based cancer therapies. *J Clin Oncol*, **20**, 3906–27.

Semenza, G. L. (2002). HIF-1 and tumor progression: pathophysiology and therapeutics. *Trends Mol Med*, **8**, S62–7.

Shalaby, F., Rossant, J., Yamaguchi, T. P., Gertsenstein, M., Wu, X. F., Breitman, M. L. et al. (1995). Failure of blood-island formation and vasculogenesis in Flk-1-deficient mice. *Nature*, **376**, 62–6.

Shima, D. T. and Mailhos, C. (2000). Vascular developmental biology: getting nervous. *Curr Opin Genet Dev*, **10**, 536–42.

Soker, S., Takashima, S., Miao, H. Q., Neufeld, G., and Klagsbrun, M. (1998). Neuropilin-1 is expressed by endothelial and tumor cells as an isoform-specific receptor for vascular endothelial growth factor. *Cell*, **92**, 735–45.

Suchting, S., Heal, P., Tahtis, K., Stewart, L. M., and Bicknell, R. (2005). Soluble Robo4 receptor inhibits in vivo angiogenesis and endothelial cell migration. *Faseb J*, **19**(1), 121–3.

Sullivan, D. C. and Bicknell, R. (2003). New molecular pathways in angiogenesis. *British Journal of Cancer*, **89**, 228–231.

Suri, C., Jones, P. F., Patan, S., Bartunkova, S., Maisonpierre, P. C., Davis, S. et al. (1996). Requisite role of angiopoietin-1, a ligand for the TIE2 receptor, during embryonic angiogenesis. *Cell*, **87**, 1171–80.

Tahtis, K., Lee, F. T., Wheatley, J. M., Garin-Chesa, P., Park, J. E., Smyth, F. E., et al. (2003). Expression and targeting of human fibroblast activation protein in a human skin/severe combined immunodeficient mouse breast cancer xenograft model. *Mol Cancer Ther*, **2**(8), 729–37.

Takahashi, T., Kalka, C., Masuda, H., Chen, D., Silver, M., Kearney, M. et al. (1999). Ischemia- and cytokine-induced mobilization of bone marrow-derived endothelial progenitor cells for neovascularization. *Nat Med*, **5**, 434–8.

Walton, H. L., Corjay, M. H., Mohamed, S. N., Mousa, S. A., Santomenna, L. D., and Reilly, T. M. (2000). Hypoxia induces differential expression of the integrin receptors alpha(vbeta3) and alpha(vbeta5) in cultured human endothelial cells. *J Cell Biochem*, **78**, 674–80.

Wang, H. U., Chen, Z. F., and Anderson, D. J. (1998). Molecular distinction and angiogenic interaction between embryonic arteries and veins revealed by ephrin-B2 and its receptor Eph-B4. *Cell*, **93**, 741–53.

Wilkinson, D. G. (2000). Eph receptors and ephrins: regulators of guidance and assembly. *Int Rev Cytol Int Rev Cytol*, **196**, 177–244.

Yancopoulos, G. D., Klagsbrun, M., and Folkman, J. (1998). Vasculogenesis, angiogenesis, and growth factors: ephrins enter the fray at the border. *Cell*, **93**, 661–4.

Yancopoulos, G. D., Davis, S., Gale, N. W., Rudge, J. S., Wiegand, S. J., and Holash, J. (2000). Vascular-specific growth factors and blood vessel formation. *Nature*, **407**, 242–8.

Zetter, B. R. (1998). Angiogenesis and tumor metastasis. *Annu Rev Med*, **49**, 407–24.

CHAPTER 18

Stem cells, haemopoiesis, and leukaemia

Mel Greaves

18.1 Introduction

The leukaemias, and related diseases lymphoma and myeloma, are all blood cell cancers. Because of the accessibility of this tissue, the relative ease of cell culture, and the availability of model systems with animal cells, knowledge of the cellular and molecular basis of these forms of cancer has often led the way and provided paradigms for cancer research in general. Leukaemias are different from other cancers in so far as their evolution and dissemination does not require architectural disruption and metastatic processes that are critically involved in most other cancers. This distinction may, at least in part, account for the clinical sensitivity and curability of many disseminated leukaemias, particularly in children. Despite this difference, leukaemias provide a particularly informative example of how multistep malignancy can be viewed as a parody or disruption of normal developmental processes. The key cell types in this process are those that serve as founders or stem cells for blood cell production. We refer to this process, overall, as haemopoiesis (or haematopoiesis) and it is often, for experimental or descriptive purposes, sub-divided into its two major components, myelopoiesis and lymphopoiesis, that is production of myeloid and lymphoid cells.

18.2 Haemopoietic regulation

Blood cell production is initiated during embryogenesis, in the yolk sac (embryonic erythropoiesis), and in the embryo body, in the so-called AGM (aorta, gonad, mesonephros) region. Subsequently, both myeloid and lymphoid cell production are housed first in the foetal liver, then bone marrow and (for T cells) in the thymus. During foetal life, haemopoiesis is seeded and then sustained by blood-borne stem cells. After birth and throughout life, haemopoiesis continues as a rapid and dynamic process in the bone marrow. Cell generation rates are prodigious—more than 10^{11} cells per day ($=\sim 10^{16}$ in a lifetime). This explosive and sustained rate of production can only be accommodated by an equivalent turnover and loss of cells *and* by maintenance of the stem cell pool by self-renewal.

Studies in mice in which individual cells can be genetically marked by unique (individual) chromosomal sites of retroviral insertion have provided convincing evidence for the existence of a class or population of multipotential stem cells that are the founders for all haemopoiesis. This provides us with the starting point for all haemopoietic lineage tree diagrams as shown in Figure 18.1.

Within this lineage hierarchy, the different cell types can be distinguished by their phenotypic

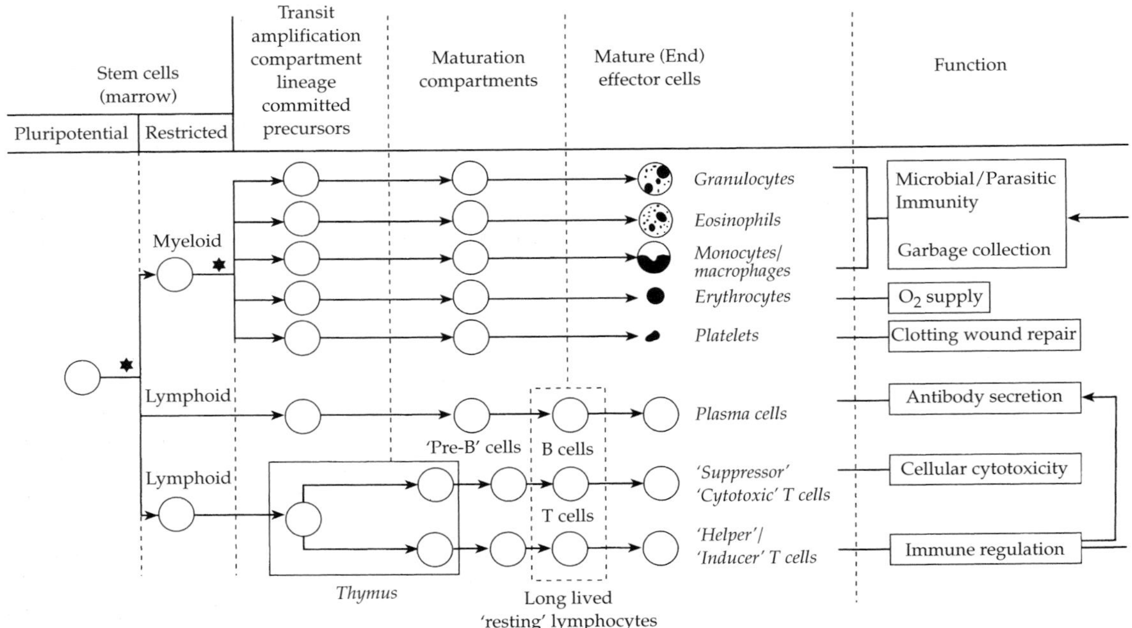

Figure 18.1 Simplified lineage hierarchy and cell function in haemopoiesis. The asterisks indicate that our understanding of developmental potentialities and the sequence or pattern of commitment at these apparent 'junctions' in the lineage tree are still very incomplete.

properties, which include some physical features (size, charge, adhesiveness), morphology (for maturing myeloid cells), antigenic markers identified with monoclonal antibodies, and by gene expression signatures (e.g. by microarray analysis or RT-PCR). Monoclonal antibodies have been especially important in this respect, both for cell type identification and physical sorting of cells. Few of these individual properties are unique to any cell type but it is possible to identify *composite* phenotypes that are. The availability of these cell markers has been extraordinarily useful, not only for experimental studies, but for practical, clinical purposes also, including differential diagnosis of leukaemia, some therapeutic strategies (e.g. toxin-tagged antibodies, see Chapter 26), and for manipulation of stem cells for gene therapy and/or transplantation purposes.

Stem cells are the most critical cells in haemopoiesis as in other tissues with continual turnover or regenerative capacity. They are also believed to be the major cellular targets for leukaemogenesis. Tissue stem cells are usually defined as cells that have two particular properties. First, they can sustain their numbers after their brief embryological spawning, and throughout the life-long postnatal period for which they are required. In haemopoiesis at least, this challenge is met by small numbers of stem cells taking turns at proliferation (called clonal succession), while most remain quiescent and out of cell cycle (G_0). Also, proliferative cycles of stem cells can generate daughter cells that themselves have stem cell properties and can return to dormancy (so-called self-renewal cycles). Second, proliferating stem cells can generate daughter cells that undergo both substantial further cell cycling and differentiation or maturation into functional, mature cells.

The divergent developmental options or fates for haemopoietic stem cells are illustrated in Figure 18.2. Note that in addition to proliferation and maturation down a lineage, cells may have to choose to differentiate down one lineage out of several available, or may choose, or be persuaded, to opt out and die. The latter fatality occurs by apoptosis or programmed cell death. Apoptosis is a critical component of haemopoiesis helping to maintain, homeostatically, population numbers within appropriate limits, and, additionally in lymphopoiesis, to facilitate the process of stringent

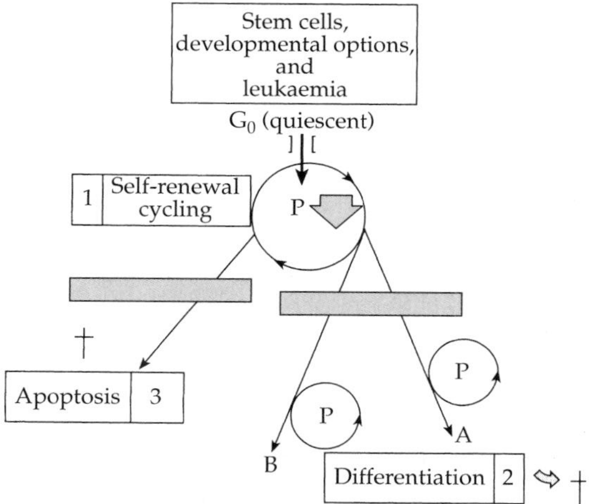

Figure 18.2 Developmental options for stem cells. Haemopoietic stem cells normally reside out of mitotic cycle (in G_0 or quiescent). When activated to undergo proliferation (P), there are three developmental options: (1) self-renewal, (2) differentiation, and (3) apoptosis or cell death (†). Disruption of any one (or all) of these three pathways by loss of function (▭) or constitutive activation (⇩) can contribute to the development of leukaemia.

clonal selection that occurs both during the production of T and B lymphocytes and in subsequent immune responses. Apoptosis is now recognized as an essential part of almost all developmental processes and many physiological responses. Two important corollaries are therefore not so surprising. First, that multiple genes, mostly of ancient evolutionary origin as evidenced by studies in yeast and nematode worms, are involved in regulating cell death; second, that genes involved in apoptosis may be altered or mutated in leukaemia and other cancers. A further and perhaps less obvious consequence of these developmental arrangements is that changes in the vulnerability to physiological cell death in leukaemic cells may have a major impact on the sensitivity of these cells to the common therapeutic agents that are given to patients (see Section 18.7; Chapter 24).

18.2.1 Molecular rules of the game

We are still ignorant of some of the basic molecular processes in haemopoiesis, but remarkable insights have been gained in recent years. These are important since they may pinpoint and help us to understand the molecular defects underlying leukaemias. With respect to DNA *replication* and *proliferation*, it is clear that the fundamental rules are laid down in a complex, multilayered, genetic circuitry occupied by interacting proteins and enzymes (predominantly kinases and phosphatases). These ground rules are of very ancient evolutionary origin, conserved and shared by different cell types and tissues. Primarily, what differs between cell types, other than some details of the circuit wiring, are the ligands and corresponding cellular receptors that regulate the process. In this respect each cell type lives in its own sensory world equivalent to the 'merkwelt' of an animal species! Similarly for *apoptosis*, a basic set of genes encoding particular proteins appears to have been invented early in evolution and, although the circuitry becomes elaborated and refined with further evolutionary developments, the ground rules remain largely intact. For apoptosis, key components for both haemopoietic and other cell types include a family of related proteins including BCL-2, BAX, and BCLx which form complexes that, depending upon their composition or stoichiometry, can impede or facilitate apoptosis. How they achieve this is not understood. Other critical proteins in blood cell apoptosis include FAS and FAS ligand and those that contribute to a cascade resulting in activation of a protease that degrades other proteins and cellular membranes, plus one or more endonucleases that can break up DNA to give the nucleosomal fragments, DNA-staining profiles, and nuclear morphology that are characteristic of apoptosis in both blood cells and most other cell types.

Differentiation is in one sense a lineage- or cell type-specific process, but even here there is common and evolutionarily conserved territory. The current view is that key differentiation decisions in haemopoiesis (as elsewhere) involve the initiation and stabilization of a unique programme of gene expression. Control of this process exists, in principle, at two levels. First, the genes involved operate in sequential cascades with positive and negative feedback loops exercised by the protein products that they encode. Second, selective activation of genes, which is the key to the process, is believed to occur through the dynamic formation of stable transcription complexes. These are heterodimeric or polymeric assemblies of proteins which bind to DNA and, as a consequence, are able to modify chromatin or DNA structure, accessibility, and the enzyme-mediated process of gene transcription. Third, cell surface receptors, interfacing with the cellular environment, regulate the process, often by initiating phosphorylation cascades that modify transcription factor complexes. Cell types in haemopoiesis come to exist and differ in their phenotypes as a consequence of their unique constellations of transcription factors empowered to regulate gene activity positively or negatively. This process is constrained by the ancestry of the cell (i.e. by prior genetic decisions) and is regulated by the cell's unique receptor profile—itself the product of a similar genetic decision-making or differentiation process. Finally, as might have been anticipated, the processes of proliferation, differentiation, and apoptosis are integrated into a network as alternative pathways for cell fate. Many of these decisions operate during the G_1 phase of the cell cycle and all are modulated or regulated by signals derived by means of cell surface receptors detecting changes in the local environment of the cells. Receptors may be triggered by soluble ligand released either locally or systematically, or by secreted ligands bound and compartmentalized by adjacent stromal cells and/or their cell surface-associated intracellular matrix components, such as heparan sulphate. Heterotypic cell–cell interactions between blood cells and vascular, lymphatic, and tissue stromal cells play a critical role in myelopoiesis and lymphopoiesis, regulating cell fate through the three major pathways alluded to above. In addition they control cell positioning and migration by selective adhesion (Figure 18.3).

Discovering which particular transcription factors are involved in the derivation of particular cell types is difficult. Biochemical identification of proteins binding to control regions (promoters, enhancers, locus control regions) of genes that have lineage-specific expression (e.g. in haemopoiesis: haemoglobin, immunoglobulin, myeloperoxidase) provides candidates whose function can be further assessed by gene transfection assays. Gene knock-out (by homologous recombination) provides an alternative strategy for identifying essential transcription factors and the developmental stages at which they operate. Figure 18.4 is a summary profile of some of the key players in haemopoiesis identified by the knock-out approach. No doubt, more remain to be discovered and many transcription factors appear to have modulating, non-essential, or redundant functions in haemopoiesis. One striking finding in these studies has been that the genes most commonly involved as mutants in acute leukaemia are essential for normal

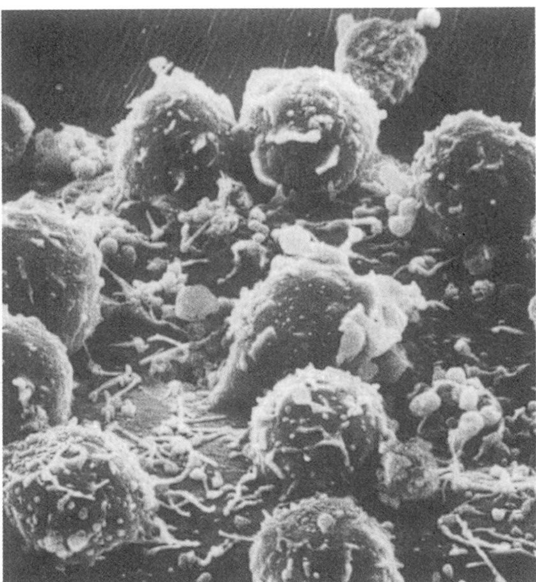

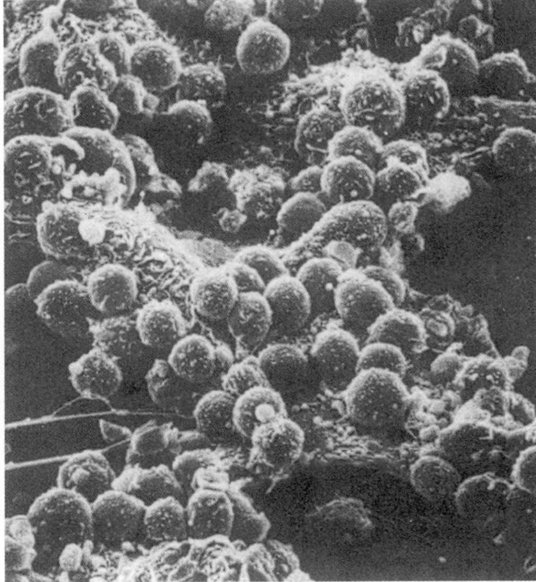

Figure 18.3 Adhesive interactions with stromal cells regulate early haemopoiesis. Stereoscan electron microscopy images of T-cell precursors binding to the surface of thymic epithelial cells. From an *in vitro* culture system believed to mimic developmental cell interactions in the thymic cortex.

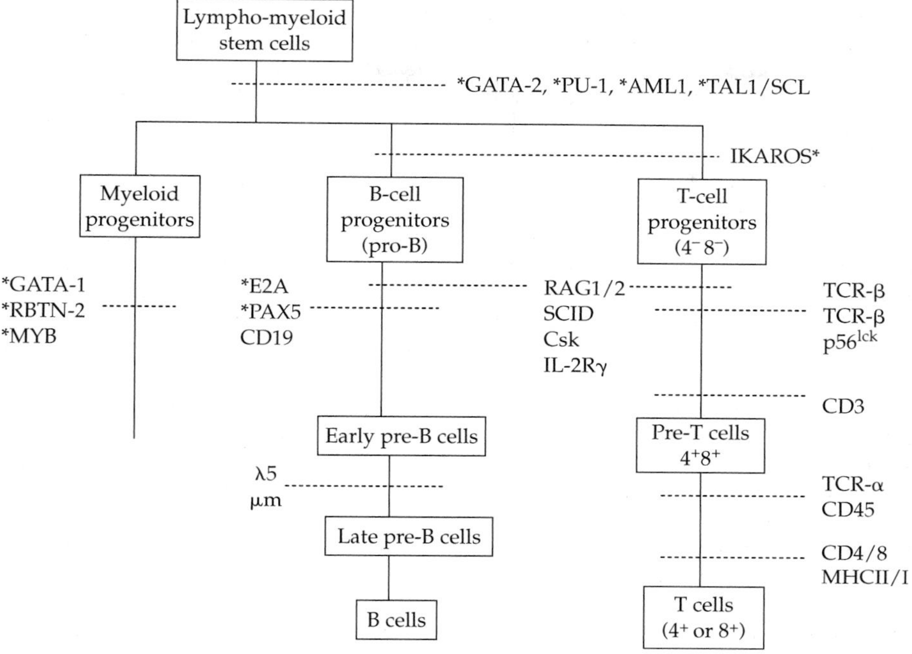

Figure 18.4 Critical regulators of haemopoiesis can be identified by 'knock-out' experiments. The diagram lists transcription factors (*) or other proteins whose function is required for defined steps in early haemopoietic differentiation (at the level indicated by the cross-bar). Differentiation beyond the level indicated is aborted in transgenic mice in which the gene has been inactivated by homologous recombination.

haemopoietic stem cell function, for example, *AML1* and other components of the core binding factor (CBF) complex, SCL (Figure 18.5). A critical unresolved issue in haemopoietic stem cell biology (and stem cell biology in general) is how the differentiating progeny of a multipotential lympho-myeloid stem cell *decides* to adopt one lineage from the many options available. It is unclear whether this choice is dictated by extracellular signals, a cell autonomous, stochastic process or a combination of these. Some evidence suggests that these cells may transit through a sequence of more simple binary choices with one of the two lineages available as a default. The mechanism of choice is assumed to involve the formation of stable transcription complexes that elicit and consolidate lineage-specific gene expression cascades or patterns. Interestingly in this context, multipotential cells, before uni-lineage commitment, express multiple lineage genes at least at low levels, in a promiscuous fashion suggesting that adoption of a lineage involves both turning-up (and consolidating) and turning-off of genes. These changes are now known to involve local alterations in

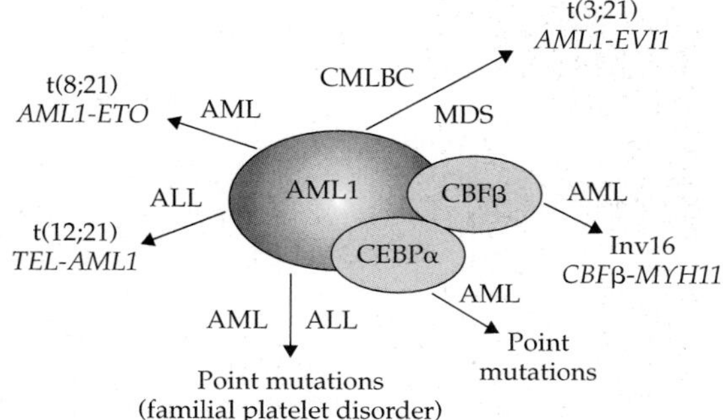

Figure 18.5 CBF transcriptional complex aberrations in leukaemia. Diagram illustrates leukaemia-associated chromosome translocations and point mutations in genes encoding each of the three major components of CBF. AML, acute myeloblastic leukaemia; ALL, acute lymphoblastic leukaemia; CMLBC, blast crisis of chronic myeloid leukaemia; MDS, myelodysplastic syndrome. AML1 is also known as RUNX1 and encodes the CBFα subunit.

chromatin acetylation, methylation, and physical accessibility. These insights derived in part from the observation that leukaemic cells in differentiation arrest often expressed bizarre or promiscuous lineage phenotypes—and that many abnormal genes in leukaemia encode altered transcriptional regulatory properties.

18.3 Leukaemia as a clonal disorder of haemopoiesis

In common with other cancers, leukaemias share a number of salient features (Table 18.1). *Proliferation* is usually continual or constitutive, though not necessarily at a fast rate in terms of cell cycle time. Very often, particularly in the acute leukaemias, *differentiation* appears to be blocked at an early stage of haemopoiesis. Cell death certainly occurs in leukaemia cell populations *in vivo* and *in vitro*, but leukaemic cells will often have an increased propensity to survive conditions of growth factor deprivation or stress that propel other cells into apoptosis. But first and foremost among these common features of leukaemia is monoclonality and its origin by means of mutation. In common with all but a few exceptional cases, leukaemias and other cancers are clonal diseases driven by mutation, that is, the leukaemic cells of any one patient all derive from a *single* mutant progenitor cell. The conventional and probably correct interpretation of this feature is that the particular mutations required to give a clone a growth advantage sufficient to produce diagnostic symptoms and pathology are exceedingly rare, so rare that they only occur in a single cell among the extraordinarily high number of stem cell divisions that occur in a lifetime.

We assume that mutations occur all the time, but that the vast majority occur either in genes that cannot confer growth advantage (i.e. neutral or deleterious) and/or in irrelevant cells. We know that leukaemias are monoclonal by long-standing observations on chromosome karyotypes and by the application of a number of immunological and molecular markers for clonal status. The formation of a leukaemic clone through mutation is not equivalent to the activation of one faulty switch in the genetic circuit. Although one mutation does initiate the process, the resultant clone is seldom stable. Over time it will, in a Darwinian fashion akin to a species, either regress or diversify by further genetic change and will be subject to competitive selection exercised by the body's own regulatory mechanisms or by therapy. This evolutionary process may be gradual or may involve relatively abrupt changes in cellular phenotype, cell behaviour, and disease pathology, as, for example, in the so-called blast crisis of chronic myeloid leukaemia. The development of leukaemic clones in this respect parallels progression in carcinoma elucidated at the molecular level by Vogelstein, Weinberg, Bodmer, and others. The underlying principle of step-wise, if chaotic, evolutionary progression was, however, first clearly enunciated by the UK pathologist Leslie Foulds in 1969 whose book on the subject remains a neglected classic (read it!). If, as we suppose, multiple mutations in different genes encoding distinct, but complementary, functions (again as in species evolution) are an invariant or inevitable component of leukaemia, then it follows from the rarity of those events that mutations will be acquired *sequentially* over an unpredictable time period. The products of this dynamic process are successive waves of dominant subclones. These essential and combinational activities set the variable timeframe, pace, and course of disease evolution in terms of pre-clinical latency, progression, drug resistance, and, for solid tumours, metastasis. In many epithelial cancers, this evolutionary process is propelled by the early acquisition of genetic instability. This does occur in leukaemia but appears to be a rarer genotypic alteration.

Table 18.1 Consistent features of leukaemic cells

Monoclonal origin
Acquired gene mutations (1-*n*)
Genetic instability, clonal diversification, and progressive subclone selection (i.e. Darwinian selection)
Dysregulation or uncoupling of critical cellular functions: proliferation, differentiation, cell death
Net growth advantage, clonal dominance, vascular and extravascular spread, and compromise of normal tissue functions (territorial hijack)

18.4 Gene culprits

From what has been outlined above on the regulation of haemopoiesis, an astute student should have no difficulty in predicting what kinds or sets of genes would be involved in leukaemia as mutants. In principle, any gene that, when mutated, can give a clone a *net* growth advantage, can initiate and/or contribute to progression of disease. Since clonal population dynamics are determined by the interplay and balance of proliferation, differentiation, and cell death, it follows that lesions in any or each of these three circuits may participate in leukaemogenesis (cf. Figure 18.2). Furthermore, in view of their complementary functions, it is not surprising that single leukaemic clones, as they evolve to more aggressive phenotypes, may acquire mutations in two or all three of these circuits. Indeed, acquisition of a complementary set of mutations may not only be advantageous to the clone, but essential for its survival, if, as is currently believed, mutations in some oncogenes (e.g. *MYC*) promoting constitutive proliferation simultaneously drive apoptosis when essential growth factors are limiting.

Although these pathological patterns are entirely predictable from first principles, it is only because the mutant genes have been cloned and sequenced and their protein functions uncovered in either a normal or abnormal context that we can present this scenario with some confidence. Table 18.2 categorizes some of the major types of gene alterations in leukaemia, their structural basis, the functions of their protein products, and leukaemia subtype associations. Note that some of these genes are involved in many forms of cancer (e.g. as cell cycle regulators) and that others have leukaemia or leukaemia subtype specificity. The most striking genetic abnormalities in this respect are the balanced chromosome translocations that give rise to chimaeric fusion genes. Such chromosomal recombinants are common also in other types of paediatric cancers, for example, soft tissue sarcomas, but are very rare in epithelial carcinomas where unbalanced chromosome breaks and deletions are the rule. The reason for this marked distinction is unclear but might relate to the common and early imposition of chromosomal instability in carcinomas. Two types of fusion genes are observed in blood cell cancers resulting in either enforced expression of one partner gene or a hybrid protein product. Very many different genes participate in these genetic liaisons but a few genes are markedly promiscuous. The gene *MLL*, related to *Drosophila trithorax*, and a master regulator of *HOX* genes in development (and haemopoiesis) can fuse with up to 50 alternative partner genes. *TEL* and *AML1*, both encoding transcription factors essential for haemopoiesis (Figure 18.4) also fuse with a multitude (>15) of different partners to create chimaeric genes encoding either novel transcriptional proteins or activated kinases. These two genes also fuse with each other to form the most common translocation-based fusion gene, *TEL-AML1*, in paediatric cancer (~25% of childhood acute lymphoblastic leukaemia (ALL)) (Figure 18.6).

Table 18.2 Diversity of molecular changes in leukaemia and related blood cell cancers

Abnormality/Genes	Function	Leukaemia/ lymphoma subtype
Reciprocal chromosomal translocations		
Dysregulation by juxtaposition to TCR-α, -β, -δ or *IGH*		
IGH-MYC	P	Burkitt's lymphoma
IGH-BCL-6	T	Diffuse (B) lymphoma
IGH-BCL-2	A	Follicular (B) lymphoma
TCR-δ-RBTN-1	T	T-ALL
TCR-β-HOX11	T	T-ALL
Unique product by gene fusion		
MLL—multiple alternative partners	T	Infant AL, secondary AML
BCR-ABL	P/A	CML, ALL
TEL-AML1	T	Bp ALL
AML1-ETO	T	AML
PML-RARAα	T	APML
Chromosomal deletions		
Loss of function		
9p-(CDK4 INHIBITOR?)	P	ALL
5q-(?)	(?)	AML
Hybrid gene formation		
TAL del = *SIL-TAL1* FUSION	T	T-ALL
Chromosomal inversions		
Dysregulation by juxtaposition		
INV14 = TCR-TCL-1	T	T-CLL
Unique product by gene fusion		
INV16 = MYOSIN(MYH11)-CBFβ	T	AML
Ploidy changes		
Hyperdiploidy	?	Bp ALL Myeloma
+8 −7	}	AML
Point mutations		
NRAS	P/A	Most subtypes
TP53	P/A	Most subtypes

P, proliferation regulation; T, transcriptional regulation of differentiation; A, apoptosis regulation; ALL, acute lymphoblastic leukaemia; AML, acute myeloblastic leukaemia; APML, acute promyelocytic leukaemia; T-ALL, thymic acute lymphoblastic leukaemia; Bp ALL, B cell precursor acute lymphoblastic leukaemia; CLL, chronic lymphocytic leukaemia; CML, chronic myeloid leukaemia.

Such a list inevitably understates the remarkable diversity of mutation that can occur. For example, in one subtype of leukaemia, ALL (the major cancer in children), over 200 different genetic abnormalities

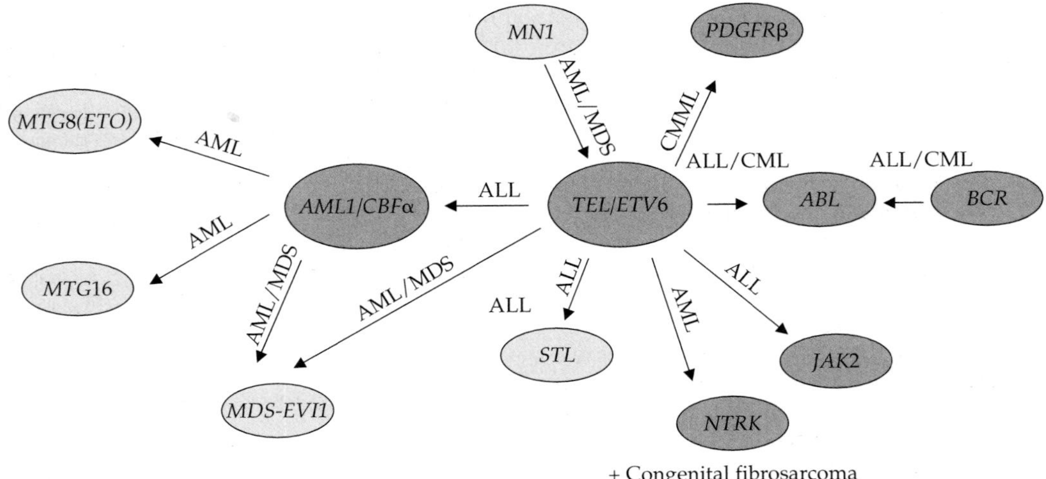

Figure 18.6 Mix and match gene fusions with *TEL* and *AML1*. Arrows indicate particular gene pairings and associated subtype of leukaemia. ALL, acute lymphoblastic leukaemia; AML, acute myeloblastic leukaemia; CML, chronic myeloid leukaemia; CMML, chronic myelomonocytic leukaemia; MDS, myelodysplastic syndrome (a form of myeloid pre-leukaemia). CBFα, core binding factor α subunit is product of *AML1/RUNX1*; *ETV6* is alternative name for *TEL*.

have been described; most are, however, relatively rare. This degree of diversity arises, we assume, because of the multiple points in the three control circuits that are rate limiting or able to perturb cell kinetics. Some changes are, however, much more common than others and these are the ones that have major clinical implications (see further).

The remarkable consistency with which these genetic lesions are associated with subtypes of leukaemia implies that they are critical components of the causal pathway of leukaemogenesis. The best evidence to support this comes from the demonstration that these same human leukaemia-associated genes, when cloned and transferred into the mouse germline or into haemopoietic stem cells, generate biologically similar leukaemias in offspring or transplant recipients, respectively. Crucially, however, leukaemia initiation in these circumstances requires additional 'secondary' mutations.

18.5 Origin of mutations and the natural history of leukaemia

Virtually all of the described mutations in leukaemia are non-constitutive or acquired. They are assumed to arise either pre- or post-natally as a consequence of either random errors in DNA replication and recombination, perhaps under conditions of proliferative stress, or as a consequence of genotoxic exposure. Different leukaemias may well have distinct aetiologies in this respect and there is considerable epidemiological evidence to support the involvement of a variety of pathways or agents, including ionizing radiation, chemicals, and microbial infection (see Chapter 2 and references given at the end of this chapter).

Except in rare cases of known medical or industrial/occupational exposure that result in leukaemia after a period of some years, or even a decade or two, we have little insight into the detailed natural history of adult leukaemia (lymphoma or myeloma). The situation is different for childhood leukaemia where considerable progress has been made. It turns out that the common chromosome translocations observed in subtypes of acute leukaemia arise predominantly before birth, during foetal haemopoiesis, that is, they are early or initiating events. The evidence for this derives from the use of fusion gene sequences as unique (patient- and clone-specific), stable and sensitive markers of the malignant clone.

In identical monozygotic twins with concordant leukaemia (i.e. both have the disease), the same unique fusion gene sequence is present, yet this fusion depends upon randomly positioned breaks in introns of the relevant genes (e.g. *TEL, AML1*) and is acquired not inherited. This outcome is only possible if leukaemia is initiated by gene fusion in a single cell in one foetus. The leukaemias are shared because twins are blood cell chimaeras in 60% of cases, a consequence of sharing a single placenta within which there are vascular anastomoses. This evidence for a pre-natal origin of acute leukaemia via chromosome translocation is directly substantiated by retrospective scrutiny, by PCR (polymerase chain reaction), of archived neonatal blood spots (Guthrie cards) of children with leukaemia (Figure 18.7). These small blood spots of 30 μl, routinely collected after birth for screening for metabolic disorders, can be shown to contain small numbers of cells with the unique fusion gene sequence subsequently present in the individual leukaemic cell. Remember again that these sequences are not inherited.

These data indicate that acute leukaemia in children is frequently initiated *in utero*, probably by the chromosome translocation itself. But, as anticipated, this single genetic event is usually insufficient for overt, clinical leukaemia. We know this because: (1) the concordance rate for leukaemia in twins is ~10% not 100%; (2) these same genes only induce leukaemia as experimental transgenes *in vivo* (in mice) if complemented by additional genetic abnormalities; and (3) functional fusion genes (e.g. *TEL-AML1*) and expanded pre-leukaemic cells occur in normal newborns that will never develop leukaemia (in fact 100 times the frequency of the

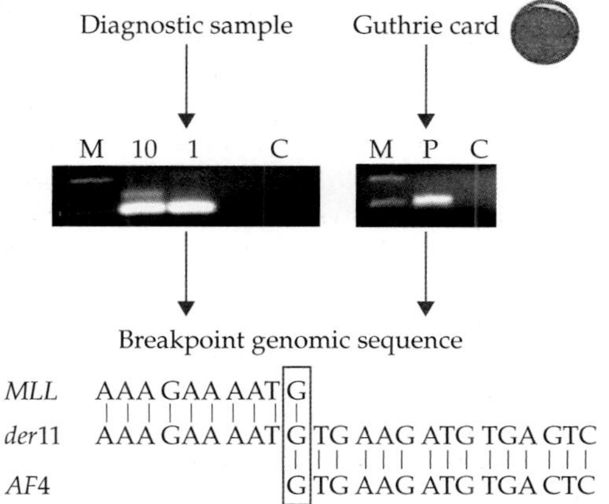

Figure 18.7 Detection of clonotypic fusion gene sequences in neonatal blood spots (Guthrie cards). Basic scheme of PCR-based test identifying same amplicon and genomic fusion sequence (*MLL-AF4* in this example) in diagnostic/leukaemic DNA and Guthrie card DNA (of same individual). M, markers; 10 and 1 = ng DNA (titration); C, control; P, patient DNA sample.

disease itself). The essential secondary genetic abnormalities will usually occur post-natally and often involve chromosomal deletions or kinase mutations. For example, most cases of childhood ALL with the *TEL-AML1* fusion have secondary deletions of the normal *TEL* allele. Other cases of childhood ALL with hyperdiploidy as an early (pre-natal) event often have secondary *FLT3* mutations. With progression of disease (and high leukaemic cell levels), additional genetic changes including *p16/CDKN2A* deletion/methylation and *TP53* mutation may occur.

18.6 Target cells in leukaemia

The morphology, immunophenotype, and mutant genes in leukaemic subsets provide an indication of the lineage and cell type that has been clonally selected in the disease. This information has, in principle, provided the framework for differential haematological and pathological diagnosis for almost a century, albeit with many biological refinements over the past two decades. But how does the leukaemic phenotype relate developmentally within haemopoiesis, to the single 'target' cell whose transformation must have initiated clonal expansion and subsequent leukaemia evolution? Factors that need to be taken into account include the stringency of differentiation arrest and the possibility that some mutant genes may directly or indirectly produce an aberrant or misleading developmental phenotype.

The phenotype of leukaemic clones may generally reflect the developmental level or window of maturation arrest within the haematopoietic hierarchy. However, both the minority clonogenic stem cells driving or sustaining the disease, and the cell type that was initially transformed by mutation can lie anywhere antecedent or 'upstream' of the maturation arrest position. More insight can be gained into this issue by physical separation of stem cells by means of their cell surface antigenic properties and assaying for the presence of chromosome translocations (e.g. by interphase fluorescence *in situ* hybridization; see Chapter 6) and by transplantation into *SCID/NOD* mice. Such experiments have usually indicated that these cells have a more primitive phenotype than the bulk of their progeny, which must therefore undergo at least limited differentiation. Another strategy to identify the developmental level of clonal expansion is to evaluate, independently of the bulk population

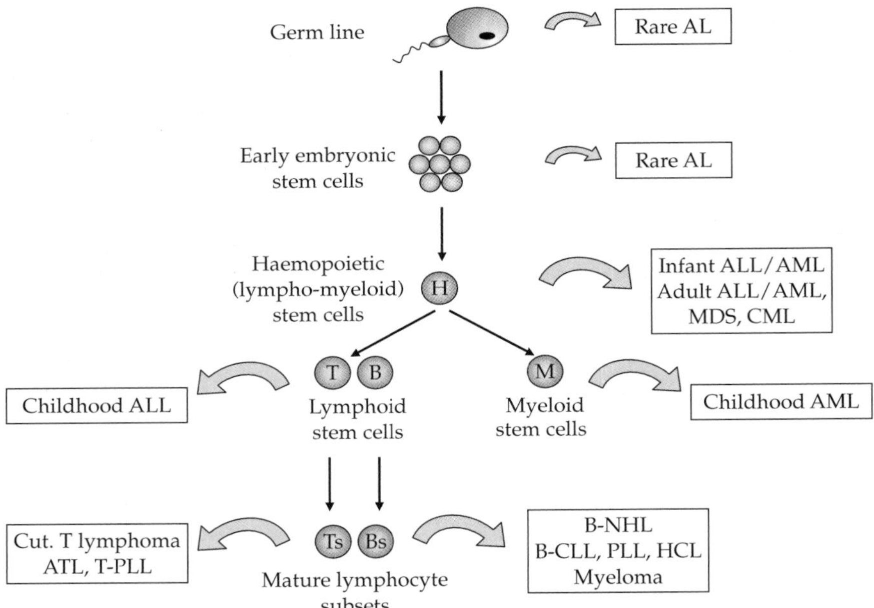

Figure 18.8 Hierarchical stem cell origins of leukaemia and related cancers. Arrows denote likely level of clonal selection for the majority of cases of leukaemia of subtype listed. AL, acute leukaemia; ALL, acute lymphoblastic leukaemia; AML, acute myeloblastic leukaemia; ATL, adult T cell leukaemia/lymphoma; cut, cutaneous; CLL, chronic lymphocytic leukaemia; HCL, hairy cell leukaemia; NHL, non-Hodgkin's lymphoma; PLL, prolymphocytic leukaemia.

phenotype, what lineages contribute to the leukaemic population, as judged by a shared clonal marker. For this purpose, cells belonging to different lineages must be identified or sorted with appropriate markers (usually monoclonal antibodies) and then interrogated for the presence of one or more of the chromosomal or molecular markers that are available as indicators of common clonal descent. When these types of analyses are performed, it is clear that many acute leukaemias, in which the population phenotype is dominated by one lineage or cell type, do, in fact, originate in dual or multilineage stem cells, with growth advantage and/or differentiation competence into different lineages being selectively expressed. The clearest example of this is with chronic myeloid leukaemia which has an overwhelmingly mature granulocytic lineage phenotype, but a multipotential lympho-myeloid stem cell origin. An important implication of these findings, paralleled in transgenic animals, is that chromosome translocation-derived fusion genes arising in multipotential stem cells have cell type-specific impacts.

It is possible to draw up a lineage map that identifies the likely developmental origins of different types of blood cell cancers (Figure 18.8). This analysis suggests that three 'tiers' of stem cells at risk exist in leukaemia and related disease: multipotential stem cells, lineage-restricted stem cells, and mature lymphoid stem cells. It is likely, though not formally proven, that most leukaemias and other cancers involve tissue stem cells responsible for embryonic morphogenesis (the paediatric tumours) or for sustained turnover (or regenerative capacity) in lymphomyeloid tissues, epithelial tissues, and endocrine organs. Mature lymphoid stem cells are, however, unusual. Despite being highly differentiated, they retain self-renewing stem cell properties and may benefit from a decade or more life span (as a clone or as individual cells residing out of cycle) with extensive proliferative potential and differentiation competence, that is, cytotoxic T-cell function or antibody secretion (see Chapters 20 and 26). There are sound reasons of immunological economy why we should preserve, for a long time, clones of cells with a memory of antigenic or infectious exposure, but this arrangement does pose an unusual risk to mature cells that is seldom, if ever, found in other tissues that do not normally indulge in clonal selection and conservation.

Considerations of precise cellular origins may seem somewhat esoteric, but they do have practical implications. Clonogenic cells residing at the various developmental levels have different inherent sensitivities to cancer drugs and radiation. Attempts to purge leukaemic clones using differentiation-linked markers (e.g. antibody), either as a purging agent or as an indicator of efficacy of other agents, require that we can identify the position of most or all clonogenic leukaemic cells within the haemopoietic hierarchy. A similar argument can be made for breast, prostate, and other cancers.

18.7 Clinical and epidemiological implications of leukaemic cell and molecular biology

The remarkable insights that have been acquired into both normal haemopoiesis and leukaemia over the past two decades have found some practical applications and have potentially profound implications for future clinical and epidemiological endeavours. Some of these applications and concepts merit special attention. First, the molecular changes that drive the disease now provide specific diagnostic markers for disease subtypes. We already know for some of these, for example, *BCR-ABL*, *MLL* gene fusions and *TP53* alterations, that, independently of other features of disease, they have a strong association with very poor prognosis in the context of currently applied therapeutic cocktails and regimes. Such cases are therefore being routinely identified and selected when possible for alternative therapies; for example, intensified chemotherapy and/or subsequent normal stem cell transplantation. Second, the molecular markers provide not only very *specific*, but very *sensitive* and *stable* clonal markers. Quantitative PCR-based methods can detect 10^{-4}–10^{-6} leukaemic cells via these unique or clonotypic markers. These methods have already provided data that is predictive of the subsequent clinical course (i.e. continued remission or relapse) for groups of patients and are being used as an important aid to patient management guiding continuation, modification, or cessation of therapy.

Chromosome translocation-generated fusion genes may be appropriate targets for selective, non-toxic therapy. This is exemplified by clinical studies with retinoid derivatives targeting retinoic acid receptor gene fusions in acute promyelocytic leukaemia (APML), histone deacetylase (HDAC) inhibitors for repression of *AML1-ETO* function in AML and, in particular, imatinib (Glivec), a selective kinase inhibitor in *BCR-ABL* positive leukaemias. Other emergent technologies can, in principle, target chromosome translocation products at the level of DNA, mRNA, or protein.

Finally, the identification of unique molecular aberrations in particular leukaemias and lymphomas may aid epidemiological investigations into aetiological or causal mechanisms. We know that the causation of blood cell cancer can involve ionizing radiation, chemicals such as benzene, and, in two cases at least, viruses—HTLV-1 in adult T-cell leukaemia and EBV in Burkitt's lymphoma. The cause(s) of most cases of leukaemia remain unknown although recent research has strongly, albeit indirectly, implicated infection in childhood ALL and maternal–foetal chemical exposures during pregnancy for infant leukaemia (with *MLL* gene fusion). These associations are further endorsed by the discovery of inherited normal alleles of genes that can increase risk. In childhood leukaemia, these include immune response genes (HLA class II), enzymes involved in folate metabolism (*MTHFR*) and an enzyme (*NQ01*) that detoxifies certain classes of genotoxic chemicals. Such molecular epidemiological studies are ongoing but already they provide potent evidence that biologically distinct subtypes of leukaemia (and lymphoma) have distinctive causes and raise the further prospect of preventative intervention.

References and further reading

Barr, F. G. (1998). Translocations, cancer and the puzzle of specificity. *Nat Genet*, **19**, 121–4.

Bonnet, D. and Dick, J. E. (1997). Human acute myeloid leukaemia is organized as a hierarchy that originates from a primitive hematopoietic cell. *Nat Med*, **3**, 730–7.

Druker, B., Sawyers, C. L., Kantarjian, H., Resta, D. J., Fernandes Reese, S., Ford, J. M. et al. (2001). Activity of a specific inhibitor of the BCR-ABL tyrosine kinase in the blast crisis of chronic myeloid leukemia and acute lymphoblastic leukemia with the Philadelphia chromosome. *N Engl J Med*, **344**, 1038–42.

Enver, T. and Greaves, M. (1998). Loops, lineage, and leukaemia. *Cell*, **94**, 9–12.

Greaves, M. (1999). Molecular genetics, natural history and the demise of childhood leukaemia. *Eur J Cancer*, **35**, 173–85.

Greaves, M. (2000). *Cancer: The Evolutionary Legacy*. Oxford University Press, Oxford.

Greaves, M. (2002). Childhood leukaemia. *Br Med J*, **324**, 283–7.

Greaves, M. F. and Wiemels, J. (2003). Origins of chromosome translocations in childhood leukaemia. *Nat Rev Cancer*, **3**, 639–49.

Greaves, M. F., Maia, A. T., Wiemels, J. L., and Ford, A. M. (2003). Leukemia in twins: lessons in natural history. *Blood*, **102**, 2321–33.

Greaves, M. F. (1997). Aetiology of acute leukaemia. *Lancet*, **349**, 344–9.

Henderson, E. S., Lister, T. A., and Greaves, M. F. (eds) (2002). *Leukemia. Seventh Edition*. Saunders, Philadelphia.

Mori, H., Colman, S. M., Xiao, Z., Ford, A. M., Healy, L. E., Donaldson, C. et al. (2002). Chromosome translocations and covert leukemic clones are generated during normal fetal development. *Proc Natl Acad Sci USA*, **99**, 8242–7.

Rabbitts, T. H. and Stocks, M. R. (2003). Chromosomal translocation products engender new intracellular therapeutic technologies. *Nat Med*, **9**, 383–386.

Reya, T., Morrison, S. J., Clarke, M. F., and Weissman, I. L. (2001). Stem cells, cancer, and cancer stem cells. *Nature*, **414**, 105–111.

Speck, N. A. and Gilliland, D. G. (2002). Core-binding factors in haematopoiesis and leukaemia. *Nat Rev Cancer*, **2**, 502–13.

Tenen, D. G. (2003). Disruption of differentiation in human cancer: AML shows the way. *Nat Rev Cancer*, **3**, 89–101.

Weissman, I. L. Stem cells: units of development, units of regeneration, and units in evolution. *Cell*, **100**, 157–68.

Wiemels, J. L., Cazzaniga, G., Daniotti, M., Eden, O. B., Addison, G. M., Masera, G. et al. (1999). Prenatal origin of acute lymphoblastic leukaemia in children. *Lancet*, **354**, 1499–503.

CHAPTER 19

Animal models of cancer

Jos Jonkers and Anton Berns

19.1 Introduction

Animal models have been invaluable in the study of human cancer, and they will undoubtedly continue to be so. Spontaneous as well as carcinogen-induced malignancies have been studied in baboons, dogs, birds, rabbits, hamsters, rats, mice, and zebrafish; even fruit flies have been instrumental in the identification of *Drosophila* tumour suppressor genes (TSGs) with orthologues involved in human cancer. Nevertheless, the mouse remains the animal of choice for several reasons. First, mice and humans have roughly the same complement of genes, and most signalling pathways are highly conserved between the two species. Indeed, tumours that either develop spontaneously or after carcinogen exposure in both mouse and human harbour mutations in the same classes of genes, indicating that similar mechanisms govern tumour development. A second reason for choosing the mouse is that many strains are available. Extensive breeding programmes employing various breeding strategies have yielded a bumper crop of isogenic, congenic, and recombinant mouse strains with broad applications in cancer research. Lastly, the possibility to modify the mouse germline has enabled us to manipulate gene expression and gene function in a controllable fashion. Especially, the latter development has dramatically increased the possibilities—and expectations—of mouse tumour models, and has paved the way for 'the modern era' of cancer research. Genetically engineered mice (GEM) have provided great insight into the functions of cancer genes, and the pathways in which they act. They have also allowed direct assessment of how cancer genes cooperate in tumorigenesis, and permitted identification of additional genes involved in tumour progression. Finally, they hold significant promise for establishing improved preclinical models.

19.2 Naturally occurring mutants and their use

Many tumour-prone strains of mice and rats have been developed over most of the twentieth century by selective breeding on the basis of a particular tumour predisposition. As a result, hundreds of inbred strains are available that can be of use in unravelling the many genetic components that can affect tumorigenesis (www.informatics.jax.org/external/festing/search_form.cgi).

19.2.1 Generating tumour-prone mouse strains by selective breeding

The creation of tumour-prone mouse strains through selective breeding began almost a century ago when William Castle and Clarence Cook Little employed consecutive generations of brother–sister matings to produce inbred or 'isogenic' strains of mice. Many of the resulting strains displayed increased susceptibility to developing spontaneous or carcinogen-induced malignancies. Examples include the lymphoma-prone AKR mice, the A, BR6, C3H, DBA, GR, and RIII strains of mice with a high incidence of mammary tumours, and the BALB/c strain with susceptibility to pristane-induced plasmacytomas.

In the mammary tumour-prone strains, the 'milk factor' was identified as the causative agent, leading to the discovery of the mouse mammary tumour virus (MMTV) and ultimately the cellular oncogenes that are activated by juxtaposed MMTV proviruses. Similarly, the susceptibility of AKR mice to T-cell lymphomagenesis was found to be causally associated with the expression of two endogenous murine Leukaemia provirus (MuLV) loci. The susceptibility of BALB/c mice to pristane-induced plasmacytomas is a more complex genetic trait, with at least five *Pctr* loci determining whether mice develop haematopoietic tumours of the plasma cell lineage in response to induction with pristane, a mineral oil, which elicits a chronic inflammatory response. The *Pctr1* locus encompasses the cyclin-dependent kinase inhibitor gene *Cdkn2a*, which encodes both p16INK4a and p19ARF products, and BALB/c mice were found to carry a rare allele of the *Cdkn2a* gene. Subsequent biological assays of the *Ink4a* and *Arf* alleles from the susceptible BALB/c and resistant DBA/2 strains pinpointed the difference to p16INK4a.

19.2.2 Generating tumour-prone mouse strains by *N*-ethyl-*N*-nitrosourea mutagenesis

Valuable additions to the long-existing tumour-prone mouse strains represent mutant mice that have been generated by random germ-line mutagenesis with *N*-ethyl-*N*-nitrosourea (ENU), followed by screening for specific tumour phenotypes. One tangible result from these mutagenesis screens is the well-known *Min* mouse. This mouse mutant carries a truncation mutation in the *Apc* TSG, which results in a high incidence of both intestinal and mammary tumours.

More recently, phenotype-driven ENU mutagenesis screens have been employed to identify mouse chromosome instability mutants using a flow cytometric peripheral blood micronucleus assay. In this way, one recessive mutation, named *chaos1*, was found to confer elevated levels of spontaneous and radiation- or mitomycin C-induced micronuclei. Although cancer susceptibility of *chaos1* mutant mice remains to be established, the data suggest that a forward genetic approach using the surrogate marker of chromosome instability as a screen might uncover new potential cancer susceptibility genes.

The completion of the human and mouse genomic sequence has enabled the design of genotype-driven screens that lead from sequence to mutants. Such screens can be performed for ENU-induced mutations in mouse embryonic stem cells, or in parallel archives of DNA and sperm from ENU-treated males. A screen of a cryopreserved library of clonal, germ-line competent ENU-mutagenized embryonic stem (ES) cells identified a large series of allelic mutations in the *Smad2* and *Smad4* TSGs by heteroduplex analysis. Similarly, a yeast-based protein truncation assay was successfully used to screen for disruption of *Brca1* or *Brca2* in offspring from ENU-mutagenized outbred Sprague–Dawley rats.

19.2.3 Mapping tumour modifier genes in tumour-prone mouse strains

Many, if not all, of the currently available tumour-prone mouse strains show 'background' effects caused by differences in the genetic make-up that modulate the effect of the engineered mutation. These effects may include differences in the number or type of tumours that arise, or the speed with which they develop. Over the past decades, several mouse models have been developed that permit identification of tumour modifier genes that are responsible for phenotypic differences in tumour susceptibility. These approaches either involve crosses between various inbred strains of mice or employ recombinant inbred, recombinant congenic, or advanced intercross strains.

The first tumour modifier gene came from investigations on phenotypic expression of the aforementioned *Min* mouse strain. The development of intestinal adenomas in these mice was found to be strongly dependent on strain background. Breeding of the *Min* allele on to a C57BL/6 background gave a strong phenotype, whereas AKR mice were resistant to *Min*-associated intestinal tumorigenesis due to the presence of a modifier of *Min* (*Mom1*) on mouse chromosome 4. Subsequent investigations highlighted the phospholipase gene *Pla2g2* as a candidate for *Mom1* by showing that the sensitive mouse strains contain a polymorphism that introduces a premature stop codon within the PLA2G2 protein coding sequence. However, PLA2G2 has not yet been shown to play a significant role in human (intestinal) tumorigenesis.

19.2.4 Mapping tumour susceptibility genes in recombinant congenic strains

One approach for systematic mapping of tumour susceptibility genes entails the generation of a series of approximately 20 recombinant congenic strains (RCSs) derived from two inbred strains that differ in their susceptibility to developing tumours. A random 12.5% of the genome of a tumour-susceptible donor strain is transferred to the relatively tumour-resistant background strain. Consequently, polygenic traits in the donor strain become separated in the 20 RCSs and can thus be studied independently. The RCS system has been used to map the chromosomal location of several *Sluc* genes, which confer susceptibility to lung cancer, and *Scc* genes, which predispose to colon cancer. Interestingly, several *Sluc* and *Scc* loci have no apparent individual effect, but show a strong reciprocal interaction, meaning that the genotype at one locus determines the effect of the allele at the second locus and vice versa. These findings demonstrate that genetic interactions are likely to play an important role in determination of tumour susceptibility. Thus far, only the colon-cancer susceptibility locus *Scc1* has been analysed in detail by positional cloning, culminating in the identification of the receptor-type protein tyrosine phosphatase *Ptprj* as the underlying gene. Interestingly, in human colon, lung, and breast cancers frequent heterozygous deletion of *PTPRJ* is found, indicating that *PTPRJ* may also be relevant to human cancer. In particular the observed allelic imbalances resulting in loss of heterozygosity, and somatically acquired missense mutations suggest that specific polymorphisms in *PTPRJ* could play a role in predisposition to cancer.

19.2.5 Mapping tumour susceptibility genes in interspecies intercross strains

One of the potential limitations of the RCS system is that the relatively limited genetic diversity between the inbred parental strains will only result in a restricted set of phenotypic differences that can be studied. An alternative approach, which has led to the detection of multiple, dominant resistance loci, has been to exploit the genetic diversity between *Mus musculus* and wild mouse strains such as *Mus spretus*. Crosses of *M. musculus* with *M. spretus* are highly resistant to carcinogen-induced tumour development in the skin, liver, colon, lung, and the lymphoid system, suggesting that *M. spretus* has multiple, dominantly acting resistance genes. This prediction was confirmed by the mapping of several loci that control resistance to skin carcinogenesis and lung tumour development. Recently, linkage analysis and haplotype mapping in interspecific crosses has led to the identification of the *Stk6* gene as a candidate skin tumour susceptibility gene. The *Stk6* allele inherited from the susceptible *M. musculus* parent was expressed at elevated levels in normal cells and preferentially amplified in skin tumours from F1 hybrid mice. Preferential amplification and increased activity in *in vitro* transformation assays was also observed for a common genetic variant in the human homologue of *Stk6* (*STK15*), suggesting that specific *STK15* variants may also play a role in human cancer susceptibility.

19.3 Chemically induced tumours

In 1915, the Japanese scientist Katsusaburo Yamagiwa tested by repeated applications of coal tar to the skin of rabbits the idea that chronic irritation causes cancer (advanced by his former teacher Rudolph Virchow years earlier). After a year, tumours appeared at the site of application in a fraction of the animals, thus providing the first direct demonstration of chemical carcinogenesis. Yamagiwa was so much delighted with their results that he composed a haiku: 'Cancer was produced. Proudly I walk a few steps'.

Since the pioneering work from Yamagiwa, many other suspected chemicals have been shown to be tumour producing in experimental laboratory animals, usually rodents. The advantage of chemically induced tumour models is that autochthonous tumours can be induced rapidly, reproducibly, and relatively inexpensively. Moreover, many parallels exist between carcinogenesis in mice and transformation of human cells. Notably, the spectrum of mutated genes in human cancers is by and large conserved in chemically induced mouse tumours. Carcinogens may produce tumours at the site of application (e.g. on the skin), at the site of absorption (e.g. the fore-stomach after oral administration), at the site of metabolic breakdown (e.g. the liver), or in the excretory organs. In some instances, a carcinogen may produce tumours in an entirely unexpected organ. For example, oral administration of the carcinogens 7,12-dimethylbenzanthracene (DMBA) and *N*-nitroso-*N*-methylurea (NMU) causes breast cancer in rats, but only when given at a particular time during puberty. If NMU is given to a pregnant animal it acts transplacentally to produce schwannomas in the offspring. Interestingly, tumours arising in these two tissues are specifically associated with activation of different oncogenes, for example, $Hras^{G12V}$ in mammary carcinomas and *Erbb2* in schwannomas.

19.3.1 Two-stage model of skin carcinogenesis

Chemical carcinogens can induce skin tumours in mice with high efficiency. A classical mouse model is the two-stage skin carcinogenesis model, in which cancer is induced by a combination of tumour-initiating and tumour-promoting agents. In this model, the first 'initiation' stage involves a single exposure of epidermal cells to carcinogens such as DMBA, resulting in a small subset of initiated cells carrying irreversible mutations in oncogenes and/or TSGs. The second 'promotion' stage involves repeated applications of non-mutagenic agents, such as the phorbol ester 12-*O*-tetradecanoylphorbol-13-acetate (TPA), that bring about important epigenetic alterations in initiated cells, facilitating their clonal expansion and leading to the formation of benign tumours or papillomas. The promotion stage is initially reversible, but leads to irreversible changes and ultimately to a progression stage, during which papillomas develop into rapidly growing invasive lesions known as carcinomas. Early studies on the two-stage skin carcinogenesis model provided evidence that activation of the *Hras* gene represents a consistent and early step in carcinogen-induced skin tumorigenesis.

The two-stage skin carcinogenesis model has been widely used to study the effects of targeted mutations in cancer-associated genes on skin tumorigenesis. In some cases, this has yielded intriguing results. For example, despite the predisposition of *Trp53* knockout mice to a broad spectrum of tumours and the occurrence of *Trp53* mutations in progressed skin tumours, p53-deficient mice do not show an increased predisposition to chemically induced skin tumours. However, progression to malignancy is greatly accelerated in the p53-deficient animals, suggesting that this gene operates primarily at the late progression stage of carcinogenesis. Another surprising result came from studies on transgenic mice expressing the E2F1 transcription factor in various epithelial tissues, including skin. Although these mice developed spontaneous skin tumours, they were found to be resistant to chemically induced skin carcinogenesis, thus demonstrating that increased E2F1 activity can either promote or inhibit tumorigenesis, depending on the experimental context. Additional experiments indicated that the tumour suppressive effect of E2F1 involves the induction of apoptosis at the promotion stage. The two-stage skin carcinogenesis model has also been instrumental in measuring the effects of telomere length on epithelial tumorigenesis. Whereas, chemically induced papilloma development in early-generation telomerase-deficient mice was comparable to wild-type animals, late-generation telomerase knockout mice, which have short telomeres, displayed a marked resistance to carcinogen-induced tumorigenesis, suggesting that anti-telomerase-based therapies could be effective in epithelial tumours.

Given the frequent activation of *Hras* in chemically induced skin tumours, the two-stage model can also be effectively used to map critical regulators of oncogenic Ras in skin tumorigenesis. An elegant example represents a study on mice that lack the Rac-specific activator Tiam1. The resistance of Tiam1-deficient mice to carcinogen-induced skin tumorigenesis highlighted an essential role for a Rac-specific activator in tumorigenesis *in vivo*, and the requirement of Tiam1 for effective skin tumour initiation implicates Tiam1 as a critical component of Ras-induced tumour formation. Tiam1 appears to be essential for survival and proliferative capacity of cells initiated with DMBA and TPA. These functions of Tiam1 are in agreement with studies that implicate Rac in the suppression of apoptosis elicited by oncogenic Ras.

19.3.2 Carcinogen-induced colon cancer models

Colorectal cancer induced by 1,2-dimethylhydrazine (DMH) or its metabolite azoxymethane (AOM) in rats or mice shows well-defined precancerous stages. A sequence of pathological changes can be observed before overt carcinomas develop, and the type and amount of altered colon epithelium depends on carcinogen dosage as well as length of treatment. Submucosal glands become dysplastic and benign polyps (adenomas) arise with increasing incidence with both dosage and time. Histologically, carcinomas can be shown to develop directly from polyps and, more rarely, from abnormal glands, indicating that these are precancerous stages in colon carcinogenesis.

Rodent models of chemically induced colon cancer are especially suitable for studying the potential role of various dietary and environmental factors in colorectal tumorigenesis. In addition, these models have been used to test the effects of chemopreventive agents such as non-steroidal anti-inflammatory drugs (NSAIDs) that function through inhibition of cyclo-oxygenase-2 (COX-2). Indeed, increased levels of COX-2 have been found in experimentally induced colon tumours in rodents. Treatment of these animals with the NSAIDs sulindac or celecoxib resulted in a significant reduction in both the number of intestinal adenomas and the total tumour volume.

19.4 Transplantation of human and animal tumours as models

Tumour transplantation models have now been used for more than 50 years, and, collectively, these studies have provided many important insights into the biological and therapeutic aspects of leukaemia and, to a lesser extent, solid cancer. Using the L1210 Leukaemia transplantation model, Skipper et al., showed that a given dose of a drug will kill a fixed fraction, not a fixed number, of widely different-sized leukaemia cell populations. This model, also known as the log-cell-kill model, is still the pre-eminent model of tumour growth and therapeutic regression. Again using L1210, Skipper showed that the emergence of drug-resistant clones within a tumour cell population may account for clinical treatment failure.

Although transplantation models have been useful for cancer research, they have serious limitations, which significantly reduce their value as models for human cancer. They do not develop spontaneously in the natural organ, nor do they have growth rates and metastatic characteristics that resemble the natural history in humans. Consequently, they do not allow us to examine the development of cancer, or to study the complex interactions between cancer and the host. These limitations are not applicable to GEM tumour models (see Section 19.6), which may therefore represent a better paradigm for human cancer development.

19.4.1 Transplantable syngeneic rodent tumours

Key to the development of transplantable tumour models was the generation in the 1920s of inbred strains of mice that allowed the successful transplantation of mouse tumours into syngeneic hosts. Several of the ensuing transplantation models have been the foundation of cancer drug development, most notably the murine L1210 and P388 leukaemia models, which were a central component of the initial drug discovery programmes employed by the National Cancer Institute (NCI). Besides leukaemia models, a number of murine syngeneic models for solid tumours have been developed. These models include different mammary adenocarcinomas (e.g. mam-16/C, mam-44), colon carcinomas (e.g. colon-26, colon-51), pancreatic adenocarcinomas (e.g. panc-02, panc-03), Lewis lung carcinoma, and the B16 melanoma model that has been widely used for metastasis studies. Furthermore, drug-resistant variants have been developed for the purpose of evaluating cross-resistance and collateral sensitivity (meaning that a drug-resistant variant displays a higher sensitivity to a specific compound than the parental model).

An apparent advantage of syngeneic mouse tumour models over the human xenograft tumour models is the histocompatability of the tumour cells with the host animal, which obviates the need for immunodeficient recipients. However, selection of variant sublines during *in vitro* or *in vivo* propagation, or genetic drift of the inbred strains from which the tumours were originally derived can cause tumour–host incompatibility, which usually results in reduced performance or excessive curability of the model. An example of the latter is a deviant line of Lewis lung carcinoma that was highly curable by agents that historically had no activity against the tumour. At least one agent was wrongly advanced to clinical trials on the strength that it was able to cure this particular Lewis lung carcinoma subline.

19.4.2 Xenotransplantation of human cancer cell lines in immunodeficient mice

With the advent of the immunodeficient nude mouse mutant, it became possible to model human cancer by xenografting of human tumour cells or tissue into mice. The ensuing success of xenotransplantation models and the ability to maintain the histological and biological identity of tumours through successive passages *in vivo* revolutionized many aspects of cancer research, including drug development. Although transplantation of tumour cells can be accomplished via several routes, subcutaneous implantation has been the predominant site for transplantation because of its simplicity and easy access to the developing tumour. Usually, between 10^6 and 10^7 tumour cells are injected into the flank of the animal. Tumours usually require a few days to several months to grow, depending on the growth rate of the cell line used. Many human tumour xenografts have been established to date, covering all common types of solid human tumours. However, an important limitation of these models is the lack of metastasis from the subcutaneous site. Although in some cases experimental metastasis can be produced by intravenous injection of cells in nude mice, this can be more efficiently achieved by orthotopic transplantation of the tumour cells, which provides the tumour cells with a more optimal environment for growth and progression. Currently, orthotopic xenograft systems have been developed for a variety of human cell lines derived from metastatic cancers of the brain, lung, breast, ovaries, colon, pancreas, prostate, and melanoma. Many of these cell lines have now been transfected with green fluorescent protein (GFP) or luciferase genes, yielding models in which cells from tumours and metastases can be imaged.

19.5 Methods to manipulate the mouse germline

In the last decades of the twentieth century, the field of mammalian genetics has been revolutionized by the development of methods for modification of the mouse germline. The first breakthrough was published in the early 1980s, when it was shown that new genes could be introduced into the mouse germline via direct pronuclear injection of exogenous DNA into fertilized one-cell mouse eggs, and that appropriate promoters could drive somatic expression of these so-called transgenes in mouse tissues. Only a few years later, a second major advance in mouse engineering was reported, namely the possibility to introduce specific mutations into endogenous genes and transmit these through the mouse germline.

19.5.1 Transgenesis

Currently, three methods exist for the generation of transgenic mice: (1) DNA microinjection of fertilized oocytes, (2) infection of pre-implantation embryos by recombinant retroviruses, and (3) gene transfer into ES cells followed by injection of transgenic ES cells into blastocysts. Whereas the latter approach has been predominantly used for the generation of targeted mutations by homologous recombination, the other two methods have spawned large numbers of transgenic mouse strains. Until now, microinjection of naked DNA has been the method of choice for generating transgenic mice, because of its high efficiency and the possibility to introduce large DNA fragments. The major drawback of this technique is the poor level of control over the manipulation, since the microinjected DNA is mostly concatemerized in head-to-tail arrays and inserted into more or less random chromosomal sites. For this reason, alternative methods have been employed that use retroviruses as gene delivery vehicles because they are able to stably integrate into the genome of infected cells. However, the generation of transgenic animals with retroviral vectors is impractical because silencing of the provirus during development results in low to undetectable levels of transgene expression. Recently, these issues have been solved by the use of lentiviral vector systems for gene delivery to one-cell embryos or ES cells. Transgenesis by lentiviral vectors overcomes many of the limitations of pronuclear injection, as it is more efficient, less invasive to the embryos, and technically less demanding. In addition, it allows transgenesis in a wide range of inbred strains that are less suitable for pronuclear injection as a result of poor yield of zygotes or fragility of the early embryos. Moreover, since this technique does not require visualization of the pronucleus, it has the potential to be extended to other animal species.

19.5.2 Inducible transgene expression

Several strategies for temporally controlled and reversible transgene expression *in vivo* were developed during the 1990s , and more refinements and/or alternatives will undoubtedly follow in the years to come. Only a few systems have been successfully applied in mouse tumour models because many approaches suffer either from leakiness (i.e. unwanted expression in the absence of the inducer) or from poor inducibility (i.e. insufficient expression in the presence of the inducer). Currently, the best-characterized and most versatile inducible approaches use the tetracycline (tet)-mediated expression systems. These systems rely on the specific, high-affinity binding of the *Escherichia coli* tet repressor protein (tetR), or its derivatives, to the *tet* operator (*tetO*) sequences (Figure 19.1(a)). When tetR is fused to the herpes simplex virus VP16 activation domain, the hybrid tetR/VP16 protein becomes a powerful tet-responsive transactivator (tTA). In the absence of tet or its analogues, the tTA protein binds *tetO* and initiates transcription from artificial promoters containing these sequences. Binding of tTA to tet, or its analogue doxycycline (dox), results in a conformational change that disrupts DNA binding and inactivates transcription. This so-called tet-off system has been invaluable in addressing many biological problems where a tightly regulated genetic switch is desirable. A second tet-regulated system employs a mutant tetR protein that only binds to *tetO* sequences in the presence of doxycycline. Fusion of this mutant to VP16 produced a reverse tTA (rtTA) protein that requires drug interaction to bind *tetO* sequences and activate transcription. This tet-on system has proven less effective in transgenic animals, where in most cases induction kinetics are slow and the fold induction is modest.

An important advantage of tet-inducible mouse models is the excellent oral bioavailability and lack

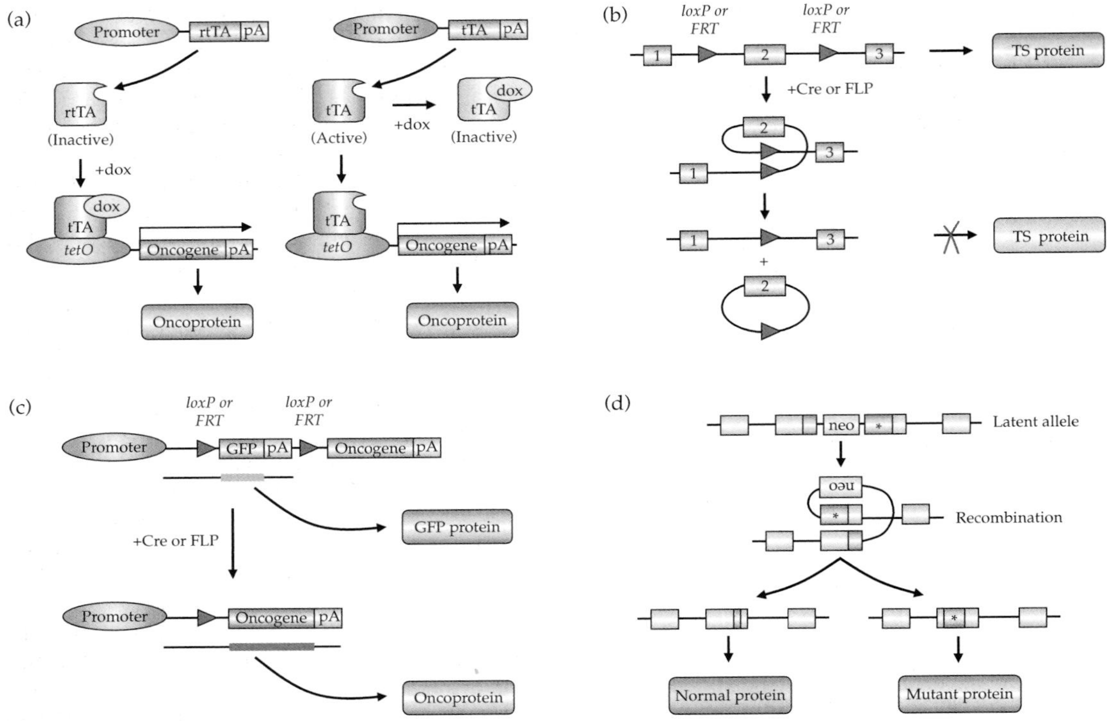

Figure 19.1 Methods for regulatable and conditional gene expression in the mouse. (a) Tet-regulatable gene expression. Tet-on systems employ a tet-inducible transactivator (rtTA; left panel). In these systems, the rtTA binds to *tetO* sequences and activates transcription only in the presence of dox. Tef-off systems use a tet-repressible transcriptional transactivator (tTA; right panel). In the absence of doxycyline (dox), tTA binds specifically to a tetO sequence, and activates transcription. Upon binding to dox, tTA undergoes conformational changes that result in loss of sequence-specific DNA binding. (b) Cre/loxP or FLP/FRT recombination-mediated gene inactivation can be accomplished by inserting loxP or FRT recombinase recognition sites around exon 2, in a direct orientation. Expression of the Cre or FLP recombinase enzymes will catalyze recombination between the recognition sites, resulting in juxtaposition of exons 1 and 3, and excision of the intervening sequence that includes exon 2. The recombination event results in gene inactivation if the deleted exon is essential for proper gene function. (c) Cre/loxP or FLP/FRT recombination-mediated gene activation can be achieved by using a floxed transcriptional terminator (e.g. a *GFP* reporter gene) to insulate the oncogene from a promoter. In the absence of the recombinase enzyme, the reporter gene is expressed and the oncogene behind the polyadenylation (pA) signal remains silent. Upon recombinase-mediated excision of the reporter gene, the oncogene is placed under direct control of the promoter. (d) Stochastic activation of a latent allele through spontaneous recombination can be accomplished by engineering a silent mutant allele in which a terminator (e.g. the *neo* marker gene) separates two copies of an exon with an activating mutation in the latter (indicated by an asterisk). Within mouse tissues, spontaneous recombination occurs either within or between chromosomes during cell division. Occasionally, this will result in the excision of *neo* from the engineered locus and the concomitant production of a functional wild-type or mutant allele, depending on the exact site of recombination.

of toxicity of doxycycline. On the other hand, the system is binary, and requires cross-breeding to produce mice bitransgenic for the tet-regulatable transgene and the tetracycline transactivator expressed from a tissue-specific promoter. Bitransgenic mice containing the rtTA transactivator will show tissue-specific expression of the tet-regulatable transgene following administration of doxycycline, whereas bitransgenic mice carrying the tTA transactivator will constitutively express the tet-regulatable transgene in specific tissues unless doxycycline is provided.

Other studies have utilized fusions between the protein of interest and the tamoxifen-responsive hormone-binding domain of the oestrogen receptor (ER^T), allowing activation of the hybrid protein by treatment with the anti-oestrogen tamoxifen or its derivative 4-hydroxytamoxifen. Compared to tet-regulatable models, this system offers the advantage of post-transcriptional control and obviates the need for cross-breeding different lines due to the presence of a single mutant allele rather than two. However, it is difficult, if not impossible, to predict whether fusing a particular protein to the ER^T domain results in a hybrid protein that shows good inducibility while retaining all of its original functions.

19.5.3 Gene targeting in ES cells

Gene targeting exploits the potential to create defined mutations via homologous recombination in ES cells, which have the capacity to contribute to all cell lineages including the germline. The procedure for the generation of mice that have been genetically modified using gene-targeting strategies is essentially the same, regardless of the specific targeting strategy, and involves injection of the targeted ES cells into blastocysts, which are transferred to the uterus of a pseudopregnant foster mother. The resulting chimeric mice are then mated with wild-type mice, and germ-line transmission of the targeted allele is checked in the F1 offspring. After a number of backcrosses to wild-type mice—required to eliminate random mutations that accumulate in ES cells during *in vitro* culture—mice that are homozygous for the targeted mutation are produced by intercrossing heterozygous animals.

Besides the generation of 'conventional' null alleles, gene targeting has been used to create knockin alleles in which the endogenous gene is replaced by another gene (e.g. a homologue, to assess whether members of the same gene family have similar functions when expressed in the same spatiotemporal pattern). Other gene-targeting strategies have been developed for the purpose of creating subtle alterations such as point mutations, as well as complex chromosomal rearrangements such as large deletions, translocations, or inversions.

19.5.4 Engineering conditional gene mutations

In recombinase-mediated conditional gene mutation strategies, the target gene, or part of it, is flanked by recombinase recognition sites (*loxP* or *FRT*) in such a way that gene function is not compromised in the absence of the respective recombinase (Cre or Flp). In the presence of the recombinase, the intervening DNA segment is deleted when the recognition sites are placed in a direct orientation (Figure 19.1(b)). Since recombinase expression is both necessary and sufficient for catalyzing recombination between the recognition sites, the system is tight in the absence of the recombinase. The bacteriophage P1 Cre/*loxP* recombinase system is currently the most widely used in mammals. Several mouse strains with conditional knockout alleles (dubbed 'floxed' alleles because exons are flanked by *lox*P sites) have been generated (www.mshri.on.ca/nagy/floxed.html). Similarly, strains have been created in which conditional activation of transgenes or knockin alleles can be induced by Cre-mediated removal of a *loxP*-flanked transcription termination sequence located between the promoter and the protein-coding sequence (Figure 19.1(c)). Finally, conditional translocations can be engineered through insertion of *loxP* sites into non-homologous chromosomes to prime them for Cre-mediated translocation.

In all conditional mouse mutants, the Cre recombinase can be introduced via intercrosses with Cre transgenic mice or via somatic delivery using Cre-encoding viruses, naked DNA, or purified Cre protein. Compound mutants harbouring multiple conditional alleles can be bred without compromising viability, and the rapidly growing list of Cre transgenics (www.mshri.on.ca/nagy/Cre-pub.html) permits an unsurpassed degree of flexibility in tissue-specific and time-controlled switching. Therefore, this technology can be expected to foster the development of many different mouse models.

19.5.5 Engineering latent mutations

A novel strategy for generating oncogene-initiated mouse tumour models is to create latent mutant alleles that become expressed only upon somatic recombination *in vivo*. This strategy is a modification of the so-called 'hit-and-run' targeting procedure, that has been designed to introduce subtle mutations in ES cells. The first step of this procedure is performed in ES cells, and involves the generation of a partial gene duplication at the target locus via insertion of the targeting vector (Figure 19.1(d)). The second step is based on the resolution of the duplication by recombination between the duplicated homologous sequences (via single reciprocal intrachromosomal recombination or unequal sister chromatid exchange), resulting in removal of the vector sequences and one complement of the duplication from the target locus. This second step occurs stochastically *in vivo*, after generation of mice from the targeted ES cells, and will occasionally result in the production of a functional wild-type or mutant gene in a stochastic fashion throughout the animal.

19.6 Genetically engineered mouse tumour models

Oncogene-expressing transgenic mice or conventional TSG knockout mice have yielded many cancer-prone mouse strains and thus provided important insights into the role of particular genes and their mutations in tumorigenesis, the cooperation of individual mutations, and the multistep process of cancer. Nevertheless, this first generation of GEM tumour models is now being replaced by second-generation GEM models utilizing conditional gene expression. These models do not suffer from limitations that are often encountered in conventional mutants such as embryonic lethality or the prevalent formation of tumours outside the tissue of interest. Moreover, they allow us to study malignant transformation in the context of the appropriate non-mutated microenvironment. It is conceivable that combining multiple conditional mutations, as they are known to occur in human cancer, may yield mouse tumours with characteristics that more closely resemble the natural history in humans. Already a significant number of conditional and regulatable mouse tumour models have been developed over the past few years (Table 19.1). An excellent, comprehensive website on GEM models of human cancer is maintained by the Mouse Models of Human Cancer Consortium (MMHCC) at the NCI (http://emice.nci.nih.gov/).

19.6.1 Constitutive oncogene-expressing transgenic mice

A major advance in cancer research occurred in 1984 when tumour-prone mice were successfully produced from oocytes injected with oncogenes. Expression of the T antigen (Tag) oncogene from simian virus 40 (SV40) in brain epithelium caused brain tumours and expression of a *Myc* transgene in the mammary gland led to breast cancer. These two studies showed that transgenic studies allow definitive tests of candidate oncogenes and dominant-negative forms of TSGs. Moreover, the initial steps in tumour development could now be studied in diverse cell types within the living animal, as the initiating mutation in the multistep process of cancer is conferred by the expression of the transgene. During the preneoplastic phase, any direct effects of the transgene on cell growth or differentiation can be studied, and potential collaboration between oncogenes in tumour development can be explored by introduction of a second gene via cross-breeding of different oncogene-expressing transgenic strains or via somatic gene delivery.

An excellent example of how transgenic mouse tumour models can be used to study the stepwise progression of cancer is the RIP (rat insulin II promoter)-Tag model of insulinoma, in which the RIP is used to drive expression of SV40 Tag in pancreatic β-cells of the islets of Langerhans. RIP-Tag mice undergo tumorigenesis through defined stages that coincide with shifts in proliferation, apoptosis, and angiogenesis. Pancreatic islets, which all express the SV40 Tag, are at first morphologically normal and do not show hyperplasia. However, after 3–4 weeks hyperplastic islets begin to appear stochastically, displaying β-cell hyperproliferation and features of dysplasia and carcinoma *in situ*. Angiogenic islets arise from hyperplastic islets by switching on angiogenesis in the normally quiescent islet capillaries, after which a small fraction progresses to solid tumours. The first step in the process, the induction of hyperproliferation, appears associated with activation of the insulin-like growth factor II (Igf2). The second step, comprising the angiogenic switch, is accompanied by the expression of the matrix metalloproteinase MMP-9. The well-characterized RIP-Tag model is ideally suited for studying the effects of deregulated expression of cancer genes at specific tumour stages. For example, inactivation of E-cadherin by expression of a dominant-negative inhibitor in RIP-Tag animals accelerated the transition from adenoma to invasive carcinoma.

Another powerful application of oncogene-expressing transgenic mice is the identification of cooperative effects between oncogenes by genetic complementation of transgenic mouse strains that overexpress two different genes in the same target cell. The utility of this approach was first demonstrated by Philip Leder and coworkers some 16 years ago. By generating bitransgenic animals, they showed that co-expression of $Hras^{G12V}$ and *Myc* in mammary epithelial cells, resulted in an earlier appearance and a higher frequency of mammary tumours, as compared to expression of either of the

Table 19.1 Conditional and inducible mouse tumour models

Tumour type	Mutations[a]	References
Tumour models using Cre/loxP or FLP/FRT recombination systems		
AML	*AML1-ETO*	*Cancer Cell*, **1**, 63–74
Colorectal adenoma	*Apc*	*Science*, **278**, 120–3
Lens tumour	SV40 Tag	*PNAS*, **89**, 6232–6
Liver haemangioma	*Vhl*	*PNAS*, **98**, 1583–8
Lung adenocarcinoma	*Kras*	*Oncogene*, **20**, 6551–8 *Genes Dev.*, **15**, 3243–8
Mammary adenocarcinoma	*Brca1 (Trp53)*	*Nat Genet*, **22**, 37–43
Mammary adenocarcinoma	*Brca2, Trp53*	*Nat Genet*, **29**, 418–25
Mammary adenocarcinoma	*Brca2*	*Oncogene* **20**, 3937–48
Mammary adenocarcinoma	*Erbb2*	*PNAS*, **97**, 3444–9
Mammary adenocarcinoma	*Pten*	*Development* **129**, 4159–70
Medulloblastoma	*Rb, Trp53*	*Genes Dev*, **14**, 994–1004
Pituitary tumour	*Rb*	*Oncogene*, **17**, 1–12
Schwannoma	*Nf2*	*Genes Dev*, **14**, 1617–30
Skin papilloma	*Ccnd1*	*Cancer Res*, **62**, 1641–7
Tumour models using latent alleles		
Lung adenocarcinoma, lymphoma, skin papilloma	*Kras*	*Nature*, **410**, 1111–16
Tumour models using *in situ* retroviral gene delivery		
Glioma	*Erbb2 (Cdk4, Cdkn2a)*	*Genes Dev*, **12**, 3675–85
Glioma	*Pdgf (Cdkn2a)*	*Genes Dev*, **15**, 1913–25
Glioma	*PyV-mT*	*Am J Pathol*, **157**, 1031–7
Glioblastoma	*Kras, Akt*	*Nat Genet*, **25**, 55–7
Tumour models using regulatable oncogenes		
Islet-cell adenocarcinoma	*Myc*	*Cell*, **109**, 321–34
Lymphoma, leukaemia	*Myc*	*Mol Cell*, **4**, 199–207
Lymphoma	*BCR-ABL*	*Nat Genet*, **24**, 57–60
Lung hyperplasia	*Fgf7*	*J Biol Chem*, **275**, 11858–64
Lung adenocarcinoma	*Kras (Cdkn2a, Trp53)*	*Genes Dev*, **15**, 3249–62
Mammary adenocarcinoma	*Myc*	*Nat Med*, **7**, 235–9
Mammary adenocarcinoma	*Erbb2*	*Cancer Cell*, **2**, 451–61
Mammary adenocarcinoma	*Wnt1 (Trp53)*	*Genes Dev*, **17**, 488–501
Melanoma	*Hras (Cdkn2a)*	*Nature*, **400**, 468–72
Osteogenic sarcoma	*Myc*	*Science*, **297**, 102–4
Salivary gland hyperplasia	*SV40 Tag*	*Science*, **273**, 1384–6
Skin hyperplasia	*Erbb2*	*Oncogene*, **18**, 3593–607
Skin papilloma	*Myc*	*Mol Cell*, **3**, 565–77

[a] Mutations include conditional TSG knockouts and conditional oncogenes. Conventional mutations are shown between brackets.

transgenes alone. Since this landmark study, many cooperative effects have been demonstrated in bitransgenic animals. An alternative route to identify genes that contribute to tumorigenesis in oncogene-expressing transgenic mice is their identification by retroviral insertional tumorigenesis (see Section 19.8.2).

19.6.2 Germline TSG knockouts

Targeted disruption of TSGs in the mouse germline has been the method of choice to establish the normal function of these genes and to create animal models for the tumour-predisposing conditions that are known in man. Indeed, many familial cancer syndromes have been modelled in mice by introducing targeted mutations in the corresponding TSGs. Examples include mouse models for retinoblastoma (*Rb*), Li-Fraumeni syndrome (*p53*), familial adenomatous polyposis (FAP) coli (*Apc*), hereditary non-polyposis colon cancer (*Msh2*), ataxia telangiectasia (*Atm*), Cowden disease (*Pten*), neurofibromatosis type 1 (*Nf1*), neurofibromatosis type 2 (*Nf2*), Wilms' tumour (*Wt1*), von Hippel-Lindau disease (*Vhl*). In fact, all of these mouse strains are tumour-prone when heterozygous for TSG expression, and demonstrate loss of the remaining wild-type allele in tumours. However, only few heterozygous TSG knockouts recapitulate faithfully all clinical features of the cognate human syndrome. For example, heterozygous *Rb* knockout animals develop pituitary cancer rather than eye tumours, and *Nf2*-hemizygous mice do not develop schwannomas but mainly osteosarcomas. In addition, it was often not possible to generate homozygous mutant mice for many TSGs due to lethal developmental defects. Therefore, conditional knockout alleles have been generated (see below).

19.6.3 Conditional TSG knockouts

Several studies have employed recombinase-mediated gene disruption to produce tissue-specific knockouts for a number of TSGs, including *Apc, Brca1, Brca2, Nf1, Nf2, Pten, Rb,* and *Vhl*, and in doing so they induced tumour phenotypes similar to those seen in humans. Illustrative examples are the different mouse models that have been created to mimic the human breast and ovarian cancer syndromes associated with germ-line mutations in *BRCA1* or *BRCA2*. Attempts to produce mouse mammary tumour models using germ-line *Brca1* or *Brca2* knockouts met with little success. Brca1- and Brca2-deficient embryos died *in utero*, and, unlike humans, heterozygous mice were not tumour-prone. Mice homozygous for hypomorphic mutations in *Brca1* were viable, but developed many different types of tumours with long latencies, including only a small proportion of mammary tumours. Similarly, homozygous mutants carrying a hypomorphic *Brca2* allele developed lymphomas rather than mammary tumours. In contrast, conditional mutation of either gene in mouse mammary gland epithelium promotes mammary tumorigenesis. In addition, synergistic tumour suppressor activity of *Brca2* and *p53* in mammary tumorigenesis could be demonstrated by tissue-specific inactivation of both genes simultaneously.

Other examples of TSGs that have been conditionally mutated to avoid embryonic lethality are *Apc, Nf2,* and *Vhl*. Colon-specific inactivation of a floxed *Apc* allele following adenoviral transduction of Cre-induced adenomas similar to those seen in FAP, and Schwann cell-specific deletion of *Nf2* resulted in the formation of schwannomas similar to the human disorder. Liver-specific mutation of *Vhl* led to vascular histopathologies, but no tumours. Interestingly, liver tumours did develop in aged *Vhl* heterozygotes, generated by recombination of the floxed *Vhl* allele in the germline, indicating that the reduced lifespan of the liver-specific *Vhl* knockout mice prohibited the formation of liver tumours.

Even when TSG deficiency does not compromise viability, tissue-specific gene disruption might be required to avoid a strong bias for tumour development outside the tissue of interest. A good example is the *Trp53* TSG. Whereas *p53* is mutated in a broad spectrum of human tumours, p53-deficient mice develop mainly lymphomas and sarcomas. Although mammary tumours could be produced from p53-deficient mice by orthotopic transplantation of mammary gland epithelium into syngeneic wild-type animals, it has been impossible to assess the tumour suppressor activity of *p53* in most other tissues from *Trp53* knockouts. Two studies have used conditional *Trp53* knockouts to avoid unwanted tumorigenesis. In addition to the aforementioned mammary tumour model based on epithelial inactivation of *Brca2* and *Trp53*, a medulloblastoma model was produced by Cre-mediated deletion of *Rb* and *Trp53* in the cerebellar external granular layer (EGL) cells.

19.6.4 Conditional activation of oncogenes

Similar to conditional TSG inactivation, recombinase-mediated tissue-restricted activation of oncogenes can be achieved by employing a transcriptional terminator flanked by recombinase target sites to separate a tissue-specific promoter from the oncogene. This approach was first used by Lasko et al., to create an oncogenic mouse strain that expressed SV40 Tag in the eye lens upon Cre-mediated activation, resulting in the formation of lens tumours. Following a similar strategy, two models have been developed for conditional expression of $Kras^{G12D}$. One study employed transgenic mice in which Cre expression caused juxtaposition of $Kras^{G12D}$ to the broadly active actin promoter; the second study used a knockin strategy to achieve Cre-induced $Kras^{G12D}$ expression under normal physiological control. Both models employed adenovirus-mediated Cre delivery, which provides two clear advantages over transgenic Cre expression. First, the number of lung tumours could be controlled by limiting the multiplicity of infection. Second, the introduction of Cre via a single infection serves as the initiating agent, thus synchronizing tumour onset and progression. Indeed, the resulting tumour lesions shared many features with human non-small cell lung cancer. Other published examples of mouse tumour models based on Cre-mediated oncogene activation include models for Erbb2-induced mammary tumours, skin tumours induced by cyclin D1, and a model for acute myeloid leukaemia (AML) based on conditional expression of an AML1–ETO fusion protein.

19.6.5 Conditional translocations

Conditional translocations can also be induced by site-specific recombination. Using the Cre/*loxP* system, *loxP* sites can be introduced into two nonhomologous chromosomes. Expression of Cre can then be performed *in vitro* to permit selection for the translocation event. Alternatively, somatic translocation can be induced by Cre expression *in vivo*. The feasibility of this concept was recently demonstrated by Forster et al., who generated a mouse model of human *MLL-ENL* translocation-associated leukaemia by engineering *de novo* reciprocal chromosomal translocations. Developmentally regulated Cre-mediated interchromosomal recombination between the *Mll* gene on mouse chromosome 9 and the *Enl* gene on chromosome 17 creates reciprocal chromosomal translocations that cause myeloid tumours due to the expression of an Mll–Enl fusion protein. Hence, these so-called translocator models may effectively recapitulate naturally occurring human cancer-associated translocations.

19.6.6 Mice carrying latent mutant alleles

Johnson et al., have employed a smart 'hit-and-run' strategy to produce a mouse model for Kras-induced sporadic cancer. The endogenous *Kras* allele was targeted to create a latent $Kras^{G12D}$ allele that becomes stochastically expressed in somatic cells following spontaneous intrachromosomal recombination. The low but substantial incidence of $Kras^{G12D}$ expression gives rise to scattered cells that—at least initially—express the mutant gene under normal physiological control. In this model, oncogene activation occurs at random, thereby mimicking the sporadic occurrence of *Kras* mutations in many different human cancer types. Indeed, these mice developed, in addition to early-onset lung tumours, multiple extrapulmonary tumours, and preneoplastic lesions, including thymic lymphomas, cutaneous papillomas, and aberrant crypt foci of the colon. It should be stressed that although this approach effectively models sporadic gene mutation, it does not feature any control over gene expression.

19.6.7 Inducible oncogene expression

Several oncogenes have been expressed in transgenic mice in a regulatable fashion and, collectively, these experiments have taught us some important lessons. Most importantly, in nearly all instances, oncogene expression appears to be essential not only for tumour initiation but also for tumour maintenance. The examples are manifold: melanomas in Cdkn2a-deficient mice with dox-induced $Hras^{G12V}$ expression in melanocytes underwent complete regression upon dox-withdrawal, lung tumours required continued expression of tet-regulatable $Kras^{G12D}$ and lymphomas regress rapidly following shut-off of *Myc* or *BCR-ABL*. Similar observations have been reported for several other models with inducible oncogene expression (Table 19.1). The almost universal need for sustained oncogene expression to support tumour maintenance shows that there is little or no redundancy within the set of complementing mutations that have accumulated in end-stage tumours, and implies that targeting a single oncogenic pathway may have a profound therapeutic effect. This notion has been extended even further by recent observations in a transgenic mouse model of *Myc*-induced osteogenic sarcoma, showing that even the brief inactivation of a single oncogene might be sufficient to result in the sustained loss of a neoplastic phenotype. These remarkable findings suggest that it might be possible to treat certain cancers by only briefly or intermittently inactivating an oncogene. The observation that, following *Myc* inactivation, immature osteogenic tumours differentiated into mature osteocytes, has led to the hypothesis that, at least in some cases, brief oncogene inactivation might revoke tumorigenesis by inducing cellular differentiation and concomitant changes in the epigenetic programme, resulting in a non-permissive differentiative state. If the oncogene becomes reactivated in this non-permissive differentiative state, the cells could fail to proliferate and, instead, undergo apoptosis.

However, some caution, is in order because in a few settings mice showed only partial tumour regression or even relapse. An early example is a salivary gland tumour model based on tet-repressible expression of SV40 Tag. Inhibition of Tag expression caused complete reversion of ductal hyperplasias in young mice up to the age of four months, but not in mice of seven months and older. The observation that the non-regressing lesions remained polyploid in the absence of Tag suggests that these cells somehow acquired mutations that obviated the need for Tag expression. Similar mechanisms may be responsible for the development of BCR-ABL-independent leukaemia in a tet-repressible *BCR-ABL* transgenic line, and non-regressing tumours in a tet-repressible Myc lymphoma model.

Mouse tumour models with controllable oncogene expression have also been instrumental in assessing the direct effects of initiation or termination of oncogene expression in the target cells or the tumour, respectively. In most cases, shut-off of oncogene expression causes rapid apoptosis in the tumour cells, but also paracrine effects have been observed. For example, abrogation of $Hras^{G12V}$ expression in malignant melanomas triggered apoptosis in both tumour cells and endothelial cells, suggesting that the tumour-promoting activities of $\mathrm{Hras}^{\mathrm{G12V}}$ are in part non-cell-autonomous.

19.6.8 RCAS-TVA-based retroviral gene targeting

An entirely different method to create mouse tumour models employs replication-competent avian leucosis retroviral vectors (RCAS) to deliver genes to somatic cells *in situ*. This approach takes advantage of the fact that normal mice cells lack the TVA receptor, required for retroviral entry, and are therefore resistant to avian virus infection. Tissue-specific expression of the retroviral receptor in transgenic animals renders the particular tissue susceptible to transduction with RCAS viruses. Retroviral gene delivery to TVA-expressing cells is achieved by local injections of RCAS-producing cells or viral particles *in situ*. As the infected murine cells do not produce infectious virus, they remain susceptible to reinfection. Therefore, different oncogenes can be introduced in the same cells, rendering the system particularly useful for studying oncogene cooperation in tumorigenesis. RCAS—TVA-based retroviral gene delivery has been used extensively to model gliomagenesis in mice (see Table 19.1). Recently, this system has also been used to produce a mouse ovarian tumour model by *in vitro* transduction of TVA-expressing primary ovarian cells with different oncogenes, followed by transplantation of infected cells into immunodeficient recipient mice.

The RCAS—TVA technology will continue to be a valuable tool in producing mouse tumour models. It is potentially a fast and flexible system because new oncogenes can be produced readily as retroviral particles and injected into any TVA-expressing transgenic mouse strain. Moreover, existing RCAS vectors and TVA-expressing mice can be used in all possible combinations, and thus represent an excellent resource for the scientific community. A number of RCAS vectors and TVA strains are listed at http://rex.nci.nih.gov/RESEARCH/basic/varmus/tva-web/tva2.html.

19.7 How far do animal models resemble human cancer?

An ideal mouse tumour model should develop few tumours with high penetrance and short latency, allowing for tumour progression analysis within a short time span. In doing so, it should mimic a range of pathobiologic, genetic, etiologic, and therapeutic characteristics of its human counterpart. Finally, the model should permit non-invasive and quantitative measurement of tumour growth and dissemination, rendering it suitable for preclinical studies. Arguably, no single animal tumour model will recapitulate every aspect of its human counterpart, but rather mimic some of the more relevant features. In view of the rapidly increasing number of available systems, it is imperative for researchers to select the model that is best suited for answering their specific questions.

19.7.1 Validating animal models of human cancer

In order to determine for which applications a given model is particularly suited, it is necessary to assess the extent to which a given animal tumour model resembles the natural history and clinical responses of human disease. Proper validation should therefore include histopathologic, molecular genetic, etiologic, as well as therapeutic features. As this is evidently an arduous and time-consuming task, it is fortunate that technologies for performing comparative histopathological and molecular analysis have greatly improved over the past years. Tissue microarrays and increasing numbers of antibodies for immunohistochemical characterization have enhanced both the quality and the throughput of histological analyses. In addition, molecular profiling of tumours has been propelled by the development of new genomewide analysis tools such as array-based gene expression profiling and comparative genomic hybridization (CGH). While these molecular approaches have only recently been established for the mouse, their importance for validating mouse tumour models is already underscored by a recent study, documenting marked similarities in gene expression changes between carcinogen-induced mouse liver tumours and human hepatocellular carcinomas.

19.7.2 Humanizing murine cancer with telomerase deficiency

The replicative potential of human cells is limited by progressive telomere shortening, which ultimately results in enforced senescence. To overcome this, cancer cells must somehow upregulate telomerase activity. Mouse telomeres are relatively long and, therefore, telomerase induction is not necessary for murine tumour development. To investigate whether differences in telomere biology also limit the capacity to model human cancer in mice, DePinho and colleagues generated a mouse strain lacking telomerase activity. Through repeated backcrossing, they were able to produce mice with short telomeres, displaying an increased incidence of spontaneous tumours. Late-generation telomerase-deficient mice with a single disrupted copy of *Trp53* showed a shifted tumour spectrum with a high percentage of carcinomas, a tumour type rarely observed in telomerase-proficient *Trp53* heterozygous mice. Importantly, this high incidence of carcinomas mimics the preferential development of epithelial cancers in older people.

In conclusion, it would be desirable to eliminate differences in telomere biology between humans and mice by generating mouse models with 'humanized' telomerase activity. Theoretically, this could be accomplished by replacing the relevant mouse genes or transcriptional control elements with their human counterparts, although it might be difficult to predict which genes or control elements need to be exchanged, and whether the gene-swap will have adverse pleiotropic effects. If successful, this approach may yield models that effectively mimic the telomere crisis, as well as the subsequent telomerase activation during tumour formation, as occurs frequently in human cancer.

19.7.3 Humanizing murine drug and carcinogen metabolism

Another important challenge is the elimination of physiological differences in carcinogen and prodrug metabolism between humans and mice. Thus, replacing the murine xenobiotic-sensing receptors and metabolizing enzymes such as PXR/SXR (pregnenolone X receptor/steroid and Xenobiotic receptor), phase-I cytochromes P450, and phase II transferases, with their human counterparts may yield mice with 'humanized' drug and carcinogen metabolism. These mice might yield tumour models that more faithfully mimic the metabolism of anticancer drugs and thereby their therapeutic effects in preclinical studies, and at the same time provide more accurate information on the potential carcinogenicity of compounds in cancer risk assessment studies. An early example of this approach is provided by Xie et al., who introduced a transgene encoding the human SXR into mice lacking the murine orthologue, the PXR, thereby creating 'humanized' transgenic mice that are responsive to human-specific xenobiotic inducers such as the antibiotic rifampicin. These mice represent an important step towards a humanized rodent toxicological model.

19.8 Tumour models in preclinical research

19.8.1 Large-scale drug screening in tumour transplantation models

Spurred on by the recognition that systemic cancer could respond to treatment with systemic drugs such as alkylating agents and antifolates, several anticancer drug discovery programmes were initiated in the mid-twentieth century. In 1955, when the NCI set up the Cancer Chemotherapy National Service Center (CCNSC) to implement a national drug development programme, based on the P388 and L1210 murine transplantation models. Leukaemias were selected as the initial systems in which potential anticancer agents would need to demonstrate activity before further development. The reason for this selection was that murine leukaemia and lymphoma models were relatively inexpensive and allowed for a throughput that kept pace with the supply of new compounds. Unfortunately, the P388–L1210 screen displayed a strong bias towards compounds with preferential activity against rapidly growing leukaemias and no specific activity against solid tumours. For this reason, the initial NCI screen was changed to a two-stage system, in which inactive compounds were first excluded in a prescreen using the inexpensive, high-throughput, highly sensitive P388 leukaemia model before more rigorous testing against a panel of transplantable murine and human tumour models for common human solid tumours such as melanoma, lung, colon, and breast cancer. Not surprisingly, the bias against drugs active in solid tumours but not in leukaemia remained, due to the P388 prescreen. For example, fewer than 2% of all compounds active against P388 showed significant effects in Lewis lung or colon adenocarcinomas. Even worse, preclinical activity of drugs in the xenograft models of solid tumours was found to have limited predictive value for clinical activity in patients with these diseases. As a result of this, the NCI screen evolved into its present configuration, an *in vitro* stage-I screen in which compounds are tested against a panel of 60 tumour cell lines representing the most common solid tumours, followed by a more refined *in vivo* stage-II screen utilizing xenografts of the most sensitive cell lines in nude mice.

The pros and cons of anticancer drug screening in transplantation models are nicely illustrated by the history of development of paclitaxel, also known as taxol. Already in the 1960s, paclitaxel had been isolated as the active compound in *Taxus brevifolia* bark extracts, which were found to have cytotoxic activity. However, there was little interest in further development of paclitaxel, as it exhibited only moderate *in vivo* activity against the P388 and L1210 murine leukaemia models. This changed with the introduction of new assays for activity against solid tumours, which led to the observation of strong activity against the B16 melanoma model, as well as against several human tumour xenograft models. Following the elucidation of its unique mechanism of action in promoting microtubule bundling and clinical trials in the 1980s, paclitaxel has now become an important drug for treatment of breast and ovarian cancers.

19.8.2 Intervention studies in conventional GEM tumour models

As we have argued before, transplantation models for preclinical testing of anticancer drugs have proven to be relatively poor predictors of tumour response in humans. By definition, transplanted tumours do not evolve *in situ* and lack the appropriate cellular interactions with the host microenvironment. Such limitations are absent in spontaneous tumours arising in mice with defined tumour-predisposing mutations.

Many studies have used spontaneous tumour models to test the responses of conventional anticancer drugs, and thus explored the parallels between these models and human cancer patients. Examples include the evaluation of retinoic acid (RA) and As_2O_3 treatment in transgenic models of acute promyelocytic leukaemia (APL), and the assessment of doxorubicin and paclitaxel in mammary tumour-prone *Myc* and *Ras* transgenic mice. Initial studies have also evaluated the chemopreventive effects of retinoids, NSAIDs, or selective COX-2 inhibitors in spontaneous tumour models.

Seminal studies using lymphoma-prone *Myc* transgenic mice have elegantly shown how GEM tumour models can be used to uncover the mechanisms and cellular pathways that influence treatment outcome. In the first instance, these mice were used to study the therapeutic effects of various cytostatic drugs, including cyclophosphamide, adriamycin, maphosphamide, and docetaxel. Subsequent experiments in which *Myc* overexpression was combined with mutations in apoptotic pathway-components (e.g. *Trp53*, *Cdkn2*, or *Bcl2*) showed marked effects on the therapeutic responses and suggested that anti-apoptotic mutations confer chemoresistance, at least in lymphoid malignancies. Besides apoptosis, a cellular senescence programme controlled by p53 and p16INK4a also contributes to the treatment outcome, since mice harbouring tumours capable of senescence but not apoptosis had a substantially better post-therapy prognosis than those harbouring tumours with defects in both processes.

Already several targeted therapies have been evaluated in spontaneous tumour models.

Published examples include the use of the epidermal growth factor receptor inhibitor AG-1478 in an *Erbb2* transgenic mammary tumour model, the FRAP1 inhibitor CCI-779 in *Pten*$^{+/-}$ mice, and evaluation of farnesyl transferase inhibitors (FTIs), which target Ras activity, in several GEM tumour models. Interestingly, FTI-mediated antitumoral effects were observed in most—but not all—models, underscoring the notion that distinct genetic lesions can influence therapeutic responses. The well-defined and reproducible angiogenic switch in pancreatic islet tumours in RIP-Tag transgenic mice has been used to test the effects of angiogenesis inhibitors. The antitumoral efficacy of angiogenesis inhibitors in this model was very modest compared to the impressive effects observed in the Lewis lung carcinoma transplantation model, underscoring the differences between spontaneous tumour models and xenograft models.

19.8.3 Intervention studies in conditional GEM tumour models

Although conventional transgenic and knockout mouse models of cancer have been instrumental in testing therapeutic intervention and chemoprevention strategies, conditional tumour models represent another step forward in preclinical research. Conditional gene mutation allows a titratable, time-controlled, and tissue-restricted induction of a mutagenic 'pulse', which will induce the synchronized formation of a single generation of tumours. Therefore, subsequent therapeutic intervention may actually result in full remission. The latter is especially feasible in tumour models that employ conditional gene switching induced by somatic delivery of the recombinase, such as the lung tumour models employing Cre-mediated expression of *Kras*^{G12}.

The utility of GEM models in preclinical research may improve even further when they are combined with non-invasive bio-imaging techniques. This permits longitudinal monitoring of tumour onset, progression, and response to therapy, and may thus be effectively used for evaluating the efficacy of cancer prevention and treatment strategies. The resulting preclinical models will be ideally suited for testing therapies that interfere with the pathways that are downstream of the conditional tumour-initiating mutations. Several bio-imaging systems have been developed. They include nuclear methods such as magnetic resonance imaging (MRI), X-ray computed tomography (CT), single photon emission computed tomography (SPECT), and positron emission tomography (PET), as well as ultrasound, fluorescence imaging, and bioluminescence imaging. Some of these approaches have already been used successfully in conditional and regulatable mouse tumour models. For example, MRI was used to monitor tumour appearance and regression in a mouse lung cancer model with tet-inducible expression of *Kras*^{G12D}. Another study used luciferase-based bioluminescence imaging (BLI) to monitor tumour development in a conditional mouse model of Rb-dependent sporadic pituitary cancer. In this way, pituitary tumour growth response to doxorubicin treatment could be quantified by BLI of anesthetized mice injected with luciferin. BLI might well be the system of choice for preclinical screening of anticancer drugs, as it is relatively inexpensive and well-suited for high-throughput imaging of many animals.

19.8.4 Drug-target validation studies in GEM tumour models

Appropriate mouse models are needed for evaluation of the growing number of potential therapeutic targets that are identified through mutational analysis of mouse and human tumours, as well as from other screens. Here, the central question is whether targeting the specific mutation—or the affected pathway—will cause tumour stasis or regression. As discussed in Section 19.6.7, mouse tumour models with regulatable oncogene expression may be used to address this question and thus provide conceptual proof for therapies targeted against the individual oncogene or the corresponding pathway.

Conventional knockout mice lacking specific oncogenes have also been used for evaluating potential drug targets. For example, cyclin D1-deficient mice have been used to measure the impact of cyclin D1 loss on mammary tumorigenesis induced by tissue-specific overexpression of *Erbb2*, *Hras*^{G12V}, *Myc*, or *Wnt1* in transgenic mice. Whereas, cyclin D1 deficiency protected against mammary tumorigenesis initiated by *Erbb2* or *Hras*^{G12V}, it did not affect tumour formation induced by *Myc* or *Wnt1*, suggesting that human breast cancers with activated Erbb2 or Ras pathways may be highly susceptible to anti-cyclin D1 therapy. A similar critical role was observed for cyclin D2 in BCR–ABL-induced proliferation and malignant transformation of haemopoietic cells *in vitro*.

19.8.5 Drug-target validation studies in upcoming mouse models

Systematic anticancer drug discovery in mouse models has a number of disadvantages, some of which have been reviewed above. On the other hand, the advantages of genetically well-defined tumorigenesis are also evident, as is well illustrated by the intervention studies described above for various transgenic and knockout models. Indeed, drug development will increasingly focus on well–defined targets in the expectation that this will have less side effects with a similar or higher efficacy. However, a good target does not have to be a deregulated oncogenic protein. It could well be a normal cellular constituent that in the context of the mutations in the tumour has become of critical importance for survival of the tumour cells. An ideal target validation method would encompass the inducible silencing of such target genes by RNAi. There is little doubt that this is an important new avenue for drug-target validation: the use of inducible *RNAi* transgenes, efficiently introduced into the germline of mice by lentiviral vectors. This method may well constitute a generic approach for target validation, as it will permit us to assess whether disabling one or more specific gene products will contribute to tumour eradication. Once the suitability of a particular target is manifest, one can immediately focus on intervention strategies to downregulate the human counterpart. This would bypass some of the important disparities that exist between mouse and man. Furthermore, it would permit focusing on development of drugs that specifically act on the human target with its own demands for specificity, stability, and pharmacokinetic properties.

19.9 Use of animals to identify genes involved in cancer

In Section 19.2.3, we have already discussed the utility of laboratory mouse strains for mapping and identification of tumour modifier genes. However, somatic mutations that are causally related to tumour onset and progression can also be mapped and identified in cancer-prone mouse strains. A growing array of tools is becoming available for mutational analysis of murine tumours. No doubt they will lead to the discovery of many new cancer genes and corresponding pathways, among which are potential therapeutic targets and diagnostic markers for human cancer.

19.9.1 Genomewide detection of genetic alterations

Additional genetic events occurring throughout cancer evolution can now be studied at various different levels with ever greater sensitivity. A range of novel technologies is available for comprehensive analysis of genetic alterations in tumour DNA, including spectral karyotyping (SKY) for detection of gross chromosomal rearrangements including translocations, CGH for detection of chromosomal imbalances, and loss of heterozygosity (LOH) analysis. Additionally, genomewide changes in gene expression patterns associated with tumorigenesis can be measured using microarray technology. Although the latter approach has proven valuable in the identification of molecular portraits of human cancer, it should be noted that only a small number of changes in gene expression are directly related to the genetic lesions that drive tumour progression. Finally, it can be expected that progress in mouse genome informatics will speed up the identification of target genes in recurrent genetic lesions. The application of genomewide analysis tools in mapping common mutations in tumours from GEM models has already yielded initial successes. SKY and fluorescent *in situ* hybridization (FISH) analysis led to the identification of a recurrent chromosome 14 translocation in lymphomas from ATM-deficient mice, and a common chromosome 2 deletion in leukaemias from PML (promyelocytic leukaemia)–RARα (retinoic acid receptor α) and RARα–PML transgenic mice. Another example is the use of array-based CGH in the detection of regions of copy number changes in pancreatic islet tumours from RIP-Tag transgenic mice and in radiation-induced mouse lymphomas.

An additional advantage of mapping cancer genes in GEM tumour models is that it permits the identification of cancer genes that collaborate with the defined tumour-initiating mutations. In this way, it is possible to define different complementation groups in transformation. This type of analysis has been particularly successful in tumour-acceleration studies employing retroviral insertional mutagenesis in transgenic and knockout animals, as will be discussed below.

19.9.2 Tagging cancer genes by retroviral insertional mutagenesis

In 1981, Hayward and colleagues first demonstrated that the cellular *Myc* oncogene could be activated by retroviral insertions into the *Myc* locus and that this was a common event in avian lymphomagenesis. Since then, insertional mutagenesis screens with slow-transforming retroviruses such as the MMTV or MuLV have led to the identification of a large number of cellular genes that, upon aberrant expression or truncation, contribute to tumour formation. Mechanistically, insertional mutagenesis can cause deregulated expression of genes or disrupt their coding sequence, leading to altered activity or even inactivation. Because retroviral integration is a relatively random process, it has a reach comparable to that of chemical mutagenesis screens. There are, however, a few important differences. First, insertional mutagenesis and chemical carcinogenesis will not necessarily yield the same genes. Retroviral insertions will not cause point mutations or large deletions and, consequently, genes that require such mutations for (in)activation will not be tagged by retroviruses. Second, insertional mutagenesis differs from chemical carcinogenesis in that it leaves a unique sequence tag and, therefore, permits the swift identification and characterization of the genes involved in conferring the selective advantage to the cell.

When a particular locus has acquired retroviral insertions in two or more independently induced tumours, this locus is named a common insertion site (CIS). Insertional mutations in a CIS are almost invariably of oncogenic significance because the possibility of this happening by chance alone is extremely low. Moreover, the majority of retrovirus-induced tumours contain integrations at more than one CIS, implying that the affected genes in these CIS can collaborate in tumorigenesis. Nowadays, polymerase chain reaction (PCR)-based retroviral tagging strategies are being used for rapid analysis of large numbers of retroviral integration sites, resulting in large data sets of retroviral insertional mutations mapped to the mouse genome sequence. The accumulation of retroviral insertion sites into a single database, such as the retroviral tagged cancer gene database (RTCGD) database maintained at the NCI (http://rtcgd.ncifcrf.gov/), enables the detection of rare, but still tumorigenic, retroviral targets. In addition, the current data sets already hold a wide variety of retroviral targets, illustrating the capacity of retroviral insertional mutagenesis to hit most common signalling pathways.

The reach of retroviral insertional mutagenesis has been further expanded by screens in cancer-prone mice with a defined tumour-initiating mutation, thus permitting the identification of genes that collaborate with the initiating lesion in tumour formation. Seminal examples include insertional mutagenesis in Eμ-*Myc* transgenic mice to identify genes that cooperate with *Myc* overexpression in B-cell lymphomagenesis, screens in MMTV–*Wnt1* transgenics to study oncogene cooperation in mammary tumorigenesis, and retroviral infection of *Cdkn2a*-deficient mice to screen for loci that can participate in tumorigenesis in collaboration with loss of the *Cdkn2a*-encoded tumour suppressors p16INK4a and p19ARF. Conversely, retroviral 'complementation tagging' can be employed by insertional mutagenesis in oncogene-deficient mice for the purpose of uncovering genes and pathways that can substitute for the ablated oncogene in tumorigenesis. A current limitation is that insertional mutagenesis screens can only be used for a small number of tissues, since all current strategies employ slow-transforming retroviruses that have a distinctive tissue specificity. More versatile (retro)transposon systems that can be activated on demand in the tissue of choice might enable insertional mutagenesis screens in a much broader range of tumours, and development of such systems is eagerly awaited.

19.10 Summary

The laboratory mouse has proven a long-time corner stone of cancer research. Natural mouse strains have been invaluable for elucidating the nature of chemical carcinogenesis, and a range of tumour transplantation models have been used for screening countless numbers of potential anticancer agents. In addition, a first generation of GEM models has provided important insights into the activities of cancer-promoting oncogenes and tumour-suppressing genes in normal development and disease. However, notwithstanding their importance for cancer research, these conventional model systems have serious limitations, and this is why researchers are creating more sophisticated tumour models that should reflect human disease more faithfully. Numerous technological advances have spawned new models that have been successfully used for investigating biological processes important in tumorigenesis, such as oncogene dependence, genomic instability, and tumour–host interactions. These second-generation models also permit the generation of highly specific tumours with high penetrance and short latency. By introducing multiple-defined mutations in a small number of cells, sporadic cancer can be induced that closely resembles the human condition. In this way the contribution of individual mutations to tumour onset and progression can be assessed with great precision. Furthermore, new bio-imaging technologies will greatly facilitate accurate measurement of tumour growth and regression in response to therapeutic intervention. In parallel with these improvements in model building, rapid progress is being made in the development of new technologies for characterization of the resulting tumours and tools for the identification of cancer-promoting mutations. No doubt these efforts will ultimately yield novel pathways that are critical for tumorigenesis and consequently represent potential targets for therapeutic intervention. Finally, the application of versatile-inducible *RNAi* transgenes will allow a completely new way of validating drug targets in a generic and efficient fashion. This will increase the success rate and shorten the phase of drug development.

Further reading

Artandi, S. E. and DePinho, R. A. (2000). Mice without telomerase: what can they teach us about human cancer?, *Nat. Med*, **6**(8), 852–5.

Balmain, A. (2002). Cancer as a complex genetic trait: tumor susceptibility in humans and mouse models. *Cell*, **108**(2), 145–52.

Balmain, A. and Harris, C. C. (2000). Carcinogenesis in mouse and human cells: parallels and paradoxes. *Carcinogenesis*, **21**(3), 371–7.

Berns, A. (1999). Turning on tumors to study cancer progression. *Nat. Med*, **5**(9), 989–90.

Berns, A. (2001). Cancer. Improved mouse models. *Nature*, **410**(6832), 1043–4.

DePinho, R. A. (2000). The age of cancer. *Nature*, **408**(6809), 248–54.

Felsher, D. W. (2003). Cancer revoked: oncogenes as therapeutic targets. *Nat. Rev. Cancer*, **3**(5), 375–80.

Fisher, G. H., Orsulic, S., Holland, E., Hively, W. P., Li, Y., Lewis, B. C. et al. (1999). Development of a flexible and specific gene delivery system for production of murine tumor models. *Oncogene*, **18**(38), 5253–60.

Hakem, R. and Mak, T. W. (2001). Animal models of tumor-suppressor genes. *Annu. Rev. Genet*, **35,** 209–41.

Hahn, W. C. and Weinberg, R. A. (2002). Modelling the molecular circuitry of cancer. *Nat. Rev. Cancer*, **2**(5), 331–41.

Hann, B. and Balmain, A. (2001). Building 'validated' mouse models of human cancer. *Curr. Opin. Cell Biol*, **13**(6), 778–84.

Jonkers, J. and Berns, A. (2002). Conditional mouse models of sporadic cancer. *Nat. Rev. Cancer*, **2**(4), 251–65.

Lewandoski, M. (2001). Conditional control of gene expression in the mouse. *Nat. Rev. Genet*, **2**(10), 743–55.

Mikkers, H. and Berns, A. (2003). Retroviral insertional mutagenesis: tagging cancer pathways. *Adv. Cancer Res*, **88,** 53–99.

van der Weyden, L., Adams, D. J., and Bradley, A. (2002). Tools for targeted manipulation of the mouse genome. *Physiol Genomics*, **11**(3), 133–64.

van Dyke, T. and Jacks, T. (2002). Cancer modeling in the modern era: progress and challenges. *Cell*, **108**(2), 135–44.

Weissleder, R. (2002). Scaling down imaging: molecular mapping of cancer in mice. *Nat. Rev. Cancer*, **2,** 11–18.

Relevant websites

Biology of the mammary gland: http://mammary.nih.gov

Cre transgenics database: mshri.on.ca/nagy/Cre-pub.html

Floxed genes database: mshri.on.ca/nagy/floxed.html

Mouse Genome Informatics (MGI): http:// informatics.jax.org

Mouse Models for Human Cancer Consortium (MMHCC) homepage: http://emice.nci.nih.gov

Mouse tumour biology (MTB) database: http://tumor.informatics.jax.org/FMPro?-db = TumorInstance& -format = mtdp.html-view

Mouse Retroviral Tagged Cancer Gene Database (RTCGD): http://rtcgd.ncifcrf.gov

Online version of Lee Silver's 'Mouse Genetics': http://informatics.jax.org/silver

TVA homepage: http://rex.nci.nih.gov/RESEARCH/basic/varmus/tva-web/tva2.html

CHAPTER 20

The immunology of cancer

Peter C. L. Beverley

20.1 Organization of the immune system

20.1.1 Structure and cells

Animals or men born without a properly functioning immune system suffer from multiple infections and usually die at an early age. However, it was proposed, as long back as the turn of the twentieth century by Paul Ehrlich, that the immune system might also prevent, or at least delay, the growth of many tumours. This chapter examines the function of the immune system in relation to cancer.

The cells of the immune system (white cells or leucocytes) are found throughout the body because they circulate in the blood stream and also migrate into tissues, particularly at sites of inflammation. Leucocytes are also found in specialized organs, the thymus, spleen, lymph nodes, and bone marrow (Figure 20.1). From tissues, leucocytes migrate via afferent lymphatics to lymph nodes, which are widely distributed. From lymph nodes, leucocytes may enter the blood stream directly or traffic through efferent lymphatics to the thoracic duct and thence to the venous blood (Figure 20.1). All the cells of the immune system originate from self-replacing stem cells in the bone marrow, as do red blood cells and platelets. Three major types of leucocytes may be distinguished (Chapter 18). Lymphocytes are small round cells with scanty cytoplasm. They mediate adaptive immunity, the

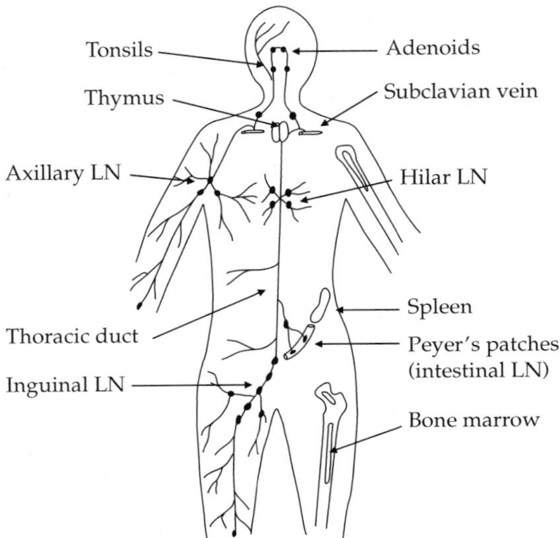

Figure 20.1 Anatomy of the lymphoid system. The immune system is distributed throughout the body. Afferent lymph-containing cells and soluble antigen drains to local lymph nodes. When an immune response takes place, cells leave the local node and migrate in efferent lymph to further lymph nodes, into the thoracic duct and thence to the blood. They may enter the spleen through the blood and effector cells enter non-lymphoid tissues. Plasma cells may go to the bone marrow to secrete antibody. The bone marrow is also the site of production of B- and T-cell precursors. Immature B cells go directly from the bone marrow to peripheral lymph nodes and the spleen. T-cell precursors go to the thymus and undergo selection before migrating to peripheral lymphoid organs.

main subject of this chapter, are responsible for immunological memory, and are long-lived. Macrophages and dendritic cells (DCs) are larger mononuclear cells with more cytoplasm. These cells are actively phagocytic and endocytic. They play a key role in the interaction between innate and adaptive immune responses. Polymorphonuclear leucocytes (granulocytes) have lobed nuclei and granular cytoplasm. They are short-lived cells that are phagocytic and also carry out many effector functions by exocytosis of granule contents.

20.1.2 Innate immunity

The innate immune system functions as the first line of defence in immune responses and includes both cells and soluble molecules. The key property of the innate immune system is that it can recognize conserved molecular structures of microorganisms. To do this it uses pattern recognition receptors

Table 20.1 Pattern recognition receptors

Receptor	Pathogen-associated molecular pattern
TLR2	Bacterial lipoproteins, Peptidoglycan Some bacterial lipopolysaccharides Lipoarabinomannan (*Mycobaterium tuberculosis*) Phosphatidylinositol dimannoside (*M. tuberculosis*)
TLR3	dsRNA of many viruses
TLR4	Some bacterial lipopolysaccharides Heat shock protein 60 F glycoprotein of respiratory syncytial virus
TLR5	Bacterial flagellin
TLR9	CpG DNA
Immunoglobulin FcγRs	Pentraxin-opsonized zymosan, serum amyloid P, C-reactive protein, immunoglobulin coated particles
Complement receptor 1 (CD35)	Complement opsonized bacteria and fungi
Complement receptor 3 (CD11b–CD18)	Complement opsonized bacteria and fungi
Complement receptor 4 (CD11b–CD18)	*M. tuberculosis*
Serum mannan binding protein	Mannan of yeasts
Mannose receptor	Mannosyl/fucosyl residues, *Pneumocystis carinii, Candida albicans*
Scavenger receptor	Apoptotic cells, Gram + cocci, lipoteichoic acid
MARCO	*E. coli*
MER	Apoptotic thymocytes
PSR	Apoptotic cells
CD36	Apoptotic granulocytes
CD14	*Pseudomonas aeruginosa*

Many receptors function in concert. Several Toll-like receptors (TLRs) form homo- and hetero-dimers and TLR 2 also interacts with CD14 to recognise lipopolysaccharide.

such as Toll-like receptors, that are expressed on macrophages and DCs or as soluble serum proteins; for example, complement components and mannan binding protein (Table 20.1). Recognition of conserved molecular structures by pattern recognition receptors delivers a 'danger signal' to the immune system that activates non-specific effector mechanisms, such as the complement cascade or production of cytokines by macrophages and DCs. However, the recognition of conserved pathogen structures also leads to activation of adaptive immunity, mediated by thymus-derived (T) and bone-marrow derived (B) lymphocytes (Section 20.1.6) (Medzhitov and Janeway, 1997). Key cells in mediating the interaction between the innate and adaptive immune systems are macrophages and DCs, which detect 'danger signals' and are found in almost every tissue.

20.1.3 Adaptive immunity

Adaptive or specific immunity is the function of lymphocytes, of which there are two main classes. B lymphocytes mature in the marrow and then migrate directly to the spleen and lymph nodes. They are then ready to react to foreign substances (antigens). T lymphocytes migrate from the bone marrow to the thymus where they mature before migrating to the peripheral lymphoid organs (spleen and lymph nodes). These two types of lymphocytes although morphologically very similar (in the resting state, small round cells with a high nuclear to cytoplasmic ratio), can be readily distinguished by their differing cell surface phenotypes; that is, the array of glycoproteins carried in the lipid bilayer of the cell surface membrane. T and B lymphocytes also have very different functions, although they interact during most immune responses, but they share two key properties: specificity, conferred by clonally distributed, somatically rearranged receptors, and immunological memory. A third type of lymphocyte, the natural killer (NK) cell, shares many phenotypic properties with T cells but does not express clonally distributed receptors or immunological memory. These cells are probably best regarded as a component of the innate immune system (see below).

20.1.4 B lymphocytes and antibody

The principal function of B lymphocytes is to synthesize and secrete antibodies. When these cells are stimulated by encountering a foreign antigen, they first go through several cycles of cell division and then differentiate into specialized antibody secreting cells called plasma cells, as well as memory B cells. Antibodies are globular glycoproteins (hence immunoglobulins) found in the blood plasma. Prototypic antibody molecules consist of two heavy (H) and two light (L) chains. The H and L chains are each divided into two portions, the N-terminal portion (approximately 110 amino acids) being termed the variable part and the remaining portion (approximately 330 or 110 amino acids for H and L chains, respectively) being termed the constant part (Figure 20.2). The constant part of the H chain determines the biological function of the molecule and differences in the amino acid sequence of the constant part of the H chain, the class of the immunoglobulin (Ig) molecule. There are five immunoglobulin classes with properties that are summarized in Table 20.2. IgM and IgD are found on the membrane of resting B lymphocytes and act as receptors for antigen. When B cells are stimulated they first secrete IgM. Later, most B cells switch to secreting IgG, A, or E. IgG is the main class present in the blood and is a monomer of the basic four-chain immunoglobulin molecule. In man there are four subclasses of IgG termed IgG1, IgG2, IgG3, and IgG4, which have closely related H chains. In the mouse and rat there are corresponding IgG subclasses called IgG1, IgG2a, IgG2b, and IgG3. IgA is specialized for protection of mucous membranes and can be transported across

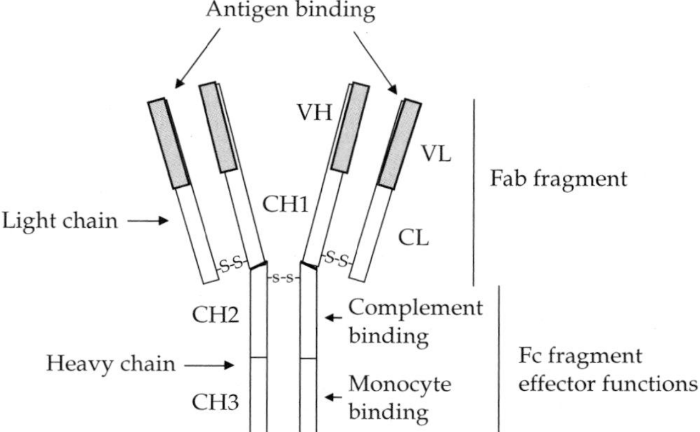

Figure 20.2 An immunoglobulin molecule. The structure of a typical IgG molecule is shown. The variable parts of the heavy and light chains (VH and VL) make up the antigen binding site. The constant domains (CH2 and CH3) of the heavy chains are responsible for the biological functions of the antibody.

Table 20.2 Properties of human immunoglobulins

Property	IgG	IgM	IgA	IgD	IgE
Molecular weight	150,000	900,000	400,000	180,000	190,000
Concentration in serum (mg/ml)	10	1	2	0.03	<0.001
Relative amount in secretions	Low	Low	High	Very low	Low
Crosses placenta	Yes	No	No	No	No
Complement fixation	Yes	Yes	No	No	No
Transport across epithelia	No	No	Yes	No	Yes
Allergic reactions	No	No	No	No	Yes
Fc binds to cells	Yes	Yes	Yes	No	No

Antibodies can kill cells by complement fixation and recruit macrophages and NK cells via Fc receptors, that can kill tumour cells.

epithelia. IgE is a minor component of serum but plays an important role in allergic reactions. The function of IgD is not known.

The immune system can produce specific antibodies (able to bind with high affinity) to almost any antigen encountered. This is because each B-lymphocyte clone synthesizes and secretes a different immunoglobulin molecule. This variability is achieved by several mechanisms. These include selection from a large pool of variable (V) genes, random joining of V genes to minigenes coding for diversity (D) and joining (J) segments, random combination of heavy and light chains and somatic mutation (Kocks and Rajewsky, 1989; Schatz et al., 1992). This allows for the production of millions of different antigen binding sites.

When an animal encounters an antigen, for example, a virus, many B cells are stimulated. Each B cell has surface immunoglobulin with a different specificity and the secreted immunoglobulin of each cell has the same specificity as the membrane-bound immunoglobulin. Each B cell divides to produce a clone of daughter cells. During this clonal expansion, somatic mutation occurs in the V regions of the heavy and light chains and cells secreting higher affinity antibody are selected so that antibody affinity increases. Since many B cells bind the antigen the serum of the immunized animal contains a mixture of the antibodies produced by many clones. A second contact with the same antigen elicits a greater and more rapid antibody response (immunological memory). Antibodies can bind to molecules in solution or attached to a surface and generally recognize structures (epitopes) that are dependent on the conformation of the target molecule. This is in contrast to T cells (see Section 20.1.6).

20.1.5 Monoclonal antibodies

Antisera made by animals in response to an antigen are the product of many different clones (polyclonal) of B lymphocytes and individual antibodies react with many different sites (epitopes) on the antigen. If the antigen is complex, as are bacterial or mammalian cells, it may be very difficult to determine exactly which molecules of the cell the antibodies are directed towards. For many years this hampered efforts to produce antibodies which would distinguish between tumour and normal cells, but in 1975, Kohler and Milstein devised a method for immortalizing single antibody-secreting B lymphocytes by fusing them to a plasma cell tumour (myeloma) to produce a hybrid cell (hybridoma). All the progeny of such a hybridoma cell produce identical (monoclonal) antibody molecules (for further details see Chapter 26). The ability to produce unlimited quantities of homogenous antibody, combined with molecular engineering methods to alter the properties of the monoclonal antibodies, has had a major impact in many areas of biology (Winter and Milstein, 1991).

20.1.6 How T lymphocytes recognize antigen

The T cell receptor (TCR) for antigen consists of two protein chains similar to the light chains of immunoglobulin (Davis and Bjorkman, 1988). Receptor diversity is generated by similar mechanisms to those in B lymphocytes (described in Section 20.1.4) except that there is no somatic mutation. While soluble antigen can bind to the surface immunoglobulin of B cells to stimulate a response, soluble antigen does not stimulate T cells. T cells always 'see' antigen in association with self-molecules. These are membrane glycoproteins coded in a region of the genome called the major histocompatibility complex (MHC). This name derives from the work showing that the same gene products are responsible for the rejection of organ grafts, a reaction known to be initiated by T lymphocytes. Thus, in both the response to foreign pathogens and tissue grafts, T lymphocytes recognize and respond to MHC antigens, although in one case foreign

MHC and in the other self-MHC + antigen. The antigen is recognized as an 8–12 amino acid peptide. These peptides lie in a cleft in the MHC molecules and the TCR binds to the complex of MHC + peptide (Bjorkman et al., 1987). That only small fragments of antigens are recognized implies that larger molecules must be broken down (processed) before T cells can recognize them.

There are two distinct antigen processing pathways (Figure 20.3). In the first, proteins produced within a cell are broken down to peptides by a complex of proteolytic enzymes known as the proteasome. These are then transported into the endoplasmic reticulum where they become associated with newly synthesized MHC class I molecules and the complex is transported to the cell surface (endogenous processing). All nucleated cells can carry out endogenous processing. Peptides bound to MHC class I molecules stimulate cytotoxic T cells, which carry a co-receptor molecule, the CD8 glycoprotein, which binds to MHC class I. The second type of antigen processing is carried out by specialized antigen presenting cells (APCs) such as DCs, macrophages, and B cells. Antigens are taken up by these phagocytic cells and degraded in endosomes to peptides (exogenous processing). In a specialized post-endosomal compartment the peptides bind to MHC class II molecules and the complexes are transported to the cell surface. Peptides presented by MHC class II molecules are recognized by T cells called helper cells, which carry on their surface the CD4 glycoprotein, which acts as a co-receptor binding to MHC class II.

In principle, any protein molecule that is turned over within a cell or enters an APC by endocytosis could stimulate CD8 or CD4 T cells. How the immune system discriminates between exogenous molecules, originating from microorganisms, and self-molecules such as those originating from a tumour, is an important issue for tumour immunotherapy. It is discussed below (Sections 20.1.8, 20.2.1, and 20.2.2).

20.1.7 The function of T cells

When naïve T lymphocytes first encounter an antigen they undergo clonal expansion, so that the frequency of antigen-specific T cells may increase by several logs to as high as one in a hundred cells or

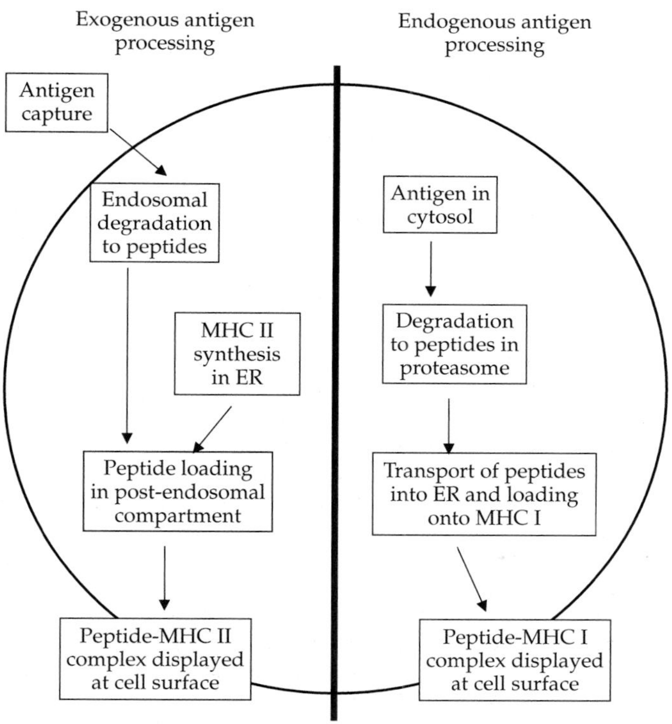

Figure 20.3 Mechanisms of antigen processing. Exogenously processed antigens are taken up from the extracellular milieu and degraded in endosomes. Peptides resulting from proteolytic degradation are loaded into newly synthesised MHC class-II molecules in a specialized post-endosomal compartment. In contrast, endogenous antigens are broken down by proteasomes in the cytosol and resulting peptides are transported into the rough endoplasmic reticulum to become associated with MHC class-I molecules.

more. As there is no somatic mutation the affinity of the TCR remains the same. T cell memory therefore resides in increased numbers of specific T cells. Memory cells are also qualitatively different from naïve T cells.

In contrast, to B lymphocytes, T cells do not secrete their receptor in measurable amounts but mediate their functions by other means. Table 20.3 lists some activities of CD4 and CD8 T cells. Some of these are carried out by T cells alone and involve direct cell to cell contact; for example, virus-infected cells carrying peptide–MHC complexes derived from endogenous processing of viral antigens, are killed by CD8 cytotoxic cells. This type of T cell may also be important in the response to tumours.

In contrast, many other functions involve other cell types as well as the responding T cells, with the T cells controlling the responses of the other cell types. Most often these immunoregulatory functions are carried out by CD4 T helper cells. Thus, helper T cells can stimulate B lymphocytes to secrete antibody or macrophages to become phagocytic and cytocidal.

These functions are mediated by cytokines (Fitzgerald et al., 2001). These act as local hormones within the immune system and have powerful effects on the growth and differentiation of their target cells (Chapter 14, Table 20.4). One of the best-characterized cytokines is interleukin-2 (IL-2) which is produced by activated T cells and can stimulate both the producing cell (autocrine stimulation) and other T cells (paracrine stimulation) to divide. Only T cells, which have been first stimulated by contact with antigen, express receptors for IL-2. IL-2 can be used to grow antigen-activated T cells *in vitro* and it is possible to grow a very large number of cells from a single T cell. This is known as an IL-2-dependent T cell clone and is the T cell equivalent of a monoclonal antibody producing hybridoma.

In contrast to IL-2, which promotes T cell growth, other cytokines induce differentiation into effector cells. IL-4, 5, and 6 together regulate the proliferation of B lymphocytes after stimulation by antigen and their differentiation into high rate antibody secreting cells. Although all the T lymphocytes produce a multiplicity of cytokines, there is a tendency for CD4 T cells to produce larger amounts of those with effects on growth and differentiation such as IL-2, 3, 4, 5, and 6 while CD8 T cells produce more effector cytokines such as interferon-γ (IFN-γ). Interferons have complex effects but an important function is the induction of expression of MHC molecules, which increases the efficiency of antigen presentation. T cells also produce and respond to chemokines, a large family of cytokines that bind to a family of related seven transmembrane-spanning chemokine receptors. Chemokines are produced by diverse cells, including epithelial cells, macrophages, and DCs, and lymphocytes. Their most important function is to control the migration of leucocytes into tissues and lymphoid organs.

Table 20.3 T-lymphocyte functions

	Cells involved	
	CD4	**CD8**
In vivo		
Delayed type hypersensitivity	++	+/−
Graft rejection	++	++
Tumour rejection	++	++
Graft versus host response	++	++
Protection against viral and fungal infection	++	++
Protection against bacterial infection	++	+
Help for antibody responses	++	−
In vitro		
Antigen binding (tetramers)	+/−	++
Mixed lymphocyte		
responses—proliferation	++	+
—cytotoxicity	+/−	++
Proliferation to mitogens	++	++
Proliferation to soluble antigens	++	−
Cytotoxicity against specific antigens (in association with MHC)	+/−	++
Production of cytokines	++	+

There is specialization among T cells with regard to cytokine production. Thus, naïve T cells produce mainly Il-2 while primed or memory T cells produce a wider range of cytokines. Among primed CD4 cells there are two major types. Th1 cells produce IL-2 and IFN-γ while Th2 cells produce IL-4, 5, and 6. While Th1 cells are particularly effective at inducing macrophage activation and maturation of cytotoxic effector cells, Th2 cells are most effective in inducing antibody production by B lymphocytes (Swain and Reth, 1994).

20.1.8 T cell assays

Since the frequency of antigen-specific cells among naïve T cells is very low, in practice detection of a T cell response indicates that immunization (priming) has occurred. In primed populations the frequency of antigen-specific cells may be as high as a few per cent. This has made it possible to detect antigen-binding T cells directly using the MHC-tetramer method. In this technique, 8–10mer peptide epitopes are bound to soluble recombinant MHC class-I molecules. The MHC molecules have a biotin tag and four molecules are bound by fluorochrome-labelled streptavidin. This tetrameric complex of MHC-peptides binds to TCRs with sufficient avidity to allow direct visualization and enumeration of antigen binding cells (McMichael and O'Callaghan, 1998). The method is limited by the need to know the target peptide and the MHC allele to which it binds. In man the responses of human leukocyte antigen (HLA-A2) donors have been well studied since ~40% of European and American donors have this allele. Methods for direct visualization of helper CD4 T cells have, so far, been less successful, partly because of technical problems in engineering MHC class II–peptide complexes and partly because CD4 T responses are often more diverse in their target epitopes than those of CD8 cells.

All other methods for detection of antigen-specific T cells depend on the response of the cells to antigen presented by APCs (an *in vitro* boost). Cytokines produced by antigen-stimulated cells (e.g. IFN-γ, IL-2, or IL-4) can be detected in the supernatant of the cultures by enzyme-linked antibody assays (ELISA assays). Alternatively, after a period of culture, cytokine-producing T cells are detected by staining with fluorochrome-labelled monoclonal antibodies after permeabilizing the cells. Cytokine-producing cells can also be detected by ELISPOT assays, in which secreted cytokine is captured by an antibody bound to the surface of the culture vessel and detected by a second enzyme-linked antibody. The former assay is readily combined with surface staining to determine what sort of cell is secreting the cytokines while the sensitivity of the ELISPOT assay allows for detection of low frequencies of responding cells.

Two other assays are often used. Memory CD4 T cells stimulated by antigen, undergo rapid clonal proliferation and this can be detected by pulsing the cultures with tritiated thymidine. CD8 T effector cells, which develop in culture from CD8 memory cells, are usually detected by their ability to kill target cells. Target cells are generally labelled with ^{51}Cr and killing is detected by release of the isotope into the culture supernatant.

20.1.9 Self-tolerance

Immune responses generate powerful effector mechanisms capable not only of combating micro-organisms but also of causing acute tissue damage as shown by the rapid destruction of foreign tissue grafts. There must therefore be mechanisms, which prevent development of immune responses to self-antigens (self-tolerance) (Kruisbeek and Amsen, 1996). For T lymphocytes induction of self-tolerance occurs in the thymus. T cell precursors first express the TCR in the thymus and if the receptor has a high affinity for self-antigens expressed on thymic antigen presenting cells, the developing T cells die. T cells which leave the thymus are therefore generally self-tolerant but there are additional 'fail safe' mechanisms in the periphery which prevent the development of damaging autoimmunity (see Sections 20.2 and 20.3).

The mechanisms of tolerance induction and maintenance in B cells are probably similar, with tolerance induction occurring during B cell development in the bone marrow and 'fail safe' mechanisms operating on mature B cells in lymphoid tissues. An additional safety mechanism for B cells is that development of high affinity antibody requires signals delivered to the B cells by CD4 T helper cells. Without self-reactive T cells, damaging B cell autoreactivity is unlikely to develop.

20.2 The immune system and cancer

20.2.1 Immune surveillance

In early attempts to demonstrate immunity to tumours, tumours were transplanted from one animal to another. The transplants were rejected and this was taken as evidence of immunity to the tumour. Later it was recognized that these experiments demonstrated transplantation immunity directed against MHC antigens. When genetically homogenous inbred animals (mice) became available it became possible to investigate tumour immunity and it was shown that if an animal was immunized with a tumour and was challenged with a graft of the same tumour, the graft was rejected. A graft of a different tumour was not, showing that the animal was specifically immune to the immunizing tumour.

At about the same time Burnett (1973) and later Thomas (1982) put forward the theory of immune surveillance against tumours. They proposed that tumours arose frequently and that the majority are eliminated by the immune system. Burnett summarized his view of immune surveillance as follows: (1) most malignant cells have antigenic qualities distinct from those of the cell type from which they derive, (2) such antigenic differences can be recognized by T cells and provoke an immune response. If this view is correct it follows that, (3) the incidence of malignant disease should be greatest in periods of relative immunological inefficiency, particularly in the perinatal period and old age, (4) immunosuppression whether genetic or induced by drugs, radiation, infection, or other causes should increase the incidence of cancer, (5) spontaneous regression of tumours may occur and evidence of an immune response should be apparent in these cases, and (6) large-scale histological examination of common sites of cancer should reveal a higher proportion of tumours than become clinically apparent. Burnett also suggested ways in which the theory of surveillance might be tested experimentally. Thus, immunosuppressive agents should facilitate the transfer of tumours, or damage to the T cell immune response produced by surgical removal of the thymus might lead to increased tumour incidence.

At first sight, a variety of clinical and experimental data do seem to be in accord with the surveillance theory. In man, some tumours show a higher incidence in the first few years of life than in early adulthood and the incidence, but of different tumour types, then rises progressively with increasing age (see Chapter 1). The incidence of tumours is also greatly increased in immunosuppressed individuals who are treated with immunosuppressive drugs to prevent rejection of the grafted kidney (Sheil, 1998). However, a closer examination does not support the surveillance hypothesis. The age incidence of tumours is as well explained by many other theories of cancer causation as by immunosurveillance. Tumours are caused by genetic changes in their cells of origin. These changes might be expected to occur either as errors during periods of rapid cell division (early life) or when external causes (carcinogens) have had time to take effect as in later life. The data derived from immunosuppressed individuals are similarly less straightforward to interpret when examined more closely. Although there does seem to be a slight increase in the frequency of most tumours, there is a disproportionate increase in a few tumour types (Table 20.5). The relative risk of suffering from some rare tumour types may be increased more than 1000-fold in immunosuppressed compared to normal individuals. An experiment in mice provided a possible explanation for these results.

Table 20.4 Functions and origins of cytokines

Cytokine	Function	Origin
Interleukin-1α and β	Pyrogenic response	Activation of T cells, many cells
IL-2	Growth of T cells	T and NK cells
IL-3	Growth of haemopoietic stem cells	T cells
IL-4	Growth and differentiation of T and B cells. Inhibition of Th1 cells	DC, T cells
IL-5	B-cell differentiation and granulocyte function	T cells
IL-6	B-cell differentiation but many other effects also	DC, many other cells
IL-7	Growth of B cells and T-cell survival	Many cells
IL-10	Inhibition of Th1 cells	DC, Th2 cells
IL-12	Induction of IFN-γ	DC, Th1 cells
IL-15	Growth of T cells	Many stromal cells
Chemokines (e.g. IL-8, rantes MIP-1α, SLC)	Chemotaxis of lymphocytes, granulocytes, and macrophages	A large family of peptides produced by many cell types
Type-1 interferons	Inhibition of viral replication	Most cells
INF-γ	Increase of MHC expression Inhibition of viral replication	T and NK cells
Tumour necrosis factor-α TNF-α	Necrosis of tumours, pyrogenic	Many cells
TNF-β	Cytotoxic *in vitro*	Many cells
Leukaemia inhibitory factor	Inducer of myeloid differentiation	Many cells
CSFs	Growth and maturation of progenitor cells	Various

When a large group of mice were treated from birth with anti-lymphocyte serum (raised in rabbits), their T cell immunity was greatly depressed. The mice did not develop large numbers of spontaneous tumours but when they inadvertently became infected with polyoma virus (see Chapter 13) a number of them developed multiple tumours of a type characteristically caused by this virus (Nehlsen, 1971). Similarly, the lymphoid tumours seen in transplant recipients (Table 20.5) contain both DNA and proteins of the Epstein–Barr virus (EBV), a herpes virus implicated in the cause of Burkitt's lymphoma (a B-cell tumour seen in parts of Africa) and nasopharyngeal carcinoma (see Chapter 13). The virus can also immortalize normal human B lymphocytes *in vitro*. These findings suggest, therefore, that the most important role of the immune system in tumour protection may be in preventing the spread of potentially oncogenic viruses.

This view agrees with experimental and clinical data on EBV, an ubiquitous infectious agent in human populations. Following infection the virus is carried lifelong and the individual also has lifelong immunity. Under normal circumstances, immune CD8 cytotoxic T lymphocytes can be demonstrated *in vitro* and there is thus a balance between virus production and the immune response, while in immunosuppressed individuals the immune system is unable to prevent virus spread. The T cells of such individuals cannot kill EBV-transformed B cells *in vitro*, and virus can often be isolated from body tissues and secretions such as saliva.

Table 20.5 Immunosuppression and tumours

Tumour type	Relative risk	Virus involved
Kaposi's sarcoma	>1000	HHV8
Lymphoma		
Of the brain	>1000	EBV
Non-Hodgkin's lymphoma	7.4	EBV
Endocrine tumours	320	—
Skin carcinoma	40	Papillomaviruses
Liver carcinoma	30	Hepatitis B
Leukaemia	6.4	HTLV 1
Cervix carcinoma	4.2	Papillomaviruses
Digestive system carcinoma	2.6	—
Respiratory system carcinoma	2.1	—
Breast carcinoma	1.1	—

Although the relative risks of Kaposi's sarcoma and brain lymphoma are very high, the majority of immunosuppressed patients do not get these tumours since they are very rare in non-suppressed individuals. In contrast, most transplant patients eventually acquire skin tumours since, although the relative risk is lower, these are much commoner tumours in normal individuals. HTLV 1 causes adult T-cell leukaemia only.

Several other viruses have now been implicated in causing human tumours and the risk of acquiring these tumours is generally increased in immunosuppressed patients (Table 20.4). Although worldwide virally induced tumours are a major cause of cancer, since hepatitis B virus and papillomaviruses infect millions of individuals, there are also many cancers where no viral involvement can be detected.

If it is accepted that immune surveillance operates principally against oncogenic viruses, what is the role of the immune system in relation to other tumours? Evidence from experimental animals (see Sections 20.2.1 and 20.3.1) suggests that there are immune responses to many tumours and the slight increase of relative risk for tumours with no known viral involvement would support this (Table 20.4). However, the fact that most tumours grow and kill the host, suggests that the immune response is probably a late event and in most cases is unable to prevent tumour outgrowth. Nevertheless, that there is an immune response suggests that tumours do contain antigens recognized as foreign by the immune system. If this is the case it should be possible to boost immunity to them by deliberate immunization.

20.3 Cell-mediated immune responses to cancer

20.3.1 Tumour antigens detected by immune cells in animals

It has been demonstrated repeatedly that laboratory animals can be immunized against tumour cells. In the case of virus-induced tumours, immunity is usually cross-reactive so that animals immunized with one tumour are generally immune to all other tumours induced by the same virus. Immunity can be transferred to other animals by immune cells and not serum and is mediated by T cells. In several such systems the target viral gene products have been identified. These results suggest that immunization against viral gene products should be a useful strategy for human tumours where viruses are known to be involved.

In contrast for experimental tumours induced by carcinogens, immunity is tumour-specific

(Section 20.2.1) and the nature of the tumour antigens remained obscure until the pioneering work of Boon and his colleagues (Boon et al., 1994). An established mouse tumour, which had become non-immunogenic following repeated passage in mice, was used for the experiments. Tumour cells were treated *in vitro* with a mutagenic chemical and variant tumour cell sublines obtained, which would no longer grow *in vivo* (unless very large numbers of cells were injected), because they induced a strong cytotoxic T cell response. Boon then set out to clone the tumour antigen of one such non-tumorigenic (tum-) subline, the P91A tumour, using the following strategy. Mice were immunized with P91A tumour cells and an IL-2-dependent cytotoxic T cell clone generated (Section 20.1.7) which would kill P91A cells but not the parental (unmutated) P815 tumour. Parental tumour cells were then transfected with a DNA library from P91A and the transfectants tested with the cytotoxic T cells to determine which expressed the P91A tumour antigen. The transfected DNA was then recovered from a clone of tumour cells recognized by the anti-P91A IL-2-dependent cytotoxic T cell clone. Fragments of the recovered DNA were sub-cloned repeatedly in a similar fashion, until a single gene was recovered that could transfer the P91A target antigen for the IL-2-dependent cytotoxic T cells to parental P815 tumour cells. The gene and its homologue in the parental tumour were then sequenced and found to differ by a single point mutation. This experiment firmly established that mutations in genes in a tumour cell can lead to a host immune response to the mutated gene product.

However, Boon used the same strategy to clone the tumour antigens from several other similar mouse tumours. Surprisingly, in several of these the gene in the tum-variant tumour cells was found to be identical to that in the parental tumour line (or DNA from normal cells of the same inbred strain of mice). In this case the mouse appears to be responding to a completely normal self-gene product. So far the evidence suggests that this is because the tumour antigen gene product is expressed at a higher level in the tumour cells than in normal tissues and can therefore stimulate an immune response. Presumably, in tumours with increased expression of normal gene products, the mutagen applied to the tumour has induced mutations that affect the level of transcription or translation of the gene without altering the sequence of the expressed protein.

20.3.2 Human tumour antigens detected by immune cells

Immune responses to human tumours are usually detected following an *in vitro* boost in which lymphocytes are stimulated with tumour antigen in culture. Both CD4 and CD8 T cells can be stimulated by appropriately pulsed APCs and the generation of effector cells in the cultures can be measured by the assays described in Section 20.1.8. For these cultures it is necessary that the T cells and APC are genetically matched. In practice, in humans they usually come from the same individual.

This constraint means that most experiments in man have taken a similar form. Lymphocytes from peripheral blood, tumour-draining lymph nodes, or extracted from the tumour itself (tumour infiltrating lymphocytes or TILs) are co-cultured with APCs and tumour cells, which have been irradiated or mitomycin treated to prevent their growth. T cells can be cloned from these polyclonal populations by limiting dilution in the presence of antigen (tumour cells), APC, and IL-2. The difficulty of obtaining lymphocytes and viable autologous tumour cells for this *in vitro* boosting procedure has dictated that most work has been carried out on tumours which can be disaggregated easily or grow well in tissue culture. In spite of these limitations evidence for tumour-specific response of CD4 or CD8 T cells has been obtained for a number of human tumour types, including lung, ovary, and renal carcinoma, and melanoma. Because melanoma grows well *in vitro* and the tumours are often superficial and can be easily biopsied, a great deal of work has been carried out on this tumour. Several target antigens have been identified by Boon and his colleagues, employing a similar strategy to that used for the cloning of murine tumour antigens (Boon et al., 1994).

CD8 cytotoxic T cell clones specific for an autologous melanoma tumour cell line were generated following *in vitro* boosting. One of these was used to clone its target antigen. Repeated exposure of the autologous melanoma cell line to the cytotoxic T cells eventually generated a tumour variant lacking the target antigen, which could not be killed by the cytotoxic T cells. A cosmid DNA library was then prepared from the original tumour and transfected into the tumour antigen negative variant. Transfectants were screened for the presence of the antigen using the cytotoxic T cell clone. From a transfectant expressing the tumour antigen, the cosmid was recovered and after further sub-cloning a previously unknown melanoma antigen gene (MAGE) was identified. The target epitope in MAGE is restricted by the MHC class-I allele, HLA-A1. The first MAGE gene has now been shown to be a member of a new gene family whose function is as yet unknown. MAGE 1 has only been detected in the testis among normal tissues tested but mRNA for MAGE 1, 2, or 3 is frequently detected in melanomas, lung cancers, and some other tumours. Interestingly, the MAGE 1 gene in melanoma cells is identical to that in non-tumour DNA of the patient. This is true also for another antigen recognized by T cells in melanoma, the enzyme tyrosinase. Like MAGE, tyrosinase has a restricted tissue distribution in normal cells.

Many other groups have now identified antigens detected by T cells in human cancers. Some of these are also recognized by antibodies from the same patients (see Section 20.4). These data indicate that many cancer patients make T and B cell responses to diverse molecules of tumour cells, the majority of which are unaltered but overexpressed antigens. Nevertheless, most tumours continue to grow in the face of this response so that either the response must be too small or ineffective, or tumours must develop effective escape mechanisms.

Table 20.6 Costimulation of T cells

T-cell receptor/ligand	APC receptor/ligand
Ig superfamily molecules	
CD2	CD58/CD48
CD4	MHC class II
CD8	MHC class I
CD28	CD80/CD86 (B7.1/B7.2)
CD152 (CTLA 4)	CD80/86 (B7.1/B7.2)
TNFR and TNF family molecules	
CD27	CD70
CD30	CD153
CD134 (Ox 40)	Ox 40 L
CDw137L (4-1BBL)	CDw137 (4-1BB)
CD154	CD40
Ig superfamily and integrin family	
CD54 (ICAM-1)	CD11a/CD18 (LFA-1)
CD11a/CD18 (LFA-1)	CD54 (ICAM-1)
Cytokines and chemokines	Cytokine and chemokine receptors
Cytokine and chemokine receptors	Cytokines and chemokines

The interaction between T cells and APC is reciprocal. APC activate T cells and in turn T cells promote differentiation and activation of APC. Some co-stimulatory cell surface molecules and cytokines are expressed by both cell types. Most of the immunoglobulin (Ig) superfamily molecules are involved in activation or inhibition of T cells. The TNF and TNF receptor family molecules appear to direct the pathway of differentiation of T cells.

20.3.3 T cell responses to human tumour antigens

The existence of immune responses to mostly unaltered self-antigens in cancer patients poses several questions. In particular, how is it that cancer patients make such responses while normal individuals do not and how are responses to these antigens initiated?

In an immune response to a pathogenic microorganism, the antigen is introduced into the body along with 'danger signals' that stimulate pattern recognition receptors. DCs and macrophages at the site of entry take up the microorganisms and begin to process antigens from them. At the same time the 'danger' signals initiate migration of dendritic cells to the draining lymph nodes and upregulation of MHC and co-stimulatory molecules. In the lymph node the DCs present antigen and lymphocytes and deliver costimulatory signals to T cells (Table 20.6) (Barclay et al., 1997). DCs also produce multiple cytokines, which also play a role in the activation of T cells. Rapid T cell clonal expansion occurs in the node followed by the exit of activated T cells from the node and the migration of these cells back to the site of inflammation. T helper cells enter B cell follicles and provide help for B cells that have responded to soluble antigen, that has also reached the node in the afferent lymph (Figure 20.4). Initially IgM and later IgG, IgA, and IgE are produced. Antigen-specific cells also migrate to distant lymph nodes and the spleen while high-rate antibody-secreting plasma cells also home to the bone marrow.

Several aspects of responses to microorganisms differ from the situation in normal tissues or a tumour. The most obvious is that although antigens from normal or tumour cells may be taken up by APCs when cells die, this is not normally accompanied by delivery of a 'danger signal'. There is thus no reason why DC should either migrate to draining lymph nodes or upregulate costimulatory molecules. In addition it is possible that the majority of cells that escape deletion in the thymus are of too low affinity to respond to self-antigens under normal circumstances.

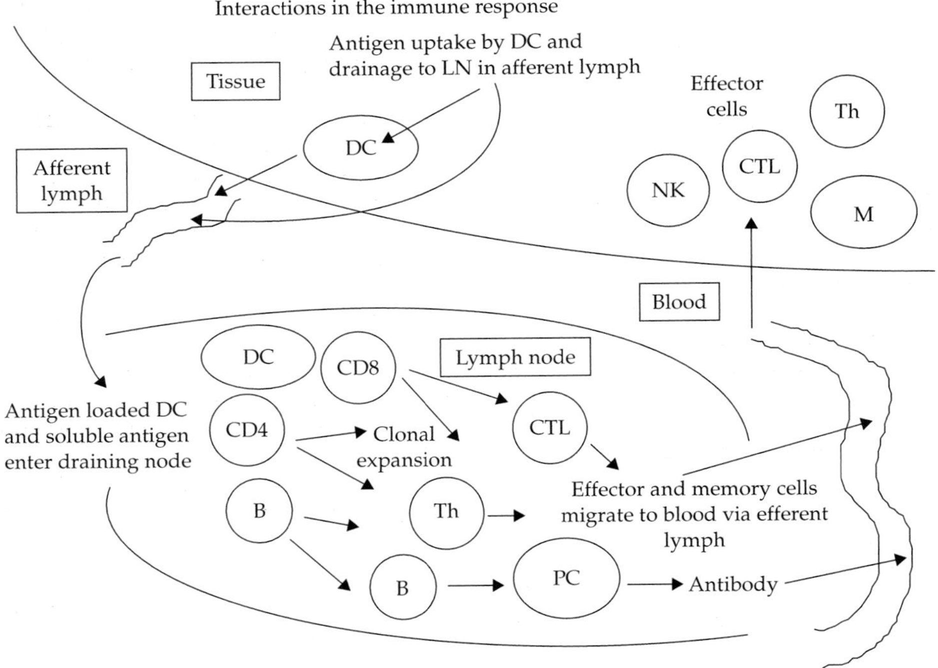

Figure 20.4 Interactions in an immune response. Antigen is taken up by DCs, which migrate to the draining lymph node. Soluble antigen also reaches the node in the afferent lymph. In the node, DCs present antigen to CD4 and CD8 T cells and B cells encounter soluble antigen. Clonal expansion of T and B cells takes place and cytotoxic T lymphocyte (CTL) and T-helper effector and memory cells are generated. B cells develop into plasma cells (PCs). Effector cells leave the node and migrate via lymph and blood to the original site of antigenic stimulation.

Of course in normal tissues or tumours, lymphocytes could interact directly with tissue or tumour cells rather than specialized APCs. However, this type of interaction has been demonstrated to result in inactivation of T cells rather than activation. Inactivation results because the tissue or tumour cells lack the costimulatory molecules present on APC and do not produce the cytokines needed for efficient T cell activation (Lanoue et al., 1998). How then, can tumours activate a specific immune response?

Experiments in mice suggest that CD4 and CD8 antitumour responses are generated not by direct contact of tumour cells and lymphocytes but only after uptake of tumour material by APCs (so-called cross-priming) (Girolomi and Ricciardi-Castagnoli, 1997). This implies that some exogenous material must enter the endogenous antigen-processing pathway and this has been shown to occur. Nevertheless, the problem of the source of danger signals required to initiate a response remains. However, as the tumour grows it often outgrows its blood supply leading to anoxia and cell death. This may cause sufficient local inflammation that activation of APC occurs. An important contributory factor is the production of stress proteins (heat shock proteins) in tumour cells. These act as an internal 'danger signal' and may also transfer bound peptide antigens to APCs (Przepiorka and Srivastava, 1998).

The foregoing discussion indicates why antitumour immune responses may be a late and suboptimal event. Early on in tumour growth no 'danger signals' will be generated and because few cells are dying little antigen will enter APCs. Any lymphocyte entering the tumour and encountering tumour cells directly will be inactivated because of the lack of co-stimuli. Only when the tumour has reached a size when cells die and a stress response is generated will 'danger signals' be produced. Even this may be suboptimal and furthermore the frequency and affinity of potential responder T cells may be low due to thymic selection. Given these handicaps, it may not be surprising that most tumours outrun the immune response and kill their host.

20.3.4 Unrestricted cytotoxicity

In early human experiments in which patients' lymphocytes were cultured with live tumour target cells, outgrowth of colonies of tumour cells was often inhibited (colony inhibition). In the early experiments the inhibition of growth appeared to be tumour type-specific so that lymphocytes from a patient with lung cancer could inhibit the growth of all lung cancer cell lines but not that of other tumour types. When more extensive controls were included in the assays the specificity appeared less clear-cut and it emerged that lymphocytes from normal individuals were often as inhibitory to tumour cell lines as were those from cancer patients. Subsequent experiments suggest that two different types of cytotoxic activity may have been detected in the earlier experiments. Finn and colleagues have shown that T cells from breast cancer patients, repeatedly boosted *in vitro* with breast cancer cells expressing the polymorphic epithelial mucin (PEM) develop PEM-specific but genetically unrestricted cytotoxicity (Jerome et al., 1993). PEM has an extracellular domain mainly consisting of a 20 amino acid sequence repeated many times. It is suggested that because this is a large repetitive array, it may bind to the TCR without the need for MHC presentation.

A second type of cytotoxicity detected in the early experiments is NK activity (Takasugi et al., 1973). NK cells have a characteristic phenotype. They are larger lymphocytes than most T and B cells and contain cytoplasmic granules (large granular lymphocytes). They share surface antigens with T lymphocytes and also with monocytes but do not express the TCR. Instead, NK cells express receptors that are members of two families of molecules, either immunoglobulin-like (killer immunoglobulin-like receptors or KIRs) or lectin-like (covalent dimers of CD94 and NKG2 family members) in structure (Lopez-Botet and Bellon, 1999). These molecules do not undergo somatic rearrangement like immunoglobulin itself or the TCR, so that a relatively small number of ligands may be recognized. The receptors are expressed on sub-populations of NK cells and on some activated T cells. It is clear that at many MHC class I molecules are ligands for NK receptors and that ligation of the receptors can have either activating or inhibitory effects on NK or T cells (KIR originally stood for killer inhibitory receptor).

The existence of KIRs provides an explanation for the early observation that NK cells often efficiently killed target cells with low or no expression of MHC class I, since these cannot deliver an inhibitory signal. That NK cell function is clearly regulated by contact with self-MHC molecules and that NK cells produce abundant IFN-γ-and other cytokines has led to suggestions of several roles. These include acting as a rapid early response system for viral infections (since many viruses downregulate MHC antigens) a role in regulating haemopoiesis and as part of the innate immune system in activating adaptive immune responses. Because they kill many tumour cell lines and recognize cells with low expression of MHC *in vitro* they have also been suggested to play a role in immune surveillance.

20.4 Human tumour antigens detected by antibodies

A great deal of effort has been devoted to attempts to use antibodies to detect new antigens on human tumours (see also Chapter 26). A unique genetic change in a cell might lead to the expression of a new antigen unique to that tumour—a tumour-specific antigen. Such an antigen may provoke a host response but the development of antibodies to it may only be useful to the tumour-bearing individual because the same antigen is not found in other tumours, even of the same type. More useful from the point of view of diagnosis or immunotherapy are tumour-associated antigens. These are antigens present on or in all tumour cells of a particular type but not found on normal cells. In tumours caused by viruses, proteins coded by the viral genome are effectively tumour-associated because they are generally found only in very rare normal cells, for example, some lymphomas have EBV antigens and one type of T cell leukaemia has antigens of the human T leukaemia virus (HTLV 1) while cervical tumours express papillomavirus genes.

Early attempts to reveal tumour-associated antigens used sera either from tumour patients or from animals deliberately immunized with human tumours. Both types of study have considerable problems. Sera from tumour patients might appear to be ideal reagents but in practice they often have in them antibodies capable of reacting with many types of cells. These include antibodies to blood groups, histocompatibility antigens, and autoantibodies that react with normal as well as tumour cells. Antisera raised in animals, usually rabbits, have similar problems. The rabbit antiserum 'sees' many antigens on a human tumour cell but the majority of these are present on normal cells also. Such sera therefore require extensive absorption to render them specific for tumour cells and it is not surprising that reports of successful production of specific heteroantisera are few in number, nor have they in general been particularly useful in tumour diagnosis or therapy. Some exceptions are mentioned below.

When monoclonal antibodies were developed, many investigators realized that monoclonal antibodies might provide reagents for detecting molecular differences between cell types and, indeed, mouse monoclonal antibodies can distinguish between human leucocytes and all other human cells, between T and B lymphocytes, or between different subpopulations of T lymphocytes. The molecules identified by these monoclonal antibodies are differentiation antigens (antigens present on one cell type but not in another or expressed at a particular stage of maturation) (see Chapters 18 and 26). In many cases they have been shown to be involved in functions associated with the particular cell type. These results suggested that it should be possible to produce monoclonal antibodies, which could distinguish between tumour and normal cells. Differences have indeed been recognized but so far there is no convincing evidence of a specific tumour-associated antigen.

Prior to the monoclonal era, polyclonal antisera raised in rabbits identified a number of antigens that initially appeared to be tumour-associated. Two examples are carcinoembryonic antigen (CEA), and common acute lymphoblastic leukaemia antigen (CALLA). CEA is a glycoprotein abundantly present in most colon carcinomas. Initially, the antigen was not thought to be present in normal colonic epithelium but was found in embryonic gut. Later, when more sensitive monoclonal antibodies were developed, CEA was shown to be present in the normal colon and in many other tumours as well as colon cancer. CEA is also found in serum. These findings are characteristic of many 'tumour-associated antigens'. First, the antigens are not truly tumour-associated and often not tumour type-specific either. Second, there is a quantitative difference in expression between tumour and normal tissue. This means that measurement of tumour antigen level (in the case of CEA by a radioimmunoassay of serum levels) can be a useful diagnostic or follow-up procedure. However, the distinction between a positive and negative result is arbitrary and both false positives and false negatives can occur (Moertel et al., 1993). CEA is really an example of a common category of molecules; differentiation antigens that are expressed at different levels on many epithelial cells and overexpressed in some epithelial tumour cells.

CALLA also appeared at first to be a tumour-associated antigen. However, once monoclonal antibodies to the molecule were produced it was discovered that a small proportion of cells in normal bone marrow expressed the antigen. Subsequently it was shown that these were developing B lymphocytes and that CALLA is transiently expressed on cells early in the B lymphocyte lineage. CALLA is therefore another normal differentiation antigen. Nevertheless, it is a useful molecule in leukaemia diagnosis since CALLA-positive cells are not normally found outside the bone marrow. Furthermore, CALLA-positive leukaemias have a relatively good prognosis (Chapter 18).

While the advent of monoclonal antibody technology led to the definition of numerous antigens of tumours, for example, over 40 different antigens in melanomas (Herlyn and Koprowski, 1988), none of these antigens, immunogenic in rats or mice, proved to be truly tumour-associated. More recently, a new method termed SEREX (serological analysis of tumour antigens by recombinant cDNA expression cloning) has allowed the definition of tumour molecules recognized by the host antibody response. In this method cDNA expression libraries are prepared from fresh tumour specimens, packaged into phages and expressed in *Escherichia coli*. Recombinant proteins expressed during growth of bacterial colonies are transferred to nylon membranes. The membranes are then probed with serum from the autologous patient which have been absorbed with normal tissues and diluted. Antibody binding is detected with an enzyme linked anti-human IgG antibody to ensure that only molecules to which the patient has made a specific and strong response are detected. Positive spots are characterized by recovering and sequencing the phage insert from the relevant bacterial colony (Chen et al., 2000). Using this method a large number of antigens recognized by host B lymphocytes have been identified. The sequences of these are available in a database of over 1000 entries (www2.licr.org/cancer/immuno-DB/index.html).

The SEREX approach has provided many new targets for immunotherapy and cancer diagnosis and in general it has confirmed what was already established with polyclonal or monoclonal antibodies raised in non-human species. Thus, most SEREX-defined antigens are expressed in some normal tissues as well as one or more tumour types (cancer-testis antigens show one of the most restricted distributions). Many antibodies are directed to molecules that are overexpressed in tumour cells compared to the corresponding normal tissue. Antigens coded by mutated genes have only rarely been detected by antibodies. Finally, and perhaps unsurprisingly since the presence of IgG antibodies implies a CD4 T cell response, several molecules in the SEREX database have also been identified as the targets of T cell responses (an example is the MAGE antigen first defined by Boon).

20.5 Immunodiagnosis

Ideal reagents for immunodiagnosis or immunotherapy would discriminate absolutely between tumour and normal cells. In addition they would distinguish between benign and malignant tumours. However, as discussed earlier, most if not all antibodies raised against tumours identify differentiation antigens. Nevertheless, these can be useful in cancer diagnosis because they identify the origin of a cell and panels of monoclonal antibodies are used in pathology and haematology laboratories to help in the identification and classification of tumours. For example, in the diagnosis of acute lymphoblastic leukaemia (see Chapter 18) antibodies have allowed clear distinctions to be made between T and B cell forms of the disease, which have a very different prognosis and respond differently to conventional chemotherapy. Identification of bad prognosis patients is important because it is sensible to try new forms of therapy in individuals with little chance of survival with current treatment.

Monoclonal antibodies are also useful in identifying the origin of tumour cells when this is difficult by conventional histological methods: antibodies to differentiation antigens (Table 20.7) can usually identify the origin of metastatic tumour cells even if these are cytologically undifferentiated. This has important implications for the management of the patient because secondary carcinoma is often chemotherapy-resistant while lymphoid tumours are often sensitive.

Table 20.7 Antibodies for identification of undifferentiated tumours

Tumour type	Tissue of origin	Antibody specificity
Carcinoma	Epithelia	Cytokeratins
Sarcoma	Connective tissue	Vimentin
Neuroblastoma	Nervous tissue	Neuro filaments
Glioma	Glia	Glial fibrillary acidic protein
Myosarcoma	Muscle	Desmin
Leukaemia/lymphoma	Leucocytes	CD45

Monoclonal antibodies are also being used in attempts to localize tumours *in vivo* for both diagnosis and therapy. For both diagnosis and therapy, specificity is all important. Radiolabelled antibodies used for diagnosis may reach a tumour but inevitably are also taken up non-specifically by organs such as the liver and the spleen. Similarly, the antibodies used for therapy and labelled with isotopes, toxins, or prodrugs may reach tumours but also other organs, which they may damage. These problems are discussed in Chapter 26.

20.6 Problems facing immunotherapy

20.6.1 Introduction

Immunotherapy is treatment by immunological means. In active immunotherapy the tumour bearer's own immune system is stimulated to respond to the tumour while in passive immunotherapy, immune cells or their products are given. Immunotherapy may also be specific or non-specific. Specific active immunotherapy aims to stimulate only a response to the tumour or deliver passively agents such as monoclonal antibodies that target the tumour. Non-specific therapy boosts all immune responses, for example, through the use of cytokines or lymphokine activated killer (LAK) cells. Many of these forms of immunotherapy are considered in detail in Chapters 14, 26, and 27. This section will therefore deal mainly with the principles underlying and problems facing, attempts to use active immunization.

Experimental evidence suggests that CD4 and CD8 T cells and antibody may all play a role in effective immunotherapy in different animal tumour models. However, generally T cells appear to play a major role in immunity to solid tumours, while antibodies are more effective against leukaemia or lymphoma. Most active immunization has therefore sought to induce strong cellular immune responses, which have been shown to be capable of eliminating large tumour masses in experimental animals and humans (Melief, 1992; Heslop et al., 1994). An additional reason for doing so is that the target antigens need not be cell surface molecules, since processed peptide epitopes reach the cell surface to be recognized by T cells (Figure 20.4).

20.6.2 Induction of antitumour immune responses: antigens and adjuvants

For immunization against tumours, what antigen to use is the first problem to be faced. Although increasing numbers of tumour antigens are being defined by SEREX, using T cell clones or by sequencing peptides eluted from tumour MHC antigens, individual tumours vary in antigen expression. This means that for any tumour type it would be sensible if possible, to immunize against several antigens (as is the case for most vaccines against microorganisms). As yet this is rarely possible in humans so that in practice most human experiments have taken one of two approaches. Either immunization is with antigens known to be well expressed on most tumours of a particular type, including CEA for colon cancer, PEM in breast cancer, and MAGE in melanoma (see Sections 20.3.2, 20.3.4, and 20.4 and Chapter 27). Alternatively, whole tumour cells are used. Irrespective of the antigen used, the aims of immunization will be to induce a strong CD4 and CD8 T-cell response against the chosen antigen(s).

One problem that particularly applies to immunization against tumours rather than microorganisms, is the possibility that damaging responses to self-antigens might be induced. As discussed above, most tumour-associated molecules are unaltered self-molecules, often expressed, though usually at a lower level, in normal tissues as well as tumours. That this is a real problem is shown by experiments in which mice undergoing successful immunotherapy against a melanoma became de-pigmented (Srinivasan et al., 2002) and patients have exhibited vitiligo (de-pigmentation) while undergoing anti-melanoma immunotherapy (Wankowicz-Kalinska et al., 2003). This particular side effect is not life-threatening but autoimmune responses to other antigens might be. Selection of antigens as target for immunotherapy should therefore take into account the tissue distribution of the antigens. It is a disadvantage of the use of whole tumour cells as antigen that it is impossible to control which antigens the host responds to.

The recognition that 'danger signals' were essential for initiation of immune responses has provided an explanation for why an immune response might be a late event in the evolution of a tumour (Section 20.3.3). This and recognition that tumour cells lacked co-stimuli such as CD80 or CD40 led to experiments in which tumour cells were transduced with genes coding for costimuli or cytokines (effectively internal 'danger signals'). However, evidence that immune responses to tumours are induced following uptake of tumour antigens by APC (cross-priming, see Section 20.3.3), suggests that optimal strategies for induction of antitumour responses should target tumour antigens to APCs. This has led to immunotherapy based on the use of antigen-loaded and activated DCs (Adams et al., 2000 and see Chapter 27). For this it is necessary that the DCs are MHC-matched with the patient, in practice usually autologous, and obtaining sufficient DCs is laborious, technically demanding, and expensive. Alternative means of targeting DC *in vivo* are being explored. Interestingly, giving antigen plus granulocyte monocyte colony stimulating factor (GM-CSF), a cytokine that is chemoattractant for DCs, has been shown to be an effective means of immunization (Pardoll, 1998). In effect, such a strategy mimics the release of cytokines, induced at a site of inflammation by 'danger signals', that leads to accumulation of inflammatory cells. A similar effect can be achieved by the use of adjuvants. These are substances that potentiate immune responses in several ways. They provide 'danger signals', often delivered by incorporated bacterial products, they often provide a slow release depot of antigen and their physicochemical properties, for example, particulate materials, may promote entry of antigen into the cytosol and endogenous antigen processing.

At present very few adjuvants are licensed for human use and the most well-established, aluminium salts, favour Th2 responses. However, new adjuvants are becoming available (Moingeon et al., 2002) and new immunization strategies are being developed to induce strong and long-lasting cellular (CD4 and CD8) responses. To date, the so-called prime/boost regimes appear to be one of the most effective (Irvine et al., 1997). In this method the antigen is first presented in one form, often as DNA, and the subjects are boosted with antigen presented in a different form, often in recombinant vaccinia or adenoviruses. These induce inflammation ('danger signals') and a large secondary immune response is induced and effector cells produced.

Whatever the target antigen and means of immunization are, it is important that both CD4 and CD8 responses are induced concurrently, as recent evidence has shown that CD8 memory cells, induced in the absence of CD4 help, do not respond to secondary stimulation (Shedlock and Shen, 2003). This dictates that the antigen should contain epitopes able to stimulate both sorts of T cells. Whole recombinant proteins or tumour cells are therefore more likely to be effective than CD8 target epitopes alone, which have been used in some human experiments (see Chapter 27).

20.6.3 Escape mechanisms

Mechanisms for escaping from immune responses are not confined to tumours. Almost, if not all, microorganisms have escape mechanisms and these are often similar to those found in tumours. Microorganisms and tumours may be immunosuppressive and these effects may be general or local. Many tumour-bearing patients show depressed immune responses and defects in signalling through the TCR and its associated CD3 complex have been demonstrated (Agrawal et al., 1998). The cause of this effect is unclear but may be due to cytokines such as transforming growth factor-β (TGF-β) and vascular endothelial growth factor (VEGF), often produced by tumours, which have been shown to have suppressive effects on lymphocytes. Furthermore, there is a complex relationship between tumours, their microenvironment, and the immune system, that may facilitate tumour growth and metastasis as much as preventing it (Coussens and Werb, 2002).

A major escape mechanism of tumours, also found in microorganisms, is interference in antigen presentation. More than half of all tumours show abnormalities in MHC class-I expression, ranging from downregulation of a single allele to loss of all class-I molecules, and diverse molecular mechanisms for this have been demonstrated (Bontkes et al., 1998). Clearly, however effective an antitumour immunization regime may be, it will be ineffective if the target epitopes can no longer be presented to effector T cells by the tumour cells. The common finding of loss of some HLA alleles in tumours suggests that antigen binding to as many different HLA molecules as possible should be used for immunization. Since HLA loss increases with tumour progression, active immunization is likely to be most effective if instituted as early as possible in the course of the disease. As yet this is seldom possible since conventional surgery, radiotherapy, or chemotherapy usually take precedence over unproven modalities such as immunotherapy.

20.7 Conclusions

T-cell cloning and the SEREX methodology have defined many tumour-associated molecules. Gene profiling is further defining what molecules are expressed or overexpressed in tumours. These are powerful techniques for defining how tumour cells differ from normal cells. Nevertheless, immunotherapy faces many difficulties but there have been some encouraging results.

Perhaps surprisingly in view of the results of experiments with antibodies against solid tumours in mice, initial results of trials with monoclonal antibodies against human colon cancer have been encouraging (Riethmuller et al., 1998). This may be because the antibodies are targeted to minimal residual disease, in other words single cells, which are more accessible to antibodies than large tumour masses. Harnessing cell-mediated responses is more difficult. While cytokines have powerful effects on host responses, so far they have been relatively disappointing (Chapter 14). Whether combining cytokines or other co-stimuli with tumour cells, recombinant antigens, or DNA, for use as vaccines, will lead to effective immunotherapies remains to be seen. The frequent development of escape mechanisms in tumours suggests that immunotherapy will always be a race against time and that it should be applied as early in tumour evolution as possible and in conjunction with other (non-immunosuppressive) debulking therapies.

There is one area in which immunology will contribute to cancer treatment, or rather prevention. A number of viruses play a role in the induction of tumours including hepatitis B virus in liver cancer, EBV in Burkitt's lymphoma and nasopharyngeal cancer, human papilloma viruses (HPVs) in genital tumours, and HTLV-1 and 2 in some lymphoid tumours (see Chapter 13). Prophylactic immunization against these and perhaps other as yet undiscovered agents is likely to prevent or reduce the incidence of these tumours. Already there is evidence that widespread use of hepatitis B vaccine in endemic areas can reduce the incidence of liver cancer (Lee et al., 1998). Much effort is being expended on vaccines for EBV and HPV and trials of HPV vaccines are showing encouraging results (Koutsky et al., 2002). As is the case with infectious disease, prophylactic immunization rather than treatment may be the most direct contribution of immunologists to the reduction of cancer mortality.

References

Adams, M., Jasani, B., Colaco, C. A. L. S., and Mason, M. D. (2000). Dendritic cell approaches to therapy. In (Eds. P. L. Stern et al.) *Cancer Vaccines and Immunotherapy*. Cambridge University Press, Cambridge, UK, p. 237–55.

Agrawal, S., Marquet, J., Delfau-Larue, M. H., Copie-Bergman, C., Jouault, H., Reye,. F. et al. (1998). CD3 hyporesponsiveness and in vitro apoptosis are features of T cells from both malignant and non-malignant secondary lymphoid organs. *J Clin Invest*, **102**, 1715–23.

Barclay, Brown, Law, McKnight, Tomlinson, and van der Merwe (eds.) (1997). *The Leucocyte Antigen Factsbook*. Academic Press, London.

Bjorkman, P. J., Saper, M. A., Samroui, B., Bennett, W. S., Strominger, J. L., and Wiley, D. C. (1987). Structure of the human histocompatibility antigen, HLA-A2. *Nature*, **329**, 506–12.

Bontkes, H. J., Walboomers, J. M. M., Meije, C. J. L. M., Helmhorst, T. J. M., and Stern, P. L. (1998). Specific HLA class I downregulation is an early event in cervical dysplasia associated with clinical progression. *Lancet*, **351**, 187–8.

Boon, T., Cerottini, J.-C., van den Eynde, B., van der Bruggen, P., and Van Pel, A. (1994). Tumour antigens recognised by T lymphocytes. *Ann Rev Immunol*, **12**, 337–66.

Burnett, F. M. (1973). Implications of cancer immunity. *Aust NZ J Med*, **3**, 70–7.

Chen, Y. T., Scanlan, M. J., Obata, Y., and Old, L. J. (2000). Identification of human tumour antigens by serological expression cloning (SEREX). In (Eds., S. A. Rosenberg et al.) *Principles and Practise of Biologic Therapy of Cancer*, 3rd edn. Williams and Wilkins, Philadelphia, pp. 557–70.

Coussens, L. M. and Werb, Z. (2002). Inflammation and cancer. *Nature*, **420**, 860–7.

Davis, M. M. and Bjorkman, P. J. (1988). T-cell antigen receptor genes and T-cell recognition. *Nature*, **334**, 395–402.

Fitzgerald, O'Neill, Gearing, and Callard (eds.) (2001). *The Cytokine Factsbook*. Academic press, London.

Girolomi, G. and Ricciardi-Castagnoli, P. (1997). Dendritic cells hold promise for immunotherapy. *Immunol Today*, **18**, 102–4.

Herlyn, M. and Koprowski, H. (1988). Melanoma antigens: immunological and biological characterisation and clinical significance. *Ann Revi Immunol*, **6**, 283–308.

Heslop, H. E., Brenner, M. K., and Rooney, (1994). Donor T cells to treat EBV-associated lymphoma. *New Engl J Med*, **331**, 517–20.

Irvine, K. R., Chamberlain, R. S., Shulman, E. P., Surman, D. R., Rosenberg, S. A., and Restifo, N. P. (1997). Enhancing efficacy of recombinant anticancer vaccines with prime/boost regimens that use two different vectors. *J Natl Cancer Inst*, **89**, 1595–601.

Jerome, K. R., Domenech, N., and Finn, O. J. (1993). Tumor-specific cytotoxic T cell clones from patients with breast and pancreatic adenocarcinoma recognise EBV-immortalized B cells transfected with polymorphic epithelial mucin complementary DNA. *J Immunol*, **151**, 1654–62.

Kocks, C. and Rajewsky, K. (1989). Stable expression and somatic hypermutation of antibody V regions in B cell differentiation. *Ann Rev Immunol*, **7**, 537–60.

Koutsky, L. A., Ault, K. A., Wheeler, C. M., Brown, D. R., Barr, E., Alvarez, F. B. et al. (2002). A controlled trial of a human papillomavirus type 16 vaccine. *New Engl J Med*, **347**, 1645–51.

Kruisbeek, A. M. and Amsen, D. (1996) Mechanisms underlying T-cell tolerance. *Curr Opin Immunol*, **8**, 233–44.

Lanoue, A., Bona, A., von Boehmer, H., and Sarukhan, S. (1998). Conditions that induce tolerance in mature CD4+ T cells. *J Exp Med*, **185**, 405–14.

Lee, M. S., Kim, D. H., Kim, H., Lee, H. S., Kim, C. Y., Park, T. S. et al. (1998). Hepatitis B vaccination and reduced risk of primary liver cancer among male adults: a cohort study in Korea. *Int J Epidemiol*, **27**, 316–19.

Lopez-Botet, M. and Bellon, T. (1999). Natural killer cell activation and inhibition by receptors of MHC class I. *Curr Opin Immunol*, **11**, 301–7.

McMichael, A. J. and O'Callaghan, C. A. O. (1998). A new look at T cells. *J Exp Med*, **188**, 1367–71.

Medzhitov, R. and Janeway, C. A. (1997). Innate immunity: impact on the adaptive response. *Curr Opin Immunol*, **9**, 4–10.

Melief, C. J. M. (1992). Tumour eradication by adoptive transfer of cytotoxic T lymphocytes. *Adv Cancer Res*, **58**, 143–57.

Moertel, C. G., Fleming, T. R., Macdonald, J. S., Haller, D. G., Laurie, J. A., and Tangen, C. (1993). An evaluation of the carcinoembryonic antigen (CEA) test for monitoring patients with resected colon cancer. *J Am Med Assoc*, **270**, 943–7.

Moingeon, P., deTaisne, C., and Almond, J. (2002). Delivery technologies for human vaccines. *Br Med Bull*, **62**, 29–44.

Nehlsen, S. L. (1971). Immunosuppression, virus and oncogenesis. *Transpl Proc*, **3**, 811–13.

Pardoll, D. (1998). Cancer vaccines. *Nat Med*, **4**, 525–31.

Przepiorka, D. and Srivastava, P. (1998). Heat-shock protein–peptide complexes: potential as cancer immunotherapeutic agents. *Mol Med Today*, **4**, 478–84.

Riethmuller, G., Holz, E., Sclimok, G., Schmiegel, W., Raab, R., Hoffken, K. et al. (1998). Monclonal antibody therapy for resected Dukes' C colorectal cancer: seven-year outcome of a multicenter randomized trial. *J Clin Oncol*, **16**, 1788–94.

Schatz, D. G., Oettinger, M. A., and Schlissel, M. S. (1992). V(D)J recombination: molecular biology and regulation. *Ann Rev Immunolo*, **10**, 359–98.

Shedlock, D. and Shen, H. (2003). Requirement for CD4 T cell help in generating functional CD8 T cell memory. *Science*, **300**, 337–9.

Sheil, A. G. (1998). Cancer in immune-suppressed organ transplant recipients: aetiology and evolution. *Transpl Proc*, **30**, 2055–7.

Srinivasan, R., Houghton, A. N., and Wolchok, J. D. (2002). Induction of autoantibodies against tyrosinase-related proteins following DNA vaccination: unexpected reactivity to a protein paralogue. *Cancer Immunother*, **19**, 2–8.

Swain, S. L. and Reth, M. (1994). Lymphocyte activation and effector functions. *Curr Opin Immunol*, **6**, 355–489.

Takasugi, M., Mickey, M. R., and Terasaki, P. I. (1973). Reactivity of lymphocytes from normal persons on cultured tumour cells. *Cancer Res*, **33**, 2898–902.

Thomas, L. (1982). On immunosurveillance in human cancer. *Yale J Biol Med*, **55**, 329–32.

Wankowicz-Kalinska, A., Le Poole, C., Van Den Wijngaard, R., Storkus, W. J., and Das, P. K. (2003). Melanocyte-specific immune response in melanoma and vitiligo: two faces of the same coin? *Pigment Cell Res*, **16**, 254–60.

Winter, G. and Milstein, C. (1991). Man-made antibodies. *Nature*, **349**, 293–9.

CHAPTER 21

The molecular pathology of cancer

Tatjana Crnogorac-Jurcevic, Richard Poulsom, and Nicholas R. Lemoine

21.1 Introduction

Molecular pathology is the study of basic mechanisms involved in pathogenesis of diseases at the molecular level. In addition to 'classical' examination of the morphology of diseased tissues and cells, it is now starting to embrace novel techniques of molecular biology that will enable us to reveal the origin and the development of the disease processes by examining the nucleic acids and proteins.

Molecular pathology has a special role in both clinical oncology and translational research. It is crucial not only in determining the tumour type and establishing tumour grade and stage (for details see Chapter 1), but is now starting to be instrumental in deciphering novel biomarkers for early cancer diagnosis, in patient stratification for individualized treatment ('tailored therapy') and determining biomarkers with a prognostic value.

In this chapter, we will first outline the principles of tissue preparation and processing that are necessary for their adequate preservation for subsequent analysis, and then give an overview of several techniques used in molecular oncology.

21.2 Preparation and processing of tissues and cells

Tumour classification is still largely based on determining the site of the tumour origin and its appearance under the microscope, the latter being the product not only of the neoplastic cells themselves but also the surrounding mesenchymal stromal elements. Optimal analysis of patients' samples can, however, only be undertaken if the specimens are correctly handled. The outline of typical specimen processing is shown in Figure 21.1.

In order to prevent autolysis and preserve fine structural characteristics of the tissues for subsequent analysis, the process of fixation of tissues should be performed as soon as they are removed. This is usually achieved through the mechanism of protein cross-linking by suspending the tissues in a volume of fixative at least 10 times larger than that of the specimen. There are several types of fixative, being either chemical (such as aldehydes, alcohols, oxidizing agents, mercurials, and picrins) or physical (heat). By far the most commonly used in histopathology practice is 4% formaldehyde (10% formalin). As lipids are largely lost during aldehyde fixation, mercuric chloride fixation should be used where it is important to demonstrate fat; for carbohydrates, alcohol-based fixatives are employed. Methanol, ethanol, or acetone are primarily used for fixing frozen sections and in the analysis of cytological smears.

After fixation, the sample is dehydrated in alcohol gradients (70%, 95%, 100%) and ethanol is then removed with xylene ('clearing'). The prepared

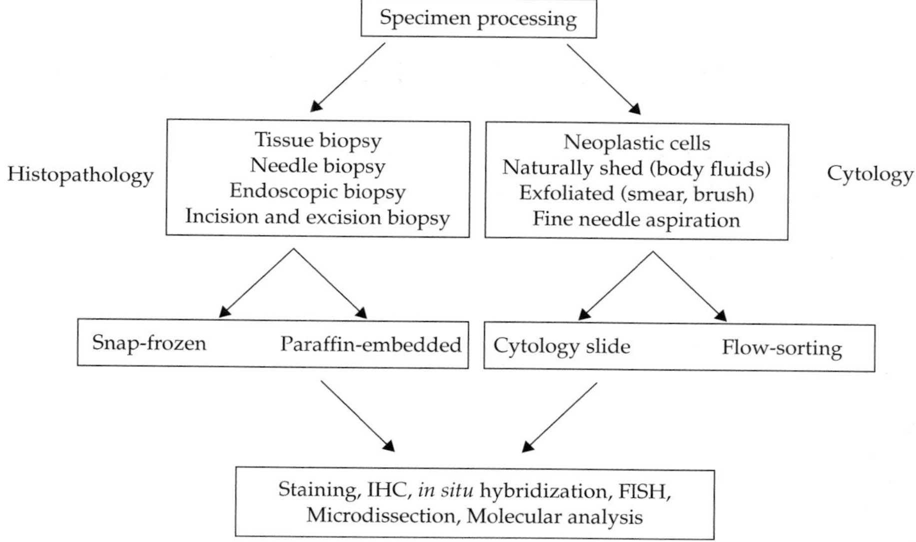

Figure 21.1 Schematic representation of specimen processing (IHC, immunohistochemistry; FISH, Fluorescence *in situ* hybridisation).

tissue is now ready for the embedding procedure, which is regularly performed using paraffin wax (paraffin wax is not miscible with water and dehydrating agents), which is cheap, provides adequate support to the tissue, and is easy to section. Once embedded in paraffin wax, the tissue can then be cut on a microtome with a disposable metal blade to produce sections of 4 μm (lymph nodes, renal biopsies) to 7 μm (majority of other tissues), which are usually adequate for most diagnostic purposes with light microscopy. For high resolution light microscopy and ultrastructural studies under the electron microscope, alternative embedding media need to be used, such as epoxy or acrylic resins. Ultra-thin section (0.5–1 μm) cutting is then performed on an ultramicrotome using a glass or diamond knife.

If rapid production of sections is required for urgent diagnosis, unfixed tissues can be snap-frozen. It is usually performed in solid carbon dioxide ('cardice'), carbon dioxide gas in aerosol spray, or by dropping the piece of tissue into isopentane that has been pre-cooled to −160°C by immersion into liquid nitrogen (−190°C). The frozen tissue can now be embedded in OCT and sectioned on a cryostat, or stored at −80°C or in liquid nitrogen. Obtaining and storing freshly frozen tissues is also crucial for the isolation of high-quality nucleic acids and proteins (particularly when analysis of activation status is anticipated), usually required for research purposes.

Neoplastic cells can be shed spontaneously into blood and other body fluids, or can be obtained by brushing, scraping, lavage, or aspiration. Cytology therefore has an increasing role in the diagnosis of human tumours because it is now possible to obtain cells from virtually any site in the human body with remarkable accuracy using advanced radiological techniques employing CT (computerized tomography) scanning, ultrasound, and nuclear magnetic resonance (NMR). Suction can be applied to a fine bore needle placed even in a relatively inaccessible tumour and cells aspirated from it. For cytological analysis, the cells can either be fixed in alcohol or allowed to dry rapidly on a glass slide which enables the cells to adhere strongly. A wide range of stains that are used in histopathology as well as immunocytochemical procedures are equally applicable to cytological preparations and, although the number of the cells per sample is usually relatively small, non-specific background staining is usually low.

For most cytology laboratories the largest proportion of specimens comprise cervical smears (for detailed description refer to Chapter 29).

21.3 Histochemistry

Before staining of the slides carrying tissue sections can be performed, the embedding process has to be reversed by passing the slides through xylene, alcohol gradients, and water ('deparaffinisation') in order to remove the paraffin wax from the tissue and allow water-soluble dyes to penetrate the sections. For most human tumours, histopathologists can establish site of origin, grading, staging, and subclassification of tumours, crucial for accurate diagnosis, just by looking at the conventional Haematoxylin and Eosin stained sections.

Haematoxylin was traditionally obtained from the heartwood of the tree *Haematoxylin campechianum* (grown in the Mexican state of Campeche), but has nowadays been exchanged for a synthetic variant. It is not a stain itself, but rather its oxidation product, haematein. Haematein is anionic, with a poor affinity for the tissue without the presence of a metal ion like iron, tungsten, or most commonly, aluminium (Mayer's, Cole's, Harris's haematoxylin, etc). These complexes have a net positive charge and thus enable binding to the nuclear chromatin. When the section is washed under alkaline buffers or tap water, the initial red colour is changed into the familiar blue stain mainly confined to the nuclei. Eosins (Eosin Y, Eosin B, and Ethyl eosin) are xanthene dyes that stain the cell cytoplasm and most connective tissue fibres in varying shades of pink, orange, and red. More complex classifications can be made using additional dyes that highlight different cellular or extracellular matrix components, such as van Gieson for collagen, Reticulin/silver method for reticulin fibres, Masson's trichrome for skeletal muscle, Periodic acid-Schiff (PAS) for glycogen, Congo red for amyloid, and Alizarin red for calcium salts.

21.4 Immunohistochemistry

Immunohistochemistry (IHC) has had a major impact on the practice of histopathology. In principle, tissue sections or cell smears are treated with an antiserum or purified antibodies to a specific protein and the binding site is identified by a marker which may be a coloured or a fluorescent dye, a heavy metal (especially for electron microscopy), a radioactive label, or an enzyme. Markers are usually attached to the antibodies and may be visualized directly or by a subsequent reaction.

Again, the detection of certain antigens is highly dependent on fixation and processing, and the availability of tissue fixed in a variety of fixatives is valuable. Some antigens can only be detected after the pre-digestion of the sections with enzymes (e.g. chymotrypsin/trypsin) that will break protein linkages and expose the target epitope(s). This procedure of antigen retrieval can also be achieved by heating in a microwave oven in citrate buffer.

Table 21.1 Selected immunohistochemistry panels for the diagnosis and characterisation of Tumours

General Panel
CD45 (Leukocyte common)
Desmin
Vimentin
CK8
CK18
CEA (carcinoembryonic antigen)
NSE (neuron-specific enolase)
EMA (epithelial membrane antigen)
HMB45 (Melanoma-specific antigen)
Lymphoma Panel
CD45 (Leukocyte common)
CD15 (Hodgkin's cells)
CD20 (B-cells)
CD3 (T-cells)
Bcl-2
Sarcoma Panel
Factor VIII
α-1 antitrypsin
Actin
Desmin
Germ Cell Panel
α-FP (alpha fetoprotein)
HCG (human chorionic gonadotropin)
PLAP (placental alkaline phosphatase)
HPL (human placental lactogen)
Mesothelioma Panel
CEA (carcinoembryonic antigen)
CK18
Calretinin
Thrombomodulin
Neuroendocrine Panel
NSE (neuron-specific enolase)
Chromogranin A
Synaptophysin
Proliferation Panel
Ki67
PCNA (proliferating cell nuclear antigen)

A wealth of commercially available antibodies has greatly expanded the role of IHC in the molecular diagnosis of tumours (Table 21.1). Detection of surface, intracellular, and extracellular proteins, locally secreted proteins and hormones, tumour classification, distinction of reactive from neoplastic cells as well as determination of the functional status of proteins (for instance, phosphorylated versus unphosphorylated (Ng et al., 1999) has now been made easy and fast, especially if performed in automatic staining machines.

Where morphological diagnosis of tumour is unclear, immunohistochemical analysis may allow subclassification with a considerable degree of accuracy. The initial screen would use a broad range of differentiation antigens to classify the tumours into epithelial, mesenchymal, and lymphoreticular/haemopoietic lineages, and within these broad groups, sequentially subclassify with increasingly restrictive panels of antigens to determine the phenotype of the cells (see Table 21.1).

Many high grade lymphomas were undoubtedly misdiagnosed as anaplastic carcinomas before the advent of IHC, and since the response of high grade lymphomas to treatment is now very good, this is a critical distinction. It is also a relatively straightforward one, that can be achieved using a small panel of antibodies that recognize lymphoid-restricted antigens such as leukocyte common antigen (CD45) or B- and T- cell markers (CD10, CD20, CD23 or CD2, CD3, CD43, respectively) or epithelial cell markers such as cytokeratins (CK8, CK18, CK19) and epithelial membrane antigen (EMA). If necessary, a further subset of more restricted antigens can either confirm a tentative diagnosis or subclassify a tumour even further. This can be important, as many tumours actually lose their high differentiation antigens during progression and may only retain a limited detectable phenotype.

Neoplastic cells may not only lose certain differentiation antigens but can also acquire others during neoplastic progression. Examples of so-called aberrant expression, that is, the detection of an antigen not expected in that particular lineage, are now readily identified by IHC. Cytokeratin expression, for example, previously thought to be restricted exclusively to epithelial lineages, may be detected in different types of cells, including reticular cells in lymph nodes, chondrocytes, plasma cells, smooth muscle cells, rhabdomyosarcomas, and malignant fibrous histiocytomas. Markers of mesenchymal lineages such as vimentin, while strongly expressed in most sarcomas and malignant melanomas, may also be expressed in some carcinomas, especially those of renal, pancreatic, and ovarian origin, as well as in carcinomas that assume a spindle cell morphology. MUC1, which is an epithelial membrane antigen, can also be found on plasma cells and some lymphoreticular cells and their neoplasms. It is therefore essential to assemble wide-ranging antibody screens with expected positive and negative results, preferably with more than one positive for each lineage or subtype. In addition, the resulting phenotype also needs to be in an agreement with a plausible clinical interpretation.

IHC has proved successful in determining the status of several tumour suppressor genes, like *TP53* and *RB*, and numerous studies have confirmed their prognostic relevance in various tumours. Antibodies against cell cycle proteins like cyclins D1 and E have been used in the evaluation of breast and squamous cell carcinomas, and immunoreactivity to the anti-apoptotic molecule BCL2 (which is upregulated in a number of tumours) can indicate unresponsiveness to therapeutic regimes and poor prognosis (Sjostrom et al., 2002).

There are some lineage-specific antigens that may identify a particular cell type with great accuracy. Examples of such antigens include thyroglobulin, parathormone, peptide hormones from neuroendocrine tumours such as calcitonin in medullary carcinomas of the thyroid gland, or endothelial antigens such as CD31, CD34, and Factor VIII-related antigen. In addition to lineage markers, immunohistochemical analysis can also highlight structural alterations in neoplasia which can be useful for assessment of tumours. To give an example, staining of the basement membrane-restricted antigens type IV collagen and laminin can delineate the basement membrane around *in situ* carcinomas. As tumours become invasive, they tend to lose the ability to form basement membranes (or it is degraded at the point of invasion) and thus, potentially, this analysis can distinguish between *in situ* and invasive cancers.

One drawback of immunohistochemistry is that both monoclonal and polyclonal antibodies can recognize more than one epitope, or a similar epitope on related or unrelated molecules, which may give rise to cross-reactivity. So-called 'non-specific' staining may also arise when antibodies bind to other tissue components. These problems are sometimes encountered, especially when antibodies raised to a particular target have only been investigated in a very restricted field. When applied in the wider sphere of diagnostic pathology, the antibodies being exposed to a whole range of potential targets in many complex tissues, problems with specificity may then become evident. Unless one is aware of this potential problem (i.e. through knowledge of data on reactivity with a wide range of normal and neoplastic tissues), misinterpretation can arise. There is also a whole range of potential artefacts owing to inappropriate fixation, endogenous pigments, endogenous enzymes activating the detection systems, and physical artefacts in the tissues or reagents that may give rise to false positive and false negative reactions. All of these problems can only be solved by experience and repetition of results with a range of appropriate controls, and in the case of novel monoclonal and polyclonal antibodies by corroboration with another antibody recognizing the same or a related molecule. Western blot analysis (immunoblotting) that combines protein gel electrophoresis, filter transfer, and detection by specific antibody, is another method of assessing protein expression and quantification. In addition to providing data on the presence and relative abundance of a particular protein, it also gives an indication of potential cross-reactivity if several bands are identified.

21.5 *In situ* hybridization

Detecting mRNA expression

In situ Hybridization (ISH) can provide crucial information about where a specific mRNA is expressed and has been applied successfully in a great variety of cancer applications.

The generally preferred method for detecting mRNAs in routinely fixed paraffin-embedded materials uses riboprobes. These are single stranded RNA molecules synthesized by *in vitro* transcription using a DNA-directed RNA polymerase (SP6, T3, or T7), sufficient nucleoside tri-phosphates (including a labelled base) and a suitable DNA template. Templates contain lengths of double-stranded DNA bearing a sequence for RNA polymerase binding and initiation, followed by sequence that is specific to the target RNA. A riboprobe capable of binding to an mRNA must be 'antisense'; that is, an RNA version of the non-coding strand. Usually, templates are made from plasmid DNA linearized using a restriction endonuclease. Alternatively, specific cDNA fragments can be amplified by RT/PCR using primers containing RNA polymerase sequences, for example (Frantz et al. 2001).

Riboprobe *in situ* hybridization offers greater specificity and sensitivity than other ISH methods using oligonucleotides or cDNA fragments because more reporting labels can be hybridized specifically to each target. Isotopic and non-isotopic riboprobes can be used, each having advantages and disadvantages that have been discussed in detail (Poulsom, et al. 1998). The value of non-isotopic riboprobe methods in studies intended to screen for sites of expression is severely limited by the fact that peak sensitivity is dependent upon individual cell type and fixation conditions, and permeabilization conditions usually need to be 'titrated' for individual blocks and even cell types within a block. Signal amplification methods, for example, using tyramide deposition to increase the number of signal-forming sites derived from each probe, have been evaluated rigorously, yet isotopic ISH is more sensitive. *In situ* PCR amplification has been used effectively to increase ease of detection but is not robust enough for screening purposes and can be prone to PCR errors (Steel et al., 2001).

Conventional formalin-fixed paraffin wax-embedded tissues are suitable for ISH, and are preferable in several ways to frozen tissue samples. Re-blocking of small fragments of tissue from one wax block to another does not usually cause problems, and tissue arrays made using needle biopsies of suitable donor blocks are a convenient way to survey large numbers of cases for population studies of mRNA expression (Figure 21.2(a)). Frozen tissues may give good mRNA labelling but are awkward to store and handle and, above all, give poor morphology. Cell cultures can be studied as cytospins or directly if grown on glass slides, or by sectioning wax-embedded plugs of agarose cast around cells pelleted in microfuge tubes.

Certain cell types have well deserved reputations for non-specific binding of probes. Eosinophils frequently show non-specific binding despite the fact that their granules are rich in RNases. Stratified squamous epithelium in the skin can give high background, and melanin can confuse, although in reflected light, melanin is brownish unlike the bright silver grains.

ISH is an excellent technique for revealing the cell types that express the highest levels of the target, compared to surrounding tissue, and can readily identify just a few cells that express a target at moderate levels, even when a northern blot is negative. Conversely, if a target is expressed widely at moderate levels, for example, GAPDH, the impression may be simply that of a generally grainy high background, even though a northern blot of homogenized tissue would be strongly positive.

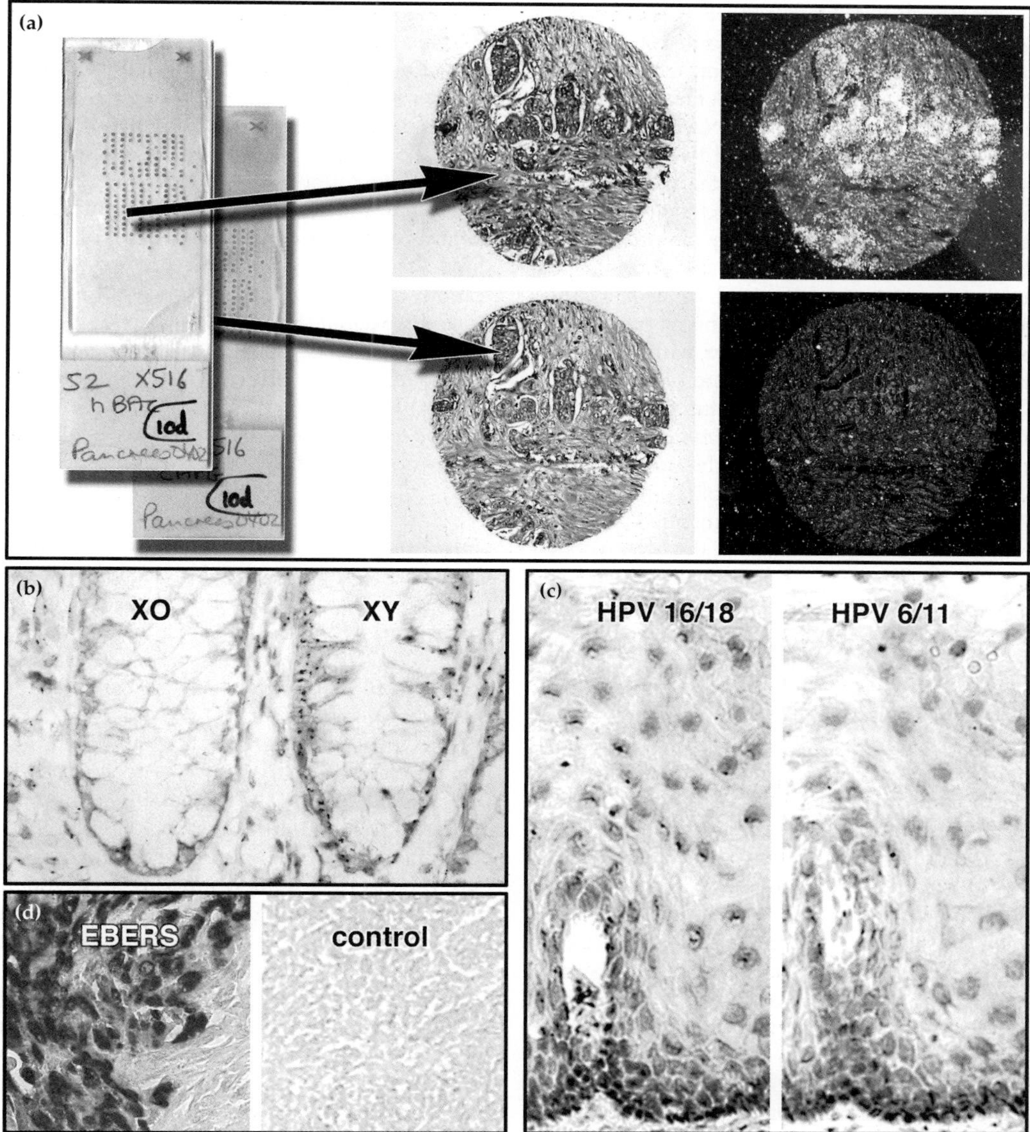

Figure 21.2 (a) Riboprobe detection of mRNAs in sections of tissue microarrays. Cores of formalin-fixed paraffin embedded pancreatic tissue are hybridized to a ^{35}S-labelled control probe for β-actin (top row) and a test probe (lower row): conventional and reflected-light dark field images demonstrate the presence of abundant β-actin mRNA, seen as autoradiographic silver grains, supporting that the test mRNA was truly absent. (b) DNA probe detection of regions of the Y chromosome in colorectal tissue. *Conventional* sections of tissue from an X0 : XY chimaeric patient reveal the clonality of crypts (c.f. Novelli et al 1996). Cosmid DNA was labelled then detected using an indirect protocol, resulting in intense dark brown deposits over positive nuclei. (c) Oligonucleotide cocktail detection of specific subtypes of human papilloma virus in conventional sections of cervix. Commercial probe cocktails labelled with fluorescein were hybridized then detected using an anti-fluorescein; peroxidase conjugate that generates a dark brown deposit over infected nuclei (several nuclei labelled with the HPV 16/18 probes, none with the HPV 6/11 probes). (d) Peptide Nucleic Acid (PNA) probe detection of abundant EBV-encoded RNAs (EBERs) in a conventional section of nasopharyngeal carcinoma. Commercial PNA probe cocktail labelled with fluorescein were hybridized then detected using an anti-fluorescein alkaline phosphatase conjugate that generates a dark purple deposit over the cytoplasm of cells with latent infection. The negative control section was hybridized with 'random' fluorescein-labelled PNAs.

The entire isotopic ISH procedure, from labelling probes and cutting sections through to dipping, takes 4–5 days, plus autoradiographic exposure time (2–3 days for abundant mRNA targets, 10 days for a moderately abundant mRNA target; prolonged exposure times are limited by background grain formation that depends on many variables). Autoradiographic silver grains are easily seen by conventional microscopy if they are clustered above cells, but a much more sensitive impression of the pattern of expression and of background graininess (due to irrelevant binding of probe) can be obtained using epi-illumination without transmitted light (Figure 21.2). This type of imaging is easy to achieve using a microscope designed for metallurgical studies, where the image is formed only from light reflecting up from the specimen (off the silver grains). Condenser block dark-field imaging is rarely satisfactory. Phosphor imaging has been tested as an alternative to the high resolution images produced by dipped emulsion autoradiography; at present it offers low spatial resolution but does allow quantification of the amounts of hybridization.

Patterns of expression derived from using several riboprobes on near serial sections can be compared and used to establish that specific, differential patterns of labelling occurred. To establish that there was hybridizable mRNA within all cell types within a section, a probe to β-actin can be used (Figure 21.2(a)). If there is no detectable actin, it is possible that all mRNA in the specimen has degraded and no useful information can be obtained from that specimen. Signals from β-actin mRNA are usually strongest over vascular smooth muscle cells and the centres of inflammatory cell aggregates, and are variable between other cell types. In contrast, the levels of signal produced by a probe to the 'housekeeping gene' GAPDH are less variable and thus difficult to distinguish from a high background.

Detecting mRNA and protein expression

Sites of expression of an mRNA can conflict with expectations, often because the protein is secreted and taken up elsewhere. For example, immunohistochemistry for gelatinase-A (MMP-2) in blocks of breast carcinoma indicates that this metalloproteinase is expressed principally in the tumour epithelium, yet the mRNA is localized principally to stromal cells with low or undetectable levels of gelatinase-A mRNA in the tumour epithelium (Poulsom et al. 1993). Thus, ISH and IHC are methods that complement each other, revealing different aspects of the gene's expression. ISH can be applied to look for sites of potential synthesis as soon as a sequence has been cloned, much more quickly than a specific antibody can be produced, indeed ISH can sometimes be used to help validate a candidate antibody.

Some applications require comparison of the patterns of expression of mRNA and protein on the same histology section, and protocols have been recently developed that accomplish this in sections of conventional blocks and tissue microarrays. Experience of combined IHC/ISH is relatively limited. Generally the distributions revealed are not significantly different from those seen using the methods singly, but this should be established for each study.

Detecting cytogenetic abnormalities in routine specimens

Chapter 6 describes several molecular cytogenetics methods that can be applied to the study of cancer. Some of the basic DNA ISH techniques can be applied to clinical specimens whether 'fresh' or archived, allowing further insight into the nature of the individual case.

DNA probes to specific regions of the genome can be labelled by a variety of techniques (many pre-labelled probes are available commercially) and used to look for the presence of highly specific abnormalities. This may be relevant to diagnosis and/or prognosis, as in Ewing's sarcoma and neuroblastoma where specific gains or losses of regions of the genome can readily be established by fluorescence ISH (FISH).

In breast cancer, the decision whether trastuzumab (Herceptin) could rationally be included in treatment, hinges on the level of expression in tumour cells of ERBB2. Overexpression of this receptor confers a selective advantage to the cells (that can be blocked by the antibody drug), and is usually driven by amplification of the gene. FISH is the preferred method for establishing *ERBB2* amplification, although chromogenic ISH (CISH) methods are thought to have advantages (Gupta et al., 2003). There is debate over the merits of IHC protocols to reveal the level of protein as these give variable levels of detection and correlation with FISH data (Bartlett et al., 2003).

In a research setting, important information concerning the mechanism of formation of early adenomas has been obtained using CISH; a probe for Y chromosomes was used on colorectal tissues taken from an individual who had XO/XY chimaerism (Figure 21.2(b)), and it was possible to establish that all cell types within individual crypts were clonal, that small adenomas were polyclonal (Novelli et al., 1996) and that the pattern of growth of these early lesions is from the crypt bases.

Detecting specific infectious agents in routine specimens

DNA and Peptide Nucleic Acid (PNA) probes can been used to establish the presence of viral sequences in tissue sections. For example, probe cocktails are available (www.innogenex.com) that can not only show the presence in cervical epithelium of Human Papilloma Virus (HPV), but also indicate which subtypes are present (e.g. Figure 21.2(c)). This can indicate whether the HPV infection is likely to present significant risk of neoplastic progression.

Another example is detection of Epstein Barr virus expressed RNAs (EBERs), which are highly abundant during latent infection in nasopharyngeal carcinoma cells and are readily demonstrated using PNA probes labelled with fluorescein (Dako www.dako.co.uk) and detected with anti-fluorescein-enzyme conjugates (Figure 21.2(d)). Recently, ISH methods have been used in a kit to detect *Helicobacter pylori* in biopsy specimens and simultaneously establish whether the bacteria found are likely to be resistant to the antibiotic clarithromycin (creaFAST® H. PYLORI TEST KIT; www.oxoid.com/uk/). This is relevant to cancer prevention as the relative risk of developing gastric adenocarcinoma is up to fourfold greater in patients infected with *H. pylori*. The World Health Organization has categorized *H. pylori* as a class I, or definite, carcinogen.

21.6 Tissue microdissection

Each organ is a complex three-dimensional structure and each tissue is composed of various cell types that can elicit different responses in different pathological states. Therefore, to delineate the precise mechanism and the chronology of the events in various diseases, isolation of pure population of cells often becomes a prerequisite.

Several microdissection techniques have been developed, starting with manual or micromanipulator-guided needle dissection under the ordinary light microscope to modern automated systems such as Leica (see www.leica-microsystems.com), PALM (www.palm-microlaser.com) or the laser capture microdissection (LCM) system from Arcturus (www.arctur.com). They all allow efficient procurement of defined cell populations from whole tissue sections and the unique possibility to study tumour biology at DNA, RNA and protein level from a single isolated cell (Figure 21.3).

Independent of which dissection method is applied, great care has to be taken throughout the (microdissection) procedure to avoid degradation of both nucleic acids and proteins, and a set of rules and protocols therefore need to be developed and validated in each laboratory and for each individual tissue type.

As the least sensitive to degradation, microdissected DNA has been used as a template for several molecular techniques, such as PCR, loss of heterozygosity (LOH), comparative genomic hybridization (CGH), CGH array, and spectral karyotyping (SKY) analyses to investigate genomic profiles in cancer.

A far smaller number of studies have been performed using RNA prepared from microdissected material. In addition to 'low-throughput' methods for gene expression such as RT-PCR or QRT-PCR, RNA prepared from dissected tissue can also be used in the context of 'high-throughput' oligo or cDNA array analysis. As for this kind of study RNA has to be of very high quality, only freshly (snap)-frozen tissue blocks should be used as a source of material. The tissue definition in frozen tissues is not very well preserved, and it is sometimes difficult to identify the particular cell type. It is possible, however, to perform immunohistochemical staining on the frozen sections just prior to microdissection ('Immuno-LCM')(Fend et al., 1999), which greatly expands the ability to study gene/protein expression in heterogenous tissue.

In addition to difficulties in obtaining high quality RNA, microdissection technique also suffers from the inherent problem of limited quantity of recovered material. PCR-based amplification procedures have recently been superseded by the method of linear amplification. This utilizes an oligo dT primer combined with the T7 RNA polymerase promoter for the cDNA synthesis reaction, and T7 RNA polymerase to amplify the cDNA. This results in several hundred-fold amplified antisense RNA (aRNA). Since the T7

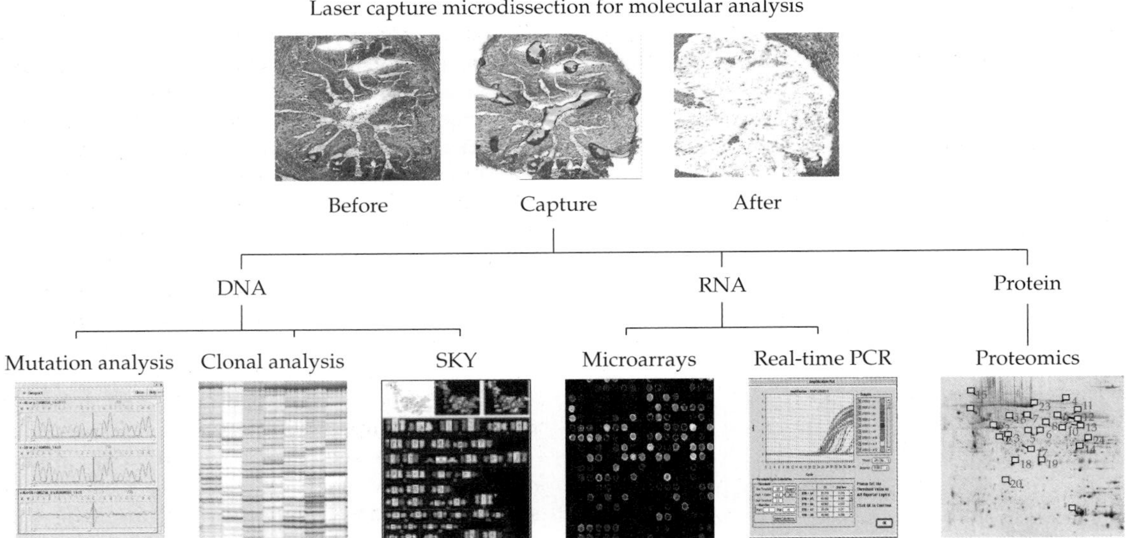

Figure 21.3 Illustration of laser capture microdissection and the utility of subsequently isolated material in molecular analysis (see also Plate 4).

RNA polymerase promoter is highly specific, it is believed that the aRNA is truly representative of the founder RNA population. Microdissected material from a variety of tumours such as breast, colorectal, oral, gastric, pancreatic, and squamous cell carcinoma of the head and neck has been employed successfully in profiling experiments (Leethanakul et al., 2000; Crnogorac-Jurcevic et al., 2002). As a result of such experiments, an increase or decrease in expression of a number of tumour cell-specific genes (representing all aspects of cell life, such as metabolism, signal transduction, cell cycle, development, immunity, and cell death), many of which have not been previously associated with the malignant process, have been discovered.

As most pathology laboratories possess large archives of paraffin-embedded tissue blocks, which are extremely valuable for retrospective studies when supported with clinical data, there have been several attempts to recover RNA from paraffin blocks for gene expression studies. Unfortunately, the time from surgical excision to fixation, fixation procedure, and RNA half-life were all shown to have effects on the quality of the RNA obtained. Although QRT–PCR analysis of small amplicons (60–100 bp) can often be successfully performed, the application of such degraded RNA for large-scale differential gene expression profiling is still under scrutiny.

Analysis of proteins from microdissected material is presented with even more difficulties due to the inability to apply amplification procedures to protein material. However, as proteins are the final 'players' in the lives of cells, and their abundance does not always follow the RNA expression levels, obtaining the pattern of protein expression in normal and pathological states, that is, normal and cancer specimens, becomes crucial. In addition to 2D-gel analysis followed by mass spectrometry, the profiling of microdissected cancer can now be performed on antibody and a variety of other protein arrays, as well as used for the pattern analysis by SELDI-TOF (Surface Enhanced Laser Desorption/Ionization—Time of Flight) mass spectrometry (Petricoin et al., 2002).

In summary, microdissection has proved to be a very powerful technique in cancer research. It enables isolation and study of tumour cells at various stages of cancer progression, distinguishing between distinct tumour types, helps in establishing the role of stromal cells surrounding tumour, and allows capture of invasive cells breaking from the primary tumour (Zhu et al., 2003). Furthermore, combining microdissection technology with large-scale functional genomic and proteomic analysis (see Chapter 22) offers the genuine possibility of gaining real insight into cellular processes in healthy and diseased states.

21.7 Tissue microarrays

Tissue microarrays are named by analogy to DNA microarrays, but instead of DNA elements, small tissue core biopsies are deposited on the glass microscopic slides in a precise and regular manner. The method was recently developed in the laboratory of Olli Kallioniemi at NIH in Bethesda (Kononen et al., 1998). Construction of tumour tissue microarrays is a straightforward procedure. After defining the type of the array one wants to construct, depending on what the aims and purposes of the studies are, it begins with a careful examination of tumour paraffin blocks by a trained pathologist. Morphologically representative regions of each individual tumour are selected and cylindrical 0.6 mm core biopsies from the donor blocks are transferred into the new recipient paraffin block.

The idea stems from a multiblock sausage that Battifora described in 1986 as a method of wrapping 100 rods of tissue each 1 mm thick in a sheet of mammalian small intestine that was then embedded in a paraffin block (Battifora, 1986). The major applications of this tissue block were to test different antibodies and routinely monitor the sensitivity of immunohistological procedures between different laboratories. However, the major drawback was the inability to precisely locate each rod of tissue, which was achieved in Kallionemi's tissue microarray by a pattern-forming spotting of circular tissue core biopsies. Its advantages also include increased capacity, negligible damage caused to the donor tissue blocks, and the possibility for automated construction and analysis of microarrays. The major question of whether the minute tissue cores of heterogeneous tumours that comprise each tissue array are truly representative of their donor tumours was addressed in several studies and the results obtained on small core biopsies were in general shown to be highly similar to the data obtained on large sections (Nocito et al., 2001). In an attempt to determine antigen survival and the potential for using very old archival tissue for the construction of TMAs, Camp et al., have arrayed in succession cases of breast cancers dating from 1932 and from each following decade to the present. Interestingly, their data have demonstrated that many proteins retain their antigenicity for more than 60 years (Camp et al., 2000). Equally important, the correlation between phenotypes and clinical outcome was proven not to be significantly different between microarrays and standard full sections. However, in all the studies, loss of cores during the experimental procedures is in the range of 10–20%, which can be compensated for by arraying larger numbers of cores.

Tissue microarrays permit a high throughput analysis of multiple targets, not only at the protein level but also at the DNA and RNA levels. It can be used for gene amplification surveys by fluorescence *in situ* hybridisation (FISH), *in situ* hybridization (ISH) to reveal the cellular localization and relative level of expression of specific genes and in immunohistochemical analysis of localization and expression of their protein products (see Figure 21.3).

Virtually all kinds of tissues or cells can be converted to a microarray format and the design of the array can vary depending on the experimental assays envisaged. For example, arrays containing cores from multiple tumour types (multi-tumour TMA) can be used for analysis of expression of various molecular markers across the spectrum of neoplastic diseases, tumour progression TMAs can be used to investigate molecular alterations in different stages of tumour growth and development, and 'patient outcome' TMAs, containing samples from patients for whom clinical follow-up data are accessible, can be utilized to look at molecular markers with prognostic significance. These kinds of studies have already been described for oestrogen and progesterone receptors, p53, and HER2 in breast cancer, vimentin in kidney cancer, and cyclin E expression in urinary bladder cancer (Moch et al., 1999; Richter et al., 2000; Nocito et al., 2001).

Thus, the tissue microarray approach provides a novel method for rapid screening of multiple genes/proteins and multiple tumours with the same methodology, thereby leading to a less biased analysis of various cancer types. In summary, it seems that TMA studies may replace most large-section studies in the near future and will greatly accelerate the translation of basic research findings to clinical application.

21.8 Molecular imaging

Molecular imaging is a rapidly emerging research discipline for the visual representation, characterization, and quantification of biological processes at the cellular and subcellular levels within intact living organisms. Much of what presently requires invasive tissue sampling for molecular pathological assessment could be replaced by *in vivo* imaging methods that reflect specific cellular and molecular processes, for example, gene expression, or more complex molecular interactions such as protein–protein interactions. Already technology is available to follow trafficking and targeting of cells in experimental animals and the systems can be scaled up to allow clinical application. Many centres are now using molecular imaging to image drug (and gene therapy) effects at the molecular and cellular level in man without the need for tissue biopsies.

Optical imaging

Optical imaging techniques represent an extension of fluorescence microscopy through the development of targeted bioluminescence probes, near-infrared fluorochromes, activatable near-infrared fluorochromes, and red-shifted fluorescent proteins (Mahmood et al., 1999; Weissleder and Mahmood, 2001). Multiple probes with different spectral characteristics could potentially be used for multi-channel imaging, analogous to *in vivo* karyotyping. Optical imaging also allows for a relatively low-cost alternative to studying reporter gene expression in small animal models (see below).

Charged coupled device (CCD) detectors are used for optical bioluminescence imaging of light-emitting proteins (for instance, encoded by the Firefly or Renilla luciferase enzyme genes, or the bacterial *lux* genes) in small animals. The latest generation of bioluminescence image acquisition systems using rotating CCD cameras and multiple views of the same animal with a single CCD camera allow volumetric imaging, enhanced when combined with novel red-shifted luciferases that have better tissue penetration. At present there is no equivalent imaging modality suitable for human studies, thus preventing direct translation of developed methods for clinical use.

In fluorescence imaging, an excitation light of one wavelength is used to illuminate a living subject, and a CCD camera collects an emission light of shifted wavelength. Cells tagged with fluorescently labelled antibodies or those in which expression of the green fluorescent protein (GFP) gene is introduced can be followed by this technique. Wild-type GFP emits green (509 nm) light when excited by violet (395 nm) light. The variant EGFP has a shifted excitation spectrum to longer wavelengths and has increased (35-fold) brightness. Between 1000 and 10,000 fluorescently labelled cells in the peritoneal cavity of a mouse can be imaged on its external surface. Fluorescence imaging can be used as a reporter in both live and fixed cells/tissues and no substrate is required for its visualization. The use of the near-infrared (NIR) spectrum in the 700–900 nm range maximises tissue penetration and minimises autofluorescence from non-target tissue. This is because haemoglobin and water, the major absorbers of visible and infrared light respectively have their lowest absorption coefficients in the NIR region.

Radionuclide imaging

Positron emission tomography (PET) records high-energy γ-rays emitted from within the subject. Natural biological molecules can be labelled with a positron-emitting isotope that is capable of producing two γ-rays through emission of a positron from its nucleus, which eventually collides with a nearby electron to produce two 511,000-eV γ -rays at $\sim 180^\circ$ apart. Positron-emitting isotopes frequently used include ^{15}O, ^{13}N, ^{11}C, and ^{18}F, the latter being used as a substitute for hydrogen. Gamma-emitting isotopes (e.g., ^{99}mTc, ^{111}In, ^{123}I, ^{131}I) can also be used for imaging living subjects using gamma cameras which, when rotated around the subject (in single photon emission computed tomography, SPECT), can allow production of tomographic images. Positron-emitting isotopes can usually be substituted readily for naturally occurring atoms, and therefore PET is a more robust technique than SPECT for imaging most molecular events. The spatial resolution of most clinical PET scanners is $\sim$6–8 mm^3, but higher-resolution clinical brain scanners have been developed approaching resolutions of $\sim$3 mm^3.

Recently, small animal micro-PET scanners have been developed. These systems typically have a spatial resolution of $\sim$2 mm^3, but the newer generation systems have a resolution of $\sim$1 mm^3 (Price et al., 2001). Development of molecular imaging assays with PET is particularly attractive because of the potential to validate them in cell culture and small animal models prior to using the same reporter probe in clinical PET scanners. The ability to perform translational research from a cell culture setting through preclinical animal models to clinical applications is one of the most unique and powerful features of PET technology.

Magnetic resonance imaging

The principle underlying MRI is that unpaired nuclear spins, called magnetic dipoles (such as hydrogen atoms in water and organic compounds), align themselves when placed in a magnetic field. In an MRI scanner, there is a strong magnet that produces a magnetic field surrounding the subject under investigation. There are also 'coils' within the magnet to produce a gradient in this magnetic field in the X, Y, and Z directions. The magnet also contains a radiofrequency coil that can produce a temporary radiofrequency pulse to change the alignment of the spins. Following the pulse, the magnetic dipoles return to their baseline orientation, which is detected (also by the radiofrequency coil) as a change in electromagnetic flux (radiofrequency waves in the range 1–100 MHz). Dipoles in different physicochemical environments (fat- or hydrocarbon-rich compared to aqueous) will have different relaxation times and, thus, generate different MR signals. The addition of chemical agents that change the MR signal intensity near these abnormalities may also be used to enhance signal differences and to further highlight the abnormality. For instance, paramagnetic metal cations such as chelated gadolinium or dysprosium, or superparamagnetic nanoparticles can be used as targeted or smart probes. MRI has two particular advantages over techniques that involve the use of radionuclides or optical probes: higher spatial resolution that approaches that of microscopy (micrometres rather than several millimetres) and the fact that physiological/molecular and anatomical information can be extracted simultaneously. Micro-MRI is likely to have a substantial influence in molecular pathology, and particularly for developmental biology, in imaging of transgenic animals, and in tracking of cell traffic.

The major disadvantage of MRI is that it is several orders of magnitude less sensitive than radionuclide and optical techniques, which offer higher levels of sensitivity for imaging relatively low levels of reporter probe: as low as 10^{-12} mole/l of radiolabelled substrate for PET, and probably in the femtomolar range for bioluminescence imaging. However, there are ways of increasing the signal-to-noise ratio in micro-MRI when imaging small animals, and thus achieving near microscopic resolution. These include working at relatively high magnetic fields (4.7–14 T), using customized hardware and software, and using much longer acquisition times during imaging.

Another example of the use of magnetic resonance in imaging is magnetic resonance spectroscopy (MRS), in which characteristic imaging spectra, composed of specific resonance frequencies absorbed by a small volume of a sample or tissue, are obtained from the tissue subjected to magnetic resonance. These spectra depend on the molecular composition of the sample or tissue. The most useful nuclei for MRS are hydrogen, phosphorus, sodium, and, to a lesser extent, carbon. Hydrogen MR spectroscopy has a greater signal-to-noise ratio and better spatial resolution than phosphorus spectroscopy. The most interesting MR spectral components in living subjects are those of metabolites and amino acids; for example, choline, creatine, N-acetyl aspartate (NAA), lactate, myoinositol, glutamine and glutamate, lipids, leucine, and alanine. There are increasingly important applications for MRS in molecular imaging. For example, MRS has been used in mice to demonstrate the feasibility of monitoring expression of the cytosine deaminase transgene in tumours (Stegman et al., 1999).

21.9 Concluding remarks

Conventional histopathology is changing rapidly. Technology to explore the ultrastructure of cells and implementation of IHC has improved morphological analysis of cells and tissues. Advanced new techniques in molecular biology that are now being implemented in cancer research will soon result in a comprehensive and holistic understanding of the molecular pathogenesis of malignant disease. Implementation of new molecular markers as biomarkers for diagnosis, screening, and therapy will soon accompany routine techniques used in traditional pathology in our management not just of cancer patients but also those at risk of the disease. In addition to techniques described in this chapter, several other 'post-genomic era' approaches that are likely to find its use in molecular pathology in the near future are described in Chapter 22.

References

Bartlett, J., Mallon, E., and Cooke, T. (2003). The clinical evaluation of HER-2 status: which test to use? *J Pathol*, **199**, 411–7.

Battifora, H. (1986). The multitumor (sausage) tissue block: novel method for immunohistochemical antibody testing. *Lab Invest*, **55**, 244–8.

Camp, R. L., Charette, L. A., and Rimm, D. L. (2000). Validation of tissue microarray technology in breast carcinoma. *Lab Invest*, **80**, 1943–9.

Crnogorac-Jurcevic, T., Efthimiou, E., Neilsen, T., Terris, B., Blaveri, E., Jones, M. et al. (2002). Expression profiling in microdissected adenocarcinomas of the pancreas. *Oncogene*, **21**, 4587–94.

Fend, F., Emmert-Buck, M. R., Chuaqui, R., Cole, K., Lee, J., Liotta, L. A. et al. (1999). Immuno-LCM: laser capture microdissection of immunostained frozen sections for mRNA analysis. *Am J Pathol*, **154**, 61–6.

Frantz, G. D., Pham, T. Q., Peale, F. V., Jr., Hillan, K. J., Ostenstadt, B., Wist, E. et al. (2001). Detection of novel gene expression in paraffin-embedded tissues by isotopic in situ hybridization in tissue microarrays. *J Pathol*, **195**, 87–96.

Gupta, D., Middleton, L. P., Whitaker, M. J., and Abrams, J. (2003). Comparison of fluorescence and chromogenic in situ hybridization for detection of HER-2/neu oncogene in breast cancer. *Am J Clin Pathol*, **119**, 381–7.

Kononen, J., Bubendorf, L., Kallioniemi, A., Barlund, M., Schraml, P., Leighton, S. et al. (1998). Tissue microarrays for high-throughput molecular profiling of tumor specimens. *Nat Med*, **4**, 844–7.

Leethanakul, C., Patel, V., Gillespie, J., Shillitoe, E., Kellman, R. M., Ensley, J. F. et al. (2000). Gene expression profiles in squamous cell carcinomas of the oral cavity: use of laser capture microdissection for the construction and analysis of stage-specific cDNA libraries. *Oral Oncol*, **36**, 474–83.

Mahmood, U., Tung, C. H., Bogdanov, A., Jr., and Weissleder, R. (1999). Near-infrared optical imaging of protease activity for tumor detection. Radiology, **213**, 866–70.

Moch, H., Schraml, P., Bubendorf, L., Mirlacher, M., Kononen, J., Gasser, T. et al. (1999). Identification of prognostic parameters for renal cell carcinoma by cDNA arrays and cell chips. *Verh Dtsch Ges Pathol*, **83**, 225–32.

Ng, T., Squire, A., Hansra, G., Bornancin, F., Prevostel, C., Hanby, A. et al. (1999). Imaging protein kinase Calpha activation in cells. *Science*, **283**, 2085–9.

Nocito, A., Kononen, J., Kallioniemi, O. P., and Sauter, G. (2001). Tissue microarrays (TMAs) for high-throughput molecular pathology research. *Int J Cancer*, **94**, 1–5.

Novelli, M. R., Williamson, J. A., Tomlinson, I. P., Elia, G., Hodgson, S. V., Talbot, I. C. et al. (1996). Polyclonal origin of colonic adenomas in an XO/XY patient with FAP. *Science*, **272**, 1187–90.

Petricoin, E. F., Zoon, K. C., Kohn, E. C., Barrett, J. C., Liotta, L. A., Fend, F. et al. (2002). Clinical proteomics: translating benchside promise into bedside reality. *Nat Rev Drug Discov*, **1**, 683–95.

Poulsom, R., Hanby, A. M., Pignatelli, M., Jeffery, R. E., Longcroft, J. M., Rogers, L. et al. (1993). Expression of gelatinase A and TIMP-2 mRNAs in desmoplastic fibroblasts in both mammary carcinomas and basal cell carcinomas of the skin. *J Clin Pathol*, **46**, 429–36.

Poulsom, R., Longcroft, J. M., Jeffery, R. E., Rogers, L. A., Steel, J. H., Ostenstadt, B. et al. (1998). A robust method for isotopic riboprobe in situ hybridisation to localise mRNAs in routine pathology specimens. *Eur J Histochem*, **42**, 121–32.

Price, P., Mahmood, U., Tung, C. H., Bogdanov, A., Jr., and Weissleder, R. (2001). PET as a potential tool for imaging molecular mechanisms of oncology in man. *Trends Mol Med*, **7**, 442–6.

Richter, J., Wagner, U., Kononen, J., Fijan, A., Bruderer, J., Schmid, U. et al. (2000). High-throughput tissue microarray analysis of cyclin E gene amplification and overexpression in urinary bladder cancer. Am J *Pathol*, **157**, 787–94.

Sjostrom, J., Blomqvist, C., von Boguslawski, K., Bengtsson, N. O., Mjaaland, I., Malmstrom, P. et al. (2002). The predictive value of bcl-2, bax, bcl-xL, bag-1, fas, and fasL for chemotherapy response in advanced breast cancer. *Clin Cancer Res*, **8**, 811–16.

Steel, J. H., Morgan, D. E., and Poulsom, R. (2001). Advantages of in situ hybridisation over direct or indirect in situ reverse transcriptase-polymerase chain reaction for localisation of galanin mRNA expression in rat small intestine and pituitary. *Histochem J*, **33**, 201–11.

Stegman, L. D., Rehemtulla, A., Beattie, B., Kievit, E., Lawrence, T. S., Blasberg, R. G. et al. (1999). Noninvasive quantitation of cytosine deaminase transgene expression in human tumor xenografts with in vivo magnetic resonance spectroscopy. *Proc Natl Acad Sci USA*, **96**, 9821–6.

Weissleder, R. and Mahmood, U. (2001). Molecular imaging. *Radiology*, **219**, 316–33.

Zhu, G., Reynolds, L., Crnogorac-Jurcevic, T., Gillett, C. E., Dublin, E. A., Marshall, J. F. et al. (2003). Combination of microdissection and microarray analysis to identify gene expression changes between differentially located tumour cells in breast cancer. *Oncogene*, **22**, 3742–8.

Further reading

Bancroft, J. D. and Stevens, A. (1999). Theory and Practice of Histological Techniques. Forth Edition, Churchill Livingstone, pp. 1–766.

Polak, J. M. and Van Noorden, S. (1997) Introduction to Immunocytochemistry, Second Edition. BIOS Scientific Publishers, NY, BIOS pp. 1–141.

CHAPTER 22

From transcriptome to proteome

Silvana Debernardi, Rachel A. Craven, Bryan D. Young, and Rosamonde E. Banks

22.1 Introduction

The rapid advance of the Human Genome Project is leading to the identification of the 30,000–35,000 genes that make up our genetic complement. The combination of this sequence information and associated bioinformatic tools together with technological advances in both nucleic acid-based microarray technology and proteomic technologies has opened up the possibility of highly parallel and complementary approaches to investigations of the cancer cell. Currently, microarray technology makes analysis of the 'transcriptome', that is the mRNA species present in the cells, unrivalled in terms of its high-throughput nature and vast numbers of genes which can be examined simultaneously. However, 'proteomics', that is the analysis of the 'proteome' or the proteins expressed in a given tissue or cell type complements such approaches by being able to integrate both genetic and epigenetic effects in terms of the information provided and additionally can provide information about features such as post-translational modifications of proteins which may be important in their function. Thus the two approaches may be regarded very much as complementary, each with its own inherent advantages and limitations, but both with the ability to impact significantly on cancer research. The volume of literature in both areas is now so large that that writing a single chapter encompassing both is a significant challenge and can only be regarded as an introduction to the area. The two approaches in turn are briefly described, explaining the underlying technological options and using selected examples from leukaemias and lymphomas in particular for the RNA analysis and various cancers for the proteomics sections, to illustrate their potential impact.

22.2 The transcriptome

22.2.1 Microarray analysis of cancer

Using microarrays it is now possible to investigate the transcriptional status of virtually every gene in a tissue sample, leading to the concept of the expression profile or signature for a given tissue or tumour type. This approach is yielding highly detailed patterns that are characteristic of the cancer cell. Many aspects of cancer biology, including disease classification, chemosensitivity, and prognosis can now be interpreteted in terms of these expression profiles (Alizadeh et al., 2001). It is important to appreciate that current expression array technology has not yet achieved full coverage of the human genome and therefore in the future we can expect even more detailed and informative maps of the cancer cell to emerge.

Since cancer itself involves the deregulation of gene expression, microarrays are becoming particularly valuable in the characterization of such aberrant disruptions and have already demonstrated that previously unknown disease subtypes can be distinguished by their unique expression profiles. In one of the earliest investigations, Golub et al. (1999) demonstrated that expression profiling could be used to distinguish reliably between acute myeloid leukaemia (AML) and acute lymphocytic leukaemia (ALL). Since then, the expression profiles of many types of human cancer have been investigated, including colon (Notterman et al., 2001; Lin et al., 2002; Zou et al., 2002), brain (MacDonald et al., 2001; Pomeroy et al., 2002), breast (Perou et al., 2000; Hedenfalk et al., 2001; Sorlie et al., 2001; van 't Veer et al., 2002), ovary (Wang et al., 1999; Welsh et al., 2001*b*; Jazaeri et al., 2002), kidney (Takahashi et al., 2001), prostate (Dhanasekaran et al., 2001; Welsh et al., 2001*a*; LaTulippe et al., 2002), and gastric (Hippo et al., 2002). Many of these studies aim to define new classes with prognostic and diagnostic relevance and to increase our knowledge of the mechanisms underlying the biology of these diseases. The pathological diagnosis and classification of human neoplasia is currently based on well-defined morphological, cytochemical, immunophenotypic, and clinical criteria. A molecular classification can take advantage of such prior knowledge but would also have the potential to define new subgroups with greater prognostic and therapeutic significance and could offer many advantages over conventional classification methods.

In addition to their role in cancer classification, microarrays are becoming fundamental to cancer therapeutics and to novel target discovery. At its simplest level, expression profiling when applied to primary cancer tissues may identify genes with previously unsuspected high levels of expression. The protein or the function associated with such high expression levels could then become a novel therapeutic target. Expression profiling can also be used in a direct manner to assess the response of cells to bioactive compounds. Since the mode of action of many compounds is not always apparent, this pharmacogenomic approach is yielding valuable information about their likely modes of action.

22.2.2 Microarray technology

Microarrays for expression profiling are systematic arrays of cDNA or oligonucleotides of known sequence that are spotted or synthesized at discrete loci on a glass or silicon surface. They allow the simultaneous analysis of large numbers of genes at a high resolution following the hybridization of labelled cDNA or cRNA derived from the samples to be examined. The amount of hybridized signal is proportional to the level of gene expression in the original sample. A number of different microarray systems are currently in use, which all use either oligonucleotides (20–30mers or 60mers) or longer gene sequences (approx. 0.2–1 kb). There are two basic types of array technology, the spotted microarrays and the high-density oligonucleotide arrays.

Spotted arrays

This type of array is created by robotically spotting pre-synthesized single-strand or double-strand cDNAs onto glass slides. Genes are represented by single fragments, greater than several hundred base pairs in length. Sequences to be printed are chosen either from databases (GenBank, dbEST, and UniGene), or from full-length cDNA or expressed sequence tag (EST) libraries, and clone collections. They are usually polymerase chain reaction (PCR) amplification products generated using vector-specific primers and printed onto glass slides as spots at defined locations. Spots are about 200 μm in size and about the same distance apart. With this technique, arrays consisting of more than 30,000 cDNAs can be fitted onto the surface of a conventional microscope slide. Because of potential variability in the amount of sequence spotted, cDNA microarrays are always hybridized with a mixture of two differently labelled cDNAs generated from two different RNA sources, one of which acts as a control. In general, it is advantageous to use a control RNA sample that is related to the experimental sample. The ratio between the signal intensities in the two scanning channels (red : green) is a reliable measure of the relative amount of specific mRNAs in each sample.

Target labelling with different fluorescent dyes (Cy3 and Cy5) can result in different efficiency of incorporation, and it is therefore advised to perform reciprocal labelling of the same sample with both dyes. In addition, replicate samples from independent experiments should be used as control for experimental variation. This results in four hybridizations (two replicate samples, two replicate hybridizations with reciprocal labelling) performed for each experimental point and therefore requires four chips to be used. In the case of tumour samples, where material can be limiting, the number of tumours chosen for the study should be high enough to allow statistically significant conclusions.

Oligonucleotide arrays

This type of array, pioneered by Affymetrix, consists of sets of oligomers synthesized *in situ* on glass wafers using a photolithographic process. Synthetic linkers modified with photochemically removable protecting groups, are attached to a glass surface. Light is directed through a mask to deprotect and activate selected sites, and protected nucleotides are coupled to the activated sites. Photolithography allows the construction of arrays with high information content, with about 500,000 probe locations or features, within 1.28 cm^2. Each single square feature harbours millions of identical oligonucleotides and a single 1.28 cm^2 array contains a probe set for approximately 40,000 human genes and ESTs. Genes are represented by 10–20 different 25-mer oligonucleotides, chosen most often from the 3′ end of the transcript and designed to uniquely represent the gene. For each oligonucleotide designed with a perfect match to a transcript, there is an identical one except for a base mismatch at the central position. The presence of a mismatch allows cross-hybridization and local background to be estimated and subtracted from the matched signal. A software algorithm is used to integrate the oligonucleotide signals into a single signal for the region of each gene. The current chip, U133A, produces signals from approximately 22,000 regions. A significant difference between this type of array and cDNA arrays is that a control RNA sample is not necessary, simplifying the probe preparations and hybridizations.

RNA preparation

The isolation of good quality RNA from the cells under investigation is critical to achieving success in expression profiling. The minimum amount for an oligonucleotide array profiling is approximately 5 μg, while considerably more is required for spotted cDNA arrays. Consideration must also be given to the clonal purity of the sample under investigation. Some cancers are available in an almost pure state, with very few contaminating normal cells, for example, high white cell count leukaemias or surgically removed clonal tumours such as retinoblastoma. In many cases, however, there will be a level of contamination with non-malignant cells. In such a sample it is possible that a 'virtual dissection' could be performed in the computer by clustering and identifying those gene groups whose expression can be attributed to normal 'host' cells, taking advantage of the patterns of expression of the subset of genes that are cell type-specific (Alizadeh et al., 2001). A second approach involves the isolation of tumour cells by laser capture microdissection (LCM). This technique can procure pure population of cells from specific microscopic regions of tissue sections, in one step, under direct visualization. No degradation is observed but the quality of the RNA depends on the procedures used to harvest and preserve the original tissue. Immediate cryopreservation and cryosectioning of the specimens is the standard for high-quality preservation. Since the yield of RNA is low from such procedures, some form of amplification is required before expression profiling can be considered.

Data analysis strategies

Data produced by a microarray assay consist of a list of genes and corresponding values that represent relative RNA transcript levels. All this information must be analysed by data-mining techniques to correlate and group the data in a meaningful manner and to generate hypotheses on possible cellular pathways, gene functions, and drug targets. This is a very active area of research (Slonim, 2002) the details of which are beyond the scope of this chapter. Three basic steps for an efficient and effective data analysis are necessary: data normalization, data filtering, and pattern identification. To compare expression values directly, it is necessary to apply some sort of normalization strategy to the data, either between paired samples or across a set of experiments. To 'normalize' in the context of expression profiles means to standardize the data to be able to differentiate between real (biological) variations in gene expression levels and variations due to the measurement process (Quackenbush, 2002). Gene expression data can be then subjected to a variation filter, which excludes uninformative genes, that is, genes showing minimal variation across the samples, and genes expressed below or above a user-defined threshold. This step facilitates the search for partners and groups in the data that can be used to assign biological meaning to the expression profiles, leading to the production of straightforward lists of increasing or decreasing genes or of more complex associations with the help of sophisticated clustering and visualization programs. Hierarchical clustering, traditionally used in phylogenetic analysis for the classification of organisms into trees, in the microarray context is applied to genes and samples. The length of a branch containing two organisms can be considered as a measure of how different the organisms are. It is possible to classify genes and experiments in a similar manner, clustering those whose expression patterns are similar into nearby places in a tree. Such mock-phylogenetic trees are often referred to as dendrograms. If the data entered into the clustering is unselected this analysis is usually referred to as 'unsupervised'. An unsupervised hierarchical analysis is often the first form of analysis and is used to establish in an unbiased manner the relationships in a dataset. Complex datasets are often difficult to visualize and therefore mathematical techniques of data reduction such as principal component analysis or multidimensional scaling can be used to reduce and display the data in an easily visualized manner.

22.2.3 Cancer classification by expression profiling

Although genome-wide expression profiling is being applied to many types of cancer, it has had the greatest impact in the study of haematological malignancies (Staudt, 2003). These cancers are particularly well-suited to this approach since a great deal of phenotypic, morphological, and clinical information already exists for leukaemias and lymphomas. Through national trials, the link between clinical outcome and certain pathological features such as cytogenetics has been well established. Furthermore, the availability of relatively pure populations of cells cryopreserved as part of such trials means that retrospective analysis to link expression profiles to a whole variety of clinical features can be performed.

Lymphoma

Expression profiling has been particularly informative in the study of diffuse large-B-cell lymphomas (DLBCLs) which are the most common lymphomas in adults (Lossos and Levy, 2003). The fact that only 40% of patients can be cured, has been taken to suggest that this type of lymphoma actually consists of heterogeneous subtypes with differing responsiveness to chemotherapy. Attempts in the past to define new subgroups on the basis of morphology have failed, largely due to variations in diagnostic reproducibility. Recently, several studies have shown that expression profiling can be used to discern subgroups within DLBCL and furthermore can yield important prognostic information (Alizadeh et al., 2000; Rosenwald et al., 2002; Shipp et al., 2002).

In one of the earliest attempts to profile this disease a chip was specifically created to contain genes of relevance to lymphocyte biology, known as the 'Lymphochip' (Alizadeh et al., 2000). Since the germinal centre B cell is thought to be the origin of DLBCL it was therefore used as a source of cDNA clones. Also, libraries derived from DLBCL, follicular lymphoma, mantle cell lymphoma, and chronic lymphocytic leukaemia (CLL) were used to supply further clones. Finally, genes important in B- and T-cell activation and general cancer cell biology were included. In this way the chip was biased in advance towards questions related to lymphoma biology. In this study, the expression profiles from 96 normal and malignant lymphocyte samples, including DLBCL, CLL, follicular lymphoma (FL), and normal resting and activated B cells were examined. It was evident using unsupervised cluster analysis, that the tumour samples clustered into three separate groups each representing the three main tumour types. Furthermore, the CLL and FL groups were clustered next to resting B-cell samples, reflecting the low proliferation rate of these disease types. Another feature of this study was the identification of clusters of coordinately regulated genes, referred to as signatures, associated with particular biological functions. For example, signatures for germinal centre B cells, for proliferation and for activated B cells were identified. Using such signatures it was possible to show that DLBCL appeared to consist of two predominant types, 'germinal centre B-like DLBCL' and 'activated

B-like'. Significantly, patients with the former type of DLBCL had a better overall survival than those with the latter.

Recently, a follow-up study of a larger number (240) of DLBCL samples demonstrated that a third class of this disease could be discerned (Rosenwald et al., 2002). This 'type 3' class of DLBCL did not express high levels of the genes from the activated B-like or the germinal centre-like signatures. Indeed, the heterogeneity of expression within this third subgroup indicated that it might consist of more than one type of diffuse large B-cell lymphoma. Interestingly, two genetic events common in diffuse large B-cell lymphoma, the t(14;18) chromosome translocation which activates the *BCL2* gene and the *REL* amplification, occur exclusively in the germinal centre B-cell like group of DLBCL. This reinforces the view that the subgroups identified by expression profiling probably arise from distinct forms of malignant transformation. The variability in patient survival following chemotherapy suggests that expression profiling could have an important role in stratifying patients. By searching for genes with expression patterns that are correlated with survival it was possible to construct a predictor set of 17 genes. It thus appears that a relatively small number of genes is necessary for outcome prediction in DLBCL, although such models will require to be tested on larger numbers of patients.

In the above studies, certain *a priori* assumptions were made concerning lymphoma biology which dictated the choice of clones to be arrayed. However, as arrays increase in their coverage it is becoming less important to have prior biological insight into the disease. For example, another study used an unbiased array to acquire expression profiles and used supervised learning methods to derive an outcome model that is independent of previous assumptions (Shipp et al., 2002). Expression profiles for 6817 genes in 58 DLBCL biopsies were compared with the profiles obtained from 19 biopsies of FLs. FLs are related to DLBCLs and can evolve over time to display similar morphological features, although they have different natural histories and therapeutic responses. Also a proportion of DLBCLs have the t(14;18) translocation which is typical of FLs. It was therefore of interest to determine whether these two classes of lymphomas could be reliably discriminated using the profiles of what is now a relatively small number of genes. A weighted voting algorithm designed to calculate the weighted combination of informative genes was used to distinguish DLBCL from FL. When such a model is trained and evaluated with the same samples, there is a statistical problem of overestimating the prediction accuracy. This problem can be addressed by the 'leave one out' cross-validation method in which one sample is withheld and the remainder used to train a gene expression model which is used to predict the class of the withheld sample. The entire process is repeated until all samples have been predicted. In this study, 91% of the tumours were correctly predicted as DLBCL or FL using a 30 gene model.

A similar approach was adopted to determine if the expression profiles could successfully predict patient outcome within the DLBCL group of patients. The patients were divided into two classes; those cured of their disease and those with fatal or refractory disease, and the weighted voting algorithm with cross-validation testing was applied. A model consisting of only 13 genes was found to have the highest accuracy and thus confirmed that at diagnosis a gene expression signature predictive for patient outcome does exist.

The transformation of FL to a more aggressive DLBCL has been examined by expression profiles (Lossos et al., 2002). When the gene expression profiles of transformed DLBCL and their previous FL were compared, no genes were observed to increase or decrease their expression in all of the cases of histological transformation. However, two different gene-expression profiles associated with the transformation process were defined, one in which *MYC* and genes regulated by *MYC* showed increased expression and one in which these same genes showed decreased expression. Furthermore, there was a striking difference in gene-expression profiles between transformed DLBCL and *de novo* DLBCL, because the gene-expression profile of transformed DLBCL was more similar to their antecedent FL than to *de novo* DLBCL. This study demonstrates that transformation from FL to DLBCL can occur by alternative pathways and that transformed DLBCL and *de novo* DLBCL have very different gene-expression profiles that may underlie the different clinical behaviours of these two types of morphologically similar lymphomas.

Chronic lymphocytic leukaemia

The CLL is the commonest leukaemia in humans and has a generally indolent clinical course. The molecular mechanisms underlying this disease have yet to be fully established. The presence of somatic mutations in the immunoglobulin genes appears to define a subgroup of this disease which evolves only slowly and requires little clinical intervention (Hamblin et al., 1999). By contrast, the absence of such mutations appears to define the subgroup that has a more progressive clinical course requiring earlier clinical intervention. There were, therefore, *a priori* reasons to suppose that expression profiling could be used to distinguish such subgroups. However, gene-expression profiling has shown that CLL cells express a common gene-expression signature which differentiates this disease from other lymphoid malignancies and from normal lymphoid subpopulations (Klein et al., 2001, Rosenwald et al., 2001). It was possible to identify approximately 160 genes whose levels of expression were significantly different between the two subtypes. The most discriminating gene was identified as *ZAP-70*. It may therefore be possible to use *ZAP-70* as a surrogate marker for the presence of immunoglobulin gene mutations in the future analysis of CLL (Crespo et al., 2003).

Acute leukaemias

Acute leukaemias of both the myeloid and lymphoid lineages are particularly characterized by the presence of chromosome translocations. Most of the frequently occurring translocations have been molecularly cloned and the resultant gene fusions identified. It is apparent that many of the genes disrupted by this class of event have the hallmarks of transcriptional regulators and by implication, the resultant clonal expansion of cells could have distinct expression profiles. It is also known that there is a strong link between the karyotype of the leukaemia cell and the prognosis of the disease in the patient. For example, in adult AMLs, patients with leukaemias bearing the translocations t(8;21), t(15;17), or the inv(16) belong to better risk subgroup (Grimwade et al., 1998). Similarly, AML with a normal karyotype or translocations affecting 11q23 belong to the intermediate risk group and those with complex karyotypes or −5 or −7 belong to the worst risk group. Childhood and infant ALLs with the t(9;22) or 11q23 rearrangements are known to belong to the poor risk group (Pui et al., 1991).

An extensive study by Yeoh et al. (2002) determined the expression profiles of the leukaemic blast cells from 360 paediatric ALL patients. Unsupervised hierarchical cluster analysis was used to demonstrate that the major translocations that create the E2A-PBX1, BCR-ABL, TEL-AML1 fusions, and the *MLL* gene rearrangements result in distinctive expression profiles. Furthermore, both hyperdiploidy (>50 chromosomes) and T-cell ALL also had distinctive profiles. It was therefore possible to find groups of genes with a significant level of expression associated with each cytogenetic group. An important conclusion from this study was that the profiles did not appear to represent a specific differentiation stage of the leukaemic blasts. For example, the E2A-PBX1 translocation is strongly associated with ALLs of the pre-B-cell immunophenotype. However, the expression profile appears to be specific for the E2A-PBX1 lesion and not the pre-B immunophenotype. In fact, in this study it was not possible to define expression profiles specific for the different immunophenotypically defined stages of B-cell differentiation. This contrasts with the findings for DLBCLs discussed above.

This study also identified a novel subgroup of ALL which was defined by the high expression of a group of genes which included *LHFPL2*, a member of the LHFP-like gene family. Significantly, the *LHFP* gene has been found to be fused to the *HMGIC* gene in a case of lipoma (Petit et al., 1999) and it could be speculated that the upregulation seen is due to unsuspected chromosomal translocation. In addition to uncovering previously unsuspected genetic events, this study also illustrated that some leukaemias could have been misclassified using conventional means. For example, four cases of ALLs were classified by expression profiling as belonging to the TEL-AML1 subgroup although they had appeared to lack the fusion transcript in a previous analysis. However, on closer examination one case was found to have the TEL-AML1 fusion by Fluorescence *in situ* hybridization (FISH), while the other three had translocations affecting 12p, the location of the *TEL* gene. Expression profiling may thus prove more effective in defining the underlying genetic abnormalities than conventional methods. A further interesting observation was that there appears to exist a distinct TEL-AML1 subtype, characterized by 20 genes, which could predict those individuals who would ultimately progress towards a secondary AML. These findings suggest that some individuals with ALL have a genetic predisposition to develop secondary AML.

It has become clear that AMLs also have highly distinct expression profiles which are strongly linked to the karyotype (Virtaneva et al., 2001; Armstrong et al., 2002; Schoch et al., 2002; Debernardi et al., 2003). The major recurrent chromosomal abnormalities in AML are the t(8;21), t(15;17), inv(16), and 11q23 rearrangements and each of these have been associated with a distinctive expression profile. Approximately 20–40% of AMLs have a normal karyotype and have been shown to have a distinctive upregulation of certain members of the class I homeobox A and B gene families (Debernardi et al., 2003). This finding suggests that this subgroup is not just a product of failed cytogenetics and moreover, that they may have a common underlying genetic lesion. It is well established that cytogenetics is an important predictor of risk in AML (Grimwade et al., 1998) with t(8;21), t(15;17), and inv(16) signifying a good risk while 11q23 and a normal karyotype indicate intermediate risk. An example of how 28 leukaemias could be segregated into these two risk groups using expression profiling is shown in Figure 22.1. It can be seen that a relatively small number of genes are required to place a leukaemia into either the low-risk or the intermediate groups. It has been shown that only 145 genes are required to segregate AMLs into their major recurrent cytogenetic classes (Debernardi et al., 2003).

It thus appears that for both ALL and AML the major determinants for the expression profiles are the karyotypic abnormalities, particularly recurrent chromosomal translocations. In this form of cancer, at least, cellular phenotype seems to have a lesser role in determining the profiles. The ability to determine the karyotype solely from the expression profile would offer many advantages and could in the future become the standard diagnostic approach for this disease.

22.2.4 Tumour origin and evolution by expression profiling

The diagnosis of cancer at an early stage in its development is a priority for modern cancer medicine since it generally leads to a better clinical outcome. However, even with early diagnosis there will be individuals in whom the disease recurs and

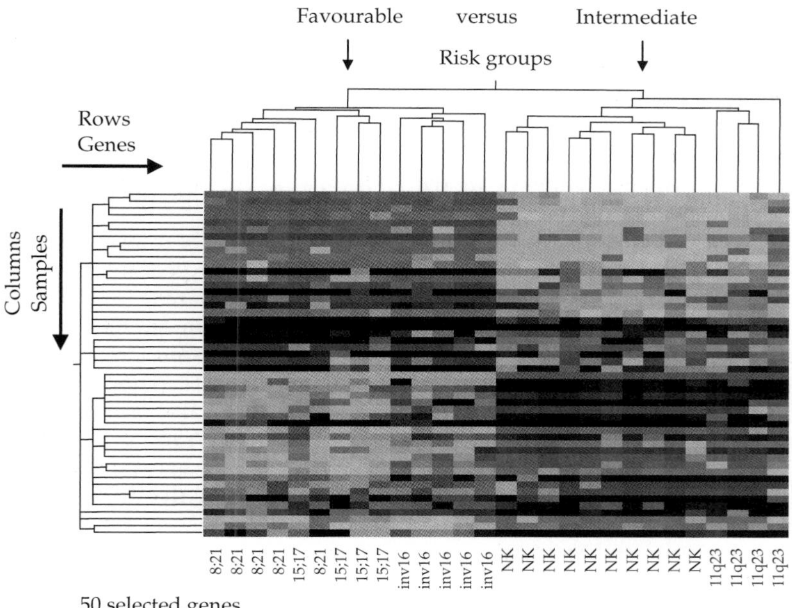

Figure 22.1 Cytogenetic risk groups in AML: favourable versus intermediate risk groups hierarchical cluster of the 50 genes selected to be the more predictive in the two class comparison performed. Each column represents a sample, and each row represents a single gene. Expression levels are normalized for each gene, where the mean is 1. Expression levels greater than the mean are shown in red and levels less than the mean are in green (see also plate 5).

evolves into a metastatic form. It is therefore a priority to investigate whether expression profiling could identify markers indicative of the likelihood that a tumour will further evolve.

To investigate this issue in breast cancer, a cohort of patients with tumours smaller than 5 cm and who had no lymph-node metastasis and were aged under 55 years were investigated by expression profiling (van 't Veer et al., 2002). This group of patients did not receive additional treatment and were followed for at least five years. The patients were separated into two groups: those who developed metastasis at less than five years and those who were free of metastasis for more than five years. A supervised analysis was performed on the expression profiles of primary tumours from these patients. A total of 231 genes that correlated with this parameter were identified and by further analysis a discriminatory set of 70 genes was identified, which showed 81% accuracy when tested in a leave-one-out cross validation analysis of the training set. This study indicates that expression profiling can be used to derive valuable clinical information from the primary tumour, which can influence clinical strategies. Another study has used expression profiling to discriminate between medulloblastomas with and without metastasis (MacDonald et al., 2001). In a similar manner, the genes identified correctly predicted metastasis status in 72% of the tumours using a leave-one-out cross validation approach. This study implicated the platelet-derived growth factor receptor (PDGFR) and the RAS/MAPK pathways in the development of metastasis.

These studies demonstrate that there are features in the expression profiles of primary tumours that can be used to predict the course of the disease. This implies that properties such as the likelihood of metastasis developing could be diagnosed from an analysis of the primary tumour and this may form the basis for clinical treatment decisions.

As well as predicting likely tumour evolution, expression profiling also has a role in the determination of the tissue of origin for tumours which are not well characterized. Several genome-wide expression profiling studies have been reported which attempt to define tumour- and tissue-specific profiles. Ramaswamy et al. (2001) performed expression profiling of 140 tumours representing 14 common tumour types. A step-by step-analysis was performed in order to define a set of genes identifying each of the 14 tissues separately. When a new sample was analysed its profile was compared with that of each of these 14 profiles and was assigned to the class it most resembled. In this analysis, six of eight metastasis samples were classified correctly. It was notable that samples that were not correctly classified were described histologically as poorly differentiated adenocarcinomas. This could be interpreted to suggest that poorly differentiated carcinomas represent a distinct class rather than being related to a differentiated class but with reduced expression of genes. In another study (Su et al., 2001) expression profiling for 10 tumour types was performed and demonstrated 75% accuracy on metastasis sample predictions. In both of these studies, site of origin of metastatic samples could be predicted, suggesting that expression profiling may have an important application in classifying tumours of an unknown origin.

It is becoming apparent that tumours which arise from germline mutations may have a different expression profile from their sporadic counterparts. For example, women who have a germline mutation in the *BRCA1* gene frequently develop breast and/or ovarian cancer. Such tumours have been shown to have distinct expression profiles (Hedenfalk et al., 2001; Jazaeri et al., 2002). Interestingly, some examples of sporadic breast cancer have been identified which have a *BRCA1* mutant profile and were subsequently shown to have a methylated *BRCA1* promoter (Hedenfalk et al., 2001).

22.2.5 Cancer therapeutics

Many aspects of cancer therapeutics are being influenced by expression profiling (Gerhold et al., 2002). By examining a series of carefully characterized tumour profiles it may be possible to identify genes with significant upregulation in that tumour type. This approach has been used to identify potential pharmacological targets in prostate cancer (Welsh et al., 2001*a*). In addition to suggesting new targets, expression profiling can also be used to dissect the response to anticancer drugs already in use. STI571 (Gleevec) is a tyrosine kinase inhibitor of the ABL protein and is highly effective against chronic myeloid leukaemias (CMLs). For reasons that are not understood, it is much less effective against a related form of Leukaemia Ph + ALL. Expression profiles obtained from 19 pretreatment Ph + ALL samples were obtained and were analysed in relation to the patients' response to STI571 (Hofmann et al., 2002). A set of 95 genes were identified whose expression could be used reliably to predict sensitivity to STI571. Thus, pretreatment profiling of Ph + ALL would have considerable clinical value and may be an approach which could be extended to the use of other signal transduction modifying drugs.

Expression profiling can be of particular value where the agent being investigated is known to affect gene expression directly. Trichostatin (TSA) is an inhibitor of histone deacetylases and thus alters gene expression by modification of chromatin structures. Rapid cellular responses to TSA have been mapped using expression profiling (Chambers et al., 2003). As well as single compound studies, the integration of the cellular responses to many pharmacological agents across a wide panel of cell lines can now be considered. NCI60 is a panel of 60 human cell lines used by the National Cancer Institute Development Therapeutics Program to screen anticancer agents (Weinstein et al., 1997). There have been several studies which sought to link the known susceptibility of the NCI60 panel to a variety of compounds with the expression profiles of the untreated cell lines (Butte et al., 2000; Scherf et al., 2000). An algorithm for the prediction of the chemosensitivity of cell lines has been developed and showed that at least for a subset of compounds this approach was feasible (Staunton et al., 2001). Recently, the drug-induced expression profiles in human neuronal cells have been used to generate a predictor of drug efficacy (Gunther et al., 2003). We can anticipate that linking pre-therapy profiles to known drug-induced profiles could eventually lead to individualized therapeutic strategies.

22.3 Proteomics

Gene-expression profiling at the mRNA level can now be realistically complemented with analysis of the proteome, that is the protein complement expressed by a cell type or tissue. By definition, the proteome is a dynamic entity that reflects both genetic and epigenetic influences (Wilkins et al., 1996). Although protein-based studies cannot currently match the scale, sensitivity and throughput of mRNA analysis, there are a number of fundamental advantages of studies at the protein level (Banks et al., 2000). There is not always good correlation between the levels of mRNA and protein present in the cell (Anderson and Seilhamer, 1997) due, for example, to regulation of gene expression at the translational level or effects on protein stability such as rapid turnover produced by selective ubiquitination of proteins leading to their degradation by the proteasome. Therefore, biomarkers identified at the protein level will not necessarily mirror those at the mRNA level. In addition, multiple protein forms can be generated from expression of a single gene. Studies at the protein level can yield data regarding protein isoforms resulting from alternative splicing, which is not necessarily available from mRNA-based analysis. Furthermore, the proteome has an additional level of complexity in the form of post-translational modifications such as glycosylation and phosphorylation that is obviously not apparent at the mRNA level. Potentially, therefore, the proteome contains a wealth of biomarkers that would not be revealed by analysis of the transcriptome. In the clinical setting, particular utilities of proteins include their use as biomarkers in biological fluids or as drug targets for therapeutic intervention. Development and application of a number of technologies to study the proteome, collectively referred to as proteomics, that are capable of global analysis of proteins in biological samples, has therefore been the subject of intensive study.

Proteomic-based approaches fall into two major classes: expression proteomics and cell map or functional proteomics (Blackstock and Weir, 1999). Expression proteomics is largely concerned with differential analysis, which includes comparisons aimed at the discovery of novel biomarkers, but also encompasses descriptive studies cataloguing the complement of proteins expressed by a cell or tissue or present in a biological fluid. Marker identification employs techniques that can be used in comparative analyses of population groups to identify markers for diagnostic and prognostic use, and to discover potential therapeutic targets and markers for tailoring treatment. Generally, such approaches need to have the sensitivity to permit profiling of large numbers of proteins but as they are preliminary screens they do not necessarily need to be high-throughput. This is distinct from the requirements for downstream validation of potential markers/targets, which necessitates the analysis of large numbers of samples. Cell map or functional proteomics on the other hand considers aspects of protein function. These studies include mapping physical interactions with other proteins and protein complexes and roles played in cellular pathways as well as protein localization. Studies on an enormous scale are required to assimilate this information and a number of systematic analyses have been reported that begin to address these issues, both in model systems such as the budding yeast *Sacharomyces cerevisiae* and in higher eukaryotes (Gavin et al., 2002; Ho et al., 2002).

22.3.1 Samples for analysis—cell lines, tissues, and biological fluids

Tissue samples are a powerful resource and have been used extensively for the identification of cancer-associated biomarkers and targets. A large number of studies have analysed whole tissue extracts. However, because of problems associated with tissue heterogeneity, measures have also been taken to enrich relevant minority cell type(s) or areas of particular pathology from whole tissue prior to analysis. This has been achieved in a number of ways including positive or negative selections using antibodies (Reymond et al., 1997; Sarto et al., 1997; Page et al., 1999), physical purification of relevant cell types (Franzén et al., 1995), or if relatively small amounts of material are required for analysis, laser-assisted microdissection techniques such as laser capture microdissection (LCM) (Craven and Banks, 2001).

Biological fluids have also been analysed as they potentially contain proteins shed or secreted from tumours; ultimately such molecules can be used as the basis for powerful non-invasive screening tools. When analysing biological fluids, an important consideration is the large dynamic range of protein expression ($>10^{10}$ in plasma (Anderson and Anderson, 2002)), which represents a significant challenge and may necessitate fractionation of samples prior to analysis. A number of protocols have been developed for the removal of abundant serum proteins such as albumin and immunoglobulins to facilitate investigation of significantly lower abundance molecules (Pieper et al., 2003; Wang et al., 2003).

In studies using patient material, sample collection and storage must be standardized to ensure consistency and must be sufficiently rapid to minimize protein degradation and maintain sample integrity. The choice of sample groups for comparative analyses must also be considered. Criteria must be defined to identify control samples such as matched normal tissue(s) or biological fluids from controls or patients with benign disease or to select patients with good or poor prognosis. The size of groups for comparative analysis is also important as it must account for disease heterogeneity.

Many studies elect to use primary or established cell lines in the study of cancer biology. The growth of enriched cell populations in culture overcomes problems such as tissue heterogeneity and serum contamination that can arise when analysing whole tissue. Furthermore, cell lines are obviously irreplaceable in studies analysing human cell behaviour, for example, in studies investigating mechanisms of drug action and resistance to chemotherapy. However, the issue of *in vitro* culture artefacts should always be taken into account and appropriate validation used. For example, RAGE-1 mRNA is expressed in a high percentage of established renal cancer cell lines but is detected much less frequently in renal tumour samples (Gaugler et al., 1996; Neumann et al., 1998). Similarly, a comparison of fresh, low-grade bladder transitional cell carcinoma (TCC) tissue with short-term cultures showed protein profiles to be generally similar but a significant number of differences in protein expression were noted (Celis et al., 1999).

22.3.2 Proteomic-based approaches

Several technical approaches have been (and continue to be) developed for the global analysis of protein expression and these will be discussed below. In each case a small number of specific, and where possible cancer-related, examples are given to illustrate their potential.

Two-dimensional polyacrylamide gel electrophoresis

Two-dimensional polyacrylamide gel electrophoresis (2D-PAGE) remains the central protein separation tool in proteomic analysis, separating proteins sequentially on the basis of two independent characteristics. In the first dimension, isoelectric focussing separates proteins on the basis of their charge, usually using an immobilized pH gradient (IPG) strip. On application of a current, proteins migrate in the pH gradient until they reach the point at which they have no net charge (their isoelectric point or pI), giving a discrete band for each protein species. This step is then followed by SDS-PAGE, in which proteins are separated on the basis of their molecular weight. Protein detection following 2D-PAGE is usually achieved by silver staining, although alternatives such as Coomassie staining and, more recently, fluorescent stains such as Sypro Ruby can also be employed. Alternatively, metabolic labelling of cells or tissue samples prior to protein extraction allows detection by autoradiography. Using this technology, up to 2000 proteins can be visualized in a single standard format gel and many isoforms of proteins can be resolved. The technique is reproducible, allowing direct comparison of the profiles of a series of samples. Quantitative or semi-quantitative analysis of the data is then possible. In most cases this involves comparison of a series of 2D-gel images to look for reproducible differences in protein expression between two or more sample classes. This process generally employs sophisticated gel analysis software to select candidate biomarkers that can then be identified and validated on a larger sample set (Banks et al., 2000).

Identification of proteins of interest is generally achieved by mass spectrometry. Proteins are digested with an enzyme, usually trypsin, and the masses of the resulting peptides are determined by mass spectrometry. The peptide masses, which together constitute a peptide mass fingerprint characteristic for a particular protein, can be compared with a theoretical digest of proteins in a database to identify the protein of interest. Alternatively, tandem MS–MS approaches can be used, where collision-induced fragmentation spectra of particular peptides can be interpreted to give information on the peptide sequence (Aebersold and Mann, 2003).

The approach of 2D-PAGE and mass spectrometry has been applied in a number of cancer-related research projects. These include differential expression profiling studies which compare normal and tumour samples (whole tissue extracts, LCM-procured samples, biological fluids, and cell lines) with the aim of identifying novel biomarkers as well as studies using cell lines to investigate cell behaviour, for example, alterations in response to drug treatment.

In a study looking for biomarkers for renal cell carcinoma (RCC), comparative analysis of whole tissue extracts of patient matched normal kidney cortex and RCC tissues by 2D-PAGE, Unwin et al. (2003*a*) identified 32 proteins whose expression was significantly higher in tumour samples (Figure 22.2) and 41 proteins whose level decreased. The upregulated proteins included a number of glycolytic enzymes reflecting the Warburg effect; Mn-superoxide dismutase, annexins I, II, and IV, and the angiogenic factor thymidine phosphorylase/platelet-derived endothelial cell growth factor (TP/PD-ECGF). Expression of TP by tumour cells was confirmed by LCM combined with western blotting and by immunohistochemistry (Unwin et al., 2003*b*), confirming other studies.

The studies of TCC and squamous cell carcinoma (SCC) of the bladder carried out by Celis and coworkers are two of the most systematic and comprehensive analyses carried out to date (Celis et al., 1999*b*). In their work on SCC, often using ^{35}S-metabolic labelling of fresh tissue samples, a number of differentially expressed proteins were identified including several keratins, PA-FABP, galectin 7, stratifin, and psoriasin (Ostergaard et al., 1997). By probing serial sections of bladder tissue with antibodies to some of these molecules, a process the authors termed 'immunowalking', clear changes associated with carcinogenesis were readily visualized (Celis et al., 1999*a*). Analysis of urine samples identified psoriasin as a putative urinary marker for SCC (Ostergaard et al., 1999).

Serum samples have also been analysed by 2D-PAGE. Sera from breast cancer patients and controls were analysed by 2D-PAGE following removal of albumin and IgG by affinity chromatography (Rui et al., 2003). Hsp27 and 14–3-3σ were found at higher levels in cancer patients and normal sera, respectively. Used in combination to analyse a masked set of sera, these biomarkers could discriminate all 69 cancer patient samples and 34 of 35 control samples.

Analysis of 2D-gels can be time-consuming and represents a rate-limiting step in 2D-PAGE based approaches. This problem has been circumvented, at least in part, by introduction of an alternative approach, 2D-differential gel electrophoresis (2D-DIGE) (Tonge et al., 2001). Samples to be compared are labelled with spectrally resolvable fluorescent dyes and electrophoresed on a single gel, allowing comparison of two samples without any need for gel matching. Although not yet used extensively due to cost and limited availability of the technology, successful examples illustrating its potential include comparison of an immortalized luminal epithelial cell line with a derivative over-expressing ERBB2 as a model for studying ERBB2-mediated transformation in breast cancer (Gharbi et al., 2002).

Although 2D-PAGE has been used in a large number of comparative analyses that have successfully detected alterations in gene expression,

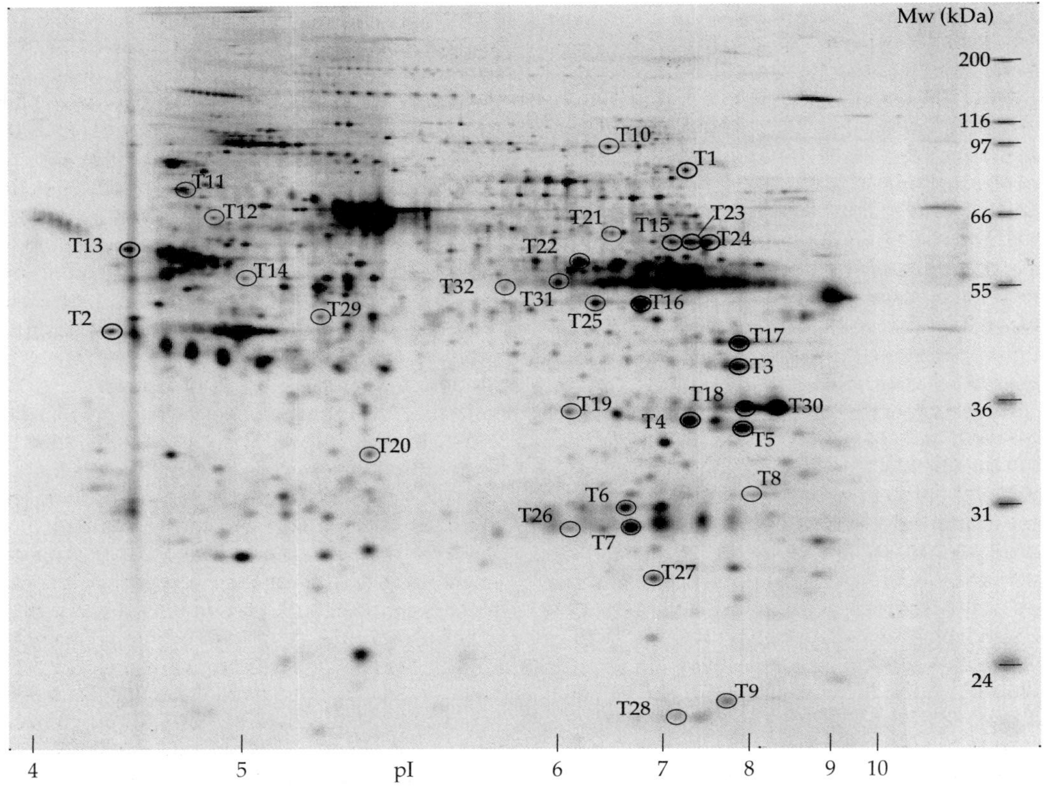

Figure 22.2 Example of a silver-stained analytical 2D-gel (pH 3–10 NL) containing 30 μg human RCC tissue showing locations of 32 protein spots which are present in significantly higher amounts in RCC tissue when compared with normal kidney cortex. Reproduced from Unwin et al. (2003*a*) with permission from Wiley VCH.

the nature of the proteins identified clearly shows that the approach is naturally biased towards the most abundant proteins present in a sample. This is partly due to the fact that the studies published to date have adopted the simplest protocol, analysing whole cell or tissue lysates using broad-range pH gradients (pH 3–10 and pH 4–7). Two distinct strategies can be used to allow the study of less abundant molecules. First, the complexity of the sample can be simplified prior to analysis. This can be achieved by fractionating total cell lysates, for example, on the basis of affinity chromatography or by using more complex protein extraction protocols such as differential detergent extraction, subcellular fractionation, or purification of particular protein complexes. Second, samples can be analysed using zoom gels with increasingly narrow pH gradients for isoelectric focussing. Narrow range pH unit IPG strips have been developed for both the acidic and basic pH ranges, allowing increased resolution of proteins (Hoving et al. 2000; Wildgruber et al., 2000). Free-flow isoelectric focussing can be incorporated to prefractionate samples prior to 2D-PAGE, improving the quality of the separation and efficiency of sample use (Zuo and Speicher, 2002). With these strategies there is the potential to considerably increase the proportion of the proteome studied, although this obviously necessitates the use of large amounts of sample. Limitations of the technology should also be considered, with problems being encountered for the profiling of specific classes of proteins such as membrane proteins and proteins at the extremes of pI and molecular weight. It is likely that many of these problems will be overcome with continued technological advances such as the use of specialized detergents for solubilizing membrane proteins (Luche et al., 2003).

Mass spectrometry

A number of studies have explored the use of mass spectrometry in combination with alternative protein and peptide separation strategies to overcome some of the limitations of 2D-PAGE (Aebersold and Mann, 2003). Free–flow electrophoresis, a liquid-based isoelectric focussing strategy, was used to resolve a cytosolic extract of the colorectal carcinoma cell line LIM1215 into 96 fractions which were each separated by SDS-PAGE. Bands were then excised, digested with trypsin, and analysed by mass spectrometry (Hoffmann et al., 2001). In a parallel study, sub-cellular fractionation was used to prepare a membrane-enriched fraction, which was separated by SDS-PAGE. A total of 284 proteins were identified including 92 membrane proteins (Simpson et al., 2000). In a similar approach, peptides can be separated by multidimensional liquid chromatography and analysed by mass spectrometry (MUDPIT). This strategy has allowed hundreds of proteins to be identified in whole cell lysates including low-abundance proteins and multi-spanning membrane proteins (Washburn et al., 2001).

Although these mass spectrometry-based approaches can be used to develop comprehensive descriptions of proteins present in a particular sample, as mass spectrometry is not quantitative, they are largely descriptive. The presence of a peak in only one sample class can theoretically be used to identify differences between samples. For example, such a strategy was successfully used on plasma membrane enriched fractions from breast cancer cell lines to identify novel proteins with cancer-specific membrane associations that were confirmed by downstream analysis (Adam et al., 2003). The use of stable isotope labelling, as illustrated by the use of isotope coded affinity tags (ICAT) (Gygi et al. 1999), has allowed mass spectrometry to be used quantitatively. In this approach, samples are labelled on cysteine residues using an ICAT reagent consisting of a thiol-specific reactive group and the affinity tag biotin, separated by a linker that can be a light or heavy version depending on the substitution of eight hydrogens for deuterium. Samples to be compared are individually labelled with either the heavy or light ICAT reagent prior to being mixed for digestion, (multidimensional) chromatography and mass spectrometry. Each peptide then appears as a doublet in the resulting spectrum, with the peaks separated by 8 Da. The ratio of the signal intensities of the two peaks is proportional to the relative level of the peptides and therefore the relative expression level of the parent protein in the two samples. A variety of cancer-related studies have used this approach. For example, a study comparing myc-null rat cells with myc-positive cells using ICAT and LC-MS/MS (Shiio et al., 2002) identified 528 proteins, 177 of which were differentially expressed. These changes involved a large number of functionally related proteins and included downregulation of adhesion molecules, actin binding proteins, proteases, and proteins in the Rho pathway, and upregulation of protein synthesis pathways, and anabolic enzymes.

Surface-enhanced laser desorption ionization mass spectrometry

Surface-enhanced laser desorption ionization mass spectrometry (SELDI) is an alternative protein profiling tool that has received much attention recently (Merchant and Weinberger, 2000). In this approach, subsets of proteins from a sample are selectively bound to ProteinChip arrays as a result of their specific interactions with particular array surface chemistries such as ion exchange and immobilized metal affinity chromatography. After addition of an energy absorbing matrix, bound proteins are then analysed by time of flight mass spectrometry, generating a spectral profile of the sample under investigation. SELDI is most suited to the study of low-molecular weight proteins (<20 kDa) making it complementary to a 2D-PAGE based approach. In addition, SELDI is sensitive in the femtomole to attamole range, making it ideal for profiling small quantities of protein samples. A number of clinical studies have employed this technique, including several analysing cancer patient samples, with the majority adopting a computer-based profiling strategy to delineate patient groups, rather than attempting to identify individual peaks. Identification of peaks is possible either using antibodies, on-chip purification, and digestion followed by mass spectrometry or, by associated tandem mass spectrometry, although this still remains technically challenging.

Several preliminary investigations have described analysis of cell and tissue extracts using SELDI. One of the pilot studies, which reported analysis of extracts prepared from LCM-procured cell populations from different normal and tumour tissue types, illustrated the feasibility of using SELDI to generate tissue- and cancer-specific spectral profiles

(Paweletz et al., 2000). Consistent differences were readily observed between the profiles of normal and tumour epithelial cells for both oesophageal and prostate cancers. The use of SELDI for profiling tissues appears promising but awaits further validation. A number of studies that have analysed biological fluids including serum, urine, and nipple aspirates, with the aim of generating patterns or signatures that can discriminate between cancer and control samples using computational models have generated very promising results. One of the most prominent studies has been in the development of a potential screening tool for ovarian cancer (Petricoin et al., 2002). Sera from 50 ovarian cancer patients and 50 controls were analysed using SELDI and the data used to develop an iterative searching algorithm. Analysis of a blind set of samples correctly predicted 50/50 ovarian cancer patients including 18 with stage I disease, a result that has obvious implications for the early detection of cancer. Of the controls, 63/66 were also correctly assigned. In studies investigating the possibility of developing a classifier for prostate cancer, serum samples from patients with prostate cancer were compared with sera from patients with benign prostatic hyperplasia and healthy controls using SELDI (Adam et al., 2002; Qu et al., 2002). A training set of 326 samples was used to develop a complex boosting decision tree algorithm capable of predicting sample class (Qu et al., 2002). Analysis of a test set of 60 further samples was able to achieve 100% sensitivity and specificity, again highlighting the potential of the approach. Studies have also been carried out to focus on patients with marginally raised prostate-specific antigen (PSA) levels (4–10 ng/ml) with promising initial results (Petricoin et al., 2002*b*). Studies such as those described here clearly show the potential of SELDI as a profiling tool. Long-term longitudinal multicentre studies are now required to fully test the robustness of the approach and consider aspects of sample handling, quality control, generation of spectra, and data normalisation and analysis. However, SELDI undoubtedly holds much promise for translational research.

Protein arrays

Analytical or expression protein microarrays have the potential to study large numbers of proteins simultaneously and will theoretically be able to achieve the scale of mRNA profiling experiments (MacBeath, 2002). Such arrays require the generation of a large bank of ligands or capture molecules such as antibodies, affibodies, or aptamers, with high affinity and specificity that are stable in an array format. Antibodies are the most obvious choice of capture molecules and although there are issues regarding antibody availability, potentially these can be solved by the use of resources such as phage display or ribosome display. The use of such libraries rather than antibodies to proteins of known identity has the additional advantage that it does not bias the approach to well-studied proteins. Furthermore, the use of single framework recombinant antibody fragments engineered to possess high on-chip stability may overcome the poor performance of many antibodies in an array format (Steinhauer et al., 2002). The sensitivity of antibody arrays remains an issue and the development of novel detection systems is likely to receive much attention.

Antibody arrays employing a sandwich enzyme-linked immunosorbent assay (ELISA) strategy (i.e. using capture antibodies specific for particular molecules and detection antibodies coupled, directly or indirectly, to a detection system) for profiling of cytokines have received the most attention. To investigate the mechanism of tumour suppression of glioblastoma by connexin 43 expression, Huang and coworkers studied the production of 43 cytokines using an antibody array (Huang et al., 2002). Monocyte chemoattractant protein-1 (MCP-1) was found to be significantly downregulated by connexin 43 expression, a finding confirmed by western blotting of immunoprecipitated MCP-1. In another study, a 51-feature array was used to profile cytokines secreted from dendritic cells in response to maturation agents (Schweitzer et al., 2002). In this case, the use of rolling circle amplification afforded a 1000X improvement in sensitivity over fluorescent detection alone. The use of such arrays to profile patient samples is likely to increase enormously in the near future.

In what will probably become a more prevalent strategy for protein profiling, antibody arrays have been probed with labelled protein extracts rather than using a second detection antibody. In a study examining alterations in protein expression induced in LoVo colon carcinoma cells upon radiation treatment, samples were labelled with Cy3 or Cy5 and applied to an array containing 146 antibodies to proteins involved in stress response, cell cycle progression, and apoptosis (Sreekumar et al., 2001). A number of apoptotic regulators were found to be upregulated, changes that were confirmed by immunoblotting. Using a slightly different detection strategy, in a study examining SCC of the oral cavity, LCM-procured samples (2500–3500 cells) of epithelium or stroma from normal, carcinoma *in situ*, and invasive cancer were analysed using an array containing 368 antibodies to cell signalling molecules, intra- and extracellular matrix proteins, cell cycle proteins, and growth factors and their receptors (Knezevic et al., 2001). Extracts were biotinylated and detected with avidin AMP and a colorimetric detection system. Changes, which were confirmed by western blotting and immunohistochemistry, included an increase in the level of retinoic acid receptor α (RARα) in the stroma surrounding progressing epithelium.

Protein arrays are also being employed in the study of protein function by identifying protein interactions. Such arrays rely on the expression, purification, and arraying of a large number of proteins in a native state, which represents a significant technical challenge. The feasibility of creating proteome chips is illustrated by the generation of an array consisting of 5800 proteins from the budding yeast *S. cerevisiae* (Zhu et al., 2001). In higher eukaryotes this will be facilitated by generation of libraries of expression constructs such as the Unigene set assimilated from a human foetal brain cDNA library (Cahill, 2001) and the FLEXGene (full length expression ready) repository (Brizuela et al., 2002). A number of studies have demonstrated that protein arrays can be used to investigate protein–protein and protein–small molecule interactions (MacBeath and Schreiber, 2000).

22.3.3 High-throughput marker validation

Putative biomarkers are often identified in comparative analyses of limited numbers of samples. Downstream validation of candidate molecules on larger sample sets is then required, which necessitates the use of high-throughput techniques and often relies on antibody-based approaches or approaches such as SELDI, as described earlier. Immunoassays are an obvious choice of method for marker validation. SELDI-based immunoassays can be employed as illustrated by the measurement of levels of PSMA in the serum of patients with benign and malignant prostate disease using antibody-coated ProteinChip arrays (Xiao et al., 2001). Immunohistochemistry is also used extensively with tissue arrays to allow simultaneous analysis of a large number of patient samples (Chapter 21). In addition, reverse arrays have recently been established as a high throughput alternative to western blotting.

Reverse arrays constructed using total cell or tissue lysates from a series of samples which are then probed with antibodies do not provide information about the form of a protein present but allow quantitative profiling of a range of antigens in large numbers of samples simultaneously. Paweletz and coworkers investigated the use of LCM-procured samples in reverse arrays and were able to detect the loss of annexin I in oesophageal cancer (Paweletz et al., 2001). This study went on to show increased levels of phosphorylated Akt and suppression of apoptosis (reduced cleavage of PARP and caspase 7) in prostate intraepithelial neoplasia (PIN) and invasive prostate cancer compared to normal prostate epithelium.

22.3.4 Post-translational modifications

The systematic study and characterization of post-translational modifications, especially protein phosphorylation and glycosylation, is an area of research that is beginning to receive a great deal of attention in proteomics-based studies. A number of gel-based approaches can be used to study protein phosphorylation, such as radiolabelling using γ-^{32}P or -^{33}P ATP followed by 2D-PAGE and autoradiography or 2D-PAGE combined with immunoblotting using antibodies specific for phospho-amino acids. An alternative strategy has been developed involving use of SH2 domains, a family of protein modules that bind particular classes of tyrosine-phosphorylated peptides, in far Western blotting. Results from a pilot study that examined a range of tumour cell lines indicated that SH2 profiling may be useful for molecular classification, including discrimination of closely related cell lines that differ in their chemosensitivity (Machida et al., 2003). Enrichment of phosphoproteins by immunoprecipitation (Gronborg et al., 2002) can be carried out prior to such analysis in combination with 2D-PAGE, for example, in studies of the effects of interferon alpha (IFNα) and interleukin2 (IL2) on lymphocytes (Stancato and Petricoin, 2001). Alternatively, protocols have been developed for derivitization of phosphorylated amino acids to facilitate isolation of phosphopeptides and incorporation of stable isotopes to allow comparative analysis by mass spectrometry, as has been applied in the analysis of inhibition of BCR-ABL fusion protein by STI571 in CML cells (Bonenfant et al., 2003).

Similarly, in studies of glycosylation, 2D blots can be probed with lectins or lectins can be used to affinity purify glycoproteins prior to analysis. Following the observation that strong binding of *Helix pomatia* agglutinin (HPA) to tissue sections was associated with aggressive breast cancer, 2D blots were probed with HPA as a first step in identifying the glycoproteins involved (Dwek et al., 2001). Stable isotope labelling has also been developed for analysis of glycoproteins by mass spectrometry. Glycoproteins were bound to a solid support using hydrazide chemistry and, following peptidolysis, stable isotope labelling on α-amino groups was carried out using heavy (d4) or light (d0) reagents. *N*-linked glycopeptides were then released enzymatically and analysed by μLC-MS/MS (Zhang et al., 2003). The value of the method as a specific enrichment strategy was clearly illustrated with analysis of serum and membrane fractions of the prostate cancer cell line LNCaP.

22.3.5 Screening for tumour antigens

Analysis of the protein profile of tissues and fluids is one strategy that can be adopted to identify tumour antigens that may be used to elicit an immune response as part of a therapeutic strategy. Several studies have now used the alternative strategy of examining the antibody repertoire of cancer patients on the basis that aberrant expression or cancer-specific protein forms may generate a humoral response and identify potential tumour antigens. SEREX (serological identification of antigens by recombinant expression cloning) is one such approach, where patient sera are used to probe an expression library generated from cDNA isolated from tumour tissue. This has identified a number of potential tumour-associated antigens in several cancer types (Sahin et al., 1997). Protein arrays represent a distinct analytical tool in such proteomic studies, both for identification of novel antigens and also, where the identity of the antigens are known, as an assay platform for the demonstration of autoantibodies that may be useful diagnostically. The analysis of a series of well-characterized sera from patients with autoimmune diseases using an array containing 196 autoantigens (proteins, peptides, and nucleic acids) and a fluorescent-based detection system is an excellent example of the use of this technology (Robinson et al., 2002). The results showed precise correlation with data obtained using more standard techniques. Preliminary data collected using an array generated from denatured recombinant proteins, identified antibodies to UM2 in sera from prostate cancer patients but not healthy controls (Sreekumar and Chinnaiyan, 2002). There is likely to be extensive interest in the development and use of such arrays to profile the sera of cancer patients.

A distinct strategy that has been adopted to identify tumour antigens is to use patient sera in immunoblotting of 2D-PAGE separated tissue or cell line extracts. In one of the earlier studies, proteins extracted from neuroblastoma tissues and cell lines were separated by 2D-PAGE and analysed by immunoblotting using sera from patients with neuroblastoma or other solid tumours and sera from healthy controls (Prasannan et al., 2000). Eleven of twenty-three of the neuroblastoma patients and one patient with a primitive neuroectodermal tumour had reactivity to a 50 kDa protein identified as β-tubulin isoforms I and III. Interestingly, the antibodies did not recognize β-tubulin found in normal brain tissue. A number of other studies have reported similar analyses of sera from patients with a range of tumour types and although many of the antigens identified are not as prevalent within the population groups examined, the approach holds much promise for identification of potential biomarkers. This has the advantage over SEREX of potentially identifying antigens whose reactivity is dependent on post-translational modifications or epigenetic influences.

22.4 Conclusion

This chapter has provided an introduction to what have rapidly become expanding and promising areas of investigation, not just in cancer but also in other biological fields. It is readily apparent that these approaches can contribute not only to translational and applied research of direct clinical relevance but also in producing new insights into the biology of cancer. In addition to the technological challenges, largely solved in the case of the transcriptome but still the area of massive investment in proteomics, the wealth of data arising from such experiments provoke new challenges in biostatistical and bioinformatic handling of the data to ensure the most efficient data mining and robust interpretation of the results, and also the infrastructure needed to follow up the large number of genes or proteins of potential interest arising from each experiment.

References

Adam, B. L., Qu, Y., Davis, J. W., Ward, M. D., Clements, M. A., Cazares, L. H. et al. (2002). Serum protein fingerprinting coupled with a pattern-matching algorithm distinguishes prostate cancer from benign prostate hyperplasia and healthy men. *Cancer Res*, **62**, 3609–14.

Adam, P. J., Boyd, R., Tyson, K. L., Fletcher, G. C., Stamps, A., Hudson, L. et al. (2003). Comprehensive proteomic analysis of breast cancer cell membranes reveals unique proteins with potential roles in clinical cancer. *J Biol Chem*, **278**, 6482–9.

Aebersold, R. and Mann, M. (2003). Mass spectrometry-based proteomics. *Nature*, **422**, 198–207.

Alizadeh, A. A., Eisen, M. B., Davis, R. E., Ma, C., Lossos, I. S., Rosenwald, A. et al. (2000). Distinct types of diffuse large B-cell lymphoma identified by gene expression profiling. *Nature*, **403**, 503–11.

Alizadeh, A. A., Ross, D. T., Perou, C. M., and van de Rijn M. (2001). Towards a novel classification of human malignancies based on gene expression patterns. *J Pathol*, **195**, 41–52.

Anderson, L. and Seilhamer, J. (1997). A comparison of selected mRNA and protein abundances in human liver. *Electrophoresis*, **18**, 533–7.

Anderson, N. L. and Anderson, N. G. (2002). The human plasma proteome: history, character, and diagnostic prospects. *Mol Cell Proteomics*, **1**, 845-67.

Armstrong, S. A., Staunton, J. E., Silverman, L. B., Pieters, R., den Boer, M. L., Minden, M. D. et al. (2002). MLL translocations specify a distinct gene expression profile that distinguishes a unique leukemia. *Nat Genet*, **30**, 41-7.

Banks, R. E., Dunn, M. J., Hochstrasser, D. F., Sanchez, J. C., Blackstock, W., Pappin, D. J. et al. (2000). Proteomics: new perspectives, new biomedical opportunities. *Lancet*, **356**, 1749–56.

Blackstock, W. P. and Weir, M. P. (1999). Proteomics: quantitative and physical mapping of cellular proteins. *Trends Biotechnol*, **17**, 121-7.

Bonenfant, D., Schmelzle, T., Jacinto, E., Crespo, J. L., Mini, T., Hall, M. N. et al. (2003). Quantitation of changes in protein phosphorylation: a simple method based on stable isotope labeling and mass spectrometry. *Proc Natl Acad Sci USA*, **100**, 880–5.

Brizuela, L., Richardson, A., Marsischky, G., and Labaer, J. (2002). The FLEXGene repository: exploiting the fruits of the genome projects by creating a needed resource to face the challenges of the post-genomic era. *Arch Med Res*, **33**, 318–24.

Butte, A. J., Tamayo, P., Slonim, D., Golub, T. R., and Kohane, I. S. (2000). Discovering functional relationships between RNA expression and chemotherapeutic susceptibility using relevance networks. *Proc Natl Acad Sci USA*, **97**, 12182–6.

Cahill, D. J. (2001) Protein and antibody arrays and their medical applications. *J Immunol Methods*, **250**, 81–91.

Celis, A., Rasmussen, H. H., Celis, P., Basse, B., Lauridsen, J. B., Ratz, G. et al. (1999). Short-term culturing of low-grade superficial bladder transitional cell carcinomas leads to changes in the expression levels of several proteins involved in key cellular activities. *Electrophoresis*, **20**, 355–61.

Celis, J. E., Celis, P., Ostergaard, M., Basse, B., Lauridsen, J. B., Ratz, G. et al. (1999*a*). Proteomics and immunohistochemistry define some of the steps involved in the squamous differentiation of the bladder transitional epithelium: a novel strategy for identifying metaplastic lesions. *Cancer Res*, **59**, 3003–9.

Celis, J. E., Ostergaard, M., Rasmussen, H. H., Gromov, P., Gromova, I., Varmark, H. et al. (1999*b*). A comprehensive protein resource for the study of bladder cancer. http://biobase.dk/cgi-bin/celis. *Electrophoresis*, **20**, 300–9.

Chambers, A. E., Banerjee, S., Chaplin, T., Dunne, J., Debernardi, S., Joel, S. P. et al. (2003). Histone acetylation-mediated regulation of genes in leukaemic cells. *Eur J Cancer*, **39**, 1165–75.

Craven, R. A. and Banks, R. E. (2001). Laser capture microdissection and proteomics: possibilities and limitations. *Proteomics*, **1**, 1200–4.

Crespo, M., Bosch, F., Villamor, N., Bellosillo, B., Colomer, D., Rozman, M. et al. (2003). ZAP-70 expression as a surrogate for immunoglobulin-variable-region mutations in chronic lymphocytic leukemia. *N Engl J Med*, **348**, 1764–75.

Debernardi, S., Lillington, D. M., Chaplin, T., Tomlinson, S., Amess J., Rohatiner A. et al. (2003). Genome-wide analysis of acute myeloid leukemia with normal karyotype reveals a unique pattern of homeobox gene expression distinct from those with translocation-mediated fusion events. *Genes Chromosomes Cancer*, **37**, 149–58.

Dhanasekaran, S. M., Barrette, T. R., Ghosh, D., Shah, R., Varambally, S., Kurachi, K. et al. (2001). Delineation of prognostic biomarkers in prostate cancer. *Nature*, **412**, 822–6.

Dwek, M. V., Ross, H. A., and Leathem, A. J. (2001). Proteome and glycosylation mapping identifies post-translational modifications associated with aggressive breast cancer. *Proteomics*, **1**, 756–62.

Franzén, B., Hirano, T., Okuzawa, K., Uryu, K., Alaiya, A. A., Linder, S. et al. (1995). Sample preparation of human tumors prior to two-dimensional electrophoresis of proteins. *Electrophoresis*, **16**, 1087–9.

Gaugler, B., Brouwenstijn, N., Vantomme, V., Szikora, J. P., Van der Spek, C. W., Patard, J. J. et al. (1996). A new gene coding for an antigen recognized by autologous cytolytic T lymphocytes on a human renal carcinoma. *Immunogenetics*, **44**, 323–30.

Gavin, A. C., Bosche, M., Krause, R., Grandi, P., Marzioch, M., Bauer, A. et al. (2002). Functional organization of the yeast proteome by systematic analysis of protein complexes. *Nature*, **415**, 141–7.

Gerhold D. L., Jensen R. V., and Gullans S. R. (2002). Better therapeutics through microarrays. *Nat Genet*, **32** (Suppl.), 547–51.

Gharbi, S., Gaffney, P., Yang, A., Zvelebil, M. J., Cramer, R., Waterfield, M. D. et al. (2002). Evaluation of two-dimensional differential gel electrophoresis for proteomic expression analysis of a model breast cancer cell system. *Mol Cell Proteomics*, **1**, 91–8.

Golub, T. R., Slonim, D. K., Tamayo, P., Huard, C., Gaasenbeek, M., Mesirov, J. P. et al. (1999). Molecular classification of cancer: class discovery and class prediction by gene expression monitoring. *Science*, **286**, 531–7.

Grimwade, D., Walker, H., Oliver, F., Wheatley, K., Harrison, C., Harrison, G. et al. (1998). The importance of diagnostic cytogenetics on outcome in AML: analysis of 1,612 patients entered into the MRC AML 10 trial. The Medical Research Council Adult and Children's Leukaemia Working Parties. *Blood*, **92**, 2322–33.

Gronborg, M., Kristiansen, T. Z., Stensballe, A., Andersen, J. S., Ohara, O., Mann, M. et al. (2002). A mass spectrometry-based proteomic approach for identification of serine/threonine-phosphorylated proteins by enrichment with phospho-specific antibodies: identification of a novel protein, Frigg, as a protein kinase A substrate. *Mol Cell Proteomics*, **1**, 517–27.

Gunther, E. C., Stone, D. J., Gerwien, R. W., Bento, P., and Heyes, M. P. (2003). Prediction of clinical drug efficacy by classification of drug-induced genomic expression profiles in vitro. *Proc Natl Acad Sci USA*, **100**, 9608–13.

Gygi, S. P., Rist, B., Gerber, S. A., Turecek, F., Gelb, M. H., and Aebersold, R. (1999). Quantitative analysis of complex protein mixtures using isotope-coded affinity tags. *Nat. Biotechnol*, **17**, 994–9.

Hamblin, T. J., Davis, Z., Gardiner, A., Oscier, D. G., and Stevenson, F. K. (1999). Unmutated Ig V(H) genes are associated with a more aggressive form of chronic lymphocytic leukemia. *Blood*, **94**, 1848–54.

Hedenfalk, I., Duggan, D., Chen Y., Radmacher, M., Bittner, M., Simon, R. et al. (2001). Gene-expression profiles in hereditary breast cancer. *N Engl J Med*, **344**, 539–48.

Hippo, Y., Taniguchi, H., Tsutsumi, S., Machida, N., Chong, J. M., Fukayama M. et al. (2002). Global gene expression analysis of gastric cancer by oligonucleotide microarrays. *Cancer Res*, **62**, 233–40.

Ho, Y., Gruhler, A., Heilbut, A., Bader, G. D., Moore, L., Adams, S. L. et al. (2002). Systematic identification of protein complexes in *Saccharomyces cerevisiae* by mass spectrometry. *Nature*, **415**, 180–3.

Hoffmann, P., Ji, H., Moritz, R. L., Connolly, L. M., Frecklington, D. F., Layton, M. J. et al. (2001). Continuous free-flow electrophoresis separation of cytosolic proteins from the human colon carcinoma cell line LIM 1215: a non two-dimensional gel electrophoresis-based proteome analysis strategy. *Proteomics*, **1**, 807–18.

Hofmann, W. K., de Vos, S., Elashoff, D., Gschaidmeier, H., Hoelzer, D., Koeffler, P. H. et al. (2002). Relation between resistance of Philadelphia-chromosome-positive acute lymphoblastic leukaemia to the tyrosine kinase inhibitor STI571 and gene-expression profiles: a gene-expression study. *Lancet*, **359**, 481–6.

Hoving, S., Voshol, H., and van Oostrum, J. (2000). Towards high performance two-dimensional gel electrophoresis using ultrazoom gels. *Electrophoresis*, **21**, 2617–21.

Huang, R., Lin, Y., Wang, C. C., Gano, J., Lin, B., Shi, Q. et al. (2002). Connexin 43 suppresses human glioblastoma cell growth by down-regulation of monocyte chemotactic protein 1, as discovered using protein array technology. *Cancer Res*, **62**, 2806–12.

International Lymphoma Study Group (1997). A clinical evaluation of the International Lymphoma Study Group classification of non-Hodgkin's lymphoma. The non-Hodgkin's lymphoma classification project. *Blood*, **89**, 3909–18.

Jazaeri, A. A., Yee, C. J., Sotiriou, C., Brantley, K. R., Boyd, J., and Liu, E. T. (2002). Gene expression profiles of BRCA1-linked, BRCA2-linked, and sporadic ovarian cancers. *J Natl Cancer Inst*, **94**, 990–1000.

Klein, U., Tu, Y., Stolovitzky, G. A., Mattioli, M., Cattoretti, G., Husson, H. et al. (2001). Gene expression profiling of B cell chronic lymphocytic leukemia reveals a homogeneous phenotype related to memory B cells. *J Exp Med*, **194**, 1625–38.

Knezevic, V., Leethanakul, C., Bichsel, V. E., Worth, J. M., Prabhu, V. V., Gutkind, J. S. et al. (2001). Proteomic profiling of the cancer microenvironment by antibody arrays. *Proteomics*, **1**, 1271–8.

LaTulippe, E., Satagopan, J., Smith, A., Scher, H., Scardino, P., Reuter, V. et al. (2002). Comprehensive gene expression analysis of prostate cancer reveals distinct transcriptional programs associated with metastatic disease. *Cancer Res*, **62**, 4499–506.

Lin, Y. M., Furukawa, Y., Tsunoda, T., Yue, C. T., Yang, K. C., and Nakamura, Y. (2002). Molecular diagnosis of colorectal tumors by expression profiles of 50 genes expressed differentially in adenomas and carcinomas. *Oncogene*, **21**, 4120–8.

Lossos, I. S. and Levy, R. (2003). Diffuse large B-cell lymphoma: insights gained from gene expression profiling. *Int J Hematol*, **77**, 321–9.

Lossos, I. S., Alizadeh, A. A., Diehn, M., Warnke, R., Thorstenson, Y., Oefner, P. J. et al. (2002). Transformation of follicular lymphoma to diffuse large-cell lymphoma: alternative patterns with increased or decreased expression of c-myc and its regulated genes. *Proc Natl Acad Sci USA*, **99**, 8886–91.

Luche, S., Santoni, V., and Rabilloud, T. (2003). Evaluation of nonionic and zwitterionic detergents as membrane protein solubilizers in two-dimensional electrophoresis. *Proteomics*, **3**, 249–53.

MacBeath, G. (2002). Protein microarrays and proteomics. *Nat Genet*, **32** (Suppl. 526–32), 526–532.

MacBeath, G. and Schreiber, S. L. (2000). Printing proteins as microarrays for high-throughput function determination. *Science*, **289**, 1760–3.

MacDonald, T. J., Brown, K. M., LaFleur, B., Peterson, K., Lawlor, C., Chen, Y. et al. (2001). Expression profiling of medulloblastoma: PDGFRA and the RAS/MAPK pathway as therapeutic targets for metastatic disease. *Nat Genet*, **29**, 143–52.

Machida, K., Mayer, B. J., and Nollau, P. (2003). Profiling the global tyrosine phosphorylation state. *Mol Cell Proteomics*, **2**, 215–33.

Merchant, M. and Weinberger, S. R. (2000). Recent advancements in surface-enhanced laser desorption/ ionization-time of flight-mass spectrometry. *Electrophoresis*, **21**, 1164–77.

Neumann, E., Engelsberg, A., Decker, J., Storkel, S., Jaeger, E., Huber, C. et al. (1998). Heterogeneous expression of the tumor-associated antigens RAGE-1, PRAME, and glycoprotein 75 in human renal cell carcinoma: candidates for T-cell-based immunotherapies? *Cancer Res*, **58**, 4090–5.

Notterman D. A., Alon U., Sierk A. J., and Levine A. J. (2001). Transcriptional gene expression profiles of colorectal adenoma, adenocarcinoma, and normal tissue examined by oligonucleotide arrays. *Cancer Res*, **61**, 3124–30.

Ostergaard, M., Rasmussen, H. H., Nielsen, H. V., Vorum, H., Orntoft, T. F., Wolf, H. et. al. (1997). Proteome profiling of bladder squamous cell carcinomas: identification of markers that define their degree of differentiation. *Cancer Res*, **57**, 4111–7.

Ostergaard, M., Wolf, H., Orntoft, T. F., and Celis, J. E. (1999). Psoriasin (S100A7): a putative urinary marker for the follow-up of patients with bladder squamous cell carcinomas. *Electrophoresis*, **20**, 349–54.

Page, M. J., Amess, B., Townsend, R. R., Parekh, R., Herath, A., Brusten, L. et. al. (1999). Proteomic definition of normal human luminal and myoepithelial breast cells purified from reduction mammoplasties *Proc Natl Acad Sci USA*, **96**, 12589–94.

Paweletz, C. P., Gillespie, J. W., Ornstein, D. K., Simone, N. L., Brown, M. R., Cole, K. A. et. al. (2000). Rapid protein display profiling of cancer progression directly from human tissue using a protein biochip. *Drug Develop Res*, **49**, 34–42.

Paweletz, C. P., Charboneau, L., Bichsel, V. E., Simone, N. L., Chen, T., Gillespie, J. W. et. al. (2001). Reverse phase protein microarrays which capture disease progression show activation of pro-survival pathways at the cancer invasion front. *Oncogene*, **20**, 1981–9.

Perou, C. M., Sorlie, T., Eisen, M. B., van de Rijn, M., Jeffrey, S. S., Rees C. A. et al. (2000). Molecular portraits of human breast tumours. *Nature*, **406**, 747–52.

Petit, M. M., Schoenmakers, E. F., Huysmans, C., Geurts, J. M., Mandahl, N., and Van de Ven, W. J. (1999). LHFP, a novel translocation partner gene of HMGIC in a lipoma, is a member of a new family of LHFP-like genes. *Genomics*, **57**, 438–41.

Petricoin, E. F., Ardekani, A. M., Hitt, B. A., Levine, P. J., Fusaro, V. A., Steinberg, S. M., et al. (2002). Use of proteomic patterns in serum to identify ovarian cancer. *Lancet*, **359**, 572–7.

Petricoin, E. F., III, Ornstein, D. K., Paweletz, C. P., Ardekani, A., Hackett, P. S., Hitt, B. A. et al. (2002*b*). Serum proteomic patterns for detection of prostate cancer. *J Natl Cancer Inst*, **94**, 1576–78.

Pieper, R., Su, Q., Gatlin, C. L., Huang, S. T., Anderson, N. L., and Steiner, S. (2003). Multi-component immunoaffinity subtraction chromatography: An innovative step towards a comprehensive survey of the human plasma proteome. *Proteomics*, **3**, 422–32.

Pomeroy, S. L., Tamayo, P., Gaasenbeek, M., Sturla, L. M., Angelo, M., McLaughlin, M. E. et al. (2002). Prediction of central nervous system embryonal tumour outcome based on gene expression. *Nature*, **415**, 436–42.

Prasannan, L., Misek, D. E., Hinderer, R., Michon, J., Geiger, J. D., and Hanash, S. M. (2000). Identification of beta-tubulin isoforms as tumor antigens in neuroblastoma. *Clin Cancer Res*, **6**, 3949–56.

Pui, C. H., Frankel, L. S., Carroll, A. J., Raimondi, S. C., Shuster, J. J., Head, D. R. et al. (1991). Clinical characteristics and treatment outcome of childhood acute lymphoblastic leukemia with the t(4;11)(q21;q23): a collaborative study of 40 cases. *Blood*, **77**, 440–7.

Qu, Y., Adam, B. L., Yasui, Y., Ward, M. D., Cazares, L. H., Schellhammer, P. F. et al. (2002). Boosted decision tree analysis of surface-enhanced laser desorption/ ionization mass spectral serum profiles discriminates prostate cancer from noncancer patients. *Clin Chem*, **48**, 1835–43.

Quackenbush, J. (2002). Microarray data normalization and transformation. *Nat Genet*, **32**(Suppl.), 496–501.

Ramaswamy, S., Tamayo, P., Rifkin, R., Mukherjee, S., Yeang, C. H., Angelo, M. et al. (2001). Multiclass cancer diagnosis using tumor gene expression signatures. *Proc Natl Acad Sci USA*, **98**, 15149–54.

Reymond, M. A., Sanchez, J. C., Hughes, G. J., Günther, K., Riese, J., Tortola, S. et al. (1997). Standardized characterization of gene expression in human colorectal epithelium by two-dimensional electrophoresis. *Electrophoresis*, **18**, 2842–8.

Robinson, W. H., DiGennaro, C., Hueber, W., Haab, B. B., Kamachi, M., Dean, E. J. et al. (2002). Autoantigen microarrays for multiplex characterization of autoantibody responses. *Nat Med*, **8**, 295–301.

Rosenwald, A., Alizadeh, A. A., Widhopf, G., Simon, R., Davis, R. E., Yu, X. et al. (2001). Relation of gene expression phenotype to immunoglobulin mutation genotype in B cell chronic lymphocytic leukemia. *J Exp Med*, **194**, 1639–47.

Rosenwald, A., Wright, G., Chan, W. C., Connors, J. M., Campo, E., Fisher, R. I. et al. (2002). The use of molecular profiling to predict survival after chemotherapy for diffuse large-B-cell lymphoma. *N Engl J Med*, **346**, 1937–47.

Rui, Z., Jian-Guo, J., Yuan-Peng, T., Hai, P., and Bing-Gen, R. (2003). Use of serological proteomic methods to find biomarkers associated with breast cancer. *Proteomics*, **3**, 433–9.

Sahin, U., Tureci, O., and Pfreundschuh, M. (1997). Serological identification of human tumor antigens. *Curr Opin Immunol*, **9**, 709–16.

Sarto, C., Marocchi, A., Sanchez, J. C., Giannone, D., Frutiger, S., Golaz, O. et al. (1997). Renal cell carcinoma and normal kidney protein expression. *Electrophoresis*, **18**, 599–604.

Scherf, U., Ross, D. T., Waltham, M., Smith, L. H., Lee, J. K., Tanabe, L. et al. (2000). A gene expression database for the molecular pharmacology of cancer. *Nat Genet*, **24**, 236–44.

Schoch, C., Kohlmann, A., Schnittger, S., Brors, B., Dugas, M., Mergenthaler, S. et al. (2002). Acute myeloid leukemias with reciprocal rearrangements can be distinguished by specific gene expression profiles. *Proc Natl Acad Sci USA*, **99**, 10008–13.

Schweitzer, B., Roberts, S., Grimwade, B., Shao, W., Wang, M., Fu, Q. et al. (2002). Multiplexed protein profiling on microarrays by rolling-circle amplification. *Nat Biotechnol*, **20**, 359–65.

Shiio, Y., Donohoe, S., Yi, E. C., Goodlett, D. R., Aebersold, R., and Eisenman, R. N. (2002). Quantitative proteomic analysis of Myc oncoprotein function. *EMBO J*, **21**, 5088–96.

Shipp, M. A., Ross, K. N., Tamayo, P., Weng, A. P., Kutok, J. L., Aguiar, R. C. et al. (2002). Diffuse large B-cell lymphoma outcome prediction by gene-expression profiling and supervised machine learning. *Nat Med*, **8**, 68–74.

Simpson, R. J., Connolly, L. M., Eddes, J. S., Pereira, J. J., Moritz, R. L., and Reid, G. E. (2000). Proteomic analysis of the human colon carcinoma cell line (LIM 1215): development of a membrane protein database. *Electrophoresis*, **21**, 1707–32.

Slonim, D. K. (2002). From patterns to pathways: gene expression data analysis comes of age. *Nat Genet*, **32** (Suppl.), 502–8.

Sorlie, T., Perou, C. M., Tibshirani, R., Aas, T., Geisler, S., Johnsen, H. et al. (2001). Gene expression patterns of breast carcinomas distinguish tumor subclasses with clinical implications. *Proc Natl Acad Sci USA*, **98**, 10869–74.

Sreekumar, A. and Chinnaiyan, A. M. (2002). Using protein microarrays to study cancer. *Biotechniques*, **33**, S46–S53.

Sreekumar, A., Nyati, M. K., Varambally, S., Barrette, T. R., Ghosh, D., Lawrence, T. S. et al. (2001). Profiling of cancer cells using protein microarrays: discovery of novel radiation-regulated proteins. *Cancer Res*, **61**, 7585–93.

Stancato, L. F. and Petricoin, E. F., III (2001). Fingerprinting of signal transduction pathways using a combination of anti-phosphotyrosine immunoprecipitations and two-dimensional polyacrylamide gel electrophoresis. *Electrophoresis*, **22**, 2120–4.

Staudt, L. M. (2003). Molecular diagnosis of the hematologic cancers. *N Engl J Med*, **348**, 1777–85.

Staunton, J. E., Slonim, D. K., Coller, H. A., Tamayo, P., Angelo, M. J., Park, J. et al. (2001). Chemosensitivity prediction by transcriptional profiling. *Proc Natl Acad Sci USA*, **98**, 10787–92.

Steinhauer, C., Wingren, C., Hager, A. C., and Borrebaeck, C. A. (2002). Single framework recombinant antibody fragments designed for protein chip applications. *Biotechniques*, (Suppl. 38–45), 38–45.

Su, A. I., Welsh, J. B., Sapinoso, L. M., Kern, S. G., Dimitrov, P., Lapp, H. et al. (2001). Molecular classification of human carcinomas by use of gene expression signatures. *Cancer Res*, **61**, 7388–93.

Takahashi, M., Rhodes, D. R., Furge, K. A., Kanayama, H., Kagawa, S., Haab, B. B. et al. (2001). Gene expression profiling of clear cell renal cell carcinoma: gene identification and prognostic classification. *Proc Natl Acad Sci USA*, **98**, 9754–9.

Tonge, R., Shaw, J., Middleton, B., Rowlinson, R., Rayner, S., Young, J. et al. (2001). Validation and development of fluorescence two-dimensional differential gel electrophoresis proteomics technology. *Proteomics*, **1**, 377–96.

Unwin, R. D., Craven, R. A., Harnden, P., Hanrahan, S., Totty, N., Knowles, M. A. et al. (2003*a*). Proteomic changes in renal cancer and co-ordinate demonstration of both the glycolytic and mitochondrial apsects of the Warburg effect. *Proteomics*, **3**, 1620–32.

Unwin, R. D., Harnden, P., Pappin, D., Rahman, D., Whelan, P., Craven, R. A., et al. (2003*b*) Serological and proteomic evaluation of antibody responses in the identification of tumor antigens in renal cell carcinoma. *Proteomics*, **3**, 45–55.

van 't Veer, L. J., Dai, H., van de Vijver, M. J., He, Y. D., Hart, A. A., Mao, M. et al. (2002). Gene expression profiling predicts clinical outcome of breast cancer. *Nature*, **415**, 530–6.

Virtaneva, K., Wright, F. A., Tanner, S. M., Yuan, B., Lemon, W. J., Caligiuri, M. A. et al. (2001). Expression profiling reveals fundamental biological differences in acute myeloid leukemia with isolated trisomy 8 and normal cytogenetics. *Proc Natl Acad Sci USA*, **98**, 1124–9.

Wang, K., Gan, L., Jeffery, E., Gayle, M., Gown, A. M., Skelly, M. et al. (1999). Monitoring gene expression profile changes in ovarian carcinomas using cDNA microarray. *Gene*, **229**, 101–8.

Wang, Y. Y., Cheng, P., and Chan, D. W. (2003). A simple affinity spin tube filter method for removing high-abundant common proteins or enriching low-abundant biomarkers for serum proteomic analysis. *Proteomics*, **3**, 243–8.

Washburn, M. P., Wolters, D., and Yates, J. R., III (2001). Large-scale analysis of the yeast proteome by multidimensional protein identification technology. *Nat Biotechnol*, **19**, 242–7.

Weinstein, J. N., Myers, T. G., O'Connor, P. M., Friend, S. H., Fornace, A. J., Jr., Kohn, K. W. et al. (1997). An information-intensive approach to the molecular pharmacology of cancer. *Science*, **275**, 343–9.

Welsh, J. B., Sapinoso, L. M., Su, A. I., Kern, S. G., Wang-Rodriguez, J., Moskaluk, C. A. et al. (2001*a*). Analysis of gene expression identifies candidate markers and pharmacological targets in prostate cancer. *Cancer Res*, **61**, 5974–8.

Welsh, J. B., Zarrinkar, P. P., Sapinoso, L. M., Kern, S. G., Behling, C. A., Monk, B. J. et al. (2001*b*). Analysis of gene expression profiles in normal and neoplastic ovarian tissue samples identifies candidate molecular markers of epithelial ovarian cancer. *Proc Natl Acad Sci USA*, **98**, 1176–81.

Wildgruber, R., Harder, A., Obermaier, C., Boguth, G., Weiss, W., Fey, S. J. et al. (2000). Towards higher resolution: two-dimensional electrophoresis of *Saccharomyces cerevisiae* proteins using overlapping narrow immobilized pH gradients. *Electrophoresis*, **21**, 2610–16.

Wilkins, M. R., Sanchez, J. C., Gooley, A. A., Appel, R. D., Humphery-Smith, I., Hochstrasser, D. F. et al. (1996). Progress with proteome projects: why all proteins expressed by a genome should be identified and how to do it. *Biotechnol Genet Eng Rev*, **13** (19–50). 19–50.

Xiao, Z., Adam, B. L., Cazares, L. H., Clements, M. A., Davis, J. W., Schellhammer, P. F. et al. (2001). Quantitation of serum prostate-specific membrane antigen by a novel protein biochip immunoassay discriminates benign from malignant prostate disease. *Cancer Res*, **61**, 6029–33.

Yeoh, E. J., Ross, M. E., Shurtleff, S. A., Williams, W. K., Patel, D., Mahfouz, R., et al. (2002). Classification, subtype discovery, and prediction of outcome in pediatric acute lymphoblastic leukemia by gene expression profiling. *Cancer Cell*, **1**, 133–43.

Zhang, H., Li, X. J., Martin, D. B., and Aebersold, R. (2003). Identification and quantification of N-linked glycoproteins using hydrazide chemistry, stable isotope labeling and mass spectrometry. *Nat Biotechnol*, **21**, 660–6.

Zhu, H., Bilgin, M., Bangham, R., Hall, D., Casamayor, A., Bertone, P., et al. (2001). Global analysis of protein activities using proteome chips. *Science*, **293**, 2101–5.

Zou, T. T., Selaru, F. M., Xu, Y., Shustova, V., Yin, J., Mori, Y., et al. (2002). Application of cDNA microarrays to generate a molecular taxonomy capable of distinguishing between colon cancer and normal colon. *Oncogene*, **21**, 4855–62.

Zuo, X. and Speicher, D. W. (2002). Comprehensive analysis of complex proteomes using microscale solution isoelectrofocusing prior to narrow pH range two-dimensional electrophoresis. *Proteomics*, **2**, 58–68.

CHAPTER 23

Local treatment of cancer

Ian S. Fentiman

23.1 Introduction

Cancer exerts its damaging effects upon patients by the destruction caused by growth and invasion at the primary site and secondly by similar damage caused at distant sites as a result of metastatic spread. For many cancers it is clear that local growth continues for some time before metastasis occurs. This presents therapists with 'a window of opportunity' during which the removal or complete destruction of the cancer at the primary site can result in complete cure. The traditional local modalities of treatment for cancer with surgery or radiotherapy therefore retain a critically important role in treating cancer patients. When used effectively early in the course of the cancer they may be curative and surgery is still the treatment that produces most cancer cures. Used later in the course of the disease they may still achieve effective 'local control' by eradicating or reducing the tumour at the primary site and this may produce real benefits for patients, even though ultimately they may succumb to the effects of metastasis.

For these two key goals of cure and local control to be achieved without harming the patient they have to be very carefully targeted. When a surgeon removes the primary cancer it is essential that it is completely 'radically' resected but it is also essential to limit the damage to surrounding normal tissues and the consequent harm to the patient. Recent years have seen great strides in the ability of cancer surgeons to resect primary cancers completely while minimizing the damage to the patient by the use of advanced surgical techniques and in particular tissue reconstruction and microvascular surgery. Radiotherapy has also seen dramatic advances in the ability of the clinical oncologist to accurately target radiotherapy into the volume within which the primary tumour sits with greatly improved control over the amount of normal tissue irradiated. These advances come from the use of sophisticated cross-sectional imaging to accurately delineate the tumour and then ever increasing shaping of the radiation fields to miss vital normal structures.

During the last two decades local treatments have been supplemented by the use of 'adjuvant' systemic treatments. The concept here is simple. If local treatment can irradicate the primary tumour at a time when only tiny quantities of micro-metastatic disease exist, then the use of drug therapies at that time may greatly increase the chance of cure. Small quantities of micro-metastatic disease, probably in an active proliferative phase, may be irradicated by drug therapies while larger quantities of metastatic disease may not be because of the increased number of cells that must be killed and the difficulty of drugs in penetrating established tumour masses. This concept of adjuvant therapy, has been shown to be valid in many kinds of cancer and most importantly in breast cancer and colorectal cancer, two of the most commonest cancers in the Western world, where the addition of adjuvant systemic chemotherapy can significantly increase cure rates in patients whose primary tumours have been removed but who are known, because of the characteristics of those primary tumours, to be at high risk of micro-metastatic disease. An important clinical facet of adjuvant therapy, which always has to be weighed very carefully in the balance by clinicians, is the difficulty of identifying which patients in fact have micro-metastatic disease. These difficulties mean that adjuvant treatments are often given on 'the balance of probabilities' to patients in whom the risk of micro-metastatic disease is substantial, even though it may be in too small a quantity to be visible on scans or detectable by biological or biochemical tests. Inherent in this approach is the fact that some patients may receive adjuvant chemotherapy, based on probabilities, who do not in fact have metastatic disease at all. Trials can show that patients benefit *on average* but it may not be possible at the current state of practice to indicate precisely which patients within an overall group will benefit individually.

Surgery is the oldest form of treatment for cancer. Whereas it was once the only modality offering a chance of cure for solid tumours, it has now become integrated in a multidisciplinary approach seeking to maximize local control of disease and minimize the likelihood of distant dissemination. The aim of surgery is to achieve complete local extirpation of cancer and also to determine the stage of disease by removing lymph nodes draining the site of the tumour. Originally this was based on an *en-bloc* resection of both primary and lymph node basin such as a radical mastectomy for breast cancer. However, these operations involved extensive damage to normal tissues and nowadays in many cases this can be avoided by a judicious combination of surgery and radiotherapy.

In future cancer surgery will continue to change. Modern technologies make it possible for a great deal of surgery to be done through small incisions using endoscopic techniques. Robotic surgery and even surgery carried remotely using robotics and telemetric transfer are all feasible. Their place in cancer surgery has to be very carefully and critically evaluated. The basic principle that a radical resection is likely to be associated with cure has to be retained. Clinical trials comparing new surgical techniques are in progress.

For radiotherapy, high-energy X-ray beams, generated from linear accelerators have a range of energies and tissue penetration depths. Radiation induces double strand breaks in DNA that are repaired less effectively by malignant cells than by their normal counterparts. Treatment is given in multiple fractions for curative treatment to limit the dose delivered in each fraction and thereby to minimize long-term damage or late effects in the normal body tissues.

The development of appropriate fields for therapy with the appropriate energy is a highly complex exercise known as planning. Medical physicists and clinicians work together to outline the field to be treated and estimate the doses of radiation to be received in each part of that field. Traditional planning involved plain X-rays and lead blocks to shape fields. Modern planning involves multi-leaf collimators and the use of intensity modulation. Computerized tomography and magnetic resonance imaging are essential elements in modern radiotherapy techniques.

Using the UICC system of staging, based on T (Tumour), N (Nodal status), and M (Metastases), produces a complex classification. The TNM system remains the international standard but many clinicians use simpler schemes bringing the TNM staging together into groups. A simpler scheme such as the Manchester system places patients in four stages of disease and is useful in determining

Table 23.1 Staging of cancers at diagnosis, treatment and prognosis

Stage	Description	Treatment	Prognosis
I	Small primary No nodal involvement No distant metastases	Surgery ± RT Sometimes systemic therapy	Often good
II	Small/medium primary Local nodal involvement No distant metastases	Surgery Systemic therapy Sometimes primary systemic therapy	Sometimes good
III	Locally advanced No distant metastases	Primary systemic therapy RT	Usually poor
IV	Distant metastases	Palliation with Systemic therapy ± RT ± Surgery	Dire

both treatment and prognosis. An outline of the staging is given in Table 23.1. Various common solid tumours will be considered in relation to the role of local treatment and how this meshes with systemic therapy.

23.2 Skin cancers

The skin is the commonest site of malignancy and there are three major types, each derived from a different precursor cell. The most frequent lesion diagnosed is a basal cell carcinoma, also known as a rodent ulcer, derived from the epidermal basal layer and these are often located on the face. Although locally invasive these lesions do not give rise to distant metastases and so local treatment (complete excision) is curative. Inadequate treatment, however, will mean that further local invasion will occur and this can be life-threatening if affecting a vital organ.

Squamous cell carcinomas (SCC) are derived from basal keratinocytes, often in sun-damaged areas where actinic keratoses are found. Unlike rodent ulcers SCC may metastasize to regional nodes or distant sites but only in <5% of cases. SCC developing from actinic keratoses is unlikely to metastasize but those arising from long-standing areas of skin inflammation, burns or chronic sinuses are more likely to be aggressive. In the majority of cases wide excision is curative.

The least common but most aggressive of skin cancers is melanoma, derived from melanocytes. Risk factors for melanoma include fair skin, sunlight exposure, multiple benign naevi, and prior diagnosis of melanoma. There is genetic predisposition and mutations in the *CDKN2A* gene, which prevent expression of p16, have been implicated. There are subtypes of melanoma: superficial spreading, nodular, lentigo maligna, and acral lentiginous but the former type comprises 70% of lesions.

Staging is based on the Breslow tumour thickness (height from granular layer to maximum depth of invasion) and the Clark level of invasion (extent of dermal penetration). The major prognostic determinant is the thickness of the lesion rather than the depth of invasion. Whenever possible the histological diagnosis of a suspected melanoma is made by wide excision to avoid cutting into the lesion and risking the shedding of viable tumour emboli. The melanoma is excised down to the deep fascia and required tumour-free margins are dependent upon the tumour thickness.

Because melanoma spreads to regional lymph nodes many surgeons carried out *en-bloc* nodal resection. This can deal with the local problem of tumour relapse but in many cases the nodes were negative and the dissection led to lymphoedema if axillary or inguinal nodes were cleared. Because of this the technique of sentinel node biopsy has developed to stage disease and reduce morbidity. The sentinel node is the first port of call for lymphatic fluid draining from a tumour and hence the first site at which tumour metastases may be found. The concept was applied by Morten, using a marker dye to identify the lymphatic basin of malignant melanomas (Morten et al., 1992). Dye is injected at the site of the lesion and lymphatics can be identified by eye and the sentinel node(s) resected. Provided that these are tumour-free no further nodal dissection is necessary.

Because of the high risk of distant metastases many agents have been tested as both adjuvants and for the treatment of advanced melanoma, mostly without success. High dose interferon-α2b has some effect as an adjuvant but there are no proven chemotherapy regimens. For management of metastatic melanoma the only agent with some effect is dacarbazine (DTIC) but the median response duration is short (3–6 months). The lack of effective therapies has prompted extensive work into biological approaches including antibodies against melanoma antigen ganglioside (GM2), polyvalent melanoma vaccine, and adoptive immunotherapy using dendritic cells.

23.3 Breast cancer

Apart from skin malignancy, breast cancer is the commonest tumour in Western European women, affecting 1 woman in 10, and is responsible for the majority of deaths in middle aged females. Invasive breast cancer is predominantly ductal in origin and almost invariably evolves from non-invasive disease, ductal carcinoma *in situ* (DCIS). In DCIS the ducts are filled with malignant cells without any breach in the basement membrane. The central cells undergo necrosis and then calcification. It is this microcalcification which is picked up on mammography and 20% of screen detected cases are DCIS. Almost invariably patients with DCIS are asymptomatic, although occasionally they may have a lump or a nipple discharge.

What used to be a rare condition is now relatively common. Depending on growth rate and morphology

DCIS is subdivided by pathologists into low, intermediate, and high grade. Although not life-threatening, unless DCIS is completely excised it is very likely to recur and progress to invasive disease: those with high grade DCIS are most likely to develop invasive cancer and this is usually also of high grade. The standard treatment was mastectomy and it was paradoxical that women with invasive breast cancer were offered breast conserving treatment whereas those with non-life-threatening DCIS were undergoing mastectomy. For this reason, in the 1980s, trials were set up to determine whether, after a complete excision of DCIS there was a benefit from breast irradiation or tamoxifen.

These trials have shown that radiotherapy does reduce the likelihood of recurrence of DCIS and progression to invasive cancer. Tamoxifen may have some effect in those with estrogen receptor positive (ER+) DCIS. What also emerged is that in many screen-detected cases DCIS is too extensive for complete wide excision so that a mastectomy is necessary. The challenge is to find novel therapies that can prevent progression and reduce the number of mastectomies for DCIS.

Breast cancer is probably the most feared malignancy in women despite the fact that more women in the United States now die of lung cancer as a result of smoking. The mortality rate from breast cancer is falling, partly as a result of earlier diagnosis from public awareness and screening but also from the judicious use of effective adjuvant therapies. The standard form of breast conservation therapy, confirmed in many prospective randomized trials, is wide excision of tumour, axillary lymph node clearance and breast irradiation. Many attempts have been made, with varying success, to minimize the extent of local intervention in the hope of reducing side-effects while maintaining good local control of disease.

It is generally agreed that the aim of surgery is to achieve tumour-free excision margins both in terms of invasive and non-invasive disease. In some cases the extent of surgery may be reduced providing that a radiotherapy boost is given to the tumour site, although a boost trial suggested that this was only necessary in younger women (Bartelink et al., 2001). If no radiotherapy is given to the breast even after complete excision there is an increased risk of relapse at the tumour site, which may be as high as 40%. Various studies have and are examining the role of radiation to the affected quadrant of the breast, and with refinement this may be effective, particularly in older women. For various reasons women aged >65, who comprise 50% of the cases of breast cancer, have a disproportionately high cancer-specific mortality (60% of all deaths). It is likely that many otherwise fit older women are offered suboptimal treatments and not offered radiotherapy when it is appropriate.

Because older women are more likely to have ER+ cancers, many have been treated with tamoxifen alone. Several trials have indicated that this leads to an unacceptably high rate of local progression and may also be responsible for more deaths. An EORTC trial comparing wide excision with tamoxifen for women aged ≥70 years showed that although there were more relapses in the former group, the mortality rate was the same (Fentiman et al., 2003). Wide excision plus tamoxifen may be an appropriate safe alternative to mastectomy in older women with ER+ breast cancer.

The prognosis in patients with operable breast cancer is determined by three main factors: tumour size, tumour type, and axillary node status and these have been combined in the Nottingham Prognostic Index (NPI) (Galea et al., 1992). The NPI score is derived as follows:

$$\begin{aligned}\text{NPI} = {} & 0.2 \times \text{tumour size} \\ & + \text{lymph node stage} \\ & \quad (1 = -\text{ve}, 2 = 1\text{–}3\text{nodes} + \text{ve}, \\ & \quad\ 3 = 4 + \text{nodes} + \text{ve}) \\ & + \text{histological grade} \\ & \quad (1 = \text{grade I}, 2 = \text{grade II}, 3 = \text{grade III})\end{aligned}$$

Based on the score, patients can be placed into prognostic categories as shown in Table 23.2.

Of these factors the most important is the axillary nodal status, not just positive or negative but the number of involved nodes. For this reason axillary clearance has been central to the treatment and staging of early breast cancer but its invariable use has been challenged. In >50% of cases the nodes are negative so that the patient could be said to have had an unnecessary operation which may be

Table 23.2 NPI score and prognosis

Group	Score	10 year survival
Excellent prognostic group	<2.4	95%
Good prognostic group	2.5–3.4	85%
Moderate prognostic group	3.4–5.4	70%
Poor prognostic group	>5.4	18%

followed by complications such as arm swelling (lymphoedema, numbness paraesthesiae pain from sensory nerve division and restriction of shoulder movement. For these reasons the sentinel node technique was adapted by Giuliano for staging patients with breast cancer (Giuliano, et al., 1994). Studies are underway to determine the suitability of this for general surgical use.

Before replacing axillary clearance with sentinel node biopsy it is important to be aware that the technique has a sensitivity of between 85% and 98%. If the axilla is under-staged the patient may be under-treated both locally and systemically since many oncologists in Europe would not give adjuvant cytotoxic chemotherapy to all node negative cases. Sentinel node biopsy will not work when lymphatic vessels or nodes are replaced with tumour and so the procedure has to be carried out with great care and selection.

For patients with primary tumours >4 cm, or with multifocal disease mastectomy is generally recommended because breast conservation therapy leads to an increased rate of breast relapse and often an unsatisfactory cosmetic outcome. For some women with large but operable primary tumours mastectomy may be an almost unacceptable option so that they will opt for primary systemic therapy (neo-adjuvant or up-front therapy). The aim is to shrink the tumour so that breast-conserving surgery is possible and this can be achieved in up to 95% of cases. For the few women with progressive or static disease a change of systemic therapy will be needed but some of these patients have a very poor prognosis because of their chemo-resistant disease. Local treatment is usually based on a combination of surgery and radiotherapy to try and achieve local control.

23.4 Lung cancer

Lung cancer is one of the commonest malignancies in men and kills more individuals than any other malignancy. More than 80% of cases are the result of smoking and the overall 5-year survival is only 15%. There are 2 main subtypes: small cell lung cancer (SCLC) and non-small cell lung cancer (NSCLC). The former is usually inoperable at diagnosis and treated with systemic therapy whereas NSCLC may be surgically resectable. NSCLC comprises four main histological types adenocarcinoma (50%), SCC (35%), large cell carcinoma (10%), and bronchoalveolar (5%).

Treatment depends upon the stage of the cancer and the performance status of the patient. As a result of smoking many of these patients have long-standing lung and heart disease. It is pointless resecting a tumour and surrounding normal tissue when the patient has such poor lung function that after surgery they would be unable to breath spontaneously. More than 50% of patients with NSCLC have inoperable disease at presentation and only 15% survive 5 years. Of those with stage I disease, 50% are alive at 5 years compared with 30% of those with stage II disease.

Originally thoracic surgeons removed the entire lung on the affected side (pneumonectomy) but this was associated with substantial mortality and nowadays the lobe or segment is removed (lobectomy/segmentectomy). The latter is associated with an increased likelihood of local relapse and illustrates the essential problem in surgical oncology: more extensive resections are associated with better tumour control but more morbidity and mortality, whereas lesser surgery may be responsible for more local relapses when attempting to cause fewer immediate problems for the patient. Because of the high mortality rate in resectable cases a variety of adjuvant treatments are being tested including cisplatin and etoposide.

23.5 Prostate cancer

This is the second commonest cancer in males, particularly affecting older men: over 80% of cases are diagnosed after age 65. Despite this, only 10% of men with prostate cancer die of the disease. This is the paradox of prostatic cancer: autopsy examination of men aged 70–79 reveals prostate cancer in 39% and this rises to 43% in those aged ≥80. Although the disease is present it is not causing many patients any problems and will not be responsible for their death.

Age is the major risk factor but there is also an increased risk in those with a family history of either prostatic or breast cancer. Vegetarians are at decreased risk and vitamins A and E may have a protective effect. Patients may be asymptomatic but the commonest complaint is difficulty with micturition, straining to start, frequency, and nocturia. All these can arise from benign prostatic hypertrophy as well as malignancy.

Many prostate tumours are hormone sensitive and the presence of dihydrotestosterone receptor is associated with response to androgen deprivation.

Unlike breast cancer the presence of either oestrogen or progesterone receptors does not relate to endocrine responsiveness. Androgen induces the production of a prostatic secretory glycoprotein, prostate-specific antigen that can be used with caution to screen for disease and monitor response.

The diagnosis is based on digital rectal examination and core needle biopsy. Prostate specific antigen (PSA) is elevated in serum, as is prostatic acid phosphatase. Both of these markers are not specific to malignancy and will be elevated after manipulation of the prostate by digital examination. If the disease is confirmed histologically other tests include transrectal ultrasound, radioisotopic bone scan ^{111}In-capromab pendetide (Protascint scan). The latter test uses antibodies to PSA, linked to ^{111}In in order to determine whether there has been spread to the lymph nodes.

Various grading tests for prostatic cancer have been devised but that in most widespread use is the Gleason system (Gleason et al., 1974). This divides tumours into five grades as shown in Table 23.4. The likelihood of progression and death within 15 years, if untreated, is also shown and among those with Gleason 5 grade tumours, discovered incidentally at surgery for presumed benign prostatic hypertrophy, 60–87% will die from prostate cancer. This has great importance since screening programmes for prostate cancer are being advocated and it is most important that asymptomatic individuals are not overtreated: those with low grade lesions may have a survival similar to that of age-matched controls without malignancy.

Patients selected for radical prostatectomy will be those with clinically localized tumours with 4/5 Gleason score and raised PSA levels who have a predicted life-expectancy of >15 years. The surgery aims to remove prostate, seminal vesicles, ampullae of vasa deferentia, and achieve tumour-free margins but this is not achieved in over 25% of cases. Lymph nodes are dissected for staging rather than therapeutic purposes and PSA levels >20 ng/ml are almost invariably associated with nodal involvement. Complications include impotence and urinary incontinence in up to 20% of cases. In a large series of 1153 patients treated by radical prostatectomy at the Mayo Clinic the 10 year survival was 75% with only 10% of cases dying of metastatic disease (Zincke et al., 1994).

The selection of patients for radical surgery remains highly controversial. Many surgeons believe that radical surgery carries the highest chance of cure, although the evidence that this is the case when compared either to radiation therapy or to a policy of careful follow-up in order to detect which patients have disease that will progress remains incomplete. Patterns of practice differ across the world with a greater enthusiasm for radical surgery in general in the United States, although a growing trend in this direction in Western Europe. Alternatives to radical therapy include observation or radical radiotherapy which can be delivered by external radiation beams or by implanting radioactive sources into the prostate in a process called brachytherapy. Both can produce control of small primary tumours without the need for radical resection of the prostate and associated tissues but still with significant local morbidity for the patient resulting from the effects of high doses of radiation. Randomized trials comparing radiation therapy with surgery have proved very difficult to deliver and currently new efforts to complete this work are being made in the United States and in Europe. The techniques involved in radiotherapy are critically important to good clinical outcomes. Usually the whole pelvis is irradiated with a boost to the prostate: a randomized

Table 23.3 Dukes staging of colorectal cancers (Dukes, 1932)

Dukes stage	Description	5-year survival (%)
A	Confined to bowel wall	85–95
B	Through bowel wall	60–80
C	Spread to lymph nodes	30–60

Table 23.4 Gleason grading for prostate cancer and survival

Grade	Description	15-year mortality (%)
1	Well-differentiated with uniform gland pattern	4–7
2	Well-differentiated with pleomorphic glands	6–11
3	Moderately differentiated with irregular acini or well-defined papillary or cribriform structures	18–30
4	Poorly differentiated with fused glands invading stroma	42–70
5	Poorly differentiated with minimal or no gland formation and central necrosis in tumour masses	60–87

trial showed that there is no benefit from pelvic node irradiation (Asbell et al., 1998). Long-term side effects may include for some patients rectal discharge, tenesmus, bleeding, and stricture, together with chronic cystitis, urethral stricture and impotence so the choice of therapy and its delivery are critically important.

To improve results, total androgen blockade with Goserelin and Flutamide has been used to shrink the tumour before radiation. Several clinical trials have shown that this reduces relapse rates and lowers mortality from prostate cancer. As with breast cancer, post-radiotherapy with a gonadotrophin releasing hormone analogue has been shown to also decrease both relapse and death from disease.

23.6 Colo-rectal cancer

Cancers of the large bowel are the third commonest tumour in both men and women and are responsible for >17,000 deaths annually in Britain. More than half the cases have rectal tumours, usually in the middle third. Of colonic cancers, half occur in the sigmoid (left side) and one quarter in the caecum and ascending colon (right side). The typical history is of a change in bowel habit sometimes associated with blood stained faeces. On the right side of the colon (caecum/ascending colon) the bowel contents are relatively fluid so that the cancer is less likely to cause obstruction but may cause symptoms of anaemia as a result of blood loss.

Approximately 25% of cases are the result of a genetic predisposition such as familial adenomatous polyposis (FAP) and hereditary non-polyposis colorectal cancer (HNPCC), but the majority have sporadic disease. Other risk factors include high animal fat diets, low vegetable intake, prior history of cholecystectomy, and ulcerative colitis. There will be a second synchronous tumour in about 5% depending on the rigorousness of the pre-operative work-up.

Unfortunately up to 15% of colorectal cancers are unsuspected until the patient presents with bowel obstruction. Such individuals may be very sick and are likely to be operated on as an emergency by a relatively inexperienced surgeon. Sometimes the correct treatment is to relieve the obstruction with a temporary colostomy before preparing the patient for subsequent elective surgery to resect the tumour. To reduce the numbers of patients presenting with bowel obstruction and to diagnose more early colon cancers population screening has been suggested, either faecal occult blood testing (FOBT) or colonoscopy in high risk cases. There is evidence that from large trials that FOBT may reduce mortality by up to 20% (Kronborg et al., 1996).

The investigation of a patient with suspected large bowel cancer includes double-contrast barium enema and flexible fibre-optic colonoscopy, an endoscope technique with a flexible endoscope that can visualize the whole colon. Rectal and sigmoid tumours may be visualized and biopsied with a sigmoidoscope, a shorter rigid or flexible scope which visualizes only the lower bowel. If a cancer is identified a biopsy is taken for confirmation and colonoscopy is carried out to exclude a second tumour. A CT scan is performed to determine whether hepatic metastases are present.

Cuthbert Dukes described the classical staging for colorectal cancer (Dukes, 1932). This relatively simple scheme does separate patients into different prognostic groups as shown in Table 23.3 but its applicability will depend upon the assiduousness of both the surgeon and the pathologist. Knowledge of the molecular genetics of colorectal cancer may also aid prognostic classification. Malignancy is characterized by an accumulation of genetic abnormalities due to hypermutability: 80% of colorectal cancers have chromosome instability and microsatellite stability (MSS). These tumours are aneuploid with K-*ras* mutation and loss of heterozygosity (LOH) at loci of *APC* and *p53* genes (Kinzler and Vogelstein, 1996). The other 20% of cancers have microsatellite instability (MSI) that can be high (MSI-H) or low (MSI-L). These tumours are diploid without LOH or K-*ras* mutation but with inactivation of genes including *TGF-α, IGF2r, and CDX2* (Jass et al., 1998).

The principles of surgery are to resect the tumour and surrounding normal bowel when possible together with its draining lymphatics which are associated with the arterial blood supply and to fashion non-leaking anastomoses of the bowel ends, avoiding a permanent colostomy whenever possible. When the disease is locally advanced and non-resectable, preoperative radiotherapy may render the tumour operable. For elective surgery the patient will need pre-operative counselling particularly if a colostomy is necessary on a temporary or permanent basis.

For rectal cancers the standard treatment used to be an abdomino-perineal excision of rectum (APER) which left the patient with a permanent colostomy. The situation has changed in the past 20 years and now up to 75% of patients are treated with sphincter sparing excision of the rectum and anastomosis of the colon to the anal canal, so avoiding the need for a colostomy. Sometimes a colonic pouch may be made to reduce urgency and frequency of defaecation. Carrying out a total mesorectal resection to completely remove the tumour and surrounding soft tissues reduces risk of local relapse significantly (Heald and Ryall, 1986).

Approximately 80% of colon cancers are operable and as many as 95% of rectal tumours, with an operative mortality of 5%. The overall 5-year survival is 50% so that surgery alone is unable to cure a substantial number of patients with colorectal cancer, although it may greatly improve quality of life by preventing or relieving bowel obstruction. The role of post-operative versus pre-operative radiotherapy is under investigation in clinical trials. Additionally the combination of radiotherapy and chemotherapy is being tested but there is, as yet, no consensus.

It is, however, clear that treatment with adjuvant chemotherapy after surgery does improve survival in those with Dukes' B and C colon tumours (i.e. those with more invasive primaries or lymph node metastases) (Buyse et al., 1988). The single agent which has been shown to be effective is 5-fluorouracil (5FU) but it has to be given for prolonged periods (6 months). Efficacy is improved by the addition of folinic acid (FA) possibly by levamisole but 5-FU plus FA is superior to 5-FU plus levamisole. Since the major site of distant metastases is the liver, 5-FU has been given via the portal vein and this may lead to an improvement in 5-year survival (Liver Infusion Meta-Analysis Group, 1997). Newer drugs including crinotecan and oxaliplatin are beginning to find a place in the treatment of colorectal cancer.

23.7 Conclusions

Other local treatments

While surgery and radiation therapy are by far the most widely used local treatments for cancer and the most effective, other approaches do exist. Ultrasonic destruction and radiowave destruction of individual metastasis, usually in the liver, have been widely applied but do not have a routine role in many centres. Photodynamic therapy in which patients are treated with drugs which are retained in tumours and sensitize them to light and then the tumours are locally exposed to intensive light sources can be very useful for superficial accessible tumours, most commonly in the lung. Cannulation of the blood supply of tumours to be followed by the introduction of agents which reduce blood flow either pharmacologically or physically (embolisation) can be useful ways of reducing a primary tumour either for palliation or to render surgery easier. Embolization can be particularly useful to reduce bleeding from tumours when radical surgery is not possible.

Surgery and radiotherapy remain mainstays of the effective treatment of cancer to irradicate the primary tumour with intent to cure the patient either by these local treatments alone or by combining these treatments with systemic drug therapies which will irradicate micro-metastatic disease. For patients who are not curable, surgery and radiotherapy can have great value to reduce the symptoms and loss of function that can result from primary cancer. They are likely to remain important parts of cancer treatment for many years to come, probably increasingly supplemented by our ability to generate combined modality approaches of which they will be a key part.

References

Asbell, S. O., Martz, K. L., Shin, K. H., Sause, W. T., Doggett, R. L., Perez, C. A. et al. (1998). Impact of surgical staging in evaluating the radiotherapeutic outcome in RTOG 77-06, a phase III study for T1BN0M0 (A2) and T2N0M0 (B) prostate carcinoma. *Int J Radiat Oncol Biol Phys*, **10**, 401–9.

Bartelink, H., Horiot, J. C., Poortmans, P., Struikmans, H., Van den Bogaert, W., Barillot I. et al. (2001). Recurrence rates after treatment for breast cancer with standard radiotherapy with or without additional radiation. *N Engl J Med*, **345**, 1378–87.

Buyse M., Zeleniuch-Jacquotte A., and Chalmers T. C. (1988). Adjuvant therapy of colorectal cancer. Why we still don't know. *JAMA*, **259**, 3571–8.

Cancer Research UK Cancerstats Monograph (2004). ed. J. R. Toms.

Dukes, C. E. (1932). The classification of cancer of the rectum. *J Path Bact*, **35**, 323–32.

Fentiman, I. S., van Zyl, J., Karydas, I., Chaudary, M. A., Margreiter, R., Legrand, C. et al. (2003). Treatment of operable breast cancer in the elderly: a randomised clinical trial EORTC 10850 comparing modified radical mastectomy with tumourectomy plus tamoxifen. *Eur J Cancer*, **39**, 300–8.

Galea, M. H., Blamey, R. W., Elston, C. E., and Ellis, I. O. (1992). The Nottingham Prognostic Index in primary breast cancer. *Breast Cancer Res Treat*, **22**, 207–19.

Giuliano, A. E., Kirgan, D. M., Guenther, J. M., and Morton, D. L. (1994). Lymphatic mapping and sentinel lymphadenectomy for breast cancer. *Ann Surg*, **220**, 391–401.

Gleason, D. F., Mellinger, G. T., and The Veterans Administration Cooperative (1974). Prediction of prognosis for prostatic adenocarcinoma by combined histological grading and clinical staging. *J Urol*, **111**, 58–64.

Heald, R. J. and Ryall, R. D. H. (1986). Recurrence and survival after mesorectal excision for rectal cancer. *Lancet*, **i**, 1479–82.

Jass, J. R., Do, K. A., Simms, L. A., Iino, H., Wynter, C., Pillay, S. P. et al. (1998). Morphology of sporadic colorectal cancer with DNA replication errors. *Gut*, **42**, 673–9.

Kinzler, K. W. and Vogelstein, B. (1996). Lessons from hereditary colorectal cancer. *Cell*, **87**, 159–70.

Kronborg, O., Fenger, C., Olsen, J., Jorgensen, O. D., and Sondergard, O. (1996). Randomised trial of screening for colorectal cancer with faecal occult blood test. *Lancet*, **348**, 1467–71.

Liver Infusion Meta-Analysis Group. (1997). Portal vein chemotherapy for colorectal cancer: a meta-analysis of 4000 patients in 10 studies. *J Natl Cancer Inst*, **89**, 497–501.

Morten, D. L., Wen, D. R., Wong, J. H., Economou, J. S., Cagle, L. A., Storm, F. K. et al. (1992). Technical details of intraoperative lymphatic mapping for early stage melanoma. *Arch Surg*, **127**, 392–9.

Zincke, H., Bergstralh, E. J., Blute, M. L., Myers, R. P., Barrett, D. M., Lieber, M. M. et al. (1994). Radical prostatectomy for clinically localized prostate cancer: long-term results of 1,143 patients from a single institution. *J Clin Onco*, **12**, 2254–63.

CHAPTER 24

Chemotherapy

D. Ross Camidge and Duncan I. Jodrell

24.1 Introduction

The term chemotherapy, under its broadest definition, covers any therapeutic intervention utilizing chemicals and includes the use of any pharmaceutical compound. However, in common oncological parlance, the term is taken to relate to the administration of cytotoxic drugs, often with significant side effects, to patients as part of the treatment of malignant disease. This chapter will concentrate on the scientific and clinical basis of using these traditional cytotoxic drugs to 'kill' malignant cells. Newer agents will also be discussed briefly to highlight the very significant changes in cancer drug discovery, development, and administration that are underway.

24.2 Mechanisms of action and resistance to traditional cytotoxic drugs

The site of action of almost all traditional cytotoxic drugs is the cellular DNA or the processes associated with this DNA (Figure 24.1). Drugs may interact directly with the DNA, intercalating between the bases (e.g. anthracyclines, actinomycin D), chemically altering the structure of DNA (adduct formation) (e.g. alkylating agents, mitomycin C, platinum compounds) or substituting the bases with analogous structures (e.g. 5-fluorouracil, cytarabine, gemcitabine). Drugs may deplete the pool of bases required for DNA (and RNA) synthesis (e.g. 5-fluorouracil, methotrexate, 6-mercaptopurine, 6-thioguanine). They may interact directly with various DNA-associated proteins such as topoisomerase I (e.g. irinotecan, topotecan) or topoisomerase II (e.g. etoposide). They may affect the microtubules that organize the chromosomes during mitosis (e.g. vinca alkaloids, taxanes).

For most cytotoxic drugs used clinically, although many of their main cellular sites of action have been identified, the precise mechanisms underlying their ability to kill cells often remain obscure. For example, cisdiamminedichloroplatinum (cisplatin) is used widely in the treatment of gynaecological, testicular, gastro-intestinal, and lung cancers. Following intra-cellular aquation, a highly reactive species is generated which binds covalently to macromolecules including DNA. Binding to DNA leads to predominantly intrastrand cross-links between adjacent guanines in the major groove of the DNA helix (interstrand guanine cross-links, direct DNA-protein cross-links, and

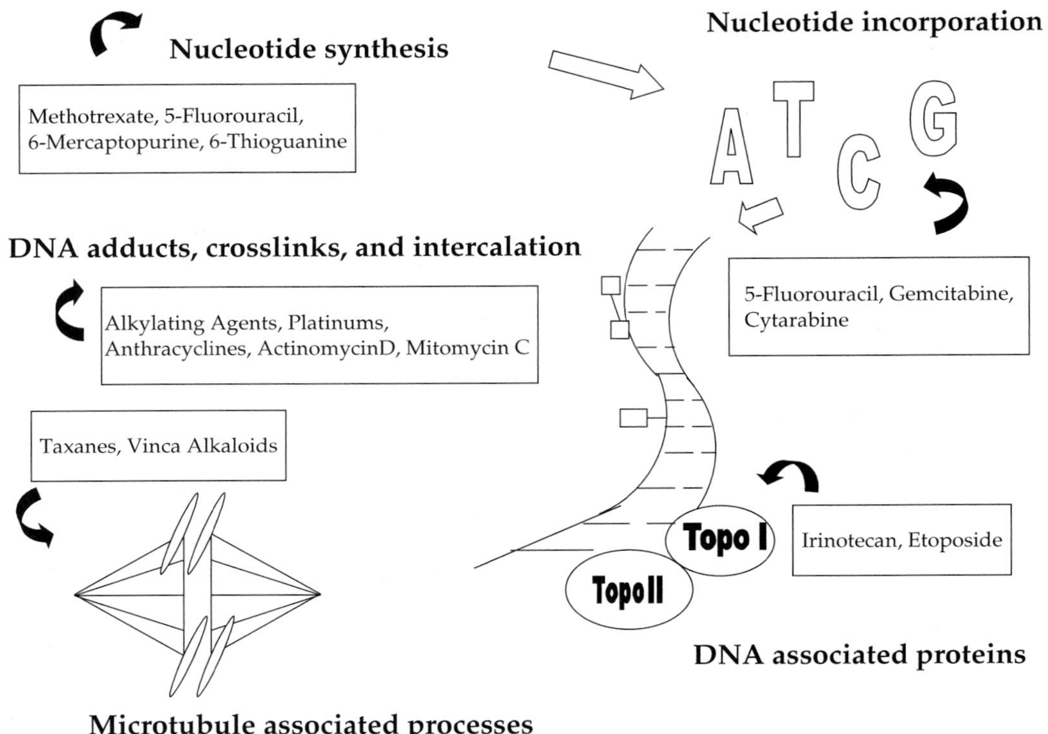

Figure 24.1 Cellular sites of action of traditional cytotoxic drugs. Many anticancer drugs have more than one site of action within the cell. The link between site of action and ultimate cellular outcome (e.g. cell cycle arrest, necrosis, or apoptosis) for most traditional cytotoxic drugs is often obscure.

adenine cross-links also occur, but at a much lower frequencies) (Raymond et al., 2002). Although it is not yet known which of these adducts is the most relevant to cytotoxicity, studies have shown that inactivation of the mismatch repair (MMR) genes *MLH1* and *MSH2* by mutation or by promoter methylation are associated with cellular resistance to cisplatin *in vitro* (Kelland, 2000). Hence, DNA-protein interactions—in the form of the MMR machinery—clearly have some role in transducing cisplatin's effects on DNA into phenotypic change. Whether the MMR complex predominantly institutes futile cycles of DNA repair at adduct sites producing single strand DNA breaks, or whether some direct signaling of, for example, the p53-dependent apoptotic pathway following adduct 'recognition' by the MMR complex is at present unclear.

In addition to DNA adduct formation and the potential role of the MMR complex in transducing this, like many other chemotherapeutic agents cisplatin may have multiple other actions within the cell that contribute to cell kill. For example, the distorting effect of platinum adducts on the helix induces binding of a range of different proteins to the surrounding area including TATA-binding protein, human upstream binding factor, high mobility group proteins 1 and 2, and sex-determining region Y protein. These proteins may trigger p53 directly, and/or the effect of DNA distortion in misdirecting these proteins to areas of DNA to which they are not normally bound ('molecular decoying') may also be significant (Hurley, 2002). In vitro 'DNA-independent' apoptotic signals, reflecting the fact that the majority of cisplatin within the cell is bound to protein and not to the DNA, have also been described (Raymond et al., 2002).

In addition to mediating sensitivity to certain cytotoxic drugs, active DNA damage recognition and repair mechanisms can also be involved in resistance to DNA-damaging drugs. For example,

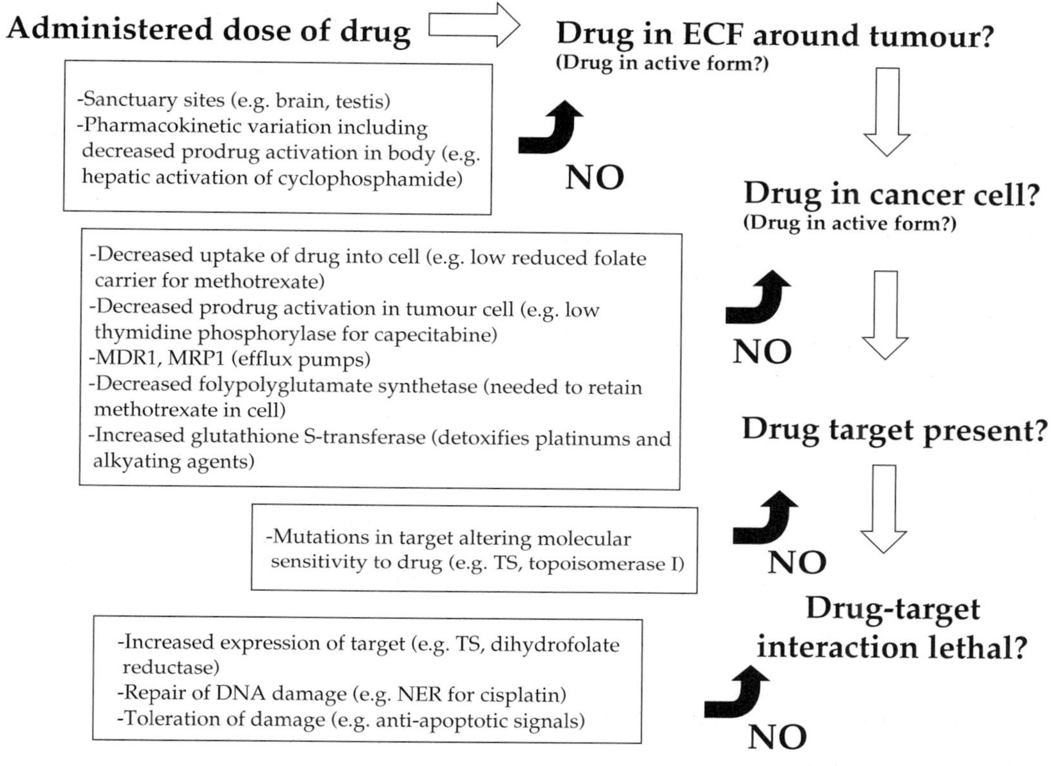

Figure 24.2 Mechanisms of innate and acquired resistance to traditional cytotoxic drugs.

increased tumour expression of ERCC1—a critical nucleotide-excision repair (NER) gene—has been shown to correlate with clinical drug resistance for platinum-containing chemotherapy regimes in gastric, ovarian, colorectal, and non-small cell lung cancer (Reed, 1998).

Drug resistance in cancer is common. Some tumours are inherently unresponsive to cytotoxic chemotherapy (e.g. renal carcinoma). Others may respond well initially but relapse rapidly with drug-resistant disease (e.g. small cell lung cancer). Many factors have been implicated in cellular resistance and these mechanisms may be drug or class specific (e.g. mutations of the cellular target or alterations in specific aspects of drug uptake and metabolism) or they may be associated with cross-resistance to a number of different drug classes (e.g. through the altered expression of drug efflux pumps that recognize drugs with related physico-chemical properties but different pharmacological targets—such as p-glycoprotein (mdr-1) and multi-drug resistance associated protein 1 (MRP1)—or anti-apoptotic signals such as p53 mutations and bcl-2 over-expression). Further examples of cellular mechanisms of cytotoxic drug resistance are given in Figure 24.2.

Even though cytotoxic drugs may have the same cellular target, they may interact with that target in different ways. For example, topoisomerase II is an enzyme that unwinds the supercoils of DNA by cutting, rotating, and rejoining the helix during replication, recombination, transcription, and chromosomal separation. Etoposide and doxorubicin are both topoisomerase II poisons that are used clinically. Each stabilizes one or more of the different 'cleavable complex' conformations of DNA and topoisomerase II, inducing double-strand breaks in the helix as the enzyme stalls part way through unwinding. Doxorubicin intercalates between the bases in DNA prior to interacting with the enzyme and stabilizes the cleavable complex formed before DNA processing (CC1). Etoposide, on the other hand, is not a DNA intercalator and only interacts with the DNA when it is already complexed with topoisomerase II, stabilizing the cleavable complexes formed both before and after DNA processing (CC1 and CC2). There is evidence that the sensitivity of cancer cells to topoisomerase II poisons may be directly proportional to their topoisomerase II content, as the enzyme functions not only as the target for these drugs but also as the primary effecter of the DNA damage (Kellner et al., 2002). In contrast to etoposide and doxorubicin, dexrazoxane acts on the same enzyme but as a catalytic inhibitor rather than as a poison and does not induce direct DNA breaks because it acts at other stages of the topoisomerase II enzymatic cycle than the cleavable complexes. As a consequence of this, overexpression of the topoisomerase enzyme is associated with reduced rather than enhanced antitumour activity of dexrazoxane *in vitro*. The clinical role of the catalytic inhibitors as cytotoxics is still being defined. In line with their different mechanisms of action, mutations in topoisomerase II associated with *in vitro* drug resistance to topoisomerase II poisons and to catalytic inhibitors cluster around different regions of the molecule (Kellner et al., 2002).

Pharmacokinetic factors also contribute towards mechanisms of resistance (Figure 24.2). For example, it is important to realize that for many anticancer drugs the administered form of the drug is not necessarily the active form. Variability in, for example, levels of activating or inactivating enzymes in the host tissues and/or in the tumour can lead to significant additional inter- and intra-individual variation in terms of normal tissue toxicity and antitumour efficacy from such drugs. Drugs in clinical use, which require metabolic activation include 5-fluorouracil (5-FU), capecitabine, cyclophosphamide, ifosfamide, and irinotecan. For example, 5-FU is inactive until metabolized to various active fluoronucleotides and fluoronucleosides within the cell. The most important 5-FU anabolites are 5-fluoro-2′-deoxyuridine-5′-monophosphate (FdUMP), the triphosphate of FdUMP (FdUTP), and 5-fluorouridine-5′-triphosphate (FUTP). FdUMP inhibits thymidylate synthase (TS), a key enzyme in *de novo* pyrimidine synthesis, leading to dTTP depletion, an unbalanced intracellular nucleotide pool and ultimately the formation of single-strand DNA breaks (although the precise mechanisms underlying these breaks are at present unknown). FUTP can also be incorporated directly into RNA, and FdUTP into DNA (Longley et al., 2003).

In addition to activation, metabolism is also important with regard to drug inactivation. For example, 5-FU is catabolized by dihydropyrimidine dehydrogenase (DPD) and cleared rapidly from the body. Therefore, administration of 5-FU by a bolus (short) injection leads to a high maximum concentration (Cmax) in the plasma, but a short duration of exposure. From animal and human studies this pharmacokinetic profile appears to favour FUTP incorporation into RNA. In contrast, continuous infusion regimes with low Cmax but prolonged exposure appear to favour TS inhibition. The TS inhibition of bolus regimes can be increased by the co-administration of 5-formyltetrahydrofolate (folinic acid), a reduced folate co-factor for TS that enhances 5-FU binding to the enzyme. These are examples of 'schedule dependency', whereby the administration of a drug by different schedules results in distinct biochemical effects and clinical outcomes. For example, the different dose limiting toxicities for 5-FU with the three different regimes are: bolus—leucopenia; bolus with folinic acid—leucopenia and mucositis; continuous infusion—palmar-plantar erythema. The tumour responses seen in patients with colorectal cancer are enhanced when folinic acid is added to bolus 5-FU (compared to bolus dosing alone) or by prolonged exposure schedules (compared to bolus dosing), supporting the notion that TS inhibition is the more important mechanism of action clinically.

Drug resistance may lead to lack of response at the time of treatment (when second line therapy using a different class of agent may be initiated) or, following an initial response the tumour regrows. On regrowth, a decision may be made whether to retreat with the same regimen or switch to second line therapy. This decision is usually based on the initial response to the drug and to the specific drug-free interval. With ovarian cancer and platinum therapy, for example, progression or relapse within 6 months of responding to platinum treatment tends to correlate with platinum resistant disease on retreatment. In contrast, progression or relapse more than 6 months after completion of platinum therapy tends to correlate with platinum sensitive disease on retreatment.

One explanation of the importance of drug-free interval in predicting sensitive and resistant disease relates to multiple populations of mutated cells existing in tumours. If relapse or progression occurs early it is presumed that the clones that were resistant to the drugs are likely to be the ones that are repopulating the tumour. The longer the time without a specific drug's selection pressure on resistant clones, the more likely it is that sensitivity to that drug will recur. For example, a number of ovarian cancers that progressed on platinum therapy have been documented as 'regaining' platinum sensitivity following a period of time on taxane treatment (Kavanagh et al., 1995).

24.3 Therapeutic principles of traditional cytotoxic chemotherapy

All of the targets for traditional cytotoxics in malignant dividing cells are also expressed within normal dividing cells. The cells in the normal human body which turnover most rapidly and therefore are those most impacted upon by traditional cytotoxics are those of the bone marrow, skin, hair follicle, and gastrointestinal mucosa. Acutely, there may be little difference between the damage sustained by the tumour and by these sensitive tissues from treatment. The essence of using traditional cytotoxics as therapy is therefore to produce an outcome differential between host and tumour that favours tumour cell death. One key to establishing such a differential between tumour and host is to exploit differences in their cellular ability to repair damage. Malignant cells tend to have impaired DNA damage repair machinery compared to normal cells. If treatment is given intermittently, subsequent doses can be timed to occur when the host has recovered but the tumour has not, gradually widening the differential cell kill. For each dose of chemotherapy it is thought that a constant fraction rather than an absolute number of malignant cells are killed (Skipper hypothesis).

Different normal tissues recover from a dose of chemotherapy at different rates. The most clinically relevant normal tissue is the bone marrow. The various circulating components of blood have different lifespans, being in order: white blood cells (1–3 days), platelets (10 days), and red blood cells (120 days). Although requirements for red blood cell transfusions are not uncommon after prolonged courses of chemotherapy, acutely it is the platelet and white cell counts that determine the timescales of intermittent dosing. The neutrophils are the most important white cells as their numbers correlate closely with the ability to fight off bacterial infections—the major risk factor from short-term immunosuppression. Most traditional cytotoxics produce nadir neutrophil counts between 7 and 10 days (conventionally a dose followed by a period of recovery is referred to as a cycle and cycle days are numbered in sequence from the first day of administration of the myelosuppressive chemotherapy). By day 21 the neutrophil count has usually recovered and so 3-weekly cycles of treatment are common. If, for whatever reason, the patient's neutrophil or platelet count has not recovered by the date of the next due cycle—age, previous chemotherapy, malignant bone marrow infiltration, bone marrow irradiation, and general malnutrition are all common reasons for blunted haematological stem cell responses—then two options are available. First, treatment may be delayed to allow further recovery (and, if the delay is very prolonged, particularly if it is associated with complications or significant non-haematological toxicities, then subsequent cycles may be given at a reduced dose). Second, bone marrow support may be utilized with transfusions (red cells, platelets, or peripheral blood stem cells), or haematological growth factors (erythropoetin, GCSF or GMCSF—viable platelet growth factors are still in development at present). Increasing haemoglobin levels with recombinant growth factor support has been associated with improved outcomes and/or better quality of life among patients undergoing radiotherapy, chemotherapy, and chemoradiotherapy (Littlewood, 2001). Randomized trials have proven the effectiveness of colony stimulating factors such as GCSF in the prevention and/or management of treatment-related neutropenic complications and in the maintenance of dose intensity (cf. Section 24.5) but direct associations between their use and improvements in response rate or survival have been more elusive (Dale, 2002).

24.3.1 Therapeutic settings

For all malignancies, treatments can be divided into those given with radical intent (i.e. with the potential for cure) and those given with palliative intent (i.e. to prolong life or reduce symptoms but with no potential to cure). Testicular tumours, lymphomas, leukaemias, and many solid tumours of childhood all have high cure rates from traditional cytotoxic chemotherapy alone, even when there is extensive disease. For certain types of localized solid tumours (e.g. breast and colon cancers), traditional cytotoxics have also been proven to increase the cure rate when administered

Table 24.1 Hypothetical reasons why overt metastatic disease is less likely to be curable with traditional cytotoxics than micrometastatic disease

1. Drug penetration into larger tumours may be poorer
2. Oxygen tension required for the activity of certain drugs (e.g. anthracyclines) in larger tumours may be lower
3. Percentage of proliferating cells in cycle in larger tumours may be lower
4. Patients with overt metastatic disease may have poorer performance status and fail to tolerate standard chemotherapeutic drug doses
5. Overt metastatic disease may be accompanied by obvious (e.g. liver dysfunction due to tumour infiltration) or more subtle (e.g. paraneoplastic) deleterious effects on drug pharmacokinetics
6. Larger tumours contain larger numbers of cells and, through the accumulation of mutations, resistant clones are more likely to exist (Goldie–Coldman hypothesis)

immediately after potentially curative surgery. However, these same cancers are incurable with chemotherapy when in the metastatic setting. Why micrometastatic and overt metastatic disease should differ so much in their apparent chemosensitivity is unclear, but some hypothetical reasons are outlined in Table 24.1.

Treatment relating to localized or early disease can be subdivided by its temporal relationship to the surgery. Treatment that is given soon after surgery, when there is no residual cancer detectable, to increase the chances of a cure is referred to as adjuvant treatment (because it is considered an *adjunct* to the surgery). Treatment that is administered prior to surgery is referred to as neo-adjuvant treatment. The aims of neo-adjuvant chemotherapy include reducing the bulk of the primary tumour (to make the surgery easier or less mutilating, rendering inoperable tumours operable and, just as with adjuvant chemotherapy, the early treatment of micro-metastatic disease (see further)). Neoadjuvant treatment has one major advantage over adjuvant treatment, in that if the cancer is not responding to the drugs then it may be detected and the drugs changed or the chemotherapy abandoned. Adjuvant treatment, on the other hand, is entirely directed against micro-metastatic disease, which, by definition, is undetectable. Therefore it is never known at the time of adjuvant therapy whether an individual patient is responding to the treatment or not. Conversely, a disadvantage of neoadjuvant treatment is that if complications of treatment occur or, as above, if no response is achieved then the definitive anticancer treatment of surgery will have been delayed. Some patients (and surgeons) also find it hard psychologically postponing their surgery to undergo neoadjuvant treatment.

For malignancies in which surgery does not play a definitive therapeutic role, terms such as adjuvant and neoadjuvant are inappropriate and a different therapeutic terminology is required. For example, leukaemias are often treated sequentially through 'remission induction' (analogous to neoadjuvant), 'consolidation' (analogous to adjuvant), and 'maintenance' chemotherapy (no real solid tumour equivalent at present).

Classically, new cytotoxic drugs have been introduced into clinical practice in a defined order, being tested initially in advanced disease after all other established treatments have failed. Adjuvant or neoadjuvant treatment is usually studied only after efficacy has been established in the advanced disease setting first.

Traditional cytotoxics can also contribute to radical treatments when given concurrently with radiotherapy ('chemoradiotherapy') in either the neoadjuvant setting (e.g. for down-staging rectal carcinoma) or as definitive anticancer treatments in their own right (e.g. for anal carcinoma). In these situations the chemotherapy acts as a radiosensitizer enhancing the effects of the radiation on both normal and malignant tissues. The drugs most commonly used for this purpose are 5-FU, gemcitabine, and cisplatin. The mechanisms of radiosensitization have been investigated, but the precise mechanisms of radiosensitization remain unknown (Lawrence et al., 2003). *In vitro*, cells are particularly resistant to radiotherapy when they are in S phase, yet cell cycle arrest at G1 before S phase prevents radiosensitization by both 5-FU and gemcitabine, indicating that inducing increased S phase radiosensitivity may be important.

Despite our increasing knowledge of mechanisms of drug sensitivity and resistance, a major predictor of outcome from treatment remains the 'fitness' of the patient which is conventionally recorded as the Performance Status (PS). This may be because either low PS is a surrogate for poor prognosis disease and/or it is harder to administer therapeutic doses of cytotoxic to patients with a low PS (Andreyev et al., 1998). The two most commonly used methods of ranking PS are the ECOG and Karnofsky systems (Table 24.2).

Table 24.2 Patient performance status scales

Karnofsky Performance Status	
100	Normal, no complaints, no evidence of disease
90	Able to carry on normal activity, minor signs, or symptoms of disease
80	Normal activity with effort, some signs, or symptoms of disease
70	Cares for self, unable to carry on normal activity or to do work
60	Requires occasional assistance from others but able to care for most needs
50	Requires considerable assistance from others, frequent medical care
40	Disabled, requires special care and assistance
30	Severely disabled, hospitalization indicated; death not imminent
20	Very sick, hospitalization necessary, active supportive treatment necessary
10	Moribund
0	Dead
ECOG Performance Status	
0	Asymptomatic
1	Symptomatic, fully ambulatory
2	Symptomatic, in bed $< 50\%$ of day
3	Symptomatic, in bed $> 50\%$ of day but not bedridden
4	Bedridden
5	Dead

24.3.2 Early and late side effects of cytotoxic chemotherapy

Drug side-effects may reflect either the primary antiproliferative action of the drug (e.g. myelosuppression with alkylating agents), some less well understood but predictable toxicological effect (e.g. palmar-plantar erythema with infusional 5-FU) or they may be entirely idiosyncratic (e.g. radiation recall dermatitis with anthracyclines). Side-effects may occur 'early'–within a few hours or days of the initial administration of the chemotherapy, or 'late'—weeks into treatment, or months, or even years after treatment has finished (Table 24.3). Early side-effects are common and usually temporary (although they can occasionally be long-lived—for example, platinum-induced peripheral neurotoxicity). Late onset side-effects are relatively rare, not least because of the generally short life-span of many oncology patients, but if they occur they are usually permanent and can be disabling.

In addition to dose adjustments and dose delays many supportive measures exist to minimize either the chances of developing, or the severity of side-effects (Table 24.4). In general, using such measures, it should be possible for many patients to experience a reasonable quality of life while on treatment and relatively uncommon for treatment to be curtailed due to unmanageable toxicity.

Table 24.3 Examples of early- and late-side-effects of traditional cytotoxic chemotherapy (and the class of drugs or specific drug associated with each side-effect)

Early side-effects
Nausea (anthracyclines, cisplatin, alkylating agents)
Alopecia (anthracyclines, alkylating agents, taxanes)
Myelosuppression (anthracyclines, taxanes, alkylating agents)
Diarrhoea (5-FU, irinotecan)
Mucositis (5-FU, etoposide, methotrexate)
Peripheral neurotoxicity (cisplatin, taxanes)
Ototoxicity (cisplatin)
Nephrotoxicity (cisplatin)
Discolouration of urine (anthracyclines)
Late side-effects
Cardiotoxicity (anthracyclines)
Myelodysplasia/acute leukaemia (alkylating agents, etoposide)
Premature menopause (alkylating agents)
Infertility (alkylating agents)
Pulmonary fibrosis (bleomycin, mitomycin C)

Table 24.4 Examples of supportive measures to minimize traditional cytotoxic chemotherapy side effects

Side effect	Supportive measure
General	
Nausea and vomiting	Antiemetics (e.g. 5HT3 antagonists, corticosteroids)
Myelosuppression	Haematological growth factors
Mucositis/gastritis/diarrhoea	Mouth washes/proton pump inhibitors/loperamide
Alopecia	Scalp cooling
Specific	
Haemorrhagic cystitis (cyclophosphamide, ifosfamide)	MESNA
Encephalopathy (ifosfamide)	Methylene blue
Cardiotoxicity (anthracyclines)	Dexrazoxane
Sterility (alkylating agents)	Sperm banking, emergency IVF with embryo freezing

24.4 Traditional cytotoxic drug discovery: from bench to bedside

The compound screening approaches that have been used, until recently, to discover and develop potential anticancer drugs have been successful in identifying agents that are inherently cytotoxic. Following optimization of a promising compound preclinically, clinical drug trials are then undertaken. With traditional cytotoxics this progresses through three distinct phases (I, II, and III), to produce evidence of tolerability and efficacy (both absolute and comparative) sufficient to allow the drug to be licensed for clinical use and marketed. Post-licensing studies are also often performed and these are referred to as phase IV trials.

24.4.1. Pre-clinical screens and drug optimisation

Screening models to select anticancer agents for evaluation in clinical trials have been developed since the late 1940s (Goodman and Walsh, 2001). In addition to private initiatives, national institutions, for example the US National Cancer Institute (NCI), have taken a leading role in setting up high throughput screening systems. Compounds are derived from academic or industrial research, from developments in organic chemistry, isolates from fermentation broths and cultures, or extracts of higher order plants and animals.

In 1955, the NCI's screen included just three transplantable rodent malignancies: Sarcoma 180, Carcinoma 755, and Leukaemia L1210. In 1975, a pre-screen involving murine leukaemia P388 was instituted and successful compounds then progressed to testing against human tumours grown as xenografts in immunodeficient congenitally athymic nude mice.

Assessments of anti-cancer activity in *in vivo* models are usually based on assessing the volume of a tumour over a given period of time following implantation, with and without the screened chemical. If the tumour is allowed to establish itself first, before the animal is exposed to the screened chemical, then tumour regression rather than growth inhibition may also be assessed. The reasons for a particular tumour model or line being included or excluded from a screening programme relate to their performance. For example, the rodent tumours used in the initial plant screening programme of the NCI—out of which came paclitaxel, irinotecan, and topotecan—were very sensitive to tannins and had to be substituted because of unacceptably high false positive rates (Goodman and Walsh, 2001).

The latest NCI screening programme consists of an initial *in vitro* human tumour cell line assay comprising up to 60 different cell types (Johnson et al., 2001). In this assay, cells are fixed after incubation with or without drug and then stained with Sulforhodamine B (a protein-binding dye). The dye is solubilized and read spectrophotometrically to reveal relative cell growth or viability. After success in the cell line assay an intermediate screen of tissue culture cells grown in hollow fibres in mouse peritoneal or subcutaneous spaces takes place before compounds are finally tried on a panel of xenografts.

Although such screening programmes have been vital in identifying clinically useful anticancer agents, it is important to remember that malignant cells grown *in vitro* or as xenografts become selected for and/or induced to develop various cellular characteristics that may not have been present in the original tumour. As such, the responses of established cell lines and xenografts to any screened chemical can differ significantly from those of cancers in clinical situations (Johnson et al., 2001).

Following the identification of a compound of interest in the *in vitro* and *in vivo* screens, considerable further work is required before a new chemical entity can be administered to humans. Synthetic chemistry is required to investigate minor modifications in structure that may enhance activity or patent life (a strong commercial position is often required to justify the huge costs associated with drug discovery and development). Physicochemical analyses are also required to assess whether the chemical entity will be 'druggable' (i.e. whether it will be stable, whether it will be soluble under physiological conditions, etc). Synthetic routes suitable for large-scale commercial synthesis of the compound rather than simply for the small quantities needed for laboratory work must also be developed. Pharmacokinetic (PK) studies are required using different routes of administration (intravenous or oral, for example) to determine each compound's absorption (for oral preparations), distribution, metabolism, and excretion. These PK studies have a significant impact on the compound selected and on the route and scheduling of administration chosen for subsequent clinical trials. The determination of routes of excretion also helps to guide whether the drug will have to be given with particular care in those with liver or kidney dysfunction.

The cytotoxic nature of many of the drugs discovered to date means that the most effective clinical dose is often close to the dose that is tolerable due to normal tissue toxicity (referred to as a narrow therapeutic margin). Therefore one tenet of cytotoxic drug development has been to determine the maximum tolerated dose (MTD) in animals. In rodents the MTD for cytotoxic drug development is usually considered to be the LD_{10}—the dose, for any given route/schedule of administration, at which 10% of the animals die. In non-rodent toxicology studies of cytotoxic agents, lethality studies are not usually undertaken to determine an LD_{10} and therefore the definition of the MTD is more subjective. At present, in the United Kingdom, non-rodent studies are not necessary to obtain regulatory approval for early clinical trials with novel cytotoxic agents. In addition to providing an approximation of the dose that will be the MTD in human studies, detailed toxicological studies also act as a guide to the specific toxicities that may be expected in man (allowing decisions to be made as to whether these would or would not be acceptable). Highly specialized toxicology studies providing information on particular issues that cannot be confirmed in human trials, such as teratogenicity and the drug's effects on fertility are also performed. Positive 'signals' in either of these would not necessarily preclude the development of a cytotoxic agent in cancer patients, but the information is useful in determining the full implications of treating humans with the drug.

If a chemical entity does manage to get over all of the 'hurdles' of pre-clinical development, it may then proceed to being developed as a potential therapy in human clinical drug trials.

24.4.2 Phase I: 'First in man' (safety and tolerability)

Having established the toxicities for a promising compound's given route and schedule of administration in animals, one-tenth of the rodent equivalent LD_{10}, appropriately scaled between species, is most commonly used as the starting dose for human trials (Eisenhauer et al., 2000). Scaling dose from animals to man (allometric scaling) tends to be done on the basis of body surface area (BSA), that is dosage per square metre, as this correlates with differences between species in basal metabolic rate, blood volume and glomerular filtration rate (GFR) better than body weight (Gurney, 1996).

In a phase I study the goal is to characterize the safety and tolerability of the new compound and establish the MTD for man. Phase I studies of non-oncology drugs are often performed in healthy volunteers, but the highly toxic, sometimes genotoxic, nature of traditional cytotoxics means that all human trials of these drugs, including phase I studies, are usually only performed in cancer patients.

Classically, cohorts of three patients receive multiple courses of the new drug with regular toxicological and PK assessments. After a defined period of time on treatment, provided the toxicities experienced by the last cohort were acceptable, a new cohort is recruited and treated at the next highest dose. Toxicities are recorded according to a defined grading system developed by the NCI called the Common Toxicity Criteria, or from March 2003 the Common Terminology Criteria for Adverse Events (CTC). Using these criteria (http://ctep.cancer.gov) toxicities can be graded formally as 0, 1, 2, 3, or 4 (roughly corresponding to absent, mild, moderate, severe or life-threatening, respectively).

As the MTD is neared additional patients are recruited into the cohorts to further characterize the dose levels. The human MTD is taken as the dose at which a third or more of patients in a dose cohort (usually 2 out of 6) develop pre-defined 'dose limiting' toxicities (DLTs)—often taken as any grade 3 non-haematological toxicity or grade 4 haematological toxicity (severe myelosuppression that either lasts for more than 5 days or is associated with complications such as infection). The acceptance of more severe haematological than non-haematological toxicities is because haematological toxicities are seen with many traditional cytotoxics and considered manageable using modern supportive techniques. In addition, in certain situations, the absence of haematological toxicity may be associated with underdosing of cytotoxic drugs (cf. Section 24.5).

Having identified the MTD, the dose level immediately below is nominated as the recommended dose to take through to the phase II studies. The number of patients required for a phase I study cannot be accurately predicted in advance, but usually about 20–30 patients are involved.

The methods used for dose escalation between cohorts in a phase I study are evolving. Classically, the commonest method has been the so-called modified Fibonacci approach, loosely based on a historical mathematical sequence of gradually reducing fractional changes. This approach allows large dose escalations at the beginning of a trial but more caution at higher doses when the anticipated MTD is being approached and toxicities are appearing. This rigid approach does mean that many patients will be treated at dose levels that are sub-therapeutic, particularly if the predicted human MTD based on preclinical animal data is inappropriately low. Newer rapid dose escalation models with only single patients at the lowest doses, with or without continual reassessment methods such as those based around Bayesian statistics to 'fine tune' the dose levels from the observed toxicity or pharmacokinetic data are therefore becoming popular.

Entry criteria for Phase I trials usually demand a reasonable level of fitness from the patients and all tumour types are eligible, as safety and tolerability rather than efficacy are the primary endpoints. It is important that patients are counselled as to these end-points and do not assume that they are receiving drug treatment in a schedule or at doses associated with optimal anticancer activity. In light of the resulting low chance of an individual responding in a phase-I study, patients recruited into these studies have usually exhausted all other conventional therapies for their disease.

24.4.3 Assessing efficacy in clinical trials

Clinical trials in oncology have strict criteria for assessing anticancer efficacy to allow decisions to be made about the development of a particular drug or drug combination. Separate groups of endpoints apply to clinical trials performed in the adjuvant, neoadjuvant, and advanced disease settings. In clinical trials, as cancer is a life-shortening disease, the standards for assessing efficacy relate to survival. In the advanced disease setting, absolute survival is considered the most important and is usually expressed as the median survival time, assessed using Kaplan/Meier statistics. In the adjuvant and neoadjuvant settings, absolute survival may also be chosen as the most important endpoint but it is often quoted as the proportion of patients alive at a fixed time point that depends on the natural history of the disease—that is, the timepoint beyond which relapse and death is considered unlikely—for example, 3 years for small-cell lung cancer or 5 years for colorectal cancer. Cancer free survival (also referred to as disease free survival) is another common endpoint that is assessable at an earlier time point than absolute survival—important when survival with metastatic disease may be prolonged due to the nature of the underlying disease (e.g. in breast cancer) or due to the impact of any subsequent 'salvage' chemotherapies.

Objective response rate (ORR) is a surrogate marker of efficacy that is commonly used in both the advanced disease and in the neoadjuvant trial setting. Using clinical or radiological measurements of tumour size before and after treatment any given change can be categorized into a complete response (CR), a partial response (PR), stable disease (SD), or progressive disease (PD). The ORR of a treatment is conventionally taken as the percentage of patients who achieve either a complete or a partial response, defined using either the WHO or RECIST (response evaluation criteria for solid tumours) schemes (Table 24.5).

Outwith clinical trials, since much of the treatment of patients with advanced cancer is palliative, disease stabilization, especially if it is associated with a meaningful reduction in symptoms is usually thought of as sufficient to consider the therapy successful. The details of how chemotherapy impacts on, for example, the paraneoplastic

Table 24.5 Criteria for evaluating tumour responses

WHO (1979)—Evaluation of target lesions based on product of perpendicular dimensions (cross-sectional area) of each lesion

- **Complete Response** (CR): Disappearance of all target lesions
- **Partial Response** (PR): At least a 50% decrease in the product of the longest perpendicular dimensions of target lesions,taking as reference the baseline product
- **Progressive Disease** (PD): At least a 25% increase in the product of the longest perpendicular dimensions of target lesions, taking as reference the baseline product, or the appearance of one or more new lesions
- **Stable Disease** (SD): Neither sufficient shrinkage to qualify for PR nor sufficient increase to qualify for PD, taking as reference the baseline product

RECIST (2000)—Evaluation of target lesions based on sum of longest dimensions (LD) of separate lesions

- **Complete Response** (CR): Disappearance of all target lesions
- **Partial Response** (PR): At least a 30% decrease in the sum of the LD of target lesions, taking as reference the baseline sum LD
- **Progressive Disease** (PD): At least a 20% increase in the sum of the LD of target lesions, taking as reference the smallest sum LD recorded since the treatment started, or the appearance of one or more new lesions
- **Stable Disease** (SD): Neither sufficient shrinkage to qualify for PR nor sufficient increase to qualify for PD, taking as reference the smallest sum LD since the treatment started

cytokine environment, to explain improvements in quality of life when there is no tumour shrinkage are unknown. However, quality of life, formally assessed using structured general and disease specific questionnaires, is becoming increasingly recognised as a valuable trial endpoint in its own right.

24.4.4 Phase II (absolute efficacy)

In a phase II study the efficacy of the drug is assessed in patients at the recommended dose established in the phase I study. A single tumour type in the advanced setting is chosen for each study and many phase II studies may be undertaken for any given new agent. Traditional phase II cytotoxic studies are not controlled, whereas placebo controls are almost universal in the phase II studies of non-oncology drugs.

Dose adjustments in phase II are allowed—both dose reductions and, increasingly, dose escalations (based on the absence of toxicity)—to ensure that patients are treated close to their 'individual' MTD. Efficacy in phase IIs is largely assessed by the ORR (Table 24.5), often via a 2 stage approach (Simon 2 stage design): X patients are treated initially with a further Y patients being treated providing a response is seen in the first stage. If a certain total number of responders are seen when accrual is complete, the values of X and Y aim to minimise the number of patients required to assign activity to a drug at a minimum specified ORR (e.g. 20%) and a given statistical probability of this assessment being correct (e.g. $p < 0.05$). Randomized phase IIs or so-called phase IIb studies investigating different doses, schedules, or combinations of treatment in larger numbers of patients with less stringent statistical criteria than in traditional phase III trials may also be undertaken. These may be stand-alone studies that inform subsequent phase III studies or, if designed properly, when preliminary findings are favourable, phase IIb studies may be extended directly into phase III studies by recruiting sufficient patients to allow more robust statistical comparisons.

24.4.5 Phase III (comparative efficacy)

Phase III studies compare the efficacy of new drugs with established standard therapies in patients with the same tumour type and stage of disease. Therapy in either the advanced disease or adjuvant setting may be assessed. Treatments are assigned randomly and large numbers of patients may be required to detect small differences in outcome with robust statistical significance (e.g. at p values of < 0.05, or less if multiple comparisons are involved).

24.5 Getting the dose and schedule right

For most cancer therapeutics, the narrow therapeutic margin between efficacy and toxicity has led to the desire to administer doses that are 'individualized' and, historically, the patient's BSA has been used for this purpose. However, for the majority of cytotoxic drugs the evidence supporting this clinical practice is debatable (Gurney, 1996) as there is often poor correlation between BSA-based dosing and the plasma concentration profiles achieved. Reasons for this include inherited and induced inter- and intra-patient variation in drug-specific metabolizing enzymes and transporters (Innocenti and Ratain, 2002), and variations in the patients' body composition in terms of fat, muscle, or oedema. Therapeutic drug monitoring, involving increasing or decreasing the amount of drug given to an individual, based on repeated blood sampling, to achieve target plasma concentrations is an alternative method of dosing. However, due to the complexities of sample collection and analysis associated with its implementation, it has not been adopted widely, except in the monitoring of methotrexate concentrations after high-dose therapy to guide folinic acid rescue. Dose calculation methods are used based on clearance estimates from a physiological variable, but only for one drug—carboplatin. Carboplatin is almost entirely cleared as the parent compound by glomerular filtration with minimal tubular excretion or absorption. A simple formula (the Calvert equation) exists for predicting the dose of carboplatin required to produce a given area under the time-concentration curve (AUC) from the patient's GFR: Dose in $\text{mg} = \text{AUC}\ (\text{GFR} + 25)$.

However they are derived, using plasma exposures to guide dosing is only ever useful if there is a clear relationship between the PK profile of the drug and its toxicity (effect on normal tissue) and/or efficacy (effect on tumour). Plasma concentrations are a surrogate for drug concentration in the tumour and concentrations of drug within the particular tissues may be more relevant. Techniques such as microdialysis and Positron Emission

Tomography (PET) scanning using customized radio-isotopes have been used for this purpose, but it is unlikely that such techniques could ever be applied to routine clinical practice.

Given the marked genetic heterogeneity of tumour as opposed to normal tissues, it is not surprising that positive PK correlations are more frequently noted for toxicity than for efficacy (Gurney, 1996). The PK parameter that has been shown to correlate most commonly with anti-proliferative toxicity, that is, myelosuppression, is the AUC. In contrast, for certain toxicities, such as the cardiomyopathy associated with anthracycline use, the total cumulative dose and Cmax are more relevant (Keefe, 2001).

In future, specific inherited predispositions relating to pharmacokinetic and pharmacodynamic variability may be screened for in advance. For example, phenotypic inactivity in thiopurine methyltransferase (TPMT) was found to be present in 71% of acute lymphoblastic leukaemia patients with bone marrow intolerance to 6-mercaptopurine (Innocenti and Ratain, 2002). 6-mercaptopurine doses are now modified on the basis of TPMT genotype on a routine basis at certain centres. In contrast, DPD—the major 5-FU metabolizing enzyme—is completely or partially deficient in 0.1% and 3–5%, of patients, respectively, yet a normal DPD phenotype is present in from 33—66% of cases of severe 5-FU toxicity (Innocenti and Ratain, 2002), indicating that the basis of toxicity variation for many chemotherapy drugs may be multi-factorial.

When PK-efficacy correlations have been noted for certain drugs they have generally been in highly chemosensitive malignancies, such as with methotrexate in acute lymphoblastic leukaemia (Gurney, 1996; Evans et al., 1998).

Dose-tailoring using a toxicity endpoint such as myelosuppression as a surrogate for efficacy, escalating drug doses to achieve particular depths or durations of haematological nadirs, has been advocated for a number of different malignancies and cytotoxic drugs largely based on retrospective correlations between nadir counts and response rates (Gurney, 1996). This practice cannot be applied easily to the use of drugs in combination and it rests on the assumption that the dose–response curves for bone marrow and tumour are similar, which may or may not be true depending on the drug and tumour involved. However, the principle of avoiding underdosing should be taken as just as important as that of avoiding overdosing in optimal anticancer treatment.

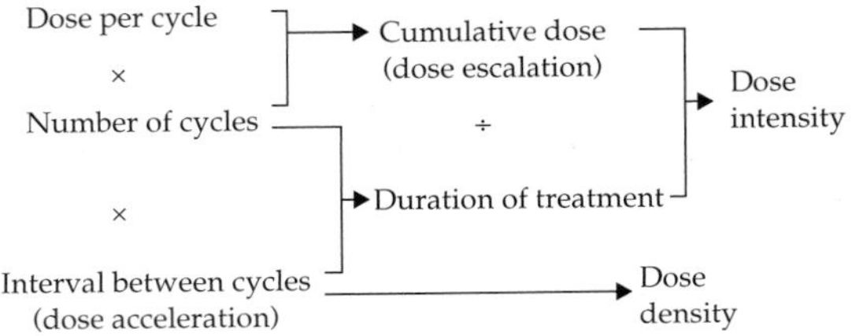

Figure 24.3 Parameter relationships relevant to dose and schedule of chemotherapy drugs with multiple cycles of treatment. Of note, increases in dose intensity may be achieved by either dose escalation and/or dose acceleration.

Different parameters of dosing have been described in an attempt to define the most effective method of delivering cytotoxic drugs over multiple cycles of treatment. These relate to the size of each individual dose, the total or cumulative dose administered, the dose intensity (cumulative dose ÷ treatment duration), and the frequency of individual dosing events (dose density) (Figure 24.3).

With regard to dose, certain drugs show log-linear dose–response curves *in vitro* over a wide range of concentrations (e.g. melphalan), while others show responses that plateau after relatively small concentration increments (e.g. paclitaxel). These differences would suggest that some cytotoxics may produce greater anticancer effects when given to patients at higher doses (provided that the patients could be supported through the toxicities of the procedure), while other drugs, which are already at the ceiling of their activity, will show very little change in efficacy with dose escalation.

In 'high dose' chemotherapy regimes, using drugs such as melphalan, the normal bone marrow function is completely ablated and transplantation using either autologous peripheral blood stem cells or bone marrow, is required to 'rescue' the patients. While some improvements in outcome have been shown for haematological malignancies such as multiple myeloma or non-Hodgkin's lymphoma, there remains no proven benefit of such extremes of dose escalation in comparison to standard dose regimes, for the majority of solid tumours tested so far, including breast and small cell lung cancer (Tjan-Heijen et al., 2002).

Dose intensity, in contrast to dose escalation, is measured in dose/unit time (e.g. mg m^{-2} $week^{-1}$), recognizing that, in addition to the effect of dose per se, gaps between doses may allow tumour repopulation, reducing treatment efficacy. Clinically, increasing the dose intensity of various solid tumour regimes with growth factor support has been investigated, but convincing evidence of improvements in outcome is minimal, indicating that we may already be close to the optimal dose intensity for many regimes (Tjan-Heijen et al., 2002; Savarese et al., 1997).

Dose density has been suggested recently as an additional therapeutic concept to address the importance of dosing frequency, partly because of the increasing awareness of the higher fraction of cells cycling in experimental than in clinical tumours. As such, each chemotherapy dose may be killing a far greater percentage of cells in the experimental system than the equivalent single dose in a slower growing human tumour. Therefore more frequent dosing than conventionally used in human anticancer regimes (dose acceleration) may be preferential.

For a single chemotherapy drug, one extreme of increasing the dose density is to deliver the drug by continuous infusion (aaaaaa versus A..A..). This is particularly relevant for phase specific drugs ensuring exposure to cells at the relevant stage of the cell cycle. The impact of such scheduling changes on the pharmacological action of 5-FU has already been discussed. Etoposide is another phase specific drug and its efficacy in small cell lung cancer has clearly been shown to be better with lower doses given by repeated dosing compared to a single large dose (Joel et al., 1994).

Chronomodulation is a particular continuous infusion technique that uses variable rate pumps (aaAAaa versus aaaaaa) in an attempt to exploit the different circadian rhythms in normal and malignant cells of target (e.g. DNA synthesis) and metabolizing enzyme activities (e.g DPD for 5-FU) to minimize chemotherapeutic toxicity and maximize efficacy (Levi et al., 1997).

The optimal treatment duration ('number of cycles') is likely to vary between tumour types, between different drug combinations and in different therapeutic settings. For example, there is considerable debate in the advanced disease setting over whether a pre-defined number of cycles should be given, or whether treatment should continue until disease progression. In favour of a defined number of cycles is the avoidance of cumulative toxicities of treatment and the fact that as the maximum response may be achieved after a defined number of cycles only *a priori* resistant clones are being exposed to further therapy. In contrast, treatment until progression may be maintaining control over any surviving sensitive clones. Neither argument is well proven. In practice, 4–8 cycles, with assessments of benefit after every 6–12 weeks tends to be standard practice in the United Kingdom, but in Europe and the United States more prolonged treatment is usual.

Combinations of cytotoxic drugs with non-overlapping mechanisms of action (to limit the effects of drug resistance) and toxicity are often used in oncology. Within a single cycle, drugs may be given in a particular order. One mechanistic reason for a preferred sequence of administration within a cycle relates to the phase-specificity of certain drugs (Table 24.6). For example, paclitaxel stabilizes microtubule assembly and is most active during the M phase of the cell cycle. Cisplatin is non-phase specific (being able to form adducts in all phases of the cell cycle), but produces cell cycle arrest at the G2/M checkpoint. If cisplatin is given before paclitaxel in experimental models there is antagonism of anticancer efficacy, but not if it is given after paclitaxel (Shah and Schwartz, 2001).

When different drugs are being used in different cycles of treatment a range of sequencing options are available. Myelosuppressive and non-myelosuppressive drugs may be alternated to allow greater bone marrow tolerability. Alternatively, blocks of treatment involving several cycles of the same drug followed by several cycles of a different drug may be used. For example, in a trial of adjuvant treatment for breast cancer, where A represented doxorubicin and B represented a double cycle of CMF (cyclophosphamide, methotrexate and 5-FU), the intercycle sequence of

Table 24.6 Non Phase-specific and Phase-specific Cytotoxic Drugs

Non phase-specific	Phase-specific
Platinum compounds	Taxanes (M phase)
Alkylating agents, for example, cyclophosphamide	Vinca alkaloids (M phase)
Anthracyclines (as multiple actions in addition to topoisomerase II inhibition)	Topoisomerase I inhibitors, for example, irinotecan (S phase)
	Etoposide (S phase)
	Nucleoside analogues, for example, gemcitabine (S phase)

AAABBB was found to be significantly more effective than the sequence ABABAB with 10 year survival rates of 58% versus 44%, respectively (Bonadonna et al., 1995). The theoretical reasons for this relate to tumours being heterogeneous populations of cells. When the sequencing is AAABBB, cells sensitive to drug A, but resistant to drug B do not have time to regrow between the first three cycles and are reduced to a level when absolute cell kill may be achieved. Cells sensitive to drug B, but resistant to drug A will have continued to increase in number during this period of time but when the three cycles of B are given, the same reduction in these cells should happen and absolute cell kill still be achieved. In contrast, when the sequencing is ABABAB each sensitive population of cells is exposed to only half the dose intensity, allowing repopulation, such that the levels necessary for absolute cell kill are never achieved.

24.6 The future: new targets, new drugs, and new approaches

In the post-genomics era, anticancer drug discovery, development, and administration are changing. Advances in the understanding of cancer biology have led to the identification of many novel drug targets. Pharmaceuticals are now screened against these targets rather than looking for crude cell turnover or tumour growth delay effects straight away. Such highly targeted approaches have significant implications regarding the allocation of treatments to patients. For example, if it is shown that the presence of a given target correlates with drug activity or the absence of the target implies resistance then pretreatment diagnostic tests may need to be developed hand in hand with each new drug.

Many of the targets being considered reflect deregulated control of cell growth and division. Re-establishment of control of these processes with drugs such as signal transduction inhibitors may be associated with far fewer side-effects than traditional cytotoxics (although non-specific and idiosyncratic side-effects may still occur). Therefore, it is likely that optimal effects will be achieved at doses lower than the MTD. There are several consequences of this. First, in drug development a readout of effect that changes in samples taken from the subject pre- and post-drug (e.g. in blood or tissue biopsies)—a pharmacodynamic biomarker—may be required for each new drug to determine the biologically effective dose. Second, the starting dose in man may become based on allometric scaling using lower animal toxicological endpoints such as the No Observable Adverse Effect Level rather than the MTD. Third, well tolerated, non-genotoxic agents may allow early clinical trial work to be performed in healthy volunteers rather than in patients, speeding up the drug development process considerably. Fourth, as many of the new drugs are orally bioavailable, in addition to having low toxicity, more prolonged treatment regimens than with traditional cytotoxic agents may become possible (especially in the adjuvant setting). As such, a shift of emphasis in safety assessments from acute to chronic side-effects will become necessary. Finally, if preclinical models suggest that early disease is the most sensitive cancer stage for any of these novel therapies (as is becoming clear), trials in the adjuvant setting may become acceptable immediately after proof of low toxicity and high tolerability in phase I studies, that is, without the need to show efficacy in the advanced disease setting first.

Although some of the newer targets being developed for anticancer therapy are associated with cancer cell survival, and interference with these targets should therefore cause cell death and tumour shrinkage, it is anticipated that many of the newer targeted therapies will primarily be cytostatic. As such, tumour response may be an inappropriate endpoint for clinical development decisions with these drugs. More relevant clinical endpoints in the future may therefore become disease stabilization and/or changes in the biology of tumours detected using modalities such as PET scanning or through tissue or blood derived biomarkers. However, all of these potential endpoints will have to be validated prospectively against the 'hard' endpoints of survival or quality of life at some point if they are ever to be considered true surrogates.

How all these new agents will be combined with traditional cytotoxics and with other anticancer modalities, such as hormonal agents and radiotherapy, will also have to be investigated, but many of the basic principles learned from traditional cytotoxics will undoubtedly inform the development of these novel agents in the future.

References and further reading

Andreyev, H. J., Norman, A. R., Oates, J., and Cunningham, D. (1998). Why do patients with weight loss have a worse outcome when undergoing chemotherapy for gastrointestinal malignancies? *Eur J Cancer*, **34**, 503–9.

Bonadonna, G., Zambetti, M., and Valagussa, P. (1995). Sequential or alternating doxorubicin and CMF regimens in breast cancer with more than three positive nodes. Ten-year results. *JAMA*, **273**, 542–7.

Dale, D. C. (2002). Colony-stimulating factors for the management of neutropenia in cancer patients. *Drugs*, **62**(Suppl 1), 1–15.

Eisenhauer, E. A., O'Dwyer, P. J., Christian, M., and Humphrey, J. S. (2000). Phase I clinical trial design in cancer drug development. *JCO*, **18**, 684–92.

Evans, W. E., Relling, M. V., Rodman, J. H., Crom, W. R., Boyett, J. M., and Pui, C. H. (1998). Conventional compared with individualized chemotherapy for childhood acute lymphoblastic leukaemia. *NEJM*, **338**, 499–505.

Goodman, J. and Walsh, V. (2001). The story of taxol: nature and politics in the pursuit of an anticancer drug. Cambridge University Press, Cambridge.

Gurney, H. (1996). Dose calculation of anticancer drugs: a review of the current practice and introduction of an alternative. *J Clin Onc*, **14**, 2590–611.

Hurley, L. H. (2002). DNA and its associated processes as targets for cancer therapy. *Nat Rev Cancer*, **2**, 188–200.

Innocenti, F. and Ratain, M. J. (2002) Update on pharmacogenetics in cancer chemotherapy. *Eur J Cancer*, **38**, 639–44.

Johnson, J. I., Decker, S., Zaharevitz, D., Rubinstein, L. V., Venditti, J. M., and Schepartz, S. et al. (2001). Relationships between drug activity in NCI preclinical in vitro and in vivo models and early clinical trials. *BJC*, **84**, 1424–31.

Joel, S. P., Shah, R., and Slevin, M. L. (1994). Etoposide dosage and pharmacodynamics. *Cancer Chemother Pharmacol*, **34**(Suppl), S69–75.

Kavanagh, J., Tresukosol, D., Edwards, C., Freedman, R., Gonzalez de Leon, C., and Fishman, A. (1995). Carboplatin reinduction after taxane in patients with platinum-refractory epithelial ovarian cancer. *J Clin Onc*, **13**, 1584–8.

Keefe, D. L. (2001). Anthracycline-induced cardiomyopathy. *Semin Oncol*, **28**(4 suppl. 12), 2–7.

Kelland, L. R. (2000) Preclinical perspectives on platinum resistance. *Drugs*, **59** (Suppl 4), 1–8.

Kellner, U., Sehested, M., Jensen, P. B., Gieseler, F., and Rudolph, P. (2002). Culprit and victim—DNA topoisomerase II. *Lancet Oncol*, **3**, 235–43.

Lawrence, T. S., Blackstock, A. W., and McGinn, C. (2003). The mechanism of action of radiosensitization of conventional chemotherapeutic agents. *Sem Rad Onc*, **13**, 13–21.

Levi, F., Zidani, R., and Misset, J-L. (1997). Randomised multicentre trial of chronotherapy with oxaliplatin, fluoruracil, and folinic acid in metastatic colorectal cancer. *Lancet*, **350**, 681–6.

Littlewood, T. J. (2001). The impact of hemoglobin levels on treatment outcomes in patients with cancer. *Semin Oncol*, **28**(suppl 2), 49–53.

Longley, D. B., Harkin, D. P., and Johnston, P. G. (2003). 5-fluorouracil: mechanisms of action and clinical strategies. Nat Rev Cancer, **3**, 330–8.

Raymond, E., Faivre, S., Chaney, S., Woynarowski, J., and Cvitkovic, E. (2002). Cellular and molecular pharmacology of oxaliplatin. *Mol Cancer ther*, **1**, 227–35.

Reed, E. (1998). Platinum-DNA adduct, nucleotide excision repair and platinum based anti-cancer chemotherapy. *Cancer Treat Rev*, **25**, 331–44.

Savarese, D. M. F, Hsieh, C.-C., and Stewart, F. M. (1997). Clinical impact of chemotherapy dose escalation in patients with haematologic malignancies and solid tumours. *J Clin Onc*, **15**, 2981–95.

Shah, M. A. and Schwartz, G. K. (2001). Cell cycle-mediated drug resistance: an emerging concept in cancer therapy. *Clin Canc Res*, **7**, 2168–81.

Tjan-Heijnen, V. C. G., Wagener, D. J. T, and Postmus, P. E. (2002). An analysis of chemotherapy dose and dose-intensity in small-cell lung cancer: lessons to be drawn. *Ann Oncol*, **13**, 1519–30.

CHAPTER 25

Radiotherapy and molecular radiotherapy

Anne Kiltie

25.1 Radiotherapy

Radiotherapy is the use of ionizing radiation (IR) to treat malignant diseases, by damaging and killing tumour cells, for tumour cure or palliation of symptoms. Radiotherapy may also be used in certain benign conditions such as keloid scars, hyperostotic new bone formation, and hyperthyroidism.

Treatment with radiotherapy has different aims in different clinical situations. *Radical* radiotherapy, as in head and neck cancer or bladder cancer, involves using radiotherapy to cure the tumour. It may be combined with chemotherapy before, during, or after radiotherapy as in lymphoma, rectal cancer, and anal cancer. *Adjuvant* radiotherapy, for example, following surgery in breast cancer or soft tissue sarcoma, is given to eradicate residual microscopic disease usually at a slightly lower than radical dose. *Palliative* radiotherapy is administered in short courses with lower doses, for example, for bone metastases to treat pain or spinal cord compression, to shrink tumour masses or relieve symptoms such as bleeding.

Radiotherapy is a local treatment aiming to achieve local control or cure of locally confined tumours. Radiotherapy may impact on metastases-free survival due to increased local control but it cannot treat micrometastatic disease already present elsewhere in the body.

Radiotherapy may be administered as external beam radiotherapy with X-rays or gamma rays, in sealed radioactive sources (e.g. prostate brachytherapy), or unsealed sources (e.g. orally administered radioiodine for thyroid cancer or thyrotoxicosis, intravenous strontium-89 for bone metastases from prostate or breast cancer). In external beam radiotherapy, the X-ray or gamma ray beams are targeted at the tumour to damage and kill the tumour cells. Inevitably, surrounding normal tissues are also affected resulting in the early and late side effects of radiotherapy. In modern radiotherapy, the X-ray beams are 'accelerated' to megavoltage levels by a linear accelerator (Figure 25.1) to allow deeper penetration into the tissues with relative sparing of skin and superficial tissues, thus minimizing side effects at these sites. Where the skin surface or subcutaneous tissue dose needs to be higher than the dose deeper within the body (e.g. skin tumours) conventional (orthovoltage) X-rays or electrons are used (Figure 25.2).

A rim of normal tissue (margin) must also be treated with the tumour for a number of reasons. First, there may be areas around the gross tumour volume (GTV), as seen on diagnostic imaging such as CT scanning, containing microscopic deposits of disease which need to be included in the treatment volume, so part of the margin is added to take this into account (clinical target volume, CTV). Second, the patient may not be set up exactly in the same position each day and the tumour itself may move within the patient (e.g. the prostate gland may move due to rectal filling with gas and faeces). Hence the precise location of the tumour relative to the X-ray beam may alter on a daily basis. Therefore a margin is added for error in set-up, which is combined with the CTV to form the planning target volume (PTV) (Figure 25.3).

The process of planning radical radiotherapy involves imaging the patient, usually by CT scanning, and making several small permanent reference marks called tattoos on the patient. Using this information the GTV, CTV, and PTV are defined and the treatment is planned by physicists/dosimetrists using a number of X-ray beams. These are chosen to encompass the PTV with at least 95% of the dose, avoiding unnecessary areas of overdose and considering the normal structures included in the X-ray beams to minimize normal tissue toxicity. The beam data is then transferred to the linear accelerator and extrapolated to the patient with reference to the tattoos.

The patient is then treated usually once a day, 5 days per week for 4–7 weeks, to a dose predetermined by the radiotherapist. Dose is determined from past experience of tumour curability and normal tissue tolerance. It has long been observed that tumours vary in their radiosensitivity. Therefore lymphomas which are very radiosensitive require relatively low doses for cure,

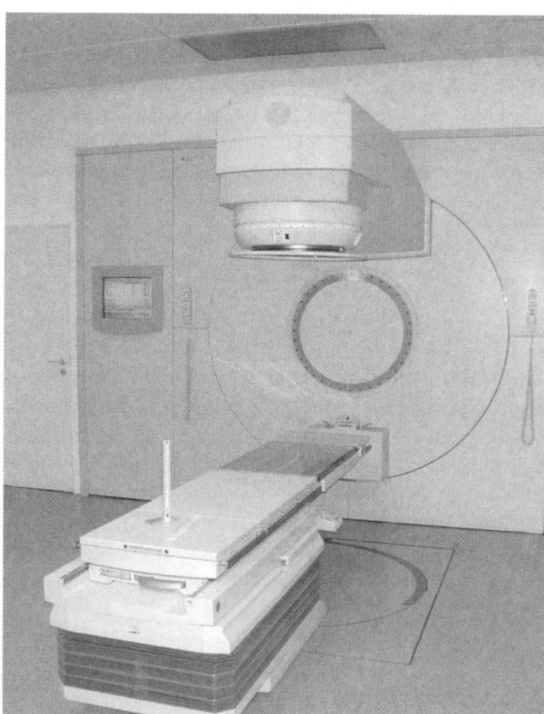

Figure 25.1 A linear accelerator.

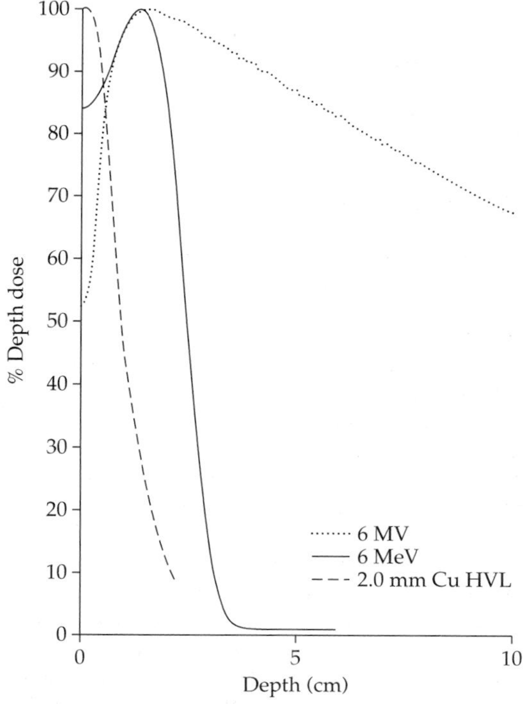

Figure 25.2 Depth dose curves for 100 kV (orthovoltage) photons (2 mm Cu HVL), 6 MeV electrons, and 6 MV (accelerated) photons.

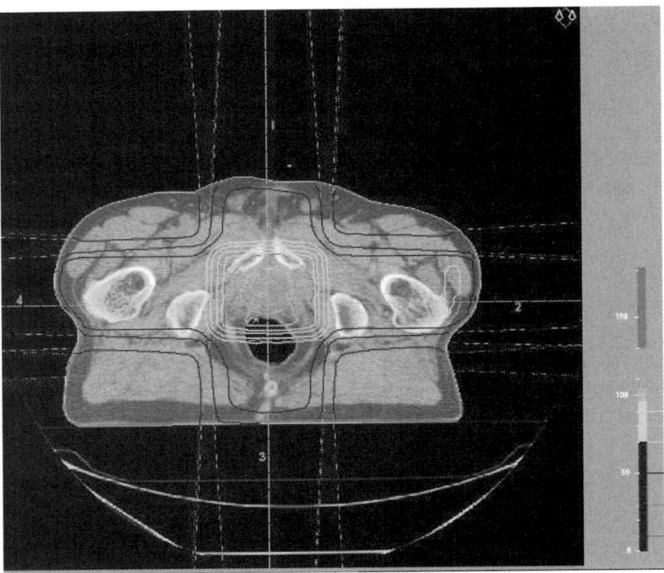

Figure 25.3 Cross-sectional image of a 4-field prostate plan. Inner (white) ring represents the GTV, and outer (grey) ring represents PTV, surrounded by white and black isodose lines (95% isodose line is innermost).

while sarcomas are relatively radioresistant and require larger doses. Some normal tissues, such as the salivary glands, are extremely sensitive to radiation due to apoptosis of serous cells, while muscle is relatively radioresistant.

Following radiotherapy tumours do not shrink immediately but do so over weeks or months. The inclusion of normal tissues in the treatment beam inevitably results in side effects which depend on the site treated and the patient's normal tissue sensitivity. Early side effects, one or two months following radiotherapy, are due to cell death in fast turnover cells such as those of the skin, gut, and bone marrow. These include skin reddening, soreness, and even ulceration, diarrhoea, and anaemia if sufficient bone marrow is irradiated. Late side effects, occurring more than 6–9 months following treatment, are due to damage and cell death in slow turnover tissues, such as subcutaneous tissues, nerves, muscle, and blood vessels, disruption of blood supply and inflammatory reactions mediated by cytokine release. These effects include fibrosis, telangiectasia, cataract formation, organ atrophy, sterility, and also cancers due to DNA mutations.

25.2 Classical radiobiology

Classical radiobiology is the science of the action of IR on living things. The field has developed from empirical observations to encompass *in vitro* and *in vivo* experimental studies of radiation effects using tissue culture methods, transplantable solid tumours in animal models, and xenografts of human tumours. It is largely a descriptive science, which frequently uses mathematical models, but does not provide mechanistic information on radiation effects (see Steel, 2002). However, it has allowed the optimization of radiation treatments such as altered fractionation schedules. Only more recently has work been undertaken to understand IR actions at the molecular level.

25.2.1 Clonogenic cell survival

IR damages cells, particularly their DNA, which if not repaired adequately may result in cell death. Although some specialized cells die through a process known as apoptosis, most cells die a mitotic (clonogenic) cell death, whereby the cell continues to metabolize nutrients but cannot reproduce itself and ultimately dies. This prevents transmission of damage to future generations of cells.

Experimentally, in the 'clonogenic assay', single cells are irradiated to doses around 1–10 Gy (a gray is the SI unit of absorbed dose of radiation) and then plated onto dishes, along with a control dish of unirradiated cells, and incubated in growth medium at 37°C for 1–3 weeks. The cells are then stained and the number of 'colonies' of more than 50 cells are counted and expressed as a fraction of the

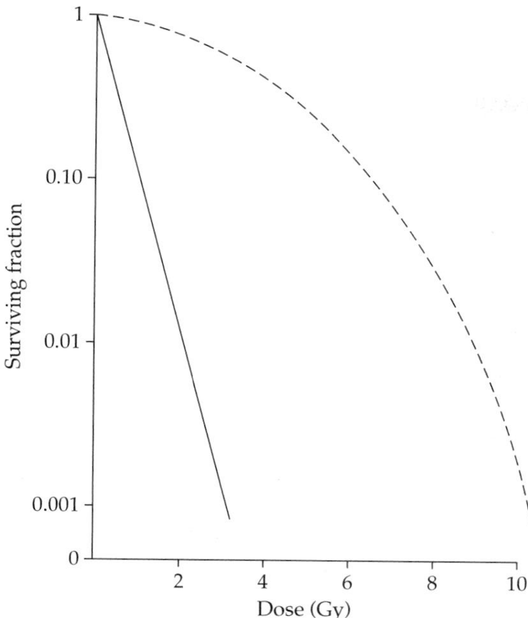

Figure 25.4 Clonogenic cell survival curves for a radioresistant (stippled line) and radiosensitive (solid line) cell line.

number of colonies on the control dish. Colonies are cells which have replicated from an individual cell, that is such cells have *not* undergone reproductive cell death. The data are plotted on a semi-logarithmic *cell survival curve* (Figure 25.4). More radiosensitive cell populations have lower proportions of surviving cells for each dose point. Using this assay, cells from the clinically highly radiosensitive ataxia–telangiectasia patients were found to be abnormally radiosensitive, as were cells from patients with other radiosensitive syndromes (e.g. Nijmegen breakage syndrome and ligase IV deficiency). Variation in cellular radiosensitivity has also been shown among normal individuals but the assay is not sufficiently robust to predict clinical radiosensitivity accurately enough to individualize treatment.

25.2.2 The therapeutic ratio

The greater the radiation dose the greater the proportion of patients achieving a given level of tumour control. This may be represented as a sigmoid dose–response curve of dose versus tumour control probability. The dose–response curve for

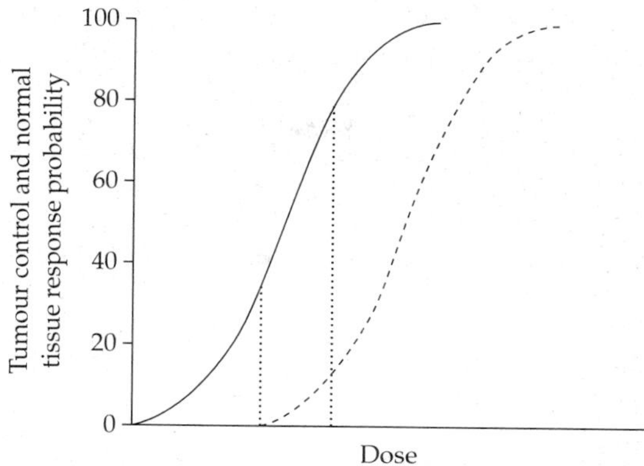

Figure 25.5 The therapeutic ratio. Solid sigmoid curve represents the tumour control probability curve; stippled curve represents the normal tissue response probability curve.

late effects in normal tissues lies to the right, so for each dose there is a higher probability of tumour control than severe late effects (Figure 25.5). To eliminate the chance of severe late effects completely, a dose would have to be chosen with a very low tumour control probability. As uncontrolled tumour usually results in death, this situation is clearly unacceptable. Higher doses result in higher incidences of severe late effects, but increased probability of local tumour control. A 5% significant late morbidity rate is usually considered acceptable and the dose set accordingly. This dose is therefore limited by those patients who manifest severe late effects.

The distance between the tumour control and severe late effects probability curves may be increased, thus increasing the 'therapeutic ratio', by altering various conventional radiotherapy parameters, such as the *treatment volume, fractionation schedule*, and *beam quality* (see Steel, 2002 for more details). Also, if the 10% most radiosensitive patients could be identified and excluded from receiving conventional treatment, at doses where only radiosensitive patients experience late effects, no such effects would occur and the therapeutic ratio would increase.

25.2.3 Additional tumour-related factors

Additional specific tumour-related factors exist over those relating to normal tissue radiation responses. Tumour cells, like normal tissues, vary in their intrinsic cellular radiosensitivity. A study of the clonogenic assay in human tumours (Fertil and Malaise, 1985) found evidence of a correlation between surviving fraction after 2 Gy (SF_2) and clinical response. Lower SF_2s were found in clinically sensitive tumours, such as lymphoma, myeloma, and neuroblastoma, compared with higher than average SF_2s in radioresistant tumours such as melanoma, osteosarcoma, glioblastoma, and renal carcinoma.

Oxygen is also an important factor in tumour radiation response. Tumours usually develop their own blood supply but they often grow more quickly than the rate of new vessel formation, resulting in hypoxic areas where cells may be viable for some time before dying of necrosis. Alternatively, previously hypoxic cells may become oxic on the death of other cells and can then resume cell division. Oxygen is a radiation sensitizer. Cells irradiated with X-rays in the absence of oxygen need three times the dose of radiation for a given level of cell killing compared to cells irradiated in the presence of oxygen. Therefore hypoxic cells are more radioresistant than oxic cells. Most of the cells surviving a fraction of radiotherapy will be hypoxic but these become reoxygenated as the radiotherapy course proceeds and the hypoxic fraction falls to near its starting value.

25.2.4 Improving the therapeutic ratio

One of the aims of classical radiobiology has been to identify treatment regimens which either reduce normal tissue toxicity for a given tumour control rate or increase the tumour control rate for a given level of normal tissue toxicity, thus increasing the therapeutic ratio. Temporal or physical factors may be modified as in altered fractionation schedules (including gaps in treatment, which are detrimental to local control), alterations to the dose rate, or the use of high linear energy transfer (LET) radiation. Alternatively, biological or chemical factors may be used, such as hypoxic cell sensitizers or chemotherapy used concurrently with radiotherapy.

Compared with a single dose of radiation, fractionation increases the therapeutic ratio by sparing normal tissues through sublethal damage repair and by increasing tumour damage by reoxygenation and reassortment of cells to a more sensitive phase of the cell cycle. Additional improvements compared to conventional 2 Gy/fraction radiotherapy schedules may be achieved by altering the fractionation. Fraction size may be reduced and the number of fractions increased with an increased overall dose in *hyperfractionated* radiotherapy, which decreases late effects but increases local control, or the overall treatment time may be reduced (*accelerated* radiotherapy) usually by delivering more than one fraction per day, to reduce the time for tumour cell repopulation which accelerates after 28 days. CHART is a combination of hyperfractionated and accelerated treatment given on consecutive days and in lung cancer results in improved survival over conventionally fractionated treatment.

Experimentally, overcoming hypoxia in tumours increases the therapeutic ratio, for example, by using mizonidazole (an hypoxic cell sensitizer) or tirapazamine (which is only activated at low oxygen tension). Chemotherapy may be given during a fractionated course of radiotherapy (*concurrent chemoradiation*) to improve radiotherapy efficacy without increasing the toxicity to a level obtained merely by increasing the radiation dose. Some chemotherapy agents inhibit the repair of DNA damage (e.g. gemcitabine which inhibits DNA synthesis, hydroxyurea which stops replication, and cisplatin which causes damage which inhibits DNA synthesis and transcription), while others selectively kill subpopulations of tumour cells in radioresistant cell cycle phases, leaving a synchronized population of sensitive cells.

25.3 DNA damage and repair

25.3.1 Ionizing radiation-induced DNA damage

At the megavoltage energies used in radiotherapy, X-ray photons interact randomly with matter mainly via the photoelectric effect and pair production. In the photoelectric effect an X-ray photon interacts with a tightly bound inner shell electron of an atom of the absorbing material, resulting in ejection of the electron and a filling of the vacancy by an outer shell electron with release of a photon. In pair production the incoming photon interacts with the atomic nucleus and disappears, forming two new particles, a negatron (an ordinary electron) and a positron, which excite and ionize other atoms in the absorbing material (Meredith and Massey, 1977).

One gray of radiation produces approximately 150,000 such nuclear ionization events, deposited sparsely or in clusters. Radiation may directly ionize atoms in critical cellular targets or may act indirectly by interacting with other atoms or molecules in the cell, especially water, to produce free radicals, which then damage critical targets (Figure 25.6). For X-rays and gamma-rays the latter process predominates (up to 70%). An X-ray photon interacts with water to form H_2O^* by excitation or H_2O^+ and an electron by ionization. Then H_2O^* can form a hydroxyl radical ($OH^\bullet$)(as can H_2O^+ on reaction with water) and a hydrogen radical. These 'free radicals' are very reactive and chemically unstable, and can transfer excess energy to other molecules thus breaking chemical bonds, leading to alterations in molecular structure such as DNA base damage or strand breaks.

DNA is thought to be the major critical target for ionizing radiation-induced cell death and mutation, although membrane damage is implicated in many biological responses to radiation. A variety of DNA

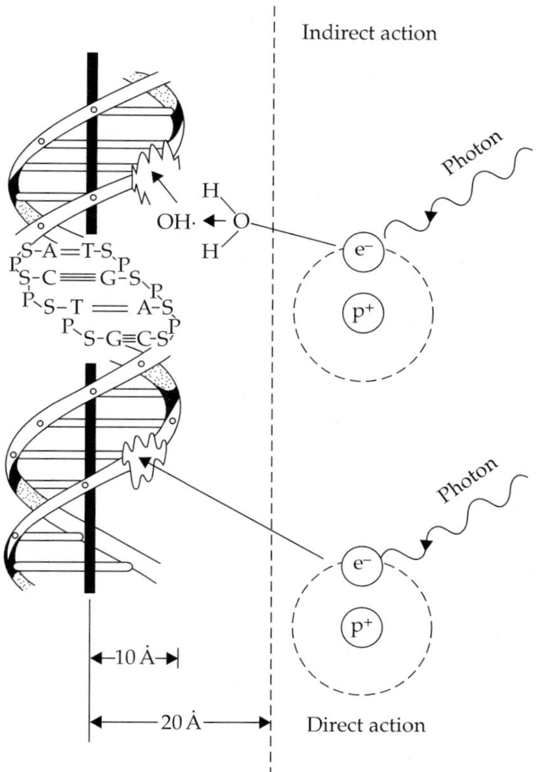

Figure 25.6 Direct and indirect actions of ionizing radiation (from Hall, 1988, with permission).

lesions are induced by ionizing radiation, at the following rate of lesions per gray of radiation per human cell: 40 DNA double-strand breaks (DSB), 500–1000 single-strand breaks (SSB), 1000–2000 base damages, 800–1600 sugar damages, 30 DNA–DNA cross links, and 150 protein-DNA cross links. Two particular features of ionizing radiation-induced DNA damage are, first, the structure of the DNA ends present at sites of strand breaks and, second, the formation of locally multiply damaged sites (LMDS) where damages, such as oxidized bases, AP sites (apurinic/apyrimidinic sites), and single strand breaks, are clustered due to closely occurring ionization events. The chemical structures at the 3′-ends of IR-induced DNA strand breaks are blocking residues, namely 3′phosphates and 3′phosphoglycolates, which cannot prime DNA polymerase and cannot be ligated by DNA ligases during repair. These blocking residues are also produced by radiomimetic drugs such as bleomycin and calicheamicin. LMDS are unique to ionizing radiation, arising because a single radiation energy deposition event can produce several free radicals in water around the DNA in close proximity, and present potential challenges to the DNA repair systems.

IR-induced DSB comprise two SSB lesions which occur directly opposite each other or in close proximity on each strand of DNA, due to two cleavages in the sugar phosphate backbone. DNA DSB are thought to be the most important IR-induced lesions; if left unrepaired such lesions are lethal, while misrepair can produce mutations, chromosome losses, or rearrangements which may lead to cellular transformation and loss of growth control.

25.3.2 Repair of ionizing radiation-induced DNA damage

Cells have specialized, highly efficient repair pathways for repairing DNA damage induced by ionizing radiation. Free radical-induced DNA damage such as oxidized bases, AP sites, and SSB are repaired by the base excision repair (BER) pathway, while DSB are repaired by homologous recombination (HR) and non-homologous end-joining (NHEJ).

The process of repairing oxidized bases by BER (Klungland et al., 1999) involves recognition of the damage by a DNA glycosylase and removal of the damaged base to form an AP site. The DNA backbone is then cleaved by the AP lyase activity of the glycosylase to leave an SSB with a 3′phosphate or modified sugar. A 5′AP endonuclease then hydrolyses the phosphodiester bonds at the AP sites and removes the 3′ blocking groups resulting in a single base gap, which is filled by a DNA polymerase using the undamaged partner strand as a template. Finally DNA ligase I or III rejoins the DNA backbone.

While ionizing radiation may produce a DSB when two SSBs are generated in close proximity on opposite strands of the DNA by a single ionization event, the frequency of DSBs may be increased during enzymatic processing of two closely opposed oxidatively damaged lesions, such as damaged bases or AP sites (Wallace, 1998). The lesion on the first strand is converted to an SSB by the recognizing enzyme but whether the lesion on the second strand is converted to an SSB also, thus resulting in a DSB, depends on the distance from the first lesion. Second strand incision occurs if the lesions are at least three bases apart (the exact number depends on the enzymes and base lesions involved). If an SSB is produced on the first strand within 1 bp distance of the second strand lesion, the DNA glycosylase cannot cleave the second lesion. It may be that when lesions are close together, distortion of the sugar-phosphate backbone prevents binding of the enzyme to the DNA (Figure 25.7). Therefore DNA glycosylases may increase the DSB frequency and hence lethality of IR to the cell. If a DSB is not formed, the lesions are repaired which may be mutagenic if DNA polymerase has to insert a base opposite the remaining lesion.

The 3′ blocking groups, 3′phosphate and 3′phosphoglycolate, are removed at the sites of SSB by the 5′AP endonuclease APE1 but APE1 is poor at removing 3′phosphoglycolates from single stranded 3′-overhangs at DSB, as is MRE11. Additional factors are therefore required for removal and recently the protein hTdp1 has been implicated in this process in man (Inamdar et al., 2002). If such blocking groups are not removed this results in failure of DSB repair and increased toxicity of radiation.

In BER the undamaged strand acts as a template for the polymerase but with a DSB there is no complementary strand of DNA to act as a template so the cell must use different repair mechanisms, namely HR or NHEJ (Figure 25.8) (reviewed by Jackson, 2002).

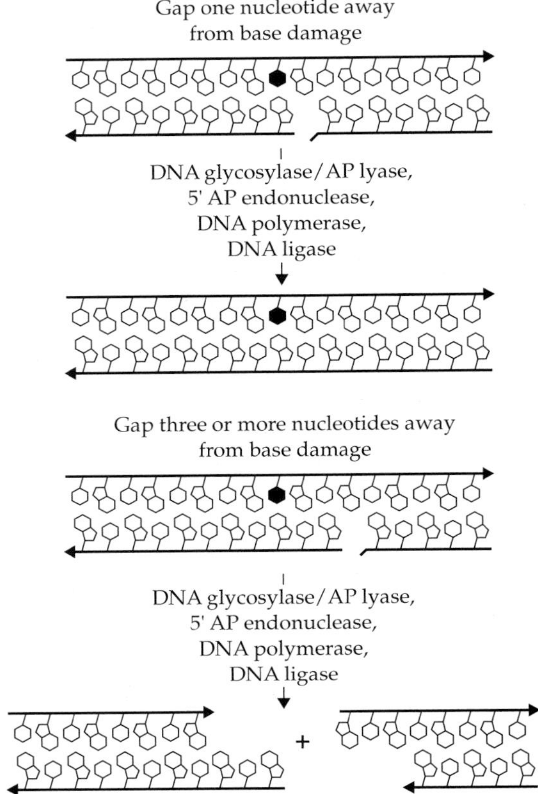

Figure 25.7 Base excision repair processing of LMDS (from Wallace, 1998, with permission). When the gap is 1 nucleotide away from the base damage the lesion is repaired; when the gap is at least 3 nucleotides away from the base damage the enzymatic processing results in DSB formation.

NHEJ is the dominant process in mammalian cells and occurs in G0 and G1/early S phase. NHEJ is a low-fidelity pathway which does not use a template and often results in small DNA deletions or additions. The Ku70/Ku80 heterodimer recognizes the DNA strand breaks and recruits other proteins for NHEJ including the DNA-PK catalytic subunit (DNA-PKcs), which has serine–threonine kinase activity, and possibly the MRE11/RAD50/NBS1 (MRN) complex, whose exonuclease activities may be required for trimming back DNA strands to areas of micro-homology, before a DNA polymerase fills any gaps and the XRCC4/ligase IV heterodimer seals the breaks, by forming a phosphodiester bond.

Recently HR has been found to be important in mammalian cells in late S phase/G2. HR is a high-fidelity repair pathway which requires

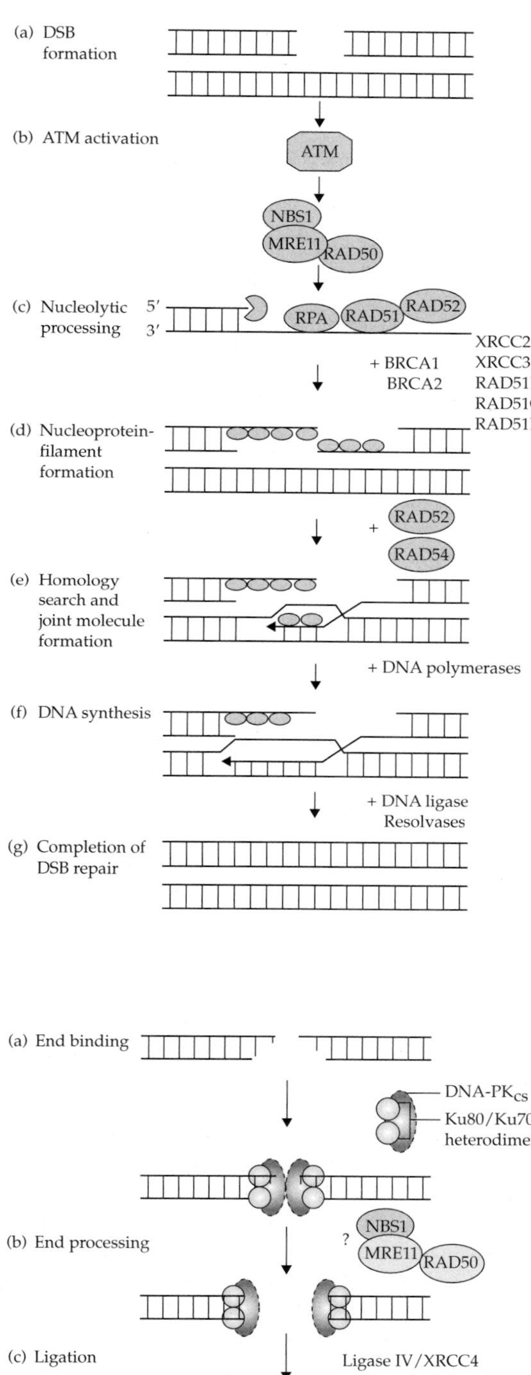

Figure 25.8 HR (top) and NHEJ (bottom) (from van Gent et al., 2001, with permission). See text for details.

extensive homology between the DSB region and a template from which repair is directed (usually the sister chromatid). In HR the DNA ends are resected by the nucleolytic processing of the MRN complex, RAD52 then binds to the single stranded end, followed by recruitment of RPA, RAD51-BRCA2, BRCA1, and RAD54 to the DNA. RAD51 forms a nucleoprotein filament on the exposed strand and initiates the search for homologous sequences on the undamaged partner DNA molecule before the damaged molecule invades the other DNA duplex via a strand exchange reaction. The 3′end of the damaged molecule is extended by a DNA polymerase prior to ligation by DNA ligase I. The cross-overs (Holliday junctions) are then resolved by cleavage and ligation. The RAD51 paralogues, RAD51B, RAD51C, and RAD51D, along with XRCC2 and XRCC3, help assembly of RAD51, while BRCA1 and 2 are needed for formation of RAD51 foci in response to IR. BRCA2 interacts directly with RAD51 and allows translocation of RAD51 into the nucleus; BRCA1 may indirectly influence RAD51 activity by altering chromatin structure or via its involvement in transcriptional responses to DNA damage.

The factors governing the predominance of each DSB repair pathway are not currently understood, but NHEJ predominates in G0 and G1/early S while HR commonly occurs in late S/G2 phases, where there is a greater availability of undamaged sister chromatid template. This complex process is most likely integrated with damage sensors and cell cycle checkpoints (see subsequently), and CDK1 may have a key function in regulating alternative pathways.

25.4 The cellular response to DNA damage

When a cell is damaged by ionizing radiation it attempts to survive and maintain its genomic integrity. It does this by recognizing the damage to DNA and plasma membrane lipids caused by the radiation and then activating various cellular pathways involved in genome maintenance and cell survival or activating cell death pathways when the damage is too great.

Cellular responses (reviewed by Lewanski and Gullick, 2001) include induction of early response genes (e.g. *JUN*, *FOS*, and *EGR1*), which can bind to specific DNA sequences to modulate the expression of other genes. Also, intermediate and late genes are induced, such as *TNFα, PDGF, TGFβ*, and *bFGF*, which are involved in premature terminal differentiation of fibroblasts by IR and therefore mediate fibrosis as a late response to radiotherapy. Activation of the mitogen-activated protein kinase (MAPK) cascade leads to cell survival and differentiation and many tumour cells have oncogenic mutations of the *RAS* oncogene, involved in this cascade, which are associated with cellular radioresistance. Clinical trials are underway to investigate use of farnesyl transferase inhibitors with radiotherapy to inhibit the RAS pathway. Apoptotic cell death is mediated partly via the plasma membrane-derived sphingomyelin pathway and the p53-dependent apoptotic pathway discussed below. Ionizing radiation can influence unirradiated cells by 'bystander effects' mediated by reactive oxygen species, gap junctions, cytokines, and growth factors, resulting in the same effects as in directly irradiated cells (Goldberg and Lehnert, 2002). Further discussion of these topics is outwith the scope of this chapter.

The response to DNA damage is one of the most important cellular responses to IR. The DNA damage response involves detection of the DNA damage, repair of the damage, and DNA damage signalling to the cell cycle, transcriptional and cell death machineries. A model of DNA damage detection, repair, and signalling has recently been proposed by Rouse and Jackson (2002). In this model, DNA damage is initially detected by specific repair factors, with an affinity for specific primary DNA lesions, which recognize the lesions and/or alterations in chromatin structure nearby. If the lesions are simple to repair (e.g. lesions repaired by BER) the DNA damage is rapidly reversed without activation of signalling pathways or subsequently the DNA damage response. In this instance cell division is unaffected. If repair is slower (e.g. IR-induced DSB with damaged bases at the ends) then the lesion persists and may be modified by end-processing enzymes such as nucleases. Then ATM (or other phosphatidylinositol 3-kinase-like protein kinases (PIKKs) such as DNA-PKcs or ATR) is recruited to the site of damage, to phosphorylate targets in the vicinity of the lesion resulting in DNA repair, again without activation of the DNA damage response. However, if the lesion still cannot be repaired further proteins are recruited resulting in activation of the *global DNA damage response* where, after signal transduction by the PIKK, the signal is amplified and diversified by kinase cascades and a range of downstream effectors regulate the various DNA damage responses, including cell cycle arrest, chromatin modulation, and increased repair capacity of the cell. This prevents progress through the cell cycle and facilitates repair of difficult lesions. This global DNA damage response requires several separate complexes to assemble at DNA damage sites. This model fits with the experimental observations of fast and slow components of DNA repair, where approx 80% of DSB are repaired within 30 minutes of IR. When the DNA damage is excessive or irreparable, mutations and chromosome aberrations occur which result in malignant transformation or cell death.

25.4.1 Damage sensing

The proteins responsible for DNA damage sensing are largely unknown, although the Ku70/Ku80 heterodimer is thought to be the damage sensor for NHEJ. The MRN complex is another putative damage sensor of DSB which may act via the nuclease activity of MRE11 to process the initial DNA damage to form an intermediate DNA structure, with single stranded ends, which can then initiate DNA damage signalling (D'Amours and Jackson, 2002).

25.4.2 DNA repair foci

DNA repair proteins are constitutively expressed in mammalian cells but one feature of the DNA damage response to IR is the formation of nuclear 'foci' at sites of DSB. Modification of chromatin structure can facilitate DNA repair. One component of chromatin is the histone protein H2AX. γ-H2AX foci are formed within a few seconds of IR, as a result of phosphorylation of H2AX by ATM and other PIKKs. A large amount of chromatin is involved with each DSB as one DSB induces phosphorylation of 0.03% of the total cellular H2AX (equivalent to 2 Mb pairs of DNA per DSB). Following ionizing radiation, γ-H2AX foci are formed and the recently discovered MDC1 protein aggregates at these sites followed by p53-binding protein-1 (53BP1), the MRN complex, RAD51 and BRCA1. The individual repair factors are not irreversibly bound to the DNA so other factors can later interact at the same DNA sites. The DNA damage signal is amplified by repeated cycles of H2AX phosphorylation followed by recruitment of repair factors.

In association with γ-H2AX, RAD51 foci form in response to IR-induced DNA damage at single stranded DNA tails, where they colocalize with RPA, RAD52, RAD54, BRCA1, and BRCA2 to form an HR 'repairosome' (RAD51 foci also form during S-phase and during meiotic recombination). NBS1 is another protein which interacts with γ-H2AX to form foci (D'Amours and Jackson, 2002; Tauchi et al., 2002) before recruiting a putative kinase to phosphorylate MRE11 and forming a complex with MRE11/hRAD50 which is directly bound to γ-H2AX. The MRE11/RAD50/NBS1 (MRN) complex is involved in DNA repair and checkpoint control. The MRN IR-related foci form within 10 min of IR and remain until damage is repaired. Early foci are thought to be involved in DSB processing, while the larger late foci (4–24 h) are probably involved in checkpoint signalling associated with lesions which are difficult to repair. In cells grown in tissue culture RAD51 foci and MRE11 foci do not co-localize, although NBS1 has been found to be essential for HR in higher vertebrate cells. The role of MRN in NHEJ is unclear but it does not appear essential. The NHEJ proteins Ku70 and Ku80 are found in a dispersed nuclear pattern following IR and foci have not been seen in human cells.

25.4.3 Cell cycle checkpoints

Cell cycle checkpoints control progression through the cell cycle and make up a network of signal transduction pathways which are activated by IR-induced DNA damage. By arresting the cell cycle they allow cells to repair their damaged DNA before resumption of cell division (see Chapter 9 and Samuel et al., 2002).

The ATM protein kinase is a key protein in the DNA DSB response (reviewed by Shiloh, 2003) and most of the cellular responses to IR depend on functional ATM protein. ATM activation results in modulation of numerous signalling pathways, including the G1/S, intra-S, and G2/M checkpoints. ATM responds to DSB by rapidly phosphorylating a wide range of substrates within minutes. These include: p53, MDM2, CHK1, CHK2, SMC1, FANCD2, BRCA1, NBS1, and H2AX. ATM also activates stress response genes via the stress-activated protein kinase (SAPK) cascade.

p53 is another key protein in the cellular response to IR and is involved in cell cycle arrest (via the G1 and G2 checkpoints), apoptosis, cell senescence, DNA repair, cell differentiation, and angiogenesis. A full discussion of p53 is outwith the scope of this chapter and readers are directed to reviews (Bristow et al., 1996; Dahm-Daphi, 2000; Ryan et al., 2001). p53 is important as p53 mutations are present in at least 50% of human tumours and are thought to underlie increased radioresistance, genomic instability, and rapid tumour progression. Under normal cellular conditions p53 levels are low due to its very short half-life and it exists in a relatively inactive state with poor DNA binding and transcriptional activation. However, in response to IR-induced DNA damage, levels of activated p53 rise markedly via post-translational modifications of the p53 polypeptide by phosphorylation, dephosphorylation, and acetylation (phosphorylation by ATM is thought to be a key event). Such modifications prevent binding of p53 to MDM2, which usually initiates ubiquitin-mediated protein degradation of p53, thus resulting in increased levels of transcriptionally active p53 with a prolonged half-life which results in transient or permanent cell cycle arrest. Wild type p53 also induces BAX, a protein involved in apoptosis in some cell types, and down regulates expression of the anti-apoptotic BCL2.

At the *G1 checkpoint* ATM phosphorylates p53 which activates transcription of the cyclin-dependent kinase (CDK) inhibitor p21, resulting in inhibition of CDK2 and retinoblastoma protein (pRB) phosphorylation and hence cell cycle progression. p21 activates transcription of GADD45 which blocks entry into S phase and stimulates repair (p21 is also involved in terminal differentiation of cells such as fibroblasts post-IR, probably via its regulation of TGFβ, which is the key growth factor involved in fibrosis). In an alternative pathway, ATM phosphorylates CHK2 which activates the phosphatase CDC25A which also prevents CDK2 activation. The *intra-S checkpoint* is one of the most important cellular responses to DSB as intra-S checkpoint failure results in *radioresistant DNA synthesis*. One intra-S checkpoint involves ATM-driven phosphorylation of NBS1 and the structural maintenance of chromosomes 1 protein (SMC1); the second involves ATM phosphorylating CHK2 which in turn inhibits CDC25A and hence CDK2. MDC1 is involved in the activation of intra-S phase and G2/M cell cycle checkpoints by recruiting the MRN complex to nuclear foci. At the *G2/M checkpoint* ATM phosphorylates BRCA1, CHK1, and NBS1. Phosphorylation of CHK1 results in inactivation of CDC25C, which usually removes inhibitory phosphates from CDK1; failure to activate CDK1 results in G2/M arrest. p53 is involved in the G2 checkpoint partly by CDK1 repression but also by upregulating GADD45, p21, and the 14-3-3σ protein which prevents nuclear import of CDC25C and hence prevents G2/M transition.

25.4.4 Cell death, apoptosis, and terminal differentiation

If IR-induced cellular damage is extreme, cells die rather than transmit erroneous genetic information to daughter cells. Cells die ultimately by apoptosis or necrosis. In normal cells, necrosis occurs following very high doses of IR, outside the range used in radiotherapy, but cells can die at the edge of necrotic tumour areas due to poor vascular supply.

As mentioned previously, cellular radiosensitivity is measured by the clonogenic assay. Reduced colony formation reflects cell death or cells entering permanent G1 arrest, which precedes senescence or terminal differentiation. Cells die by apoptosis during interphase or at or after the first mitosis (described as mitotic or clonogenic cell death). Apoptosis in interphase is the mode of cell death in small intestinal crypt cells, lymphocytes, thymocytes, and salivary glands and is observed in most experimental tumour systems. This mode of death involves p53, the SAPK/JNK signalling pathway, reactive oxygen species (ROS) and the plasma membrane (Verheij and Bartelink, 2000). These pathways activate caspases which are cytoplasmic cysteine proteases which cleave cellular proteins and activate a nuclease responsible for DNA fragmentation. The p53 pathway involves upregulation of BAX expression, and possibly upregulation of FAS, the CD95 death receptor. Increased levels of ROS trigger mitochondria to release caspase-activating factors. However, apoptosis in interphase is not the mechanism of cell death for solid tumours *in vivo* (except lymphomas). These are intrinsically resistant to apoptosis in interphase due to upregulation of the PI3K/AKT pathway (which promotes cell survival and prevents triggering of apoptosis), overexpression of anti-apoptotic genes such as *BCL2*, or due to the presence of mutations in the pro-apoptotic gene *BAX* (Igney and Krammer, 2002). Instead, in these tumours mitotic cell death is important (Shinomiya, 2001). This mode of death is distinguished from interphase death by the late activation of caspases 24 h after damage, transient G2/M block and downregulation of the anti-apoptotic *MAPK* and *BCL2* genes.

25.5 Clinical outcomes of radiotherapy resulting from DNA damage and cellular responses

It is hoped that in future molecular information can be used to improve radiotherapy treatments, for example by accurate prediction of outcomes (tumour response and late effects) to individualize the radiotherapy prescribed, by increasing the therapeutic ratio through intervention or by the introduction of new treatments in a scientifically rational manner.

25.5.1 Normal tissues

Normal tissue responses to radiotherapy include cell death in fast and slow turnover tissues, accelerated cellular differentiation, and vascular damage which can result in early and late side effects. Several human syndromes are associated with extreme clinical radiosensitivity, such as ataxia–telangiectasia, Nijmegen breakage syndrome, and AT-like disorder which are associated with mutations in *ATM*, *NBS1*, and *MRE11* genes respectively. These syndromes also predispose to malignancy. Patients demonstrate clinical and *in vitro* radiosensitivity and have defective checkpoint functions, although they are apparently proficient in DSB repair. DNA ligase IV deficiency has also been identified where patients have intact checkpoints but impaired DSB rejoining. One such patient had leukaemia and was extremely clinically radiosensitive. Cells from patients with germline mutations in *BRCA1* and *BRCA2* are also radiosensitive. No human defects have been identified in *DNA-PKcs* or *Ku70/Ku80*, and no individuals have been found with inactive *RAD51*, *RAD52*, or *RAD54*.

Apart from rare syndromic patients showing extreme radiosensitivity, there is a normal distribution of radiosensitivity in patients. As the 5% most severe reactors limit the dose given to the whole population, an ability to predict outcome would be advantageous. It was thought that a substantial proportion of the 5% overreactors in breast cancer might be A-T heterozygotes or patients carrying *BRCA1* or *BRCA2* germline mutations (Appleby et al., 1997; Pierce et al., 2000) but this has not proved to be the case. It is more likely that a large number of genes are involved in the normal tissue radiation response, including genes coding for DNA repair enzymes, cell cycle and proliferation proteins, cytokines, and growth factors. cDNA microarrays might be useful investigative tools, although following radiation DNA repair enzymes are not generally upregulated. Around 0.1% of the genome is polymorphic and most of the variation is due to single nucleotide polymorphisms (SNPs) of which there are probably 3 million in an individual's DNA. Some SNPs are predictive of toxicity from cytotoxic drugs, so the same may be true for radiotherapy. Functional assays such as clonogenic, DNA repair, or chromosomal (micronucleus) assays have only demonstrated weak correlations with late effects, probably reflecting the influences on late normal tissue responses other than cell death and DNA repair, including fibrosis and vascular damage. In some tumour sites there is a choice of treatment, for example, between surgery and radiotherapy, and predictive testing, by SNP analysis or other methods, may help choose the most appropriate treatment for an individual patient.

The therapeutic ratio can be increased by ameliorating late effects in patients, for example, by preventing apoptosis in sensitive normal tissues such as the parotid glands to prevent xerostomia. Prevention of p53-induced apoptosis in normal tissues has been demonstrated in mice with inactive tumour *p53* genes using pifithirin α, a chemical inhibitor of p53.

If IR-induced DNA damage is misrepaired resulting in DNA losses, additions and chromosome translocations, and the cell survives, this may result in genomic instability and cancer. This effect has been observed clinically for many years with the development of solid tumours such as breast cancer in Hodgkin's disease post-radiotherapy in the low dose areas at the treatment field edges. In Gorlin's syndrome basal cell and squamous cell carcinomas appear at the edge of the radiotherapy fields within a few years of treatment. Malignancies in radiotherapy fields have been observed not only in patients with previous malignancies and hence a likely genetic predisposition to cancer but also in patients receiving radiotherapy for benign conditions, such as, historically, scalp ring worm where patients subsequently developed skin tumours. Knowledge of the molecular mechanisms of development of genomic instability may one day enable us to prevent second malignancies occurring following radiotherapy.

25.5.2 Tumours

It is thought that the majority of cancers arise due to impaired ability to respond to or repair DNA damage which leads to genomic instability. Tumour cells have often also lost some aspect of checkpoint function, via mutation of genes coding for growth factors, and inactivators of apoptotic pathways, as well as mutations in genes promoting angiogenesis, resulting in a growth advantage. For example, loss of BRCA2 causes gross chromosomal rearrangements, spontaneous DNA breakages, and mutation due to defective HR via RAD51. Some tumour cells express higher levels of RAD51 resulting in more efficient HR and hence increased radioresistance compared to normal cells.

Human tumour cell lines exist which are deficient in DNA repair enzymes, for example, M059J (DNA-PKcs deficient glioma), Capan-1 (BRCA2 deficient pancreatic tumour), and HCC1937 (BRCA1 deficient breast carcinoma). MO59J cells are radiosensitive, with deficient NHEJ measured by pulsed-field gel electrophoresis. BRCA1 and BRCA2 deficient cells show no definite NHEJ impairment but are HR deficient and mouse xenograft tumours defective in BRCA2 are highly sensitive to IR (Abbott et al., 1998). This suggests that human tumours with DNA repair defects may be more sensitive to radiotherapy.

Tumour predictive assays are potentially useful if a tumour was particularly radiosensitive and the radiation dose could be reduced to ameliorate late effects. Again clonogenic assays, DNA repair assays, and hypoxia assays have not accurately predicted outcome probably due to the large number of pathways and hence genes involved in tumour cell death by IR, including oncogenes such as *RAS*, *RAF*, *MYC*, and genes coding for DNA repair, cell cycle, and apoptotic machinery proteins. Immunohistochemical (IHC) studies have been predictive of outcome in cohorts of patients but are not sensitive enough to be used on an individual basis. They allow stratification as for tumour stage and grade which are currently the most important prognostic variables. There are technical problems with p53 immunohistochemistry but it appears that loss of wild type p53 function results in increased radioresistance and *p53* gene mutations, which are associated with a worse prognosis. High expression of *BCL2* also results in tumour radioresistance and poor prognosis in patients after radiotherapy. Examples involving DNA repair proteins include DNA-PKcs expression and outcome following chemoradiotherapy in oesophageal cancer, Ku70 expression and clinical tumour radiosensitivity along with disease-free survival in rectal cancer, and Ku70 expression and survival following radiotherapy in cervix cancer. Tumours with low levels of expression had better outcomes, presumably because of poorer repair leading to increased radiosensitivity. Perhaps studying a range of relevant proteins with IHC, by tissue arrays, may allow prediction of outcome. This approach might be particularly useful where treatment options are available. For example, in bladder cancer patients whose tumours have low expression levels of various DNA repair exzymes (and hence would be expected to be less efficient at repairing DNA damage) might be more suitable candidates for radiotherapy than those with higher levels who would be better served with cystectomy. In rectal cancer prior knowledge of response would allow selection for pre-operative radiotherapy.

Gene expression arrays (cDNA arrays) allow investigation of large numbers of patients' genes and show variation in gene expression among tumours with similar histological features. In diffuse large B-cell lymphomas there is a very different overall survival between two such groups using this assay. Genes that would be good candidates for prediction of radiosensitivity include DNA repair genes (see *BRCA2* above) and genes related to cell cycle, growth, and differentiation. Proteomics technology may also have a role in investigation of radiosensitivity as it can provide a more accurate indicator of protein function than cDNA arrays in view of post-translational modifications.

Tumours often have mutations in tumour suppressor genes, such as *TP53* or oncogenes such as *RAS*. In terms of altering the therapeutic ratio it should be theoretically possible to restore normal function to mutant p53 in tumour cells. Use of concurrent chemoradiation, with drugs that alter DNA repair such as cisplatin or gemcitabine, aim to increase tumour cell kill without increased toxicity. It may be possible to exploit the different distribution in the cell cycle of normal cell and tumour cell populations by using agents which radiosensitize in S phase where there tends to be a higher proportion of tumour cells than normal cells. Gene therapy is still experimental but in radiotherapy it could involve the use of ionizing radiation-inducible promoters to limit gene expression or use of vectors with replicative potential limited to tumours, with targets such as ATM or DNA-PK to radiosensitize tumours.

An important future aim of molecular studies in radiotherapy is to increase the therapeutic ratio to increase tumour control and/or decrease late effects by predicting outcome on an individual basis to select the most appropriate treatment for each patient. Also they should enable development of new combined-modality treatments such as radiotherapy and concurrent biological therapies or chemotherapy in a scientifically rational manner.

Acknowledgements

I wish to thank Dr Jo Bentley, Dr Christine Diggle, and Dr Alan Melcher for critical reading of the manuscript and Mrs Jane Garrud for her medical illustration expertize.

References

* indicates review article

Abbott, D. W., Freeman, M. L., and Holt, J. T. (1998). Double-strand break repair deficiency and radiation sensitivity in BRCA2 mutant cancer cells. *J Natl Cancer Inst*, **90**, 978–85.

Appleby, J. M., Barber, J. B. P., Levine, E., Varley, J. M., Taylor, A. M., Stankovic, T. et al. (1997). Absence of mutations in the ATM gene in breast cancer with severe responses to radiotherapy. *Br J Cancer*, **76**, 1546–9.

*Bristow, R., Benchimol, S., and Hill, R. P. (1996). The p53 gene as a modifier of intrinsic radiosensitivity: implications for radiotherapy. *Radiother Oncol*, **40**, 197–223.

*Dahm-Daphi, J. (2000). p53: biology and role for cellular radiosensitivity. *Strahlenther Onkol*, **176**, 278–85.

*D'Amours, D. and Jackson, S. P. (2002). The Mre11 complex: at the crossroads of DNA repair and checkpoint signalling. *Nat Rev Mol Cell Biol*, **3**, 317–27.

Fertil B. and Malaise E. P. (1985). Intrinsic radiosensitivity of human cell lines is correlated with radioresponsiveness of human tumors: analysis of 101 published survival curves. *Int J Radiat Biol Oncol Phys*, **11**, 1699–707.

*Goldberg Z. and Lehnert B. E. (2002). Radiation-induced effects in unirradiated cells: a review and implications in cancer. *Int J Oncol*, **21**, 337–49.

Hall E. (1988). *Radiobiology for the radiologist*, 3rd edn. Lippincott, Philadelphia.

*Igney F. H., Krammer P. H. (2002). Death and anti-death: tumour resistance to apoptosis. *Nat Rev Cancer*, **2**, 277–88.

Inamdar, K. V., Pouliot, J. J., Zhou, T., Lees-Miller, S. P., Rasouli-Nia, A., and Povirk, L. F. (2002). Conversion of phosphoglycolate to phosphate termini on 3′overhangs of DNA double strand breaks by the human tyrosyl-DNA phosphodiesterase hTdp1. *J Biol Chem*, **277**, 27162–8.

*Jackson, S. P. (2002). Sensing and repairing DNA double-strand breaks. *Carcinogenesis*, **23**, 687–96.

Klungland, A., Hoss, M., Gunz, D., Constantinou, A., Clarkson, S. G., Doetsch, P. W. et al. (1999). Base excision repair of oxidative DNA damage activated by XPG protein. *Mol Cell*, **3**, 33–42.

*Lewanski, C. R. and Gullick, W. J. (2001). Radiotherapy and cellular signalling. *Lancet Oncol*, **2**, 366–70.

Meredith, W. J., Massey, J. B. (1977). *Fundamental physics of radiology*. John Wright and Sons, Bristol.

Pierce, L.J., Strawderman, M., Narod, S.A., Oliviotto, I., Eisen, A., Dawson, L. et al. (2000). Effect of radiotherapy after breast-conserving treatment in women with breast cancer and germline BRCA1/2 mutations. *J Clin Oncol*, **18**, 3360–9.

*Rouse, J. and Jackson, S. P. (2002). Interfaces between the detection, signaling, and repair of DNA damage. *Science*, **297**, 547–51.

*Ryan, K. M., Phillips, A. C., and Vousden, K. H. (2001). Regulation and function of the p53 tumour suppressor protein. *Curr Opin Cell Biol*, **13**, 332–7.

*Samuel, T., Weber, H. O., and Funk, J. O. (2002). Linking DNA damage to cell cycle checkpoints. *Cell Cycle*, **1**(3), 162–8.

*Shiloh, Y. (2003). ATM and related protein kinases: safeguarding genome integrity. *Nat Rev Cancer*, **3**, 155–68.

*Shinomiya, N. (2001). New concepts in radiation-induced apoptosis: 'premitotic apoptosis' and 'postmitotic apoptosis'. *J Cell Mol Med*, **5**, 240–53.

Steel, G. (ed) (2002). *Basic Clinical Radiobiology*, 3rd edn. Edward Arnold, London.

*Tauchi, H., Matsuura, S., Kobayashi, J., Sakamoto, S., and Komatsu, K. (2002). Nijmegen breakage syndrome gene, NBS1, and molecular links to factors for genome stability. *Oncogene*, **21**, 8967–80.

*van Gent, D. C., Hoeijmakers, J. H., and Kanaar, R. (2001). Chromosomal stability and the DNA double-stranded break connection. *Nat Rev Genet*, **2**, 196–206.

*Verheij, M. and Bartelink, H. (2000). Radiation-induced apoptosis. *Cell Tissue Res*, **301**, 133–42.

*Wallace, S. S. (1998). Enzymatic processing of radiation-induced free radical damage in DNA. *Radiat Res*, **150**(5 Suppl), S60–79.

CHAPTER 26

Monoclonal antibodies and therapy

Tom Geldart, Martin J. Glennie, and Peter W. M. Johnson

26.1 Introduction

Over the past 25 years, monoclonal antibodies (mAbs) have revolutionized experimental and diagnostic laboratory techniques. More recently they have established themselves as the most rapidly expanding class of therapeutic agents for a wide range of human diseases (Carter, 2001). Although only a few mAbs have so far been licensed for routine therapeutic use, several hundred are in clinical development, many of them aimed at treating cancer (see http://archive.bmn.com/supp/ddt/glennie.pdf). This chapter aims to give an insight into normal antibody structure and function, outline the development of therapeutic mAbs, explore their potential mechanisms of action and evaluate the mAbs currently licensed for the treatment of malignancy.

26.2 Antibody definition and structure

26.2.1 Antibody definition

Antibodies (immunoglobulins) are glycoproteins that perform a key role in the adaptive, targeted, immune response to foreign antigen. Antibodies are synthesized by B lymphocytes and expressed on their cell surface as the B-cell receptor (surface immunoglobulin). Surface immunoglobulin confers unique antigenic specificity to B cells; approximately 80,000 immunoglobulin molecules are expressed on the surface of a single B cell, each with an identical antigen-binding site. Interaction between specific antigen and surface immunoglobulin on mature naïve B cells (in the presence of T-helper cells and appropriate cytokines) will induce B-cell division, maturation and differentiation into a clonal population of memory B cells and plasma cells. Plasma cells lack membrane bound immunoglobulin, but are able to synthesize and secrete high levels of soluble mAb with identical antigen specificity to that of the parent B cell. Circulating soluble antibodies are the mediators of humoral immunity, binding foreign antigen, and neutralizing it or targeting it for elimination. Because of the unique way in which antibody diversity is generated (see Section 26.3), the immune system is capable of producing antibodies specific to virtually any antigen encountered, a property that makes antibodies immensely powerful tools for experimental, diagnostic, and therapeutic use.

26.2.2 Antibody structure

Antibodies are large 'Y' shaped glycoproteins composed of four polypeptide chains made up from two identical heavy chains combined with two identical light chains (Figure 26.1). The chains are folded into a number of distinct domains linked together by a series of covalent and non-covalent disulfide bonds. Heavy chains consist of one variable domain and three or four constant domains each representing regions of relatively variable or constant aminoacid sequence. Five types of heavy chain (grouped according to heavy chain constant region sequences) have been identified in humans; alpha (α), delta (δ), epsilon (ε), gamma (γ), and mu (μ). On the basis of these heavy-chain constant region sequences, antibodies are classified into five main classes or isotypes; immunoglobulin A (IgA), IgD, IgE, IgG, and IgM. Minor differences in the

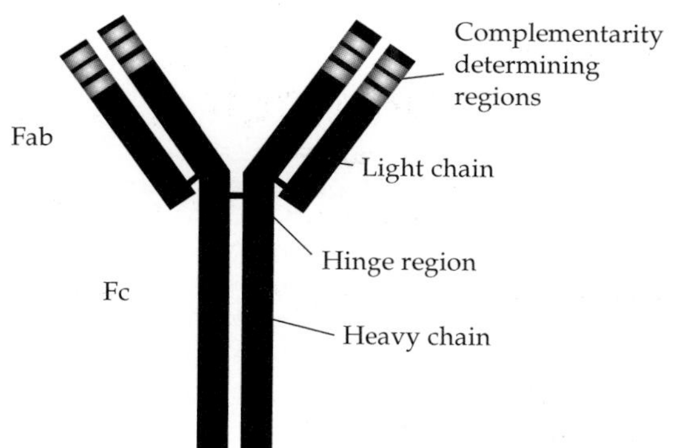

Figure 26.1 Schematic representation of an antibody.

heavy chain amino acid sequences of IgA and IgG allow further sub-classification of these antibody isotypes (IgA_{1+2} and IgG_{1-4}, respectively). Light chains are smaller and consist of one variable and one constant domain. Two types of light chain are described in humans; kappa (κ) and lambda (λ). Any two identical light chains may be combined with any two identical heavy chains to form a complete antibody monomer (e.g. IgG kappa or IgG lambda, IgE kappa or IgE lambda). IgD, IgE, and IgG are produced and secreted as monomers. IgM is expressed on the cell surface of B cells as a monomer but secreted by plasma cells as a pentamer. IgA exists primarily as a monomer but may form dimeric, trimeric, or tetrameric forms. The two arms that make up the top of the Y-shaped immunoglobulin structure are identical and are known as Fab fragments (fragment, antigen binding). Each Fab fragment is composed of one variable region and an adjacent constant region from one light chain and one heavy chain. Within each variable domain, three short polypeptide sequences show immense variability. These hypervariable regions make up the specific antigen-binding site of the antibody and are known as the complementarity-determining regions (CDRs). Intervening polypeptide sequences called framework regions act as a scaffold for the CDRs. The two Fab fragments of IgA, IgD, and IgG are joined at an area of structural flexibility known as the hinge region (replaced by an additional constant domain in IgM and IgE). Beyond the hinge region is the remainder of the antibody, the Fc fragment (fragment, crystallizable), made up from the remaining heavy-chain constant regions. The Fc fragment is responsible for mediating the immune effector functions of antibody such as opsonization, complement-mediated cytotoxicity (CDC) and antibody dependent cellular cytotoxicity (ADCC), discussed in detail below.

26.3 Generation of antibody diversity

The immune system is capable of producing antibodies with specificity for an almost infinite number of antigens. A number of mechanisms are employed by B cells in order to achieve this diversity.

26.3.1 Somatic recombination

The heavy and light immunoglobulin polypeptide chains that together make up a complete antibody molecule are encoded by the recombination of different versions of gene segments rather than a single contiguous DNA gene sequence. These gene segments are categorized and grouped into leader (L), variable (V), diversity (D), joining (J), and constant (C) sets with each set containing a number of different versions of the gene segment. During B-cell ontogeny, individual versions of these gene segments are randomly selected and brought together to form a contiguous functional gene, a process known as somatic recombination. This process allows the generation of immense antibody diversity even in the absence of exposure to specific antigen. For light chains, a complete gene results from the recombination of single V_L and J_L gene segments (together encoding for the light chain variable region) with a C_L gene (encoding for the constant region). For kappa light chains, approximately 40 versions of the V_k gene segment have been identified and these may be combined with any of five J_k gene segments and one C_k gene to form a complete kappa light-chain gene. For lambda light chains, approximately 30 V_λ gene segments, 4 J_λ gene segments and 4 C_λ gene segments have been described. Human heavy-chain genes are similar to, but more complex than, light chains, with an additional gene segment, (D_H), encoding for part of the variable region along with the V_H and J_H gene segments. About 50 versions of the heavy chain V_H gene segment have been identified, along with 27 D_H gene segments and 6 J_H gene segments. Any VDJ recombination may combine with any of the C_H genes that encode for the five different immunoglobulin isotypes. Leader (L) gene segments encode for a short leader peptide responsible for guiding the heavy or light chain through the endoplasmic reticulum; this peptide is cleaved prior to immunoglobulin assembly.

26.3.2 Somatic hypermutation

An additional process, somatic hypermutation, is employed to generate further V region diversity following the assembly of a functional antibody gene. On exposure to antigen, this mechanism allows the introduction of point mutations into the antibody V region, resulting in antibodies with varying affinity to antigen. On average, once a B cell is activated, it has the capacity to undergo a mutation once every one or two cell divisions. Following somatic hypermutation, B cells producing antibody with high affinity to specific antigen are preferentially selected for maturation into antibody forming (plasma) cells, a process known as affinity maturation.

26.4 Antibody production

26.4.1 Polyclonal antibodies

Naturally occurring, soluble antibodies are generated *in vivo* following exposure of foreign antigen to the immune system. In the laboratory, antibodies may be raised artificially by injecting antigen into an animal and collecting the resultant antibody rich serum several weeks later. This serum (also known as antiserum) will contain a heterogeneous, polyclonal mixture of antibodies. Polyclonal antibodies, by definition, are produced by the clonal populations of a number of different B lymphocytes whose surface immunoglobulin recognize any of the epitopes (specific antibody-binding sites) present on the given antigen.

26.4.2 Monoclonal antibodies

Antibodies produced from identical copies or clones of a single B lymphocyte will have identical antigen epitope specificity and are known as mAbs. In 1975, an experimental technique was devised that enabled stable and permanent production of mAb (Kohler and Milstein, 1975). This technique opened the way to the widespread introduction of mAbs into experimental, diagnostic, and therapeutic work. Köhler and Milstein's method immunizes animals, generally rodents, with an antigen of interest in order to elicit an antibody response. A cell suspension containing antibody producing B lymphocytes is then prepared from these animals' spleens and mixed *in vitro* with a myeloma (immortal B-lymphocyte tumour) cell line. The addition of polyethylene glycol to the cell suspension will result in cell–cell fusion and the generation of hybridomas—the fusion products of normal, antibody-producing B cells and myeloma cells. Through the use of myeloma cell lines that lack the ability to synthesize endogenous immunoglobulin, hybridomas may be created which secrete antibody specific to the antigen used for the original immunization and possess the immortal growth properties of the cell line. Once antibody-secreting hybridomas have been selected, they can be screened to identify and isolate those populations producing antibodies with the desired antigenic specificity. This is generally achieved by diluting out hybridoma cell suspensions to single cell dilutions which are subsequently grown up as clonal cell populations. The presence of specific antibody within the cell supernatant can be assayed by a variety of techniques such as enzyme-linked immunosorbent assay (ELISA) or radioimmunoassay. By repeat limiting dilution, truly monoclonal cell populations may be obtained thereby enabling stable and permanent production of large quantities of mAb through modern continuous tissue culture techniques.

26.4.3 Antibody humanization

The techniques of Kohler and Milstein rely on the immunization of rodents, generally mice, to derive a population of antibody producing B lymphocytes. It follows that the mAb produced by this system will be of mouse origin (murine). Although murine mAbs are of immense importance in experimental and diagnostic techniques, their use in human therapy is problematic. Murine antibodies may be highly immunogenic to humans and repeated administration commonly leads to the generation of human anti-mouse antibody (HAMA) responses. HAMA responses not only adversely affect the clinical efficacy and half-life of antibody but are also implicated in the clinical symptoms of allergy and anaphylaxis. In addition, because the Fc fragment of the mAb is of murine rather than human origin, its therapeutic administration may fail to activate appropriate immune effector functions such as CDC and ADCC, and as such prove ineffective.

Chimeric monoclonal antibodies

In an attempt to overcome the HAMA response and improve the clinical efficacy of murine-derived mAbs for human therapy, genetic engineering techniques have been developed to 'humanize' murine mAbs (Figure 26.2). Genes that encode mouse antibody variable regions specific to an antigen of interest may now be identified, cloned and inserted into a vector along with the genes encoding human immunoglobulin constant domains. Transfection of this vector into an appropriate cell line such as Chinese hamster ovary cells will result in expression of these transfected genes and synthesis of a chimeric mAb containing mouse variable and human constant regions. These cells may be screened, cloned, and expanded like conventional hybridomas to provide a stable source of chimeric mAb.

Humanized monoclonal antibodies

The humanization of murine-derived mAbs has been further developed to produce 'CDR grafted' or humanized mAbs. This approach requires the synthesis of a novel variable region utilizing gene sequence information for the three epitope specific murine CDRs combined with compatible sequences from human variable framework regions. The newly created humanized variable regions can then be linked to human constant region genes that when expressed in an appropriate cell line will produce a humanized mAb. In practice, grafting of murine CDRs alone usually results in some loss of antigen-binding affinity and a number of the original framework region aminoacid residues may also need to be retained alongside the CDRs to maintain mAb affinity.

Fully human monoclonal antibodies

The production of fully human mAbs is now possible through the use of phage display libraries or transgenic mice carrying human immunoglobulin gene loci. Phage display technology requires the isolation of gene segments encoding human variable mAb domains and their fusion to genes encoding bacteriophage coat proteins. By infecting bacteria with these transfected phages, particles containing immunoglobulin variable domain proteins will be synthesized and expressed. Phage display libraries may be built up consisting of a large collection of phages ($>10^{10}$), each expressing a variable domain specific for an individual antigen. By challenging these libraries with antigens

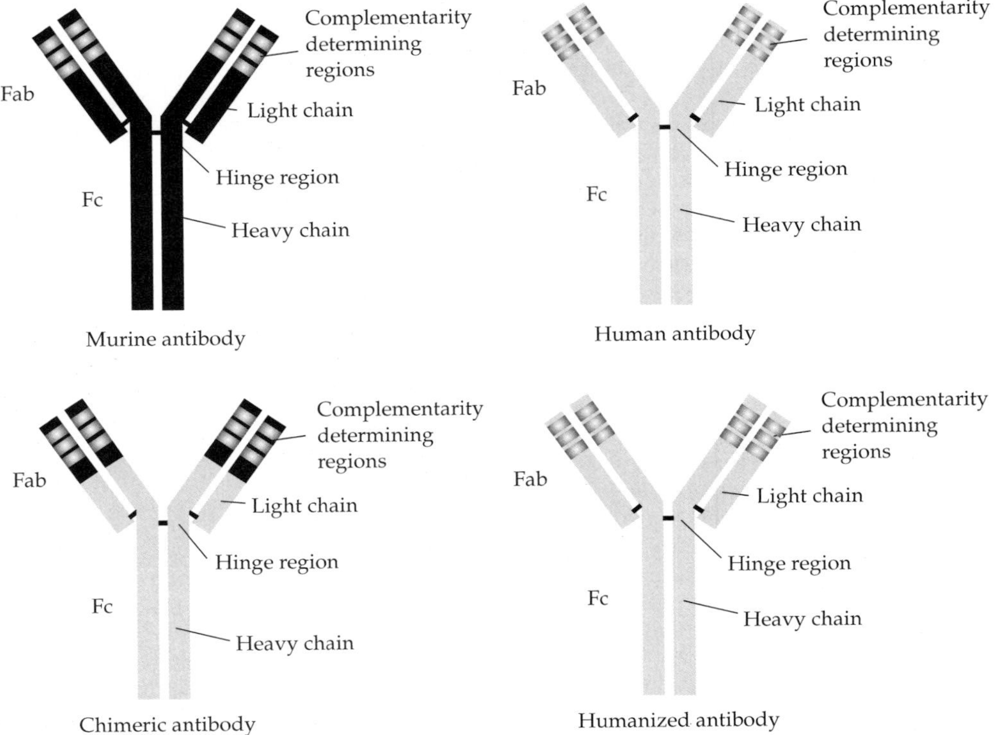

Figure 26.2 Murine, human, chimeric, and humanized antibodies.

of interest and isolating phages that express appropriate antigen-binding domains, the gene encoding the variable region of interest may be recovered from the isolated phage, joined to the remaining parts of a human immunoglobulin gene and transfected into an appropriate host cell capable of secreting the resultant fully human mAb. In addition to the fully human nature of mAbs produced through phage display techniques, other advantages of this technique include the number and diversity of mAbs that can be generated in a relatively short time-frame and the ability to use selection and screening strategies to isolate mAbs with desirable characteristics (e.g. high affinity) (Vaughan et al., 1996, 1998).

An alternative approach in development is the production of fully human mAbs utilizing transgenic animals (Jakobovits, 1995; Mendez et al., 1997). This technology requires deletion of an animal's own immunoglobulin genes and the subsequent introduction of human immunoglobulin gene segments. As a result of this genetic manipulation, antigen immunization results in the *de novo* generation of a fully human immunoglobulin which may be modified using standard somatic fusion technology to generate mAbs of any class desired.

26.5 Antibody function—mechanisms of action

Antibodies are the mediators of humoral immunity. Following the recognition of specific antigen, antibodies may trigger a number of immunological effector mechanisms that include antigen opsonization, CDC and antibody-directed cellular cytotoxicity (ADCC). In addition to these classical functions, therapeutic mAbs provide scope for additional modes of action. These include blockade or augmentation of cell signalling by tumour cells or by cells of the immune system and the delivery of a variety of cytotoxic immunoconjugates (Figure 26.3).

26.5.1 Opsonization

Opsonization describes the process whereby target cells expressing antigen are coated by specific

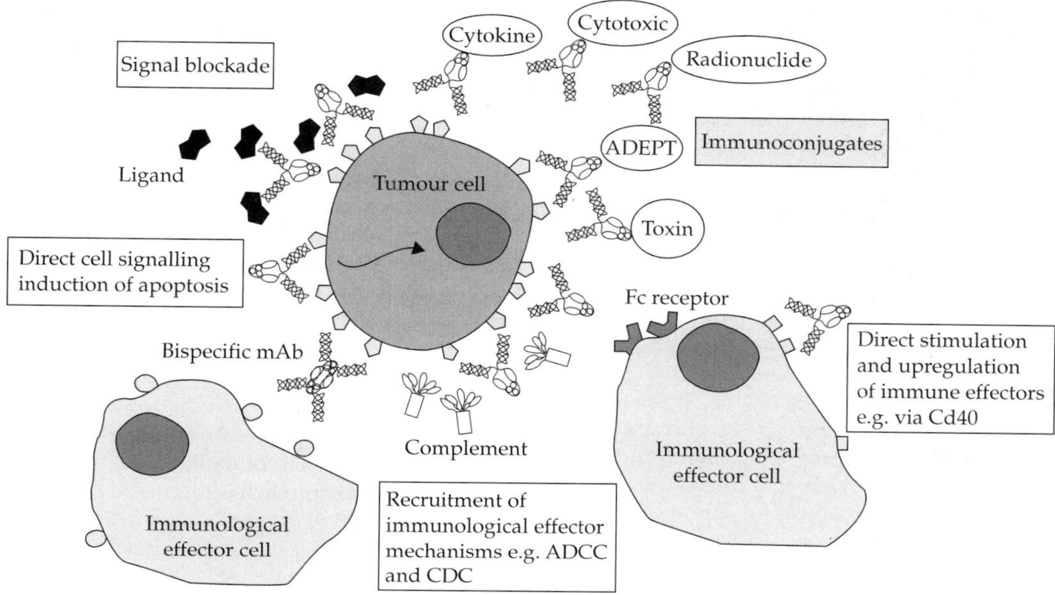

Figure 26.3 Potential mechanisms of action of therapeutic mAbs.

antibody which in turn attracts phagocytic cells such as neutrophils and macrophages. Phagocytosis of antibody coated cells is an important defence against common bacterial pathogens but is not thought to play a major role in anti-cancer mAb therapy.

26.5.2 Complement-mediated cytotoxicity

Complement is a major effector component of humoral immunity and is thought to contribute considerably to the therapeutic effect of a number of mAbs used in the treatment of cancer. Complement exists as a number of circulating serum glycoproteins which, when activated via a tightly regulated enzymatic cascade, promote the development of an inflammatory response, target cell opsonization and cell lysis. Complement can be activated through a number of pathways but the 'classical' pathway of complement activation is dependent upon the binding of antibody to target antigen. C1, a component of complement is able to bind to the Fc portions of aggregated antibodies bound to target antigen. C1 binding leads to a conformational change in C1 that converts it to an active serine protease enzyme capable of initiating the enzymatic cascade of complement activation. The end result of complement activation is the production of the membrane attack complex (MAC), a macromolecular complex able to perforate target cell membranes and cause cell death by profoundly disrupting cellular osmotic stability. In addition to MAC formation, the complement cascade leads to the generation of anaphylotoxins such as C3a, C4a, and C5a. These complement fragments play an important role in the development of an effective inflammatory response. Complement fragments such as C3b can also act as opsonins, coating antigen, and antigen–antibody complexes.

26.5.3 Antibody-dependent cellular cytotoxicity

Natural killer cells, macrophages/monocytes, neutrophils, and eosinophils lack immunological specificity and memory but express membrane receptors that recognize the Fc fragment of antibody. Fc receptor binding can effectively direct these non-antigen-specific effector cells to a target dictated by antibody specificity. Once localized to the target cell, the secretion of lytic enzymes, tumour necrosis factor and other cytotoxic substances by effector cells mediates target cell killing, a process known as ADCC. In common with CDC, ADCC is thought to contribute considerably to the therapeutic effect of many anticancer mAbs.

26.5.4 Cell signalling and blockade

Therapeutic antibodies may be raised against a variety of cell surface receptors expressed on the surface of malignant cells. Upon receptor binding, mAb can stimulate (i.e. provide growth inhibitory or apoptotic signals) or block (i.e. prevent growth signals) receptor signalling. The development of Trastuzumab (Herceptin), a humanized IgG_1 mAb directed against the extracellular domain of the HER-2/neu (c-erbB-2) epidermal growth factor receptor (EGFR) and licensed for the treatment of metastatic breast cancer is an example of this approach (see also Section 26.6).

mAbs can be also be raised against key cytokines or ligands and prevent cell–cell signalling through their elimination or by preventing their binding to target receptor. Of considerable interest are mAbs that have been developed to mimic or block ligand/receptor interactions that are capable of promoting strong cellular immune responses against tumours, irrespective of tumour antigen expression. These molecules, among others, include the immune cell co-receptors CD152 (CTLA4) and CD40. Normal signalling through CTLA4 (cytotoxic T-lymphocyte antigen 4), expressed on the surface of T cells down regulates T-cell activation. Through the development of mAbs which can bind and block CTLA-4 signalling, it appears possible to promote T-cell activation and proliferation and significantly enhance tumour cytotoxicity (van Elsas et al., 2001). The targeting of CD40 represents an alternative approach designed to augment weak tumour antigen responses. CD40 is normally expressed on antigen-presenting cells (APCs) and its stimulation by activated T-helper cells empowers APCs to present antigen to and activate responding cytotoxic T cells. Stimulation of CD40 by therapeutic mAb can effectively bypass the need for specific T-cell help and impressive results with agonistic anti-CD40 mAbs have been seen in syngeneic mouse models of malignancy (French et al., 1999). A human phase I clinical trial of a chimeric IgG_1 anti-CD40 mAb is currently underway. This approach to mAb therapy has a number of advantages over conventional tumour targeting. By selecting an antigen expressed by the immune system rather than tumour itself, a wide range of malignancies may be targeted regardless of tumour antigen expression. An additional advantage includes the potential for the development of persistent, long-term, antitumour immunological memory, a result in keeping with animal models of anti-CD40 mAb treatment, where treated animals were protected from further tumour rechallenge without the need for further mAb therapy (French et al., 1999). There are a number of unknowns with this approach, not least the worry about the induction of unwanted autoimmunity; reassuringly, this was not encountered in the published phase I trial of CD40 ligand therapy that evaluated its safety and tolerability in the treatment of a variety of malignancies (Vonderheide et al., 2001).

26.5.5 Immunoconjugates—arming mAbs

Laboratory techniques exist to allow the conjugation of a wide variety of molecules to specific antibodies and this approach is discussed below. Given careful selection of tumour antigen, this technology permits the selective delivery of an anticancer agent directly to antigen expressing tumour cells with the aim of maximizing delivery of the agent to tumour and minimizing systemic toxicity.

Immunotoxins

A variety of plant and bacterial toxins have been conjugated to mAbs and tested in pre-clinical and early phase clinical trials as potential anticancer therapies. These have included the potent ribosome inactivating proteins ricin and saporin and bacterial toxins such as *Pseudomonas* exotoxin (Pai et al., 1996; Flavell et al., 2001). These molecules are highly toxic and without conjugation and selective delivery by mAb, their systemic use would not be feasible. Plant or bacterial toxins are potentially immunogenic and antibody responses to toxin immunoconjugates have been noted. Despite selective toxin delivery, clinical trials have encountered problematic toxicity, predominately with vascular leak syndrome (Schnell et al., 2003). This syndrome, manifested by widespread oedema that may be dose limiting and severe, is thought to be secondary to toxin-mediated endothelial injury. Encouragingly, recent animal data suggest that for ricin, it may be possible to modify a short aminoacid motif in the ricin A chain and abolish vascular leak syndrome without loss of tumour cytotoxicity (Smallshaw et al., 2003).

Cytotoxic agents

A variety of conventional chemotherapy agents have been conjugated to mAbs and some of these cytotoxic immunoconjugates have been evaluated in clinical trials. Doxorubicin, an anthracycline cytotoxic in routine systemic use, has been conjugated to a mAb that recognizes the oncofetal antigen Lewis Y, expressed on many common solid tumours. Pre-clinical testing revealed promising activity but early phase clinical trials in the treatment of breast and gastric malignancies have been disappointing (Trail et al., 1993; Tolcher et al., 1999; Ajani et al., 2000). The absence of significant clinical activity may be related to the low proportion of antibody (and therefore cytotoxic drug concentration) that can effectively localize to target; in contrast to conventionally administered doxorubicin, the dose-limiting toxicities of the immunoconjugate were found to be gastrointestinal rather than haematological, a finding thought to be related to normal tissue mAb binding. Gemtuzumab ozogamicin (Mylotarg), a humanized IgG_4 mAb directed against the CD33 antigen and conjugated to the tumour antibiotic calicheamicin (an agent several hundred-fold more potent than doxorubicin) has met with more clinical success and is discussed later (Section 26.6).

Antibody-directed enzyme-prodrug therapy

An alternative approach with the aim of selectively delivering cytotoxic drug to the site of tumour is known as antibody-directed enzyme-prodrug therapy (ADEPT). This approach involves the activation of a cytotoxic prodrug at the tumour site by an enzyme that has been targeted to tumour through its conjugation to specific mAb (Figure 26.4). This approach has a number of theoretical advantages. Exceptionally high concentrations of active drug can be selectively delivered to any number of tumour sites while minimizing active drug exposure to normal tissues (and hence toxicity). In contrast to the delivery of mAb-toxin/chemotherapy conjugates, a much larger number of active cytotoxic molecules can, in theory, be generated at the tumour site by a single mAb–enzyme conjugate. The generation of high concentrations of active drug within the interstitial space of a tumour site allows for effective drug diffusion and exposure to adjacent tumour cells without the need for antibody binding (by-stander effect). This can help to overcome the limited diffusion capabilities of antibodies within tumour sites and the considerable variability in intratumoral antigen expression. However, in common with other immunoconjugates immunogenicity has been a problem. This may be overcome through the use of human(ized) mAbs and enzymes, an approach already being undertaken (Bosslet et al., 1994). A number of early phase I clinical trials have been undertaken and clinical development is ongoing (Napier et al., 2000; Francis et al., 2002). Some tumour responses have been seen but myelosuppression appears to be dose limiting, a feature likely to be related to diffusion of activated drug from the site of tumour into the systemic circulation.

Cytokines

A number of mAb immunoconjugates have been developed to target cytokines such as interleukin 2 (IL2), interleukin 12 (IL12) and granulocyte/macrophage colony-stimulating factor (GM-CSF) to the tumour micro-environment with the aim of enhancing the recipient's immune response to tumour whilst minimizing the substantial side-effects that are associated with systemic cytokine delivery (Penichet and Morrison, 2001). Promising pre-clinical results have been achieved using this approach to deliver IL2, a cytokine (normally produced by responding T helper cells) able to stimulate T cells to proliferate and become cytotoxic. Early clinical trials with IL2 immunoconjugates are ongoing.

Radioimmunotherapy

By arming antibodies with radionuclides, effective tumour cell killing may be augmented through the delivery of radiotherapy to both the target and by-stander cells (tumour cells in close proximity, but not bound by mAb) in addition to any endogenous, anti-tumour activity of the naked carrier antibody (Illidge et al., 1999). mAb-targeted radiotherapy, in common with ADEPT may overcome some of the potential problems of variable tumour antigen expression and poor mAb penetration in poorly vascularized or bulky tumours. Clinical studies in non-Hodgkin's lymphoma of ^{90}Yttrium-labelled Ibritumomab, a radiolabelled anti-CD20 mAb, have demonstrated its superior efficacy over naked mAb (Witzig et al., 2002) (see also Section 26.6). Radioimmunotherapy is also under investigation in the treatment of solid tumours. Pemtumomab (Theragyn) is a murine IgG_1 mAb that has been conjugated to the radioisotope Yttrium-90. It binds specifically to a glycoform of MUC1 (CD227), a cell surface glycoprotein overexpressed on the surface of epithelial tumour cells, including ovarian, gastric, breast, and lung. The results of

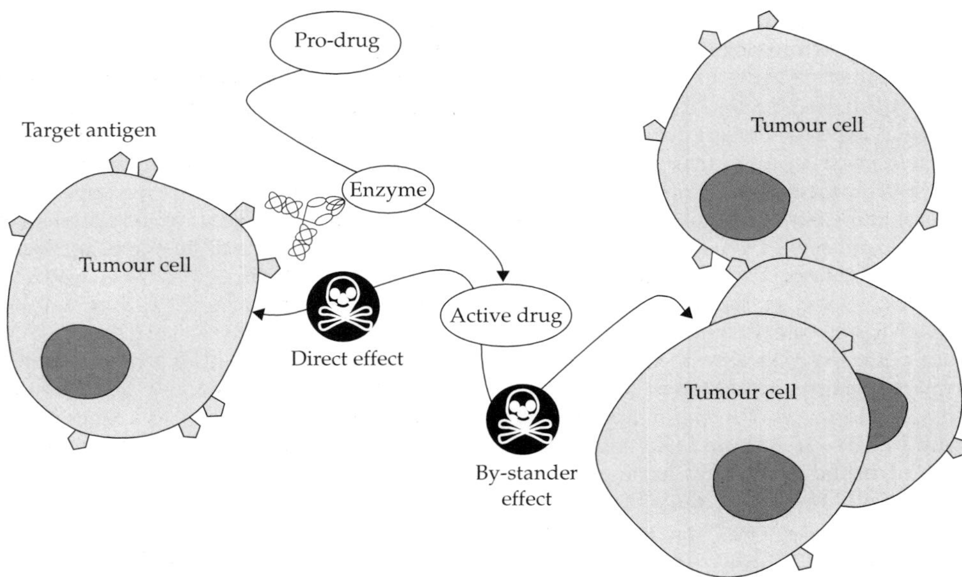

Figure 26.4 A schematic representation of antibody-directed enzyme-prodrug therapy (ADEPT) therapy. Inactive, non-toxic prodrug is converted to active drug at the site of tumour by an enzyme conjugated to mAb. Active drug is able to diffuse to adjacent tumour cells not bound by mAb (by-stander effect) in addition to a direct effect on tumour cells bound by mAb.

a recently completed large phase III study (SMART trial) evaluating its efficacy in addition to standard adjuvant therapy for epithelial ovarian carcinoma are awaited. An alternative approach to radioimmunotherapy that has been examined in early clinical trials involves the use of tumour specific mAbs conjugated to streptavidin (Cremonesi et al., 1999). Tumour-selective delivery of radionuclide can then be accomplished through its conjugation to biotin, a molecule with extremely high affinity for streptavidin.

26.5.6 Bispecific antibodies

Cytotoxic and T-helper cells are normally activated following T-cell receptor recognition of processed antigen in association with the major histocompatibility complex (MHC) displayed on the surface of APCs. mAbs have been generated that can bind to and activate the T-cell receptor independent of MHC or antigen. Bispecific antibodies, immunoglobulin constructs that can effectively bind two epitopes, have been created that combine this T-cell activating property in association with an anti-tumour mAb. In doing so, bispecific antibodies can activate and retarget cellular immune responses towards a preselected, targeted tumour antigen. T-cell activation in this situation requires effective cross-linking by antibody and by designing bispecific antibodies with only a single T-cell arm, widespread T-cell activation can be limited; only those bispecific antibodies that have bound to tumour cells and are presented in a multimeric array will effectively activate T cells. Bispecific antibodies that can target natural killer cells (via CD16/FcγRIII) and macrophages (via FcαRI/CD89) have also been designed. This approach is not limited to the recruitment of cellular immunity; in theory, bispecific antibodies can be designed to recruit and deliver an array of cytotoxic agents such as radionuclides, toxins, cytokines, and cytotoxic drugs (French et al., 1995; Koelemij et al., 1999). Although this approach has shown promising results *in vitro*, and *in vivo* animal and human studies have met with more limited success (Segal et al., 1999).

26.6 Successful antibody targeting: mAbs licensed for clinical use

A number of mAbs are now in therapeutic use for humans in the treatment of malignancy and their role is discussed below. A much larger number of mAbs are being evaluated in a range of phase I, II, and III trials.

26.6.1 Rituximab

Four mAbs currently in routine clinical use recognize cluster designation (CD) molecules expressed by a variety of haematological malignancies. Rituximab (Rituxan, Mabthera) was the first mAb to be approved for the treatment of a malignant condition. It was rapidly incorporated into clinical use and quickly became the largest selling new anti-cancer drug. Licensed for the treatment of B-cell lymphoma, it is a chimeric IgG_1 anti-CD20 mAb. CD20 is a transmembrane protein expressed on normal and malignant B cells but is absent from stem cells, plasma cells, and non-lymphoid tissue. Rituximab binds CD20 with high affinity and is thought to achieve its clinical effects through the activation of CDC, ADCC, and the induction of apoptosis (Reff et al., 1994; Shan et al., 1998; Cragg et al., 2003). Both normal and malignant B cells are targeted but the regeneration of normal B cells from pluripotent stem cells effectively leads to the selective depletion of the malignant clone. Rituximab has demonstrated efficacy in the treatment of both low and intermediate-grade non-Hodgkin's lymphoma (NHL), as a single agent or in combination with standard chemotherapy regimens. In the pivotal phase II study of Rituximab therapy for follicular NHL, response rates of 48% were achieved in relapsed disease, with minimal toxicity (McLaughlin et al., 1998). Significantly higher response rates have subsequently been demonstrated in trials of first-line therapy (Colombat et al., 2001). Retreatment with rituximab at relapse seems well tolerated and effective with a very low rate of human anti-chimeric antibody (HACA) development (Davis et al., 2000). For intermediate-grade NHL, a phase III study evaluating the treatment of diffuse large B-cell NHL in elderly patients, demonstrated that the addition of rituximab to standard CHOP (cyclophosphamide, doxorubicin, vincristine, prednisone) chemotherapy significantly improved response rates, event free survival and overall survival without an increase in clinically relevant toxicity (Coiffier et al., 2002).

26.6.2 ^{131}Iodine-Tositumomab and ^{90}Yttrium-Ibritumomab

^{131}Iodine-Tositumomab (Bexxar) and ^{90}Yttrium-Ibritumomab (Zevalin) also target the CD20 molecule but in contrast to rituximab have been conjugated to radionuclides. Both ^{90}Yttrium-labelled Ibritumomab, a murine IgG_{2a} anti-CD20 mAb (the parent mAb of Rituximab) and ^{131}Iodine-labelled Tositumomab, a murine IgG_1 anti-CD20 mAb are in use for the treatment of relapsed or refractory low-grade, follicular, or transformed B-cell non-Hodgkin's lymphoma. A randomized phase III trial of ^{90}Y-Ibritumomab against Rituximab in patients with refractory or relapsed low-grade, follicular or transformed NHL, demonstrated that the addition of a radionuclide to naked mAb significantly improved overall response rates and complete response rates (Witzig et al., 2002). Treatment with ^{90}Y-Ibritumomab was well tolerated but was associated with an increased incidence of reversible myelosuppression.

26.6.3 Gemtuzumab ozogamicin

Gemtuzumab ozogamicin (Mylotarg) is a humanized IgG_4 mAb conjugated to novel enediyene tumour antibiotic, calicheamicin. It is directed against another CD molecule, CD33, a sialic-acid-binding Ig-like lectin found on the surface of 80–90% of acute myeloid leukaemia (AML) cells and myeloid progenitor cells. It is licensed for the treatment of first relapse, CD33 expressing AML in elderly patients. In common with CD20 it is not expressed on pluripotent stem cells or normal non-haematopoietic tissues (Dinndorf et al., 1986). Calicheamicin becomes inactivated when conjugated to a mAb but is selectively reactivated within the tumour following receptor binding and antibody internalization. Calicheamicin is an extremely potent inducer of double-stranded DNA breaks (Zein et al., 1988). Remission rates of 30% have been demonstrated using Gemtuzumab ozogamicin in patients with relapsed AML although significant myelosuppression and hepatotoxicity due to veno-occlusive disease have been encountered (Sievers et al., 2001).

26.6.4 Alemtuzumab

Alemtuzumab (Campath-1H) is a humanized IgG_1 mAb directed against the CD52 antigen, a glycopeptide highly expressed on the majority of normal and malignant B and T lymphocytes but not normal stem cells. It is thought to achieve its therapeutic effects through a combination of CDC and ADCC

(Heit et al., 1986; Dyer et al., 1989; Greenwood et al., 1993). It is licensed for the treatment of patients with B-cell chronic lymphocytic leukaemia who have been treated with alkylating agents and have failed fludarabine therapy. In a large phase II study, objective response rates of 33% were seen (Keating et al., 2002). In contrast to rituximab, the treatment of B-CLL by alemtuzumab is associated with significant levels of immunosuppression and an increased risk of infective complications. A proportion of these infections are opportunistic in nature, a finding at least in part related to the T-cell depletion that results from alemtuzumab treatment. This property of alemtuzumab has been exploited in studies evaluating the effects of T-cell depletion in allogeneic bone marrow transplant grafts (Hale et al., 1998).

26.6.5 Trastuzumab

Trastuzumab (herceptin) is approved for the treatment of metastatic breast cancer and is a humanized IgG_1 mAb directed against the extracellular domain of the HER-2/neu (c-erbB-2) EGFR. HER-2/neu is overexpressed on approximately 25% of breast cancers and its overexpression correlates well with a number of adverse histological prognostic factors that include tumour grade, size, ploidy, and lack of steroid receptor expression (Slamon et al., 1987). The antibody shows moderate efficacy with a response rate of around 15% when used as a single agent in the treatment of metastatic breast cancer (Cobleigh et al., 1999). When combined with conventional cytotoxic chemotherapy, trastuzumab and has been shown to provide significant additional benefit. In the pivotal phase III trial, combination therapy resulted in significantly higher response rates, longer median duration of response, better one year survival rates and improved overall survival (Slamon et al., 2001). The effects of trastuzumab are likely to be mediated through a number of mechanisms that include signal blockade and immune effector recruitment (Sliwkowski et al., 1999; Harries and Smith, 2002) Of note, trastuzumab, particularly when used in combination with anthracycline chemotherapy, has been associated with an increased incidence of cardiac dysfunction. The basis for the observed cardiotoxicity is, as yet, not fully explained. HER-2/neu is also overexpressed on a number of other epithelial malignancies that include lung, prostate, ovary, and gastrointestinal tract and clinical trials using trastuzumab in these diseases are underway.

26.7 Antibodies in development and target antigens

In addition to those mAbs in routine clinical use, a large number of therapeutic anticancer mAbs are in pre-clinical development and many are being evaluated in clinical trials. Interest has been focused on a number of tumour antigens that include cell surface receptors, oncofetal antigens, and cellular adhesion molecules, in addition to antigens associated with tumour neovasculature. A selection of these mAbs is discussed below in relation to their target antigens.

26.7.1 Growth factor receptors

In common with HER-2/neu, HER-1 is a member of the EGFR family and the target of cetuximab (erbitux) a chimeric IgG_1 mAb. HER-1 is implicated in tumour cell invasion, proliferation, metastasis, and angiogenesis and its blockade by cetuximab is associated with clinically useful activity in a number of solid tumours (Baselga, 2001). Cetuximab has shown therapeutic efficacy as a single agent or in combination with radiotherapy or chemotherapy and its evaluation continues in phase III trials of the treatment of colorectal cancer and head and neck cancer.

26.7.2 Oncofetal antigens

Carcinoembryonic antigen (CEA) is one of the best known and most extensively studied oncofetal antigens. Oncofetal antigens are proteins normally expressed transiently during embryonic development of normal tissues that are also expressed on the surface of many malignant cells. CEA is expressed on the cell surface of many adenocarcinomas, particularly those of the gastrointestinal tract and its measurement in serum is a useful marker in the clinical management of colorectal cancer. CeaVac, a murine IgG anti-idiotype mAb, is currently being evaluated in phase III clinical trials. In contrast to other therapeutic mAbs, the approach of CeaVac is one of vaccination rather than direct mAb-mediated therapy. CeaVac is an anti-idiotype antibody that acts as an image of the true CEA antigen. It was developed by immunizing Balb/C mice with a mAb (8019) against human CEA to produce a mAb recognising the idiotype of the 8019 mAb (Bhattacharya-Chatterjee et al., 1990). Following administration, it can act as a surrogate tumour antigen and lead to the development of 'anti-anti-idiotype' antibodies that in turn recognize and bind the original tumour antigen CEA. Clinical studies have shown that administration of CeaVac is associated with the development of a potent humoral and cellular response against CEA in patients with resected colorectal cancer (Foon et al., 1999). Disappointingly, a recent phase III clinical trial has failed to show any significant survival benefit following the addition of CeaVac to 5FU-based chemotherapy for metastatic colorectal cancer, despite the development of anti-CeaVac antibodies in more than 75% of patients treated (Bhatnagar et al., 2003). Antibodies to a number of other oncofetal antigens are currently being evaluated. These include the Lewis X and Y antigens and tumour-associated glycoprotein-72, expressed on a variety of common solid tumour types.

26.7.3 Cellular adhesion molecules

A variety of antigens associated with cellular adhesion molecules have been identified as potential targets for therapeutic mAbs. Edrecolomab (panorex) is a murine IgG_{2a} mAb that recognizes Ep-Cam (17-1A antigen), an epithelial cellular adhesion molecule expressed on normal epithelial cells and various malignancies. Following the publication of a Phase III clinical trial demonstrating its efficacy as adjuvant therapy in the treatment of surgically resected Duke's C colorectal cancer, edrecolomab was licensed for this indication in Germany (Riethmuller et al., 1994). However, initial clinical optimism has been met with disappointment following the results of a subsequent, much larger European study that has shown it to be inferior to standard chemotherapy and that its addition to chemotherapy does not improve overall or disease-free survival (Punt et al., 2002). The targeting of endothelial cell adhesion molecules in an attempt to disrupt tumour angiogenesis is also under investigation. Target molecules include the integrins ($\alpha V\beta 3$/ $\alpha V\beta 5$), E-selectin, platelet/endothelial-specific cell adhesion molecule (PECAM) and vascular endothelial cadherin. Preclinical and clinical trials are in varying stages of development.

26.7.4 Tumour vasculature

Targeting tumour vasculature is an attractive alternative approach to cancer therapy with potential application to a broad spectrum of tumours. Vascular endothelial growth factor (VEGF) a potent pro-angiogenic factor produced by many types of tumour cells has been targeted by Bevacizumab, a humanized IgG_1 mAb currently in phase III clinical trials for the treatment of a variety of solid tumours. A recently reported phase III trial of Bevacizumab in the first line treatment of colorectal cancer has shown that the addition of this mAb to chemotherapy results in significantly improved survival, progression free survival, response rate and duration of response compared to chemotherapy alone (Hurwitz et al., 2003). Therapeutic mAbs against basic fibroblast growth factor (bFGF), another potent endothelial cell mitogen, are also in development.

26.8 Problems with antibody therapy

Although mAbs have shown great promise in the treatment of a cancer, a number of problems have been encountered that have limited their success. Tumour masses generally sit within a dense packing of stromal tissue, are poorly vascularized and lack a lymphatic circulation. These factors make effective delivery of mAb to target antigen difficult and represent one way in which tumours can avoid effective therapy. Tumour antigens may be internalized or shed by cells with a resultant decrease in tumour cell expression and circulating free antigen. Shed antigen is an easy target for circulating mAb, effectively reducing the quantity of mAb that can reach the malignant cell and potentially increasing mAb toxicity. If therapeutic mAb is able to penetrate tumour, the expression of a target antigen may be highly variable among cells within a tumour or within histologically related tumours in different individuals. Poor targeting of cells with low or absent antigen expression will limit response to treatment and may lead to treatment resistance. The direct arming of mAbs and utilization of the 'by-stander effect' through the development of immunoconjugates is one approach that has been taken to try and overcome the problems of poor antibody penetration and low tumour antigenicity. Antibody immunogenicity has been an additional problem encountered during the development of mAb therapy. HAMA responses are commonly encountered following multiple infusions of mouse mAbs and will adversely affect the clinical efficacy and half-life of antibody. HAMA responses are also implicated in the clinical symptoms of allergy and anaphylaxis. Chimerization, humanization and the production of fully human antibodies have dramatically reduced the incidence of this neutralizing antibody response, although the addition of cytotoxic conjugates in an attempt to improve therapeutic efficacy may once again increase immunogenicity.

26.9 Conclusions

The development of specific mAbs able to selectively target malignant cells has heralded a new era in the development of cancer immunotherapy. The production of murine mAbs, their subsequent chimerization and humanization and, latterly, the production of fully human mAbs, has allowed the development of a wide variety of generally safe, clinically useful therapies able to produce clinical benefit through a variety of mechanisms that include direct cell signalling, receptor/ligand blockade, recruitment of immunological effectors and the delivery of immunoconjugates. Given the large number of mAbs currently undergoing preclinical development and being evaluated in clinical trials, the indications for mAb therapy are set to increase dramatically.

References

Ajani, J. A., Kelsen, D. P., Haller, D., Hargraves, K., and Healey, D. (2000). A multi-institutional phase II study of BMS-182248-01 (BR96-doxorubicin conjugate) administered every 21 days in patients with advanced gastric adenocarcinoma. *Cancer J*, **6**, 78–81.

Baselga, J. (2001). The EGFR as a target for anticancer therapy—focus on cetuximab. *Eur J Cancer*, **37** Suppl 4, S16–22.

Bhatnagar, J., Carmichael, T., Cosgriff, T., Harper, W., Steward, J., Bridgewater, J. et al. (2003). A randomized, double-blind, placebo controlled phase III study of monoclonal antibody 3H1 plus 5-fluorouracil(5-FU)/ leucovorin (LV) in stage IV colorectal carcinoma. *Proc Am Soc Clin Onc*, Abstract 1041.

Bhattacharya-Chatterjee, M., Mukerjee, S., Biddle, W., Foon, K. A., and Kohler, H. (1990). Murine monoclonal anti-idiotype antibody as a potential network antigen for human carcinoembryonic antigen. *J Immunol*, **145**, 2758–65.

Bosslet, K., Czech, J., and Hoffmann, D. (1994). Tumor-selective prodrug activation by fusion protein-mediated catalysis. *Cancer Res*, **54**, 2151–9.

Carter, P. (2001). Improving the efficacy of antibody-based cancer therapies. *Nat Rev Cancer*, **1**, 118–29.

Cobleigh, M. A., Vogel, C. L., Tripathy, D., Robert, N. J., Scholl, S., Fehrenbacher, L. et al. (1999). Multinational study of the efficacy and safety of humanized anti-HER2 monoclonal antibody in women who have HER2-overexpressing metastatic breast cancer that has progressed after chemotherapy for metastatic disease. *J Clin Oncol*, **17**, 2639–48.

Coiffier, B., Lepage, E., Briere, J., Herbrecht, R., Tilly, H., Bouabdallah, R. et al. (2002). CHOP chemotherapy plus rituximab compared with CHOP alone in elderly patients with diffuse large-B-cell lymphoma. *N Engl J Med*, **346**, 235–42.

Colombat, P., Salles, G., Brousse, N., Eftekhari, P., Soubeyran, P., Delwail, V. et al. (2001). Rituximab (anti-CD20 monoclonal antibody) as single first-line therapy for patients with follicular lymphoma with a low tumor burden: clinical and molecular evaluation. *Blood*, **97**, 101–6.

Cragg, M. S., Morgan, S. M., Chan, H. T., Morgan, B. P., Filatov, A. V., Johnson, P. W. et al. (2003). Complement-mediated lysis by anti-CD20 mAb correlates with segregation into lipid rafts. *Blood*, **101**, 1045–52.

Cremonesi, M., Ferrari, M., Chinol, M., Stabin, M. G., Grana, C., Prisco, G. et al. (1999). Three-step radioimmunotherapy with yttrium-90 biotin: dosimetry and pharmacokinetics in cancer patients. *Eur J Nucl Med*, **26**, 110–20.

Davis, T. A., Grillo-Lopez, A. J., White, C. A., McLaughlin, P., Czuczman, M. S., Link, B. K. et al. (2000). Rituximab anti-CD20 monoclonal antibody therapy in non-Hodgkin's lymphoma: safety and efficacy of re-treatment. *J Clin Oncol*, **18**, 3135–43.

Dinndorf, P. A., Andrews, R. G., Benjamin, D., Ridgway, D., Wolff, L., and Bernstein, I. D. (1986). Expression of normal myeloid-associated antigens by acute leukemia cells. *Blood*, **67**, 1048–53.

Dyer, M. J., Hale, G., Hayhoe, F. G., and Waldmann, H. (1989). Effects of CAMPATH-1 antibodies in vivo in patients with lymphoid malignancies: influence of antibody isotype. *Blood*, **73**, 1431–9.

Flavell, D. J., Boehm, D. A., Noss, A., Warnes, S. L., and Flavell, S. U. (2001). Therapy of human T-cell acute lymphoblastic leukaemia with a combination of anti-CD7 and anti-CD38-SAPORIN immunotoxins is significantly better than therapy with each individual immunotoxin. *Br J Cancer*, **84**, 571–8.

Foon, K. A., John, W. J., Chakraborty, M., Das, R., Teitelbaum, A., Garrison, J. et al. (1999). Clinical and immune responses in resected colon cancer patients treated with anti-idiotype monoclonal antibody vaccine that mimics the carcinoembryonic antigen. *J Clin Oncol*, **17**, 2889–5.

Francis, R. J., Sharma, S. K., Springer, C., Green, A. J., Hope-Stone, L. D., Sena, L. et al. (2002). A phase I trial of antibody directed enzyme prodrug therapy (ADEPT) in patients with advanced colorectal carcinoma or other CEA producing tumours. *Br J Cancer*, **87**, 600–7.

French, R. R., Chan, H. T., Tutt, A. L., and Glennie, M. J. (1999). CD40 antibody evokes a cytotoxic T-cell response that eradicates lymphoma and bypasses T-cell help. *Nat Med*, **5**, 548–53.

French, R. R., Hamblin, T. J., Bell, A. J., Tutt, A. L., and Glennie, M. J. (1995). Treatment of B-cell lymphomas with combination of bispecific antibodies and saporin. *Lancet*, **346**, 223–4.

Greenwood, J., Clark, M., and Waldmann, H. (1993). Structural motifs involved in human IgG antibody effector functions. *Eur J Immunol*, **23**, 1098–104.

Hale, G., Zhang, M. J., Bunjes, D., Prentice, H. G., Spence, D., Horowitz, M. M. et al. (1998). Improving the outcome of bone marrow transplantation by using CD52 monoclonal antibodies to prevent graft-versus-host disease and graft rejection. *Blood*, **92**, 4581–90.

Harries, M. and Smith, I. (2002). The development and clinical use of trastuzumab (Herceptin). *Endocr Relat Cancer*, **9**, 75–85.

Heit, W., Bunjes, D., Wiesneth, M., Schmeiser, T., Arnold, R., Hale, G., Waldmann, H. et al. (1986). Ex vivo T-cell depletion with the monoclonal antibody Campath-1 plus human complement effectively prevents acute graft-versus-host disease in allogeneic bone marrow transplantation. *Br J Haematol*, **64**, 479–86.

Hurwitz, H., Fehrenbacher, L., Cartwright, J., Hainsworth, W., Heim, W., Berlin, J. et al. (2003). Bevacizumab (a monoclonal antibody to vascular endothelial growth factor) prolongs survival in first-line colorectal cancer (CRC): Results of a phase III trial of Bevacizumab in combination with bolus IFL (irinotecan, 5-fluorouracil, leucovorin) as first-line therapy in subjects with metastatic CRC. *Proc Am Soc Clin Onc*, Abstract 3646.

Illidge, T. M., Cragg, M. S., McBride, H. M., French, R. R., and Glennie, M. J. (1999). The importance of antibody-specificity in determining successful radioimmunotherapy of B-cell lymphoma. *Blood*, **94**, 233–43.

Jakobovits, A. (1995). Production of fully human antibodies by transgenic mice. *Curr Opin Biotechnol*, **6**, 561–6.

Keating, M. J., Flinn, I., Jain, V., Binet, J. L., Hillmen, P., Byrd, J. et al. (2002). Therapeutic role of alemtuzumab (Campath-1H) in patients who have failed fludarabine: results of a large international study. *Blood*, **99**, 3554–61.

Koelemij, R., Kuppen, P. J., van de Velde, C. J., Fleuren, G. J., Hagenaars, M., and Eggermont, A. M. (1999). Bispecific antibodies in cancer therapy, from the laboratory to the clinic. *J Immunother*, **22**, 514–24.

Kohler, G. and Milstein, C. (1975). Continuous cultures of fused cells secreting antibody of predefined specificity. *Nature*, **256**, 495–7.

McLaughlin, P., Grillo-Lopez, A. J., Link, B. K., Levy, R., Czuczman, M. S., Williams, M. E. et al. (1998). Rituximab chimeric anti-CD20 monoclonal antibody therapy for relapsed indolent lymphoma: half of patients respond to a four-dose treatment program. *J Clin Oncol*, **16**, 2825–33.

Mendez, M. J., Green, L. L., Corvalan, J. R., Jia, X. C., Maynard-Currie, C. E., Yang, X. D. et al. (1997). Functional transplant of megabase human immunoglobulin loci recapitulates human antibody response in mice. *Nat Genet*, **15**, 146–56.

Napier, M. P., Sharma, S. K., Springer, C. J., Bagshawe, K. D., Green, A. J., Martin, J. et al. (2000). Antibody-directed enzyme prodrug therapy: efficacy and mechanism of action in colorectal carcinoma. *Clin Cancer Res*, **6**, 765–72.

Pai, L. H., Wittes, R., Setser, A., Willingham, M. C., and Pastan, I. (1996). Treatment of advanced solid tumors with immunotoxin LMB-1: an antibody linked to Pseudomonas exotoxin *Nat Med*, **2**, 350–3.

Penichet, M. L. and Morrison, S. L. (2001). Antibody-cytokine fusion proteins for the therapy of cancer. *J Immunol Methods*, **248**, 91–101.

Punt, C. J., Nagy, A., Douillard, J.-Y., Figer, A., Skovsgaard, T., Monson, J. et al. (2002). Edrecolomab alone or in combination with fluorouracil and folinic acid in the adjuvant treatment of stage III colon cancer: a randomised study. *The Lancet*, **360**, 671–7.

Reff, M. E., Carner, K., Chambers, K. S., Chinn, P. C., Leonard, J. E., Raab, R. et al. (1994). Depletion of B cells in vivo by a chimeric mouse human monoclonal antibody to CD20. *Blood*, **83**, 435–45.

Riethmuller, G., Schneider-Gadicke, E., Schlimok, G., Schmiegel, W., Raab, R., Hoffken, K. et al. (1994). Randomised trial of monoclonal antibody for adjuvant therapy of resected Dukes' C colorectal carcinoma. German Cancer Aid 17–1A Study Group. *Lancet*, **343**, 1177–83.

Schnell, R., Borchmann, P., Staak, J. O., Schindler, J., Ghetie, V., Vitetta, E. S. et al. (2003). Clinical evaluation of ricin A-chain immunotoxins in patients with Hodgkin's lymphoma. *Ann Oncol*, **14**, 729–36.

Segal, D. M., Weiner, G. J., and Weiner, L. M. (1999). Bispecific antibodies in cancer therapy. *Curr Opin Immunol*, **11**, 558–62.

Shan, D., Ledbetter, J. A., and Press, O. W. (1998). Apoptosis of malignant human B cells by ligation of CD20 with monoclonal antibodies. *Blood*, **91**, 1644–52.

Sievers, E. L., Larson, R. A., Stadtmauer, E. A., Estey, E., Lowenberg, B., Dombret, H. et al. (2001). Efficacy and safety of gemtuzumab ozogamicin in patients with CD33-positive acute myeloid leukemia in first relapse. *J Clin Oncol*, **19**, 3244–54.

Slamon, D. J., Clark, G. M., Wong, S. G., Levin, W. J., Ullrich, A., and McGuire, W. L. (1987). Human breast cancer: correlation of relapse and survival with amplification of the HER-2/neu oncogene. *Science*, **235**, 177–82.

Slamon, D. J., Leyland-Jones, B., Shak, S., Fuchs, H., Paton, V., Bajamonde, A. et al. (2001). Use of chemotherapy plus a monoclonal antibody against HER2 for metastatic breast cancer that overexpresses HER2. *N Engl J Med*, **344**, 783–92.

Sliwkowski, M. X., Lofgren, J. A., Lewis, G. D., Hotaling, T. E., Fendly, B. M., and Fox, J. A. (1999). Nonclinical studies addressing the mechanism of action of trastuzumab (Herceptin). *Semin Oncol*, **26**, 60–70.

Smallshaw, J. E., Ghetie, V., Rizo, J., Fulmer, J. R., Trahan, L. L., Ghetie, M. A. et al. (2003). Genetic engineering of an immunotoxin to eliminate pulmonary vascular leak in mice. *Nat Biotechnol*, **21**, 387–91.

Tolcher, A. W., Sugarman, S., Gelmon, K. A., Cohen, R., Saleh, M., Isaacs, C. et al. (1999). Randomized phase II study of BR96-doxorubicin conjugate in patients with metastatic breast cancer. *J Clin Oncol*, **17**, 478–84.

Trail, P. A., Willner, D., Lasch, S. J., Henderson, A. J., Hofstead, S., Casazza, A. M. et al. (1993). Cure of xenografted human carcinomas by BR96-doxorubicin immunoconjugates. *Science*, **261**, 212–5.

van Elsas, A., Sutmuller, R. P., Hurwitz, A. A., Ziskin, J., Villasenor, J., Medema, J. P. et al. (2001). Elucidating the autoimmune and antitumor effector mechanisms of a treatment based on cytotoxic T lymphocyte antigen-4 blockade in combination with a B16 melanoma vaccine: comparison of prophylaxis and therapy. *J Exp Med*, **194**, 481–9.

Vaughan, T. J., Osbourn, J. K., and Tempest, P. R. (1998). Human antibodies by design *Nat Biotechnol*, **16**, 535–9.

Vaughan, T. J., Williams, A. J., Pritchard, K., Osbourn, J. K., Pope, A. R., Earnshaw, J. C. et al. (1996). Human antibodies with sub-nanomolar affinities isolated from a large non-immunized phage display library. *Nat Biotechnol*, **14**, 309–14.

Vonderheide, R. H., Dutcher, J. P., Anderson, J. E., Eckhardt, S. G., Stephans, K. F., Razvillas, B. et al. (2001). Phase I study of recombinant human CD40 ligand in cancer patients *J Clin Oncol*, **19**, 3280–7.

Witzig, T. E., Gordon, L. I., Cabanillas, F., Czuczman, M. S., Emmanouilides, C., Joyce, R. et al. (2002). Randomized controlled trial of yttrium-90-labeled ibritumomab tiuxetan radioimmunotherapy versus rituximab immunotherapy for patients with relapsed or refractory low-grade, follicular, or transformed B-cell non-Hodgkin's lymphoma. *J Clin Oncol* **20**, 2453–63.

Zein, N., Sinha, A. M., McGahren, W. J., and Ellestad, G. A. (1988). Calicheamicin gamma 1I: an antitumor antibiotic that cleaves double-stranded DNA site specifically. *Science*, **240**, 1198–201.

CHAPTER 27

Immunotherapy of cancer

Andrew M. Jackson and Joanne Porte

27.1 Introduction

Immunotherapy has the potential not only to destroy tumours but also to engender life-long immunity. Furthermore for a small proportion of tumours with viral ethiology, it may be possible to prevent malignancy by prophylactic vaccination. Immunotherapy is a most important and rapidly growing area in applied cancer research and is no longer at the fringe of biological science or restricted to *in vitro* and pre-clinical systems. Rather, immunotherapy is now being explored as a clinical option for all malignancies, and for some diseases it is already the front-line therapy of choice. This chapter brings together some of the most significant advances with promising experimental concepts, placing them in the context of our growing understanding of oncology and immunity.

27.2 Specific Immunotherapy

Antigenic-specificity is conferred by highly polymorphic receptor systems of the B-cell receptor (or antibody), the T-cell receptor (TCR), and the major histocompatibility complex (MHC). Both passive and active antibody-based immunotherapies are discussed in Chapter 26, and so this section will focus on advances relating to the cognate recognition by lymphocytes of antigen (Ag) in the context of MHC. There is an established body of evidence showing that cytotoxic T lymphocytes (CTL) are crucial for controlling tumour growth. CTL recognize small antigenic peptides when associated with cell-surface MHC (also termed human leucocyte antigen—HLA) molecules. Peptide Ag or 'epitopes', generated by cytosolic proteolysis, are transported via the endoplasmic reticulum before export to the cell surface. Numerous reports testify that animals can be immunized against tumours by exploiting the HLA/TCR interaction. However, the majority of Ag explored in these systems were, until recently, foreign (i.e. mutated, viral, or model Ag such as ovalbumin). The process of generating immunity against such foreign Ag is relatively straightforward when compared to priming T-cell responses against Ag from the majority of naturally arising tumours. Most tumours do not express truly unique Ag and therefore 'appear' to the immune system as self, indistinguishable from normal cells. Although self-reactive T and B cells are abundant in the periphery of healthy individuals they fail to react because they have low affinity, are tolerized or anergized in the periphery, or the Ag are poorly presented. Despite this, self-reactive lymphocytes are the arsenal which must be recruited for specific cancer immunotherapy. Correspondingly there is concern over the potential for autoimmune pathology in normal tissues. Indeed autoimmunity is occasionally observed with specific-immunotherapy (e.g. vitiligo in malignant melanoma patients). However, this is usually mild and self-limiting in that pathology arrests once vaccination ceases. Tumours and normal cells are poorly immunogenic and are not likely to be able to perpetuate vaccine-induced immunity, therefore autoimmunity is not presently a limiting factor for immunotherapy. Rather the lack of immunogenicity makes tumours poor targets for activating CTL responses.

27.2.1 Human tumour antigens

It was not until surprisingly recently that Boon and co-workers defined the first human tumour Ag at the molecular level and the approach they pioneered was set to revolutionize tumour immunology (van der Bruggen 1991). Cytolytic effectors, generated from patient's blood by cloning T cells in the presence of autologous tumour cells, were used to screen HLA-matched cells transfected with a cDNA library derived from the patient's tumour. Ultimately a single cDNA was identified which corresponded with the target epitope recognized by the lytic CTL clone. The cDNA derived from the melanoma antigen (MAGE) gene and contained within the translated protein was a small target peptide that bound to HLA-A1. Interestingly, when compared to normal cells, the MAGE gene from tumour cells was identical, and therefore the reason MAGE served as a tumour associated Ag (TAA) lay down-stream of genetic coding. Recently the number of defined TAA has increased and nowhere is this more evident than in melanoma research (Table 27.1). Tumour Ag are categorized according to their origin:

- **Viral**: In tumours with viral ethiology viral proteins serve as targets (e.g. HPV/cervical carcinoma). However, virally induced tumours comprise only a minor portion of cancers and Ag expressed by the bulk of malignancies are more difficult to utilize.
- **Tumour-specific mutated**: As with viral Ag, these provide a unique motif for immune recognition. Mutations exist in many proteins, for example, β-catenin, CDK-4, Hsp70, and KIAA0205. This group also includes proteins arising from translocation such as Bcr-abl. However, mutations are frequently unique to individuals and hence of limited use.
- **Tumour-specific shared**: Although not expressed by normal tissue, these are expressed on a range of tumours. Wide-spread expression makes them useful for generic vaccines. This group includes MAGE-1, BAGE, GAGE, RAGE, NY-ESO, and mucins MUC-1 and -2.
- **Differentiation**: Comprising the bulk of potentially useful TAA these lineage specific markers include tyrosinase, CEA, MC1R, MART-1/MelanA, and PSA. They are particularly useful targets when the target organ is non-essential (e.g. prostate), however, as they are not unique to tumour cells, their use carries the risk of autoimmunity against normal tissues.
- **Overexpressed**: A similar risk is associated with 'overexpressed' Ag, for example, HER2/neu, p53, PRAME, and telomerase (HTERT). Nevertheless, auto-immunity has not been a limiting factor in their use in trials to date.

As CTL recognize epitopes bound to HLA class I, the vast majority of defined Ag are restricted to class I. However, a small number of class II-restricted epitopes have been identified (e.g. for MAGE-A3, NY-ESO-1) and recent studies suggest that tumour-specific class-II 'helper' epitopes are important for optimal immunity (Marzo 2000, Su 2002). Tumour-specific $CD4^+$T cells are found in a range of malignancies including breast, colon, and malignant melanoma and the T-cell help they provide is essential for improving the quality and quantity of CTL responses. The precise role played by specific $CD4^+$T cells at the tumour site remains unclear. However, it is thought that they play a key role in the effector phase, enhancing the local expansion of specific $CD8^+$CTL at the tumour site, augmenting HLA class I expression on tumour cells, and providing memory (Hung 1998, Janssen 2003). Vaccination with tuberculin PPD or tetanus-toxoid provides help at the priming phase of CTL responses. However, only with tumour-specific help is assistance provided at effector phases. In addition, $CD4^+$T cells can lyse target cells by reacting with peptides presented by class II molecules (Manici 1999). One example is the cytolysis of MAGE-A3 expressing HLA-$DP4^+$tumours by

Table 27.1 Defined melanoma antigens and epitopes

Antigen	HLA type	Epitope
MART1	A2	AAGIGIL TV
MART1	A2	ILTVILGVL
MART1	B45	AEEAAGIGIL
MART1	B45	AEEAAGIGILT
gp100	A2	KTWGQYWQV
gp100	A2	AMLGTHTMEV
gp100	A2	MLGTHTMEV
gp100	A2	SLADTNSLAV
gp100	A2	ITDQVPFSV
gp100	A2	LLDGTATLRL
gp100	A2	YLEPGPVTA
gp100	A2	VLYRYGSFSV
gp100	A2	RMLKQDFSV
gp100	A2	RLPRIFCSC
gp100	A3	LIYRRRLMK
gp100	A3	ALNFPGSQK
gp100	A3	SLIYRRRLMK
gp100	A3	ALLAVGA TK
gp100	A24	YVFFLPDHL
gp100	Cw8	SNDGPLI
Tyrosinase	A1	HSTNGVTRIY
Tyrosinase	A1	KCDICTDEY
Tyrosinase	A2	SSDYVIPIGY
Tyrosinase	A2	YMDGTMSQV
Tyrosinase	A2	MLLAVLYCL
Tyrosinase	A24/B44	SEIWRDIDF
TRP-1	A31	MSLQRQFLR
TRP-2	A2	SVYDFFVWL
TRP-2	A2	TLBSQVMSL
TRP-2	A31/33	LLGPGRPYR
TRP-2	Cw8	ANDPIFVVL
TRP-2 6 bis	A2	ATTNILEHY
NA88-A	B13	MTQGQHFLQKV

Antigen	HLA type	Epitope
PSM	A1	HSTNGVTRIY
PSA	A1	VSHSFPHPLY
PSA	A2	FLTPKKLQCV
PSA	A2	VISNDVCAQV
MAGE-A1	A1	EADPTGHSY
MAGE-A1	A3	SLFRAVITK
MAGE-A1	A24	NYKHCFPEI
MAGE-A1	A28	EVYDGREHSA
MAGE-A1	B37	REPVTKAEML
MAGE-A1	B53	DPARYEFLW
MAGE-A1	Cw2	SAFPTTINF
MAGE-A1	Cw3/16	SAYGEPRKL
MAGE-A2	A2	KMVELVHLF
MAGE-A2	A2	YLQLVFGIEV
MAGE-A2	A24	TFPDLESEF
MAGE-A2	A24	IMPKAGLLI
MAGE-A3	A1	EADPIGHLY
MAGE-A3	A2	FLWGPRALV
MAGE-A3	A24	TFPDLESEF
MAGE-A3	A24	IMPKAGLLI
MAGE-A3	B44	MEVDPIGHLY
MAGE-A3	B53	WQYFFPVIF
MAGE-A4	A2	GLYDGMEHL
MAGE-A6	A34	MVKISGGPR
MAGE-A12	Cw7	VRIGHLYIL
BAGE	Cw16	AARAVFLAL
GAGE	A29/Cw6	YYWPRPRRY
NY-ESO-1	A2	SLLMWITQCFL
NY-ESO-1	A2	QLSLLMWIT
NY-ESO-1	A31	ASGPGGGAPR
MC1-R	A2	TILLGIFFL
MC1-R	A2	FLALIICNA

$CD4^+$ CTL specific for the MAGE-$A3_{247-258}$ peptide (Schultz 2000). However, there is a paucity of defined $CD4^+$TAA and at present only limited immunotherapeutic advances can be made.

27.2.2 Genetically enhanced T cells

Administration of tumour-specific CTL yields clinical responses but is fraught with difficulty. There is a paucity of tumour-specific T cells and obtaining sufficient quantities for treatment is almost impossible. Despite significant technological advances for *ex vivo* CTL purification (notably tetrameric-HLA complexes and magnetic selection) isolating CTL that retain viability, specificity, and lytic function remains challenging. Lastly, although it is possible to expand CTL *in vitro* and even generate immortalized T-cell lines or clones this is technically challenging, time-consuming, and has a poor success rate in most laboratories. With advances in gene-manipulation it is now possible to re-engineer T cells for adoptive transfer (reviewed Sadelain 2003). First, the antigenic-specificity is redirected by genetic introduction of physiological T-cell receptor chains or hybrid Ag receptors. Second, T cells are modified to secrete cytokines or express performance-enhancing adhesion or co-stimulatory molecules. Lastly, genetically modified T cells are engineered to incorporate unique markers to allow tracking or suicide genes for deletion.

A number of functional T-cell gene transductions have been made with constructs encoding αβ-TCR specific for human TAA. These include MART1/Melan-A, MAGE-A1, MDM2, and LMP2 (Clay, 1999; Kessels, 2001). However, there are drawbacks to the TCR-transgenic approach. To generate T cells for routine use would require engineering discrete TCR-constructs for different HLA-types and there is a risk of unwanted pairing between transgenic and endogenous TCR chains and acquisition of unknown Ag-specificity. One alternative is chimeric receptors that combine an Ag-binding motif with a transmembrane domain endowed with signalling activity for T-cell activation. Antigen-binding motifs are provided by specific single-chain variable fragments (scFv) of immunoglobulin molecules and phage-display libraries are used to redirect T-cell specificity (Willemsen, 2001). Chimeric receptors exist to a wide-range of Ag, for example, CEA, HER2/neu, PSMA, CD19 (B cell malignancies), and tumour neovasculature using chimeric receptors to VEGF-R2. For signal transduction, the majority of constructs fuse intracellular signalling domains from CD3ζ or FcεRIγ chains to the Ag-specific receptor (Ren-Heidenreich, 2002). One further refinement is the use of CD28 signalling domains (alone or in concert with CD3ζ chain) to substitute for genuine co-stimulation due to the frequent absence of CD80 on tumours (Maher, 2002). Chimeric Ag-receptors offer important advantages over physiological TCR in that they do not require Ag-processing and presentation. Components of the Ag-processing and presentation systems are frequently deregulated in malignancy rendering tumour cells able to escape immune recognition. Furthermore, chimeric receptors can be generated which recognize epitopes not normally 'seen' by TCR such as lipid and carbohydrate moieties. In contrast to TCR-constructs, chimeric receptors can be used in a broad range of patients because they are not HLA-restricted and there is no risk of unexpected receptor specificity.

27.2.3 The importance of dendritic cells

The archetypal Ag-presenting-cell (APC) is the dendritic cell (DC), of which there are several subtypes (Banchereau, 1998). DC are the immune-systems 'nerve-centre', regulating both innate and acquired aspects and balancing homeostatic tolerance with activating lymphocyte responses. Although other professional-APC exist (B cells, macrophages) these cannot match the DC at induction of naïve T-cell responses. Therefore, in order to generate effective CTL responses, TAA need to reach the cytoplasm of DC for presentation on their surface. Many immunotherapy trials have been conducted with tumour-derived material, including peptide, protein, irradiated tumour cells, and nucleic acid. One limitation with these approaches is that the material must encounter DC in order to be processed and presented appropriately. Therefore an increasing number of strategies rely on adoptive transfer of antigenically modified DC (Figure 27.1) including:

(1) loading cell-surface HLA molecules with tumour-peptides
(2) transducing DC with gene therapy vectors (viral, bacterial, plasmid DNA)
(3) fusing DC with the patient's tumour cells
(4) transducing DC with tumour-derived mRNA.

There are also a number of approaches by which Ag can be targeted to DC without *ex vivo* manipulation. These involve generating fusion molecules in which Ag is linked to a targeting molecule with specificity for DC. Targeting moieties of current interest include:

(1) antibodies to cell surface markers, for example, DEC-205, CD83. Although these structures have been used successfully to target Ag to DC they fail to deliver activating signals and hence are poorly immunogenic. Other cell-surface targets such as CD40 may provide useful signals;
(2) cytokine receptors, for example, GM-CSF which serves both to activate DC and deliver Ag to the endosomal compartment;
(3) heat shock proteins (hsp), for example, HSP60, HSP70, HSP110. Heat shock proteins are chaperones and frequently complexed with antigenic peptides. They not only deliver Ag to HLA class I but mature DC by binding to toll-like receptors (TLR) (e.g. TLR4/HSP60).

As understanding of DC increases there is growing interest in the optimal 'type' of DC and the 'stage' of maturation at which it should be used. There are several subsets or lineages of DC, the best characterized of which are myeloid/DC1 and plasmacytoid/DC2 (Figure 27.2). These differ in cell-surface phenotype, cytokine secretion, and consequently have important functional differences. Differentiation of naïve Th1 cells are preferentially primed by DC1 while Th2 cells are driven by DC2. The stage at which naïve T-cells encounter DC

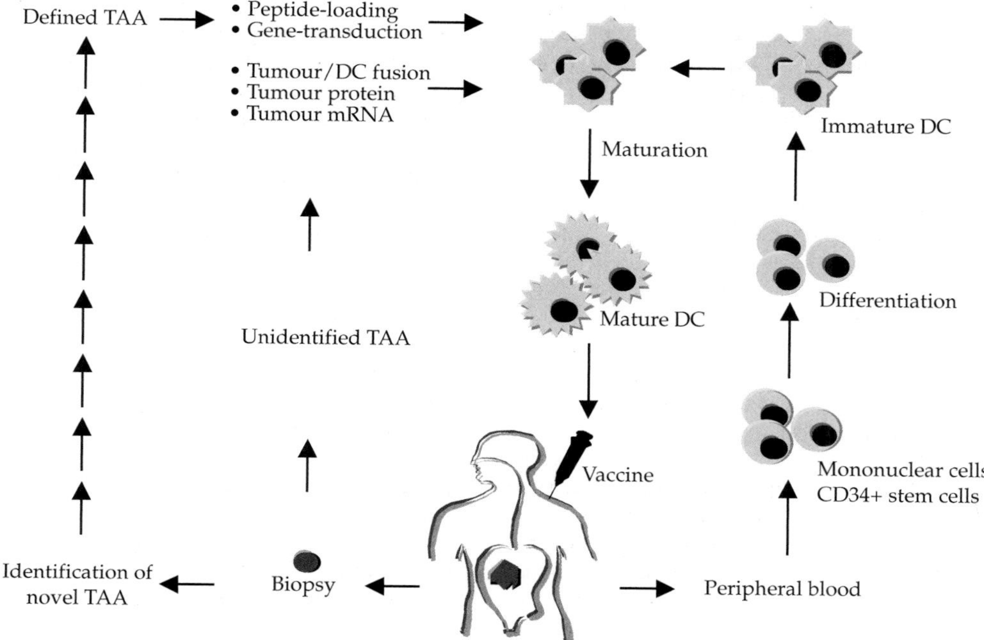

Figure 27.1 Cancer immunotherapy and DCs.

DC1-Myeloid DC
CD11c+, express TLR1, TLR2, TLR3, TLR4, DC-SIGN, DEC-205
preferentially differentiate naïve T cells into Th1
produce IL-12
CCR5, CCR7, CXCR3 lo
secrete CCR4 ligands CCL17 (TARC), CCL22 (MDC): recruit Th2 and Tr cells

DC2-Plasmacytoid DC
CD11c-, CD123+ (IL3Ra), express TLR7,TLR 9, BDCA-2
preferentially differentiate naïve T cells into Th2—elevated in asthma
specialised production of type I IFN
CCR5, CCR7, CXCR3 hi
secrete CCL3 (MIP1a): recruit Th1 and effector T-cells

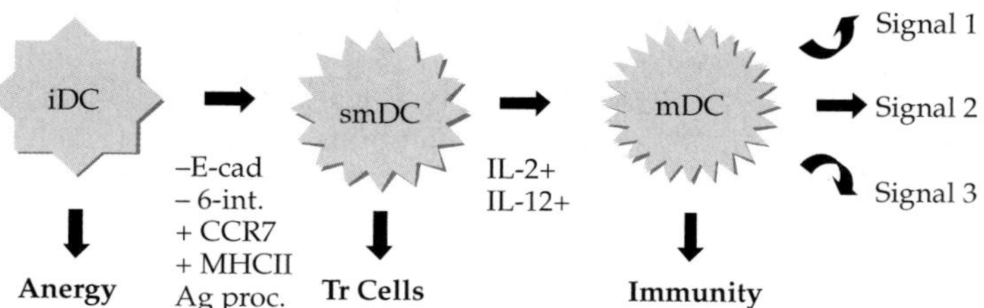

Figure 27.2 DCs subsets and maturation stage.

is critical for determining the outcome of events. Encounter with a mature DC will likely prime immunity, while encounter with immature DC leads to anergy (Figure 27.2). A key advance in our understanding is the appreciation that DC do not solely exist in 'ON' or 'OFF' states, rather they progress through intermediate stages where they are termed semi-mature DC which may bias the induction of regulatory T cells (Tr) (see Chapter 20). Therefore for cancer immunotherapy it is desirable that the DC is mature before encounter with naïve T cells, however, this presents a problem. While injection of immature DC may not prime immunity or may even induce anergy (Dhodapkar, 2001), there are concerns that full-maturation of DC impairs trafficking to lymph-nodes upon adoptive transfer. Research is underway to provide Ag-loaded DC transduced with cDNA encoding maturation factors (e.g. cytokine), such that maturation occurs after re-injection and migration to draining nodes. The route by which DC are injected also impinges upon immunity with Th1 responses only effectively arising following intradermal (i.d) or intralymphatic (i.l) delivery (Fong, 2001).

27.2.4 Peptide vaccines

Empty HLA molecules do not persist on the cell surface, however, peptides load onto HLA by competing with existing peptides. Incubating DC with TAA-peptides renders them highly efficient inducers of CTL responses *in vitro* and *in vivo*. This is one of the most extensively applied DC-based approaches to date, however, despite safety, success is limited with response rates $<20\%$. The majority of peptide trials are undertaken in melanoma, although other studies have been conducted with cervical and breast carcinoma. Marchand et al. (1999) employed the HLA-A1-restricted MAGE-$3_{161-169}$ epitope administered s.c. and i.d. to 39 melanoma patients. At the study's conclusion, 7/25 exhibited significant regression and received further rounds of vaccination. Ultimately three of these achieved complete response (CR) which was durable ($>$2 years) in two despite the absence of detectable MAGE-3-specific CTL. More recent studies used combinations of peptides restricted by a range of HLA (Scheibenbogen, 2000). The combination of cytokine adjuvant (e.g. IL-2) and peptides may offer advantages over peptide alone (Rosenberg 1998). However, significant clinical responses were achieved at the expense of detectable gp100-specific CTL raising questions regarding the mechanism of action.

There are a number of reasons why purified peptide vaccines yield disappointing results. First, in the absence of adjuvant, peptide-vaccines will at best be weakly immunogenic. Second, although peptides effectively generate CTL that kill peptide-pulsed targets in the laboratory, these CTL are of low-quality when required to destroy cells displaying endogenously processed Ag. Third, most trials have used 'immunodominant' peptides, that is, those which bind tightly and stably to HLA. However, these peptides are not ideal candidates for tumour vaccines. The choice of immunodominant peptides largely reflects the technical approaches frequently employed to identify epitopes. However, there are several reasons why peptides such as the HLA-A2-binding peptide of MART-1/MelanA are not ideal. Importantly, there may be a paucity of CTL precursors specific for immunodominant epitopes as the T-cell pre-cursors are deleted during thymic-education. Furthermore, even if a substantial pool of naïve CTL escape deletion they are likely to be tolerized in the periphery. Lastly, one important aspect of peptide selection is the antigen-processing mechanism responsible for generating the epitope. The outcome of antigen-processing is sometimes different in tumour cells compared to DC. This is because the proteasome which is largely responsible for epitope generation is modified in APC in response to pathogen-associated molecular patterns (PAMP) or pro-inflammatory cytokines, for example, IFNγ. Such 'cryptic' epitopes are therefore of little use as vaccines and there is now a requirement for identification of useful epitopes to include confirmation of their generation in tumour cells.

Because of the short half-life of peptides attention has turned to adoptive transfer of peptide-pulsed DC. The study of Thurner (1999) employed three, two-weekly injections of MAGE-$3_{161-169}$-pulsed DC (s.c and i.d. routes) followed by two other i.v. injections. CTL responses were noted in 8/11 HLA-A1 + melanoma patients and regression in 6/11 individual metastases despite overall progression. One important aspect of this type of immunotherapy is immune-escape. Thurner's study found that persistent metastases lacked MAGE-3 mRNA and infiltrating CTL, in contrast to regressing lesions. The use of multiple epitopes, restricted by more than 1 HLA molecule aims to tumour escape. Fourteen melanoma patients were immunized with 5×10^6–5×10^7 DC derived from $CD34^+$ precursors loaded with MART-1, gp100, tyrosinase, MAGE-1, and MAGE-3 peptides (depending on HLA-type) (Mackensen 2000). A number of patients displayed changes in immune status, namely peptide-specific DTH, increased CTL frequency and vitiligo, while 1/14 had no residual disease after resection of metastases.

27.2.5 Gene-modified DC vaccines

Genetically modified vaccines deliver TAA genes and provide a means to generate specific CTL responses with the option of antibody if desired. By delivering only genes encoding the particular TAA against which immunity is desired, some of the limitations and risks of other approaches are negated. No matter which approach is adopted, the vaccine must still access DC for optimal immunity. There are now a number of means by which gene-encoded TAA are introduced into DC (e.g. plasmid, virus, bacteria). All these vectors have PAMPs to deliver activating 'danger' signals transmitted via pattern recognition receptors (PRR) such as the TLR family (Underhill 2002). TLR are specific for a wide-range of danger signals used in immunotherapy including bacterial DNA (TLR9), viral RNA (TLR3), mycobacterial lipoarabinomannan (TLR2), TLR9 (CpG motifs), lipopolysaccharide, and heat-shock proteins (TLR4). Activation of TLR triggers NF-kB and MAPK signalling pathways, a crucial event to enable T-cell priming and activation.

Viral vaccines

A number of viral vectors have been generated with safe profiles for use in immuno-compromised cancer patients, for example, attenuated retrovirus, adenovirus, alphavirus, and vaccinia virus (Bonnet, 2000). However, repeated immunization with one vector is commonly limited by strong anti-vector responses. Strong anti-viral immunity can lead to lethal immune-mediated pathology and 'diverts' the focus of CTL activity away from tumours. Attenuated adenoviruses and vaccinia notably induce particularly strong immune responses, while replication defective retrovirus have been developed for safety and poxviruses have a restricted host range, do not replicate in human cells and can be given repeatedly. Many viral vectors engineered to express TAA are already in clinical trial with some success although most studies are only in phase I/II (reviewed Bonnet, 2000; Moingeon, 2001). As with peptide-vaccines, although specific CTL are frequently noted there is little correlation with objective clinical responses. Heterologous prime/boost strategies using combinations of vectors and/or route offer a more advanced approach and avoid limiting anti-vector immunity. Further advances include agents such as 'CEA-TRICOM', recombinant vaccinia, and fowlpox vectors engineered to express CD54, CD80, and LFA-3 co-stimulatory molecules as well as TAA.

DNA vaccines

Plasmid DNA-vaccines are safe, inexpensive (cheap to engineer and stable), and effective in pre-clinical models. They operate via direct transfection of DC where the TAA cDNA is expressed and processed for presentation to T cells. This can be enhanced by biolistic delivery, propelling DNA-coated gold microparticles through the skin into resident dermal Langerhans cells. Although unmethylated CpG motifs act as adjuvant and they trigger specific CTL, DNA is not as immunogenic as virus or bacteria. This may account for the somewhat disappointing clinical results with DNA cancer vaccines. A recent study with plasmid encoding CEA and HBSAg in 17 patients with colorectal metastases failed to generate CEA-specific antibodies or objective clinical responses (Conry, 2002). Studies directing immune responses against multiple epitopes from a number of TAA are currently underway. Such polyepitope DNA-vaccines have already been shown in pre-clinical models to induce a broader range of CTL-specificities and it is hoped they will address the issue of immune-escape due to antigenic modulation. A combination of DNA-prime with recombinant fowl-pox-boost (notably modified vaccinia virus Ankara—MVA) is a particularly effective way of harnessing the positive properties of both vectors (Robinson, 1999). A heterologous prime/boost trial is underway in patients with malignant melanoma using plasmid DNA/recombinant MVA both engineered to encode a polyepitope vaccine. More recently, and still at the pre-clinical stage, recombinant bacteria have been used to deliver DNA vaccines. Indeed bacteria such as *Salmonella* effectively deliver plasmid DNA directly in to APC. Specificity is provided by mammalian promotor/enhancer elements and translation is maximized by using human optimized codons (reviewed Dietrich, 1999).

Bacterial vaccines

In contrast to classical dogma, antigen from intracellular bacteria is efficiently delivered to HLA class I molecules via alternate antigen processing pathways. Intracellular bacteria are taken up and degraded in phagosomes. Intracellular bacteria (e.g. *Listeria monocytogenes, Shigella flexneri*) escape the phagosome entering the cytosol and accessing the classical class I pathway. Extracellular bacteria like

Escherichia coli also deliver to the HLA class I pathway in a variety of antigen presenting cells (Radford 2003). A more detailed discussion of the antigen processing pathways employed by bacteria is provided in Cheadle and Jackson (2002). Since the realization that bacteria deliver Ag to HLA class I and class II there has been much interest in their use as vaccines. Although there are no published bacterial anti-tumour specific vaccines in clinical trial there are promising pre-clinical results. *Salmonella typhimurium* invades the intestinal epithelium, is phagocytosed by underlying DC and primes T-cell responses. The type III secretion system that *Salmonella* uses to invade epithelium also facilitates entry of recombinant Ag to the class I pathway thus conferring protection against lethal viral challenge. Perhaps the most important advance is the development of *Salmonella*-DNA vaccines which facilitate DNA delivery to DC. Tumour protection was provided in 70% animals when DC infected by auxotrophic mutants of *Salmonella* and *Shigella flexneri* encoding melanoma Ag were used. Despite the extensive use of BCG for local immunotherapy there has been little success with recombinant mycobacteria as tumour vaccines so far. However, BCG is worthy of exploration due to its potent immunostimulatory capacity, history of safe use, and worldwide distribution network. An anti-tumour *Mycobacterium bovis* BCG vaccine was unsuccessful in generating protection against an E7 expressing tumours (Jabbar, 2000). This may be because the tumour antigen was expressed in the bacterial cytosol, whereas it has been shown that for effective cell mediated immunity Ag must be secreted or membrane bound. However, specific anti-tumour CTL responses can be generated as recently demonstrated with recombinant BCG expressing human MUC1 and IL-2 (He, 2002). In addition to whole organisms, a number of bacterial proteins are in pre-clinical evaluation. One study involves cDNA for the translocation domain II of *Pseudamonas aeroginosa* exotoxin-A fused to TAA (Hung, 2001). Domain II translocates to the cytosol from endosomal compartments thus allowing it to target HLA class I. Vaccination resulted in increased HPV E7-specific CTL, and eradication of E7-expressing tumours. Similarly, a construct where the HPV 16 protein E7 was fused to a non-haemolytic listeriolysin has been tested and shown to effectively deliver Ag to the class I pathway. Specific tumour protection has also been observed with the immunotherapeutic administration of fusions between BCG HSP65 and HPV16 E7.

27.2.6 DC/tumour hybrid vaccines

The first trial with DC-tumour hybrid cells was undertaken using allogeneic DC fused with patients' tumour cells (Kugler, 2000). Using electrofusion, hybrids were generated that presented TAA in concert with the co-stimulating capabilities of DC. Patients received up to 5×10^7 hybrids on two occasions 6 weeks apart and, with a mean follow-up time of 13 months, four patients completely rejected all metastases, one presented a 'mixed response', and two had >50% tumour mass reduction. Three of the four CRs were free of disease for up to 21 months. More recently this approach, modified by use of autologous DC, has been applied to melanoma (Krause, 2002). However, although there was evidence of anti-tumour responses it was clinically ineffective. This approach is limited by the need for large amounts of tumour cells and poor fusion rate. An alternative to generating hybrid tumour vaccines is in the form of DC pulsed with tumour lysates or killed tumour cells. In this approach, autologous DC take up tumour material by phagocytosis or pinocytosis. Among the earliest studies is that of Nestle (1998) where 16 melanoma patients were treated with either tumour-lysate pulsed DC or DC pulsed with a cocktail of peptides. Immunity to both tracer immunogen (KLH) and TAA were induced and objective responses were observed in five patients (two CR, three partial responses (PR)). In a further study, 15 neuroblastoma, sarcoma, and renal cancer patients were treated with lysate-pulsed DC without toxicity (Geiger, 2001). Tumour-specific CTL were induced in 50% of patients, marked regression of metastases in one, and stable disease of a durable nature in five (16–30 month follow-up). A recent study compared DC-tumour hybrids with DC loaded with apoptotic B-CLL tumour cells and found that endocytosed tumour cells induced stronger T-cell responses than hybrids (Kokhaei, 2003). This may be accounted for by the greater efficiency of uptake of tumour material than successful formation of DC-tumour hybrids.

27.2.7 DC/mRNA vaccines

The transduction of DC with tumour-derived mRNA avoids many of the limitations with other approaches in that it does not require defined TAA or epitope, it represents all transcribed differences between malignant and normal cells, and the process can be undertaken with minimal amounts of starting material such as those obtained by fine-needle biopsy. This is because it is possible to exponentially amplify mRNA molecules using the PCR (polymerase chain reaction) and generate large amounts of cDNA from which to produce replica mRNA molecules *in vitro*. This process typically takes only hours, compared with the time required for identification and validation of TAA (months/years). In addition, the efficiency of transduction with mRNA is superior to other methods, a fact reflected in CTL-priming and anti-tumour immunity. This approach has been explored in a number of trials where the study end-point of safety was satisfied (Su, 2003; Heiser, 2002). Furthermore, tumour specific immune responses were measured in patients with metastatic renal and prostatic disease. As discussed, one limitation of this and any other approach where professional APC must process antigen lies in the differences in antigen-processing in the target tumour cells. Most recently pre-clinical data has been published to show that transduction of DC with defined mRNA target molecules can prime naïve CTL to destroy tumour vasculature. When immunized with DC transduced with mRNA for neoangiogenic gene products (vascular endothelial growth factor (VEGF), VEGFR-receptor-2 (VEGFR-2), and Tie2 (expressed in proliferating endothelia)) CTL were stimulated, angiogenesis inhibited, and tumour development arrested (Nair, 2003). Future developments may involve generation of subtractive mRNA libraries to minimize autoimmunity or use of mRNA from allogeneic pools of tumour cells avoid the need for patient-specific tumour samples.

27.3 Non-specific immunotherapy

Although elaborate Ag-specific approaches to cancer immunotherapy receive much attention it should not be forgotten that the bulk of immunotherapy procedures are non-specific and often highly effective. Non-specific approaches encompass direct cytopathic effect of cytokines, administration of immune adjuvants (e.g. BCG), and unrestricted cellular cytotoxicity. Although these approaches are not targeted to defined TAA the vigorous immune response elicited by these treatments has often been shown to involve recruitment of Ag-specific CTL.

27.3.1 Immunotherapy with cytokines

Extensive pre-clinical studies indicated great promise for cytokine immunotherapy but this has unfortunately not yet translated into impressive clinical gains. Various practical issues have made this approach problematic, including difficulty in administering sufficient doses systemically, the lack of effective targeting systems to alleviate the need for such high doses and particularly severe toxicity. Although some of the side effects of cytokine-therapy can be managed (e.g. the use of anti-depressants to increase tolerance to both IL-2 and IFNα), more serious toxicity, such as capillary-leak syndrome observed with high-dose IL-2 therapy, is life-threatening. Presently, only a few tumour-types, including renal cell carcinoma and melanoma, are treated with cytokines. The reason why these particular tumours are more responsive than others is unclear but is thought to be due to their increased 'immunogenicity'. Furthermore, as advanced renal cell carcinoma is frequently resistant to chemotherapy and existing treatments for advanced malignant melanoma are largely ineffective, alternative and often experimental treatments are required. The bulk of cytokine-therapy has focused on administration of IL-2 and IFNα, although cytokines such as IL-4, IL-12, IFNγ, and TNFα have also been explored. A summary of traditional and contemporary approaches to cytokine therapy is presented in Figure 27.3.

Approved by the FDA at up to 6mIU/kg/dose by slow i.v. infusion, IL-2 has found particular use for advanced renal cancer. Hospitalization is often required for high-dose IL-2 (especially for i.v. routes) due to severe toxicity and many planned schedules of treatment need to be curtailed. Subcutaneous administration increases tolerability and may be administered on an outpatient basis, encouraging patients to complete schedules. Many studies show both efficacy and toxicity is route-dependent, while others show no difference between bolus and continuous infusion in terms of efficacy or toxicity. Like renal carcinoma, malignant melanoma is also highly chemo-resistant and the best available single-agent chemotherapy is dacarbazine/DTIC with only a 15–20% CR and six-month median survival. Immunotherapy with IL-2

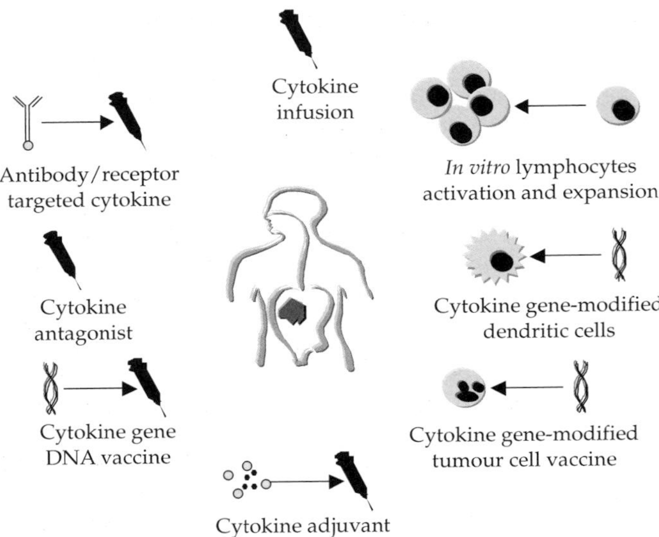

Figure 27.3 Summary of major uses of cytokine in cancer immunotherapy.

induces durable complete remission in a small proportion of patients and recently it has been proposed that combinations of IL-2, IFNα, and chemotherapy may increase survival. However, under phase III examination this proved not to be the case (Rosenberg, 1999).

IFNα is approved in Europe for renal cancer, but its side effects are serious and dose limiting. Common side effects seen with both of these cytokines include a flu-like syndrome, dry skin, and mucous membranes, and changes in mental state such as depression. Randomized trials do, however, suggest that IFNα may give increased survival, for example Pyrhonen (1999) showed a response rate of 16.5% when IFNα was given in conjunction with Vinblastine versus 2.5% with Vinblastine alone. A Medical Research Council trial comparing IFNα with medroxy-progesterone (MRC, 1999) also showed increased two-year survival from 13% to 22%.

Another cytokine, Interleukin-12, is a heterodimeric molecule required for both innate and acquired arms of immunity. It exerts its action by stimulating production of IFNγ and a host of other cytokines that in turn are directly toxic to tumour cells, are anti-angiogenic and induce Th1/CTL responses. Pre-clinical data with IL-12 demonstrated its remarkable anti-tumour properties either alone or as adjuvant for other vaccines. However, in clinical practice, excessive toxicity and modest clinical responses have rendered it of little use. One promising protocol, however, is a combination of IL-12 and anti-CD20 (Rituximab) for B-cell lymphoma (Ansell, 2002). In addition to marked changes in immune status objective responses were found in 29/43 patients and CR in eight patients who received the highest IL-12 dose. IL-12 belongs to a growing family of heterodimeric cytokines with anti-tumour potential including IL-23 and IL-27 that act at different stages in Th-cell differentiation. Although these new cytokines require investigation they may offer further opportunities for cytokine therapy with decreased toxicity.

Second generation cytokine immunotherapy

As survival benefits from cytokine-therapy are at best modest, investigations are underway to enhance efficacy with targeted approaches. If locally high concentrations needed for efficacy can be achieved then toxicity of systemic delivery can be reduced. One new product, pegylated interferon (PEG-Intron, Schering-Plough), is reported to allow 10-fold greater intra-tumoral concentration to be achieved than standard IFNα (Bukowski, 2002). The safety profile of PEG-Intron has been determined and it has demonstrable clinical activity in CML, melanoma, and renal cancer. An alternative approach is that of Bayer Corp., using targeted mutagenesis of human IL-2 to generate a variant with approximately 3000-fold increased selectivity for T cells over NK cells, relative to wild-type IL-2. The variant, 'BAY 50–4798', mobilizes and activates

T cells and inhibits metastasis in pre-clinical models with similar efficacy to standard Proleukin IL-2 but is better tolerated (Shanafelt, 2000). Whether these products exhibit a greater therapeutic index than standard cytokines in humans remains to be determined.

Cytokine gene therapy has advantages over infusion of recombinant proteins in that the levels of cytokine given are considerably lower thereby reducing toxicity, while it is possible to engineer cytokine release specific to the tumour site, thus maximizing efficacy. Vical's Leuvectin consists of an IL-2 expression plasmid complexed with a lipid delivery vehicle for intra-tumour injection. The aim is to stimulate immune responses in large and primary tumours that will also be able to travel to distant sites of metastasis. Autologous tumour-cell vaccines have also been developed. In one study 16 melanoma and sarcoma patients were treated with *GM-CSF*-gene-modified autologous tumour cells (Máhvi, 2002). Although transgene expression was demonstrated, there was little evidence of either immune or clinical responses probably due to the low levels of GM-CSF production. Allogeneic vaccines also have significant potential as illustrated by a recent study of IL-2 and lymphotactin transduced neuroblastoma cells where immune responses were noted in the majority of patients, 2/21 had CR, and one had PR (Rousseau, 2003).

Although the cytokines so far discussed have favoured tumour-destruction, certain members of the cytokine family are responsible for allowing tumours to escape immune detection (e.g. IL-10, TGFβ). Among the most important is TGFβ, an immuno-suppressive cytokine expressed by the majority of tumours. Therefore TGFβ is an important target for immunotherapy with the aim to restore normal immuno-surveillance and destroy tumour cells. Different approaches have been used to target TGFβ including specific antibodies, non-functional soluble receptors, small molecule inhibitors, and anti-sense technology. Gorelick and Flavell showed that blockade of TGFβ signalling allows the generation of anti-tumour immunity in mice which is capable of eradicating live tumour cells that are seeded subsequently, that is, memory. However, wholesale removal of TGFβ causes other problems as it has many other regulatory activities. Further research is therefore required to identify selective inhibitors that block the immuno-suppression pathways while still allowing the other key functions of TGFβ.

27.3.2 Immunotherapy with bacteria

Anecdotal reports describing use of *Streptococci* and tubercule bacilli for cancer therapy date back to the end of the nineteenth century. Coley's approach induced regression but due to serious complications an attenuated *Streptococci* and *Serratia* combination was developed (Coley, 1894). In 1928 Raymond Pearl described that it was unusual for malignancy and florid tuberculosis to co-exist and with the attenuation of *M. bovis* to give BCG the way was paved for bacterial immunotherapy. In addition to protection against leprosy and TB, BCG is the most successful cancer immunotherapy notably against *carcinoma-in-situ* of the bladder (80% CR) (Jackson, 1994; Alexandroff, 1999). Success with BCG-therapy is T- and NK-cell dependent, triggering local inflammation, and infiltration with $CD4^+$ and $CD8^+$T-cells, PMN and NK cells. Current research aims to increase the efficacy of BCG and reduce the potential for toxicity. Other non-viable mycobacteria are currently being investigated for cancer therapy including SRL172, a heat killed preparation of *M. vaccae*. SRL172 is in phase I and II trials for a variety of tumours including non-small-cell lung cancer, renal cell carcinoma, and advanced prostate cancer with some encouraging results, including changes in immune status (decreased IL-4 producing T cells), possible therapeutic benefit and mild toxicity (O'Brien, 2000; Mendes, 2002). Other bacterial products are in clinical trial including a truncated exotoxin fused with interleukin-4 for high-grade glioma (Rand, 2000). Increased IL-4 receptor expression on glioma and astrocytoma provides a degree of targeting particularly when coupled with intra-tumoural delivery. In this study 6/9 patients showed tumour necrosis and one underwent CR without neurotoxicity. The p40 outer membrane protein of *Klebsiella pneumoniae* functions as adjuvant inducing $CD8^+$ CTL independent of $CD4^+$ T-cell help (Miconnet, 2001). The p40 protein is an important technological advance as it binds preferentially to DC. Although the curative potential of live bacteria is established it has been proposed that bacterial DNA and viral RNA, rather than live organisms *per se*, are the active agent. Unmethylated CpG dinucleotides (CpG motifs) directly stimulate a variety of leucocytes including B-cells, DC, Mϕ and NK-cells and ultimately influence the generation of T-cell responses. There is also an additive effect when classical adjuvants such as IFA or alum are co-administered with CpG DNA. Indeed, recent data shows that CpG motifs directly stimulate tumour-specific CTL and current interest centres on its use as either a single-agent therapeutic or as an adjuvant to B- and T-cell vaccines.

27.3.3 Adoptive leucocyte transfer

Adoptive transfer of leucocytes has been subject to intense study for over two decades. An important advance was made when in 1982 the phenomenon of lymphokine activated killer (LAK) cells as a non-MHC-restricted activity of lymphocytes cultured with high-dose IL-2 was first described (Grimm, 1982). Since then, clinical studies have explored LAK cells with or without cytokines such as IL-2, IFNα. Although examined in a wide range of tumour-types, LAK-therapy was only minimally effective (10–20%) in renal cancer, colorectal disease, and malignant melanoma. Around the same time studies began with tumour-infiltrating lymphocytes (TIL) which were found to be up to 100-fold more effective than LAK. However, despite this the clinical results with IL-2 expanded TIL were no better than with LAK cells (Rosenberg, 1987). Both LAK and TIL immunotherapies are still being explored. A recent randomized study using TIL as adjuvant immunotherapy for 88 patients with stage III malignant melanoma failed to show significant differences in relapse-free interval or survival (Dreno, 2002). However, differences were noted in a sub-group of patients with only one involved node with increased survival in the TIL + IL-2 group versus IL-2 alone.

Natural killer (NK) cells, a large granular lymphocyte subset lacking surface antibody or TCR, have the capacity to kill tumour cells while ignoring normal cells (unless infected with certain viruses). Although NK activity is innate, their growth and cytolytic activity is readily enhanced by the action of IL-2 or IFNα. However, when used for immunotherapy these cytokines do not consistently enhance NK activity. Despite years of use, adoptive transfer of activated NK cells has not shown any clear anticancer benefit in the clinic. This may be due to poor activation, delivery, or indeed evolved tumour-escape mechanisms. In order to appreciate how tumours escape NK cell surveillance it is first necessary to understand some basic NK cell biology. The default killing programme of NK cells is effected by means of perforin/granzyme and cytokine production (e.g. IFNγ). However, for the vast majority of surveillance encounters (i.e. contact with normal cells) NK cells do not mediate destruction. This is because they express a vast array of killer cell immunoglobulin-like receptors (KIR) that regulate cytotoxicity upon interaction with HLA class I. The KIR family includes both activating and inhibitory receptors with cytoplasmic immunoreceptor tyrosine-based activating (ITAM) and inhibitory (ITIM) motifs that become phosphorylated during the process of receptor engagement. In the case of ITIM, cells expressing sufficient appropriate HLA class I molecules avoid destruction. One means by which tumour cells and virally infected cells avoid T-cell mediated recognition is downregulation of components of the HLA class I antigen-processing pathway, including class I molecules *per se* and β2-microglobulin. In order to avoid destruction by NK cells tumours also increase expression of certain *HLA*-alleles corresponding to the cognate ligand for an inhibitory KIR. More advanced approaches for the use of NK cells are therefore being devised to address tumour cell escape from NK cell mediated surveillance and cytotoxicity. One such approach is to develop long-term cell lines such as NK-92 (in phase I/II trials) which lacks KIRs yet retains its cytolytic machinery and activity (Tonn, 2001) and recent work has show that antigen-specificity can also be transferred to NK cells in a similar fashion to T cells—Section 27.2.2 (Schirrmann, 2002).

27.4 Conclusions

Immunotherapy already makes measurable contributions to the management of cancer. However, increased understanding of malignancy, immunity, recombinant DNA technology, and sequencing the human genome places us in a stronger position to make meaningful advances. In contrast to mainstream modalities (surgery, radiotherapy, chemotherapy) immunotherapy has the potential to engender life-long protection. Although immunotherapy will not supersede traditional treatments it is apparent that a combined approach delivers better results. Already immunotherapy has been successfully combined with a number of traditional modalities including; fractionated X-rays with bacterial therapy, XRT with IL-2, thalidomide-analogues with peptide vaccines, anti-angiogenic treatment with T-cell vaccines. As tumours operate a number of systems to evade immune detection (e.g. secretion of immunosuppressive compounds, antigenic-modulation, and mutation) strategies that address these offer some of the greatest potential to improve therapeutic efficacy and patient survival.

References

Alexandroff, A. B., Jackson, A. M., O'Donnell, M. A., and James, K. (1999). BCG immunotherapy of bladder cancer: 20 years on. *Lancet*, **353**, 1689–94.

Ansell, S. M., Witzig, T. E., Kurtin, P., Sloan, J. A., Jelinek, D. F., Howell, K. G. et al. (2002). Phase I study of IL-12 in combination with rituximab in patients with B-cell non-Hodgkin lymphoma. *Blood*, **99**, 67–74.

Banchereau, J. and Stenman, R. M. (1998). Dendritic cells and the control of immunity. *Nature*, **392**, 245–52.

Bonnet, M. C., Tartaglia, J., Verdier, F. Kourilsky, P., Lindberg, A., Klein, M. et al. (2000). Recombinant viruses as a tool for therapeutic vaccination against human cancers. *Immunol Lett*, **74**, 11–25.

Bukowski, R. M., Tendler, C., Cutler, D., Rose, E., Laughlin, M. M., and Statkevich, P. (2002). Treating cancer with PEG Intron: pharmacokinetic profile and dosing guidelines for an improved interferon-alpha-2b formulation. *Cancer*, **95**, 389–96.

Cheadle E. J. and Jackson A. M. (2002). Bugs as drugs for cancer. *Immunol*, **106**, 1–15.

Clay, T. M., Custer, M. C., Sachs, J., Hwu, P., Rosenberg, S. A., and Nishimura, M. I. (1999). Efficient transfer of a tumor antigen-reactive TCR to human peripheral blood lymphocytes confers anti-tumor reactivity. *J Immunol*, **163**, 507–13.

Coley, W. B. (1894). Treatment of inoperable malignant tumours by repeated inoculations of *Eprysipelas* and the *Bacillus prodigiouses. Am J Med Sci*, **108**, 183–212.

Conry, R. M., Curiel, D. T., Strong, T. V., Moore, S. E., Allen, K. O., Barlow, D. L. et al. (2002). Safety and immunogenicity of a DNA vaccine encoding CEA and hepatitis B surface antigen in colorectal cancinoma patients. *Clin Cancer Res*, **8**, 2782–7.

Dietrich, G., Gentschev, I., Hess, J., Ulmer, J. B., Kaufmann, S. H., and Goebel, W. (1999). Delivery of DNA vaccines by attenuated intracellular bacteria. *Immunol Today*, **20**, 251–3.

Dhodapkar, M. V., Steinman, R. M., Krasovsky, J., Munz, C., and Bhardwaj, N. (2001). Antigen-specific inhibition of effector T cell function in humans after injection of immature dendritic cells. *J Exp Med*, **193**, 233–8.

Dreno, B., Nguyen, J. M., Khammari, A., Pandolfino, M. C., Tessier, M. H., Bercegeay, S. et al. (2002). Randomised trial of adoptive transfer of melanoma TIL as adjuvant therapy for stage III melanoma. *Cancer Immunol Immunother*, **51**, 539–46.

Fong, L., Brockstedt, D., Benike, C., Wu, L., and Englemann, E. G. (2001). DC injected via different routes induce immunity in cancer patients. *J Immunol*, **166**, 4254–9.

Geiger, J. D., Hutchinson, R. J., Hohenkirk, L. F., McKenna, E. A., Yanik, G. A., Levine, J. E. et al. (2001). Vaccination of pediatric solid tumour patients with tumour-lysate-pulsed DC can expand specific T cells and mediated tumour regression. *Cancer Res* **61**, 8513–9.

Grimm, E. A., Mazumder, A., Zhang, H. Z., and Rosenberg, S. A. (1982). Lymphokine activated killer cell phenomenon. *J Exp Med*, **155**, 1832–41.

He, J., Shen, D., O'Donnell, M. A., and Chang H. R. (2002). Induction of MUC1-specific cellular immunity by a recombinant BCG expressing human MUC1 and secreting IL-2. *Int J Oncol*, **20**, 1305–11.

Heiser, A., Coleman, D., Dannull, J., Yancey, D., Maurice, M. A., Lallas, C. D. et al. (2002). Autologous dendritic cells transfected with prostate-specific antigen RNA stimulate CTL responses against metastatic prostate tumours. *J Clin Invest*, **109**, 409–17.

Hung, C. F., Cheng, W. F., Hsu, K. F., Chai, C. Y., He, L, Ling, M. et al. (2001). Cancer immunotherapy using a DNA vaccine encoding the translocation domain of a bacterial toxin linked to a tumor antigen. *Cancer Res*, **61**, 3698–703.

Hung, K., Hayashi, R., Lafond-Wlaker, A., Lowenstein, C., Pardoll, D., and Levitsky, H. (1998). The central role of CD4+ T cells in the antitumour immune response. *J Exp Med*, **188**, 2357–68.

Jabbar, I. A., Fernando, G. J., Saunders, N., Aldovini, A., Young, R, Malcolm, K. et al. (2000). Immune responses induced by BCG recombinant for human papillomavirus L1 and E7 proteins. *Vaccine*, **18**, 2444–53.

Jackson, A. M., and James K. (1994). Understanding the most successful immunotherapy for cancer. *The Immunologist*, **2**, 208–15.

Janssen, E. M., Lemmens, E. E., Wolfe, T., Christen, U., von Herrath, M. G., and Schoenberger, S. P. (2003). CD4+ T cells are required for secondary expansion and memory in CD8+ T lymphocytes. *Nature*. **421**, 852–6.

Kessels, H. W., Wolkers, M. C., van den Boom, M. D., van der Valk, M. A., and Schumacher, T. N. (2001). Immunotherapy through TCR gene transfer. *Nat Immunol*, **10**, 957–6.

Kokhaei, P., Razvany, M. R., Virving, L., Choudhury, A., Rabbani, H., Osterborg, A. et al. (2003). DC loaded with apoptotic tumour cells induce a stronger T-cell response than DC-tumour hybrids in B-CLL. *Leukemia*, **17**, 894–9.

Krause, S. W., Neumann, C., Soruri, A., Mayer, S., Peters, J. H., and Andreesen, R. (2002). The treatment of patients with disseminated malignant melanoma by vaccination with autologous cell hybrids of tumor cells and dendritic cells. *J Immunother*, **25**, 421–8.

Kugler, A., Stuhler, G., Walden, P., Zoller, G., Zobywalski A., Brossart, P. et al. (2000). Regression of human metastatic renal cell carcinoma after vaccination with tumor cell-dendritic cell hybrids. *Nat Med*, **6**, 332–6.

Mackensen, A., Herbst, B., Chen, J. L., Kohler, G., Noppen, C., Herr, W. et al. (2000). Phase I study in melanoma patients of a vaccine with peptide-pulsed DC generated in vitro from CD34+ hematopoietic progenitor cells. *Int J Cancer*, **86**, 385–92.

Maher, J., Brentjens, R. J., Gunset, G., Riviere, I., and Sadelain, M. (2002). Human T-lymphocyte cytotoxicity and proliferation directed by a single chimeric TCRzeta/CD28 receptor. *Nat Biotechnol*, **1**, 70–5.

Mahvi, D. M., Shi, F., Yang, N., Hank, J., Albertini, M., Schiller, J. et al. (2002). Immunisation by particle-mediated transfer of the GM-CSF gene into autologous tumour cells in melanoma or sarcoma patients. *Hum Gene Ther*, **13**, 1711–21.

Manici, S., Sturniolo, T., Imro, M. A., Hammer, J., Sinigaglia, F., Noppen, C. et al. (1999). Melanoma cells present a MAGE-3 epitpe to CD4+cytotoxic T cells in association with HLA DR11. *J Exp Med*, **189**, 871–76.

Marchand, M., van Baren, N., Weynants, P., Brichand, V., Dreno, B., Tessier, M. et al. (1999). Tumour regressions observed in patients with metastatic melanoma treated with an antigenic peptide encoden by gene MAGE-3 and presented by HLA-A1. *Int J Cancer*, **80**, 219–30.

Marzo, A. L., Kinnear, B. F., Lake, R. A., Frelinger, J. J., Collins, E. J., Robinson, BWS. et al. (2000). Tumour-specific CD4+T-cells have a major 'post-licensing' role in CTL mediated anti-tumour immunity. *J Immunol*, **165**, 6047–55.

Medical Research Council Renal Cancer Collaborators (1999). Interferon-alpha and survival in metastatic renal carcinoma: early results of a randomised controlled trial. *Lancet*, **353**, 14–7.

Mendes, R., O'Brien, M. E., Mitra, A., Norton, A., Gregory, R. K., Padhani, A. R. et al. (2002). Clinical and immunological assessment of Mycobacterium vaccae (SRL172) with chemotherapy in patients with malignant mesothelioma. *Br J Cancer*, **86**, 336–41.

Miconnet, I., Coste, I., Beermann, F., Haeuw, J. F., Cerottini, J. C., Bonnefoy, J. Y. et al. (2001). Cancer vaccine design: a novel bacterial adjuvant for peptide-specific CTL induction. *J Immunol*, **166**, 4612–19.

Miconnet, I., Koenig, S., Speiser, D., Krieg, A., Guillaume, P, Cerottini, J. C. et al. (2002). CpG are efficient adjuvants for specific CTL induction against tumor antigen-derived peptide. *J Immunol*, **168**, 1212–18.

Moingeon, P. (2001). Cancer vaccines. *Vaccine*, **19**, 1305–1326.

Nair, S., Boczkowski, D., Moeller, B., Dewhirst, M., Vieweg, J., and Gilboa, E. (2003). Synergy between tumour immunotherapy and anti-angiogenic therapy. *Blood*, **102**, 964–71.

Nestle, F. O., Alijagic, S., Gilliet, M., Sun, Y., Grabbe, S., Dummer, R. et al. (1998). Vaccination of melanoma patients with peptide- or tumour lysate-pulsed dendritic cells. *Nat Med*, **4**, 328–32.

O'Brien, M. E., Saini, A., Smith, I. E., Webb, A., Gregory, K., Mendes, R. et al. (2000). A randomized phase II study of SRL172 (*Mycobacterium vaccae*) combined with chemotherapy in patients with advanced inoperable non-small-cell lung cancer and mesothelioma. *Br J Cancer*, **83**, 853–57.

Pyrhonen, S., Salminen, E., Ruutu, M., Lehtonen, T., Nurmi, M., Tammela, T. et al. (1999). Prospective randomized trial of interferon alfa-2a plus vinblastine versus vinblastine alone in patients with advanced renal cell cancer. *J Clin Oncol*, **17**, 2859–67.

Radford, K. J., Jackson, A. M., Wang, J.-H., Vassaux, G., and Lemoine, N. R. (2003). Recombinant *E. coli* efficiently delivers antigen and maturation signals to human dendritic cells: Presentation of MART1 to CD8+T cells. *Int J Cancer*, **105**, 811–9.

Rand, R. W., Kreitman, R. J., Patronas, N., Varricchio, F., Pastan, I., and Puri, R. K. (2000). Intratumoral administration of recombinant circularly permuted interleukin-4-Pseudomonas exotoxin in patients with high-grade glioma. *Clin Cancer Res*, **6**, 2157–65.

Ren-Heidenreich, L., Mordini, R., Hayman, G. T., Siebenlist, R., and LeFever, A. (2002). Comparison of the TCR zeta-chain with the FcR gamma-chain in chimeric TCR constructs for T cell activation and apoptosis. *Cancer Immunol Immunother*, **8**, 417–23.

Robinson, H. L., Montefiori, D. C., Johnson, R., Manson, K., Kalish, M., Lifson, J. et al. (1999). Neutralising antibody-dependent containment of immunodeficiency virus challenges by DNA priming and recombinant fowl-pox virus booster immunizations. *Nat Med*, **5**, 526–34.

Rosenberg, S. A., Lotze, M. T., and Muul, L. M. (1987). A progress report on the treatment of 157 patients with advanced cancer using LAK cells and interleukin-2 or high-dose interleukin-2 alone. *N Engl J Med*, **316**, 889–97.

Rosenberg, S. A., Yang, J. C., Schwartzentruber, D. J., Hwu, P., Marincola, F. M., Topalian, S. L. et al. (1998). Immunologic and therapeutic evaluation of a synthetic peptide vaccine for the treatment of patients with metastatic melanoma. *Nat Med*, **4**, 321–27.

Rosenberg, S. A., Yang, J. C., Schwartzentruber, D. J., Hwu, P., Marincola, F. M., Topalian, S. L. et al. (1999). Prospective randomized trial of the treatment of patients with metastatic melanoma using chemotherapy with cisplatin, dacarbazine, and tamoxifen alone or in combination with interleukin-2 and interferon alfa-2b. *J Clin Oncol*, **17**, 968–7.

Rousseau, R. F., Haight, A., Hirschmann-Jax, C., Yvon, E., Rill, D., Mei, Z. et al. (2003). Local and systemic effects of an allogeneic tumour cell vaccine combininat transgenic human lymphotactin with IL-2 in patients with advanced or refractory neuroblastoma. *Blood*, **101**, 1718–26.

Sadelain, M., Riviere, I., and Brentjens, R. (2003). Targeting tumours with genetically enhanced T lymphocytes. *Nat Rev Cancer*, **31**, 35–45.

Scheibenbogen, C., Schmittel, A., Keilholz, U., Allgauer, T., Hofman, U., Max, R. et al. (2000). Phase 2 trial of vaccination with tyrosinase peptides and GM-CSF in patients with metastatic melanoma. *J Immunother*, **23**, 275–81.

Schirrmann, T. and Pecher, G. (2002). Human NK cell line modified with a chimeric immunoglobulin T-cell receptor gene leads to tumour growth inhibition in vivo. *Cancer Gene Ther*, **9**, 390–8.

Schultz, E. S., Lethe, B., Cambiaso, C. L., Van Snick, J., Chaux, P., Corthals, J. et al. (2000). A MAGE-A3 peptide presented by HLA-DP4 is recognized on tumor cells by CD4 + cytolytic T lymphocytes. *Cancer Res*, **60**, 6272–5.

Shanafelt, A. B., Lin, Y., Shanafelt, M. C., Forte, C. P., Dubois-Stringfellow, N., Carter, C. et al. (2000). A T-cell-selective interleukin 2 mutein exhibits potent antitumor activity and is well tolerated in vivo. *Nat Biotechnol*, **18**, 1197–202.

Su, Z., Dannul, J., Heiser, A., Yancey, D., Pruitt, S., Madden, J. et al. (2003). Immunological and clinical responses in metastatic renal cancer patients vaccinated with tumour RNA-transfected dendritic cells. *Cancer Res*, **63**, 2127–33.

Su, Z., Viewweg, J., Weizer, AZ., Dahm, P., Yancey, D., Turaga, V. et al. (2002). Enhanced induction of telomerase-specific CD4 + T cells using dendritic cells transfected with RNA encoding a chimeric gene product. *Cancer Res*, **62**, 5041–48.

Tonn, T., Becker, S., Esser, R., Schwabe, D., and Seifried, E. (2001). Cellular immunotherapy of malignancies using the clonal NK cell line NK-92. *J Hematother Stem Cell Res*, **10**, 535–44.

Thurner, B., Haendle, I., Roder, C., Dieckmann, D., Keikavoussi, P., Jonuliet, H. et al. (1999). Vaccination with MAGE-3 A1 peptide-pulsed mature, monocyte-derived DC expands specific CTL and induces regression of some metastases in advanced stage IV melanoma. *J Exp Med*, **190**, 1669–78.

Underhill, D. M., and Ozinsky, A. (2002). Toll-like receptors: key mediators of microbe detection. *Curr Opin Immunol*, **14**, 103–10.

van der Bruggen, P., Traversari, C., Chomez, P., Lurquin, C., De Plaen, E., van den Eynde., Knuth A. et al. (1991). A gene encoding an antigen recognised by cytolytic T lymphocytes on a human melanoma. *Science*, **254**, 1643–47.

Willemsen, R. A., Debets, R., Hart, E., Hoogenboom, H. R., Bolhuis, R. L., and Chames, P. (2001). A phage display selected fab fragment with MHC class I-restricted specificity for MAGE-A1 allows for retargeting of primary human T lymphocytes. *Gene Ther*, **8**, 1601–8.

CHAPTER 28

Cancer gene therapy

John D. Chester

28.1 Introduction

Gene therapy is a new and exciting treatment modality with potential utility in a range of diseases for which there are either no current effective treatments or in which existing treatments have had limited efficacy and/or significant toxicity. Clinical scenarios in which gene therapy is being applied include monogenic inherited disorders such as haemophilia, severe combined immunodeficiency and cystic fibrosis. Its use is also being investigated in a variety of acquired diseases, such as vascular disease (including coronary artery and cerebrovascular disease), neurological diseases such as Parkinson's disease, and infectious diseases, particularly acquired immune deficiency syndrome (AIDS). It is also appropriate for the huge collection of neoplastic conditions we call cancer.

Gene therapy involves the introduction of exogenous nucleic acids (usually DNA) into cells with a view to altering the phenotype of a diseased cell via altered patterns of gene expression. As such, it is the therapeutic application of the techniques of recombinant DNA technology or 'genetic engineering'. The exogenous nucleic acid sequences, in most cases, consist of the transcription unit of a therapeutic gene (including protein-coding exons), plus regulatory sequences controlling transcription initiation and termination. They may be intended either to replace missing/damaged cellular chromosomal DNA sequences, or to introduce novel gene products. The aim of such alterations in phenotype may be either to restore the normal phenotype or to kill the diseased cell. In principle, gene therapy can be used to induce both somatic and germline modifications, but heritable, germline mutations are currently felt to be ethically unacceptable.

Cancers are attractive targets for gene therapy. First, while an increasing number of patients with cancer can be cured by surgery or non-surgical treatment modalities such as chemotherapy, radiotherapy, and hormonal manipulation, the first presentation of many others is with disease which is incurable by existing treatments, or which relapses as incurable disease following treatment with curative intent. New and/or improved antitumour treatments are therefore urgently needed. Secondly, genetic manipulation is a rational approach to the treatment of cancer, as the aetiology of most cancers is known to involve an accumulation of multiple genetic defects.

Cancer gene therapy has the dual aims of enhancing recent improvements in cancer survival rates, achieved by existing cancer treatments, and of doing so with maximum efficacy and minimum toxicity (optimum therapeutic index). Cancer is not just one disease, and we should not expect a single gene therapy to work for all cancers. The recent rapid expansion in our understanding of the molecular bases of cancers, including the sequencing of the human genome, and early steps in the definition of individual tumour transcriptomes and proteomes, provides us with an exciting range of possibilities for targeting cancer cells. Consequently, the field of cancer gene therapy includes a wide variety of different strategies for genetic manipulation of tumour phenotype.

Like any new treatment, gene therapies which work *in vitro* in the laboratory and *in vivo* in pre-clinical animal models must undergo testing in human subjects within the controlled conditions of clinical trials. In the earliest (Phase I) stage of testing in human subjects, they must be demonstrated to be safe and have acceptable toxicity. Then (in Phase II clinical trials), they must be demonstrated to be effective, shrinking or reducing the rate of growth of tumour in at least a proportion of patients. Finally, (Phase III trials) they must be compared to existing therapies (either on their own, or in addition to existing treatments) and be demonstrated to be superior to existing treatments, either in terms of improved efficacy or equivalent efficacy but with reduced toxicity.

A gene therapy strategy is ultimately only useful if it can be used to help patients. Gene therapy has already been demonstrated to be effective in achieving long-term control/cure of non-malignant monogenic inherited diseases such as X-linked severe combined immunodeficiency (X-SCID) (Cavazzana-Calvo, 2000) and haemophilia B (Kay, 2000). This article will therefore emphasize cancer gene therapy strategies which are not only elegant attempts to manipulate tumour cell phenotype in the laboratory, but which have also already been used, or have the potential to be used, safely and effectively, in human subjects. It will discuss problems encountered, and highlight current strategies to overcome these limitations.

28.2 Components of a gene therapy strategy

A cancer gene therapy strategy should aim to solve a genuine clinical problem—either a tumour which does not have an adequate treatment using existing treatment modalities, or one in which the therapeutic index might be improved. An individualized strategy for each clinical situation should be based upon an understanding of the biological behaviour and natural history of the tumour. Each strategy has multiple components—choice of target, effector mechanism for altering the tumour cell phenotype, delivery strategy, tumour-selective targeting of transgene expression, and the nature of the effector transgene itself (Figure 28.1). Rapid

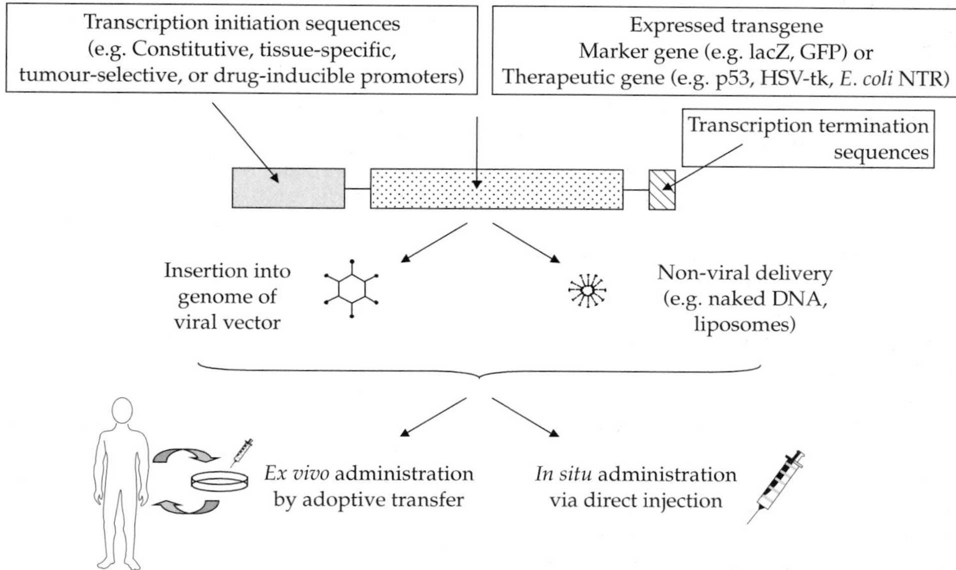

Figure 28.1 Components of a gene therapy strategy. Expression of marker or therapeutic transgenes is transcriptionally regulated by promoter sequences which may selectively target certain cell types or tumours. Gene therapy constructs are then introduced into cells either as naked DNA, complexed with lipids, or in recombinant viral vectors. Therapeutic administration of viral or non-viral vectors may be either via direct intracorporeal injection or extracorporeal modification of extracted cells, followed by their return.

developments in the field of gene therapy have resulted in a range of options for each of these components, resulting in an exciting, but potentially bewildering, array of possible gene therapies. Careful selection from a number of options for each component is necessary for successful treatment of a given tumour type. We will deal with each of the component parts of the strategy, in turn.

28.2.1 Cellular targets for gene therapy

Our improved understanding of molecular tumour biology provides a wealth of potential targets for cancer gene therapy. Therapeutic genes can be targeted to exploit the many differences between normal and tumour cells—aberrant stimulus-response signalling, loss of control of proliferation, aberrations of regulation of the cell cycle, immortalization, failure to undergo apoptosis, tumour angiogenesis, invasion, and metastasis.

In most cancer gene therapy strategies, the targets are tumour cells themselves. For example, such strategies might replace defective tumour suppressor genes, downregulate overexpressed cell surface receptors (or inhibit their kinase activity), block aberrant intracellular signalling pathways, restore the cells' capacity to undergo senescence, stimulate apoptosis or inhibit tumour angiogenesis. However, in some gene therapy strategies, normal cells, rather than tumour cells are targeted. For example, stem cells, which are sensitive to the antiproliferative effects of conventional cytotoxic drugs can be selectively protected by incorporating drug-resistance genes, permitting the use of chemotherapy in a more dose-intense fashion, without jeopardizing sensitive normal cells. Conversely, gene therapy which introduces negatively selectable markers into engrafted cells permit conditional elimination if/when they become more of a problem than a solution.

28.2.2 Effector mechanism

The nature of the biological defect to be targeted determines the means by which therapeutic transgene expression modifies tumour cell behaviour. Gene therapy strategies might aim to correct the molecular defects which result in malignant transformation. Such strategies are frequently referred to as 'gene replacement' strategies. Alternatively, where phenotypic reversal is difficult or impossible, the tumour cells may be selectively killed by the expression of so-called 'suicide genes'. In this case, the inherent inefficiency of current methods of introducing transgenes into tumour cells requires that a 'by-stander effect' must be exerted upon the surrounding majority of non-expressing tumour cells by the minority which have taken up and express the therapeutic transgene.

28.2.3 Delivery strategy

Route of delivery

Gene therapy constructs can be delivered to tumour cells in two ways. Either the transgene can be administered to the tumour *in situ*, often by direct intratumoral injection, or the transgene can be incorporated into cells *ex vivo*, with cells being extracted from the tumour-bearing animal or patient, the transgene introduced into cells extracorporeally, and the genetically modified cells returned (Figure 28.1). Depending upon whether the transgene is introduced into the target cell via a plasmid or viral vector, the process is referred to as transfection or transduction, respectively.

The *ex vivo* 'adoptive transfer' gene therapy approach works well for haematological malignancies, where circulating peripheral blood stem cells can be extracted easily and, once genetically modified and returned to the host, have a natural tropism for the bone marrow, where they can either re-populate or form a chimaera. The technique is also useful for immunotherapy, where the modified cells are cells of the immune system. However, the *ex vivo* approach has the disadvantage that the modified cells must then seek out the site of tumour growth *in vivo*, an intrinsically inefficient process. Consequently, most gene therapy strategies employed for solid tumours to date involve the *in situ* approach.

Where a tumour is localized, and has not yet metastasized, direct administration may be all that is required to effectively target the tumour. This strategy for transgene delivery is particularly suitable for superficial tumours such as subcutaneous lesions or lesions which can be visualized by endoscopic procedures, and where intratumoral injection can be performed under direct vision. A modification of this approach has been used for delivery of transgenes to muscles and peripheral nerves, whereby intramuscular delivery of naked DNA is achieved trans-dermally using a so-called 'gene gun' (see below).

Although direct intratumoral injection is useful as a model for testing efficacy, it is unlikely to make a major impact on localized cancers, prior to metastasis, where existing local treatments such as surgery and radiotherapy achieve good cure rates. Gene therapy is most likely to be of value, however, in the treatment of advanced disease, with multiple sites of disseminated metastasis. For simultaneous treatment of multiple sites of synchronous tumour growth, systemic delivery of a transgene is required. The most commonly employed route is intravascular injection (usually intravenous, but occasionally directly into arteries).

However, systemic administration imposes severe limitations on the efficiency of transgene delivery to the site(s) of tumour growth. Barriers between a systemically delivered therapeutic transgene and its target tumour site(s) include circulating antibodies and immune effector cells, non-specific adsorption in the liver, difficulties in extravasation and interactions with the extracellular matrix, let alone entry into the target cells themselves. Indeed, the small proportion of intravenously administered gene therapy vector which actually reaches tumour cells is one of the main obstacles to successful implementation of gene therapy for disseminated malignancy.

An extension of the *ex vivo* approach which is intended to overcome some of the problems of systemic delivery is to deliver the transgene inside autologous cells which have an innate ability to 'home' to sites of tumour growth (Harrington, 2002). These cell types include lymphocytes, macrophages, endothelial, haematological, and mesenchymal stem cells. The principle of 'hiding' the transgene construct within such a cell, then using the cell's natural tumour tropism to facilitate efficient delivery, followed by activated dissemination of the transgene throughout the tumour once *in situ*, has been demonstrated in xenograft models of human colon cancer using both antigen recognition (Chester, 2002) and pharmacological stimulus (Crittenden, 2003) for release of the gene therapy construct from the cellular carrier.

Gene delivery systems

For any given route of delivery, entry of the gene therapy construct into cells can be achieved by biological, chemical, or physical means. The most commonly used biological method involves the use of genetically modified viral vectors. Chemical methods involve the generation of liposomes from cationic lipids or cationic polymers. Physical methods include direct injection, hydrodynamic methods, and facilitated entry using electroporation or ultrasound treatment.

Viral vectors. The use of genetically modified viruses to facilitate transgene entry into target cells exploits millions of years of viral evolution. The transgene is incorporated within the viral genome, and thereby gains entry to the host cell. Various virus families have been assayed for use in cancer gene therapies (Thomas, 2003). Each has advantages and disadvantages, but none has all the features of an ideal viral vector: non-pathogenic; non-immunogenic; capable of production in high titre to permit saturation of target cells; packaging capacity sufficient to include coding and regulatory sequences for the transgene; and the ability to gain entry to non-dividing and proliferating cells. Therefore, the choice of viral vector depends upon the particular application, and upon whether long-term or short-term transgene expression is required. For long-term expression viral vectors must integrate within host cell chromosomes or be maintained in an episomal state with successive rounds of tumour cell division. Conversely, for short-term transgene expression, viral vectors which are not integrated, and remain episomal suffice.

No figures are available for the proportions of experimental/*in vitro*/laboratory strategies employing the various vectors, but an idea can be gained from statistics concerning the large number of gene therapy trials already under way (Gene Therapy Clinical Trials Database, 2004). About three-quarters of the more-than-900 clinical trials initiated employ viral vectors, and more than half have been retrovirus- or adenovirus-mediated.

Retroviral vectors. Retroviruses were among the first viruses to be used as gene therapy vectors. They illustrate several important principles of vector design (and their drawbacks), and nearly 30% of clinical trials to date (Gene Therapy Clinical Trials Database, 2004) have employed them, including some therapies which have resulted in cures of monogenic inherited diseases (Cavazzana-Calvo, 2000; Kay, 2000). The life cycle of retroviruses includes conversion of a single-stranded RNA genome into a double-stranded DNA 'provirus', using a virally encoded polymerase known as reverse transcriptase (RT). The double-stranded DNA becomes integrated into the host cell's chromosomes. This makes retroviral vectors particularly useful for gene therapy applications where long-term expression of the transgene is required, such as in monogenic disorders. It also allows a virally incorporated transgene to be efficiently expressed in daughter cells following mitotic cell division. However, there is a theoretical downside to this integration process. Proviral integration into the host cell's chromosomes can result in insertional mutagenesis, itself potentially resulting in malignancy. Sadly, this theoretical limitation of retrovirus-mediated gene therapy has recently been borne out in practice in clinical trials of X-SCID where two patients who have been effectively cured of their immunodeficiency have developed secondary, treatment-related leukaemias (Hacein-Bey-Abina, 2003).

Retroviral vectors used for gene therapy applications contain deletions of portions of the viral genome. This is for two reasons: first, to make the virus replication-defective—that is, the virus is able to enter the host cell, but unable to synthesise viral genome, and so unable to spread to cells other than those to which it was initially transferred; secondly to accommodate the coding and regulatory sequences of the (marker or therapeutic) transgene. As with any viral vector used to introduce exogenous genetic material, the size of the non-viral insert is limited by the packaging capacity of the virus capsid. In most cases, the viral genes encoding structural proteins are dispensable. In the case of retroviral vectors, the *env* structural genes, for example, are not required after the viral genome has become integrated and can be deleted from the gene therapy construct, making room for transgene sequences.

Deletion of viral sequences, of course, means not only that the virus is replication-defective, but also that high titres of infectious particles cannot be generated without structural capsid proteins being made available in other ways. There are two basic ways in which the deleted gene products can be made available. One is co-infection with a 'helper' virus which encodes products which can be shared with the recombinant viral vector. By deleting the packaging signals of the helper virus, production of viral particles containing only the gene therapy genome can be achieved, in theory at least. However, in practice, homologous recombination events between the gene therapy vector genome and the helper virus genome can generate wild-type genomes, containing all the necessary viral sequences for a productive infection, with spread of wild-type virus to surrounding cells. This has obvious safety implications. Multiple deletions of viral sequences in vector and/or helper virus genomes make such recombination events less likely (as multiple recombinations would be required), but a second method of providing viral gene products *in trans* is often preferred, namely the use of 'packaging' cell lines. The sequences absent from the gene therapy vector genome are stably integrated within the chromosomal DNA of immortalized tissue-culture cell lines. Transfection of these packaging cells with plasmid DNA containing the vector genome results in synthesis of retroviral ssRNA genome which can be packaged, released from the packaging cells and collected from the cell supernatant.

Retroviruses have natural tropisms for cells of certain mammalian species, based upon the nature of their *env* gene products. The so-called ecotropic retroviruses, for example, can infect only murine cells, while xenotropic viruses infect only non-mouse cells. Amphotropic retroviruses can infect both mouse and non-mouse cells. It is possible to alter the tropism of a retroviral vector by replacing the *env* genes of one retrovirus (e.g. an ecotropic one) with the *env* gene of another (e.g. an amphotropic one). In this way, the virus can enter a wider range of host cells. An extension of this principle is known as pseudotyping. The best known example involves the use of the vesicular stomatitis virus G protein, a coat protein derived from a virus of a completely different family, the rhabdoviruses.

Despite their many useful features, retroviral gene therapy vectors have several shortcomings. In addition to the phenomenon of insertional mutagenesis described above, they also have a relatively small capacity for insertion of exogenous genes and are difficult to produce in high titres. Perhaps the most significant drawback for their use in cancer gene therapy, however, is that they can only integrate into (and therefore express their transgenes from) actively dividing cells; non-dividing cells cannot express virally encoded transgenes. This is because integration of the dsDNA provirus into host chromosomes can only occur after dissolution of the nuclear membrane, during mitosis.

Lentiviral vectors. A recent promising development in retroviral gene therapy vectors has been the use of lentiviral vectors. Lentiviruses, such as the aetiological agents of AIDS, the human immunodeficiency viruses (HIV-1 and -2), are one of the subsets of retroviruses. Their genomes are more complex than those of the type C mammalian retroviruses, such as the murine leukaemia viruses, which have been previously used as retroviral vectors. The additional sequences contained within the lentiviral genome enable nuclear localization, permitting the proviral cDNA to integrate into the chromosomes of both dividing and non-dividing host cells. This represents an important improvement, increasing the proportion of tumour cells transduced by a single administration of vector.

An improvement in the safety profile of lentiviral vectors has been provided by so-called self-inactivating (SIN) vectors (Miyoshi, 1998; Zufferey, 1998). Endogenous retroviral transcription regulatory sequences are contained within the directly repeating sequences known as LTRs (long terminal repeats) at the 5′ and 3′ ends of the integrated proviral genome. The regulatory sequences in the 5′LTR control transcription of the viral genome. As a consequence of the retroviral provirus integration mechanism, inactivating mutations in the regulatory sequences of the 3′LTR are subsequently transferred to the 5′LTR of the provirus as well. Thus, after integration of SIN vectors into the host chromosome, the 5′ and 3′ LTRs are both inactivated, and transcription is only possible from exogenous, non-viral promoters, inserted into the viral genome between the LTRs.

Adenoviral vectors. Like retroviruses, the majority of adenoviral gene therapy vectors used for experimental work and in clinical trials are replication-defective. They can enter and express their transgenes, but do not undergo replication of their genome nor subsequently form intact viral particles. However, much attention has been focused recently on tumour-selective, conditionally replicating adenoviruses (CRAds) and their use as oncolytic vectors (see below).

Unlike retroviral vectors, adenoviruses can infect both dividing and non-dividing cells. This is important for cancer gene therapy as, at any given moment, only a proportion of cancer cells are undergoing cell division.

One of the principal problems of adenoviral vectors is their immunogenicity. Studies investigating the distribution of systemically administered adenoviral vectors have demonstrated that a large proportion of the total viral dose does not reach the intended tumour site. Serological studies show that the vast majority of the population has been exposed to wild-type adenoviruses and exogenous administration of adenoviral vectors can stimulate both humoral and cellular immune responses. A great deal of effort has gone into developing more advanced adenoviral vectors with reduced immunogenicity. Whereas so-called 'first-generation' replication-defective adenoviral vectors contained deletions in only the E1 early region of the genome and the dispensable E3 region, 'second generation' vectors also had deletions of the E2 and/or E4 genes, and have been shown to be less immunogenic. A natural extension of this principle is the development of so-called 'gutless' adenoviral vectors in which almost the entire viral genome is deleted, leaving only essential viral genes and packaging sequences, with other viral gene products produced *in trans*. While the packaging capacity of first generation adenoviral vectors was not greatly different from that of retroviral vectors, 'gutless' adenoviral vectors are capable of containing inserts of up to about 30 kb, well in excess of the maximum packaging capacity of retroviruses. An inevitable consequence of this large-scale deletion is that many of the viral gene products essential for assembly of viral particles must be provided *in trans* if adequate titres are to be obtained. As for other viral vector types, these 'helper-dependent' adenoviruses raise safety concerns.

Unlike retroviruses, adenoviral dsDNA does not integrate into host cell chromosomes, but remains episomal within the nucleus. This means that long-term expression from adenoviral vectors is not possible without multiple dosing, and that the dosage of replication-defective adenoviral vectors is effectively diluted as cells undergo repeated rounds of mitosis. This would be a disadvantage for gene therapy applications requiring long-term expression of the vector's transgene, but has little bearing on cancer gene therapy strategies which aim to kill tumour cells, and fits well with the intermittent dosing of established antitumour treatments. It can also be regarded as an important safety measure, both avoiding the potential for insertional mutagenesis and ensuring that any potential deleterious effects of transgene expression are time-limited.

Adenoviral vectors can gain entry into a wide range of cell types. Binding of the viral particles to the target cell surface seems to involve at least two virus–cell interactions. The first involves binding of the fibre knob proteins which project out from the viral capsid to a specific cell surface receptor, the coxsackie/adenovirus receptor (CAR). A second interaction between the penton base protein at the proximal end of the viral fibres with cell-surface integrins then leads to endocytosis via clathrin-coated pits. Unfortunately, the requirement for specific binding to CAR has limited the efficiency of cancer gene therapy, both because CAR is widely expressed in non-tumour cells and because CAR expression in tumour cells is commonly down-regulated.

A variety of techniques has therefore been adopted to improve the tumour selectivity of adenoviral vectors by re-targeting them to molecules which are either exclusively present or are overexpressed on the surface of tumour cells (Figure 28.2). One such strategy involves the use of bi-functional 'adaptor' molecules which bind to both the viral knobs and cell surface molecules which are differentially expressed on the surface of tumour cells. In each case, the two ends of a bipolar molecule must specifically attach to either the viral coat or cell surface. Thus, one 'adenobody' strategy employs an antibody against the viral knob protein covalently coupled to the epidermal growth factor (EGF) whose receptor is overexpressed on the surface of tumour cells (Watkins, 1997). An extension of this principle involves the use of 'diabodies' in which bispecific single-chain antibodies, recognizing both the viral coat and a cell surface receptor act as 'molecular bridges' between the virus and the cell surface (Nettelbeck, 2001). A similar approach involves the formation of a synthetic fusion protein composed of the extracellular domain of the CAR molecule linked, via a synthetic peptide linker sequence, to the ligand for a receptor which is overexpressed in a variety of tumours, such as EGFR (Dmitriev, 2000).

Another strategy for re-targeting adenoviral vectors to tumour cells is to modify the adenoviral knob by mutation of the adenoviral genome. Thus insertion of the characteristic integrin-binding motif arginine–glycine–aspartate (RGD) into the knob protein sequence redirects adenovirus binding away from CAR, towards the ubiquitous integrin family of transmembrane proteins (Dmitriev, 1998). Similarly, oligopeptides can be introduced into the H1 loop of the fibre knob to produce adenoviruses with altered tropism (Krasnykh, 1998).

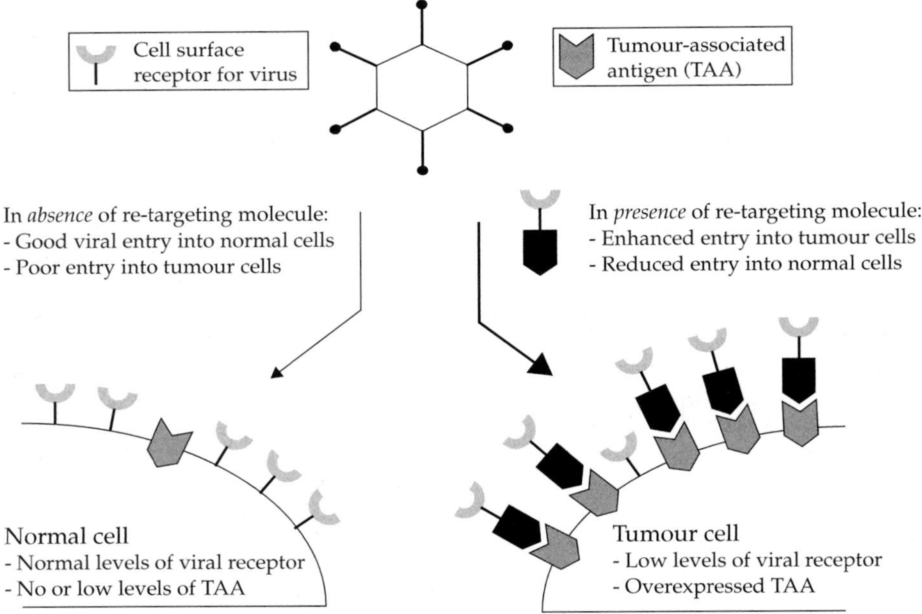

Figure 28.2 Re-targeting of adenoviral gene therapy vectors. Overexpression of Tumour-Associated Antigens (TAA) on the surface of tumour cells can be exploited to improve transduction of tumour cells by adenoviruses. In addition to re-targeting using fusion protein molecules such as those shown here (receptor: ligand fusions, 'adenobodies' and 'diabodies'), re-targeting can also be achieved by modifying or substituting the viral fibre knob proteins, as described in the text.

Adenoviruses can also be re-directed by introducing the sequences encoding the fibre knob of other adenovirus serotypes into the genome of the most commonly used serotype 5, in a manner analogous to the pseudotyping of retroviruses above.

Adeno-associated viral vectors. A family of viral vectors which have recently gained favour are the adeno-associated virus (AAV) vectors. These parvovirus vectors share many of the positive features of replication-defective adenoviruses, including stability and consequent production at high titre, broad target cell tropism (they bind via the widely expressed proteoglycan, heparan sulfate) and high-efficiency entry into both dividing and non-dividing cells. One advantage over adenoviruses is that they are non-pathogenic in humans. The AAV can exist in either latent state (in which the viral genome is predominantly episomal, with less than 10% integrated) or lytic states. For the latter, factors required for a productive infection must be provided *in trans* by co-infection with helper viruses, most commonly adenoviruses (hence their name), herpesviruses, vaccinia, or papillomaviruses. In the absence of helper virus, the vector remains in a latent state. While the requirement for helper viruses contributes to the safety of AAV vectors, which are naturally replication defective in the absence of helper functions, it also means that production at high titres require purification of AAV from helper virus capsids.

The wild-type virus integrates into the host genome, like retroviruses, but at a specific site on chromosome 19, theoretically reducing the risks of insertional mutagenesis. The ability to integrate in this site-specific fashion appears to reside in the *rep* gene, one of only two protein-coding regions in this very simple viral genome. Unfortunately, the very small (4.7 kb) size of the single-stranded DNA genome means that the transgene capacity of these vectors is very small (about 4.5 kb maximum). The more useful AAV vectors therefore have all their protein-coding portions, including the *rep* gene, deleted. Consequently, site-specific integration is abolished.

A variety of strategies has been employed to try and overcome the size-limitation of recombinant AAV vectors, including trans-splicing vectors and overlapping vectors. Both these strategies involve splitting the transgene between two separate rAAV vector genomes, followed by co-infection. In the overlapping strategy, the 5′ end of the gene is in one vector and the 3′ end in another, with the middle portion of the transgene in both. The full length transgene is then recreated in co-transduced cells by homologous recombination events. In the trans-splicing strategy, the 5′ and 3′ ends of the transgene are again in separate vector genomes, but there are no duplicated sequences. Rather, there is a splice donor sequence downstream of the 5′ end of the transgene in one vector, and a splice acceptor sequence upstream of the 3′ end in another. Thus, when both vector genomes are integrated in close proximity and in the correct orientation, intervening sequences are spliced out. Whilst these ingenious strategies work well in experimental conditions, there must be doubt about whether the necessary efficiency can be obtained in clinical situations.

Pseudotyping, incorporating the AAV-2 genome within the capsid of other AAV serotypes, has been used to alter the range of cells infected, in an analagous manner to retroviruses above. In this way, AAV vectors can be preferentially targeted to liver, brain, muscle, or retina. Re-targeting of AAV vectors has also been attempted in a similar way to that of adenoviruses above.

Herpesvirus vectors. The most frequently used herpesvirus vectors are based on herpes simplex virus-1 (HSV-1). The natural tropism of herpes simplex virus for neurones makes them particularly attractive vectors for neurally derived tumours, while the large size of their bipartite dsDNA genome (approx. 150 kb, encoding 80–90 genes) means that deletion of genes which are non-essential for HSV growth in culture permits large inserts of up to 50 kb to be incorporated easily. In this way, the vectors can carry genes controlled by complex regulatory elements, large protein-coding sequences or simultaneous delivery of multiple transgenes, either with separate transcription regulatory sequences or coordinately regulated from a single promoter, but separated by an internal ribosome entry site (IRES) sequence.

Like AAVs, once inside a host cell, HSV can either enter a lytic cycle, or can remain latent. In either case, the viral DNA does not become integrated, but remains as an intra-nuclear episome. Whereas this inability to integrate is a drawback for adenoviral vectors, it is useful for latent HSV in slow- or non-dividing neural cells, allowing protracted gene expression, particularly if transgenes are placed under the control of the promoters of the latency associated transcript (LAT) genes. Latency also prevents immune recognition, which is particularly important as a large proportion of the human population have had previous exposure to HSV.

A second category of HSV-derived gene therapy vectors are known as HSV amplicons. These are plasmid-based vectors, including bacterial origin of replication and selectable antibiotic resistance gene as in ordinary plasmids, but also incorporating an HSV viral origin of replication and packaging (α) signal, plus a transgene under the control of either a heterologous or HSV LAT promoter. Infectious HSV particles are formed in producer cells by co-infection with helper HSV lacking functional packaging signals. In principle, amplicons can accommodate exogenous inserts up to approximately 90% of the full length of the HSV genome. Unfortunately, it has proved difficult to obtain high titre stocks of these amplicon vectors.

Although HSV vectors are capable of persistent transgene expression, HSV vectors, like adenoviruses, are not transmitted to both progeny cells on mitotic cell division. Rather, rapid cell division effectively 'dilutes' the gene therapy vector. This is not a problem for members of the gamma subgroup of herpesviruses, including Epstein–Barr Virus (EBV), which can maintain an episomal state in which the viral genome is coordinately replicated along with host cell chromosomes, thereby efficiently transferring the vector genome and transgene to all progeny cells. EBV is not an ideal gene therapy vector, as it is associated with a number of human pathologies, including the lymphoproliferative disorder Burkitt's lymphoma and nasopharyngeal carcinoma. However, another member of the gamma herpesvirus family which has recently attracted attention as a potential gene therapy vector is herpesvirus saimiri (HVS), a non-pathogenic virus of squirrel monkeys. Genetically modified HVS has been demonstrated to be capable of establishing an episomal state in a variety of human tumour cell lines and of being efficiently segregated between progeny cells in rapidly proliferating cells, and of inhibiting growth of human tumour xenografts in animal models. The ability to coordinately replicate with host chromosomes has been localised to the Orf73 gene in the HVS genome (Calderwood, 2004). Incorporating this gene into other episomal vectors raises the tantalizing possibility of converting these to vectors which are capable of being efficiently passed down generations of proliferating cells.

Hybrid viral vectors. Each of the viral vector types above has its own advantages and disadvantages. It is therefore tempting to create recombinant viral vectors which combine the positive features of more than one virus type. There has been much imaginative work in the development of such hybrid vectors. Examples include adenovirus/AAV hybrids in which a pair of 145 bp AAV inverted terminal repeats (containing replication origin and packaging sequences) are contained within an adenoviral genome. The greater packaging capacity of the adenovirus allows larger inserts between the AAV inverted terminal repeats. AAV/HSV hybrids have been constructed in a similar way. This strategy also permits the restoration of AAV site-specific integration, as the rep protein can be provided outside the AAV genome without reducing the packaging capacity.

Non-viral gene delivery. The numerous recent developments in viral vectors mean that it has been easy to overlook recent important advances in physical and chemical methods of introducing therapeutic genes into cells, especially as a little over 20% of the gene therapy clinical trials involve non-viral delivery (Gene Therapy Clinical Trials Database, 2004), making this the third most commonly employed method for treating patients, behind retroviral and adenoviral vectors. Like viral vectors, transgene expression can be successfully targeted, but the absence of any viral coat proteins results in improved safety, particularly reduced immunogenicity. Non-viral methods also avoid other problems of viral vectors, such as regeneration of potentially pathogenic wild-type virus and insertional mutagenesis or oncogenesis.

Physical methods of delivery are often employed to deliver naked DNA. Naked DNA has the advantage over viral vectors that it is relatively simple and inexpensive to prepare to clinical grade, and that the genetic material itself is not immunogenic prior to expression of the transgene (though the transgene product itself may be). The absence of packaging constraints also means that there is no size limit on the transgene or its regulatory sequences. Physical delivery is particularly appropriate where the tumour target is in easily accessible bodily tissues such as skin or muscle.

The simplest form of delivery of naked DNA is injection using a needle and syringe. Recently, an alternative 'bio-ballistic' delivery mechanism has been developed. A 'gene gun' involves the delivery of plasmid DNA coated on gold particles via a pressurized jet of inert gas as an alternative needle-free mechanism for local 'injection'. In addition, the permeability of cell membranes to naked DNA may be increased by local application of ultrasound waves or by electroporation (the application of a low-strength electromagnetic field). Electroporation may be useful after systemic as well as local delivery, helping to facilitate uptake in particular areas of the body after intravenous administration. Other means of improving uptake of naked DNA after intravascular administration include rapid 'hydrodynamic injection' of a relatively large volume of DNA solution, which may act by mechanical stretching of the endothelium, or transient localised occlusion of blood vessels such as the hepatic portal vein immediately after bolus administration.

The principal chemical means of enhancing uptake of plasmid DNA is to complex the DNA with polycations. Until recently, the most common approach was to form liposomes with cationic lipids such as 1,2-dioleoyl-3-sn-phosphatidylethanolamine (DOPE) or 1,2-dioleoyl-3-(trimethylammonium) propane (DOTAP), and most of the clinical trials to date have employed this approach. More recently, *in vitro* studies have increasingly employed a second generation of cations, including polymers such as poly(L-lysine) (PLL) or polyethyleneimine (PEI), which can exist as either linear or branched polymers of varying molecular weights.

Polyethyleneimine is particularly useful because it has an extremely high density of amine groups. Release of the gene therapy construct from the endosome is facilitated by PEI, because it acts as a 'proton sponge', the influx of protons into the endosomes bringing with it water, and resulting in rupture of the endosome and release of the DNA into the cytoplasm.

Although naked DNA and DNA/liposome complexes are less immunogenic than many viral vectors, they can still generate limited immune responses. This can be minimized by the elimination of CpG motifs from the plasmid DNA or sequential intravenous injection of the DNA and liposome, immediately after one another.

Once in the nucleus, some cancer gene therapy strategies may require chromosomal integration for longer-term transgene expression. This may be facilitated by the use of bacteriophage site-specific integrase enzymes or the 'Sleeping Beauty' transposable elements within the non-virally delivered DNA construct.

For the time being, non-viral delivery is less suitable than viral vectors for the majority of gene therapy applications where the efficiency of uptake and subsequent expression is important. One way in which this gap may be closed is to incorporate, into the DNA/cation liposome or lipoplex, proteins or peptides which act as ligands for cell surface receptors. For example, the inclusion of a single-chain antibody against the transferrin receptor, generating an 'immunoliposome' has been shown to facilitate uptake of systemically delivered transgenes by tumours in preclinical animal models (Xu, 2002). A natural extension of this idea, and a potentially exciting development for future gene therapy applications is the construction of vectors which combine the best features of viral and non-viral mechanisms, so-called 'artificial virus-like particles'.

Artificial virus-like particles. Although non-viral gene delivery strategies avoid some of the pitfalls of viral vectors, they are generally less efficient in transducing target cells than viral vectors. In some gene therapy uses, this does not prove a significant obstacle to their use. For example, in immunomodulation, transduction of only a small proportion of immune system target cells can be sufficient to produce an adequate immune response. In most other gene therapy uses, however, the efficiency of transduction is of vital importance to the success of the strategy. In these cases, a combination of viral and non-viral delivery mechanisms may provide the best of both worlds. Thus, various attempts have been made to produce artificial virus-like particles (AVLPs), in which plasmid DNA is packaged within a synthetic polycation coating with specific targeting and/or improved cell entry being achieved by conjugation with eukaryotic or viral peptides known to have a role in the processes of receptor binding and internalization. Specificity in the targeting of AVLPs can be achieved by incorporating either specific ligands such as monoclonal antibodies against the transferrin receptor or relatively non-specific ligands such as peptides containing the integrin-binding RGD peptide sequence.

Tumour-selective transgene expression

To maximize the therapeutic index of cancer gene therapy strategies, the effect of the transgene must be carefully targeted, such that tumour cells, but not normal cells, are affected. Targeting can be achieved at a variety of levels—targeting of delivery to a specific anatomical location, targeting of the types of cells which a vector can enter, or targeting expression of the transgene to particular cell types or particular situations. It seems likely that the most precise targeting of tumour cells, and therefore therapies with optimum therapeutic index, will involve targeting at multiple levels. For example, a gene therapy might be targeted both to a tumour-associated antigen at the cell surface and to cells with particular patterns of transcription.

Transcriptional targeting. One of the most commonly employed mechanisms for selective targeting is to regulate the transcription of the transgene. Transcriptional regulation is the most common point at which regulation of gene expression is achieved in nature, and it is therefore convenient to exploit this for gene therapy.

Most gene therapy strategies involve a transgene which encodes a protein effector, expressed via an mRNA intermediate, which is transcribed by DNA-directed RNA Polymerase II (PolII). The site of initiation of transcription and the quantity of transcripts produced from the gene are determined by transcription regulatory sequences, known as promoters and enhancers. Promoters are almost invariably immediately 5′ (or 'upstream') of the transcribed sequences, and determine the situations in which transcription is initiated; enhancers can be found upstream or downstream of the transcription unit, sometimes at large distances, in either orientation or within introns, and greatly increase the quantity of transcripts produced. Promoters are modular entities, being composed of collections of *cis*-acting sequences, each recognized by a DNA sequence-specific transcription factor. These bind to the DNA and interact with one another, forming a transcription initiation complex with PolII (Beckett, 2001).

In this way, the initiation of transcription is tightly regulated, such that expression of the transgene product occurs only when and where intended. This targeting of transcription can be achieved in simple ways such as direct injection of the gene therapy construct into a tumour mass, under direct or endoscopic vision. In cases such as this, no temporal or spatial control of transcription is required; simply high-level expression starting immediately after injection, and only in the cells in the immediate vicinity. For gene therapy approaches such as this, a constitutive promoter is all that is required, and the most commonly used are viral promoter/enhancers such as the promoter/enhancer which controls transcription of the cytomegalovirus (CMV) immediate early region.

Tissue-specific promoters. For other strategies, however, precise spatial and/or temporal control of gene expression is required. Perhaps the most common example is the use of tissue-specific promoters. In principle, these permit systemic administration of the gene therapy construct, but transcription and subsequent steps in gene expression occur only in specific tissues. This is because the promoter region contains sequence elements which are recognized by transcription factors found only in a particular tissue (or limited subset of tissues), and without which a transcription initiation complex cannot be formed. Thus, removing the promoter region from in front of a gene which is expressed only in a particular tissue, say liver, and placing it in front of a suicide gene will, in theory, result in tissue-specific expression of the systemically delivered gene therapy construct only in liver, and not in other tissues. On this basis, the tyrosinase gene promoter has been used to restrict expression to melanocytes in the treatment of melanoma, the α_1-antitrypsin or albumin gene promoters to target liver cells for treating hepatocellular carcinoma, glial fibrillary acidic protein (GFAP) promoter to astrocytes in the central nervous system, and immunoglobulin promoters to B lymphocytes for the treatment of B-cell lymphomas such as Burkitt's lymphoma. Potential new tissue-specific promoters will hopefully become available following the completion of the sequencing of the human genome and the mass of new data becoming available on the 'transcriptome' as a result of bioinformatic analysis of results of comparative cDNA arrays (Lockhart, 1996) and SAGE (serial analysis of gene expression) data (Velculescu, 1995).

Tumour-selective promoters. Tissue-specific promoters are particularly useful for targeting metastases using a systemically delivered vector. Of course, there is the risk that normal cells in the appropriate tissue will also be damaged. This is not necessarily a problem for tissues which are 'dispensable', such as the prostate. However, for many if not most tissues, tumour-selective targeting is more important than tissue specificity. A variety of tumour-selective promoters have been identified and investigated for use in cancer gene therapy. These include the promoters for the oncofetal proteins alpha-feto protein (AFP), which is expressed in hepatocellular carcinoma and the teratoma subset of testicular cancers, and carcinoembryonic antigen (CEA) which targets colorectal and some other cancers, the prostate specific antigen gene promoter which is active in prostate cancer cells, and the thyroglobulin promoter for thyroid cancer.

Each of these promoters is useful for only one or a few tumour types. However, it would be desirable to have a single gene therapy construct with broad tumour tropism. Human telomerase permits escape from senescence and consequent cellular immortalization. It is aberrantly overexpressed in 80–90% of human tumours. Inclusion of the promoters for either the RNA or protein components of human telomerase may therefore provide a tumour-selective gene therapy strategy applicable to a wide range of tumour types (Keith, 2001).

Inducible promoters. Tissue-specific and tumour-selective promoters provide spatial regulation of therapeutic gene expression. Temporal control, and the possibility of multiple dosing of gene therapy after only a single administration of the vector, can be obtained by using inducible promoters. In strategies of this type, the addition of a small molecule is sufficient to switch transcription on or off. A variety of systems have been designed. The earliest of these systems employed inducing agents such as the heavy metal ions zinc and cadmium (metallothionein promoter) and/or glucocorticoid hormones. One of the most popular is based upon the transcriptional repressor sequences of the bacterial tetracycline metabolism operon. Modifications have been made which enable transcription to be either turned on or off by the presence of tetracycline (or its analogue, doxycycline) (Gossen, 1995; Mizuguchi and Hayakawa, 2002). Another inducible system is based on the promoter for the insect hormone ecdysone. Combinations of inducible and tissue-specific regulation have already been investigated (Chyung, 2003; Smith-Arica, 2000).

Inducible systems rely on DNA-binding proteins known as transcription factors. These are composed of two domains, one of which binds to specific promoter sequences, and the other of which interacts with other components of the transcription initiation complex. The anti-progestin or 'GeneSwitch' system involves inducible transcription in the presence of the small molecule anti-progestin drug RU486 (mifepristone). A chimaeric transcription factor binds to the GAL4 recognition sequence and activates transcription only in the presence of mifepristone.

The rapamycin-inducible 'dimerizer' system employs the same principle of bi-partite transcription factors, but the two components are encoded separately, and are brought together only in the presence of rapamycin, a macrolide antibiotic which also has immunosuppressant and anti-tumour properties (Rivera, 1996). When rapamycin is present it forms a 'bridge' between the two components, permitting initiation of transcription. This pharmacological induction of transgene expression has already been utilized in a number of preclinical gene therapy strategies, but has not yet been applied in clinical trials. In a comparison between the various inducible promoter systems, it has been suggested that the rapamycin dimerizer system is superior to tetracycline-regulatable, ecdysone-inducible and antiprogestin-inducible systems (Xu, 2003).

One of the main obstacles to the efficient use of transcriptionally targeted gene therapy is achieving appropriate levels of transcription. On the one hand, a particular problem for inducible promoters is 'leaky' transcription, whereby the transgene is transcribed at low levels in the absence of the inducing signal; on the other hand, especially in the use of tissue-specific promoters, the levels of transcription may be too low to generate adequate levels of the transgene product to achieve a therapeutic effect. A solution to the former problem is to insert transcriptional 'insulator' sequences, such as those found in the chicken beta-globin locus, or the 'gypsy' transposable element of *Drosophila*, upstream of the inducible promoter, avoiding inappropriate transcription by establishing higher order domains of chromatin structure. One potential solution to the problem of low-level tissue-specific expression is the use of the Cre/loxP system. DNA sequences placed between the recognition sequences (loxP sites) for the bacterial Cre recombinase enzyme are excised when the bacterial enzyme is expressed in mammalian cells. The problem of low levels of expression from a tissue-specific promoter can therefore be overcome by employing two constructs. One contains a high-level constitutive promoter separated from the transcription unit of the transgene by a transcription 'stop' sequence flanked by loxP sequences. In the second the Cre gene is placed under the transcriptional control of a tissue-specific promoter. In non-target tissues, neither the therapeutic transgene product nor Cre is expressed, the former because of the transcription stop sequences and the latter because of the absence of tissue-specific transcription factors. In the target tissue, however, low-level expression of Cre occurs from the tissue-specific promoter. Effective amplification of this tissue-specific expression is achieved via the catalytic activity of the Cre enzyme, which recognizes the loxP sequences flanking the transcription stop signal, removes them, and places the transgene under control of the high-level promoter. An elegant modification of this Cre/lox switching mechanism for transcriptional control enables a switch to be made between the expression of two alternative genes (Kaczmarczyk and Green, 2001).

Other promoters used in cancer gene therapy are active only in certain physiological situations. These promoters are activated in circumstances commonly seen in the tumour microenvironment. Perhaps the best example of this is the use of hypoxia-inducible promoters. Transcription of genes encoding products such as erythropoietin, vascular endothelial growh factor, carbonic anhydrase IX, glucose transporters, and glycolytic enzymes is stimulated in the presence of hypoxia, a situation which is commonly seen in large tumour bulks and which correlates both with poor prognosis and poor response to conventional treatment modalities such as chemotherapy and radiotherapy.

The potential value of gene therapy as an adjunct to existing cancer treatments has highlighted the potential importance of radiation-inducible promoters (Greco, 2002; Scott, 2000). Hypoxic tumours respond poorly to radiotherapy, even with the use of known radio-sensitizers. Combined treatment with radiotherapy plus gene therapy ('genetic radiotherapy') may allow radiotherapy to kill radio-sensitive components of a tumour at the same time as activating transcription of a cytotoxic transgene in portions of the tumour that are not sensitive to the radiotherapy itself.

While regulation of transcription at the level of transcription initiation is a commonly employed mechanism in nature, and therefore in gene therapy strategies to date, gene expression can also be regulated at a variety of other levels. Another mechanism for altering levels of transcripts available for translation, without altering the level of transcription initiation is to modify the stability of the mRNA, thereby altering the duration for which each transcript is available for translation, and the number of protein molecules generated per transcript. Certain mRNAs, such as that transcribed from the prostaglandin-endoperoxide synthase 2 (*PTSG-2*; cyclo-oxygenase 2) gene, are stabilized by the presence of AU-rich sequences in their 3′ untranslated regions. Preferential stabilization of the PTSG-2 mRNA appears to occur in tumour cells via the activated Ras/MAP kinase pathway, permitting the construction of a tumour-selective conditionally replicating adenovirus in which the adenoviral E1a protein is stabilized by the addition of the 3′ untranslated region of the *PTSG-2* gene (Ahmed, 2003).

Cell-surface targeting. Tumour cells can be selectively targeted by exploiting known differential expression patterns between tumour and normal cells. Cell surface tumour-associated antigens which are relatively overexpressed in tumour cells can be targeted via specific molecular interactions, such as the modifications of viral coat proteins or the use of 'molecular adaptors', such as those used for the re-targeting of adenoviral vectors (see above).

Oncolytic viruses. The majority of gene therapy strategies employing viral vectors use replication-defective viruses. The role of the virus is to gain entry to host cells; the therapeutic transgene is contained within the viral genome merely to enable packaging within the virus capsid, thereby exploiting the highly evolved mechanisms of viral cell entry.

Employing viruses in this way is safe, but efficiency is limited by the number of cells which take up the viral genome. The effects of the transgene product are limited to the infected cell itself and a limited number of cells in the immediate vicinity, exposed to a 'by-stander effect' (see above). Although viral vectors transduce cells with high efficiency *in vitro*, this efficiency is greatly reduced *in vivo*, where cells are organized into tissues, with tight junctions between epithelials cells, extra-cellular matrix components and secreted glycoproteins providing additional barriers to viral entry. As a result, only a small proportion of cells are transduced *in vivo* (Chester, 2003).

Another class of viral vectors, however, can replicate preferentially in tumour cells. These 'oncolytic' or 'conditionally replicating' viruses both selectively target tumours and improve the spread of transgene products from cell to cell, thereby improving the efficiency of gene therapy. The ability of these viruses to selectively replicate in tumour cells rather than normal cells has been appreciated for many decades, but until recently it has been viewed as no more than an interesting phenomenon. In the last few years, however, interest in the use of viruses themselves as anti-tumour therapies, in their own right has been rekindled, with a range of different viral families being employed as oncolytic agents (Antonio Chiocca, 2002).

Some of these viruses are oncolytic as wild-type viruses, exploiting defects in intracellular pathways which are commonly associated with the tumour phenotype. For example, Newcastle disease virus and vesicular stomatitis virus are tumour-selective by exploiting defects in the interferon-response pathways, while reovirus replication requires an activated Ras pathway, again a common feature of tumour cells. Newcastle disease virus (oncolytic strain PV701) has already been proven to be safe in a clinical trial on patients with advanced malignancy.

Other viruses are not oncolytic as wild type, but can be genetically engineered to exploit features associated with tumour cells. For example, deletion of the thymidine kinase (*tk*) gene of vaccinia virus removes the virus' ability to generate its own nucleotide precursors, thereby inhibiting viral replication. However, many tumour cells have high intracellular pools of nucleotides, compared to normal cells, and thus the *tk*-deleted vaccinia virus mutant can preferentially replicate in tumour cells.

The prototype for the recent explosion in renewed interest in oncolytic viruses was a selectively replicating adenovirus, dl1520 (ONYX-015). This virus contains a deletion in a portion of the adenovirus *E1b* early gene which encodes a 55 kDa protein product. One of the roles of this 55 kDa protein is to interact with the tumour suppressor protein p53, preventing cell cycle arrest and apoptosis, and allowing viral replication. The dl1520 adenovirus mutant was postulated to produce selective lysis in tumour cells with *p53* mutations, but not in normal cells. In normal cells the *E1b*-deleted virus would, like any replication-defective adenovirus, be unable to replicate. However, in cells with mutant *p53*, the absence of the 55 kDa protein would be irrelevant, and the virus would be able to complete its natural lytic cycle. As a large proportion of human tumours contain *p53* mutations, dl1520 therefore has oncolytic potential across a range of tumour types. Indeed, initial *in vitro* work supported this (Bischoff, 1996). Subsequent investigations reveal the situation to be more complex, with replication of dl1520 being observed in cells having wild-type *p53* sequence. This apparent anomaly can be explained in terms of the p53 molecule being only one component of a pathway with complex regulation—defects at any one of a number of points could prevent function of the pathway, and allow replication of dl1520, even if p53 itself were normal (McCormick, 2000). Whatever the precise molecular mechanism, dl1520 has been proven to be safe when administered via a variety of routes, in a variety of tumour types, and even in pre-malignant conditions. Although results when used as a single agent in patients with recurrent head-and-neck cancers were not impressive, it has proven effective in combination with cisplatin/5FU chemotherapy (Khuri, 2000). Consequently, a Phase III trial has been initiated.

The results of clinical trials with dl1520 have provoked a rush of other selectively replicating adenoviruses. Another selectively replicating adenovirus whose mechanism of action is based upon the same principles as dl1520, but which may be more efficient at lysing cells is an *E1a*-deleted adenovirus, dl922–947 (ONYX-411) (Heise, 2000). This virus, and a similar virus constructed by another group, Δ24 (Fueyo, 2000), are designed to permit replication in cells which are defective in function of the pRb (retinoblastoma) tumour suppressor gene pathway, but not in normal cells. Other adenoviruses with enhanced oncolytic activity have been obtained by 'bioselection', a process involving random mutagenesis of the viral genome, followed by serial passage in human tumour cell lines (Yan, 2003).

A development of the principles on which these selectively replicating viruses were built involves conditional expression of *E1a* or *E1b* gene products, rather than simple deletion of the genes. Thus, replacing the intrinsic viral promoter with a tissue-specific or inducible promoter will result in expression of *E1a* or *E1b* only in particular circumstances. For example, insertion of the tyrosinase promoter into an *E1a* mutant adenovirus similar to those described above results in preferential killing of melanoma cell lines, compared to non-melanoma cells (Nettelbeck, 2002). Similarly, replacing the viral promoter with the prostate cancer-specific PSA promoter in the recombinant adenovirus CV706 (previously known as CN 706, Rodriguez, 1997) resulted in selective lysis of PSA-expressing prostate cancer cells. CV706 has therefore now entered clinical trials.

Another development is to encode additional exogenous transgenes, rather than relying on oncolytic activity alone. Suicide genes such as cytosine deaminase can be inserted within the viral genome of either dl1520 or dl922–947 in an attempt to improve by-stander effect and/or immune stimulation. Results presented in poster form at a major international meeting suggest that intravenous administration of the dl922–947 derivative, ONYX-443, can inhibit the growth of human tumour xenografts in nude mice (Robinson, 2003; Shen, 2003).

Results with these conditionally replicating adenoviruses have prompted renewed interest in oncolytic viruses from other viral families. The most widely studied are the oncolytic herpesviruses G207 and NV1020. G207 has been demonstrated to be tumour-selective, both *in vitro* and *in vivo*, in a variety of tumour types.

28.2.4 Effector gene

Cancer gene therapy must aim to either control or eliminate cancer cells which have escaped normal limitations on cell growth and proliferation. This can be achieved either by selectively killing tumour cells or by limiting/reversing the malignant phenotype.

Gene replacement strategies

Loss of both copies of 'recessive' tumour suppressor genes is observed in many human tumours. In principle, the re-introduction of a single functional copy might reverse or abrogate the tumour cell phenotype. An attractive potential target for such gene replacement therapy is p53, the 'guardian of the genome', which has multiple intracellular roles as transcription factor, cell cycle regulator and inducer of DNA repair or apoptosis, in response to DNA damage. Mutations of the *p53* gene are seen in over half of all human tumours, and are often associated with poor prognosis.

A *p53* gene replacement strategy was employed in one of the first cancer gene therapy trials, a Phase I study of safety in patients with metastatic non-small cell lung cancer (NSCLC), in which the wild-type *p53* gene was transcribed from a β-actin promoter in a retroviral vector (Roth, 1996). A variety of other phase I trials have followed, mostly employing two similar adenoviral vectors (INGN201 and Sch-58500) in which the *p53* gene is expressed at high levels from a constitutively active CMV promoter. These vectors have been demonstrated to be safe in patients with advanced NSCLC, squamous head-and-neck carcinoma, breast cancer and melanoma, glioma, and muscle-invasive bladder cancer. Several of these Phase I trials showed expression of the *p53* transgene, in terms of either mRNA expression, protein expression, or biological activity of p53, such as induction of p21/WAF.

In further, Phase II, trials of INGN-201 and Sch-58500 in NSCLC, in combination with radiotherapy or chemotherapy, objective tumour response, and *p53* transgene expression were seen in more than 60% of cases. Phase II/III trials of *p53*-expressing adenoviral vectors, given intravenously or intraperitoneally in combination with systemic chemotherapy +/− radiotherapy are now under way in NSCLC, head-and-neck cancer and ovarian cancer (Gene Therapy Clinical Trials Database, 2004). A failure to demonstrate added benefit would not be entirely surprising. To completely eradicate chemotherapy- or radiotherapy-resistant tumour would require 100% efficiency of transduction and transgene expression. Even if this were possible, success would also depend upon the targeted transgene being the sole causative event and its re-introduction being capable of reversing all downstream phenotypic defects. This seems unlikely given our knowledge of the multi-stage nature of carcinogenesis. Hence, many of its proponents feel that gene therapy is most likely to be useful by killing tumour cells.

Suicide gene therapy

The most commonly used effector genes in gene therapy strategies are so-called 'suicide genes'. In their simplest form, suicide gene therapies encode proteins, such as the A subunit of *Diphtheria* toxin, which are in themselves directly toxic to cells. More commonly, the 'suicide' transgene product is not toxic in itself. Rather, the transgene encodes an enzyme which activates a non-toxic prodrug to form an active drug with cytotoxic activity. These suicide genes are usually prokaryotic or lower eukaryotic genes which either do not have homologues in human cells, or whose human homologues have far less enzymic activity.

Therefore, prodrugs can be activated selectively in transduced cells. Suicide genes of this sort are the principal component of so-called gene-directed enzyme prodrug therapy (GDEPT) or virus-directed enzyme prodrug therapy (VDEPT). The inherent safety of this mechanism is obvious. Cell killing requires both expression of the transgene and the presence of the prodrug: each component is non-toxic on its own; both are required for any effect.

One of the first prodrug activating enzymes used was bacterial cytosine deaminase (CD). The normal reaction catalysed by CD is the deamination of the pyrimidine base cytosine, to uracil. However, its substrate specificity is not limited to cytosine; it can also deaminate halogenated derivatives of cytosine, including 5-fluoro-cytosine (5FC), forming the anti-metabolite, 5-fluoro-uracil (5FU), which is an inhibitor of DNA and RNA synthesis. GDEPT strategies localize the conversion of systemically delivered 5FC so that the cytotoxic activity of 5FU is confined to cells which contain the transgene, thereby optimizing therapeutic index. Recent developments include the use of yeast, rather than bacterial CD, which has a far greater affinity for 5FC substrate, making cells transduced with yeast CD more sensitive than those transduced with the bacterial enzyme, for a given 5FC dose.

The most widely used prodrug activating enzyme, experimentally and clinically, is the Herpes Simplex Virus thymidine kinase (*HSV-tk*) gene. This activates the prodrug ganciclovir, which is a nucleoside analogue. Activation of the prodrug involves three phosphorylation steps. The triphosphate acts as a DNA replication chain-terminator, in a cell cycle S phase-specific fashion. In mammalian cells, there are no kinases capable of efficiently performing the first of these three phosphorylation steps. Ganciclovir on its own is therefore non-toxic to mammalian cells. However, gene therapy employing the *HSV-tk* gene performs the monophosphorylation with high efficiency, whereupon endogenous kinases rapidly form the di- and triphosphates.

Ganciclovir is less toxic than 5FC when administered systemically, and the efficiency of conversion of prodrug is higher. Therefore, the HSV-tk/ganciclovir system has been more widely applied in preclinical and clinical studies. However, a major limitation of the HSV-tk system is that the 'by-stander effect' (see above) is dependent upon gap junction communications between adjacent cells, a significant limitation for use in a number of tumour types with reduced expression of the connexin proteins which make up gap junctions.

The relative or absolute lack of gap junctions is less of a problem for another prodrug activating enzyme, bacterial nitroreductase (NTR). Its prodrug substrate CB1954 (5-(aziridin-1-yl)-2,4-dinitrobenzamide) is a weak monofunctional DNA-alkylating agent. Activation produces a 4-hydroxyl-amino derivative, which is a much more potent bifunctional alkylating agent. The inter-strand cross-links formed result in cytotoxicity which is independent of cell cycle phase. In other words, unlike HSV-tk ganciclovir and CD/5FC, the toxicity of the activated prodrug can affect both dividing and non-dividing cells. This is important as, at a given moment when gene therapy is delivered, a large proportion of tumour cells are either 'out of cycle' in the G0 phase or cycling slowly. Crucially, activated CB1954 is able to spread from cell to cell via diffusion, rather than requiring the presence of gap junctions (Bridgewater, 1995). Adenoviral vectors with the *NTR* gene under control of a constitutive promoter are currently in clinical trials, and preliminary results of anti-tumour efficacy are eagerly awaited.

Attention has focussed recently on improving the by-stander effect of HSV-tk. One of the methods employed has been to deliver a second prodrug activating enzyme and prodrug. However, data regarding the combination of HSV-tk/ganciclovir and CD/5FC systems is conflicting, with a couple of reports suggesting additive or synergistic effects, and another suggesting that the two systems counteract one another. Combining HSV-tk/ganciclovir with NTR/CB1954 resulted in cooperative killing (Bridgewater, 1995).

Other mechanisms which might improve the bystander effect of HSV-tk/ganciclovir include co-transduction of gap junction-deficient tumour cells with connexin genes and use of the *HSV* gene product, VP-22. This protein has the unusual ability to undergo intercellular trafficking. Fusion proteins in which VP-22 is covalently linked to GFP and the prodrug activating enzymes HSV-tk and cytosine deaminase were not only efficiently transported to neighbouring cells, but also retained function of the non-viral portion of the chimaeric protein.

Purified preparations of the C-terminal half of the VP-22 protein can also be complexed with other proteins, peptides, oligo-deoxynucleotides (ODNs), and ribozymes to form novel particles for improving the efficient delivery of gene therapy. Complexing with ODNs produces light-inducible ribonucleoprotein 'vectosomes', which are dissociated by light, releasing ODNs (Zavaglia, 2003). Although successful *in vitro* and in pre-clinical studies, this strategy is yet to be proven in published clinical trials.

Some studies investigating the bystander effect of the HSV-tk/ganciclovir system have suggested a 'distant bystander' effect, as well as a local effect seen immediately surrounding cells expressing the *tk* transgene. The observation that the distant bystander effect was delayed compared to the local one may imply an immune mechanism. Combination gene therapy strategies in which there is co-expression of prodrug activating enzymes and immuno-modulatory/cytokine genes are therefore attractive.

A novel cytotoxic strategy more akin to the 'direct' suicide gene strategies above, combines direct cytotoxicity with the stimulation of the immune system. Fusogenic membrane glycoproteins (FMGs) are viral structural proteins found in viruses such as gibbon ape leukaemia virus (GALV), vesicular stomatitis virus (VSV) and measles virus, whose normal function is to facilitate the entry of the viral genome into host cells. When expressed as transgenes, however, they can form tumour cell syncytia and induce non-apoptotic cell death both *in vitro* and in preclinical animal tumour xenograft models (Bateman, 2000). Cytotoxicity appears to be more potent than with the 'traditional' suicide genes *HSV-tk* and *CD*. Syncytium formation not only produces a form of bystander effect by the fusion (and subsequent death) of virally transduced cells with surrounding non-transduced cells, but also appears to stimulate specific anti-tumour immunity. Use of these FMGs in conjunction with conditionally replicating adenoviruses also seems to enhance cytotoxicity of the virus. Translation of promising preclinical results with these promising new gene therapy agents into clinical trials is keenly anticipated.

RNA-directed strategies

Most gene therapy strategies have relied upon effector mechanisms based around proteins, with the exogenous transgene either encoding a protein, or targeting a protein. However, gene therapy strategies can also target mRNA. For example, selective targeting of EGFR-overexpressing tumours could, in theory, be directed against the EGFR mRNA in a sequence-specific fashion (Nagy, 2003).

There are three basic types of RNA-directed gene therapy strategies: 'anti-sense' single-stranded oligo-deoxynucleotides; 'ribozymes'; and 'RNA interference' (Kurreck, 2003; Scherer and Rossi, 2003). In each case, the effector is a ss RNA gene therapy product, rather than an enzyme or antibody. All three strategies result in sequence-specific recognition (and in most cases subsequent cleavage) of mRNA transcripts. Each selectively reduces the quantity of mRNA transcripts, or blocks their translation. They are therefore particularly useful as therapies for tumours in which there is aberrant qualitative or quantitative gene expression—for example in the expression of mutated or overexpressed proto-oncogenes.

Because of this ability to reduce the level of mRNA transcripts, they are therefore sometimes referred to as 'knock-down' strategies. This is by analogy with so-called 'knock-out' transgenic mice, in which individual genes, or portions of genes, are selectively deleted from the genome, to investigate the phenotypic consequences. Similarly, anti-RNA strategies have been widely used to investigate the phenotypic effects of reducing the level of specific mRNA transcripts in the embryological development of organisms such as the nematode worm *Caenorhabditis elegans*.

While the use of RNA-directed strategies in this sense is an experimental tool, aimed at identifying molecular function, these strategies also present therapeutic possibilities. Such RNA-directed gene therapy strategies have been under investigation for many years. While elegant in principle, they have, until recently, had limited efficacy. However, the recent elucidation of the mechanism of so-called RNA interference, involving small interfering RNAs (siRNAs) or short hairpin RNAs (shRNAs) has rejuvenated interest in this type of strategy.

The first of the RNA-directed gene therapy strategies involved so-called anti-sense technology. Single-stranded oligo-deoxynucleotides (ODNs), complementary to mRNAs and introduced into cells, can reduce the level of expression of the encoded protein in one of two ways (Kurreck, 2003; Scherer and Rossi, 2003). Sequence-specific Watson–Crick base-pairing between the antisense ODN and its complementary mRNA can sterically inhibit translation of the message. Alternatively, ODNs form an RNA : DNA heteroduplex which is recognized by the cellular enzyme RNase H, with consequent mRNA cleavage. The ODN can be re-cycled to target further RNA molecules. It can thus be thought of as a co-factor for RNase H in a genuinely catalytic process. The sequence-specific nature of the ssDNA : mRNA interaction makes this a particularly attractive feature for tumour-selective targeting. The requirement for a precise match between ODN and mRNA can be exploited to differentially target the mutated mRNA of a cellular proto-oncogene.

Unlike other RNA-directed strategies, anti-sense strategies have been around sufficiently long to have entered clinical trials. Only one, for the non-cancer condition CMV retinitis has received official regulatory approval for use beyond clinical trials. Others (e.g. ISIS 2503 directed against mutated H-ras and 3521 (Affinitak) against protein kinase C) are being trialled as anti-cancer agents.

The second anti-RNA strategy involves ribozymes. These are derivatives of naturally occurring molecules found in a variety of organisms, including the ciliate protozoan *Tetrahymena thermophila*. These molecules can perform cleavage of ssRNAs, in the absence of any protein. In nature, many of these catalyse intra-molecular cleavage 'in *cis*', but they have been engineered to form *trans*-splicing ssRNA molecules about 40 nt in length with exotic names such as 'hammerhead', 'axehead', 'pseudoknot' and 'paperclip' ribozymes. Like ODNs, they bind to target mRNAs in a sequence-specific fashion, via substrate-binding sequences either side of a catalytic site which recognizes a triplet sequence in the target mRNA. The most efficiently cleaved nucleotide triplet cleavage sequence is often GUC. Of course, this requirement places limitations on the mRNA sequences which can be recognized and cleaved. Clinical trials with ribozymes have been initiated in patients with AIDS and in healthy volunteers, but not, as yet, for patients with cancer.

The third type of RNA-directed gene therapy is known as RNA interference. The so-called 'gene silencing' can be achieved via 21–23nt ssRNA effectors known as siRNAs, complementary to mRNA targets. These siRNAs are derived from short dsRNAs which are sufficiently short to avoid inducing the cellular type I interferon anti-viral response to cytoplasmic dsRNAs longer than approximately 30nt. siRNA production is via an intracellular multi-molecular complex known as RISC (RNA-induced silencing complex). Short dsRNAs can be introduced into target cells in a variety of ways, including the PolIII-mediated transcription of shRNAs or cleavage of longer dsRNAs *in vitro* by the 'Dicer' enzyme complex, but in all cases, complexing with RISC forms a final common pathway. RISC separates 21–23nt dsRNAs (with short 3′ overhangs) into single strands, and forms sequence-specific ternary complexes with mRNAs. The RISC complex then cleaves the target mRNA. siRNAs can thus be designed to target mRNAs which are over-expressed in tumours. Again, the siRNA : RISC complex remains catalytically active. *In vitro*, these reductions in transcript levels can persist for periods between several days and several weeks.

Like other RNA-directed strategies, the sequence-specific recognition of mRNAs by siRNAs provides the possibility of tumour-specific targeting. Both point mutations and gross chromosome abnormalities can be targeted. For example, it is possible to target the transcript which results from the *bcr–abl* gene fusion responsible for chronic myelogenous leukaemia (CML) and a sub-set of acute lymphoblastic leukaemia (ALL). In established and primary cell lines from CML patients, chemically synthesized siRNAs have been shown in *in vitro* experiments to reduce the levels of *bcr–abl* fusion transcripts by 87%, without affecting either of the unfused *bcr* or *abl* transcripts from the unaffected chromosomes. In addition the siRNAs were able to reduce the levels of the fusion protein by 80% and to limit the proliferation of cells (Scherr, 2003).

Whilst RNA interference offers exciting prospects for potential therapeutic strategies, and is the focus of much pre-clinical work, none of these approaches has yet reached a clinical trial. Laboratory experience suggests that the selection of target sequences is important—there appears to be an enormous variability in the efficiency with which sequences from different regions of a single mRNA achieve a gene silencing effect.

Immunotherapy

Rare observations of spontaneous regression of solid tumours such as renal carcinoma and melanoma, combined with serendipitous clinical discoveries such as the ability of Streptococcal cultures to induce regression of advanced sarcomas, have generated the hypothesis that treatment might be directed at overcoming a tumour's ability to 'escape' immune surveillance.

The complexity of the human immune system and the diversity of tumour types make for a potentially bewildering array of immunotherapy strategies. Some of these are amenable to gene therapy approaches. Gene therapy and immunotherapy can thus be thought of as overlapping subsets of anticancer treatments.

Immunotherapy is well established in the treatment of certain cancers, particularly those which respond poorly (or not at all) to established treatments (see Chapter 27). For example, exogenous administration of the cytokine interleukin-2 (IL-2), a naturally occurring component of the human immune system, either alone or in combination, can produce tumour shrinkage in a proportion of patients with advanced renal cell carcinoma.

Some immunotherapies involve only passive immunity, using 'humanized' antibodies against tumour antigens, sometimes with toxins such as ricin or radiolabels attached, or the induction of 'graft-versus-tumour' responses such as those seen with mini-allografts against renal cancer. However, it seems likely that the most successful immunotherapy strategies will involve induction of active immunity, involving the stimulation of both cellular and humoral components of the immune response.

The simplest type of active immunotherapy strategy involves attempting to generate an antitumour immune response by vaccinating with tumour-associated antigens (TAAs), expressed exclusively by tumours, or overexpressed in tumour cells compared to normal cells. In its simplest form, this need not involve gene therapy. For example, patients can be injected subcutaneously, intradermally or intramuscularly with whole cell lysates derived from tumour cells, with partially or fully purified preparations, or with synthetic peptide sequences derived from known tumour antigen sequences. However, vaccination strategies of this type are of limited clinical efficacy, due to the low efficiency of antigen presentation and/or lymphocyte activation. Gene therapy has the potential to improve the efficiency of induction of these tumour-specific immune responses. Either a single antigen can be expressed at high levels by driving its expression from a constitutive high-level promoter, or multiple epitopes can be expressed from a single gene therapy construct—so-called poly-epitopes (Smith, 2001).

'Immunogene therapies' may involve either genetic modification of tumour cells themselves *in situ*, or of cells of the immune system *ex vivo*, by 'adoptive transfer'. These genetic modifications can either be performed using naked DNA or viral vectors.

Alternatively, tumour cells can be genetically modified *in situ* by the introduction of gene therapy vectors encoding cytokine genes to stimulate non-specific activation of the immune system, or to attract antigen-presenting cells or T lymphocytes. Efficiency of these activation processes can be enhanced by co-administering genes encoding co-stimulatory molecules such as B7.

Ex vivo modification is usually of professional antigen-presenting cells such as dendritic cells, or of cytotoxic lymphocytes (CTLs). For example, TAA or cytokine genes can be introduced into dendritic cells using a variety of viral vectors, including adenoviruses and lentiviruses. *Ex vivo* modification can be of either autologous or heterologous cells. Using autologous cells obviously requires individualized treatment, which is necessarily time-consuming and expensive, whereas heterologous (allogeneic) donor cells or cell lines permits the treatment of multiple patients with the same vaccine preparation.

One role for immunogene therapy is to enhance the immune recognition of poorly immunogenic tumours. Cytotoxic lymphocytes can be genetically modified *ex vivo* so that they can be activated by antigen alone, in a major histocompatibility complex (MHC)-independent fashion. This is potentially particularly useful as many tumours have limited or absent class I MHC expression. Transgenes are introduced which encode chimeric immune receptor proteins known as 'T bodies', consisting of TAA-specific antibody sequences linked either to the transmembrane and intracellular portions of T-cell receptors, or to intracellular signalling domains.

Immunogene therapy thus represents one of the most promising categories of gene therapy, and may be particularly useful in combination with suicide gene therapy, as described above.

28.3 Gene therapy in practice

Cancer gene therapy is a new antitumour treatment modality. Along with gene therapies for other, non-malignant, conditions it is a rationally designed approach, based on sound scientific principles, and fuelled by the recent dramatic expansion in our understanding of the molecular basis of cancer. A plethora of elegant strategies has been proposed and tested for a wide variety of tumours, involving different combinations of delivery route, vectors for cell entry, intracellular targets, effector genes and tumour-targeting approaches. Like other treatment modalities, some gene therapy approaches may be applicable across a range of tumour types, and gene therapy need not be considered to be tumour site-specific.

Gene therapy is one of a class of new biological therapies which are rationally designed to exploit known molecular characteristics of disease, with selective targeting of known molecular pathologies. Molecularly-targeted biological therapies for cancer have already been shown to be safe and effective for a range of tumour types. For example, humanised monoclonal antibodies have been demonstrated in Phase III clinical trials to improve survival in subsets of breast cancer (Slamon, 2001) and colon cancer, while receptor tyrosine kinase inhibitors have been shown to be effective in chronic myelogenous leukaemia and gastrointestinal stromal tumours.

While no longer in its infancy, gene therapy should probably still be regarded as a developing treatment modality. Many of the proposed strategies have been demonstrated to work *in vitro*, and a large number have gone into clinical trials. Any new treatment entering clinical trials must be proven to be safe and effective, and, to be accepted as a new standard of care, must improve upon the therapeutic index of existing therapies, either as a replacement or as an adjunct to current treatment. The evidence to date suggests that most gene therapies have little or no immediate toxicity. Despite the recruitment of several thousand patients into more than 900 clinical trials of gene therapy to date, there has been only one acute treatment-related death reported (Assessment of adenoviral vector safety and toxicity, 2002). Some long-term toxicity is now starting to be recognised, the theoretical possibility of treatment resulting in second malignancy due to retroviral insertional mutagenesis becoming reality, with the discovery of secondary leukaemias in two non-cancer patients cured of SCID. While disappointing, and rightly a cause for reflection before pursuing these treatments further, we should not be unduly surprised or deterred. All the existing cancer treatment modalities have significant side effects and non-zero treatment-related mortality. While one of the goals of cancer gene therapy is to obtain the best possible therapeutic index, it was never likely that we could obtain both zero toxicity and 100% efficacy.

Demonstration of clinical efficacy is a time-consuming process, and given that most gene therapy strategies are still in the early stages of clinical testing (more than 60% of trials have been phase I toxicity assessments, and less than 2% phase III comparisons with standard treatments) we still have few which are proven to work. What, then, is the future for cancer gene therapy and what will be its place in future treatment of cancer? It seems likely that, like other non-surgical treatments, it is most likely to be effective in the context of minimal disease bulk. It may be that, like other 'biological therapies', gene therapy will be effective only in selected subsets of patients whose tumours exhibit precise molecular profiles. For those gene therapy strategies which do turn out to be effective, it seems likely that they will work best in combination with existing treatment modalities. It may be that these combinations are not able to eliminate a patient's cancer completely, but may be able to change it from a rapidly fatal disease to a chronic disease, similar, say, to diabetes. Certainly, gene therapy is not (and should never have been anticipated to be) a single-agent 'miracle cure' for all types of cancer. Rather, it is likely to be used as combination therapy to provide a further incremental improvement in cancer treatment success, as part of an armamentarium of cancer treatment modalities from which an appropriate patient-specific combination can be selected.

References

Ahmed, A., Thompson, J., Emiliusen, L., Murphy, S., Beauchamp, R. D., Suzuki, K. et al. (2003). A conditionally replicating adenovirus targeted to tumor cells through activated RAS/P-MAPK-selective mRNA stabilization. *Nat Biotechnol*, **21**(7): 771–7.

Antonio Chiocca, E. (2002). Oncolytic viruses. *Nat Rev Cancer*, **2**(12): 938–50.

Assessment of adenoviral vector safety and toxicity. (2002). Report of the National Institutes of Health Recombinant DNA Advisory Committee. *Hum Gene Ther*, **13**(1): 3–13.

Bateman, A., Bullough, F., Murphy, S., Emiliusen, L., Lavillette, D., Cosset, F. L. et al. (2000). Fusogenic membrane glycoproteins as a novel class of genes for the local and immune-mediated control of tumor growth. *Cancer Res*, **60**(6): 1492–7.

Beckett, D. (2001). Regulated assembly of transcription factors and control of transcription initiation. *J Mol Biol*, **314**(3): 335–52.

Bischoff, J. R., Kirn, D. H., Williams, A., Heise, C., Horn, S., Muna M. et al. (1996). An adenovirus mutant that replicates selectively in p53-deficient human tumor cells. *Science*, **274**(5286): 373–6.

Bridgewater, J. A., Springer, C. J., Knox, R. J., Minton, N. P., Michael, N. P., and Collins, M. K. (1995). Expression of the bacterial nitroreductase enzyme in mammalian cells renders them selectively sensitive to killing by the prodrug CB1954. *Eur J Cancer*, **31A**(13–14): 2362–70.

Calderwood, M. A., Hall, K. T., Matthews, D. A., and Whitehouse, A. (2004). The herpesvirus saimiri ORF73 gene product interacts with host-cell mitotic chromosomes and self-associates via its C terminus. *J Gen Virol* **85**(Pt 1): 147–53.

Cavazzana-Calvo, M., Hacein-Bey, S., de Saint Basile, G., Gross, F., Yvon, E., Nusbaum, P. et al. (2000). Gene therapy of human severe combined immunodeficiency (SCID)-X1 disease. *Science*, **288**(5466): 669–72.

Chester, J., Ruchatz, A., Gough, M., Crittenden, M., Chong, H., Loic-Cosset, F. et al. (2002). Tumor antigen-specific induction of transcriptionally targeted retroviral vectors from chimeric immune receptor-modified T cells. *Nat Biotechnol*, **20**(3): 256–63.

Chester, J. D., Kennedy, W., Hall, G. D., Selby, P. J., and Knowles, M. A. (2003). Adenovirus-mediated gene therapy for bladder cancer: efficient gene delivery to normal and malignant human urothelial cells in vitro and ex vivo. *Gene Ther*, **10**(2): 172–9.

Chyung, Y. H., Peng, P. D., and Kay, M. A. (2003). System for simultaneous tissue-specific and disease-specific regulation of therapeutic gene expression. *Hum Gene Ther*, **14**(13): 1255–64.

Crittenden, M., Gough, M., Chester, J., Kottke, T., Thompson, J., Ruchatz, A. et al. (2003). Pharmacologically regulated production of targeted retrovirus from T cells for systemic antitumor gene therapy. *Cancer Res*, **63**(12): 3173–80.

Dmitriev, I., Krasnykh, V., Miller, C. R., Wang, M., Kashentseva, E., Mikheeva, G. et al. (1998). An adenovirus vector with genetically modified fibers demonstrates expanded tropism via utilization of a coxsackievirus and adenovirus receptor-independent cell entry mechanism. *J Virol*, **72**(12): 9706–13.

Dmitriev, I., Kashentseva, E., Rogers, B. E., Krasnykh, V., and Curiel, D. T. (2000). Ectodomain of coxsackievirus and adenovirus receptor genetically fused to epidermal growth factor mediates adenovirus targeting to epidermal growth factor receptor-positive cells. *J Virol*, **74**(15): 6875–84.

Fueyo, J., Gomez-Manzano, C., Alemany, R., Lee, P. S., McDonnell, T. J., Mitlianga, P. et al. (2000). A mutant oncolytic adenovirus targeting the Rb pathway produces anti-glioma effect in vivo. *Oncogene*, **19**(1): 2–12.

Gene Therapy Clinical Trials Database. *J Gene Med* (2004). http://www.wiley.co.uk/genmed/clinical

Gossen, M., Freundlieb, S., Bender, G., Muller, G., and Hillen, W. (1995). Transcriptional activation by tetracyclines in mammalian cells. *Science*, **268**(5218): 1766–9.

Greco, O., Marples, B., Dachs, G. U., Williams, K. J., Patterson, A. V., and Scott, S. D. (2002). Novel chimeric gene promoters responsive to hypoxia and ionizing radiation. *Gene Ther*, **9**(20): 1403–11.

Hacein-Bey-Abina, S., von Kalle, C., Schmidt, M., Le Deist, F., Wulffraat, N., McIntyre, E. et al. (2003). A serious adverse event after successful gene therapy for X-linked severe combined immunodeficiency. *N Engl J Med*, **348**(3): 255–6.

Harrington, K., Alvarez-Vallina, L., Crittenden, M., Gough, M., Chong, H., Diaz, R. M. et al. (2002). Cells as vehicles for cancer gene therapy: the missing link between targeted vectors and systemic delivery? *Hum Gene Ther*, **13**(11): 1263–80.

Heise, C., Hermiston, T., Johnson, L., Brooks, G., Sampson-Johannes, A., Williams, A. et al. (2000). An adenovirus E1A mutant that demonstrates potent and selective systemic anti-tumoral efficacy. *Nat Med*, **6**(10): 1134–9.

Kaczmarczyk, S. J. and Green, J. E. (2001). A single vector containing modified cre recombinase and LOX recombination sequences for inducible tissue-specific amplification of gene expression. *Nucleic Acids Res*, **29**(12): E56–6.

Kay, M. A., Manno, C. S., Ragni, M. V., Larson, P. J., Couto, L. B., McClelland, A. et al. (2000). Evidence for gene transfer and expression of factor IX in haemophilia B patients treated with an AAV vector. *Nat Genet*, **24**(3): 257–61.

Keith, N. W., Jeffry Evans, T. R., and Glasspool, R. M. (2001). Telomerase and cancer: time to move from a promising target to a clinical reality. *J Pathol*, **195**(4): 404–14.

Khuri, F. R., Nemunaitis, J., Ganly, I., Arseneau, J., Tannock, I. F., Romel, L. et al. (2000). A controlled trial of intratumoral ONYX-015, a selectively-replicating adenovirus, in combination with cisplatin and 5-fluorouracil in patients with recurrent head and neck cancer. *Nat Med*, **6**(8): 879–85.

Krasnykh, V., Dmitriev, I., Mikheeva, G., Miller, C. R., Belousova, N., and Curiel, D. T. (1998). Characterization of an adenovirus vector containing a heterologous peptide epitope in the HI loop of the fiber knob. *J Virol*, **72**(3): 1844–52.

Kurreck, J. (2003). Antisense technologies. Improvement through novel chemical modifications. *Eur J Biochem*, **270**(8): 1628–44.

Lockhart, D. J., Dong, H., Byrne, M. C., Follettie, M. T., Gallo, M. V., Chee, M. S. et al. (1996). Expression monitoring by hybridization to high-density oligonucleotide arrays. *Nat Biotechnol*, **14**(13): 1675–80.

McCormick, F. (2000). ONYX-015 selectivity and the p14ARF pathway. *Oncogene*, **19**(56): 6670–2.

Miyoshi, H., Blomer, U., Takahashi ,M., Gage, F. H., and Verma, I. M. (1998). Development of a self-inactivating lentivirus vector. *J Virol*, **72**(10): 8150–7.

Mizuguchi, H. and Hayakawa, T. (2002). The tet-off system is more effective than the tet-on system for regulatory transgene expression in a single adenovirus vector. *J Gene Med*, **4**(3): 240–247.

Nagy, P., Arndt-Jovin, D. J., and Jovin, T. M. (2003). Small interfering RNAs suppress the expression of endogenous and GFP-fused epidermal growth factor receptor (erbB1) and induce apoptosis in erbB1-overexpressing cells. *Exp Cell Res*, **285**(1): 39–49.

Nettelbeck, D. M., Miller, D. W., Jerome, V., Zuzarte, M., Watkins, S. J., Hawkins, R. E. et al. (2001). Targeting of adenovirus to endothelial cells by a bispecific single-chain diabody directed against the adenovirus fiber knob domain and human endoglin (CD 105). *Mol Ther*, **3**(6): 882–91.

Nettelbeck, D. M., Rivera, A. A., Balague, C., Alemany, R., and Curiel, D. T. (2002). Novel oncolytic adenoviruses targeted to melanoma: specific viral replication and cytolysis by expression of E1A mutants from the tyrosinase enhance/promoter. *Cancer Res*, **62**(16): 4663–70.

Rivera, V. M., Clackson, T., Natesan, S., Pollock, R., Amara, J. F., Keenan, T. et al. (1996). A humanized system for pharmacologic control of gene expression. *Nat Med*, **2**(9): 1028–32.

Robinson, M. J. Z. J., Wang, W., Gao, Y., Zhang, S., Shen, A., Aspelund A. et al. (2003). Tumor-specific transgene expression via intravenous delivery using selectively replicating adenoviruses. *Proc Am Assoc Cancer Res*, **551**, abstract 2806.

Rodriguez, R., Schuur, E. R., Lim, H. Y., Henderson, G. A., Simons, J. W., and Henderson, D. R. (1997). Prostate attenuated replication competent adenovirus (ARCA) CN706: a selective cytotoxic for prostate-specific antigen-positive prostate cancer cells. *Cancer Res*, **57**(13): 2559–63.

Roth, J. A., Nguyen, D., Lawrence, D. D., Kemp, B. L., Carrasco, C. H., Ferson, D. Z. et al. (1996). Retrovirus-mediated wild-type p53 gene transfer to tumors of patients with lung cancer. *Nat Med*, **2**(9): 985–91.

Scherer, L. J. and Rossi, J. J. (2003). Approaches for the sequence-specific knockdown of mRNA. *Nat Biotechnol*, **21**(12): 1457–65.

Scherr, M., Battmer, K., Winkler, T., Heidenreich, O., Ganser, A., and Eder, M. (2003). Specific inhibition of bcr-abl gene expression by small interfering RNA. *Blood*, **101**(4): 1566–9.

Scott, S. D., Marples, B., Hendry, J. H., Lashford, L. S., Embleton, M. J., Hunter R. D. et al. (2000). A radiation-controlled molecular switch for use in gene therapy of cancer. *Gene Ther*, **7**(13): 1121–5.

Shen, Y. W. W., Gao, Y., Zhan, J., Shen, A., Laquerre, S., Johnson, L. et al. (2003). Anti-tumor efficacy of ONYX-411 and ONYX-443 following intravenous administration. *Proc Am Assoc Cancer Res*, 142, R738.

Slamon, D. J., Leyland-Jones, B., Shak, S., Fuchs, H., Paton, V., Bajamonde, A. et al. (2001). Use of chemotherapy plus a monoclonal antibody against HER2 for metastatic breast cancer that overexpresses HER2. *N Engl J Med*, **344**(11): 783–92.

Smith, S. G., Patel, P. M., Porte, J., Selby, P. J., and Jackson, A. M. (2001). Human dendritic cells genetically engineered to express a melanoma polyepitope DNA vaccine induce multiple cytotoxic T-cell responses. *Clin Cancer Res*, **7**(12): 4253–61.

Smith-Arica, J. R., Morelli, A. E., Larregina, A. T., Smith, J., Lowenstein, P. R., and Castro, M. G. (2000). Cell-type-specific and regulatable transgenesis in the adult brain: adenovirus-encoded combined transcriptional targeting and inducible transgene expression. *Mol Ther*, **2**(6): 579–87.

Thomas, C. E., Ehrhardt, A., and Kay, M. A. (2003). Progress and problems with the use of viral vectors for gene therapy. *Nat Rev Genet*, **4**(5): 346–58.

Velculescu, V. E., Zhang, L., Vogelstein, B., and Kinzler, K. W. (1995). Serial analysis of gene expression. *Science*, **270**(5235): 484–7.

Watkins, S. J., Mesyanzhinov, V. V., Kurochkina, L. P., and Hawkins, R. E. (1997). The 'adenobody' approach to viral targeting: specific and enhanced adenoviral gene delivery. *Gene Ther*, **4**(10): 1004–12.

Xu, L., Huang, C. C., Huang, W., Tang, W. H., Rait, A., Yin, Y. Z. et al. (2002). Systemic tumor-targeted gene delivery by anti-transferrin receptor scFv-immunoliposomes. *Mol Cancer Ther*, **1**(5): 337–46.

Xu, Z. L., Mizuguchi, H., Mayumi, T., and Hayakawa, T. (2003). Regulated gene expression from adenovirus vectors: a systematic comparison of various inducible systems. *Gene*, **309**(2): 145–51.

Yan, W., Kitzes, G., Dormishian, F., Hawkins, L., Sampson-Johannes, A., Watanabe, J et al. (2003). Developing novel oncolytic adenoviruses through bioselection. *J Virol*, **77**(4): 2640–50.

Zavaglia, D., Normand, N., Brewis, N., O'Hare, P., Favrot, M. C., and Coll , J. L. (2003). VP22-mediated and light-activated delivery of an anti-c-raf1 antisense oligonucleotide improves its activity after intratumoral injection in nude mice. *Mol Ther*, **8**(5): 840–5.

Zufferey, R., Dull, T., Mandel, R. J., Bukovsky, A., Quiroz, D., Naldini, L., et al. (1998). Self-inactivating lentivirus vector for safe and efficient in vivo gene delivery. *J Virol*, **72**(12): 9873–80.

CHAPTER 29

Screening

Peter Sasieni and Jack Cuzick

29.1 Introduction

Screening is aimed at identifying selecting a small group of individuals who are likely to benefit from some form of intervention to reduce the morbidity and mortality from cancer. Screening can take several forms, can be aimed at different populations, and can have different goals. Very often it is a multistage process in which individuals positive at one stage are referred on to a more invasive or intensive procedure to see if cancer is present. There are several pitfalls in the evaluation of the efficacy of screening modalities and it is vitally important that screening should do more good than harm, since one is approaching a healthy population and asking them to undergo a medical procedure, as opposed to the usual clinical paradigm in which an unwell patient approaches the doctor and actively seeks advice and treatment. It is sometimes useful to think of screening in terms of insurance in which many individuals have to pay a small fee in order for a few individuals to benefit.

Since screening can only identify individuals in need of treatment, it alone cannot affect the course of cancer. It is the subsequent treatment which aims to do this. In most cases this is surgical, but when an increased risk of developing cancer is found and/or pre-cancerous lesions that may recur are detected, there is increasing interest and activity in the use of agents to arrest the development of cancer.

In this chapter we review some general considerations relevant to screening, consider a number of different screening technologies, and then examine the role of screening for a number of specific cancers.

The key requirement in screening is the existence of a safe, acceptable test which discriminates well between those in need of treatment and those who do not. Sufficient knowledge of the natural history of the disease to identify at which stage early detection is likely to be important for reducing mortality and morbidity, and choice of the population to be screened are also critical. Other issues such as the age range, screening interval, and follow-up procedures are also important and can have a large impact on the cost of screening. These issues are discussed in greater detail below along with the possible methods for evaluating screening programmes.

29.1.1 Types of screening tests

Broadly speaking, one can identify three very different types of cancer screening: genetic screening, screening aimed at early diagnosis of cancer, and screening aimed at the identification of pre-cancerous lesions. The first of these, genetic screening, is a form of risk profiling and is only briefly considered in this chapter. The other two forms of screening are both designed to detect neoplasia at a point in time when it can be easily and successfully treated. Such screening could be offered either to a large subgroup of the general population (identified by age and sex) or to a small group considered to be at particularly high risk for a particular cancer. Examples include lung screening for current and ex-smokers or those exposed to asbestos; and bladder screening for those with occupational exposure to certain carcinogens.

Screening aimed at early detection of the cancer can never reduce the incidence of disease, but may reduce mortality and morbidity associated with advanced disease. For example, a reduction in breast cancer mortality has been clearly demonstrated in women who have been screened by mammography, and this is due to the fact that, in many women early detection permits the surgical removal of the lump *before* it has metastasized, so that the chances of cure are high. However, this example also illustrates the limitations of screening tests aimed at early detection, since some breast cancers metastasize at a very early stage, before they are detectable by mammography. For these women slightly earlier detection of their cancers by mammography is of little benefit.

Other screening modalities aim to detect pre-cancerous lesions. The classic example of this is cervical cytology. Here the goal is to detect precursor lesions before they become invasive, so that removal carries an almost 100% cure rate. In this case a major problem is knowing which lesions are likely to become cancerous if left untreated so as to avoid over treatment of benign lesions with no malignant potential.

These two examples illustrate the need to understand the natural history of the cancer under consideration. Screening can only be effective if lesions are detected at a time when effective treatment is still possible and in this respect the ability to detect pre-cancerous lesions is a key feature. The use of mammography is thought to reduce mortality from breast cancer by about 30% whereas estimates of the mortality reduction associated with regular cervical smears are between 70% and 90%. Opposing this, however, is the fact that screening can only be cost-effective and generally acceptable to the population if treatment, especially invasive and unpleasant treatment, is restricted as much as possible to those lesions which are destined to become cancer if left untreated. The benign to malignant ratio in open biopsies following a mammographically detected abnormality is well below one in European centres, whereas, for cervical cancer, far more pre-invasive lesions are treated than would ever become cancer. It is also worth remembering that because breast cancer is so much more common in the Western world, mammographic screening still has a greater potential for overall mortality reduction, even though the test is less effective. A perfect screening test would detect all lesions destined to become cancer at a stage before they become incurable, but would not refer for further investigation and treatment any abnormality not destined to become invasive cancer. In practice, this is never achieved and one is usually prepared to tolerate a considerable amount of overtreatment for the safety and peace of mind that the treatment of any suspicious lesions brings.

Genetic testing will develop enormously in the future as more cancer predisposing genes are found. At the moment it is limited to rare cancer-family syndromes such as familial adenomatous polyposis (FAP), where genetic testing can indicate which members of the family carry a mutation with almost 100% penetrance for colon cancer. Similar tests can now be performed on families with rare genes (*BRCA1*, *BRCA2*) predisposing to breast and ovarian cancer. Some genetic changes, such as the Li–Fraumeni syndrome (a mutation in the *TP53* gene), are also clearly linked to a high risk of many cancers and screening for this mutation imposes a severe challenge since positives must then be screened regularly for a variety of tumours. Future work will make similar tests available for other cancers that run in families and eventually allow one to test for sporadic or somatic mutations, which increase the risk of cancer, in the general population. This is already leading to difficult ethical problems regarding who should be tested and who has the right to know the results of such tests. Genetic screening will lead to a very different form of programme as it will involve whole families and populations with founder mutations. It will then require intensive follow-up of individuals testing positive, and the use of chemopreventive agents or prophylactic surgical removal of the organs at risk.

29.1.2 Safety and acceptability

Safety and acceptability are also important issues when considering the introduction of a screening test. The demands are far more acute than in a therapeutic setting, since the number of screens needed to save one life is usually measured in thousands. Thus even a low complication rate can seriously affect the risk–benefit ratio. In addition to problems occurring at the initial screen any untoward effects associated with the further investigation of false positives also need to be assessed. For example, faecal occult blood testing is certainly a safe initial screen for bowel cancer, but when rehydrated samples are assayed, the positivity rate approaches 10% per test and all of these individuals may be referred for colonoscopy, a major procedure with an appreciable complication rate.

Acceptability is a larger issue, which partly relates to safety but also includes issues of discomfort, anxiety, and cost. To a large extent, acceptability is based on prevailing social perceptions. For example, any kind of screening for bowel cancer, which requires collection of faecal material or endoscopic viewing of the bowels, will have to overcome certain taboos. A large element in achieving this will be the ability to persuade patients that the test truly protects them from cancer. This cannot be claimed until convincing large trials are completed, so the problems are particularly acute at the early stages of development of a new test. Human papillomavirus (HPV) testing provides a different example. Here there are concerns about the stigma associated with having a sexually transmitted virus and the affect this could have on a married couple. However, social taboos can be overcome, as evidenced by the high rate of attendance that is now achieved in Britain and Scandinavia following an invitation for a cervical smear or a mammogram where embarrassment, fear, and discomfort were initial barriers. Education of the public and profession about the benefits and goals of screening can make a large impact on the compliance rates and ultimately on the effectiveness of a screening programme.

29.1.3 Who should be screened?

The population chosen for screening is crucial to its success. A key issue in deciding if screening is appropriate is the amount of disease present in the population offered screening. In public health terms this means that population screening has the potential for doing the most good if directed at the major cancers. For the developed world the common cancers arise in the lung, bowel, breast, prostate, stomach (especially in Japan), and to a lesser extent ovary and bladder. For developing countries the priorities are different. For example, cervix cancer would have the highest priority in many places, liver cancer would be important in Africa and the south-east coast of China, and oesophageal cancer would rate high in parts of China, south-east Africa, and around and to the east of the Caspian Sea.

While focusing on the common cancers is helpful in deciding which sites are good candidates for screening, this is of little help unless an effective screening test exists. Less common cancers can be appropriate targets if highly effective but simple means of screening exist. Some modalities are only suitable for high-risk populations. For example, regular screening for bladder cancer by urine cytology is appropriate for workers in the dyestuff or rubber industry where the risk is increased because of exposure to chemicals known to cause bladder cancer. However, it would not be cost-effective if applied to the general population. In other cases it might be appropriate to screen the general population once, but then only apply repeated screening to a high-risk subgroup identified at the initial screen. At the other extreme is screening of the entire (male/female) population within a given age range at regular intervals. The two procedures for which this has become an established practice are cytological examination of cervical smears in women aged 25–64 every 3–5 years and mammographic imaging of the breast in women aged over 50 every 2–3 years.

29.2 Evaluation of screening

29.2.1 Evaluating the test

Screening tests are usually evaluated in terms of sensitivity, specificity, and positive predictive

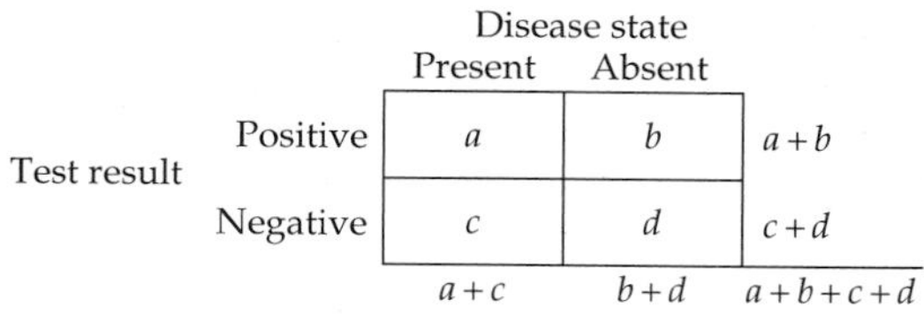

		Disease state: Present	Disease state: Absent	
Test result	Positive	a	b	$a+b$
	Negative	c	d	$c+d$
		$a+c$	$b+d$	$a+b+c+d$

Parameter	Estimated by
Sensitivity	$= a/(a+c)$
Specificity	$= d/(b+d)$
Positive predictive value	$= a/(a+b)$
Negative predictive value	$= d/(c+d)$
Detection rate	$= a/(a+b+c+d)$

Figure 29.1 Parameters used for evaluating a screening test. The values of *a*, *b*, *c*, and *d* are the number of screened individuals in a given category.

value. These quantities are computed from a 2×2 table, which classifies whether disease was present or not according to whether the test was positive or negative. The basic quantities are shown in Figure 29.1. Sensitivity is the proportion of individuals with disease who were positive on the test, while specificity gives the proportion of individuals without the disease who tested negative. Sensitivity and specificity do not depend on the prevalence of disease. A measure which also reflects this is the positive predictive value. This is defined as the probability of having disease given that the test was positive.

Calculation of these measures is often difficult. A major problem is that unless the entire population offered screening receives a full diagnostic workup, the total number of people who have the disease is not known. When a number of different screening tests are applied simultaneously, their relative sensitivities can be determined from the number of diseased individuals among those who were positive on any test. Alternatively, cancers arising within a given interval after a negative screening outcome (usually one or two years) can be used as a surrogate for false negative tests. Another problem is how to decide what constitutes a disease being present, especially when screening for precursor lesions. Also, when a multi-step screening process is applied, it may be difficult to decide at what stage the 'screening test' is positive without careful recording and reporting.

29.2.2 Potential biases

Ultimately, screening needs to be evaluated in terms of its impact on morbidity and mortality. Because of the large size and long follow-up time needed to do this properly, there has been much interest in using short-term intermediate endpoints for evaluation. These include detection rates for pre-cancerous and cancerous lesions and characteristics of the cancers detected such as size, stage, and grade. The rate of occurrence of 'interval cancers' in the period following a screen showing no abnormalities can also be used. These markers are very useful for deciding if a screening modality has promise and for tuning the finer parameters of a screening programme, such as the screening interval and age group to be offered screening. However, they can be unreliable as the only method of evaluation and need to be underpinned by clearly established mortality reductions in randomized trials.

Naïve analysis of survival rates is subject to serious biases. The most important of these are lead-time bias and length-bias. Lead-time bias refers to the fact that early detection of disease will give the appearance of better survival (from the date of diagnosis) in screen-detected cases compared to symptomatically detected cases, even when screening has no effect on the natural history of disease. In this circumstance, screening is actually detrimental to the patient who is given a death sentence and cancer label sooner, but whose disease course is unchanged. This appears to be the case for lung cancer screening by chest X-ray. In a less extreme form, where screening does some good, the apparent benefits can be exaggerated by this bias. However, it should be remembered that the effect of screening is dependant on the available treatments and new more effective treatment may make earlier detection more important. A different bias, leading to similarly exaggerated apparent benefits of screening, is known as length-bias. This is due to the fact that more slowly growing cancers, which generally have a better prognosis, are more likely to be detected by screening. The reason for this is that because of their slower growth, the time interval of potential preclinical detection by screening is longer so that their chances of being detected by screening are greater. Thus good prognosis cancers are preferentially detected by screening. An extreme form of this bias occurs when cancers are detected by screening which would not become apparent during the lifetime of the individual. This is a major problem in screening for prostate cancer.

Another approach is to compare the cancer rates of those who accept screening against those who do not. This is usually done on a case-control basis by comparing the screening histories of people who developed or died from cancer to randomly selected (age and sex matched) controls who did not. While this approach is much better than the comparison of survival times, it still suffers from the bias that the cancer risk among individuals who chose to accept screening is often different from those who refuse it, even when screening has no effect. The use of case-control studies to evaluate screening is complicated and attempts to correct this and other biases by using a third control population in an unscreened area can help to overcome these problems.

29.2.3 Randomized trials

The only truly reliable way of assessing screening procedures (or almost any medical intervention) is by means of a randomized trial. For this a population suitable for screening is identified, but only a randomly chosen proportion is offered screening. Random allocation is done at the individual level or in a large number of small units such as household, or GP practice. The cancer mortality (and incidence for screening methods designed to detect precancerous lesions) is then compared between the two randomized groups without regard to actual compliance. Low compliance will make such trials impossible and this is usually the key issue in obtaining a proper evaluation. Methods exist for estimating the treatment effect in compliers in an unbiased way, but these do not increase the power of the study (Cuzick et al., 1997).

29.2.4 Screening programmes

Once a safe, effective, and acceptable screening test is found, further efforts are needed to create a cost-effective screening programme. The costs of a screening programme depend on the frequency with which the test is offered, the age range over which screening takes place, and the policy for referral for additional tests. Less tangible costs in terms of anxiety, time, and personal expense consumed in attending a screening clinic also need to be considered. Effectiveness depends on a high compliance rate, quality control of the screening test, and appropriate treatment and follow-up for individuals found to have positive results. Regular monitoring and audit of a programme is essential to ensure that goals are met and cancer mortality is being reduced. Case-control studies looking at the screening history of individuals dying (or in some cases developing) the cancer of interest are an important part of this process. They offer an important way of continually monitoring screening programmes, not only to assess the relative protection in the years following a negative screening test, but also to evaluate other potential weaknesses such as low compliance; failure to adequately follow-up women with positive screening tests; development of cancer in women who have had abnormal screening test followed by a normal work-up; and adequacy and correct reading of screening results in women who subsequently developed cancer. Ultimately, bottom-line figures such as cost per life-year saved, need to be computed to put screening programmes into perspective and to allow comparisons between screening programmes for different cancers, screening for other diseases, and other medical interventions such as kidney transplants, etc.

29.3 Types of screening test

29.3.1 Visual inspection

The simplest form of screening requires only a visual inspection. Unfortunately, such simplistic approaches have never been demonstrated to be effective. Despite the lack of evidence in support of simple inspection, it is still considered potentially useful for control of oral cancer and melanoma. Dentists can be easily trained to look for oral plaques suggestive of carcinoma, particularly in individuals who use chewing tobacco or betel nut or are heavy consumers of alcohol (Rodrigues et al., 1998). Similarly, education of the general public and of those with a family history of melanoma in recognizing potentially invasive melanocytic lesions has been proposed as a cheap, but effective means of reducing mortality associated with melanoma. The signs that people are asked to look out for are large (>5 mm in diameter) moles with an irregular edge or variable pigmentation. Growth and change in appearance are thought to be particularly relevant (Bataille, 2003).

It has been known for well over 50 years that addition of weak acetic acid to the cervix of the uterus makes lesions stand out as white patches. The precise mechanism involved is still not fully understood, but direct visual inspection of the cervix by a nurse or midwife after application of

3–5% acetic acid has been proposed as a cheap method of screening particularly for low resource settings. Good results require appropriate training and continual retraining of the individuals carrying out the inspection, but several groups have reported reasonably high levels of sensitivity (65–90%) for detecting high-grade histological lesions (Gaffikin et al., 2003). More recently, it has been suggested that Lugol's iodine should be used to help identify neoplastic cervical lesions in a low-resource setting (Sankaranarayanan et al., 2003). More sophisticated use of technology results in magnified direct inspection (such as colposcopy for cervical screening) or use of cameras for indirect visualization of the digestive tract. Colposcopy has been proposed as a screening tool, but is generally reserved for triage of women identified by a cheaper and less-invasive screening test.

Colonoscopy is used for screening high-risk populations such as those with a strong family history of colorectal cancer. Polyps can be seen and in most cases removed during colonoscopy. Occasionally, colonoscopy will detect an occult invasive cancer, but more often polypectomy of a high-risk adenoma will prevent a future cancer. The efficacy of this approach in reducing the incidence of and mortality from colorectal cancer by more than 50% has been demonstrated in hereditary non-polyposis colorectal cancer (HNPCC) families (Jarvinen et al., 2000). Colonoscopy requires a full bowel preparation and sometimes a sedative and is felt by many to be too invasive for use in general population screening. More acceptable, is flexible sigmoidoscopy which can be more easily performed, but which only visualizes the left colon (as far as the sigmoid junction). Colonoscopy and sigmoidoscopy are discussed in greater detail in the section on colorectal screening. Endoscopy of the upper gastrointestinal tract to detect pre-cancer or early cancer of the oesophagus or stomach are generally reserved for symptomatic patients in the UK.

29.3.2 Palpation

Palpation, whether by a clinician or self-examination, has been proposed as a cheap form of screening for a number of sites, but what little evidence that does exist is not encouraging. Breast self-examination (BSE) has been widely recommended, but the evidence for efficacy is minimal coming mostly from epidemiological studies subject to potential confounding (Ellman et al., 1993; Gastrin et al., 1994; UK Trial of Early Detection of Breast Cancer Group, 1999). There have been two major randomized trials of BSE (Thomas et al., 1997, 2002; Semiglazov et al., 1999), neither of which showed any benefit on breast cancer mortality. Non-randomized studies suggest that women who practice BSE have higher rates of benign breast disease and are more likely to detect invasive tumours themselves and to have smaller tumours diagnosed at a less advanced stage (IARC, 2002). Women in the United Kingdom are encouraged to be 'breast aware', a vague term introduced to try to avoid the anxiety generated by the recommended monthly exam, while at the same time hoping to benefit from early detection. However, there is a lack of information as to whether *clinical* breast examination is useful for screening. Digital-rectal examinations are sometimes used to screen for prostate or rectal cancer, despite evidence of its poor sensitivity (Schroder et al., 1998) and young men are sometimes encouraged to check their testicles with no evidence as to whether that is worthwhile (Buetow, 1996).

29.3.3 Analysis of exfoliated cells

Cytology, the microscopic examination of cells, forms the basis of the highly successful cervical screening programmes in many countries (see below), and has also been proposed for use in screening for early breast (using nipple aspirates), bladder (using urine), and lung (using sputum) cancers. Cytology using the same Papanicolau stain used for cervical screening has been proposed as a screening test for anal cancer in gay men, but although the test seems to have reasonable sensitivity and specificity, there are a lack of suitable treatment options for men with pre-invasive disease. Cytology may be considered in screening whenever it is possible to obtain neoplastic cells through a simple, acceptable procedure that does not first require the identification of a potential cancer. Traditionally, cytology samples have been looked at microscopically for morphological features such as abnormal nuclear to cytoplasmic ratio, but the addition of immunohistochemical stains and other molecular techniques allow these same samples to be used for more precise testing. Examples include, markers of abnormal methylation in sputum, using antibodies to measure mini-chromosome maintenance protein 5 (MCM5) levels in urine (Stoeber et al., 2002), and HPV testing in cervical scrapes (see below). MCM proteins are essential for DNA replication. They are present within the nucleus throughout cell cycle, but are rapidly downregulated in differentiated cells. They can therefore be used to distinguish dysplastic cells that remain in cell cycle from differentiated cells. Another cell proliferation marker that may be useful in screening is $p16^{INK4a}$. It holds particular promise from HPV-related cervical lesions (Klaes et al., 2001). To be useful in screening, such markers would have to be present sufficiently early in the neoplastic process so as to detect cancers before they become symptomatic and sufficiently late so as not to identify very early neoplastic lesions that have little likelihood of progressing to invasive cancer.

Faecal testing for colorectal screening (see below) may be included here as it relies on material carried from an area of neoplasia to the outside of the body where it may be easily analysed. The traditional approach is to look for blood and is not strictly based on exfoliated cells. More recent attention has focused on molecular markers. For instance, Davies and colleagues showed that it is possible to retrieve colonocytes from faeces and to use immunohistochemistry to identify MCM2 (Davies et al., 2002). They found MCM2-positive cells in 92.5% of 40 patients with (symptomatic) colorectal cancer and none of 25 healthy controls. Others have successfully extracted DNA from stool samples and obtain reasonable sensitivity and specificity for colorectal cancer using a panel of markers for mutations in genes such as *KRAS*, the adenomatous polyposis coli (*APC*) gene, *TP53*, and for microsatellite instability in markers such as BAT26 (Ahlquist et al., 2000; Dong et al., 2001; Tagore et al., 2003).

29.3.4 Imaging

Generalizing the ideas of visual inspection, there are many organs that can be visualised by aid of some other form of imaging such as X-ray (e.g. mammography, discussed in detail later), ultrasound (e.g. for ovarian screening), spiral computed tomography (CT) scanning (for lung or bowel), or magnetic resonance imaging (MRI) (for breast or colon). The earliest of these technologies, X-rays, was also the first to be used in screening. But whereas low-dose X-rays have proven useful for detecting small breast tumours in asymptomatic women, trials of X-ray screening for lung cancer have had disappointing results. Although there were substantial numbers of small-screen detected tumours, the trials did not find any reduction in lung cancer mortality in those randomized to screening (Gohagan et al., 2003). Spiral CT scanning is far more sensitive than chest X-rays for detecting small tumours, and there is currently much interest in this technology for screening high-risk groups such as current or ex-smokers or those exposed to asbestos (Henschke et al., 1999, 2001; Swensen et al., 2003). The Early Lung Cancer Action Project screened 1000 current and ex-smokers over 60 years of age (Henschke et al., 1999). Non-calcified nodules were detected on baseline in 23% and malignant disease in 2.7%. Only seven of these 27 cases were detectable by chest X-ray. After three rounds of annual screening in the Mayo Clinic cohort, 69% of the 1520 individuals enrolled had at least one non-calcified nodule detected (Swensen et al., 2003). A total of 40 cases of lung cancer were diagnosed: 26 at baseline CT screen and 10 on subsequent screens; 2 cancers were detected only by sputum cytology and 2 were diagnosed between screens.

Spiral CT scanning has also been studied in the context of colorectal screening where it is usually referred to as virtual colonoscopy (Vining et al., 1994). Technologies are still improving. Previously a bowel cleansing and a muscle relaxant was required (making them less acceptable than they would be otherwise), but recent reports suggest that this may not be necessary if an oral contrast is taken in advance of the examination (Lauenstein et al., 2002). However, they are still unable to differentiate low-risk polyps and adenomas from high-risk adenomas and cancer except on the basis of size. The disadvantage of imaging is that a colonoscopy is required to excise any suspicious lesion found (typically in about 30% of all prevalent screens), whereas if endoscopy was the primary screening test, polypectomy could be carried out during the screening without need for a second examination.

Barium enemas can be used to examine the colon, but are relatively insensitive for the detection of cancer and, in particular, small polyps. The sensitivity of barium enema in a series of over 2000 cancers was 83% with little evidence of double-contrast being more sensitive than single-contrast (Rex et al., 1997). In a screening setting, its sensitivity was only 32% for small (<5 mm) adenomas and about 50% for larger adenomas (Winawer et al., 2000). Using ultrasound to screen for enlarged ovaries lacks specificity for cancer since most enlarged ovaries are due to benign cysts. Campbell et al. (1989) have conducted a screening study on 5479 volunteers aged above 40 recruited by media publicity. They performed annual trans-abdominal ultrasound for up to three years and 326 (5.9%) women were found to be positive and referred to a surgeon for laparotomy/laparoscopy. Five of these women were found to have primary ovarian cancer (all stage I) and an additional four had metastatic cancer in the ovary from a primary in the breast or colon. The positive predictive value per test was about 1.4%, which is too low when the next stage involves abdominal surgery. The false-positive rate on the first screen was 3.5%, dropping to 1.8% and 1.2% on subsequent screens. To improve the specificity, trans-vaginal colour Doppler ultrasound has been used to image blood flow. Blood-vessel formation is thought to be a good discriminant between cancer and benign cysts and early reports indicate that the test can substantially reduce the false-positive rate (Bourne et al., 1993). More recent attention has focussed on trans-vaginal ultrasound used in conjunction with CA 125 testing (Menon et al., 2000).

Because of its high incidence and mortality, screening for gastric cancer by barium X-ray is already a national programme in Japan. The aim is to screen everyone over the age of 40 every year in order to detect cancer at an earlier stage. In Miyagi Prefecture almost 3 million tests were performed between 1960 and 1988 and the test was positive in about 10% of cases leading to a recommendation for gastroscopy. The positive predictive value is reported to be 1.7% (Hisamichi et al., 1991). No randomized trials have been reported, but indications of effectiveness have been seen in time trends of mortality, cohort studies, and case-control studies (see Hisamichi et al., 1991; Maehara et al., 2000). The results from a case-control study in Miyagi Prefecture are shown in Table 29.1 (Fukao et al., 1987) and suggest a substantial benefit in the year following screening, but little benefit subsequently. Potential biases exist in all these analyses since the incidence of stomach cancer is falling in Japan and compliers may have a different risk than non-compliers.

Ultrasound has been considered for breast screening but appears to lack sensitivity. However, because it can safely be done at short intervals, it is used in follow-up and may have a role in young women who have a family history or dense breasts, which are opaque to radiology. The possibility of using MRI for breast screening has also been raised, especially in dense breasts, but this is extremely expensive and has yet to be properly validated although trials are now underway. In a series of 23 very high-risk women screened by MRI in Italy, four breast cancers were identified, none of which were detectable by mammography (Trecate et al., 2003). A review of MRI of the asymptomatic contralateral breast in 223 women with recently diagnosed breast cancer, identified 2.5% with occult invasive breast cancer and 2.5% with ductal carcinoma *in situ* (DCIS), but 32% of women would have been referred for a biopsy based on an abnormal MRI (Liberman et al., 2003).

Table 29.1 Optimal interval for screening for stomach cancer

Time since last negative result (years)	No. of cases of advanced cancer	No. of controls	Relative protection	95% CI
1	132	220	2.92	2.09–4.08
2	40	31	1.36	0.80–2.32
3	23	18	1.37	0.70–2.67
4	16	9	0.99	0.42–2.32
Never screened	156	89	1[a]	
Total	367	367		

[a] Reference category.

Source: Fukao et al. (1987).

29.3.5 Serum and urine markers

Screening using molecular markers in exfoliated cells from the site of interest usually relies on generic markers of neoplasia such as markers for cell-cycle progression (e.g. cyclin E), DNA replication (e.g. MCM), DNA synthesis (e.g. PCNA), cell-cycle control (e.g. $p16^{INK4a}$, WAF1), anti-apoptosis (e.g. BCL-2), or angiogenesis (e.g. VEGF, bFGF). By contrast, serum markers must be site-specific. The two that have received most attention are CA-125 for ovarian screening and prostate-specific antigen (PSA), which is discussed in detail under prostate screening). CA-125 is a tumour marker with an established place in monitoring tumour burden, response to treatment and recurrence in women with ovarian cancer. CA-125 is produced in the embryonal Mullerian duct and coelomic epithelium and is raised in about 80% of women with ovarian cancer, but can also be elevated when benign ovarian cysts, endometriosis, or cancers of the colon, breast, or pancreas are present, as well as in pregnancy. Early studies using a fixed cut-off of 30 U/ml for serum CA-125 reported a false-positive rate of about 1.4% in a study of 22,000 asymptomatic post-menopausal women aged over 45 and a sensitivity of 60% (Jacobs et al., 1993). Better specificity can be obtained by requiring both ultrasound and CA-125 to be positive and in this study the false-positive rate was reduced to 1.4 per 1000 when ultrasound was used as a second-stage screen (Figure 29.2). Only one of 19 true positives was lost in this manner. More recently, attention has focused on using a more sophisticated algorithm based on a woman's age and her CA-125 profile with time to determine who should receive further work-up. An algorithm, that refers women whose CA-125 levels increase over time, is being employed by the large UK Collaborative Trial of Ovarian Screening (Skates et al., 1995). Questions regarding the appropriate age and interval at which to screen are even less well understood, but most studies have focused on annual screening in women aged 40–70 years.

Neuroblastoma is the second commonest malignancy in children and accounts for about 10% of childhood cancer. In Japan neonates are screened by looking for elevated levels of the catecholamine metabolites vanillylmandolic acid (VMA) and homovallic acid (HVA) in urine at ages 3 and 6 months. Sensitivity is about 80% and about one in 8500 infants tested turn out to have neuroblastoma. Prognosis appears to be much improved by early detection (Sawada et al., 1991; Sawada, 1992) but there is no evidence of reduced incidence rates at older ages or a decrease in mortality. It is possible that the cases picked up by screening are of a different variety which would regress spontaneously and are not related to the more aggressive tumours which arise in children aged over one year (Murphy et al., 1991). The present consensus is against screening for neuroblastoma (Esteve et al., 2001; Woods et al., 1996).

29.3.6 Screening for and treatment of infections

A very different approach to cancer screening has been put forward in connection with stomach and

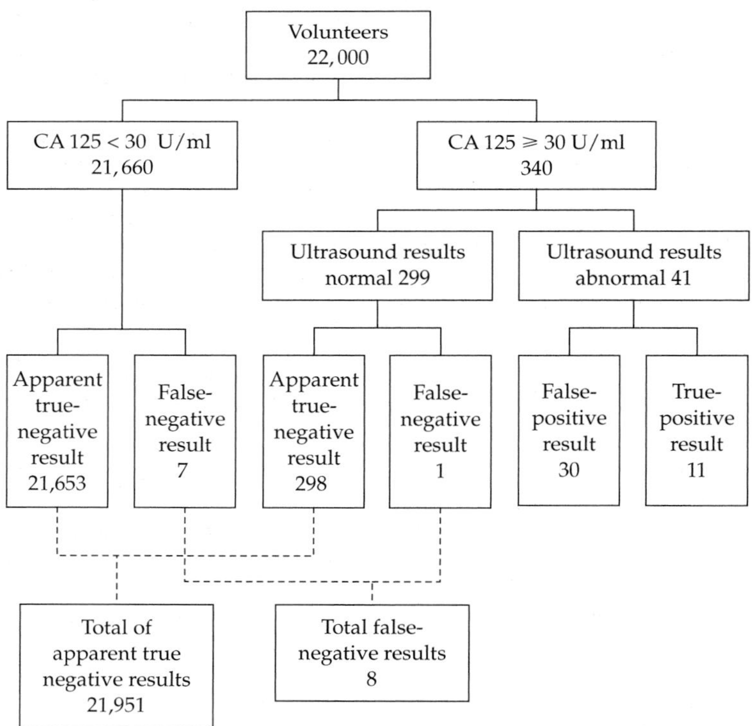

Figure 29.2 Summary of study findings in 22,000 post-menopausal volunteer women participating in a screening programme for ovarian cancer. (After Jacobs et al., 1993).

liver cancer. In both cases, cancer appears to be a rare outcome following a common asymptomatic infection and cancer could be prevented by screening for the infection and treating it in those who test positive.

Helicobacter pylori causes chronic active gastritis which can progress to chronic atrophic gastritis which is thought to be one of the early steps in gastric carcinogenesis. Relative risks for gastric cancer typically range from two-fold to eight-fold (Yamagata et al., 2000; Uemura et al., 2001; Helicobacter and Cancer Collaborative Group, 2001) and it has been estimated that about 50% of distal gastric cancers are associated with *H. pylori* (Parsonnet et al., 1996). Cancers of the gastro-oesophageal junction or gastric cardia do not appear to be related to *H. pylori*. Accurate serological tests based on IgG antibodies exist (Loy et al., 1996; Roberts et al., 2000). A systemic immune response is present in virtually all infected individuals (Glupczynski et al., 1992; Blecker et al., 1995) and commercially available IgG-based Elisa tests have sensitivities in excess of 85%. Treatment is by a proton pump inhibitor combined with two antibiotics (clarithromycin and either amoxicillin or metronidazole for one week) and eliminates infection in about 85% of patients who comply (Moayyedi et al., 2000). The prevalence of *H. pylori* is high, ranging from 80% to 90% in adults in developing countries to 30–60% in the developed world (Loy et al., 1996; Roberts et al., 2000). Thus, one option would be to treat everyone without first screening for infection. Randomized trials of the effect of *H. pylori* screening and treatment on gastric cancer incidence are in progress in China and the United Kingdom (Forman, 1998).

Hepatitis B is a primary cause of hepatocellular cancer in China, Southeast Asia, the Pacific Islands, Eskimos, sub-Saharan Africa, and the Amazon Basin, particularly where there is also exposure to aflatoxins (IARC, 1994). Chronic infection is associated with a range of liver disease and approximately 25% of carriers will eventually die from primary liver cancer (Beasley, 1982). It has been estimated that there are about 300 million chronic carriers worldwide (Ghendon, 1990). Chronic infection is most often associated with perinatal or childhood infection, and is often asymptomatic. In very high-risk areas such as West Africa, horizontal childhood infection is so likely that universal vaccination may be the most appropriate policy, but in lower prevalence areas chronic infection is more likely to be due to perinatal transmission and screening pregnant women, with selective vaccination of infants from an infected mother may be a more cost-effective strategy. A global strategy for prevention was first discussed by the World Health Organization in 1983 (WHO, 1983).

The presence of hepatitis B surface antigen (HBsAg) in asymptomatic individuals is generally taken as evidence of being in the chronic carrier state. A possible approach to screening for liver cancer is first to look for chronic carriers, who are then screened for an increased level of α-fetoprotein, which is a tumour marker for liver cancer. Further investigation by ultrasound could be useful in detecting small resectable cancers. Such an approach has been suggested by Sun et al. (1988). Another approach is to screen pregnant women (Arevalo, 1988; Stroffolini et al., 1990). Here it is the unborn infant that stands to benefit. There is ample evidence that use of hepatitis B immunoglobulin within hours of birth followed by hepatitis B vaccine on multiple occasions is effective in reducing the infection rate by more than 80% and the carrier state by more than 90% (Beasley et al., 1983*a*,*b*; Taylor et al., 1988; Schalm et al., 1989; Wainwright et al., 1989; Stevens et al., 1992; Fortuin et al., 1993). In Italy where vaccination coverage is estimated to be over 90%, from 1988 to 1994 there has been a reduction of 50% in acute hepatitis B reports in subjects aged 15–24 years (Lo Monaco et al., 1996; Mele et al., 1996). There are no reports yet on the effectiveness of vaccination on cancer rates as this will typically take about 40 years of follow-up to evaluate. However, there are ongoing studies in The Gambia (Whittle et al., 1995) and China (Xu et al., 1995).

29.4 Screening for specific cancers where widespread programmes already exist

29.4.1 Cervix cancer

The universally accepted screening method for preventing cervix cancer is cytological examination of cervical scrapes that have been smeared onto slides and stained by Papanicolaou's method. This procedure has a long history. In 1928, Papanicolaou published a report indicating that cervix cancer could be diagnosed from exfoliated cells. Working with Trout, he developed this into a screening test in the 1930s and they published their definitive work in 1941 (Papanicolaou, Trout, 1941). The war

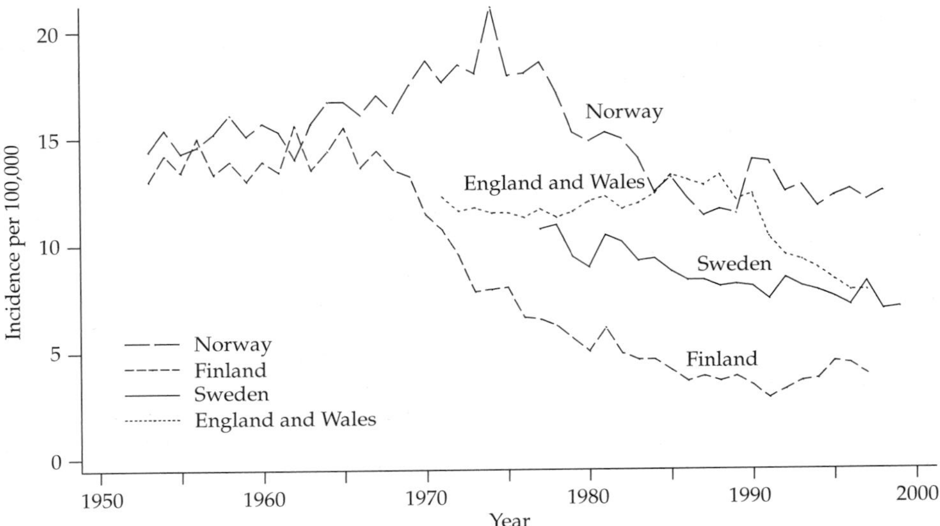

Figure 29.3 Trends in the incidence of invasive cervical cancer in Nordic countries and England and Wales: age-standardized 1950–98.

delayed initial attempts at implementation but the subsequent slow acceptance of the approach meant that large-scale field trials did not begin until the 1960s. These were turned into organized screening programmes in the Nordic countries (except Norway) during the 1960s and already by the mid-1970s large reductions in incidence and mortality were seen in these countries (except Norway) (Figure 29.3, Hakama, 1982; Läärä et al., 1987).

'Pap smear' screening is designed to detect pre-cancerous lesions. Nomenclature for these lesions varies by country and continues to change. This system is mirrored by a histopathological classification of biopsies based on the depth of cervical intra-epithelial neoplasia (CIN), which has grades 1, 2, and 3 according to whether the lesion is confined to the lower one-third, two-thirds, or greater depth of epithelium. The correspondence between cytology and histology is by no means perfect and much confusion arises when the terms are used interchangeably. In particular, low-grade cytological abnormalities are associated with a wide range of underlying lesions when biopsied and assessed by histology.

The efficacy of Pap smear screening has never been evaluated by means of a randomized trial. However, following pioneering work by Clarke and Anderson (1979) in Canada, several case-control studies have been undertaken around the work and these were collated and synthesized in an important paper (IARC Working Party, 1986). The main results are summarized in Table 29.2. Compared to unscreened women, the reduction in cancer incidence afforded by screening women aged 20–64 every five years was estimated to be 84% and this increases to 91% if screening is undertaken every three years. Little additional gain was achieved by screening more often. These results refer specifically to the low

Table 29.2 Geometric mean relative protection against cervical cancer in women with two or more previously negative smears participating in centrally organized screening programmes

Months since last negative smear	Relative proportion[a] (No. of cases)	95% confidence limits
0–11	15.3 (25)	10.0–22.6
12–23	11.9 (23)	7.5–18.3
24–35	8.0 (25)	5.2–11.8
36–47	5.3 (30)	3.6–7.6
48–59	2.8 (30)	1.9–4.0
60–71	3.6 (16)	2.1–5.9
72–119	1.6 (6)	0.6–3.5
120+	0.8[b](7)	0.3–1.6
Never screened	1.0 (reference group)	

[a] A large relative protection corresponds to a larger benefit of screening. For example, a relative protection of 10 means that the odds of developing cancer in the stated interval is one-tenth that of an age-matched woman who has never been screened.

[b] Based on figures from Aberdeen and Iceland only.

Source: IARC Working Party (1986).

risk attributed to regular negative smears, and as such evaluate the test, but not the entire programme, since some patients with abnormal smears still go on to develop cancer. Thus, these results are somewhat optimistic even if full compliance were achieved. More recently, a very large case-control study from the United Kingdom looked at the relative risk of cervical cancer following a negative smear separately in each of three age groups. The authors found that the negative predictive value was less in young women (Table 29.3) and suggested the need for more frequent screening under the age of 50 (Sasieni et al., 2003).

Successful as it has been, screening by cytology is not without its problems. It is very tedious and labour intensive, and requires subjective judgements and has a relatively low sensitivity for high-grade disease (Fahey et al., 1995; Nanda et al., 2000). Better quality slides can be made by collecting cells in a liquid medium rather than smearing them directly onto the glass slide. So-called liquid-based cytology has a number of advantages: the slides are easier to read because the cells are less clustered (they form a thin layer on the slide) and most of the debris (blood, mucus) is removed, and significantly the proportion deemed to be inadequate for evaluation is greatly reduced. There are two commercially available systems that have been evaluated in large trials and both have been deemed to be better than conventional cytology by the American Food and Drug Administration. However, the yield of high-grade smears is similar to that for conventional cytology in many studies (Payne et al., 2000). Work on automating the reading of smears has been ongoing for over 30 years (Banda-Gamboa et al., 1992) and computer-assisted systems are beginning to become available. The new systems are designed to work with liquid-based cytology. Some highlight areas needing more careful (human) analysis and others can be used to identify a proportion of slides (currently only 20%) that do not require further human analysis.

Table 29.3 Odds ratios (with 95% confidence intervals) for frankly invasive cervical cancer by time since last operationally negative cytological smear. The figures for "years since last negative smear" apply to those with two or more negative smears. To obtain odds ratios for those with just one negative smear, multiply by the given factor. For example, the odds ratio associated with a single negative smear 3.0–4.9 years previously in a woman aged 55–69 is 1.35*0.20 = 0.27

	Odds ratio (95% CI)		
Age group	**20–39 (*n* = 438)**	**40–54 (*n* = 481)**	**55–69 (*n* = 386)**
Years since last negative smear			
0–2.9	0.28 (0.20–0.41)	0.12 (0.08–0.17)	0.13 (0.08–0.19)
3.0–4.9	1.03 (0.68–1.56)	0.39 (0.26–0.58)	0.20 (0.12–0.33)
Over 5.0	2.05 (1.20–3.49)	0.72 (0.43–1.18)	0.45 (0.25–0.81)
No negative smear	1.00*	1.00*	1.00*
Number of negative smears			
One	1.03 (0.73–1.46)	1.32 (0.91–1.91)	1.35 (0.85–2.14)
Two or more	1.00*	1.00*	1.00*

* Baseline

Note: *n* is the number of cases included in the analysis, there are approximately twice as many controls.

At a more basic level, there is much interest in applying tests for human papilloma virus (HPV) in a screening context. Numerous case-control studies have shown very high odds ratios associated with HPV infection (Table 29.4, Muñoz and Bosch, 1992) and it has clearly been demonstrated that certain types of HPV (types 16, 18, 31, 33, 35, 45, 51, 52, 56) are more related to cancer and high-grade CIN than other low-risk genital types (6, 11, 42–44). The oncogenic role of the high-risk types, especially HPV 16 is also supported by much laboratory research.

One role for HPV testing may lie in its use as a second-level screen for women with borderline or mild abnormalities on cytology. Only about 20–30% of these women actually have high-grade CIN in need of immediate treatment. Initial studies (Cuzick et al., 1992, 1994; Bavin et al., 1993) suggested that testing for high-risk types of HPV on the smear material by polymerase chain reaction (PCR) might be useful in deciding which women should be referred immediately and which can be followed by cytological surveillance. More recent studies have confirmed this. HPV testing by Hybrid Capture II was performed on left over material from the original liquid-based sample in a study of just under a thousand women with a smear result of atypical squamous cells of undetermined significance (ASCUS): 40% were HPV positive and 65 women were found to have CIN 2+: the sensitivity of HPV testing was 89% (Manos et al., 1999). A randomized trial looking at management of women with ASCUS and low-grade smears collected a second cervical sample for HPV testing on

Table 29.4 Case-control studies of HPV status and invasive cervix cancer

Study	No. of cases (% positive)	No. of controls (% positive)	OR (95% CI)	Method and type
Hong Kong (Donnan et al., 1989)	30 (37)	17 (6)	9.3 (1.0–84.1)	Southern HPV-16
Uganda (Schmauz et al., 1989)	34 (50)	23 (4)	22.0 (5.1–104.3)	Southern HPV-16, -18
Latin America (Reeves et al., 1989)	721 (47)	1225 (18)	4.0 (3.3–5.0)	FISH HPV-16, -18
Pakistan (Anwar et al., 1991)	80 (69)	30 (10)	19.8 (5.8–66.8)	ISH HPV-16, -18
Japan (Anwar et al., 1991)	82 (68)	26 (19)	9.0 (3.2–25.7)	FISH HPV-16, -18
China (Peng et al., 1991)	101 (35)	146 (1)	32.9 (7.7–141.1)	PCR HPV-16, -33
Columbia (Muñoz and Bosch, 1992)	87 (72)	98 (13)	15.6 (6.9–34.7)	PCR Manos-consensus
Spain (Muñoz and Bosch, 1992)	142 (69)	130 (5)	46.2 (18.5–115.1)	PCR Manos-consensus

Abbreviations: HPV = human papillomavirus; Southern = Southern blot hybridization; FISH = filter *in situ* hybridization; ISH = *in situ* hybridization; PCR = polymerase chain reaction; OR = odds ratio; CI = confidence interval.

Table 29.5 Results of studies directly comparing HPV testing (by Hybrid Capture II) to cytology. Sensitivities and specificities are with respect to biopsy confirmed cases of CIN 2 or worse. In most studies women were referred to colposcopy if either screening test was positive

Author		Sensitivity		Specificity		Comments
	n	Cytology $\geq$ LSIL	HPV	Cytology $<$ LSIL	HPV	
Blumenthal et al. (2001)	2,199	44	80	91	61	Zimbabwe
Cuzick et al. (1999)	2,988[a]	79	95	99	95	Age $\geq$ 35 years
Schiffman et al. (2000)	8,636[b]	75	88	96	89	Conventional cytology
Hutchinson et al. (1999)[c]		84		96		LBC
Ratnam et al. (2000)	2,098	40	90	77	51	69% HC-I, 31% HC-II
Kuhn et al. (2000)	2,944[d]	78	88	94[e]	80[5]	S. Africa
Clavel et al. (2001)	2,281	68	100	95	86	Conventional cytology
	5,651	88	100	93	87	LBC
Cuzick (2003)	11,085	70	97	97	93	Age 30–60

[a] HC II on stratified sample of 1703.
[b] HC II on stratified sample of 1119.
[c] Cytology results published separately from HPV results. All women received both conventional and liquid-based cytology.
[d] HC II on stratified sample of 424
[e] Specificity differs from published value, because original paper excludes women with LSIL on histology from calculation.
Note: *n* is the number of cases included in the analysis.

average two months after the initial abnormality. They found HPV DNA (using Hybrid Capture II) in 83% of women with low-grade cytological abnormalities, and in 51% of women with ASCUS cytology. They estimated the sensitivity of HPV testing for CIN 2+ to be 96% (Solomon et al., 2001).

The larger question of the role of HPV testing as part of primary screening is also of interest. Several studies have shown that HPV testing has a much higher pick-up rate for CIN 2+ than cytology (Table 29.5). However, large trials will be needed to properly evaluate the role of HPV testing within a screening programme and these have yet to be done. It seems likely, however, that HPV-positive samples will require triaging using cytology and that HPV-positive women with normal or borderline abnormal cytology will need to be re-screened after an interval of about 12 months.

29.4.2 Breast cancer

The most fully investigated modality for early detection of breast cancer is mammography. This method is aimed at early detection of invasive cancer and so is limited by the fact that this may still be too late to affect survival. As a result, moderate benefits of the order of a 30% reduction in mortality are expected from this approach. However, because breast cancer is so common (affecting about 10% of women in the Western world) a benefit of this magnitude is well worth having and would amount to a larger reduction in the death toll from cancer in the Western world than the complete eradication of cervix cancer.

Gershon-Cohen advocated the use of X-ray screening as a screening test for breast cancer in the 1930s (Gershon-Cohen, and Colcher, 1937). However, it was not until 1964 that the first randomized trial of mammography was conducted: by the Health Insurance Plan (HIP) in New York City (Shapiro et al., 1982). Four annual mammograms were offered to 31,000 randomly selected women aged 40–64 and the remaining 31,000 unscreened women served as a control group. Clinical palpation of the breast was also undertaken at each visit in the screened group. Since then, other randomized trials have been mounted in Canada, Sweden, and Scotland, and non-randomized studies have been performed in Holland, Italy, and the United Kingdom. These data have been reviewed by an IARC working group (IARC, 2002). There is a consensus that mammography is effective in women aged 50–69 years of age and the studies overall suggest that 2–3 yearly screening can reduce breast cancer mortality by about 35% in those screened (Figure 29.4(b)). There is considerable controversy about the value of mammography from age 40 to 49 with limited evidence suggesting a reduction in mortality of about 20% (Figure 29.4(a)). There are at least three mutually non-exclusive possible reasons for this: (1) breast cancer is rare in this age group and so the absolute benefit will be less, (2) the lead-time gained by screening is shorter in younger women so that screening must be done annually to have much effect, and (3) the breast is more dense in pre-menopausal women, making imaging more difficult and limiting its application.

Using Swedish data, Tabar et al. (1992) have shown that for women under 50 the rate of cancer in the year following screening only drops to about half of that in an unscreened population, whereas in older women the rates were about 20% of control rates for the first two years after screening and rose to about half only after three years. Additionally, intermediate end-points such as the ratio of cancers detected at the first (prevalent) screen divided by the expected annual incidence rate are lower in younger women (Table 29.6). Overall the lower rates of disease and the poorer performance of the test make mammography a less-viable proposition in women as young as 40, but a good case can be made for screening from age 47 (Sasieni and Cuzick, 2003).

29.4.3 Colorectal cancer

The screening method that has received the most attention for colorectal cancer is the use of a guaiac impregnated slide to test for small amounts of blood in a stool sample. The goal of the test is to detect cancers at an early stage when they are still

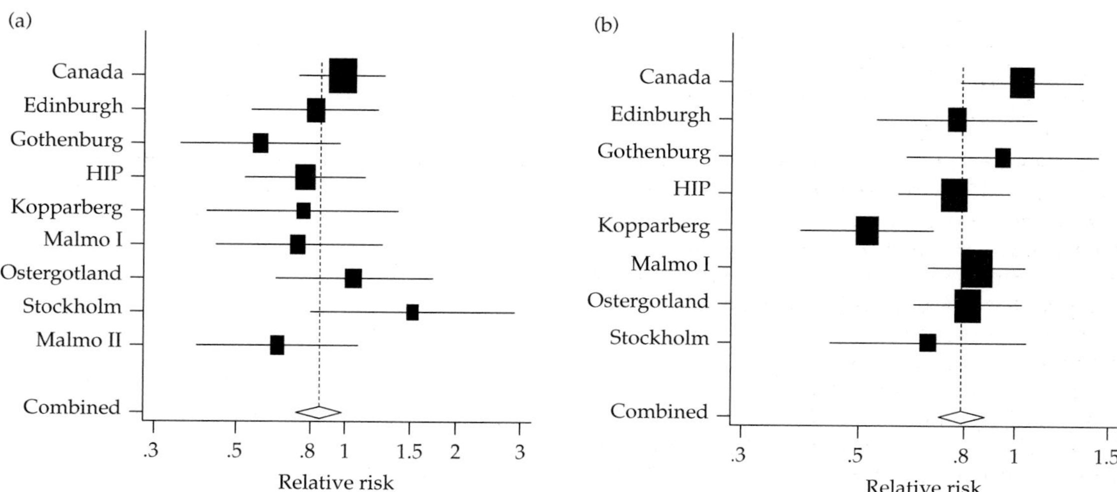

Figure 29.4 Results of randomized trials of mammographic screening on breast cancer mortality rates. (a) Data on women aged 40–49, (b) data on women aged 50–69.

Table 29.6 Prevalence to incidence ratios in screening populations by age for breast cancer

Age group (years)	Study		
	Two counties, Sweden Tabar et al. (1992)	Florence, Italy Paci and Duffy (1991)	Nijmegen, Netherlands[a] Peer et al. (1994)
40–49	1.99	0.74	1.16
50–59	2.50	2.42	3.72
60–69	3.52	3.36	
70–74	4.06	3.36	4.67

[a] Prevalence to interval cancer rate for women aged <50, 50–69, 70+.

treatable and the very good survival of Dukes' stage A cancers (better than 90% at five years) compared to colorectal cancer overall (approximately 30% at five years) suggests this could be successful. The test actually detects haeme but will react positively to any peroxidase and is not very specific. It detects blood from any lesion in the bowels as well as reacting to a number of foods (red meat, fresh fruits, and vegetables with peroxidase activity, for example, tomatoes) and aspirin-induced gastrointestinal bleeding. Dietary restriction before testing or retesting has been used to try to minimize false-positives. The sensitivity of the test is also an area for concern (Ahlquist et al., 1993) and it can be affected by vitamin C supplementation. The issue of whether or not to rehydrate samples before testing is also important. Rehydration improves sensitivity but at the expense of a large number of false-positive tests. In one trial conducted in Minnesota the positivity rate for rehydrated tests was almost 10% (Mandel et al., 1993) leading to many unnecessary referrals for colonoscopy. In that study a mortality reduction of 33% for colorectal cancer has been found for annual faecal occult blood testing (FOBT), but it is unclear whether the results can be attributed to any selective value of FOBT screening, or merely due to the fact that 38% of this group received a colonoscopy at some stage as a result of a positive test. It is possible that similar reductions in mortality could be achieved by colonoscopy and polyp removal in 38% of any population.

New tests have been developed to attempt to improve on the one (Haemoccult II) currently in use. These include an immunological test specific for human haemoglobin (Haemeselect) and a more sensitive guaiac-based test (Haemoccult-SENSA) that detects haeme-derived porphyrins, so that it can detect degraded de-ironed haemes as well as the intact haeme detected by Haemoccult II (St. John et al., 1993).

A randomized trial in Nottingham offered two-yearly FOBT (not rehydrated) to people aged 45–74. The positivity rate was 2.1% on the first round of screening and 1.2% in those rescreened within 27 months. After a median follow-up of 7.8 years, a significant 15% (95% CI 2–26%) reduction in colorectal cancer mortality was observed (Hardcastle et al., 1996). A similar screening protocol was used in a randomized trial in Denmark. The positivity rates were lower (1.0% on the first round increasing to 1.8% on the fifth round of screening), but a similar mortality reduction was observed: 18% (95% CI 1–32%) (Kronborg et al., 1996; Jorgensen et al., 2002).

Another approach to colorectal cancer screening is based on the work of Morson (1976), who proposed that most cancers arise from pre-existing adenomas. Adenomas are pre-cancerous growths, which occur throughout the bowel and have the same sub-site distribution as cancers, but occur at a younger age. Thus a better strategy to control colon cancer may be to detect and remove adenomas, since the transition time from an adenoma to a carcinoma is thought to be very long (of the order of 10–25 years), implying that screening need only be carried out very infrequently. Also since one is now preventing cancer rather than detecting it early, the potential for mortality reduction is much greater.

The FOBT detects some adenomas although the sensitivity is low. An approach specifically aimed at the detection of adenomas is to use flexible 60 cm sigmoidoscope as a screening tool. This is far less-expensive and traumatic than complete colonoscopy and approximately 60% of colorectal cancers occur in the region accessible by this instrument. To date there is limited evidence on its efficacy. Selby et al. (1992) have shown in a case-control study that mortality due to cancers within the reach of the rigid sigmoidoscope (approximately within 20 cm of the anus) was reduced by 60% for at least 10 years (Table 29.7) and similar results have been reported in two other studies (Newcomb et al., 1992; Muller and Sonnenberg, 1995). Several studies have suggested that endoscopic surveillance of the bowel greatly reduces colon cancer rates, but a direct demonstration that screening by sigmoidoscopy reduces mortality will require a large randomized trial. Such trials are underway in the United Kingdom, Italy, and the United States. Atkin et al.

(1993, 2001) argue that most of the benefit of sigmoidoscopy would accrue from a single screening test and only a small group of individuals (about 3–5% in most series) would need colonoscopy and further surveillance. A key issue is at what age this single screen should take place. Ideally, this should be after most adenomas have appeared, but few of the cancers have developed. Figure 29.5, shows that this window of opportunity is probably between ages 55 and 65. Baseline results from this trial have now been published (UK Flexible Sigmoidoscopy Screening Trial Investigators, 2002).

There are those, particularly in North America, who advocate colonoscopy for population screening at age 50 and again 10–15 years later (Detsky, 2001; Lieberman et al., 2001; Winawer and Zauber, 2001).

Table 29.7 Most recent screening sigmoidoscopy in case subjects and controls, before the diagnosis of fatal cancer within reach of the rigid sigmoidscope in the case subjects

Years before diagnosis	Case subjects ($n = 261$)	Controls ($n = 868$)	Odds ratio
	No. (%)		
1–2	4 (1.6)	27 (3.1)	0.41 (0.14–1.22)
3–4	5 (2.0)	20 (2.3)	0.74 (0.27–2.01)
5–6	5 (2.0)	30 (3.5)	0.44 (0.17–1.15)
7–8	1 (0.4)	22 (2.5)	0.11 (0.01–0.83)
9–10	1 (0.4)	21 (2.4)	0.12 (0.02–0.93)
Multiple	7 (2.6)	90 (10.3)	0.22 (0.10–0.47)
1–10	23 (8.8)	210 (24.2)	0.41 (0.25–0.69)
>10 years or, never	238	658	1[a]

[a] Reference category.

Source: Selby et al. (1992).

The obvious advantage of colonoscopy over flexible sigmoidoscopy is that it examines the proximal colon where 40% of colorectal cancers occur. The disadvantage is that those screened are required to take a laxative and consume only fluids on the day before the examination and will need several hours to recover from sedation (if used) after the examination. Additionally, colonoscopy requires a skilled endoscopist. Flexible sigmoidoscopy, by contrast, can be carried out by a specially trained nurse, requires only a couple of hours from those screened and has a lower complication rate. Quantification of the added benefit of colonoscopy is difficult. Lieberman et al. (2000) found that in 20% of 329 patients with advanced neoplasia detected on colonoscopic screening, the adenoma was located in the proximal colon and was not associated with a distal adenoma that could have been detected on flexible sigmoidoscopy. The additional impact of colonoscopy on the incidence and mortality of colorectal cancer may be different and a pilot randomized trial is in progress to address these issues (Winawer and Zauber, 2001).

29.4.4 Prostate cancer

Screening for prostate cancer provides a dilemma unique among cancer sites. The disease is exceedingly common in elderly men, but many cancers are indolent and are asymptomatic at the time of death from another cause. Indeed, autopsy studies have shown that about 10% of men aged 50 who died from other causes have a focus of invasive disease and this increases to 40% in 80-year-old men (Figure 29.6). Thus, while death from prostate

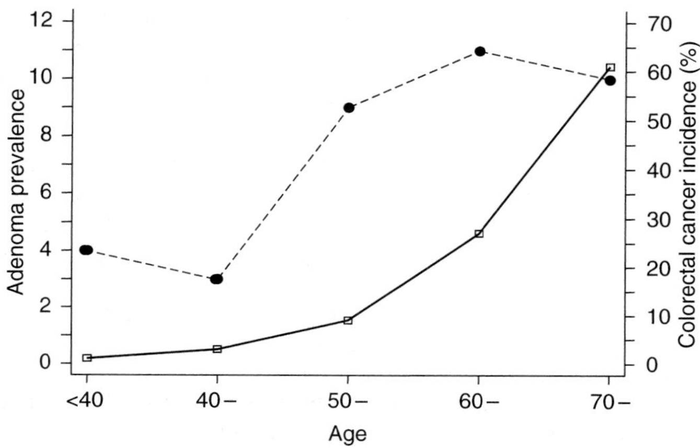

Figure 29.5 Distal adenomas detected at screening by sigmoidoscopy (●) versus colorectal cancer incidence (□). (After Atkin et al., 1993).

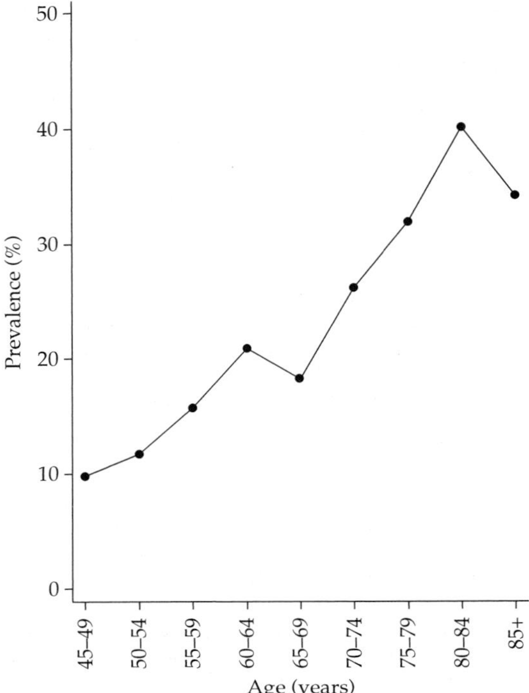

Figure 29.6 Age-prevalence curve for latent prostatic carcinoma in autopsy specimens of men dying from other causes (adjusted for area effects). (After Breslow et al., 1997).

cancer is common, being second only to lung cancer in men in many western countries, the true incidence is much higher, and the as yet unsolved problem is how to discriminate aggressive disease with lethal potential from indolent cancers that are likely to remain asymptomatic for the remainder of the patient's lifetime.

Nevertheless, prostate cancer is a significant public health problem and an obvious target for screening. Three screening modalities are currently in use. Digital rectal examination involves palpation of the prostate to detect increased size, but lacks sensitivity (Schroder et al., 1998). A blood test is also available which measures the level of PSA, a glycoprotein produced only by (both benign and malignant) prostate cells. A third method is transrectal ultrasonography, which because of its cost is usually reserved as a second-stage screen in individuals who are positive for one of the first two tests, although many clinical algorithms for combining these tests exist. PSA is well established as a tumour marker in patients with prostatic cancer, but its use as a screening test has generated much controversy. A typical cut-off for positivity is 4 ng/ml and levels above this are very common at older ages (Table 29.8). There is little doubt that this test is relatively specific for prostate disease but it is unable to distinguish benign from malignant lesions unless higher cut-off levels are used and even less able to distinguish aggressive cancers from slowly growing ones. The majority of PSA secreted into the blood becomes bound to protease inhibitors (mainly alpha anti-chymotrypsin). A low proportion of free (unbound) PSA is associated with the presence of cancer and some have suggested that the free to total ratio should be used as a secondary screening criterion: either in those with PSA levels between 2.5 and 4 ng/ml to improve sensitivity, or in those with levels between 4 and 10 ng/ml to improve specificity (Ito et al., 2003). But the cost of the additional assay and the need for more careful specimen handling make free PSA testing less attractive for screening. Others have suggested that age-specific cut-offs should be used (Gustafsson et al., 1998) or that change in PSA levels would be more useful than an absolute cut-off.

Table 29.8 Serum PSA concentrations and the incidence of prostate cancer as a function of age in 1653 men

Age group (years)	No. of men (%)	Serum PSA level: 4.0–9.9 ng/ml		Serum PSA level: 10.0 ng/ml	
		No. (%)	No. with cancer/ No. with biopsy (%)	No. (%)	No. with cancer/ No. with biopsy (%)
50–59	629 (38)	12 (2)	2/11 (18)	4 (1)	1/3 (33)
60–69	737 (45)	53 (7)	8/40 (20)	15 (2)	12/15 (80)
70–79	264 (16)	39 (15)	9/32 (28)	10 (4)	4/8 (50)
80–89	23 (1)	3 (13)	0/2 (0)	1 (4)	1/1 (100)
All	1653	107 (6)	19/85 (22)	30 (2)	18/27 (67)

From Catalona et al. (1991).

When a screening test is positive, the next step is a trans-urethral prostatic resection to obtain a biopsy. This can distinguish benign from malignant disease, but malignant cases then usually go on to a radical prostatectomy or radiotherapy. This is a major operation with non-negligible mortality and high morbidity often including incontinence and impotence. To date, no trials have been completed to show if prostate screening has any effect on mortality, although large trials are underway in the United

States (Prorok et al., 1991) and in Europe (Schroder et al., 1997). Basic questions regarding the value of radical surgical and radiotherapy treatment in early disease also have not been established.

Prostate cancer is now the most common cancer in men in the United States and there has been a large recent increase in incidence largely attributable to increased utilization of PSA screening. In 1994, it is estimated that 40% of white men aged over 65 years in the United States received a PSA test (Legler et al., 1998; Shaw et al., 2004). PSA testing was also common in the Austrian state of Tyrol, but not elsewhere within Austria and the observation that there was a significantly greater decline in prostate cancer mortality in Tyrol compared to the rest of Austria was interpreted as evidence of the effectiveness of screening (Bartsch et al., 2001). The association between the level of PSA testing and the decline in prostate cancer mortality, is unfortunately not replicated internationally. Although the incidence of advanced prostate cancer decreased in the 1990s and mortality rates have fallen in the United States (Hankey et al., 1999), similar trends in mortality have been seen in the United Kingdom, a country with little prostate screening; and mortality rates in Australia continue to increase despite widespread PSA testing (Oliver et al., 2001). These observations raise doubts about the value of currently available screening methods and the results of randomized trials are awaited with much interest.

References

Ahlquist, D. A., Wieand, H. S., Moertel, C. G., McGill, D. B., Loprinzi, C. L., O'Connell, M. J. et al. (1993). Accuracy of fecal occult blood screening for colorectal neoplasia. A prospective study using Hemoccult and HemoQuant tests. *JAMA*, **269**, 1262–7.

Ahlquist, D. A., Skoletsky, J. E., Boynton, K. A., Harrington, J. J., Mahoney, D. W., Pierceall, W. E. et al. (2000). Colorectal cancer screening by detection of altered human DNA in stool: feasibility of a multitarget assay panel. *Gastroenterology*, **119**(5), 1219–27.

Anwar, K., Inuzuka, M., Shiraishi, T., and Nakakuki, K. (1991). Detection of HPV DNA in neoplastic and non-neoplastic cervical specimens from Pakistan and Japan by nonisotopic *in situ* hybridization. *Int J Cancer*, **47**, 675–80.

Arevalo J. A. and Washington A. E. (1988). Cost-effectiveness of prenatal screening and immunization for hepatitis B virus. *JAMA*, **259**, 365–9.

Atkin, W. S., Cuzick, J., Northover, J. M. A., and Whynes, D. K. (1993). Prevention of colorectal cancer by once-only sigmoidoscopy. *Lancet*, **341**, 736–40.

Atkin, W. S., Edwards, R., Wardle, J., Northover, J. M., Sutton, S., Hart, A. R. et al. (2001). Design of a multicentre randomised trial to evaluate flexible sigmoidoscopy in colorectal cancer screening. *J Med Screen*, **8**(3), 137–44.

Banda-Gamboa, H., Ricketts, I., Cairns, A., Hussein, K., Tucker, J. H., and Husain, N. (1992). Automation in cervical cytology: an overview. *Anal Cellular Pathol*, **4**, 25–48.

Bartsch, G., Horninger, W., Klocker, H., Reissigl, A., Oberaigner, W., Schonitzer D. et al. Tyrol Prostate Cancer Screening Group. (2001). Prostate cancer mortality after introduction of prostate specific antigen mass screening in the federal state of Tyrol, Austria. *Urology*, **58**(3), 417–24.

Bataille, V. (2003). Screening for melanoma. In *Evidence-based Oncology* (Eds. C. Williams). BMJ Publishing Group, London, pp. 188–201.

Bavin, P. J., Giles, J. A., Deery, A., Crow, J., Griffiths, P. D., Emery, V. C. et al. (1993). Use of semi-quantitative PCR for human papillomavirus DNA type 16 to identify women with high grade cervical disease in a population presenting with a mildly dyskaryotic smear report. *Br J Cancer*, **67**, 602–5.

Beasley, R. P. (1982). Hepatitis B virus as the etiologic agent in hepatocellular carcinoma—epidemilogic considerations. *Hepatology*, **2**: 21S-6S.

Beasley, R. P., Hwang, L. Y., Stevens, C. E., Lin, C. C., Hsieh, F. J., Wang, K. Y. et al. (1983*a*). Efficacy of hepatitis B immune globulin for prevention of perinatal transmission of the hepatitis B virus carrier state: final report of a randomized double-blind, placebocontrolled trial. *Hepatology*, **3**, 135–41.

Beasley, R. P., Hwang, L. Y., Lee, G. C. Y., Lan, C-C., Roan, C-H. et al. (1983*b*). Prevention of perinatally transmitted hepatitis B virus infections with hepatitis B immune globulin and hepatitis B vaccine. *Lancet*, **ii**, 1099–102.

Blecker, U., Lanciers, S., Hauser, B. et al. (1995). Serology as a valid screening test for *Helicobacter pylori* infection in asymptomatic subjects. *Arch Pathol Lab Med*, **119**, 30–2.

Blumenthal, P. D., Gaffikin, L., Chirenje, Z. M., McGrath, J., Womack, S., and Shah, K. (2001). Adjunctive testing for cervical cancer in low resource settings with visual inspection, HPV, and the Pap smear. *Int J Gynaecol Obstet*, **72**, 47–53.

Bourne, T. H., Campbell, S., Reynolds, K. M., Whitehead, M. I., Hampson, J., Royston, P. et al. (1993). Screening for early familial ovarian cancer with transvaginal ultrasonography and colour blood flow imaging. *Br Med J*, **306**, 1025–9.

Buetow, S. A. (1996). Testicular cancer: to screen or not to screen? *J Med Screen*, **3**(1), 3–6.

Campbell, S., Bhan, V., Royston, P., Whitehead, M. I., and Collins, W. P. (1989). Transabdominal ultrasound screening for early ovarian cancer. *Br Med J*, **299**, 1363–7.

Catalona, W. J., Smith, D. S., Ratliff, T. L., Dodds, K. M., Coplen, D. E., Yuan, J. J. J. et al. (1991). Measurement of prostate-specific antigen in serum as a screening test for prostate cancer. *N Engl J Med*, **324**, 1156–61.

Clarke, E. A. and Anderson, T. W. (1979). Does screening by 'PAP' smears help prevent cervical cancer? *Lancet*, **ii**, 1–4.

Clavel, C., Masure, M., Bory, J. P., Putaud, I., Mangeonjean, C., Lorenzato, M., et al. (2001). Human papillomavirus testing in primary screening for the detection of high-grade cervical lesions: a study of 7932 women. *Br J Cancer*, **84**, 1616–23.

Cuzick, J., Terry G., Ho, L., Hollingworth, T., and Anderson, M. (1992). Human papillomavirus type 16 DNA in cervical smears as a predictor of high-grade cervical intraepithelial neoplasia. *Lancet*, **339**, 959–60.

Cuzick, J., Terry G., Ho, L., Hollingworth, T., and Anderson, M. (1994). Type-specific human papillomavirus DNA in abnormal smears as a predictor of high-grade intraepithelial neoplasia. *Br J Cancer*, **69**, 167–71.

Cuzick, J., Edwards, R., and Segnan, N. (1997). Adjusting for non-compliance and contamination in randomised clinical trials. *Stati Medi*, **16**, 1017–29.

Cuzick, J., Beverley, E., Ho, L., Terry, G., Sapper, H., Mielzynska, I. et al. (1999). HPV testing in primary screening of older women. *Br J Cancer*, **81**, 554–8.

Cuzick, J., Szarewski, A., Cubie, H., Hulman, G., Kitchener, H., Luesley, D. et al. (2003). Management of women who test positive for high-risk types of human papillomavirus: the HART study. *Lancet* **362**(9399), 1871–76.

Davies, R. J., Freeman, A., Morris, L. S., Bingham, S., Dilworth, S., Scott, I. et al. (2002). Analysis of mini-chromosome maintenance proteins as a novel method for detection of colorectal cancer in stool. *Lancet*, **359**(9321), 1917–19.

Detsky, A. S. (2001). Screening for colon cancer—can we afford colonoscopy? *N Engl J Med*, **345**(8), 607–8.

Dong, S. M., Traverso, G., Johnson, C., Geng, L., Favis, R., Boynton, K., et al. (2001). Detecting colorectal cancer in stool with the use of multiple genetic targets. *JNCI*, **93**(11), 858–65.

Donnan, S. P. B., Wong. F. W. S., Ho, S. C., Lau, E. M. C., Takashi, K., and Estève, J. (1989). Reproductive and sexual risk factors and human papilloma virus infection in cervical cancer among Hong Kong Chinese. *Int J Epidemiol*, **18**, 32–6.

Ellman, R., Moss, S. M., Coleman, D., and Chamberlain, J. (1993). Breast self-examination programmes in the trial of early detection of breast cancer: ten year findings. *Br J Cancer*, **68**, 208–12.

Esteve, J., Duffy, S. W., and Hill, C. (2001). Screening for neuroblastoma in children: insight gained from the modelling of various screening strategies. In *Quantitative Methods for Evaluation of Cancer Screening* (Eds. S. W., Duffy, C. Hill, J. Esteve) Arnold, London.

Fahey, M. T., Irwig, L., and Macaskill, P. (1995). Meta-analysis of Pap test accuracy. *Am J Epidemiol*, **141**(7), 680–9.

Forman, D. (1998). Lessons from ongoing intervention studies. In *Helicobacter pylori: Basic Mechanisms to Clinical Care* (Eds. Hent RH and Tytgat GNH). Kluwer, Dordrecht.

Fortuin, M., Chotard, J., Jack, A. D., Maine, N. P., Mendy, M. et al. (1993). Efficacy of hepatitis B vaccine in the Gambian expanded programme on immunization. *Lancet*, **341**, 1129–31.

Fukao, A., Hisamichi, S., and Sugawara, N. (1987). A case-control study on evaluating the effect of mass screening on decreasing advanced stomach cancer (in Japanese). *J Jpn Soc Gastroenterol Mass Survey*, **75**, 112–16.

Gaffikin, L., Lauterbach, M., and Blumenthal, P. D. (2003). Performance of visual inspection with acetic acid for cervical cancer screening: a qualitative summary of evidence to date. *Obstet Gynecol Survey*, **58**(8), 543–50.

Gastrin, G., Miller, A. B., To, T., Aronson, K. J., Wall, C., Hakama, M. et al. (1994). Incidence and mortality from breast cancer in the Mama program for breast screening in Finland, 1973–1986. *Cancer*, **73**, 2168–74.

Gershon-Cohen, J. and Colcher, A. E. (1937). Evaluation of roentgen diagnosis of early carcinoma of the breast. *JAMA*, **108**, 867–71.

Ghendon, Y. (1990). WHO strategy for the global elimination of new cases of hepatitis B. *Vaccine*, **8**(Suppl.), S129–33.

Glupczynski, Y., Burette, A., Gossens, H., DePrez, C., and Butzler, J. P. (1992). Effect of antimicrobial therapy on the specific serological response to *Helicobacter pylori* infection. *Eur J Clin Microbiol Infect Dis*, **11**(7), 583–8.

Gohagan, J., Marcus, P., Fagerstrom, R., Black, W., Kramer, B., Pinsky, P. et al. (2003). Screening for lung cancer. In *Evidence-Based Oncology* (Eds. C. Williams.) BMJ Publishing Group, London, pp. 164–72.

Gustafsson, O., Mansour, E., Norming, U., Carlsson, A., Tornblom, M., Nyman, C. R. (1998). Prostate-specific antigen (PSA), PSA density and age-adjusted PSA reference values in screening for prostate cancer—a study of a randomly selected population of 2,400 men. *Scand J Urol Nephrol*, **32**(6), 373–7.

Hakama, M. (1982). Trends in the incidence of cervical cancer in the Nordic countries. In *Trends in Cancer Incidence: Causes and Practical Implications* (Ed. K. Magnus). Hemisphere Publishing Corporation, USA, pp. 279–92.

Hankey, B. F., Feuer, E. J., Clegg, L. X., Hayes, R. B., Legler, J. M., Prorok, P. C. et al. (1999). Cancer surveillance series: interpreting trends in prostate cancer—part 1; evidence of the effects of screening in recent prostate cancer incidence, mortality, and survival rates. *JNCI*, **91**(12), 1017–24.

Hardcastle, J. D., Chamberlain, J., Robinson, M. H., Moss, S. M., Amar, S. S., Balfour, T. W. et al. (1996). Randomised controlled trial of faecal-occult-blood screening for colorectal cancer. *Lancet*, **348**(9040), 1472–7.

Helicobacter and Cancer Collaborative Group. (2001). Gastric cancer and *Helicobacter pylori*: a combined analysis of 12 case control studies nested within prospective cohorts. *Gut*, **49**, 347–53.

Henschke, C. I., McCauley, D. I., Yankelevitz, D. F., Naidich, D. P., McGuiness, G., Miettinen, O. S., et al. (1999). Early Lung Cancer Action Project: overall design and findings from baseline screening. *Lancet*, **354**(9173), 99–105.

Henschke, C. I., Naidich, D. P., Yankelevitz, D. F., McGuinness, G., McCauley, D. I., Smith, J. P. et al. (2001). Early lung cancer action project: initial findings on repeat screenings. *Cancer*, **92**(1), 153–9.

Hisamichi, S., Fukao, A., Sugawara, N., Nishikouri, M., Komatsu, S., Tsuji, I. et al. (1991). Evaluation of mass screening programme for stomach cancer in Japan. In *Cancer Screening* (Eds. A. B. Miller, J. Chamberlain, N. E. Day, M. Hakama, and P. C. Prorok), pp. 357–70. Cambridge University Press, New York.

Hutchinson, M. L., Zahniser, D. J., Sherman, M. E., Herrero, R., Alfaro, M., Bratti M. C. et al. (1999). Utility of liquid-based cytology for cervical carcinoma screening: results of a population-based study conducted in a region of Costa Rica with a high incidence of cervical carcinoma. *Cancer*, **87**, 48–55.

IARC. (2002). *Breast cancer screening*. In *IARC Handbooks of Cancer Prevention*, vol. 7 (Eds. H. Vainio, and F. Bianchini). IARC Press, Lyon.

IARC Working Party. (1986). Screening for squamous cervical cancer: duration of low risk after negative results of cervical cytology and its implication for screening policies. *Br Med J*, **293**, 659–64.

International Agency for Research on Cancer IARC (1994). *Hepatitis Viruses* (IARC Monographs on the Evaluation of Carcinogenic Risks to Humans), vol 59, IARC, Lyon.

Ito, K., Yamamoto, T., Ohi, M., Takechi, H., Kurokawa, K., Suzuki, K. et al. (2003). Natural history of PSA increase with and without prostate cancer. *Urology*, **62**(1), 64–9.

Jacobs, I., Davies, A. P., Bridges, J., Stabile, I., Fay, T., Lower, A. et al. (1993). Prevalence screening for ovarian cancer in postmenopausal women by CA 125 measurement and ultrasonography. *Br Med J*, **306**, 1030–4.

Jarvinen, H. J., Aarnio, M., Mustonen, H., Aktan-Collan, K., Aaltonen, L. A., Peltomaki. P. et al. (2000). Controlled 15-year trial on screening for colorectal cancer in families with hereditary nonpolyposis colorectal cancer. *Gastroenterology*, **118**(5), 829–34.

Jorgensen, O. D., Kronborg, O., and Fenger, C. (2002). A randomised study of screening for colorectal cancer using faecal occult blood testing: results after 13 years and seven biennial screening rounds. *Gut*, **50**(1), 29–32.

Klaes, R., Friedrich, T., Spitkovsky, D., Ridder, R., Rudy, W., Petry, U. et al. (2001). Overexpression of p16^{INK4A} as a specific marker for dysplastic and neoplastic epithelial cells of the cervix uteri. *Int J Cancer*, **92**(2), 276–84.

Kronborg, O., Fenger, C., Olsen, J., Jorgensen, O. D., and Sondergaard, O. (1996). Randomised study of screening for colorectal cancer with faecal-occult-blood test. *Lancet*, **348**(9040), 1467–71.

Kuhn, L., Denny, L., Pollack, A., Lorincz, A., Richart, R. M., and Wright, T. C. (2000). Human papillomavirus DNA testing for cervical cancer screening in low-resource settings. *J Natl Cancer Inst*, **92**, 818–25.

Läärä, E., Day, N. E., and Hakama, M. (1987). Trends in mortality from cervical cancer in the Nordic countries: association with organised screening programmes. *Lancet*, **8544**, 1247–9.

Lauenstein, T., Goehde, S., Ruehm, S., Holtmann, G., and Debatin, J. (2002). MR colonography with barium-based fecal tagging: initial clinical experience. *Radiology*, **223**, 248–54.

Legler, J. M., Fener, E. J., Potosky, A. L., Merrill, R. M., and Kramer, B. S. (1998). The role of prostate-specific antigen (PSA) testing patterns in the recent prostate cancer incidence decline in the United States. *Cancer Causes Control*, **9**(5), 519–27.

Liberman, L., Morris, E. A., Kim, C. M., Kaplan, J. B., Abramson, A. F., Menell, J. H. et al. (2003). MR imaging findings in the contralateral breast of women with recently diagnosed breast cancer. *AJR Am J Roentgenol*, **180**(2), 333–41.

Lieberman, D. A., Weiss, D. G., Bond, J. H., Ahnen, D. J., Garewal, H., and Chejfec, G. (2000). Use of colonoscopy to screen asymptomatic adults for colorectal cancer. Veterans Affairs Cooperative Study Group 380. *N Engl J Med*, **343**(3), 162–8. Erratum in: *N Engl J Med* (2000), **343**(16), 1204.

Lieberman, D. A., Weiss, D. G., Veterans Affairs Cooperative Study Group 380 (2001). One-time screening for colorectal cancer with combined fecal occult-blood testing and examination of the distal colon. *N Engl J Med*, **345**(8), 555–60.

Lo Monaco, R., Mentore, B., Rebora, M. et al. (1996). Hepatitis B vaccination coverage and epidemiology of HBV-related disease in Liguria, Italy (abstract C282). In *Proceedings of IX Triennial International Symposium on Viral Hepatitis and Liver Disease*, April 21–25. Rome: CpA, p. 272.

Loy, C. T., Irwig, L. M., Katelaris, P. H., and Talley, N. J. (1996). Do commercial serology kits for *Helicobacter pylori* infection differ in accuracy? *Am J Gastroenterol*, **91**, 1138–44.

Maehara, Y., Kakeji, Y., Oda, S., Takahashi, I., Akazawa, K., and Sugimachi, K. (2000). Time trends of surgical treatment and the prognosis for Japanese patients with gastric cancer. *Br J Cancer*, **83**(8), 986–91.

Mandel, J. S., Bond, J. H., Church, T. R., Snover, D. C., Bradley, M. G., and Schuman, L. M. et al. (1993). Reducing mortality from colorectal cancer by screening for fecal occult blood. *N Engl J Med*, **328**, 1365–71.

Manos, M. M., Kinney, W. K., Hurley, L. B., Sherman, M. E., Shieh-Ngai, J., Kurman, R. J. et al. (1999). Identifying women with cervical neoplasia: using human papillomavirus DNA testing for equivocal Papanicolaou results. *JAMA*, **281**(17), 1645–7.

Mele, A., Stroffolini, T., Sagliocca, L. et al. (1996). Control of hepatitis B in Italy (abstract 67). In *Proceedings of IX Triennial International Symposium on Viral Hepatitis and Liver Disease*, April 21–25. Rome: CpA, p. 21.

Menon, U., Talaat, A., Rosenthal, A. N., MacDonald, N. D., Jeyerajah, A. R., Skates, S. J., et al. (2000). Performance of ultrasound as a second line test to serum CA125 in ovarian cancer screening. *BJOG*, **107**(2), 165–9.

Moayyedi, P., Feltbower, R., Crocombe, W. et al. (2000). The effectiveness of omeprazole, clarithromycin and tinidazole in eradicating *Helicobacter pylori* in a community screen and treat programme. *Alimen Pharmacol Ther*, **14**, 719–28.

Morson, B. C. (1976). Genesis of colorectal cancer. *Gastroenterology*, **5**, 505–25.

Muller, A. D., and Sonnenberg, A. (1995). Protection by endoscopy against death from colorectal cancer. A case control study among veterans. *Arch Intern Med*, **155**(16), 1741–8.

Muñoz, N. and Bosch, F. X. (1992). HPV and cervical neoplasia: review of case-control and cohort studies. In *The Epidemiology of Human Papillomavirus and Cervical Cancer* (Eds. N. Munoz, F. X. Bosch, K. V. Shah, and A. Meheus), vol. 119, IARC, Lyon, pp. 251–61.

Murphy, S. B., Cohn, S. L., Craft, A. W., Woods, W. G., Sawada, T., Castleberry, R. P. et al. (1991). Do children benefit from mass screening for neuroblastoma? *Lancet*, **337**, 344–5.

Nanda, K., McCrory, D. C., Myers, E. R., Bastian, L. A., Hasselblad, V., Hickey, J. D. et al. (2000). Accuracy of the Papanicolaou test in screening for and follow-up of cervical cytologic abnormalities: a systematic review. *Ann Intern Med*, **132**(10), 810–19.

Newcomb, P. A., Norfleet, R. G., Storer, B. E., Surawicz, T. S., and Marcus, P. M. (1992). Screening sigmoidoscopy and colorectal cancer mortality. *JNCI*, **84**, 1572–5.

Oliver, S. E., May, M. T., and Gunnell, D. (2001). International trends in prostate cancer mortality in the 'PSA ERA'. *Int J Cancer*, **92**(6), 893–8.

Paci, E. and Duffy, S. W. (1991). Modelling the analysis of breast cancer screening programmes: sensitivity, lead time and predictive value in the Florence district programme (1975–1986). *Int J Epidemiol*, **20**, 852–8.

Papanicolaou, G. N. (1928). In *Procedings of the Third Race Betterment Conference*. Race Betterment Foundation, Battle Creek, Michigan, pp. 528–34.

Papanicolaou, G. N. and Trout, H. F. (1941). The diagnostic value of vaginal smears in carcinoma of the uterus. *Am J Obstet Gynecol*, **42**, 193–206.

Parsonnet, J., Harris, R. A., Hack, H. M., and Owens, D. K. (1996). Modelling cost-effectiveness of *Helicobacter pylori* screening to prevent gastric cancer: a mandate for clinical trials. *Lancet*, **348**, 150–4.

Payne, N., Chilcott, J., and McGoogan, E. (2000). Liquid-based cytology in cervical screening: a rapid and systematic review. *Health Technol Assess*, **4**(18), 1–73.

Peer, P. G. M., Holland, R., Hendriks, J. H. C. L., Mravunac, M., and Verbeek, A. L. M. (1994). Age-specific effectiveness of the Nijmegen population-based breast cancer-screening program: assessment of early indicators of screening effectiveness. *JNCI*, **86**, 436–41.

Peng, H. Q., Liu, S. L., Mann, V., Rohan, T., and Rawls, W. (1991). Human papillomavirus types 16 and 33, herpes simplex virus type 2 and other risk factors for cervical cancer in Sichuan Province, China. *Int J Cancer*, **47**, 711–16.

Prorok, P. C., Byar, D. P., Smart, C. R., Baker, S. G., and Connor, R. J. (1991). Evaluation of screening for prostate, lung, and colorectal cancers: the PLC Trial. In *Cancer Screening* (Eds. A.B. Miller, J. Chamberlain, N.E. Day, M. Hakama, and P.C. Prorok), Cambridge University Press, New York, pp. 300–20.

Ratnam, S., Franco, E. L, and Ferenczy, A. (2000). Human papillomavirus testing for primary screening of cervical cancer precursors. *Cancer Epidemiol Biomarkers Prev*, **9**, 945–51.

Reeves, W. C., Brinton, L. A., Garcia, M., Brenes, M. M., Herrero, R., Gaitan, E. et al. (1989). Human papillomavirus infection and cervical cancer in Latin America. *N Engl J Med*, **320**, 1437–41.

Rex, D. K., Rahmani, E. Y., Haseman, J. H., Lemmel, G. T., Kaster, S., and Buckley, J. S. (1997). Relative sensitivity of colonoscopy and barium enema for detection of colorectal cancer in clinical practice. *Gastroenterology*, **112**(1), 17–23.

Roberts, A. P., Childs, S., Rubin, G., and de Wit, N. J. (2000). Tests for *Helicobacter pylori* infection: a critical appraisal from primary care. *Fam Prac*, **17**(Suppl. 2), S12–20.

Rodrigues, V. C., Moss, S. M., and Tuomainen, H. (1998). Oral cancer in the UK; to screen or not to screen. *Oral Oncology*, **34**(6), 454–65.

Sankaranarayanan, R., Wesley, R., Thara, S., Dhakad, N., Chandralekha, B., Sebastian, P. et al. (2003). Test characteristics of visual inspection with 4% acetic acid (VIA) and Lugol's iodine (VILI) in cervical cancer screening in Kerala, India. *Int J Cancer*, **106**(3), 404–8.

Sasieni, P. and Cuzick, J. (2003). The UK breast-screening programme should start at age 47 years. *Lancet*, **362**(9379), 246–7.

Sasieni, P., Adams, J., and Cuzick, J. (2003). Benefit of cervical screening at different ages: evidence form the UK audit of screening histories. *Br J Cancer*, **89**(1), 88–93.

Sawada, T. (1992). Past and future of neuroblastoma screening in Japan. *Am J Pediatr Hematol Oncol*, **14**, 320–6.

Sawada, T., Matsumura, T., Matsuda, Y., and Kawakatsu, H. (1991). Neuroblastoma: studies in Japan. In *Cancer Screening* (Eds. A. B. Miller, J. Chamberlain, N. E. Day, M. Hakama, and P. C. Prorok), Cambridge University Press, New York, pp. 325–36.

Schalm, S. W., Mazel, J. A., de Gast, G. C. et al. (1989). Prevention of hepatitis B in new borns through mass screening and delayed vaccination of all infants of mothers with hepatitis B surface antigen. *Pediatrics*, **83**, 1041–7.

Schiffman, M., Herrero, R., Hildesheim, A., Sherman, M. E., Bratti, M., Wacholder, S. et al. (2000). HPV DNA testing in cervical cancer screening: results from women in a high-risk province of Costa Rica. *JAMA*, **283**, 87–93.

Schmauz, R., Okong, P., de Villiers, E. M., Dennin, R., Brade, L., Lwanga, S. K. et al. (1989). Multiple infections in cases of cervical cancer from a high-incidence area in tropical Africa. *Int J Cancer*, **43**, 805–9.

Schroder, F. H. and Bangma, C. H. (1997). The European Study of Screening for Prostate Cancer (ERSPC). *Br J Urol*, **79**(Suppl. 1), 68–71.

Schroder, F. H, van der Maas, P., Beemsterboer, P., Kruger, A. B., Hoedemacher, R., Rietbergen, J. et al. (1998). Evaluation of the digital rectal examination as a screening test for prostate cancer. Rotterdam Section of the European Randomised Study of Screening for Prostate Cancer. *JNCI* **90**(23), 1817–23.

Selby, J. V., Friedman, G. D., Quesenberry, C. P., and Weiss, N. S. (1992). A case-control study of screening sigmoidoscopy and mortality from colorectal cancer. *N Engl J Med*, **326**, 653–7.

Semiglazov, V. F., Moiseyenko, V. M., Manikhas, A. G. et al. (1999). Role of breast cancer self-examinationin early detection of breast cancer: Russia/WHO prospective randomised trial in St Petersburg. *Cancer Strat* **1**, 145–51.

Shapiro, S., Venet, W., Strax, P., Venet, L., and Roeser, R. (1982). Ten-to-fourteen year effect of screening on breast cancer mortality. *J Natl Cancer Inst*, **69**, 349–55.

Shaw, P. A., Etzioni, R., Zeliadt, S. B., Mariotto, A., Karnofski, K., Penson, D. F. et al. (2004). An ecologic study of prostate-specific antigen screening and prostate cancer mortality in nine geographic areas of the United States. *Am J Epidemiol, Dec*, **160**, 1059–69.

Skates, S. J., Xu, F. j., Yu, Y. H., Sjovall, K., Einhorn, N., Chang, Y. et al. (1995). Towards an optimal algorithm for ovarian cancer screening with longitudinal tumor markers. *Cancer*, **76**(10 Suppl), 2004–10.

Solomon, D., Shiffman, M., Tarone, R., and ALTS Study Group (2001). Comparison of three management strategies for patients with atypical squamous cells of undetermined significance; baseline results from a randomised trial. *JNCI*, **93**(4), 273–9.

St. John, D. J. B., Young, G. P., Alexeyeff, M. A., Deacon, M. C., Cuthbertson, A. M., Macrae, F. A. et al. (1993). Evaluation of new occult blood tests for detection of colorectal neoplasia. *Gastroenterology*, **104**, 1661–1668.

Stevens, C. E., Toy, P. T., Taylor, P. E., Lee, T., and Yip, H-Y. (1992). Prospects for control of hepatitis B virus infection: implications of childhood vaccination and long-term protection. *Pediatrics*, **90**, 170–173.

Stoeber, K., Swinn, R., Prevost, A. T., de Clive-Lowe, P., Halsall, I., Dilworth, S. M. et al. (2002). Diagnoisis of genito-urinary tract cancer by detection of mini-chromosome maintenance 5 protein in urine sediments. *JNCI*, **94**(14), 1071–9.

Stroffolini, T., Pasquini, P., and Collaborating Group (1990). Five years of vaccination campaign against hepatitis B in Italy in infants of hepatitis B surface antigen carrier mothers. *Italian J Gastroenterol*, **22**, 195–197.

Sun, T., Yu, H., Hsia, C., Wang, N., and Huang, X. (1988). Evaluation of sero-survey trials for the early detection of hepatocellular carcinoma in area of high prevalence. In *Screening for Gastrointestinal Cancer* (Eds. J. Chamberlain and A. B. Miller). Hans Huber, Bern, pp. 81–6.

Swensen, S. J., Jett, J. R., Hartman, T. E., Midthun, D. E., Sloan, J. A., Sykes A. M. et al. (2003). Lung cancer screening with CT: Mayo Clinic experience. *Radiology*, **226**(3), 756–61.

Tabar, L., Fagerberg, G., Duffy, S. W., Day, N. E., Gad, A., and Gröntoft, O. (1992). Update of the Swedish two-county program of mammographic screening for breast cancer. *Radiol Clin N Am*, **30**, 187–209.

Tagore, K. S., Lawson, M. J., Yucaitis, J. A., Gage, R., Orr, T., Shuber, A. P. et al. (2003). Sensitivity and specificity of a stool DNA multitarget assay panel for the detection of advanced colorectal neoplasia. *Clin Colorectal Cancer*, **3**(1), 47–53.

Taylor, P. E., Stevens, C. E., de Cordoba, S. R., and Rubinstein, P. (1988). Hepatitis B virus and human immunodeficiency virus: possible interactions. In *Viral Hepatitis and Liver Disease*. (Ed., A. J. Zuckerman). New York, Alan R Liss, pp. 198–200

Thomas, D. B., Gao, D. L., Ray, R. M., Wang, W. W., Allison, C. J., Chen, F. L. et al. (2002). Randomized trial of breast self-examination in Shanghai: final results. *JNCI*, **94**(19), 1445–57.

Thomas, D. B., Gao, D. L., Self, S. G., Allison, C. J., Tao, Y, Mahloch, J. et al. (1997). Randomised trial of breast self-examination in Shanghai:methodology and preliminary results. *JNCI*, **89** (5), 355–65.

Trecate, G., Vergnaghi, D., Bergnzi, S., De Simone, T., Fengoni, E., Costa, C. et al. (2003). Breast MRI screening in patients with increased familial and/or genetic risk for breast cancer: a preliminary experience. *Tumori*, **89**(2):125–31.

Uemura, N., Okamoto, S., Yamamoto, S. et al. (2001). *Helicobacter pylori* infection and the development of gastric cancer. *N Engl J Med*, **345**, 784–9

UK Flexible Sigmoidoscopy Screening Trial Investigators (2002). Single flexible sigmoidoscopy screening to prevent colorectal cancer: baseline findings of a UK multicentre randomised trial. *Lancet*, **359**(9314), 1291–1300.

UK Trial of Early Detection of Breast Cancer Group (1999). 16-year mortality from breast cancer in the UK Trial of Early Detection of Breast Cancer. *Lancet*, **353**(9168), 1909–14.

Vining, D., Gelfand, D., Bechtold, R. et al. (1994). Technical feasibility of colon imaging with helical CT and virtual reality. *Am J Roentgenol*, **162**(Suppl), 104.

Wainwright, R. B., McMahon, B. J., Bulkow, L. R., Hall D. B. et al. (1989). Duration of immunogenicity and efficacy of hepatitis B vaccine in a Yupik Eskimo population. *JAMA*, **261**, 2362–6.

Whittle, H. C., Maine, N., Pilkington, J. et al. (1995). Long-term efficacy of continuing hepatitis B vaccination in infancy in two Gambian villages. *Lancet*, **345**, 1089–92.

Winawer, S. J. and Zauber, A. G. (2001). Colonoscopic polypectomy and the incidence of colorectal cancer. *Gut*, **48**(6), 753–4.

Winawer, S. J., Stewart, E. T., Zauber, A. G., Bond J. H., Ansel, H., Waye, J. D. et al. (2000). A comparison of colonoscopy and double-contrast barium enema for surveillance after polypectomy. National Polyp Study Work Group. *N Engl J Med*, **342**(24), 1766–72.

Woods, W. G., Tuchman, M., Robison, L. L., Bernstein, M., Leclerc, J. M., Brisson, L. C. et al. (1996). A population-based study of the usefulness of screening for neuroblastoma. *Lancet*, **348**, 1682–87.

World Health Organisation (1983). Prevention of hepatocellular carcinoma by immunization. *Bull. World Health Organ*, **61**, 731–744.

Xu, Z. Y., Duan, S. C., Margolis, H. S. et al. (1995). Long-term efficacy of active postexposure immunization of infants for prevention of hepatitis B virus infection. United States-People's Republic of China Study Group on Hepatitis B. *J Infect Dis*, **171**, 54–60.

Yamagata, H., Kiyohara, Y., Aoyagi, K. et al. (2000). Impact of *Helicobacter pylori* infection on gastric cancer incidence in a general Japanese population: the Hisayama study. *Arch Intern Med*, **160**, 1962–8.

CHAPTER 30

Conclusions and prospects

Peter Selby and Margaret Knowles

The ultimate goal of all cancer research is to provide benefits for cancer patients, and those at risk of cancer. The immediacy of those benefits from research will vary from the long-term products of basic biomedical research through to the direct benefits to patients that come from clinical trials. The process of editing this book has allowed us to take an overview of what has happened in recent years, when new knowledge and new technologies have been firmly established and great progress has been made in translating these into real advances in prevention and treatment. This also allows for some speculation about the changes that we will see in the next three to five years.

Cancer research has benefited greatly from the general advances made in science in the last five years, not only the obvious inputs from biology and medicine but also from the strides that have been made in physics and chemistry, electronics, and computing. Without these we would not be able to present, analyse, or understand the progress in structural biology and cell and molecular biology, conduct projects like the human genome project and its genomic and proteomic successors or generate new chemical entities that may become useful drugs for cancer. E-science and Grid technology will provide the key electronic/computing contribution to cancer research in the next five years and large-scale science will allow access to very large data collection and very-large-scale computing resources but with ready access for individual scientific users.

Throughout the book there is extensive discussion of the advances made in the basic biology which underlies carcinogenesis. Although much was known five years ago about carcinogens and the identity and function of oncogenes and tumour suppressor genes, Chapters 6–8 demonstrate our increased knowledge both of the nature and interactions of the genetic abnormalities which contribute to carcinogenesis and the mechanisms which activate or inactivate these genes. To this we can now add a much more thorough understanding of how the genetic and epigenetic (Chapter 5) changes in key genes interact with each other and the tissue microenvironment to determine cell survival, cell death (Chapter 12), growth and metastasis (Chapters 5, 9, 11, and 16).

Biological and clinical outcomes depend not only on the genetic and epigenetic influences within the tumour but also upon the host response. Basic immunology has clarified the cellular interactions which underpin a specific immune response with an increasing recognition of the role of professional antigen-presenting cells and the importance of the biological context within which antigen presentation occurs (Chapters 20 and 27). Co-stimulation of immune cells with both cell surface and paracrine factors and the importance of 'danger' signals are highly relevant to the immune response to cancer cells. We are beginning to have insights into the interaction between the genetic abnormalities in cancer cells and the capacity of the immune response to eliminate them (Chapters 20 and 27).

The cancer risk of a person is determined by their genetic constitution and their exposure to environmental factors. The outcome of a cancer is also influenced by genetic polymorphisms (Chapters 2–4). Such polymorphisms influence cell proliferation, survival, apoptosis, repair, and responses to hormones and cytokines. The human genome is about 0.1% polymorphic. Our understanding of the influence of these polymorphisms remains in its infancy but the next five years will see increased understanding of the association of polymorphisms with risk, outcomes, and the interactions between genes and the environment.

In a malignant cell, multiple genetic abnormalities affect the expression of genes and determine the malignant phenotype. This is influenced by complex tissue environments. It is not surprising that experimental methods which evaluate any single abnormality or process give us only limited insights into the behaviour of a tumour, its growth, metastasis, and response to chemotherapy or radiotherapy. The new biotechnologies of genomics and proteomics have in common the ability to assay multiple changes in parallel systems rapidly. Dense arrays of oligonucleotides, genomic, and cDNAs are now available to evaluate genetic abnormalities and changes in gene expression. The presence of thousands of individual items on a dense array is now commonplace and the presence of tens of thousands is becoming commonplace. Despite early technical difficulties, these systems are now robustly generating data (Chapter 22). Frequently the greatest challenges to the experimenter are in the area of data handling, analysis, and informatics. The data generated about individual genes, clusters of genes and their relationship to biological processes, diagnosis, and clinical outcomes are summarized in (Chapters 7, 8 and 23–28).

Analysis of changes in nucleic acids, however, have limitations. The behaviour of cells, tumours and the host ultimately depends upon structures and functions carried out by proteins. While proteins are a direct consequence of gene expression, they frequently undergo post-translational changes that can have profound influences on their function and have potential use as markers and therapeutic targets in cancer. The exploitation of existing techniques and the development of new techniques which allow the evaluation of the proteome of tumours and normal tissues was therefore necessary. The ability to separate proteins on the basis of charge and size using two-dimensional gel electrophoresis has been available for several decades. However the application of modern computing and image analysis of two-dimensional gels and of mass spectrometry to fingerprint and sequence proteins has increased their utility. These techniques remain at the heart of much of modern proteomics but are laborious and require highly developed laboratory bench skills. They are being supplemented, although not yet replaced, by alternative mass spectrometric approaches to fractionate proteins based on their charge, size, or conformation to generate protein profiles and identities. Diagnostic and prognostic advances are likely from proteomics and therapeutic advances should follow (Chapter 22). These new technologies are reaching a level of reliability and utility which allows applications in many laboratories. Frequently the limiting stages of the experiment are the availability of well preserved, numerous and well characterized tissue samples and clinical data. Large amounts of data are becoming available and require advances in informatics to analyse these in large numbers of patients.

Molecular and cellular studies will remain central to cancer research but there will be increasing use of rodent models in coming years, both to evaluate tumour growth and spread and its underlying biology as well as to evaluate novel therapeutic approaches. The relevant biological questions are discussed in Chapters 16 and 18, the model systems in Chapter 19 and the therapeutic opportunities in Chapters 23–28.

The claim that cancer research will deliver scientifically sound, rational, and non-toxic treatments for cancer patients is not new. However, it can now be claimed that this goal is being delivered, albeit on a limited front. The most prominent recent example was the development of a selective inhibitor for the tyrosine kinase which is the product of the *BCR–ABL* translocation which characterizes chronic myeloid leukaemia. This treatment proved effective and remarkably non-toxic. The spectrum of activity of the drug (Imatinib, Glivec, STI571) extends to a limited number of other kinases which are commonly found in other rare cancers, particularly gastrointestinal stromal tumours, a rare subtype of intra-abdominal sarcoma. Effective treatment, although less successful than in chronic myeloid leukaemia, has resulted. Similar concepts underpinned the development of drugs which inhibit epidermal growth factor (EGF) receptor. Significant antitumour effects resulted but clinical benefits proved to be modest. Re-examination of the molecular biology and pharmacology of EGF receptor and its inhibition suggests that only some specific forms of receptor are true targets for the drug, although when present the response rates are high. Nevertheless there are reasons for optimism that the knowledge of carcinogenesis and cancer biology which we have summarized in this book will increasingly generate new targets for anticancer drugs which will avoid the lack of selectivity and therefore the toxicity which remains a characteristic of current cancer pharmacology.

Perhaps less prominent, but equally promising, have been the successes using chimeric and humanized monoclonal antibodies for cancer treatment. These are summarized in Chapter 26 and in several cases real and substantial benefits for patients are now demonstrated. In B-cell lymphoma anti-CD20 antibodies, in breast cancer antibody to Her2/neu receptor and in colorectal cancer antibodies to VEGF (vascular endothelial growth factor) have all been shown to benefit patients in randomized prospective trials. It is now almost 30 years since the discovery of monoclonal antibodies, a sobering reflection of the slow progress of translational research to date.

The promise of immunotherapy based on increasing knowledge of cellular immunology remains, but the evidence for the success of cancer vaccines is still rather slender as summarized in Chapter 27. Vaccines based on protein and peptide vaccination, DNA vaccination and cellular vaccines involving antigen-presenting cells are all capable of producing remissions in some patients, particularly those with malignant melanoma and renal cancer. Cytokine therapies produce remissions consistently in a proportion of patients with melanoma and renal cancer (Chapter 14). Unfortunately, the effects so far are infrequent with no more than 20% of patients benefiting in most studies. The literature is inconsistent, which is a reflection of the complexities of the technologies involved and of the biological systems being studied. There is enough preliminary data from translational research in vaccines to suggest that it is worth pursuing this field of enquiry but none of these approaches have yet established themselves as routine for patients in large prospective randomized trials.

The technologies which underpin modern clinical research were developed in the 1970s and 1980s and particularly depend upon the careful design and conduct of prospective randomized trials. After preliminary work on small numbers of patients to demonstrate safety and detect toxicity (Phase 1) investigations move on to establish that a new treatment has activity against cancer in general or a particular group of cancers (Phase 2) and then this new approach, either alone or in combination, is compared to standard therapy in a Phase 3 trial. The last decade has seen significant developments in clinical research and its methodologies.

The availability of specific drug targets requires the restriction of treatments to patients whose tumours express those targets. The trend towards the conduct of early clinical trials in patients in whom targets are present and shown to be expressed will increase. Also, it will no longer be sufficient to demonstrate that a treatment can be safely given to patients before evaluating its effectiveness. It will increasingly be necessary to demonstrate that the administration of the candidate treatment actually inhibits the defined target against which it was developed. Pharmacological and biological monitoring of treatments will therefore have to become more sophisticated and will be an essential element in future early clinical trials.

In large Phase 3 randomized perspective trials, careful definition of targets will be necessary. Integrating large clinical databases with biomedical databases is a massive challenge for clinical investigators and scientists in bioinformatics and biostatistics. Organizing research on this scale within modern health care services is in itself a special and considerable challenge. Producing technical and organizational solutions to the conduct of research of this complexity and on this scale is quite difficult; changing the culture of clinicians, managers, and the funders of health care may be considerably more difficult.

What predictions are possible for the next five years? Genomic and proteomic analyses of malignant tissues will yield huge amounts of data. Carefully analysed patterns of genetic abnormalities, gene expression, and proteins will allow new approaches to diagnosis, categorization, and prognosis for tumours. Genotyping will allow more accurate identification of people at risk of cancer and estimations of best treatment choices and likely outcomes. The identification of new targets and the exploitation of existing ones, will result in several new and effective drug and vaccine developments. These will eventually be focussed on relatively small groups of patients who adequately express the target and/or activate and tolerate the treatment.

There is no doubt that our knowledge of the cellular and molecular biology of cancer will continue to grow rapidly, making it even more difficult to encompass in one book.

Index

Note: Page numbers in *italics* refer to Figures and Tables.